General Pathology

General Pathology *5th Edition*

J. B. WALTER TD MD MRCP (Lond.) FRCPath
Department of Pathology, Banting Institute, University of Toronto, and Departments of Medicine and Pathology, Toronto General Hospital, Toronto, Canada

M. S. ISRAEL MB ChB MRCP (Lond.) FRCPath DCP
Department of Pathology, Institute of Basic Medical Sciences, Royal College of Surgeons of England, and Lewisham Group Laboratory, London, England

CHURCHILL LIVINGSTONE
EDINBURGH LONDON AND NEW YORK 1979

CHURCHILL LIVINGSTONE
Medical Division of Longman Group Limited

Distributed in the United States of America by Churchill Livingstone
Inc., 1560 Broadway, New York, N.Y. 10036, and by associated
companies, branches and representatives throughout the world.

First Edition 1963
Second Edition 1965
Third Edition 1970
Fourth Edition 1974
Italian translation 1977
Fifth Edition 1979
    Reprinted 1983
    Reprinted 1984

ISBN 0 443 01890 1

British Library Cataloguing in Publication Data
Walter, John Brian
    General pathology.—5th ed.
    1. Pathology   2. Medicine
    I. Title   II. Israel, Martin Spencer
    616   RB111   78-41014

Printed in Great Britain by Butler and Tanner Ltd., Frome and London

Preface

For over a hundred years pathology has been one of the keystones of medicine, and as an academic subject it has been taught as part of the medical curriculum to prepare the student for the more nebulous clinical programme that completes his training. Unfortunately the practice of pathology has come to be relegated to the full-time pathologist and clinical medicine to the specialised clinician. This separation of pathological practice from the direct care of the patient is quite artificial, and indeed is unnecessary and undesirable. Recently this cleavage has been bridged, and the process is being accelerated by the advances that have taken place during the last two decades in clinical pathology, namely cytology, biochemistry, haematology, and microbiology. Even the isolation of histopathology, surely the last bastion of the non-clinical medical pathologist, has eroded before the advancing techniques of needle biopsy and the various types of endoscopy. Diseases even of previously inaccessible organs like the kidneys, pancreas, and central nervous system can now be adequately investigated during life and their progress mapped with precision. The necropsy has ceased to be the final event of revelation, but has rather assumed the role of an epilogue to a drama already well documented. Nevertheless, the epilogue quite frequently provides engaging and disquieting twists to the story—but it is no longer the major part of the record of the tale itself.

Pathology is the scientific study of disease: it follows the morbid process from its inception to its termination and it investigates the lesions produced. Wherever possible it uses accurate measurement, for the scientific method demands reproducible data. Thus, the size of a cancer cell, its content of DNA, its characteristics in tissue culture, and the life span of the patient in whom it is found can all be measured; all these considerations fall within the scope of pathology. The subject is therefore the concern of clinicians no less than pathologists, a fact well attested by the many valuable contributions made to pathology by clinicians and to clinical medicine by pathologists. The medical graduate whose practice is restricted either to the bedside or the laboratory can be sure of having only an incomplete and unbalanced understanding of medicine.

The fifth edition of *General Pathology* is our continued effort to provide an account of the fundamental processes of pathology in relationship to medical practice. A full understanding of the subject involves the disciplines of morbid anatomy, biochemistry, haematology, microbiology, physiology, and clinical medicine; all these aspects of disease process are dealt with in this book, and in particular we have tried to give a careful description of the basic pathological processes, for both these and the terms that are commonly used to describe them are a constant source of difficulty to the beginner. We do not aim at giving a comprehensive account of recent advances; many fine books and reviews are available for such information.

Five years have now elapsed since the last edition, and although no outstanding breakthroughs in medicine have been evident, the many advances that have been recorded have necessitated a complete revision. Worn-out type and aged blocks have required that the whole text be reset, and we have taken advantage of this situation to recast the book. Three entirely new chapters have been added; in Chapter 33, Some Disorders of Metabolism, the section on glucose metabolism includes an account of diabetes mellitus and the glycogen-storage diseases; an account of gout and the porphyrias follows. Chapter 34, Disorders of Nutrition, encompasses the important topics of starvation, the role of vitamins, and the malabsorption syndrome. Chapter 35, Disturbances of Endocrine Function, includes a section on the APUD system of cells. The topic of calcium metabolism has been expanded and added to the existing section on heterotopic calcification: this now constitutes a new Chapter 36. The remaining new addition to the book is Appendix 4 which is devoted to the HLA histocompatibility antigens.

Over 150 illustrations have been added, either to replace unsatisfactory figures or to provide new material. Sections in which major revision has been necessary are those describing the chemical mediators of acute inflammation, the granuloma, the bactericidal mechanisms in polymorphs in relationship to immunity, immunology, viral diseases (especially the section on the oncogenic viruses and the viruses of hepatitis), rickettsial and chlamydial infections, and the pathogenesis of amyloidosis.

Among numerous topics which have either been expanded or introduced for the first time are the techniques and uses of freeze etching, horseradish-peroxidase staining, gel-filtration chromatography, banding of chromosomes, counter-current electrophoresis, the structure and function of the cell membrane, the Golgi complex, microtubules and microfilaments, Noonan's syndrome, myelin figures, unscheduled DNA synthesis, DNA repair, the metabolism of mucoproteins, the chemical composition of collagen, the collagenases, the functions of macrophages, axial regeneration in amphibians, regeneration of muscle, the tissue reactions in leprosy, silicosis, and asbestosis, the Jarisch–Herxheimer reaction, apoptosis, the anion gap, the platelet release reaction, the pathogenesis of atheroma, vasculitis, the Prinzmetal type of angina pectoris, mountain fever, and the clonal origin of tumours.

There have been two other departures from our previous custom. SI units have been introduced for the first time, since these are commonly used in many parts of the world. The traditional units have been retained for readers who are unfamiliar with the new nomenclature. The references at the end of each chapter have been rigorously scrutinised, and most of those over 10 years old have been omitted. The old references can easily be obtained from the previous editions and standard texts of pathology, as well as from the current reviews. For the first time the full title of each reference has been included, and it is hoped that this will stimulate the reader to consult the material cited and adopt a critical approach.

J.B.W., Toronto, Canada
M.S.I., London, England

1979

Acknowledgements

We wish to thank W. B. Saunders Company of Philadelphia for generously allowing us to use over 45 illustrations from *An Introduction to the Principles of Disease* by one of us (J.B.W.). The great majority of the specimens illustrated are from the Wellcome Museum of Pathology, and we are grateful to the President and the Council of the Royal College of Surgeons of England for permission to reproduce them. In accordance with their wishes each is acknowledged at the end of the caption, and their catalogue number is indicated. A number of specimens illustrated are from the Boyd Museum, University of Toronto, and we thank Dr E. Farber of that institution for permission to use these.

We are indebted to a number of colleagues for providing valuable criticisms and for assisting in the realms of their particular expertise: Dr Y. Bedard (Toronto), for electron microscopy, Dr G. T. Simon (Toronto), for electron microscopy, Professor J. L. Turk (London) for his views on the granuloma, and Dr G. C. R. Morris (London) for electrolyte balance and renal failure. We thank Dr Leslie P. Spence for reviewing the section on virology; many of the new electronmicrographs of viruses have been provided by Micheline Fauvel of his department of virology at the Toronto General Hospital. We are grateful to Professor A. Fonnesu (Florence) for his helpful criticism, and also for allowing us to use material (especially Figures 33.4 and 33.5) that he added in the Italian translation of the Fourth Edition of *General Pathology*. We are particularly indebted to Mrs Mary Crookston for her continued help in writing Chapter 55 on Blood Grouping and Blood Transfusion. We owe special gratitude to those who have given us unpublished material or have allowed us to modify their original published work. Each figure is acknowledged separately under its caption.

Our thanks are due to Mrs Sonja Duda, librarian at the Banting Institute, Toronto, for valuable help in obtaining references, and to Mr A. A. Silcox and Mr J. T. Manders of the Royal College of Surgeons of England, London, for help with photomicrography.

Contents

Appendices

Chapter 1. Introduction

Pathology, the scientific study of disease processes, has its roots deeply implanted in medical history. The earliest observers, from Celsus (about 30 B.C.–A.D. 38) to Morgagni in the eighteenth century, based their work upon the naked-eye appearances of diseased individuals and organs. Only as the technique of microscopy improved was the Germanic School of Pathology, headed by Virchow (1821–1905), able to investigate changes at a cellular level.

In France, Pasteur, using the microscope, laid the foundation of the science of bacteriology, while later on the German dye industry enabled Koch, Ehrlich, and Domagk to extend this knowledge and open the era of chemotherapy. Advances in pathology thus have been closely related to advances in technology. This in no way belittles the efforts of inspired experimenters like Jenner, who in England pioneered the way to active immunisation.

Nowadays technological advances are occurring so rapidly that no doctor can hope to have a working knowledge of all the methods that are available. Nevertheless, it is by utilising all these complex techniques that problems are fully investigated. The student of medicine should therefore have some understanding of the techniques which are available, and the type of problem which they might be able to solve. In this way investigators conversant with many different disciplines are brought together to their mutual benefit.

TECHNIQUES AVAILABLE IN PATHOLOGY

MICRODISSECTION

Apparatus is available for dissecting cells. In this way the nucleus can be removed, and the effect of this on the deprived cell observed (p. 13). Micropipettes can be inserted into the capillaries, and microelectrodes placed in single nerve cells or fibres. More recently, microbeams of ultraviolet light, or Laser rays (*L*ight *A*mplification by *S*timulated *E*mission of *R*adiation), have been used to produce damage in a particular part of a cell.

The micromanipulation of embryos can produce some interesting results. Thus the developing eggs from two pregnant mice of different strains can be removed and made to adhere to each other *in vitro*. If reimplanted into a pseudopregnant female, the combined embryo can develop into one animal called an allophenic mouse. In this the two cell types form clones* of varying numbers in different organs. When hair colour is involved, roughly equal numbers of melanocytes of both genotypes are produced. If black and white strains of mice are used, the allophenic progeny have a series of trans-

*A clone is a group of cells of like hereditary constitution which has been produced asexually from a single cell. The word is derived from the Greek *klon* meaning a cutting used for propagation.

verse bands like a zebra![1] It has been suggested that even in the normal animal mutations could lead to the production of clones of different genetic constitution. Furthermore, even if all the cells of an individual have the same genotype, some could exhibit a separate phenotype due to suppression of certain genes. Perhaps some type of clonal segregation can account for the irregular and patchy distribution of the lesions seen in some human diseases.[2]

MICROSCOPY

The Light Microscope

The light microscope has two disadvantages:

(*a*) Its *resolution* is limited by the wavelength of light. The ability to distinguish between two adjacent points is called the resolving power. In theory resolution should be possible up to a distance of half the wavelength of the light used, but in practice using green light the resolving power of the microscope is about 250 nm.† Thus, only the largest viruses (the poxviruses) can be seen with a good optical microscope. The shorter the wavelength of the light used the better is the resolution, and with ultraviolet light it can be improved two to three times. It is important to distinguish between *visibility* and *resolution*. Particles as small as 75 nm may be visible, but no detailed structure can be resolved. A simple analogy illustrates this difference. If an open book is placed at a distance from the eyes, the writing can easily be distinguished as such, i.e. it is visible, but it may be quite impossible to recognise individual letters because their details cannot be resolved.

(*b*) Living tissue is transparent, and the homogeneity in optical density of its components hides its detailed structure. Staining techniques must therefore be used to see cellular details, but these must almost invariably be performed on dead fixed tissue. It is possible to stain cells by supravital techniques, e.g. the mitochondria of living leucocytes can be stained by Janus green, but even this damages them rapidly so that the cells soon lose their motility and begin to die.

Three techniques have been developed to overcome these difficulties in examining living cells.

Dark-ground illumination relies upon the fact that objects placed in a beam of light may be seen by the rays which they reflect in much the same way that dust particles are rendered visible by a shaft of sunlight. The method finds particular application in the demonstration of organisms which cannot be readily stained, e.g. *Treponema pallidum* (Fig. 1.1).

Phase contrast microscopy takes advantage of the different refractive indices of various parts of the cell. These differences are converted into differences in optical density. In this way

†1 mm = 1000 μm, 1 μm = 1000 nm.

Figure 1.1
Dark-ground method for demonstrating *Treponema pallidum*. This came from a hanging-drop preparation of fluid from a chancre. It was illuminated by the dark-ground method. (*Photograph by courtesy of Dr. Marta Marschalko and the late Professor Kiraly, Institute of Dermatology and Venereology, Semmelweis Medical School, Budapest, Hungary.*)

living cells can be examined; the method is commonly used in virology (see Figs. 22.8 and 22.9).

Interference microscopy works on a different principle. The light that passes through the microscope is split into two beams. The light passing through the specimen is retarded, and interferes with the light of the other beam when the two are recombined in an image plane. The method finds little application in routine pathology.

Examination of Fixed Tissues[3]

Paraffin section technique. This is the most commonly used routine method of examination. Tissue is fixed, dehydrated in graded alcohols, cleared in xylol, chloroform, or other solvent which is miscible with both alcohol and wax, and finally embedded in paraffin wax.

Fixation. Fixation is a complex process which involves killing the cells rapidly and inhibiting the enzymatic processes of autolysis. Macromolecules are stablised and aggregated, proteins are denatured, and some active groups, e.g. $-NH_3^+$ of protein and $-PO_4{-}^-$ of nucleic acid are exposed. The cell's membranes are altered in such a way that stains can penetrate into the cell and its organelles.

Formaldehyde, as a 10 per-cent aqueous solution called formalin, is the most useful, cheap, and commonly-used fixative. It penetrates tissue with ease and will therefore fix large specimens. It reacts by forming bridges between adjacent $-NH_2$ groups in the side-chains of proteins and in phospholipids. Only substances which are rendered insoluble, such as proteins, or which become attached to insoluble substances, such as nucleic acids, can be made visible by subsequent staining. Small soluble molecules, such as Na^+, glucose, and urea, cannot be localised with any degree of precision by present-day methods.

Frozen section technique. The paraffin-wax technique removes certain chemicals, e.g. fat, and alters others, e.g. enzymes and antigens. To meet this difficulty the cryostat has been developed: in essence this is a microtome with which sections are cut at $-30°C$. This is achieved by having the microtome enclosed in a refrigerator. The sections of frozen fresh material thus obtained are so little damaged that they are suitable for histochemical study. They may also be stained with haematoxylin and eosin, and the method can be used for quick examination of tissue. Some hospitals employ the me-

thod for the routine examination of surgical material, but the sections, although adequate for diagnosis, are nevertheless of poor quality.

STAINING TECHNIQUES FOR DEMONSTRATING CELL STRUCTURE[4,5]

Although many of the staining methods of histopathology have been developed empirically, some general principles can be discerned. There are three types of staining method:

Solution of lipid-soluble dyes in the liquid lipid of cells or tissue.

Staining of tissue by chemical union of coloured or chromogenic substances to reactive loci.

Coloration of added reagents by reactive loci (commonly enzymic) of tissue.

Each of these will be considered in more detail. It should be noted that those methods that are designed to demonstrate specific chemicals in cells or tissues fall within the domain of the sub-specialties of *cytochemistry* or of *histochemistry* respectively.

Lipid Soluble Dyes

An alcoholic solution of a lipid-soluble dye, such as Sudan III or Oil Red O, when applied to a frozen tissue section, will rapidly pass into cellular lipid droplets and thereby colour them. Similarly osmium tetroxide will dissolve in liquid lipid; it is then reduced by ethylenic double bonds to black lower oxides. Osmium tetroxide also acts as a fixative, and in this role finds particular application in electron microscopy (see p. 4).

Staining of Tissue by Chemical Union of Coloured or Chromogenic Substances to Reactive Loci of Cells

The attachment by chemical union depends on one of three mechanisms:

(*a*) electrostatic attraction of dye to oppositely charged tissue loci;

(*b*) precipitation of charged colloids on to oppositely charged tissue loci;

(*c*) covalent union to reactive sites.

(*a*) **Electrostatic attraction of dyes to oppositely-charged tissue loci.** *Acidophilic (positively-charged) tissue loci.* The principal cationic loci are the $-NH_3^+$ groups of basic amino acids. These can be demonstrated by anionic dyes such as eosin, picric acid, and acid fuchsin. If careful, controlled techniques are used, combinations of these dyes will stain cytoplasm and connective tissue selectively. Thus in Van Gieson's stain, picric acid stains cytoplasm and muscle yellow, whereas collagen takes up the red acid fuchsin.

Basophilic (negatively-charged) tissue loci. These include the $-PO_4{-}^-$ groups of nucleic acids, $-SO_4{-}^-$ of polysaccharides, and the $-COO^-$ of uronic and amino acids. The union of cationic dyes with the last group is tenuous and, in practice, the dyes stain nucleic acids, polysaccharides, and some acidic lipids. Important members of this group are methylene blue, Azur A (formed by the oxidation of methylene blue), pyronin, and methyl green. As with the anionic stains, combinations of dyes can produce differential staining. Thus in Leishman's stain DNA is stained violet by Azur A, RNA of cytoplasm and nucleoli is coloured blue by methylene blue, and cytoplasmic protein including haemoglobin is tinted red by eosin (p. 601). The most useful cationic dye is derived from haematoxylin, a dye extracted from a tree. By oxidation haematein is produced, and this when mordanted with Al^{3+}, Cr^{3+}, or Fe^{3+} forms a useful deep purple, positively-charged dye, commonly referred to as 'haematoxylin' and used in combination with eosin.

(b) Precipitation of charged colloids on oppositely charged tissue loci. A good example of this method is Hale's colloidal iron stain. Positively-charged colloidal iron is precipitated and bound to sulphate esters and uronic acids of polysaccharides. The bound ferric ions are converted to Prussian blue by the addition of potassium ferrocyanide.

(c) Covalent union of coloured or chromogenic substances to reactive tissue loci. Reactive loci in the cell can be demonstrated by combining them covalently with coloured compounds. Two examples will be considered.

Periodic Acid-Schiff (PAS) reaction. When periodic acid is applied to a section, many carbohydrate components are oxidised to aldehydes. Aldehydes produce a red colour with Schiff's reagent (a solution of basic fuchsin decolorised by sulphurous acid). Therefore, if Schiff's reagent is applied to the treated section, the parts containing carbohydrate are stained red. The periodic acid-Schiff reaction is useful for the demonstration of glycogen, ground substance, and epithelial mucus. Glycogen can be differentiated from the others by pretreating the section with diastase, which removes it.

Feulgen stain. Tissue is treated with hydrochloric acid followed by Schiff's reagent. The reaction depends upon the hydrolysis by hydrochloric acid of the purine-deoxyribose linkages in the DNA molecule. The pentose-phosphoric acid complex which is released has a free aldehyde group, which can be detected by Schiff's reagent. Nuclei and chromosomes are therefore coloured magenta. The method is specific for DNA.

Coloration of added reagents by reactive loci of tissue. Some reactive loci, commonly enzymatic, can convert added reagents into coloured or opaque material. If this material is precipitated, the reaction product is located at, or very close to, the original locus. Several examples of this technique will be described:

(*a*) *Enzymatic localisation.* The demonstration of an enzyme is well illustrated by the method used for alkaline phosphatase. The section is placed in a solution of the substrate *4-glycerophosphate* in the presence of calcium. The enzyme splits off phosphate, and this forms calcium phosphate which is invisible. Addition of cobalt nitrate converts it into cobalt phosphate, and ammonium sulphide changes this to black cobalt sulphide.

Although the amount and situation of the black sulphide is indicative of the amount and site of the phosphatase originally present, it is evident that errors can creep in at each of the stages: glycerophosphate → calcium phosphate → cobalt phosphate → cobalt sulphide. The X-ray microscope demonstrates these stages very well.[6, 7] This instrument takes radiographs of sections using X-rays generated at 5 to 10kV. The rays are absorbed by elements of high atomic number, and as in the conventional full-size radiographs show up deposits of calcium. Figure 1.2 shows how the original calcium phosphate is localised, whilst there has been considerable diffusion by the time the last step is reached. The X-ray microscope can, of course, be used on unstained tissues to show deposits of calcium as well as other structures.

Histochemical techniques are of value in many areas of pathology: nowhere are they of more value than in the study of disease of the muscles.[8] Two major types of muscle fibre can be identified, and the changes that take place in disease can be studied (Fig. 1.3). Histochemical techniques may also be applied to the study of cells by electron microscopy (see Fig. 2.6, p. 16).

(*b*) *Perls's Prussian-blue reaction for haemosiderin.* Acid is applied to the tissue to release Fe^{3+} from haemosiderin. Next, potassium ferrocyanide is applied; this reacts with the Fe^{3+} to form blue ferric ferrocyanide (Fig. 1.4).

(*c*) *Reduction of silver nitrate to metallic silver.* Some loci, such as those present on melanin granules and in the cells of Kultschitzky, which are called *argentaffin*, can reduce silver nitrate to metallic silver, and are thereby blackened.

Argyrophilic loci bind silver but do not reduce it. Subsequent treatment of the tissue with a reducing agent leads to the precipitation of metallic silver. This silver impregnation method is useful for demonstrating reticulin fibres and spirochaetes (**Fig. 1.5**).

(*d*) *Metachromasia.* Some tissue components have the property of taking up certain dyes and so altering the dye's structure, usually by polymerisation, that the colour is changed. This is called metachromatic staining, and is a property exhibited by the granules of mast cells and by some acid mucopolysaccharides (p. 60). Dyes of the thiazine group are commonly used, and toluidine blue is the best known. It stains most tissues blue, but metachromatic material is coloured purple or even red.

Immunological Techniques in Histochemistry

The highly specific binding of antibody to antigen can be utilised to great advantage in histochemistry. The antibody can be labelled with fluorescein; when it is applied to a section, it will become fixed to the appropriate antigen. This can be detected by examining the section under ultraviolet light. An alternative method is to apply unlabelled antibody to the section, thoroughly wash, and then detect the site of antibody attachment by using a second labelled anti-immunoglobulin (Coombs's reagent). This method is known as the *sandwich technique*, and has many advantages. Thus with each layer there is an amplification effect that renders the detection of specific fluorescence easier. Also commercial labelled Coombs's reagent can be purchased, whereas labelling of specific antibody must be done by the investigator himself. Sometimes complex multilayered techniques are used with each layer adhering to a specific receptor site of the previous reagent.

Labelling of antibodies can be done in other ways.

Radioactive isotopes can be used in conjunction with autoradiography both for light and electron microscopy (p. 9). A more recent histochemical method utilises *horseradish peroxidase*.[9, 10] This enzyme splits hydrogen peroxide, and the released oxygen produces a brown oxidation deposit with 3-3'-diaminobenzidine. Since osmium tetroxide reacts with this end-product to form an electron-dense chelate, the method can be modified for use in electron microscopy. The peroxidase system can be used in several ways. The enzyme can

Figure 1.2
(*a*) Historadiograph of rat kidney after incubation of the section with
β-glycerophosphate in the presence of calcium chloride. The deposits
of calcium phosphate indicate the site of alkaline phosphatase activity.
(*b*) Section treated as (*a*) above, but the calcium phosphate has been
converted into cobalt phosphate by the action of cobalt nitrate.
(*c*) Final treatment with ammonium sulphide converts the cobalt
phosphate into cobalt sulphide. The historadiograph shows that there
has been considerable diffusion, and that the distribution of the radio-
opaque material no longer corresponds accurately to that of the
alkaline phosphatase. Cobalt sulphide is black, and is visible under the
light microscope. However, it is evident that a radiograph at stage (*a*)
gives a clearer indication of the actual distribution of the enzyme.
× 150. (*From Photograph by courtesy of Dr. A. J. Hale. Published
previously in Hale, A. J.* (1961), J. biophys biochem. Cytol., **11**, 488)

(a)

be attached to the appropriate antibody, and the method then
involves one step. Usually it is more convenient to use a
multiple sandwich technique with the last reagent being an
antibody to peroxidase. The addition of the horseradish peroxidase followed by 3-3′-diaminobenzidine and hydrogen peroxide produces the brown reaction product. This can be
detected by routine light microscopy and the preparation is
permanent, an advantage over the fluorescent techniques.

The immunoperoxidase technique can be used for many
purposes, and has been employed to detect spirochaetal antigen, pituitary hormones, α-fetoprotein, and hepatitis antigen
(HBsAg).

The Electron Microscope[11]

The electron microscope resembles the light microscope
except that a stream of electrons is used instead of light, and
electromagnetic fields instead of glass lenses. Its resolving
power is 0·6 to 0·7 nm.* By its use viruses can be seen with
ease, and our knowledge of detailed cell and tissue structure
has increased enormously (see Ch. 2). The electron microscope of current design has, however, three disadvantages.

1. Only very small pieces of tissue can be examined; 1 to 2
mm blocks are usual. Orientation of the specimen under the
electron microscope is aided by first preparing 'thick' sections;
these are about 1 μm thick as compared with the 60nm
normally used in electron microscopy. The sections are stained
with toluidine blue and examined under the light microscope.

2. The tissue must be examined in a vacuum—living cells
cannot therefore be used.

3. Tissue must be fixed immediately, preferably *in vivo*, if
artefacts are to be avoided. This must be borne in mind if it is
proposed to examine human surgical material.

The most widely-used fixative is *osmium tetroxide*; this also
acts as a stain by virtue of the increased electron scattering
power of the tissue components after the deposition of osmium. Osmium tetroxide fixes unsaturated lipids and phospholipids well, but protein components are poorly preserved,
and prolonged fixation causes considerable damage to the
specimen. Penetration of the tissue is slow, particularly if it
has been prefixed by aldehyde.

Glutaraldehyde is a commonly-used fixative that fixes protein well but lipids very poorly. Cytoplasmic organelles, e.g.

(b)

(c)

*For comparison the diameter of a globular protein of molecular
weight 80 000 daltons is 6 nm, glucose is 0·5 nm, and water 0·28 nm.

Figure 1.3
Myosin ATPase reaction in skeletal muscle. The routine reaction for ATPase clearly separates muscle fibres into two groups. Type I fibres are lightly stained, and type II fibres are heavily stained. The insert shows normal muscle with the characteristic checkerboard appearance. The fibres are of equal size. Compare this with the muscle from a case of type-I spinal muscular atrophy (Werdnig-Hoffmann disease), which is also shown. Many of the fibres are atrophic, and both types of fibres are affected (1) and (2). A few type I fibres are hypertrophied (1), whereas type II fibres are of normal size. (*Photographs by courtesy of Dr. Dawna L. Armstrong.*)

Figure 1.5
Smear from syphilitic lesion stained by a silver-impregnation method. The field is crowded with *Treponema pallidum*. (*Photograph by courtesy of Dr. Marta Marschalko and the late Professor Kiraly, Institute of Dermatology and Venereology, Semmelweis Medical School, Budapest, Hungary.*)

Figure 1.4
Section stained for haemosiderin by the Prussian-blue method. The section shows a massive deposition of haemosiderin in the liver cells. The pigment is stained brilliant blue by this method, but appears black in the photograph. The detailed structure of the liver cells is not well shown. The tissue was from a patient with haemochromatosis. ($\times$ 380).

microtubules and microfilaments, are well preserved. Prolonged fixation causes less damage than with osmium tetroxide, an asset when dealing with human biopsy material that has to be transported to the laboratory. *Formaldehyde* penetrates tissue very rapidly but fixes it slowly. Proteins, e.g. enzymes, are less damaged than by glutaraldehyde, and it is therefore used as a fixative in histochemical studies. Glutaraldehyde can also be used, but osmium is quite unsuitable. Potassium permanganate was used as a fixative, but has largely been replaced by glutaraldehyde.

Double fixation. It is now a common practice to combine several fixatives in the hope of bringing together their various virtues. A popular method is to use glutaraldehyde as a primary fixative and follow this by 'post-fixation' in osmium tetroxide. *Universal fixative* contains formaldehyde and glutaraldehyde; an advantage is that tissue can remain in it with little damage. Regardless of the fixative used, sections can usefully be stained by a salt of a heavy metal; alkaline lead hydroxide and uranyl acetate are the ones most often used.

Although fixation is essential if cellular details are to be examined, remarkably good results can be obtained with poorly fixed material under some circumstances. Thus even formalin-fixed tissue embedded in paraffin wax can be examined usefully by electron microscopy. In this way melanosomes or neurosecretory granules can be identified in tumour cells if it is desired to re-investigate the nature of a tumour in old surgical material (see p. 310).

Histochemistry. Whereas in light microscopy the final reaction product of a histochemical stain is coloured, in electron microscopy it contains a heavy metal and is therefore electron-dense (see Fig. 2.6). Another approach is to conjugate ferritin with protein; in this way intracellular antigens and antibodies may be localised[12] (see p. 152).

Methacrylate was the first embedding medium to gain popularity, but this plastic tends to disintegrate in the electron beam and artefacts are produced. It has therefore been replaced by more stable plastics, e.g. araldite and epon, and pictures of much higher quality can now be obtained. Two other developments of electron microscopy are of note:

Replication. A surface can be examined by making a replica of it, e.g. with a carbon film, and then examining the replica with the electron microscope. The technique is commonly combined with freeze fracturing.[13] Tissue is frozen to the temperature of liquid nitrogen, placed in a vacuum chamber, and fractured with a special knife. The surface so exposed is sprayed immediately with evaporated platinum and carbon from an angle of 45°, and the replica so formed is strengthened by further deposition of carbon applied vertically. The tissue itself is dissolved away, and the replica is studied by transmission electron microscopy. The process is known as *fracture replication.* If the fractured tissue surface is partially freeze-dried, ice is sublimated, and a deeper surface is revealed. This process is referred to as 'etching'. A replica is subsequently made in this process of 'freeze-etching'. When tissue is fractured, the lines of cleavage tend to follow membranes, and indeed may actually split the unit membranes (p. 14). Hence these techniques have been of greatest value in the study of cell membranes.

Negative staining. The method consists of embedding the particles to be examined in a layer of electron-dense material, e.g. containing sodium phosphotungstate or a uranium salt, so that the objects stand out against a dense background. Viruses and amyloid fibres have been usefully studied by this technique (Figs. 22.1 and 2 and 48.6 and 7).

Instruments with a high accelerator voltage are now available, and by their use it has been possible to photograph living bacteria. Although useful in metallurgy, their contribution to biological knowledge has so far been small.

Scanning electron microscope. This instrument works on a different principle from the conventional transmission electron microscope: a very fine beam of electrons is focused to a point and made to scan the surface of the specimen. The secondary electrons scattered from the surface are collected and amplified. The current so generated is used to modulate the brightness of a television tube which is scanned in synchronicity with the electron beam scanning the object. The method is useful for examining the surfaces of objects, and the pictures so obtained have a remarkable three-dimensional effect (Fig. 1.6). Micro-organisms, red cells, and intestinal epithelium have been studied with advantage.

THE ULTRACENTRIFUGE

The tremendous centrifugal force that can be applied by this machine is utilised to separate mixtures of large molecular chemicals. The present-day instrument can develop a centrifugal field sufficient to spin down partcles as small as 1 nm. The velocity with which sedimentation occurs can be measured, and the ratio:

$$\frac{\text{Sedimentation velocity}}{\text{Centrifugal field}}$$

is called the Sedimentation Constant. It is measured in Svedberg units (S).

Figure 1.6
Scanning electron micrograph showing the sinuses of a haemolymph node of a rat. Trabeculae are seen crossing the sinuses, and in this mesh-work there are macrophages surrounded by red cells which are being phagocytosed. The sinus-lining cells cannot be discerned, but the groups of red cells forming a rosette around each macrophage are clearly seen and one of them is indicated by an arrow. (*Photograph by courtesy of Drs. C. Nopajaroonsri, S. C. Luk and G. T. Simon*)

The ultracentrifuge has been used to separate mixtures of proteins; it was in this way that the macroglobulins were identified (see Ch. 49).

The various components of cells can also be separated and examined by physical and chemical means. If cells are disrupted either physically or by ultrasonic vibration, the cell membranes, nuclei, mitochondria, and ribosomes can be isolated in a fairly pure state after centrifugation. By analysing these fractions the results of histochemistry may be correlated with those of the well-established procedures of chemistry. The many enzyme systems of mitochondria have been investigated in this way. The granules in cloudy swelling have been isolated and identified as altered mitochondria. (See p. 52.)

CHEMICAL AND PHYSICAL ANALYSIS OF SUBSTANCES OF BIOLOGICAL INTEREST

It is beyond the scope of this book to deal with this subject. It is sufficient to note that methods are available which have led to the complete analysis of substances as complex as the insulin molecule (51 amino-acid residues), the enzyme ribonuclease (124 amino-acid residues), and more recently immunoglobulin. X-ray diffraction techniques have revealed the complex folded structure of a large molecule like myoglobin. Modern methods of chemical analysis combined with automation have made it possible to estimate the concentration of a large number of chemical substances in a small quantity of body fluid, e.g. blood. With the SMA-12 AutoAnalyzer, which is routinely used in large centres, it is currently possible to estimate the concentration of 12 substances from a single sample of blood. It is often cheaper to obtain this *biochemical profile* than to make individual chemical estimations.

The techniques of immunology have been of great value in the identification and assay of proteins. The radio-immunoassay method has been adapted to measure the blood levels of certain peptide hormones, e.g. insulin, glucagon, TSH, and ACTH, which are present in picograms or nanograms per ml.* The method depends upon the ability of unlabelled hormone to inhibit, by simple competition, the binding of labelled hormone (e.g. with ^{131}I or ^{125}I) by specific antibody. The hormone content of an unknown sample is determined by comparing the degree to which it inhibits the binding of labelled antigen with the inhibition produced by a series of standard solutions containing known amounts of hormone. The reagents required are therefore pure hormone, labelled hormone, and specific antibody. The amount of labelled hormone bound to antibody is determined after separating it from the free labelled hormone. This separation is done by electrophoresis or by chemical means.

Two other methods have found particular application in pathology:

Electrophoresis

If a mixture of proteins is placed in an electric field at a known pH, individual proteins move at particular rates dependent to a great extent upon their size and charge. The test is conveniently performed on filter paper, starch or other gel, or cellulose acetate strip, the choice depending upon the nature of the substances being investigated. After passing an electric current for a suitable time the strip is dried, and the separated proteins are stained with a simple dye, e.g. light green. Figure 1.7 shows a typical electrophoretic separation of the plasma proteins. Combined with the agar-diffusion technique, electrophoresis has proved invaluable in separating protein mixtures (see Fig. 1.8 and caption).

Chromatography[14]

Chromatography is an important technique for separating pure substances from mixtures. The chromatographic system consists of two immiscible phases, a *stationary phase* which is fixed and granular, and a *moving phase* which flows through the interstices of the stationary phase. The moving phase is fluid (liquid or gas), and its movement is effected by gravity, applied pressure, or capillarity. The stationary phase is usually a finely divided insoluble solid.

Chromatographic separation depends on the fact that different substances follow the moving solvent at different rates. All these substances must be soluble in the moving phase, but some become distributed on the surface (adsorption) or throughout the interior (partition) of the particles of the stationary phase (Fig. 1.9). Those substances whose distribution favours the moving phase pass more rapidly through the chromatogram than those which favour the stationary phase. If the column is sufficiently long, a complete separation of

Figure 1.7

Cellulose acetate electrophoresis of serum. On the left electrophoretic strips from 8 separate sera are shown. The anode is on the left, and the dense band that has moved furthest to the left is due to albumin. No. 8 is normal serum, whereas Nos. 4 and 7 show a diffuse increase in the γ-globulins; each shows the picture of a polyclonal gammopathy. No. 1 shows a dense band in the γ-globulin area; the density of the bands of strip No. 1 is depicted in graphic form on the right. The various serum proteins are in the same relative positions on both the strip and the graph. The sharp spike in the γ region is characteristic of a monoclonal gammopathy. (*Reproduced, with permission, from Hall, C. A.: Gammopathies. In Halsted, J. A. (Ed.) (1976) The Laboratory in Clinical Medicine, p. 493. Philadelphia: Saunders.*)

substances between successive bands of pure solvent can be achieved, as is seen in Figure 1.8.

There are three main types of chromatography: (*a*) *column chromatography*, in which liquid passes down through particles of solid packed in a glass tube; (*b*) *paper chromatography*, in which an organic solvent moves by capillary action through the pores of filter paper, the fibres of which contain a little water; (*c*) *thin-layer chromatography*, which resembles (*b*) except that the stationary phase in the form of a gel or plastic sheet, is made to adhere to a glass up which the solvent moves by capillarity.

Paper or thin-layer chromatography has found great use in the separation of amino acids and sugars in a solution such as urine. Each component moves at a specific rate along the paper depending on the solvent, so that the ratio

$$\frac{\text{Distance travelled by component}}{\text{Distance travelled by solvent}},$$

or the R_f value, is a constant for each component under the conditions of the test. After allowing the solvent to move a certain distance the paper is dried, and the area occupied by the component is 'developed' by spraying the paper with a chemical that reacts with that component, e.g. ninhydrin turns purple with amino acids. If a series of known substances are run in parallel with the unknown components, their R_f values

---

*1 milligram = 1000 micrograms (g). 1 microgram = 1000 nanograms (ng). 1 nanogram = 1000 picograms (pg).

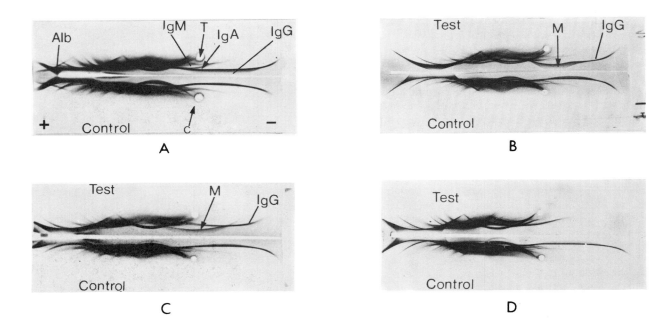

Figure 1.8
Immunoelectrophoresis of serum. This method entails the separation of the proteins by electrophoresis in a gel, and then demonstrating each fraction by means of a precipitin reaction using an antibody.

Sera (test and control) are placed in the two cups in a sheet of agarose gel. Albumin has a strong negative charge, and γ-globulin has a weak negative charge. The application of an electric field results in a tendency for the proteins to move towards the anode. Their actual movement, however, is determined not only by their molecular size and charge but also by a flow of water towards the cathode due to the phenomenon of electro-osmosis. This is due to a negative charge on the gel itself, and as the gel is fixed, so its tendency to move towards the anode actually results in a movement of water to the cathode. The weakly charged γ-globulins are thus carried towards the cathode.

The separated plasma components are demonstrated by placing antiserum to whole plasma down the central strip. From there the antibodies diffuse to form precipitin lines with each separated serum protein. A stain to accentuate these lines has been used.

A. The IgG band is heavier than that of the control and is closer to the central strip. Serum tested here was from a case of systemic lupus erythematosus with polyclonal hypergammaglobulinaemia. The IgA and IgM bands are well shown. *B.* An M protein is present and distorts the normal IgG band (from a case of multiple myeloma with an IgG M protein). *C.* An M protein is present and is in the position of the normal IgA band; note how the normal IgG band crosses the M protein (from a case of multiple myeloma with an IgA M protein). *D.* Note the deficiency of the IgG band (from a case of congenital hypogammaglobulinaemia). (*Photograph by courtesy of Dr. K. C. Carstairs.*)

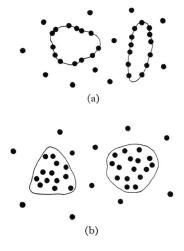

Figure 1.9
Distribution of a substance between moving and stationary phases (*a*) adsorption and (*b*) partition mechanisms. (*Eastoe, J. E.* (1964), Ann. roy. Coll. Surg. Engl., **35,** 234)

can be compared. In this way an unknown component can be identified.

Column chromatography is used to separate and purify the individual components of a solution containing a mixture. In *ion-exchange chromatography*[15] a cellulose resin is packed into the column, and proteins are bound in varying degree to the particles by electrostatic forces. The diffusion of small molecules into the pores of a gel from which large molecules are excluded because of their size forms the basis of *gel-filtration (exclusion) chromatography.*[15] The original starch gel has now been replaced by standardised cross-linked dextran known as *Sephadex.* Many grades are available and vary in the degree of cross-linkage—this determines the upper limit of size of molecule that can enter the pores. Gel-forming beads are allowed to swell in water, and are then packed in the column. Large molecules cannot enter the beads, and so pass rapidly through the column. Small particles enter the beads and pass slowly through the column. The method has found great use in the separation and purification of proteins; in general they appear in the column eluent in order of decreasing molecular size (Fig. 1.10).

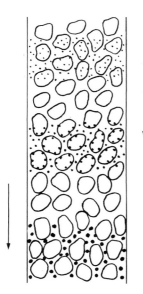

Figure 1.10
Gel filtration or exclusion chromatography.
Molecules of three sizes are seen being separated by passage down a column of gel beads. Large molecules are excluded from the beads, and pass rapidly through the column. Small molecules enter the beads, and pass slowly down the column.

FLUORESCENT TRACING TECHNIQUES[16]

The ability of certain compounds to convert the energy of ultraviolet light into visible light can be utilised in various ways. Fluorescent dyes, e.g. auramine, have been used to stain tubercle bacilli, which are then easily visible under the ultraviolet microscope. The use of the fluorescent dye quinacrine for Q-banding of chromosomes and for demonstrating the Y body is described in Chapter 3.

Fluorescein and lissamine rhodamine B can easily be attached to protein molecules. Labelled antibodies are widely used in immunopathology (see p. 152).

RADIOACTIVE ISOTOPES

The radioactive isotopes are treated by living cells in the same way as the normal elements. Their radiation can be detected by suitable counters, and they may usefully be employed as labels in a wide range of fields. Clinically, thyroid function can be investigated by estimating the distribution of an administered dose of radioactive iodine in the plasma and over the thyroid gland. Radioactive chromium can be attached to the red cells, and their length of survival estimated (see Ch. 52). The clearance of a small quantity of injected radioactive sodium from the skin has been used to measure blood flow. In the experimental animal many compounds can be tagged and their metabolism followed, e.g. albumin.

The introduction of the man-made element *technetium* has revolutionised the use of radioactive isotopes in humans. This element emits gamma radiation only, and is therefore safer to use than isotopes that emit other more damaging radiations. It has a half-life of six hours. When injected intravenously with pyrophosphate, technetium is taken up selectively by the bones, probably by the osteoid tissue. Using this technique the whole skeleton can be surveyed, and the method now augments radiography in the detection of bony lesions, particularly metastatic carcinoma. If the technetium is attached to aggregated albumin, it becomes concentrated in the lung; an estimate of the blood flow through this organ is thereby obtained. By various techniques it is now possible to scan many other organs; it is particularly useful in the investigation of lesions in the liver and the thyroid gland.

Autoradiography

The isotopes can also be used at a microscopic level. By placing a section of tissue on a photographic film, subsequent photographic development will reveal the site of isotope localisation as a series of black grains. As an example of the value of this it is found that tritiated thymidine given to a cell is incorporated into its nucleus. This may therefore be used as an indicator of DNA synthesis (see Fig. 1.11).

PHOTOGRAPHY

Apart from the value for record purposes photography plays an important role in many other fields. It is essential in ultraviolet, electron, and X-ray microscopy. The ultrafast films now available have made high-speed cine photomicrography possible, and blood flow can be examined from films shot at 7600 frames per second (the 'normal' is 24 per sec.). Time-lapse cine photography, on the other hand, has made it possible to 'speed up' the movement of living cells grown in tissue culture. This technique, as yet but little used, has provided interesting information on the behaviour of phagocytes, lymphocytes, and tumour cells.

TISSUE CULTURE[17]

Tissues of various types can be cultured outside the body with comparative ease. The usual surface employed is glass or plastic, and the tissues can be grown in test-tubes, medicine-flat bottles, flasks, or simply on the surface of a cover-slip inverted over a slide with a hollow depression.

There are two types of tissue culture: (*a*) *cell culture*, in which the cells of an organ or tumour are allowed to grow out. The organ is first cut up into small fragments which are then digested with trypsin at 37°C until there is complete disintegration. The cells derived from the tissue are centrifuged, suspended in a liquid growth medium that usually contains serum and a balanced salt solution, and allowed to sediment in a container; they rapidly become attached to the surface, and within a few days multiplication is sufficient to cause it to be covered with a monolayer of confluent cells. Another method consists of attaching a tissue fragment, or explant, to the glass surface, adding a growth medium, and then waiting for an outgrowth of cells from it. Cell culture is an extremely important technique for cultivating viruses, and is described in Chapter 22. Its use in cancer research has proved disappointing except in the study of tumours of nervous tissue, where the cells growing out sometimes differentiate into specific elements, e.g. astrocytes or ganglion cells, thus allowing the tumour to be more easily classified. (*b*) *Organ culture*, in which a fragment of tissue is grown on a grid so that there is no cellular outgrowth, but the organ is kept as normal

(a)

(b)

Figure 1.11
DNA localisation. Autoradiograph of a Feulgen-stained anaphase figure in a squash preparation of the root tip of *Allium cepa* fed with tritiated thymidine. (*a*) Photographed at the level of the section to show the chromosomes. (*b*) The same cell photographed at the level of the photographic emulsion. The labelled thymidine has been taken up by the cell and incorporated into the DNA. Note how the silver dots correspond to the chromosomes. × 3200. (*Photographs by courtesy of Dr. P. B. Gahan*)

histologically as is possible. Limb buds, eye rudiments, and bones have been studied while growing in an artificial medium, and their differentiation observed. The effect of vitamin A on the skin of chick embryos has been investigated in this way (see Ch. 34).

The culture of human cells has yielded much information.[18] Some normal human cells, e.g. fibroblasts, can be sustained in tissue culture for about 50 generations. Serially propagated mammalian cells do not necessarily carry out the same specific functions as when situated in the organ from which they were isolated. However, enzyme studies on human cell cultures have shed some light on the genetic enzyme defects seen in some diseases, and have proved to be useful in the antenatal diagnosis of some inherited diseases (p. 44).

Another interesting aspect of cell culture is the technique of making two somatic cells fuse to form a common cell. Sometimes the stimulus of a virus infection has been used, and the mononuclear hybrid cell may be capable of proliferation. For example, hybrid cells between a human cell line and a mouse cell line have been obtained.[19] Another method of combining DNA from two cells is based on the finding that

certain DNA viruses, such as polyoma and S.V. 40, can add new genes to cells in culture when these are infected.[20] The viral DNA can become incorporated in the host's DNA and reproduce with the host-cell chromosomes. Sometimes the descendants of these infected cells can be stimulated to synthesise infectious virus particles again, and, in the case of the polyoma virus infecting mouse cells, the infected virus particles contain mouse genes.[21]

Tissue culture has played a useful part in adding to our knowledge of cellular metabolism, but its use is greatly limited by the fact that the cells are surviving in a completely abnormal environment; the vascular arrangement of the living body is replaced by a synthetic fluid medium which bathes the tissue.

It is certain from this bewilderingly large number of specialised techniques at our disposal that many of the intimate secrets of cellular physiology are now being revealed. Nevertheless, it is still as true as ever that the most important investigation into the nature of disease is based on a careful study of the patient.

REFERENCES

1. MINTZ, B. (1967) Gene control of mammalian pigmentary differentiation, 1. Clonal origin of melanocytes. *Proceedings of the National Academy of Sciences of the United States of America*, **58**, 344.
2. MINTZ, B. (1969) In *Clinical Delineation of Birth Defects, Birth Defects: Original Article Series*, ed. Bourne, G. H. Vol. 5, no. 1, p. 11. New York: Academic Press.
3. HAM, A. W. (1972) In *Histology*, 7th edn, p. 3 *et seq*. Philadelphia: Lippincott.
4. PEARSE, A. G. E. (1968 and 1970) *Histochemistry, Theoretical and Applied*, 3rd edn, Vols 1 and 2. London: Churchill.
5. DIXON, K. (1970) In *An Introduction to the Biology of the Skin*, ed. Champion, R. H., Gillman, T., Rook, A. J. & Sims, R. T. p. 35. Oxford: Blackwell Scientific Publications.
6. ENGSTRÖM, A. V. & FINEAN, J. B. (1967) In *Biological Ultrastructure*, 2nd edn, p. 9. New York: Academic Press.
7. TSALTAS, T. T. (1967) In *Methods and Achievements in Experimental Pathology*, Vol. 2, p. 30. Chicago: Year Book Medical Publishers.

8. DUBOWITZ, V. & BROOKE, M. H. (1973) *Muscle Biopsy: A Modern Approach*. Philadelphia: Saunders.
9. AFROUDAKIS, A. P., LIEW, C.-T. & PETERS, R. L. (1976) An immunoperoxidase technic for the demonstration of the hepatitis B surface antigen in human livers. *American Journal of Clinical Pathology*, **65,** 533.
10. MESA-TEJADA, R., PASCAL, R. R. & FENOGLIO, C. M. (1977) Immunoperoxidase: a sensitive immunohistochemical technique as a 'special stain' in the diagnostic pathology laboratory. *Human Pathology*, **8,** 313.
11. WEAKLEY, B. S. (1972) *A Beginner's Handbook in Biological Electron Microscopy*. Edinburgh: Churchill Livingstone.
12. SINGER, S. J. (1959) Preparation of an electron-dense antibody conjugate. *Nature (London)*, **183,** 1523.
13. STOLINSKI, C. & BREATHNACH, A. S. (1975) *Freeze-Fracture Replication of Biological Tissues*, 173 pp. London: Academic Press.
14. GORDON, A. H. & EASTOE, J. E. (1964) *Practical Chromatographic Techniques*. London: George Newnes.
15. FAHEY, J. L. & TERRY, E. W. (1967) In *Handbook of Experimental Immunology*, ed. Weir, D. M., p. 23 *et seq*. Oxford: Blackwell.
16. NAIRN, R. C. (1976) *Fluorescent Protein Tracing*, 4th edn. Edinburgh: Churchill Livingstone.
17. PAUL, J. (1975) *Cell and Tissue Culture*, 5th edn. Edinburgh: Churchill Livingstone.
18. KROOTH, R. S. (1969) Genetics of cultured somatic cells. *Medical Clinics of North America*, **53,** 795.
19. WEISS, M. C. & GREEN, H. (1967) Human-mouse hybrid cell lines containing partial complements of human chromosomes and functioning human genes. *Proceedings of the National Academy of Sciences of the United States of America*, **58,** 1104.
20. WESTPHAL, H. & DULBECCO, R. (1968) Viral DNA in polyoma — and SV40 — transformed cell lines. *Proceedings of the National Academy of Sciences of the United States of America*, **59,** 1158.
21. WINOCOUR, E. (1968) Further studies on the incorporation of cell DNA into polyoma-related particles. *Virology*, **34,** 571.

Chapter 2. The Normal Cell

The importance of the cell as the basic building unit of the body has been recognised since the microscope was first applied to the analysis of biological material. This is scarcely surprising, because simpler forms of life like the amoeba consist entirely of one cell. In 1858 Virchow published his famous treatise on 'Cellular Pathology', and since then our concept of many diseases has been centred on abnormalities in cellular behaviour or appearance. No attempt will be made to describe in detail the various types of cells which are present in the body, for such descriptions are available in standard text-books of histology. In this chapter the over-all structure and function of the mammalian nucleated (eukaryotic) cell are described.

The majority of cells in the human body are not disposed separately, but are grouped together to form tissues or organs. Traditionally two types of cells are distinguished—those of the epithelia and those of the connective tissue.

Epithelial cells cover surfaces, e.g. skin, or line cavities, e.g. the mouth, and in these situations they are essentially protective in function. Some covering epithelia may also perform a secretory function: the respiratory epithelium, for instance, secretes mucus.

In addition to covering extensive surfaces, the secretory type of epithelial cell may be arranged to form glands, which may be simple, like the mucous glands of the colon, or more elaborate, like those of the breast and pancreas. In the endocrine glands secretion is absorbed directly into the blood stream, and in some situations, e.g. pituitary, no tubular or acinar spaces are present. A feature common to all epithelial cells is that they are closely contiguous to one another. This is evident on light microscopy, and even under the electron microscope these cells appear to be separated by only a thin layer of low electron density which is about 15 nm in width.

Connective tissue cells are the other cell type present in the body. These are usually widely separated from each other by a zone containing much ground substance, and in which there are embedded collagen fibres. This type of connective tissue, typified by tendon, bone, cartilage, and fibrous tissue, is primarily supportive in function. Other connective tissue cells have been endowed with a specialised cytoplasm either for contraction (muscle fibres) or conduction (nerve cells).

This classification of cells into 'epithelial' and 'connective tissue' is not as simple as is sometimes assumed. The flattened 'endothelial' cells which line blood and lymph vessels are usually considered to be connective tissue, although they are, in fact, performing a covering function. The same may be said of the mesothelial cells lining the pleura and peritoneum, and those of the synovium.

Under abnormal conditions such cells may assume an 'epithelial' appearance. Squamous metaplasia has been described in the pleura, and some pleural and synovial tumours have a frankly adenocarcinomatous appearance. It must be accepted that the distinction between epithelial and connective tissue cells is not as rigid as used to be supposed.

This is not merely of academic interest. Its implications are obvious when it is remembered that an important component of the classification of tumours is their tissue of origin (see p. 310).

STRUCTURE OF CELLS

Although the different cells of the body possess striking features which readily distinguish them one from another, all are built upon a similar basic plan. This is to be expected, because in spite of their diversity of structure and function, each is in fact remarkably independent. Each receives a supply of oxygen and foodstuff from the blood stream, with which it must produce its own structural components and secretions and from which it must release energy required for mechanical, chemical, or electrical work. Each possesses an outer limiting membrane and within its protoplasm there is another limiting membrane which encloses the nuclear material. Most cells possess a single nucleus which is centrally placed. The basal nuclei of some columnar epithelial cells and the eccentric nucleus of the plasma cell are obvious exceptions. Cells with more than one nucleus are called *giant* or *multinucleate cells*. The osteoclast is an example of such a cell found normally in the body. To this may be added the syncytiotrophoblast of the placenta. Striated muscle fibres may be regarded as multinucleate cells with specialised cytoplasm. Giant cells are not infrequently found in pathological lesions: these are listed in Table 2.1 (see also pp. 127 and 337).

TABLE 2.1   Types of giant cell

Damaged striated muscle fibres

1. Regenerating sarcolemmal cells in damaged voluntary muscle.
2. Aschoff giant cell in heart muscle (? fused myocardial macrophage).

Tumour giant cells

1. Giant-cell tumours, e.g. of bone, poorly differentiated astrocytoma (glioblastoma multiforme), choriocarcinoma, Hodgkin's disease (Sternberg-Reed cell), etc.
2. Giant-cell variants of many tumours, e.g. carcinoma of lung and kidney.

Fused cells due to virus infection

1. Epithelial giant cells, e.g. in herpesvirus infections.
2. Connective tissue, e.g. Warthin-Finkeldey giant cells of measles.

Fused macrophages

See Table 11.1.

The nucleus forms an essential part of all living mammalian cells. The technique of microdissection has shown that after removal of the nucleus, respiratory activity may continue for two or three days, but the cell dies inevitably soon afterwards. Introduction of a nucleus from another cell may, however, ensure its continued life. Under some circumstances an enucleated cell can continue to grow and differentiate for many months. The messenger RNA already in the cytoplasm is responsible for this.[1] In the human the only non-nucleate cells are platelets and erythrocytes; both have a limited existence and neither is capable of reproduction. The extranuclear protoplasm, or cytoplasm, contains a number of bodies (*organelles*): some of these can be seen with the light microscope, but others are recognisable only by means of the electron microscope. The most conspicuous structures are the mitochondria, the endoplasmic reticulum and its associated ribosomes, lysosomes, and a variety of granules or vacuoles which are present in many specialised cells, e.g. eosinophils (Figs. 2.1 and 2.2).

Figure 2.2
Rat liver cell showing the main features of a cell as revealed by electron microscopy. The nucleus is bounded by the nuclear membrane (nm) in which there is a nuclear pore (np). A nucleolus is present in the part of the nucleus which is included. In the cytoplasm there are mitochondria (m) with cristae, lysosomes (ly), and rough endoplasmic reticulum (rer). The tissue was fixed in osmic acid and embedded in epon-araldite mixture. × 10 000. (*Photograph by courtesy of Dr. Y. le Beux*)

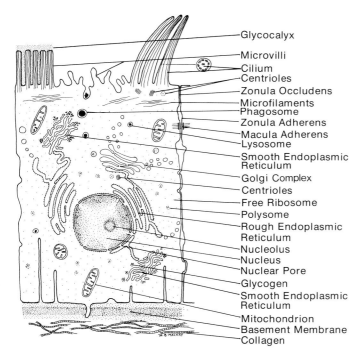

Figure 2.1
Diagrammatic representation of a hypothetical typical epithelial cell. The free surface of the cell has projecting microvilli, which on the left are arranged regularly to form a brush border. In the centre the villi are irregular, and micropinocytotic-vacuole formation is depicted. On the right cilia are shown. The cell adjoins its neighbours with some interdigitation of their plasma membranes; one junctional complex is shown. The nucleus contains one nucleolus, and is surrounded by a double-layered membrane. Between the nucleus and the free border is the cell centre, or centrosome, and adjacent to this is one Golgi complex. There are two centrioles lying at right angles to each other. The base of the cell rests on a basement membrane, and adjacent to this collagen fibres are shown. The plasma membrane, like the other membranes of the cell, has a trilaminar structure. Ribosomes are scattered free in the cell cytoplasm, and are also attached to the rough endoplasmic reticulum and the outer nuclear envelope. (*Drawn by Margot Mackay, Department of Art as Applied to Medicine, University of Toronto*)

The increasing complexity which the electron microscope reveals has brought morphology more into line with function. The numerous complicated biochemical reactions that are known to occur in the cell could hardly be reconciled with a cytoplasm as devoid of structure as it appears by light microscopy of H. and E. sections.

THE CELL MEMBRANE[2-4]

The *cell membrane*, or *plasma membrane*, is an extremely important structure, since it forms the interface between the cell cytoplasm and the interstitial tissue fluids or in lower forms of life, the exterior. Its functions may be listed: movement; cell recognition; cell growth; adhesion; transfer function.

Cell Movement[2]

The amoeboid movement and phagocytic activity of white blood cells are well known, but apart from this, an examination of living cells by phase contrast microscopy reveals the cell surface to be in constant movement. The undulating surface of the macrophage is particularly characteristic. Folds of the membrane have been observed to entrap a droplet of fluid by a process known as *pinocytosis*.

Cell Recognition

The membranes of the cell, including the plasma membrane, are associated with the antigens by which the body is able to recognise its own cells and tolerate them. Cells from another individual are regarded as aliens, and are attacked by the immune response which they provoke.

Receptor function. Many agents act on cells at specific points, or *cell receptors*. Thus influenza viruses attach themselves to specific receptors on the red-cell envelope (p. 267). Likewise drugs and hormones act on their own receptors. The presence of these specific receptors on particular cells is indeed the explanation of how hormones act only on their target cells and not on other cells. The mechanism of action of many non-steroid hormones is of great interest. The attachment of the hormone to its receptor activates the enzyme adenylate cyclase, which is situated in the cell membrane. This enzymatic activation causes ATP, which is present in abundance on the inner side of the cell membrane, to be converted into adenosine 3′,5′-cyclic phosphate—a nucleotide more widely known as *cyclic AMP* or simply *cAMP*.[5,6] This important compound has many actions. Thus in a liver cell acted upon by adrenaline, the formation of cAMP leads to the activation of a phosphorylase that converts glycogen to glucose: this is then released from the cell. In other instances cAMP acts on the nucleus and stimulates the expression of some particular genetic information (Fig. 2.3). In this way cAMP acts as a *second messenger* for the action of glucagon, thyrotrophic hormone, ACTH, and other hormones. Insulin also acts *via* a specific cell membrane receptor, but another nucleoside, guanosine 3′,5′-cyclic phosphate or cGMP, is its second messenger. With the steroid hormones the specific cell receptors are in the cytoplasm (see Ch. 35).

Figure 2.3
The second-messenger concept.
Many hormones act first by becoming attached to specific receptor sites on the membranes of target cells. Thus, adrenal cells have receptors that 'recognise' adrenocorticotrophin. The enzyme adenylate cyclase is activated in the cell membrane and passes into the cytoplasm where it catalyses the formation of cyclic AMP, which acts as a second messenger. In some cells it leads to enzyme activation. Thus, in the liver phosphorylase is activated and leads to the formation of glucose from glycogen. This is a mechanism by which adrenaline leads to the release of glucose from the liver cell. Cyclic AMP appears to act also by stimulating the expression of genetic information. It may therefore be regarded as a type of chemical switch that turns on the cell to perform specific functions. (*Drawn by Anthony J. Walter.*)

Cell Growth

The phenomenon of contact inhibition (see p. 111) is a function of the cell surface. Some procedures, e.g. treatment with proteolytic enzymes, appear to alter the cell membrane and also remove components involved in the control of the cell growth. In this way cell cultures can be obtained, although normal diploid cells can grow for only a limited time before they die (see p. 28). Malignant transformation may so alter the cell surface that it abolishes the control of cell growth. This involves the exposure of previously hidden receptor sites; it is of interest that viruses can produce the same effect.

Cell Adhesion

The cell membrane is concerned with adhesiveness, which is a factor that induces cells of like constitution to stick together. If the cells of an embryo are separated from each other and are then allowed to come together again, they aggregate to form organs and tissues. At first sight this would seem to indicate that differentiated cells have specific surface sites for recognition and adhesion. However, an alternative hypothesis is that differential adhesion is determined by the quantity and distribution of the sites of adhesion available. Groups of cells therefore strive to attain an arrangement that is thermodynamically most favourable.[7] This affinity which cells have for their own kind must be an important mechanism in the development and maintenance of the architecture of multicellular animals. But not all cells behave in this manner. The cells of the blood do not normally exhibit adhesiveness, nor to any great extent do malignant cells, for they are able to infiltrate freely into the surrounding tissues.

Transfer Function

All substances which enter or leave the cell protoplasm must cross the cell membrane, and the properties of this membrane are responsible for the peculiar chemical composition of the cytoplasm.

Chemicals soluble in organic solvents enter cells much more readily than do those which are water soluble. The absorption of some substances is related to enzymatic activity occurring at or near the cell surface. How chemicals cross the membrane and the factors which regulate their passage can be understood only in relationship to the structure of the membrane itself, for as in other realms of pathology, structure and function are interdependent.

Membrane structure in relation to function. Electron microscopy has shown an intact membrane some 7·5 nm in width, which at high magnification of suitably prepared material can be resolved into two electron-dense laminae with an intervening clear space. This trilaminar structure, as first described by Robertson, is known as a *unit membrane*, and it appears to have no pores such as have been postulated to explain the observed permeability of the cell membrane.

Substances are transported across the cell membrane either by bulk transfer or by diffusion. *Bulk transfer* involves the processes of phagocytosis, pinocytosis (previously described), and micropinocytosis. In *micropinocytosis* small invaginations of the cell membrane (Fig. 2.4), the *caveolae intracellulares*, become nipped off to form vesicles. In this way small quan-

Figure 2.4
Radioautograph of mouse jejunum.
The mouse was killed one hour after the instillation of radioactive iron in its stomach. The silver grains (arrows) represent radioactive iron that has been absorbed into the cell. The course of this radioactive material can be followed by examining animals killed at different times after being fed with labelled iron. Note the regular arrangement of the microvilli, which form the brush border of light microscopy. This arrangement appears to be adapted for absorption. An endocytotic vesicle is clearly shown (end). A junctional complex with its desmosome (des) is seen near the free border of the two epithelial cells depicted in this illustration. Figure 2.7 shows details of this complex. Mitochondria (m) and rough endoplasmic reticulum (rer) can be identified but are shown more clearly in other figures ($\times 16\,000$). (*From Bedard, Y. C.: Ultrastructural and Radiographic Studies on Iron Absorption in the Mouse. University of Toronto Ph.D. Thesis, 1972.*)

tities of fluid or particulate matter may be imbibed by a process that resembles pinocytosis but on a small scale. Indeed, the processes of phagocytosis, pinocytosis, and micropinocytosis are commonly grouped together as *endocytosis*, in contrast to *exocytosis*, in which the contents of membrane-bound vacuoles (e.g. secretions) are liberated at the cell surface by fusion of the cell membrane with the vacuolar membrane. The contents of endocytotic vacuoles are still membrane bound and not in the cytoplasmic ground substance proper. The fusion of the vacuole with a primary lysosome containing lytic enzymes results in the formation of a *secondary lysosome*, *phagosome*, or *heterophagosome*, and the digestion of its contents may result in their being released by diffusion into the substance of the cell.

The formation of micropinocytotic vesicles on one side of a cell and their discharge from another surface by exocytosis, is one postulated mechanism whereby substances may cross a cellular barrier, e.g. blood-vessel endothelium. The process is known as *cytopempsis*.

The *passive diffusion* of small ions across the cell membrane and the sodium pump are described on page 22.

In *active transport* there is the passage of chemicals across the cell membrane against a physico-chemical gradient, and the mechanism requires the expenditure of energy[8] Amino-acid transport is a good example, and is of great importance in the intestine and the renal tubules. Sometimes a single transport mechanism may serve a single amino acid. Thus a selective defect in the transport system for tryptophan in the intestine causes the *blue-diaper syndrome*. Unabsorbed tryptophan is broken down to indols by bacteria in the intestine. These are absorbed and excreted in the urine. The formation of indigo leads to the staining of the infant's diapers. Sometimes a single transport mechanism involves a group of amino acids; thus there is a failure to reabsorb cystine, lysine, ornithine, and arginine in the kidney in the classical type of *cystinuria*.

It is generally accepted that the cell membrane is made up of a lipid–protein combination but the details of its construction are not known. Davson and Danielli introduced the concept of a bimolecular lipid leaflet with two layers of lipid molecules having their polar (hydrophilic) ends turned outwards, and being covered by protein. This concept of a lamellar structure fits well with the observed electron microscope appearance of an approximately 7·5 nm thick trilaminated membrane. Analysis of the protein component of cell membranes has indicated that about 25 per cent of the protein is present as α-helix and there is no β-structure.* Calculations based on this and of the polar residues available indicate that the Davson and Danielli model is not a stable configuration.

The current concept of the cell membrane is that it is composed of two layers of structurally asymmetrical lipid molecules with their hydrophilic polar heads turned outwards (Fig. 2.5). Globular proteins form an integral part of the membrane and are bonded by hydrophobic interaction with lipid. These proteins are thus floating in a sea of lipid, thereby forming a *fluid mosaic*.[9] The proteins can move laterally, and while some are exposed only on one side of the membrane, others traverse it completely. These transmural proteins probably correspond to the intramembranous particles seen in freeze-fracture electronmicroscopic preparations.

The proteins of the cell membrane are heterogeneous—some act as antigens, while others are specific receptors for hormones, lectins, viruses, etc. Others have transport or enzymatic functions (Fig. 2.6). The cell receptors are probably linked to the microtubules and microfilaments of the underlying cytoplasm. The microtubules connecting one receptor with the next could be regarded as forming a cytoskeleton anchoring respective receptors. The microfilaments, on the other

*The *primary structure* of the protein is the order in which the individual amino acids are linked on the peptide chain. Orderly folding of this chain, such as the formation of a right-handed α-helix, is referred to as *secondary structure*. The peptide chains can also be held by adjacent chains to form sheet-like structures, β structures, or no structures at all (a random coil). Proteins whose major secondary structure is in the alpha form are elastic: keratin is a good example. Proteins that have extensive β structure, such as fibrin, are not readily extensible, since the polypeptide chains are already fully extended. *Tertiary structure* is the result of the interaction between active groups lying in the side chains of the amino acids. Disulphide bonds are the most important linkages involved. *Quaternary structure* is the association of individual monomers to form dimers, trimers, tetramers, etc.

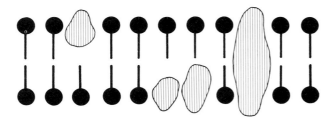

Figure 2.5
Diagrammatic representation of the plasma membrane.
The membrane is shown as a double layer of phospholipid molecules with their hydrophilic (water-loving) ends pointing outward and their hydrophobic (water-hating) ends facing inward. Globular proteins are partially or completely embedded in the lipid. This concept of a fluid lipid bilayer with embedded protein was described by Singer and Nicolson (Science, 1972, *175*, 720). It is believed that the carbohydrate side-chains of the protein molecules form the glycocalyx, which is illustrated in Figure 2.7. (*Drawn by Margot Mackay, Department of Art as Applied to Medicine, University of Toronto.*)

Figure 2.6
Detail of the plasma membrane of a HeLa cell with much surface activity in the form of profuse filamentous microvilli. After staining for enzymes splitting adenosine triphosphate, dense reaction-product has been deposited with close precision at the cell membrane, indicating that the enzymes are localised there, presumably for the supply of energy requirements. × 55 000. (*Electron micrograph by courtesy of Professor M. A. Epstein and Dr. S. J. Holt*)

hand, could act as contractile elements, so that the receptors could move within the cell membrane. That such movement can occur is well known, for after the attachment of antibodies or lectins to their specific receptors on the cell membrane, the receptor–ligand complexes aggregate to form groups called clusters, patches, or caps according to their size. These complexes may then enter the cell by endocytosis. In this way receptors may be removed from the cell surface. The most extensively studied phenomenon has been the capping that follows the attachment of lectins. These substances attach to sugar groupings and cause red-cell agglutination. Concanavalin A and *Ricinus communis* agglutinin are the two most often used.

The importance of this transmural linkage of receptor sites to the cytoskeletal system of microtubules and microfilaments is not known, but it has been investigated extensively in the hope that it might be related to the control of cell growth, and that abnormalities might be found to explain the behaviour of cancer cells.

In summary, the plasma membrane is a complex lipoprotein structure. It can consume energy and change its shape in response to stimuli. It contains protein molecules which are heterogeneous, some being responsible for the receptor sites, other for antigenicity, enzyme activity, etc.

Projections from the Cell Surface

Cilia, e.g. of respiratory epithelium, and flagella, e.g. of spermatozoa, are easily recognisable under the light microscope. Electron microscopy also reveals a very characteristic structure. Cilia contain nine peripherally-placed electron-dense bundles of microtubules: each bundle consists of two microtubules arranged in cross-section like a figure-of-eight. These ciliary filaments terminate in the basal plate opposing which there is another plate*; this is part of the basal body, a hollow, cylindrical structure with nine peripherally-arranged triplets of microtubules. This basal body resembles the structure of the centriole. The microtubules of the cilia are extensions of the innermost two of the triplets of the basal body. In the centre of each cilium there is a pair of single filaments. Flagella resemble cilia closely.

The electron microscope has revealed projections, or *microvilli*, on cells, which are not readily visible by light microscopy (see Fig. 2.6). The function of the microvilli is probably related to absorption; certainly the well-marked villus formation in the renal tubules and small intestine appears to subserve this function. It forms the 'brush border' seen by light microscopy.

Relationship of Cells to Each Other

Epithelial cells are generally closely applied to each other, but even then there is an electron-lucent area of 15 to 20 nm between their adjacent cell membranes. This is probably due to a covering of mucopolysaccharide which may well prove to be an important component of the external cell membrane itself. The free surface of epithelial cells is also covered by an additional coat, the *glycocalyx*, which on high-resolution electron microscopy can be seen to be filamentous (Fig. 2.7). The degree of indentation of one cell into another varies according to the tissue.

Cell Junctions.[10] Adjacent cells exhibit specialised junctional areas that subserve two important functions. (1) They enable cells to *adhere* to their neighbours, and can be adapted to form a seal to prevent substances passing between them.

*The precise manner in which the cilia terminate in the basal body varies in different species.

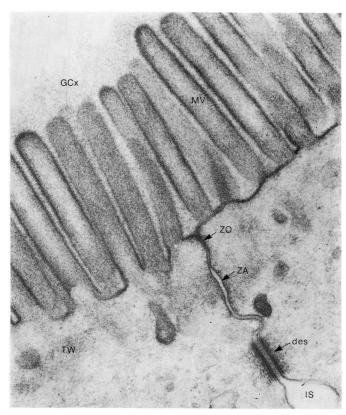

Figure 2.7
Details of the luminal surface of an absorptive cell of the human small intestine.
The apical cell membrane is thrown into regular microvilli (MV). There is a fuzzy covering, which is termed a *glycocalyx* (GCx). One junctional complex is shown. It consists of three parts: (1) The tight junction, or *zonula occludens* (ZO), which is an area where the plasma membranes of the two adjacent cells appear to fuse. "Zonule" means an encircled band or girdle; the zone forms an effective seal between adjacent cells. It is an area where one cell can communicate with adjacent ones. (2) The *zonula adherens* (ZA), which is an area where the cell membranes are closely applied to each other but are not fused. Filaments of the terminal web are concentrated at this area. (3) The *desmosomes*, or *maculae adherentes* (des), which are complex structures and are button shaped. Numerous microfilaments converge on the desmosomes. Where junctional complexes are not present, there is a space between adjacent cells (IS = intercellular space). (× 56 000). (*Photograph by courtesy of Dr. Y. C. Bedard.*)

This is particularly important in the intestinal epithelium (Fig. 2.7) and in the endothelial lining of blood vessels. (2) They form areas of close contact through which cells can *communicate* with each other. Most cells do not live in isolation; they co-operate, and co-ordinate their activities with those of their neighbours. How this is brought about is poorly understood, but the phenomena of peristalsis, contact inhibition (p. 111), and tissue induction may well be regulated by mechanisms that involve cell junctions. One might speculate that these structures are also important in the organised processes of embryogenesis, repair, and regeneration, as well as in the disorganised proliferation of neoplasia.

Three types of cell junction may be described:
The occludens type (*tight junctions*). The trilaminar membranes of the two adjacent cells come into intimate contact and

their outer leaflets appear to fuse. Many epithelial cells and some endothelial cells have this type of junction. It forms a band or girdle encompassing the cells at their free borders (Fig. 2.7). This is called the *zonula occludens.** An incomplete band is called a *macula occludens.**

*The nexus** or *gap junction*. At this type of junction the two trilaminar membranes are separated by an electron-lucent gap of 2 nm. The space contains structures that cross from one cell to the other, and through which electrical impulses and small ions can pass. The gap junctions are thought to be important in heart and smooth muscle, so that a wave of contraction can pass from cell to cell. Their function in other cell types is unknown.

The adherens type of junction. In this type of junction the cell membranes are separated by a gap of about 20 nm, which is filled with electron-lucent material that appears to glue the cells together. The *zonula adherens* forms a band around intestinal cells, and together with the zonula occludens and desmosome constitutes the *junctional complex* (Fig. 2.7). The *macula adherens,** or *desmosome*, is a button-like structure best seen in epidermis. The tonofilaments that converge on it do not cross from one cell to the next (Fig. 2.7).

In connective tissue the space between individual cells is considerably greater, and it usually contains fibres, e.g. collagen and elastic, as well as ground substance.

THE CELL NUCLEUS

The Nuclear Membrane or Envelope

The nucleus is bounded by the nuclear envelope which under the electron microscope can be resolved into two membranes, each about 7·5 nm in width, and separated from each other by a space (the perinuclear cistern) 40 to 70 nm wide (Fig. 2.8). The outer lamina is studded with ribosomes, and is continuous with the endoplasmic reticulum from which it is produced at the completion of mitosis. The inner lamina is reinforced on its internal aspect by a layer of filamentous material called the 'fibrous lamina'. The two layers of the nuclear envelope are continuous with each other around the edges of the nuclear pores, which appear as circular holes 50 nm in diameter. Whether there is free communication between the nucleus and cytoplasm through these pores is undecided. High-resolution electron micrographs indicate that there is a membrane across each pore.

Nuclei are generally circular or oval in shape, but they may show indentations, especially when the ultra-thin sections used in electron microscopy are examined. They are particularly well marked in contractile cells (such as muscle) when examined in the relaxed state. Invaginations of the nuclear envelope can lead to the formation of pseudo-inclusions. This is a well-known feature of malignant melanoma cells, and should not be mistaken for intranuclear viral inclusions. Indeed, irregular folding of the nuclear membrane is seen in many actively dividing cells both in regeneration and neoplasia.

The principal components of the nucleus are the chromatin, the nucleolus, and the nuclear sap, or nuclear matrix, in which they are suspended.

*Zonule means a girdle or band; a macule is a spot; a nexus is a bond or connexion.

Figure 2.8
Liver cell showing part of its nucleus (Nuc) and cytoplasmic organelles.
Mitochondria (m) with their cristae (Cr) are shown along with rough endoplasmic reticulum (rer) to which are attached ribosomes (r). Smooth endoplasmic reticulum (Ser) is associated with glycogen granules (Gly). Some ribosomes appear free in the cytoplasm and are forming rosettes (rr). Note also the nuclear membrane (NucM) surrounding the nucleus ($\times 24\,000$). (*Photograph by courtesy of Dr. Y. C. Bedard.*)

Chromatin

The nuclear material takes the form of long threads (*chromosomes*), of which each somatic cell contains 46—comprising 22 pairs of autosomes and one pair of sex chromosomes (p. 39). Only at mitosis can these chromosomes be seen, and in the interphase nucleus—i.e. between mitoses—the chromosomes merely contribute acidic substances to the nucleus that make it stain with basophilic dyes like haematoxylin (and methylene blue in the Romanowsky technique). This blue material is called *chromatin*. In the interphase nucleus, some chromatin (*heterochromatin*) appears as areas of deep staining and is thought to represent those regions of the chromosomes which remain condensed and relatively inert metabolically. The remainder of the nucleus is lightly stained, and the dispersed chromatin material (*euchromatin*) is in an active form. It follows that the actual morphology of the nucleus varies considerably from one cell to another, and that an assessment of function can be made from nuclear structure. In active cells, e.g. neurons, the nucleus is vesicular and very little heterochromatin is present. Heterochromatin is more abundant in epithelial cells, and gives the nucleus a stippled appearance. In inactive cells, e.g. lymphocytes and late normoblasts, the heterochromatin occupies much of the nucleus which therefore appears deeply basophilic. In the mature plasma cell the heterochromatin is disposed close to the nuclear membrane in clumps to produce the cart-wheeled, or clock-faced, appearance so typical of this cell.

Sex chromatin, or Barr body. The Barr body is most easily demonstrated in squamous epithelial cells, and in prac- tice scrapings from the buccal mucosa are commonly used. It appears as a demilune on the nuclear membrane and represents an inactivated X chromosome (Fig. 2.9). It follows that the number of Barr bodies present in a normal diploid cell is one less than the number of X chromosomes present. Hence the cells of a normal male have no Barr body (and are 'chromatin negative'), whereas those of the female possess one (and are 'chromatin positive').

Another site for the investigation of sex chromatin is the neutrophil leucocyte in the peripheral blood. In this situation it is disposed as a drumstick attached to the side of the nucleus (Fig. 2.10). About 3 per cent of leucocytes in females exhibit drumsticks.

Y-chromatin. The chromatin of the Y chromosome can now be made visible in the interphase nucleus by staining with quinacrine and examining the cell under ultraviolet light (see p. 40).

Deoxyribonucleic Acid

Deoxyribonucleic acid (DNA) is the essential genetic material of the nucleus and is confined to the chromosomes. Chromosomes are in fact made up of DNA (about 20 per cent), RNA (about 10 per cent), and protein (about 70 per cent). The last consists of approximately equal parts of histone and acidic chromosomal proteins.

DNA is a polymer of molecular weight around $6-10 \times 10^6$ daltons* composed of a long chain of monounits, or nuc-

*A *dalton* is the weight of one hydrogen atom.

Figure 2.9
The Barr body. Nucleus of a cell from a female buccal mucosal smear showing the sex chromatin mass on the nuclear membrane. Stained by orcein acetic. (*Photograph by courtesy of Dr. Nigel H. Kemp*)

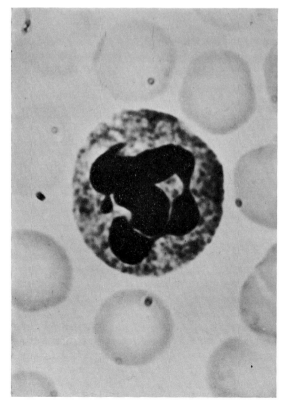

Figure 2.10
Polymorphonuclear neutrophil leucocyte from a normal female subject showing the drumstick appendage to the nucleus. The film has been stained by a Romanowsky technique. × 3000. (*Picture by courtesy of Dr. Nigel H. Kemp*)

leotides (Base—Sugar—Phosphate). The deoxyribose molecules are linked together by a phosphate: a base is attached to each sugar. The common bases are either purines (adenine and guanine) or pyrimidines (thymine and cytosine). As a result of X-ray diffraction studies Watson and Crick have proposed a structure which fits in remarkably well with our concept of DNA as a self-reduplicating genetic material. They proposed that the molecule is composed of two polynucleotide chains spiralled round a common axis (see Fig. 2.11). The bases are directed inwards towards the axis, and the two chains are linked by hydrogen bonds between a purine and a pyrimidine. They showed that only adenine could pair with thymine, and guanine with cytosine.

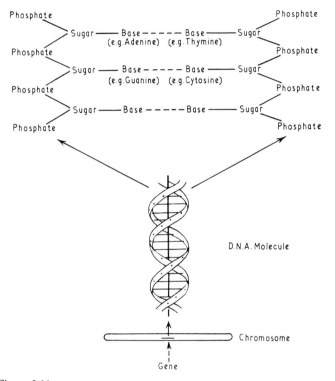

Figure 2.11
Suggested chemical structure of DNA. The two polynucleotide chains are united by their bases, the order of which constitutes the genetic code. (*After Watson, J. D. and Crick, F. H. C.* (1963), Narure (*Lond.*) **171**, 737)

Role of the Nucleic Acids as Genetic Material[11]

The DNA in the nucleus contains genetic information which is passed *via* RNA into the cytoplasm where it is utilised in the manufacture of proteins (often enzymes) of exact composition.

The order of the bases in DNA constitutes the genetic code, a sequence of three bases corresponding to a single amino acid. A type of RNA (*messenger RNA*, or mRNA) is made in the nucleus in the presence of DNA-dependent RNA polymerase, or transcriptase, for the process is called *transcription*, and the mRNA is modelled on one of the polynucleotide chains of DNA which acts as a template. The base sequence of the RNA is thus complementary to that of DNA, i.e. cytosine corresponds with guanine, etc. This mRNA passes

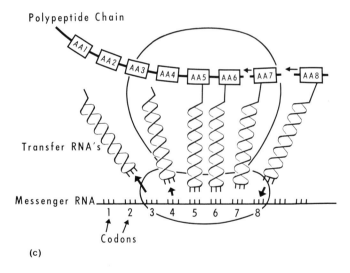

Figure 2.12
Schematic model of protein synthesis. In (*a*) and (*b*) a long single-stranded molecule of messenger RNA (mRNA) is seen associated with a group of ribosomes to form a polysome. As each ribosome moves along the mRNA, an ever-growing polypeptide chain is produced. In (*c*) a single ribosome is depicted as a combination of two particles of unequal size. The sequence of bases of the mRNA forms triplets, or codons, which for the sake of clarity are drawn as groups of three upright lines. Each molecule of transfer RNA (tRNA) is composed of a long thread bent on itself to form a helical structure. At one end of the molecule there is a particular amino acid (AA1, AA2, etc.), and at the other end, where it is bent on itself, there are three unpaired bases which form an anti-codon. Each codon of the mRNA is "recognised" by a corresponding anticodon of a tRNA. In this way specific amino acids are added to the polypeptide chain in a specific linear sequence determined by the mRNA, which is itself modelled on the nuclear DNA. (*Drawn by the Department of Art as applied to Medicine, University of Toronto: after Warner, J.R. and Soeiro, R. (1967), New Engl. J. Med.* **276,** 613; *and Nirenberg, M. W. (1965), in* The Living Cell, *San Francisco and London: Freeman*)

into the cytoplasm and becomes associated with a group of ribosomes (a *polysome*). Here protein synthesis occurs. Each triplet of the RNA base order is responsible for one amino acid.* As the ribosomes 'read along' the RNA molecule, successive amino acids are added to an ever-increasing polypeptide chain. In this way a protein of exact composition is built up; secondary and tertiary structure are presumably a consequence of this. The actual addition of each amino acid is effected by another type of RNA (*transfer RNA*, or tRNA), a separate form of which exists for each of the amino acids. The process is complex and is described as *translation*, for the code of the DNA finally appears legible in the form of a polypeptide chain (Fig. 2.12). It should be noted that mRNA molecules are 10 to 15 per cent longer than would appear necessary for the actual coding of their message. The extra portions, e.g. runs of poly A, appear to play a part in the regulation of translation and in the stability of the messenger.

Thus the genetic code of DNA consists of triplets, or *codons*, which determine the insertion of particular amino acids in the peptide chain. The sequence of the codons is colinear with the sequence of amino acids. The codons responsible for a whole peptide chain form a group called a *cistron*. It is believed that a number of cistrons are grouped together to form a larger unit, the *operon*,[12] which is described below. The actual code has been investigated by various means. Synthetic polyribonucleotides have been prepared and can act as mRNA in cell-free preparations containing ribosomes, suitable substrates, and a source of energy. Thus a polynucleotide containing uridine only (poly U) leads to the formation of phenylalanine. Hence the code for this amino acid is UUU.

Although it is well established that the encoded message of DNA is passed on to RNA, it is also known that the reverse can occur. Several RNA tumour viruses contain a DNA polymerase activity which can lead to the formation of specific nuclear DNA (p. 378).

Relationship of DNA to Genes

It is apparent that DNA provides the chemical basis for the inheritance of characteristics which are described as genes (Ch. 3). The nucleotide sequence of a length of DNA comprises a gene whose message is first transcribed into mRNA and then translated into a polypeptide chain of specific amino-acid sequence.

Control of gene action. It is evident that each nucleated cell of the body contains the necessary information for the manufacture of every protein of which the body is composed. That they do not do so all the time is evidence that there is some very adequate control mechanism. Thus erythroid cells manufacture haemoglobin, plasma cells immunoglobulin, etc.

The degree of permanence with which genetic information is repressed when cells differentiate has been the subject of much speculation. A fertile adult frog can develop from the implantation of an intestinal-cell nucleus of an adult frog into an enucleate ovum.[13] It would seem that in this instance none

---

*With 4 bases, 64 triplets are possible, but as only about 20 amino acids have to be coded, some duplication occurs. The code is therefore said to be degenerate. Thus UUU and UUC both correspond to phenylalanine. It is thought that the code is universal, i.e. the same for all organisms. The code is written in terms of the order of bases in mRNA.

of the DNA in the differentiated cell is irreversibly repressed. If this is true, it is not surprising that under abnormal circumstances cells produce substances which are alien to their accustomed products. This occurs in metaplasia and neoplasia. An excellent example is the secretion by certain cancer cells of hormones which normally are produced only in the very specialised cells of the endocrine glands. The production of α-fetoprotein by some hepatomata is another example (p. 388).

The control of gene action is poorly understood, but is being actively investigated at the present time. Some genes lead to the production of proteins which are enzymes, or which are used in the metabolism of the cell. These are termed *structural genes*. In certain bacteria it has been found that a group of genes are closely linked, and either function together or are completely repressed, i.e. no mRNA is produced. The mechanism of control is also under genetic influence, and Figure 2.13 illustrates a scheme of this based on that proposed by Jacob and Monod. Each group of genes, or *operon*, is controlled by a closely associated gene called the *operator gene*. This itself is regulated by another gene, the *regulator gene*, which through its own mRNA leads to the production in the cytoplasm of a protein (*repressor substance*) which suppresses the operator gene. The regulator gene may itself be inhibited, and in that event the operator is derepressed and the genes of the operon are allowed to act; mRNA is produced and protein synthesis proceeds (Fig. 2.13).

The model is derived from a study of prokaryotic cells, particularly *Escherichia coli*. In eukaryotic, or nucleated, cells the situation is different. Instead of a single naked strand of bacterial DNA, the DNA in chromosomes is in the form of a double helix and is associated with protein and RNA. It has been estimated that in most differentiated cells less than 5 per cent of the genetic material is expressed at any one time, i.e. only a very limited region of the genome is being transcribed. Since histones are known to inhibit both DNA and RNA synthesis, it has been suggested that the histone component is the important repressor chemical, and that its removal—perhaps by a derepressor RNA—leads to derepression of the genes. However, it now seems more likely that the acidic

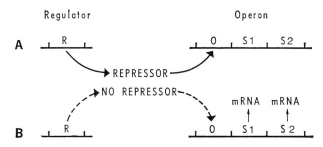

Figure 2.13
The regulator-operator hypothesis. A. The regulator gene (R) forms a repressor substance which acts through the cytoplasm to repress the operator gene (O). When O is thus inhibited, the structural genes (S1 and S2) in its operon cannot form mRNA. B. If the regulator gene cannot form repressor substance, or if the repressor does not reach the operator gene, the operator is *derepressed* and S1 and S2 are then able to produce mRNA. (*Diagram redrawn from Thompson, J. S. and Thompson, M. W. (1966), Genetics in Medicine. Philadelphia and London: Saunders. The hypothesis is that of Jacob, F. and Monod, J. (1961), J. molec. Biol.* **3,** 318)

proteins ('chromosomin'), being more heterogeneous by possessing both species and tissue specificity, play, in conjunction with RNA, a major role in the regulation of genetic information. [14,15]

The complexity of the subject is apparent when it is appreciated that in every cell, every gene is under continuous control and so regulated that the requirements of the body are met. This applies not only during adult life but also during the complex processes of development. The ovum provides an excellent example of how protein synthesis can be inhibited, only to be switched on suddenly by the event of fertilisation.

Effect of antibiotics on nucleic-acid metabolism. Certain antibiotics have a very specific action on nucleic-acid metabolism, which can be used therapeutically as well as in investigative work. Mitomycin C, which has antitumour and antibacterial activity, inhibits DNA synthesis, while RNA and protein synthesis are unaffected. Actinomycin D, on the other hand, inhibits DNA-dependent RNA polymerase activity by binding to DNA, and mRNA production is therefore stopped by its action. Streptomycin and puromycin block the transfer of amino acids from tRNA to the polypeptide chain, whereas chloramphenicol, which also inhibits protein synthesis, probably acts by preventing mRNA from binding to the ribosomes.

Replication of DNA. The DNA molecule has been observed to uncoil, and it is believed that each half can act as a template for the manufacture of another half. The enzyme concerned is called DNA polymerase. In this way the exact order of the bases is faithfully copied during cell division.

The amount of DNA is constant in all resting cells (the 2 n amount), whereas there is only half this amount in the germ cells (n). However, there are exceptions to this rule. In normal liver with increasing age some cells are found with nuclei containing abnormal, multiple amounts of DNA, i.e. 4 n, 8 n, and 16 n amounts. These are called *polyploid* nuclei, and in essence occur in cells that have replicated their genetic material, but have been blocked in the G_2 phase of the cell cycle and have not proceeded to mitosis. The increase in nuclear DNA is accompanied by an increase in cell mass. Polyploidy is also a feature of hypertrophied muscle, and is encountered in megaloblasts (Ch. 52).

Cells may contain an amount of DNA that is not an exact multiple of the normal amount. This condition is termed *aneuploidy*, and is a feature of malignant cells.

It can be seen that by measuring the amount of DNA in a tissue, an estimate can be made of the number of cells present. Likewise the amount of DNA which appears on a surface can be used to estimate the number of cells which are exfoliated. Thus it has been calculated that from 20 to 50 million cells are shed from the human small intestine each minute.[16]

DNA, together with RNA, is thus the material responsible for the appearance of chromatin of the cell nucleus. It is basophilic and stains dark blue with H. and E. Methyl green stains DNA green, and this is a selective reaction. Feulgen's method (p. 3) is also specific for DNA. It can furthermore be recognised by being depolymerised by specific enzymes (deoxyribonucleases), after which the stains mentioned above are all negative. It has a characteristic absorption of ultraviolet light of 260 nm wavelength, and can in this way be estimated quantitatively, since the amount of light absorbed is proportional to the amount of DNA present. (RNA has the same optical properties, and must be distinguished by some other form of separation.)

Nucleoli

The nucleus frequently contains one or more round bodies known as nucleoli. There may be a surrounding condensation of chromatin to form the *nucleolus-associated heterochromatin.* The nucleoli contain *granules* 15 nm in diameter, and *fibrils* which are 5 nm in diameter and of variable length. Together these are concentrated to form an electron-dense network (fibrillo-granular meshwork, or *nucleolonema*) which encloses spaces of low electron opacity called the *pars amorpha* (Fig. 2.14). The nucleolus appears to be the site of RNA formation, and it is thought that the fibrillar component is the precursor of the granules. The latter closely resemble the ribosomes of the cytoplasm, but whether they migrate into the cytoplasm is not clear. Although the precise role of the nucleoli in RNA metabolism is unclear, their presence in a cell is related to activity. Thus cells which are active metabolically, e.g. neurons, regenerating cells, and malignant cells, often have large and sometimes numerous nucleoli with a prominent granular component (Fig. 2.15).

Ribonucleic acid. RNA occurs in the cell in various forms. Its basic structure is similar to that of DNA in that it consists of a polynucleotide chain. However, uracil (the naturally-occurring uridine base) is present instead of thymine. mRNA, previously described, is single-stranded and has a short life, while tRNA is double-stranded (Fig. 2.12). RNA is the principal component of the ribosomes (p. 25) as well as the granular and fibrillar components of the nucleoli. RNA can be recognised by the action of specific enzymes (ribonucleases) which break it down, and also by its selective red staining with pyronin. Methyl green and pyronin are generally used together: the nucleus stains green and the cytoplasm and nucleoli red.

THE CYTOPLASM

Chemical Composition

The cytoplasm is composed largely of water. There is also about 8 per cent of protein. The contents differ from the extracellular fluid in several important respects. There is a high concentration of potassium, magnesium, and phosphate which contrasts with the sodium, chloride, and bicarbonate found in the extracellular fluids. The osmotic pressure within the cells (exerted principally by protein, potassium, magnesium, and phosphate) is equal to that of the extracellular fluid (exerted by sodium, chloride, and bicarbonate).

Water and chloride diffuse readily across the cell membrane, but potassium and sodium do so comparatively slowly, potassium diffusing about one hundred times faster than sodium. Others, phosphate and protein, do not diffuse at all. The net negative charge of protein and phosphate within the cell is balanced by potassium. In a passive diffusion system the result would be a greater concentration of ions within the cell than outside it, and the cell would swell. However, there is a mechanism in the cell membrane which actively excludes sodium. This is the *'sodium pump'*, which requires ATP for its operation. The ultimate source of energy is mitochondrial cell

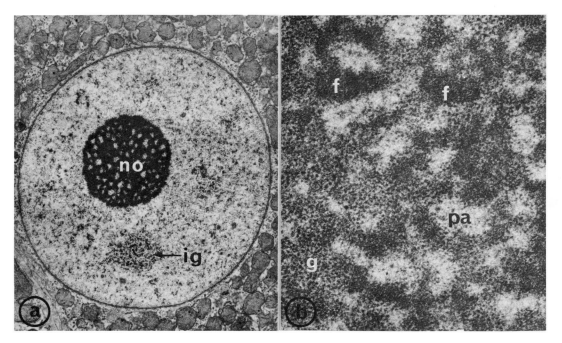

Figure 2.14
Nucleolar structure of the hepatocyte. (*a*) This shows the nucleus of a rat hepatocyte of an animal given ethionine. The nucleolus (no) is large, deeply staining, and shows the nucleolonema as a dense network enclosing spaces of low opacity called the pars amorpha. ig interchromatin granules. Uranyl acetate. ×7500. (*b*) A higher magnification of a nucleolus similar to that shown in (*a*). The fibrillar (f) and granular (g) components are seen, and together surround clear spaces the pars amorpha (pa). Lead hydroxide. ×45 000. (*Photographs by courtesy of Dr. Katsumi Miyai*)

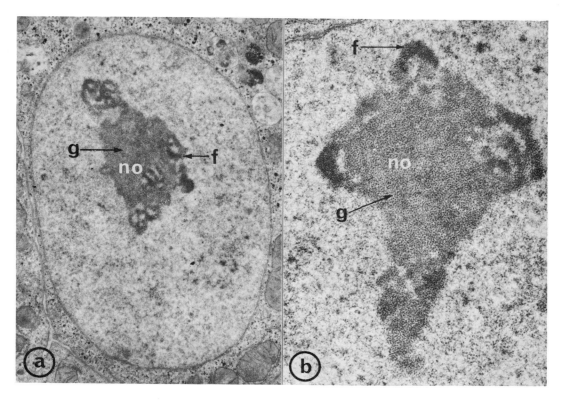

Figure 2.15
Nucleolar structure in a malignant cell. (*a*) This shows the nucleus of a hepatoma cell. The tumour was induced in a rat by the administration of ethionine. The nucleolus is enlarged and irregular in size, and has an abundant granular component (g). The fibrillar zones (f) of the nucleolus are distinct and form a twisted rope-like pattern. Chromatin is inconspicuous. Lead hydroxide. × 6300. (*b*) A higher power of a nucleolus similar to that shown in (*a*). The abundant granular component is obvious. Lead hydroxide. × 43 750. (*Photographs by courtesy of Dr. Katsumi Miyai*)

respiration; it follows that damage to these organelles is characterised by cell swelling (p. 52). In severe illnesses, such as heart failure and hepatic failure, there is an increase in the cell-membrane permeability. Potassium leaves the cells and sodium enters them. This has been called the '*sick-cell syndrome*', and is evident biochemically as hyponatraemia (p. 568).[17]

Cytoplasmic DNA.[18,19] The presence of DNA in the cytoplasm is well established. Some is present in the mitochondria and directs protein synthesis *via* specific tRNA. In trypanosomes a mass of DNA at the end of a giant mitochondrion forms the kinetoplast. DNA is also present in the mitochondria of mammalian cells, and this has given rise to the concept, popular but not necessarily true, that mitochondria originally evolved from intracellular symbionts. Likewise the chloroplasts of *Euglena* may be symbiotic algae.

Other forms of cytoplasmic DNA are known. These may act as infective agents, e.g. bacteriophage and resistance transfer factor, and can replicate in the cytoplasm and act as genetic material. These agents are known as *episomes*, or *plasmids*. Their presence can alter the functions of a cell. Thus the production of toxin by *Corynebacterium diphtheriae* and colicines by *Esch. coli*, the antibiotic sensitivity of bacteria, and even the sex of certain moulds are determined by these agents. They have been extensively studied in bacteria and protozoa,

and undoubtedly also occur in the higher forms of life. One can speculate about their importance in explaining some types of inheritance, certain aspects of the immune response, and the development of tumours.

Formed Structures (or Organelles)

Mitochondria. Situated in the cytoplasm of nearly all cells there are oval or rod-shaped bodies known as mitochondria (Fig. 2.16). They are plentiful in actively metabolising cells, but sparse in others. Under the electron microscope the mitochondria are seen to have a smooth outer limiting membrane and an inner electron-dense membrane, which is folded into incomplete septa, or cristae, which subdivide the mitochondria into compartments. Both membranes can be resolved into double structures like the 7·5 nm outer cell membrane. The cristae form plates which project into the mitochondrion, and in some cells form complete septa. High-resolution electron microscopy has revealed the presence of subunits, 8 to 10 nm in diameter, which are attached to the inner membrane by narrow stalks. In some cells the inner membrane is folded to produce blind-ending tubules rather than plates. This is quite common in certain protozoa, but in the human being mitochondria containing tubular cristae occur mostly in cells involved in cholesterol metabolism and

Figure 2.16
Liver cell mitochondrion. The organelle is surrounded by an outer membrane with a second, inner membrane close within it: the inner membrane is folded into shelf-like cristae which protrude into the interior. ×52500. (*Photograph by courtesy of Professor M. A. Epstein*)

in the manufacture of steroids. Mitochondria have been observed to divide by transverse fission, but there is considerable diversity of opinion as to whether they can also be formed from other cytoplasmic constituents.

The chemical composition of mitochondria is very important. The matrix contains the enzymes of the Krebs cycle, while the electron-transport and oxidative-phosphorylation enzymes form molecular assemblies in or on the inner mitochondrial membrane covering the walls and cristae. The Krebs cycle is a system whereby products of carbohydrate, fat, and protein metabolism are oxidised to produce energy, which is stored in the form of the high energy bonds of ATP, and is utilised whenever the cell performs any kind of work, whether mechanical, osmotic, or biosynthetic (Fig. 2.17). Mitochondria are therefore plentiful in actively metabolising cells, e.g. muscle. Furthermore, the complexity of their internal structure is a reflection of their activity; numerous cristae point to great activity. The mitochondria are thus intimately concerned with energy production, and are amongst the first structures to show the effects of the many adverse conditions which may affect the cell.

Mitochondria are sparse in some malignant tumours, a fact no doubt related to the predominance of glycolysis over respiration as a means of energy production in many neoplasms.

Lysosomes. Lysosomes are rounded, membrane-bound organelles which contain lytic enzymes that are active at a low pH, i.e. acid phosphatase, esterases, deoxyribonuclease, and the proteolytic enzymes previously grouped under the heading 'cathepsins'. The lysosomal enzymes are formed in the rough endoplasmic reticulum and pass into the Golgi complex where they are packaged. They are released from the maturing face of the Golgi complex as *primary lysosomes*. Membrane-bound material in the form of *heterophagosomes* formed as a result of endocytosis, or as *autophagosomes* (or *cytolysomes*) containing damaged or worn-out cell components, fuse with the primary lysosomes to form *secondary lysosomes*. These bodies present a variety of appearances. They contain foreign, ingested material or fragments of cell membrane with cell receptors combined with their specific ligand. They may contain recognisable cell components—mitochondria, endoplasmic reticulum, etc. (Figs 2.18 and 2.19). Sometimes they contain lipid which assumes the form of the concentric laminations of myelin figures (Fig. 2.20). Eventually the lysosomes contain only indigestible material, and they remain as *residual bodies* containing lipofuscin. These are the wear-and-tear pigments of light microscopy.

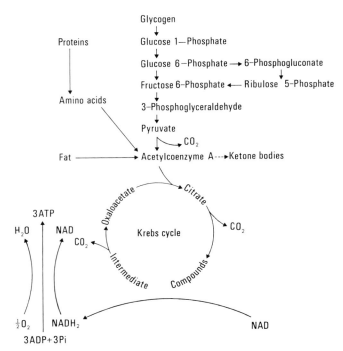

Figure 2.17
Outline of the metabolic pathways concerned in energy production. The whole process in the oxidation of glycogen to CO_2 and water can be considered as occurring in two phases. The first, or anaerobic, phase results in the formation of pyruvate, and is known as glycolysis. The second, or aerobic, phase is the Krebs cycle. Products of carbohydrate, fat, and protein metabolism are fed into the Krebs cycle *via* acetylcoenzyme A. Several enzymic reactions of the Krebs cycle involve the reduction of NAD to $NADH_2$. Reoxidation of $NADH_2$ by the cytochrome system is coupled with phosphorylation of ADP to ATP, viz.

$$NADH_2 + \tfrac{1}{2}O_2 + 3ADP + 3Pi \rightarrow NAD + H_2O + 3ATP.$$

The hexose monophosphate shunt, or pentose–phosphate pathway, leads to the formation of ribulose phosphate and is an alternative pathway in certain cells. It is an aerobic process, and in addition to its products re-entering the glycolytic sequence, sugars of 4–7 carbon atoms are formed and utilised in various synthetic processes. *Key:* NAD—Nicotinamide adenine dinucleotide. $NADH_2$—Dihydronicotinamide adenine dinucleotide. Pi—Inorganic phosphate. ADP—Adenosine diphosphate. ATP—Adenosine triphosphate.

The stability of the lysosomal membrane can be increased by the action of cortisol, and this may be a factor in the protective action of this hormone against the effects produced by ultraviolet light and bacterial endotoxin. Vitamin A, on the

Figure 2.18
Various types of lysosome. (*a*) A lysosome (ly) in a normal parenchymal liver cell. Lead hydroxide. × 43 750. (*b*) Membrane-bound structures containing ferritin granules. These are sometimes called siderosomes (so). G — Golgi complex. Lead hydroxide. × 22 400. (*c*) A cytolysome (cly) in a normal rat hepatocyte containing small fragments of the rough-surfaced endoplasmic reticulum (er). Lead hydroxide. × 46 200. (*d*) A cytolysome (cly) containing structures which are probably degraded mitochondria. Lead hydroxide. × 17 900. (*Photographs by courtesy of Dr. Katsumi Miyai*)

other hand, has the converse effect and causes the release of lysosomal enzymes. Thus, if administered to a rabbit there is softening of the cartilages so that the ears collapse. A similar effect follows the injection of the enzyme papain, because it has the same action on cartilage as does the released lysosomal enzymes.

Lysosomal digestion plays a part in the removal of unwanted cells during embryonic development. For example there is a great increase in lysosomal enzyme activity in the tail during the metamorphosis of the tadpole *Xenopus laevis*. Interestingly enough, regression of the tail can be accelerated by administering vitamin A and retarded by cortisol. In starvation the formation of cytolysomes is probably a factor in the mobilisation of cell constituents.

The enzyme defects that result in the abnormal accumulation of substances in cells, e.g. in the gangliosidoses and type II glycogen-storage disease, can be regarded as lysosomal abnormalities (p. 37 and p. 431). The role of the lysosomes in cell degeneration and necrosis is described in Chapter 4.

Microbodies. Microbodies are membrane-bound, rounded organelles characterised by their content of oxidases (such as urate oxidase) and catalase, an enzyme which acts on hydrogen peroxide and liberates oxygen. For this reason they have been called peroxisomes. Microbodies often contain an electron-dense nucleoid; this probably contains the urate oxidase. Both the enzyme and the nucleoid are absent in human cells (p. 432). The origin and function of microbodies are at present ill-defined, but the catalase is probably responsible for protecting cells against the damaging effect of peroxide.

The rough endoplasmic reticulum. Situated in the cytoplasm of all cells there are a series of membranes which include between them a complex series of intercommunicating tubes, vesicles, and cisterns. The secretion of some glandular cells, e.g. pancreas, appears between these membranes, and such cells show a well-developed rough endoplasmic reticulum, as the system of membranes is called. Situated on the membranes there are granules about 15 nm in diameter and rich in RNA. These are the *ribosomes*, and they give this component of the endoplasmic reticulum a rough appearance (Fig. 2.8). The rough endoplasmic reticulum is particularly well developed in cells engaged in the manufacture of protein for export, e.g. pancreatic acinar cells and plasma cells.

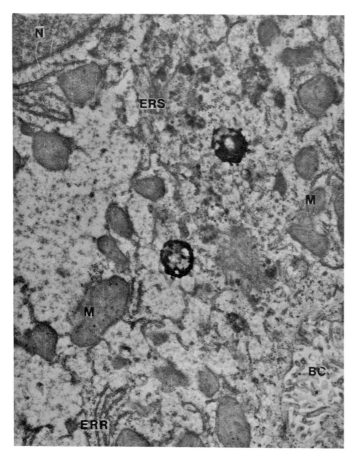

Figure 2.19
Rat liver cell. Survey of cytoplasm stained for acid phosphatase. The nucleus (N) lies in the top left corner and a bile canaliculus (BC) in the bottom right. The cytoplasm contains mitochondria (M) and both rough (ERR) and smooth (ERS) endoplasmic reticulum. The specific localisation of heavy stain in two lysosomes indicates that these bodies are the storage site for the hydrolytic enzyme acid phosphatase. × 23 000. (*From S. J. Holt and R. M. Hicks* (1961), J. biophys. biochem. Cytol. **11,** 47.)

Ribosomes are also found lying free in the cytoplasm, either separately or in the form of polysomes. Again their function is related to protein synthesis, but here it is for use within the cell. They are therefore abundant in actively growing cells, e.g. normoblasts and tumour cells.

The endoplasmic reticulum and its associated ribosomal granules cannot be distinguished in the paraffin sections used in routine pathology. The RNA content, however, is distinguishable by its basophilia with haematoxylin and its red staining with pyronin. For this reason the cytoplasm of cells actively engaged in protein synthesis is blue or mauve in H. and E. sections. Plasma cells are an excellent example of this, for immunoglobulin (a glycoprotein) is formed in the rough endoplasmic reticulum. Sometimes the accumulation of glycoprotein is so excessive that the cisterns of the rough endoplasmic reticulum become greatly dilated and contain masses that are visible on light microscopy. These take the form of refractile, eosinophilic, PAS-positive, spherical objects either solitary or forming grape-like clusters in the cell cyto-

plasm. They are called *Russell bodies*, and must not be mistaken for fungi in sections of chronic inflammatory tissue. The rough endoplasmic reticulum of nerve cells may be visible as the *Nissl granules*.

Smooth endoplasmic reticulum. In some parts of the cell the endoplasmic reticulum also forms a complex lattice of tubules which has no attached ribosomes and therefore appears smooth. The smooth and rough elements of the endoplasmic reticulum are continuous with each other and also with the outer lamina of the nuclear membrane.

The smooth endoplasmic reticulum has been related to the following functions:

Drug metabolism. Following the administration of barbiturates and other toxins there is an increase in the smooth endoplasmic reticulum of the liver cells. This appears to be an adaptive response to ensure detoxification (see Figure 4.6).

Steroid and cholesterol metabolism.

Carbohydrate metabolism. In the liver glycogen synthesis occurs in close relationship to smooth endoplasmic reticulum (Fig. 2.21).

Muscle contraction. In striated muscle, specialised smooth endoplasmic reticulum is important in the release and recapture of calcium ions during contraction and relaxation of the fibres.

Undulating tubules.[20] These are groups of tubular structures that have been described in both normal and abnormal cells. The best known are seen in the renal endothelial cells in systemic lupus erythematosus. It has been suggested that these are paramyxoviruses, but this is unproven.

The Golgi complex or apparatus. The Golgi complex is best developed in exocrine glandular cells, and is usually situated close to the nucleus on the side nearest to the lumen. It stains poorly in H. and E. sections, appearing as a clear zone (negative image). On electron microscopy it is seen to consist of a series of flattened sacs and vesicles often arranged in curved stacks.

A major function of the Golgi complex is the modification and packaging of material synthesised in the rough endoplasmic reticulum. It is possible that the membranes of the rough endoplasmic reticulum are directly continuous with those of the Golgi complex. However, it is more likely that material in the rough endoplasmic reticulum is pinched off in smooth, covered vacuoles (*transport vesicles*), which pass to the forming face of the Golgi complex (this is generally on the convex surface). The membrane of the vesicle fuses with that of the Golgi complex, and its contents pass through the stacks, being finally released from the maturing face of the Golgi complex as membrane-bound vacuoles (Fig. 2.22). During its passage through the stacks the material may be condensed, sulphated (e.g. the glycoproteins of ground substance), or combined with carbohydrate. The vacuoles leaving the maturing face of the Golgi complex can be of many varieties, according to the cell type. Some are secretory vacuoles, others contain mucopolysaccharide or tropocollagen, others are primary lysosomes, while others again pass to the cell surface and by fusing with the cell membrane, contribute material to it. Melanosomes are yet another variety of vesicle formed in the Golgi complex.

Microtubules and microfilaments. High-resolution electron microscopy has revealed that most cells contain fibrillar material which is composed of either thin filaments or tubules.

Figure 2.20
Myelin figures in spleen.
Many platelets (PL) are seen lying free in a splenic sinusoid (S). One platelet (arrow) has been engulfed by a phagocytic cell. Note the numerous myelin figures in some reticulo-endothelial cells. × 25 000. The insert shows the typical laminated appearance as seen under higher magnification. The spleen was from a patient with thrombotic thrombocytopenic purpura. (*Photographs by courtesy of Dr. G. T. Simon.*)

Their composition, structure, and function probably vary from one cell type to another and only a brief description will be given here.

Microtubules. These are tubular structures about 25 nm in diameter. Their centres are composed of material of low electron density, and they therefore appear as hollow tubes. The outer dense wall is actually composed of approximately 13 longitudinal filamentous subunits with a distance of 5·5 to 6 nm between them. Microtubules are composed of protein subunits called tubulin, and can undergo rapid break-down and re-assembly. This re-assembly is inhibited by the alkaloids colchicine and vinblastine. In some cells, e.g. diatoms, the microtubules appear to provide rigidity, acting as a cytoskeleton, and they may be responsible for the relatively fixed shape of some cells, e.g. blood platelets and podocytes. Another function of the microtubules is that of assisting the transport of material within the cell; they serve to direct secretory granules, e.g. containing insulin, to the cell surface prior to exocytosis. Their function in relationship to cell receptors has already been described (see p. 15). The filaments of the spindle at mitosis are composed of microtubules, and therefore colchicine inhibits mitosis at the metaphase.

Microfilaments. Most cells also contain long filamentous structures about 6 to 8 nm in diameter. Bundles of these are clearly seen in squamous epithelial cells, and are known as tonofibrils. They also form bundles or sheets closely apposed to the cell membrane, and here form the terminal web. Actin, myosin, and tropomyosin have been identified in

Figure 2.21
A perinuclear store of glycogen in a liver cell of a rat poisoned with ethionine. Glycogen (g) is mainly in the form of rosettes of particles, but occasional solitary particles are also present. Vesicular profiles of smooth endoplasmic reticulum are intermingled with glycogen particles. ly—lysosome, nu—nucleus. Lead hydroxide. × 23 150. (*Photograph by courtesy of Dr. Katsumi Miyai.*)

Figure 2.22
The Golgi complex (Golgi apparatus) and its possible functions.
This diagram depicts the Golgi complex as a series of flattened sacs from which numerous vacuoles arise. Some vacuoles contain secretory material that has been synthesised in the endoplasmic reticulum. Some vacuoles appear to be empty and travel to the cell surface where their membranes fuse with the cell membrane. Other vacuoles contain lytic enzymes and become primary lysosomes. These fuse with autophagosomes or heterophagosomes to form secondary lysosomes. Undigested material remains in residual bodies. (*Drawn by Margot Mackay, Department of Art as Applied to Medicine, University of Toronto.*)

microfilaments, and it is believed that these structures are contractile and perform important functions in cell movement, as well as in the movement of structures, such as granules, within the cell itself. Cytochalasin B, a fungal metabolite, disrupts microfilaments. This agent therefore inhibits the phenomenon of capping (see p. 16). Tertiary amine anaes-

thetic agents, like procaine, disrupt both microtubules and microfilaments.

Centrioles. A centriole is a cylindrical body, about 150 nm long, which on transverse section shows nine evenly-spaced triplets of microtubules. Each cell contains at least two centrioles, each at right angles to the other and situated in an area of the cytoplasm called the centrosome. This is close to the nucleus and is partially surrounded by components of the Golgi complex. Before mitosis the centrioles replicate, and each pair migrates to the opposite poles of the nucleus. Their function is to form or orientate the microtubules that constitute the spindle in mitosis. Some cells contain many centrioles, for example the megakaryocyte can contain as many as 40. Furthermore, the basal bodies of the base of cilia and flagella are morphologically identical with centrioles. Their function is again concerned with movement—this time in relation to the microtubules of the cilia and flagella.

Cell Ageing[21-23]

Although some cell clones can be cultivated indefinitely, there seems little doubt that normal diploid cells have a limited life in isolated tissue culture. Human embryonic fibroblasts have a finite capacity of 40 to 60 population doublings before they die. This has been termed *clonal ageing*, and the senescence that is exhibited by cells may explain why life itself is finite. Thus the Galapagos tortoise can live for up to about 175 years, and its embryonic fibroblasts can undergo 90 to 125 doublings; the corresponding figures for the mouse are 3·5 years and 14 to 28 doublings. The factors responsible for clonal ageing are not understood. Errors in DNA replication (somatic mutation) or abnormal structural protein formation due to errors in transcription or translation have been suggested but not proven. Malignant cells do not show the phenomenon, and indeed all established cell lines are malignant, e.g. HeLa cells.

An immortal clone of amoeba may be converted into a mortal one by suitably manipulating the environment, and the change may reside in either the cytoplasm or the nucleus.[24] Whether ageing is the end-result of a programmed genetic sequence or whether it is due to the effects of random chemical damage is not known.[25]

THE CELL CYCLE

The cell cycle is reckoned to begin at the completion of one cell division (mitosis) and to end at the completion of the next division. The time taken for one cell cycle is the *generation time*.

Immediately following cell division the cell enters the first resting, or G_1 phase. The length of this phase is the most variable component of the cell cycle. Sometimes a cell may remain in this state for a long period; it is then described as having entered the G_0 phase. It may later return to the cell cycle, or else become so fully differentiated as to become incapable of further mitosis. There are some cells, notably the neuron, which cannot undergo mitosis.

The G_1 phase is followed by a synthesis, or S, phase, during which the DNA of the nucleus replicates. There then follows a short gap, the G_2 phase, before the beginning of mitosis.

MITOSIS

The mechanism whereby somatic cells divide is a complicated process in which the nuclear material is reduplicated, and then carefully divided into two equal parts, which reform the nuclei of the two daughter cells (Fig. 2.23).

During the period between mitoses (*interphase*) the chromosomes are present in the nucleus as long drawn-out threads. These are not visible as such using the light microscope, but in areas along the thread there is sufficient coiling for the condensation of material to render these areas recognisable as the heterochromatin of the nucleus (p. 18). Each chromosome is thought to contain many DNA molecules rather than a single long one.

Following the G_2 phase, each chromosome is seen to have divided longitudinally into two *chromatids* which are held together by a *centromere*. The chromosomes show coiling along their length; in this way they become shorter and thicker, and therefore visible. The cell has now entered into the first phase of mitosis—the *prophase*. Meanwhile in the centrosome the microtubules become arranged so as to form the spindle fibres which converge on a dense body adjacent to the centrioles. The centrioles move away from each other to opposite poles of the cell, and in this way the *spindle* is formed. Its microtubules are attached to the centromeres, and each centriole looks like a star, or *aster*.

Concurrently the nucleoli and nuclear membrane disappear. The cell is now in *metaphase* with the split chromosomes being arranged along a plane which bisects the cell (the 'equatorial plate').

During the next phase (*anaphase*) the centromeres divide, and each set of chromatids (now called chromosomes) is guided by the fibrils of the spindle to either pole of the cell.

The final stage (*telophase*) involves division of the cytoplasm of the cells, and the reconstitution of the nucleoli and nuclear membrane of each daughter cell.

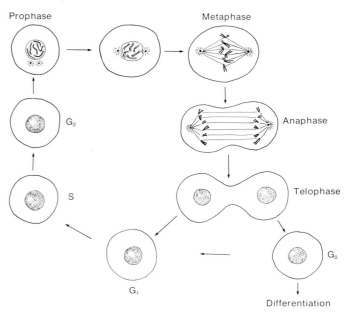

Figure 2.23
The cell cycle. DNA reduplication occurs during the synthesis stage (S). This is followed by a short resting stage (G_2) before the cell enters mitosis. Following division the daughter cells may enter the second resting stage (G_1) before recommencing DNA synthesis. Other daughter cells can pass into a resting phase (G_0), and after a period can either re-enter the cell cycle or become differentiated and cease to be capable of mitosis.

In prophase the individual chromosomes become visible—for the sake of clarity only six are shown, but the normal human cell contains 46. Each chromosome has already split into two chromatids. In metaphase the chromosomes are arranged along the equatorial plate, and the spindle is fully formed. In anaphase, the chromatids, now called chromosomes, move apart. In telophase the daughter nuclei reform, and the cytoplasm divides to produce two new cells each with the amount of DNA corresponding to the normal number of chromosomes.

It can be readily understood how during mitosis each chromosome reduplicates itself exactly, and each daughter cell contains an identical quota of nuclear material. It is presumed that each DNA molecule (and gene) is also reduplicated exactly. Should an error occur during mitosis such that an abnormal gene is produced, the process is called a *somatic mutation*. It is possible that cancer develops in this way.

MEIOSIS

In the testis the primitive spermatogonia on the basement membrane of the seminiferous tubules divide by mitosis to form *primary spermatocytes*. The next division is called meiosis, and is complex. Although each chromosome divides into two, the chromatids do not separate as in mitosis, but instead behave as a single structure. The double chromosomes line up on the equatorial plate to form 23 pairs. During this phase corresponding pairs of maternal and paternal chromosomes (actually four chromatids) come closely together, develop breaks, and exchange homologous segments. This process is called *crossing over*, and the points of junction of the exchanged segments on the newly-constituted chromosome are

Figure 2.24
Diagrammatic representation of spermatogenesis. Only the sex chromosomes
are shown. The primary spermatocytes
are depicted at the onset of meiosis with
the chromosomes already divided.

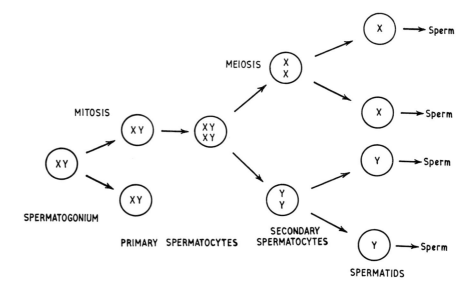

Figure 2.24
Diagrammatic representation of spermatogenesis. Only the sex chromosomes
are shown. The primary spermatocytes
are depicted at the onset of meiosis with
the chromosomes already divided.

called *chiasmata*. The importance of crossing over is that it allows a complete admixture of maternal and paternal genes in the developing gamete.

The chromosomes then separate and the cell divides. Each *secondary spermatocyte* contains 22 autosomes and one sex chromosome: each of these is still a double structure. It should be noted that as there is no fixed arrangement of the chromosomes on the spindle, each daughter cell contains a mixture of maternal and paternal chromosomes selected at random. Nevertheless, each cell possesses only one of each pair.

Each secondary spermatocyte divides once more, and it is at this stage that the chromatids actually separate. The two *spermatids* so formed thus contain 22 autosomes and one sex chromosome. This is the n, or haploid, number, and the cells contain only half the normal amount of DNA. The meiotic division and the one that follows it are called the two *maturation divisions*. The spermatids do not divide further, but develop into *spermatozoa* (Fig. 2.24).

In the ovary the process is very similar, the oöcyte undergoing two maturation divisions, the first (meiosis) before and the second after ovulation. With each division, however, the cytoplasm is divided unequally between the daughter cells with the result that only one survives, and the other, the shrunken *polar body*, dies. Actually the two polar bodies themselves divide before they die. The sex chromosomes in the oöcyte are equal in size because they are both X* (Fig. 2.25).

Thus each ovum and sperm contains 23 chromosomes, and with fertilisation the 2n, or diploid, number of 46 is restored.

*The female of the human species is described as the homogametic sex, because she produces only one type of gamete (X). The male (XY) is heterogametic. This rule applies to all mammals. However, in birds and reptiles the converse is true, and different letters are used as a reminder of this difference. The female is heterogametic (ZW) and the male homogametic (ZZ). In the other vertebrates (fish and amphibians) the situation is confusing, since it varies according to species and even race. Some species even change sex or are hermaphrodite.[26]

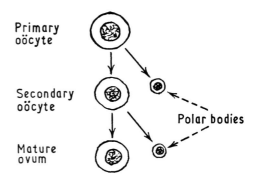

Figure 2.25
Diagrammatic representation of oögenesis.

The pairs of chromosomes in the normal cell are important, because it is on them that the pairs of factors, or genes, are situated (see p. 32). It is noteworthy that only at meiosis do the chromosomes actually pair off.

Non-disjunction. At either of the two maturation divisions a pair of chromosomes may fail to separate, in which case both are drawn into one of the daughter cells. This is called non-disjunction. Thus, if the sex chromosomes are involved, abnormal secondary spermatocytes or oöcytes can be formed, one spermatocyte, for instance, containing XY/XY and the other O. If the next division is normal, two types of spermatozoa are produced, one with no sex chromosome and the other with XY. If there is also non-disjunction at the second division, then gametes with XXYY, XYY, XXY, X, Y, or O can be produced. Such defects of gametogenesis can give rise to gross defects in the resulting offspring. When the autosomes are involved the zygote usually dies, or is produced as a macerated fetus. Abnormalities in the sex chromosomes are, however, often compatible with long life.

It is evident that during the formation of the gametes there is ample opportunity for rearrangement of the genetic material. The extraordinary plasticity of the process of sexual reproduction is demonstrated by the fact that one human being is unlike any other. Errors may, however, occur. Faults in DNA synthesis result in *mutations*, while failure of the chromosomes to separate (*non-disjunction*) leads to an abnormal number of chromosomes. Breakage of chromosomes or chromatids is a common phenomenon, and although the broken ends may rejoin immediately, they may also join in other ways. In *deletion* there is loss of part of a chromosome; it may be interstitial, i.e. occurring between two breaks. In *translocation* a detached part of a chromosome becomes attached to another chromosome. *Duplication* of part of a chromosome is not uncommon, and may indeed be part of the evolutionary process. *Inversion* of a part of a chromosome can occur between two breaks. If two breaks occur in the same

chromosome, the ends may join together to form a *ring chromosome*. Chromosome breaks can be induced by *ionising radiation, certain drugs*, and by *viruses*.[27] They are also more common in three rare syndromes: ataxia telangiectasia (p. 171), Fanconi's anaemia (p. 627), and Bloom's syndrome.* Of interest is the observation that in all these conditions leukaemia or other types of malignancy are common in early life.

The next chapter deals with some of the effects of these errors.

Bloom's syndrome[28] is characterised by low birth weight, stunted growth, and a sun-sensitive telangiectatic skin disorder affecting the cheeks and nose—called the butterfly area of the face and also affected in lupus erythematosus.

GENERAL READING

HAM, A. W. (1974) *Histology*, 7th edn, 1006 pp. Philadelphia: Lippincott. An excellent reference book that co-ordinates structure with function.
LEESON, C. R. & LEESON, T. S. (1976) *Histology*, 3rd edn, 605 pp. Philadelphia: Saunders.

REFERENCES

1. Annotation (1966) Messenger and morphogenesis. *Lancet*, **2**, 1351.
2. Various Authors: Cell movement and cell contact. (1961). *Experimental Cell Research*, Supplement **8**.
3. BERLIN, R. D. *et al.* (1975) The cell surface. *New England Journal of Medicine*, **292**, 515.
4. NICOLSON, G. L. & POSTE, G. (1976) The cancer cell: dynamic aspects and modifications in cell-surface organization. *New England Journal of Medicine*, **295**, 197 and 253.
5. Leading Article (1970) Cyclic A.M.P.: the second messenger. *Lancet*, **2**, 1119.
6. PASTAN, I. (1972) Cyclic AMP. *Scientific American*, **227**, No 2, 97.
7. STEINBERG, M. S. (1964) In *Cellular Membranes in Development*, ed. Locke, M. p. 321. New York: Academic Press.
8. SCRIVER, C. R. (1969) The human biochemical genetics of amino acid transport. *Pediatrics*, **44**, 348.
9. SINGER, S. J. & NICOLSON, G. L. (1972) The fluid mosaic model of the structure of cell membranes. *Science*, **175**, 720
10. WEINSTEIN, R. S. & McNUTT, N. S. (1972) Cell junctions. *New England Journal of Medicine*, **286**, 521.
11. YCAS, M. (1969) *The Biological Code*. Amsterdam: North Holland Publishing Co.
12. STENT, G. S. (1964) The operon: on its third anniversary. *Science*, **144**, 816.
13. GURDON, J. B. & UEHLINGER, V. (1966) 'Fertile' intestine nuclei. *Nature (London)*, **210**, 1240.
14. FRENSTER, J. H. & HERSTEIN, P. R. (1973) Gene de-repression. *New England Journal of Medicine*, **288**, 1224.
15. STEIN, G. (1972) The control of gene expression in *The Pathology of Transcription and Translation*, ed. Farber, E. p. 21. New York: Marcel Dekker.
16. CROFT, D. N. *et al.* (1968) D.N.A. and cell loss from normal small-intestinal mucosa. *Lancet*, **2**, 70.
17. Leading Article (1974). Sick cells and hyponatraemia. *Lancet*, **1**, 342.
18. PREER, J. R. (1971) Extrachromosomal inheritance: hereditary symbionts, mitochondria, chloroplasts. In *Annual Review of Genetics*, ed. Roman H. L. Vol. 5, p. 361. Palo Alto: Annual Reviews Inc.
19. WOLSTENHOLME, G. E. W. & O'CONNOR, M. (Eds) (1969) *Bacterial Episomes and Plasmids*, Ciba Foundation Symposium, London: Churchill.
20. UZMAN, B. G., SAITO, H. & KASAC, M. (1971) Tubular arrays in the endoplasmic reticulum in human tumor cells. *Laboratory Investigation*, **24**, 492.
21. Annotation (1968) Mortal clones. *Lancet*, **1**, 1240.
22. BURNET, F. M. (1973) A genetic interpretation of ageing. *Lancet*, **2**, 480.
23. HAYFLICK, L. (1976) The cell biology of human ageing. *New England Journal of Medicine*, **295**, 1302.
24. MUGGLETON, A. & DANIELLI, J. F. (1968) Inheritance of the 'life-spanning' phenomenon in *Amoeba proteus*. *Experimental Cell Research*, **49**, 116.
25. Leading Article (1967) Ageing. *Lancet*, **2**, 502.
26. BEATTY, R. A. (1970) Genetic basis for the determination of sex. *Philosophical Transactions of the Royal Society of London, B*, **259**, 1.
27. NICHOLS, W. W. (1966) The role of viruses in the etiology of chromosome abnormalities. *American Journal of Human Genetics*, **18**, 81.
28. BLOOM, D. (1966) The syndrome of congenital telangiectatic erythema and stunted growth. *Journal of Pediatrics*, **68**, 103.

Chapter 3. The Cause of Disease

It is customary to regard pathology as the basis of both medicine and surgery. Certainly when the morbid anatomy and altered physiology of a patient are understood, the clinical picture falls into place, hence the popularity of the clinico-pathological conference. There is, however, a danger in regarding pathology in this light. Syndromes may be recognised, described, and named, but when once a condition acquires the distinction of becoming a 'disease', further thought on the subject often tends to stop. It would perhaps be better to remember that the characteristics of each individual and each disease are the results of the interplay of two basic factors: inherited genetic constitution and environment.

The most characteristic feature of living matter, apart from its reproductive capacity, is its ability to adapt to changing circumstances and make good any damage that may be sustained. The mechanisms involved in the protective or reparative reactions are of fundamental importance; they are of a structural or chemical nature, and may be regarded as the units from which all pathological lesions are built. The fact that certain circumstances are sufficiently common for the body's reaction to them to be regarded as 'diseases', does not detract from this concept.

Pathological processes frequently involve the body's normal responses to abnormal environmental influences. The major part of this book is, in fact, devoted to a consideration of the body's reaction to such noxious external influences as pathogenic organisms, trauma, and dietary deficiencies. Less frequently the body's response is abnormal, and in this chapter we shall first consider those abnormalities which are the result of innate errors.

THE GENETIC BASIS OF DISEASE[1]

Mendel's laws of inheritance, which laid the foundations of the science of genetics, are of great importance in the understanding of many diseases.[2] It is postulated that a particular characteristic is determined by a pair of factors, or genes, each of which is situated at a specific site, or *locus*, on one of a pair of chromosomes. Such genes, forming a pair, are called *alleles* or *allelomorphs*. They may be alike (*homozygous*) or dissimilar (*heterozygous*). The genetic make-up of an individual is called the *genotype* and the effect which is produced is called the *phenotype*.

The simplest approach to the mode of inheritance of a particular characteristic, e.g. a disease, is to consider that genes may be either *dominant* or *recessive*. A dominant gene produces its effects whether combined with a similar dominant allele or a recessive one. Recessive genes, on the other hand, produce their effects only in the homozygous condition. This may be illustrated by reference to the inheritance of the Rhesus blood groups. '*D*' may be considered as dominant, and '*d*' as recessive*:

Genotype		Phenotype (*i.e. Blood group*)
D	D	D
D	d	D
d	d	d

It is evident that if the phenotype is known, only in the case of Group d can the genotype be inferred. A person of Group D may be homozygous *DD* or heterozygous *Dd*. The actual genotype can be deduced only by investigating the whole family. The terms dominant and recessive are used in the context of a gene producing an obvious clinical effect. Heterozygotes for recessive genes can often be detected by biochemical tests (see p. 38).

Multiple alleles and co-dominance. In the above example the site, or locus, could be occupied by either *D* or *d*. In the inheritance of the ABO groups each locus may be occupied by one of three allelic genes, *O*, *A*, or *B*. O is recessive and *A* and *B* are co-dominant, i.e. both alleles are fully expressed in the heterozygote.*

Thus the possible genotypes are:

These correspond to the phenotypes:

The presence of multiple alleles is common, e.g. in the inheritance of the transplantation antigens, haemoglobin, and the many variants of some of the plasma proteins and enzymes. The occurrence of two or more genetically different classes of individuals with respect of a single trait is known as *polymorphism*.[3]†

It is convenient at this point to describe the features of those diseases inherited as either dominant or recessive characteristics.

Diseases inherited as a dominant characteristic are numerous, but none is common clinically. The skeletal system provides many of the best examples, e.g. diaphysial aclasis,

---

*It will be appreciated that the ABO and Rhesus blood groups are more complicated than this, see Chapter 55. Note that it is now conventional to depict genes in italics.

†The frequency of any one class should be greater than 1 per cent, since very rare traits can occur by mutation and their occurrence in a population does not constitute polymorphism in the sense in which this term is used. Polymorphism should be distinguished from *pleiotropism*, which means that a single aetiological factor, such as a defective gene, can produce multiple separate effects.

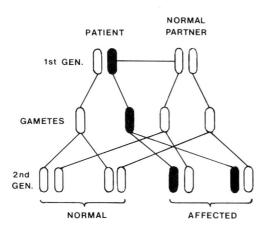

Figure 3.1

Diagram illustrating the transmission of a disease inherited as a dominant trait. One pair of chromosomes is shown for each individual, the black chromosome being the one carrying the defective gene. It will be seen that half the children of an affected patient are themselves diseased.

achondroplasia, osteogenesis imperfecta, and cleidocranial dysostosis. Other important examples are polyposis coli, neurofibromatosis, Huntington's chorea, hereditary haemorrhagic telangiectasia, and some cases of cataract. The mode of inheritance is shown in Figure 3.1.

The following features of a typical disease inherited as a dominant characteristic should be noted.

1. The disease appears in every generation of the family: i.e. one of the patient's parents should have the disease. The occasional instance of poor penetrance, e.g. in retinoblastoma, and the occurrence of a new mutant provide exceptions to this rule.

2. Unaffected members of the family need not usually fear transmitting the disease to their children. However, sometimes the disease becomes manifest only in adult life, when children

have already been produced. This is the tragedy of Huntington's chorea.

3. The affected members are usually heterozygous; therefore, if their breeding partner is normal, each of the offspring has a 50 per cent chance of being affected.

4. The disease is usually not severe enough to prevent reproduction, otherwise the affected genes would be rapidly lost from the community. In the few instances where the disease greatly diminishes the breeding potential of the sufferer, this loss is common and most cases are sporadic.

5. Some genes are lost in this way, but replacement is continuously occurring by mutation; new cases may therefore be found occasionally in previously unaffected families. An important factor in predisposing to such a mutation is an increased paternal age—this has been proved in acrocephalosyndactyly, Marfan's syndrome, and achondroplasia.

6. Affected males and females occur in equal numbers.

Diseases inherited as a recessive characteristic are frequently severe, and reduce the breeding chances of the sufferer. The mode of transmission is shown diagrammatically in Figure 3.2.

The following features should be noted.

1. The birth of an abnormal child is usually the first indication of the condition.

2. As with other Mendelian characters the chances of further members of the family being affected or passing on the trait can be calculated: the family therefore is entitled to accurate counselling.[4] Thus the chances of the next child being affected are 1 in 4. Half the offspring will be carriers. If an affected individual mates with a 'normal' partner, all the offspring will be carriers.

3. The seriousness of producing carriers should not be overemphasised. It has been estimated that we all carry 1 to 3 harmful genes. The known carrier therefore differs from the remainder of the population only in that he knows one of his genes!

4. The heterozygous carrier can often be detected because

Figure 3.2

Diagram to illustrate the transmission of a disease inherited as a recessive trait. It will be seen that the patient's parents are both unaffected heterozygotes, and that all the patient's children are likewise carriers.

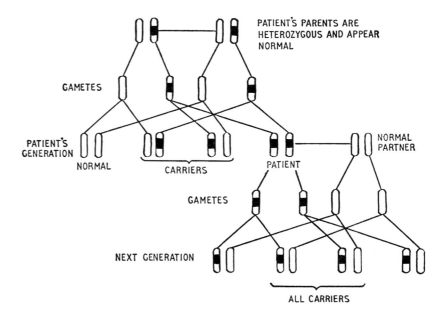

Figure 3.3
Mode of transmission of a disease like haemophilia, which is inherited as a sex-linked recessive trait. The abnormal gene is situated on the X chromosome, and therefore produces its effect in the male but not in the female except in the rare event of her being homozygous. All the patient's daughters are carriers, but all his sons are normal.

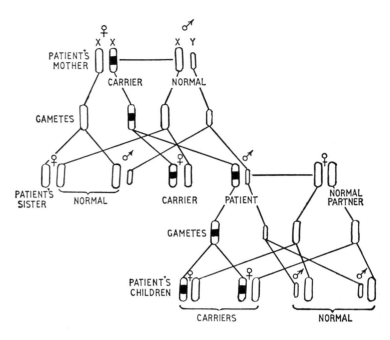

he exhibits minor stigmata of the condition, detectable either by clinical examination or biochemical investigation.

5. Particular recessive genes often tend to be more frequent in members of one family. Hence consanguineous breeding increases the risk of producing a defective offspring. This is particularly true if the recessive gene is rare in the general population. If, on the other hand, the gene is very common (e.g. that for Tay-Sachs disease in Ashkenazi Jews), the dangers of cousin marriages are little greater than those of any other union within the same ethnic group.

Some of the best-known diseases inherited as recessive characters are retinitis pigmentosa, albinism, xeroderma pigmentosum, cystic fibrosis, and Werdnig-Hoffmann disease (the progressive spinal muscular atrophy of infancy—see Fig. 1.3).

Linkage of genes. The phenomenon of crossing over has revealed the location of some genes on a chromosome. The ABO genes and those responsible for the nail-patella syndrome* are always situated close together on one chromosome. This situation of genes at loci on the same chromosome is called *linkage*. When a gene is known to be situated on one of the sex chromosomes (almost invariably the X) the phenomenon is called *sex-linkage*. The only Y-linked characteristic so far described in the human is hairy ears.

Genetic mapping. Over 200 genes have been assigned to specific human chromosomes either by linkage analysis or by other means. The most widely used technique for gene mapping is somatic-cell hybridisation. Human-rodent hybrid cells (see Chapter 1) tend to retain their rodent genome, but lose many of their human chromosomes. Different cell lines can be obtained, each carrying a few, but different, human chromosomes. Hence if the gene product can be identified in the culture, it is possible to analyse the features of several cell lines and thereby ascribe a particular gene to a single chromo-

some or even to a region of a chromosome. Thus it is now known that the *ABO* genes are situated at the distal end of the long arm of chromosome 9, whereas the *Rh* genes are on chromosome 1, and the *HLA* region is on the short arm of chromosome 6.

Diseases inherited as a sex-linked recessive characteristic (Fig. 3.3). The gene is located on the X chromosome; the female heterozygote is unaffected, since she is protected by the normal allele on the other X. In the male, however, the heterozygote is affected, since the Y does not carry the allele. Thus the disease affects males but is transmitted by the female. Father-to-son transmission never occurs. The disease may occur in the female, but this only follows the mating of an affected male with a female carrier—an unlikely event. Diseases inherited in this way are haemophilia, Christmas disease, red-green colour blindness, and often nephrogenic diabetes insipidus, congenital agammaglobulinaemia, and pseudohypertrophic muscular dystrophy. The complete list of conditions considered to be X-linked is well over 50.

Diseases inherited as a sex-linked dominant characteristic. In this case affected females convey the gene to half their sons and daughters, whereas affected males transmit it only to their daughters; there can be no male-to-male transmission. Therefore there is an excess of female victims. Familial hypophosphataemia and haemolytic anaemia due to glucose 6-phosphate dehydrogenase deficiency are examples of diseases inherited thus. The locus for the Xg blood group is on the X chromosome. The two alleles are Xg^a and Xg, and give rise to the phenotypes Xg(a+) and Xg(a−). Xg^a is dominant.

Other Features of Gene Expression[5]

Not all human inherited disease can be explained in terms of simple dominant or recessive gene action. There are many complicating factors:

Penetrance and expressivity. It may happen that a trait, although dominant, occasionally misses a generation. The trait is said to exhibit *reduced penetrance*. Another complication is

*This comprises the tetrad: absence of patellae, deformed finger nails, dislocated radial heads, and bilateral iliac bone-spurs.

seen in some families where a dominant gene produces a variable effect. Some individuals who possess it have a severe disease while others have a minor defect, or *forme fruste*, of the disease. In such instances the trait is said to exhibit *variable expressivity*. Penetrance and expressivity are closely related, but whereas penetrance is an all or none affair, expressivity is variable. Clearly when a gene produces a minor defect it is said to exhibit poor expressivity if the defect is detected, and poor penetrance if the defect is not detected.

Intermediate inheritance. When the heterozygote differs from either homozygote, the inheritance is described an intermediate. A good example is sickle-cell anaemia. The homozygote with the two sickle-cell genes has the fully developed anaemia, whereas the heterozygote carrying one defective gene and one normal allele has the mild sickle-cell trait—a state intermediate between the disease and the normal.

Sex limitation. A disease which is present only in one sex is said to be sex limited. Premature baldness may be an example, being inherited as a dominant autosomal factor, but manifest in the male and only rarely in the female.

Interaction of several non-allelic genes. Genes situated at separate loci may interact in complex ways. A good example is that of the ABO, secretor, and Lewis blood-group systems.

Multifactorial, or polygenic inheritance. Certain traits, e.g. intelligence and height, appear to be influenced by many genes, and the same may well apply to essential hypertension, diabetes mellitus, and other diseases where the line of division between disease and health is not clearly drawn. Environmental factors are almost certainly involved as well.

Genetic heterogeneity, or polymorphism.[6,7] If variants of a single phenotype can be caused by different genes the trait is said to be genetically heterogeneous. Sometimes the diseases may be distinguished from each other on clinical grounds, for example the various types of muscular dystrophy,* and the defective genes are located at separate loci. In other instances the two conditions are almost indistinguishable, e.g. types of elliptocytosis and congenital deafness. The most direct proof that different genes are involved is where two individuals with similar defects inherited as autosomal recessive characters mate and produce a normal offspring.

Many examples of genetic polymorphism are known in respect of proteins and enzymes. Thus there are at least 150 variants of haemoglobin, 78 of glucose 6-phosphate dehydrogenase, 3 of phenylketonuria, and 3 of galactosaemia. These variants could be due to defective genes at separate loci, but are usually due to the existence of multiple alleles at one locus. This raises interesting possibilities. In some patients, e.g. with galactosaemia, who are presumed to be homozygous, the phenotype is atypical. In these instances it is probable that the individual is in fact heterozygous for two abnormal alleles, in this instance the allele for the classical type of galactosaemia and that for the Duarte variant. Such a mechanism may provide the explanation for some instances of incomplete

*The Duchenne type, which is inherited as a sex-linked recessive trait and affects males only, appears in early childhood, and progresses rapidly. The limb-girdle type is an autosomal recessive, which appears at puberty and is less severe, while the facio-scapulo-humeral type is inherited as an autosomal dominant with variable expressivity, which develops in the teens and progresses slowly.

penetrance or expressivity of a particular gene. It might also explain why in some families the heterozygotes for a particular trait can be detected while in other families they are undetectable. This will occur if the test employed can detect the effects of one allele but not that of another.

Phenocopies. Characteristics can occur in the absence of the genes which are known to produce that particular effect in other families. The effects of genetic error may thus be mimicked by other factors, presumably acquired. These *phenocopies* are not inherited.

Finally it should be noted that some characteristics could be inherited from genetic material in the cytoplasm, or plasmagenes (p. 23). Such material need not be passed from one generation to the next in the precise way that mitosis determines the distribution of the nuclear genes. It is therefore no wonder that in human disease conditions are found which do not follow any simple Mendelian characteristic.

Mode of Gene Action

It is now well established that the genetic material is composed of nucleoprotein, and that the DNA component is of prime importance in transfering information from each cell to its progeny and from one generation to the next. Its triplet code provides information whereby the cytoplasm is programmed for the manufacture of protein, and a defect in a part of the DNA molecule can result in the formation of an abnormal protein. Such a defect arises by a *point mutation*, i.e. a simple substitution of one nucleotide by another. This altered codon results in a different amino acid being incorporated into the particular protein specified by the gene. Such a condition is called a *molecular disease*,[6] and many good examples are to be seen in the haemoglobinopathies.

In sickle-cell anaemia the red cells contain an abnormal haemoglobin (haemoglobin S) which precipitates at low oxygen tensions and leads to a sickle-shaped deformity of the cells. This is associated with their more rapid destruction in the body as well as their obstruction of small vessels with local infarction.

The formation of the abnormal haemoglobin is determined by an abnormal gene. Cases of sickle-cell anaemia are homozygous, whilst those with the sickle-cell trait are heterozygous; their cells contain both normal and abnormal haemoglobin. The formation of normal haemoglobin is therefore determined by the normal allele. It has been found that the differences between the two haemoglobins lie in the globin moiety. In the abnormal form a valine residue replaces the normal glutamic acid residue at the sixth position in one of the two β-polypeptide chains of the molecule.

Many other abnormal haemoglobins have been described.[7] Usually the red cells containing them are more easily destroyed and anaemia results. One rare type, haemoglobin Zurich, predisposes to severe reactions from sulphonamides, while another, haemoglobin M, leads to hereditary methaemoglobinaemia. Thus an error of one codon can lead to widespread effects.

Sometimes genetic error results in the complete failure to form a protein, e.g. analbuminaemia. In many instances the protein formed as a result of gene action is an enzyme. The concept 'one gene, one enzyme' is useful when one considers the conditions characterised by the presence of a defective enzyme. An example of this is the abnormal pseudocholinesterase which may be found in the plasma of certain individuals who in all other respects appear to be normal. These people are unduly susceptible to the action of short-acting muscle relaxant drugs, like suxamethonium, and this is of great importance to the anaesthetist.[8]

An ever-increasing number of conditions, usually inherited as Mendelian recessives, are being described in which there is an abnormality of a single enzyme. These are genetically determined biochemical lesions, or *inborn errors of metabolism*, a term coined by Sir Archibald Garrod over 50 years ago.[9] They are important, because they demonstrate how one simple biochemical error can affect many tissues and often produce severe disease. Furthermore, if they are diagnosed early enough, successful treatment may be instituted. The conditions are rare, but as noted by Harvey over 300 years ago, 'nature is nowhere accustomed more openly to display her secret mysteries than in cases where she shows traces of her workings apart from the beaten path'.*

It may be postulated that an abnormal allele can occupy the locus of a structural gene or of a gene that exercises control, such as an operator gene. When a structural gene is involved there can be one of several effects. The protein formed in the body, being of abnormal composition, may differ in chemical or physical properties. The many variants of haemoglobin are examples of this. In the case of enzymes, their specific activity may be lessened or their stability altered. It should be noted that it is technically difficult to distinguish between three possibilities:

(*a*) Less enzyme is produced and indeed there may be complete absence.

(*b*) A normal quantity of enzyme is produced but its specific activity is reduced or modified.

(*c*) The enzyme produced shows an increased lability and is rapidly catabolised.

Defective enzyme activity can therefore be due to several mechanisms, and it is not surprising that apparently simple enzyme-deficiency states, such as glucose 6-phosphate dehydrogenase deficiency, are in fact examples of complex genetic polymorphism.

A gene having a regulatory function may be defective. Thus a defective repressor gene might lead to excess formation of an enzyme. Acute intermittent porphyria may be an example of this, for there is an excess of δ-amino-laevulinic acid synthetase formation (p. 435). A defective operator gene might lead to a failure in the formation of several enzymes. The very rare *hereditary orotic aciduria* has been cited as an example, for there is a deficiency of two enzymes responsible for the *sequential* steps in the conversion of orotic acid to uridine-5'-phosphate. This is a precursor of RNA. The syndrome is characterised by retardation in infancy and a megaloblastic anaemia. Another example is sucrose intolerance, in which there is a deficiency of sucrase, maltase, and isomaltase in the gut.

It is sometimes stated that a particular germ-layer is affected, but in fact there is no known genetic error which affects

---

* '*The Works of William Harvey, M.D.*', translated by Robert Willis, p. 616, Sydenham Society, London, 1847. (Cited by Garrod, A. E., 1928, *Lancet*, **1**, 1055.)

---

one layer as a whole. One particular cell type may be affected; thus in albinism there is a failure of the melanocytes to form melanin. This affects the iris, retina, and skin, although these structures are not all formed at the same time embryologically. A genetic error therefore does not affect different processes merely because they are occurring at a particular stage of development.

Although a number of inherited diseases are explicable in chemical terms, the great majority are not. Presumably the obvious abnormalities, e.g. achondroplasia and polyposis coli, are far removed from the defective gene and its primary product. There is, however, every hope that these gaps in our knowledge will be spanned in due course, and ways will be found to foil such perverted developments.

Some Examples of Inborn Errors of Metabolism[5, 10]

Galactosaemia. This is a condition in babies who fail to thrive, have large livers, and pass galactose, amino acids, and albumin in the urine. Mental retardation, cataract, and cirrhosis of the liver ultimately develop. The defect is due usually to an absence of the enzyme galactose 1-phosphate uridyl transferase which is responsible for converting galactose 1-phosphate to glucose 1-phosphate (Fig. 3.4). It follows that galactose (from the lactose of milk) cannot be utilised; it accumulates and is excreted in the urine. Galactose itself is not toxic, but galactose 1-phosphate probably interferes with some metabolic process (possibly involving phosphoglucomutase, which converts glucose 1-phosphate to glucose 6-phosphate), which is essential for the proper development of the brain, lens, liver, and kidney. The accumulation of the sugar alcohol galactitol, formed from galactose in the lens, has been suggested as the cause of the cataracts. The avoidance of galactose in the diet from an early age may prevent the baneful effects of this abnormality.

A mild form of galactosaemia, with cataract development in childhood as its major symptom, has also been described. It is due to a deficiency of galactokinase (see Fig. 3.4).

Alcaptonuria (or Alkaptonuria). In this condition the urine contains large amounts of homogentisic acid, which causes it to darken on standing if the reaction is alkaline. Staining of the diapers may be the first sign of the disease. The condition is of little consequence except that as the

Figure 3.4
Metabolic pathway concerned in the conversion of galactose to glucose 1-phosphate.
Key: 1. Galactokinase. 2. Galactose 1-phosphate uridyl transferase. 3, UDP Galactose 4-epimerase. UDP—Uridine diphosphate. ATP—Adenosine triphosphate. ADP—Adenosine diphosphate.

Figure 3.5
Some steps in the metabolism of phenylalanine. The absence of phenylalanine hydroxylase results in phenylketonuria, of homogentisic acid oxidase in alkaptonuria, and of tyrosinase in albinism (see p. 588).

patient grows older, his cartilages and ligaments become pigmented (ochronosis, p. 588). Osteoarthritis may develop. the reason for which is not known. Alcaptonurics are unable to metabolise homogentisic acid, which is an intermediary in the metabolic breakdown pathway of tyrosine and phenylalanine (Fig. 3.5). There are, however, alternative metabolic pathways, which probably explains why no serious lesion develops. Alcaptonuria was the first human disorder found to be inherited as a Mendelian autosomal recessive characteristic, and the study of this condition led Garrod to formulate the concept of enzyme deficiency as a cause of disease.

Phenylketonuria. Between 3 and 5 persons per 100 000 of the population exhibit this condition, which commences shortly after birth, and is characterised by retardation of mental development. Other neurological abnormalities, hypopigmentation of the skin, and sometimes eczema also occur.

In the classical form of the defect there is an absence of the hepatic enzyme phenylalanine hydroxylase, which normally converts into tyrosine that dietary phenylalanine not utilised in the synthesis of protein (Fig. 3.5). Therefore the level of phenylalanine in the blood (normally up to 2 mg per dl) and cerebrospinal fluid is high. The urine contains, in addition to phenylalanine, phenylpyruvic acid, which gives a green colour with ferric chloride solution. If the disease is detected early, certainly before the age of six months, and the patient given a diet low in phenylalanine content, brain damage can be largely averted. The administration of tyrosine itself does not prevent the development of mental deterioration, so presumably phenylalanine or one of its derivatives is toxic. The condition is inherited as an autosomal recessive trait; 1 per cent of the population are heterozygotes, and can be detected by the administration of a dose of phenylalanine, when the blood level rises. This does not occur in a normal individual.

Lesch-Nyhan syndrome. This is inherited as a sex-linked recessive trait and is characterised by hyperuricaemia, gout, mental deficiency, and spastic paralysis with choreoathetosis. Its most remarkable characteristic is impulsive, uncontrollable self-mutilation of the fingers and lips. This bizarre behaviour may result in great tissue loss, and yet at autopsy no neurological structural abnormality can be found. These patients lack the enzyme hypoxanthine: guanine phosphoribosyltransferase used in the synthesis of nucleotides. In its absence there is an overproduction of uric acid. The enzyme defect can be demonstrated in cells cultured from the patients, and also in some individuals who suffer from gout only. The relationship between the enzyme defect and the other features of the Lesch-Nyhan syndrome is not understood. The disease is of great interest because of the association of a known

biochemical lesion with a specific, aggressive, destructive type of behaviour, itself a gross caricature of the type of behaviour that afflicts the human being today.

Glucose 6-phosphate dehydrogenase deficiency. Patients lacking this enzyme in their red cells are liable to develop acute haemolytic crises if they take certain drugs, e.g. primaquine, sulphones, and sulphonamides. The defect is inherited as a sex-linked factor in Black Africans and their American descendants. Another type occurs in Greeks and Sardinians, and is responsible for haemolytic reactions to the bean *Vicia faba*, as well as to drugs.

A large number of variants of glucose 6-phosphate dehydrogenase deficiency are now known. The enzyme is necessary for the conversion of glucose 6-phosphate to 6-phosphogluconate in the hexose monophosphate shunt (Fig. 2.17). On this depends the maintenance of glutathione in the reduced state in the red cell. For reasons which are not clearly understood, reduced glutathione is required for the maintenance of the integrity of the red-cell membrane particularly under the influence of certain drugs (see p. 603).

Pharmacogenetics.[8] The study of genetically determined variations in response to drugs is known as pharmacogenetics. Usually there is an increased sensitivity to a drug, and *suxamethonium sensitivity* has been described on page 36. Another example is *isoniazid sensitivity*; certain individuals lack an isoniazid acetylating enzyme and maintain a high level of unaltered drug after the administration of a test dose. They are liable to develop toxic polyneuropathy. Hereditary resistance to a drug is rare, but cases are recorded of individuals resistant to coumarin.[11] Hereditary metabolic disorders which modify drug effects form a third group. Glucose 6-phosphate dehydrogenase deficiency is a well-known example.

The glycogenoses. In the glycogenoses, or glycogen-storage diseases, glycogen accumulates in cells as a consequence of an enzyme defect. At present eight types are recognised depending upon which enzyme is affected. These conditions are described in Chapter 33.

Lysosomal enzyme defects.[12] The concept of lysosomal-storage disease, proposed by Hers in 1965, embodies the notion that because a specific lysosomal enzyme is absent, its natural substrate will accumulate in the cell. This emphasises the fact that lysosomes normally play a vital part in the removal of effete cytoplasmic components. Although rare, these diseases are of great interest because they illustrate how a simple enzyme defect can have devastating effects. Many of the diseases can be detected *in utero* by culturing fetal cell and demonstrating the defective or absent enzyme. The following groups of disease are included in the group of lysosomal-storage diseases:

1. *Glycogenoses.* Type 2 glycogen-storage disease (Pompe) is due to α-1,4-glucosidase deficiency, and glycogen granules are found in greatly enlarged secondary lysosomes.

2. *Sphingolipidoses.* This group includes Tay-Sachs disease (GM_2-gangliosidosis), metachromatic leukodystrophy, Fabry's disease (Fig. 3.6), Gaucher's disease, and Niemann-Pick disease.

3. *Mucopolysaccharidoses.* See page 61.

A careful study of these diseases has shown remarkable genetic heterogeneity. Thus, although most patients with Type 2 glycogenosis die within a few months of birth, a few

Figure 3.6
Ganglion cell in Fabry's disease.
The ganglion cell of the appendix shows numerous secondary lysosomes filled with lipid material in the form of myelin figures (myelinoid bodies). High magnification (insert) shows the typical laminated appearance of these structures. The appearances are typical of a lysosomal disease in which there is an abnormal accumulation of material within lysosomes due to the deficiency of an essential enzyme. Fabry's disease is inherited as a sex-linked recessive trait (occurs only in males), and is characterised by an accumulation of glycolipid in blood vessels and, to a lesser extent, the nervous tissues. In the skin the vascular lesions are characteristic (angiokeratoma corporis diffusum). Magnification × 4200 and 192 000. (*Photographs by courtesy of Dr. N. B. Rewcastle*).

have mild symptoms and live for years. Likewise the 'characteristic' cherry-red spot at the macula in patients with Tay-Sachs disease (a $GM2$-gangliosidosis) is also present in the $GM1$-gangliosidoses and in Niemann-Pick disease, although in these conditions the enzyme defect is different.

Many other inborn errors of metabolism are known, but they are rare and often restricted to particular families. Some are described elsewhere in this book: Wilson's disease, haemochromatosis, acatalasia, cystinuria, Crigler-Najjar syndrome.

Detection of Heterozygote Carriers[13]

In about two-thirds of the diseases inherited as recessive traits, the heterozygote carriers can be detected by a variety of tests. In some there is a low level of a particular enzyme e.g. glucose 6-phosphate dehydrogenase, whereas in others a loading dose of the appropriate substrate, e.g. phenylalanine, reveals impaired tolerance. Another method is to examine cultured skin fibroblasts. In the Lesch-Nyhan syndrome there is lack of the enzyme which converts hypoxanthine and guanine to their respective ribonucleotides. In Pompe's disease the cells lack α-1,4-glucosidase, and accumulate an excess of glycogen. In Hurler's syndrome the fibroblasts develop metachromasia as revealed by staining with toluidine blue. However, such a phenomenon is also seen in cystic fibrosis,

Marfan's syndrome, and even in normal people. No doubt defects found in cultured cells are sometimes secondary events and cannot automatically be equated with events *in vivo*.

Diseases Associated with Genetic Errors

There exist many examples of inherited characteristics which are associated with certain diseases. They are not, however, the obvious cause. The association of a particular disease with race, e.g. diabetes mellitus and Gaucher's disease in Jews, or with sex (goitres in women) is an example of this. Likewise, the ability to resist infection (innate immunity, p. 162) is an inherited characteristic, as is also the inherited liability to develop hypersensitivity (atopy, p. 178). The association of blood groups with disease has also been recognised; thus cancer of the stomach is more frequent in Group A subjects, while duodenal ulceration is more common in those of Group O. There is a relationship between certain histocompatibility antigens and disease, e.g. HLA-B27 and ankylosing spondylitis, Reiter's disease, and acute anterior uveitis,[14–16] and HLA-B8 and gluten-sensitive enteropathy and dermatitis herpetiformis[17] (see Appendix 4).

We are quite ignorant of the mechanisms involved, but undoubtedly this type of association was noted by the great clinicians of the past, who often referred to a characteristic disease 'diathesis'.

Genetic Abnormality Associated with Gross Chromosomal Abnormalities

Advances in the technique of chromosome counting have played a leading part in the elucidation of certain congenital abnormalities. It has been found that colchicine holds up mitosis at the stage of metaphase by inhibiting spindle formation. If cells are grown in tissue culture and colchicine is added to the medium, there will be an accumulation of cells with nuclei showing arrested mitosis. If these cells are placed in a hypotonic solution and squashed under a coverslip, the individual chromosomes of the dividing cells can be clearly seen after using suitable stains, e.g. Feulgen or aceto-orcein.

Each chromosome has already divided into two chromatids, which are held together by a centromere. The method of preparation tends to separate the two chromatids except where they are held by the centromere (Fig. 3.7a). If this is near the middle, they appear X-shaped and are termed *metacentric*. If the centromere is off-centre, the chromatid pair are *submetacentric*, and when near the end the pair are V-shaped and are called *acrocentric*. Human acrocentric chromosomes, except the Y, have small masses of chromatin attached by narrow stalks to their short arms. These masses are called *satellites*.

By using a photograph of a mitosis one can cut out the individual chromosomes and arrange them in pairs in order of length to form a *karyotype* (Fig. 3.7b). An international system of nomenclature was put forward by the Denver Study Group, and has subsequently been elaborated by conferences in London,[18] Chicago,[19] and Paris.[20] The pairs are numbered 1 to 22, leaving two extra chromosomes—a pair of Xs in females and an X and a Y in males (see Fig. 3.7b). The human being therefore normally has 46 chromosomes. The term *autosome* is applied to any chromosome which is one of an equal pair. In the human the only unequal pair is the XY of the male, but in practice an autosome has come to mean any chromosome other than X or Y, which are called *sex chromosomes*. Until recently it was not possible to identify every individual chromosome, since some are almost identical in configuration and length. It was therefore convenient to define seven groups: A (1–3), B (4–5), C (6–12 and the X chromosome), D (13–15), E (16–18), F (19–20), and G (21–22 and the Y chromosome). Four new staining techniques have been developed, the use of which has revealed that each chromosome has a characteristic series of transverse bands. The following methods are available:[21]

Figure 3.7a

Human chromosomes at metaphase.
Lymphocytes from the blood of a normal woman were grown in culture for 72 hours before colcemid (a colchicine derivative) was added. This chemical inhibits spindle formation so that mitoses are halted at metaphase. Two hours later a hypotonic solution was added to make the cells swell. The dispersed chromosomes were then stained with Giemsa after they had been pretreated with trypsin. This technique brings out the banding of the chromosomes.

The mitosis shown contains 46 chromosomes, each of which is a divided structure joined by a centromere. The individual chromosomes can be cut out with scissors and arranged in pairs as shown in Figure 3.7b. Such an arrangement is called a karyotype. (*Photograph by courtesy of Dr. H. A. Gardner, Division of Cytogenetics, Toronto General Hospital.*)

Figure 3.7b

Karyotype showing trisomy 18 from a stillborn male with cyclopia.
The karyotype is that of a cell with 47 chromosomes. It is evidently from a male, since there is a Y chromosome. The anomaly must therefore be of fetal origin, since the mother had a normal 46,XX karyotype. The additional chromosome No. 18 arose by nondisjunction; its manifestations were incompatible with postuterine life. (*From Lang, A. P., Schlager, M., and Gardner, H. A. (1976) Trisomy 18 and cyclopia. Teratology, 14, 195*)

1. Q—*Quinacrine fluorescent method*. After staining with quinacrine, the chromosomal bands show varying fluorescence when examined under ultraviolet light. The most brilliant fluorescence is that of the distal portion of the Y chromosome. Indeed, it is this that forms the Y body of the interphase male nucleus (Fig. 3.8).

2. G—*Giemsa methods*. The deeply staining G-bands are generally in the same location as the Q-bands. However, the method does not require fluorescent microscopy.

3. R—*Reverse banding method*. This technique reveals the reciprocal of the pattern seen with the G-banding method. Giemsa staining or fluorescent methods may be used. An advantage of R-banding is that the ends of the chromosomes are stained well.

4. C—'*centric or constitutive heterochromatin*' *method*. This method involves denaturation of DNA by alkali treatment, renaturation, and then Giemsa staining. The heavy C-bands are located near the centromeres of most chromosomes, and over the distal segment of the long arm of the Y chromosome.

Many additional banding techniques have been developed; most of them yield banding patterns similar to those of the four established methods. Others, however, reveal a different pattern (e.g. T-banding and N-banding), and these are useful under special circumstances. A recent improvement in technique has allowed the study of chromosomes in prophase: the chromosomes are elongated and show many more bands than can be resolved at metaphase. Hence subtle abnormalities in chromosomal structure can more readily be detected.

These staining methods complement each other, and their use permits the identification of each pair of human chromosomes. It is now known that minor variations in chromosomal morphology occur at relatively high, but different, frequencies in different races. These are usually associated with no obvious clinical abnormality. Some chromosomal morphological variants occur in families and are inherited. Indeed, it may ultimately be found that a person's karyotype is as individual as are the fingerprints.

The present convention for recording a karyotype is as follows: first is given the total number of chromosomes, and this is followed by the sex-chromosome complement, 46,XX or 46,XY in the case of normal individuals. Then a notation is made of any abnormalities. The addition or deletion of a whole chromosome is shown as a + or − before the symbol for the affected chromosome—thus 47,XY,+21 in the common type of Down's syndrome. If an arm of a chromosome is increased or deleted, it is shown as a + or − after the notation for the chromosome and its arm. The arms are recorded as p for short (petite) and q for long. Thus 46,XY,5p− signifies a male with a deletion affecting the short arm of number 5 chromosome (see cri du chat syndrome, p. 44). Other abbreviations are: r = ring chromosome, s = satellite, t = translocation, and i = isochromosome. When mosaicism is present all cell types are given and are separated by a diagonal line.

There is no doubt that the Barr body, or sex chromatin, described on page 18 is derived from a single X chromosome—the number of Barr bodies seen in the diploid nucleus is one less than the number of X chromosomes.

Mary Lyon has put forward a hypothesis that one of the X chromosomes in each cell of a female fetus becomes inactive

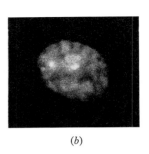

(a)   (b)

Figure 3.8

The fluorescent Y chromosome. Blood smears were air-dried, fixed in methanol, and after staining in 0.5 per cent quinacrine dihydrochloride (atebrine) and washing, were examined in ultraviolet light. The Y chromosome shows a characteristic point of fluorescence in the nuclei of the two cells shown. In (a) the blood was taken from a normal male, whilst in (b) the blood was from an individual with the karyotype 47/XYY. (*Photographs by courtesy of Dr. Peter K. Lewin. From Lewin, P. K. and Conen, P. E.* (1971), Nature, **233**, 334)

early in embryonic life. This inactivation is random, so that about half the cells carry an active maternal chromosome and an inactive paternal one, and *vice versa*. This inactive chromosome replicates later than the other chromosomes during the mitotic cycle, and its descendants follow the same pattern. Since the two chromosomes may carry different sets of X-linked genes, there may be patchiness of a visible characteristic transmitted thus, e.g. coat colour in an animal. Women heterozygous for glucose 6-phosphate dehydrogenase deficiency, an X-linked dominant characteristic, possess two races of red cells, one normal and the other enzyme deficient, and it is these latter that undergo haemolysis. Two clones have also been isolated in women with other X-linked genetic abnormalities.[22] If the characteristic is an X-linked recessive, e.g. haemophilia, it is possible that some of the cells responsible for making AHG are inactive, but the defect is masked by those that are normal. The deficiency of AHG would escape notice except under the stress of a major procedure, such as extracorporeal circulation. This demonstrates once more how tenuous is the distinction between dominant and recessive.

This hypothesis of *lyonisation of the X chromosome* is now generally accepted, but there is evidence that part of the chromosome remains functional,[23] page 42.

Chromosomal Aberrations

Chromosomal aberrations may be of two types: (*a*) *an alteration in number*, either an addition or an absence of a chromosome. This is called *aneuploidy*, as the cells do not contain an exact multiple of the haploid number. In respect of autosomes, an additional chromosome produces *trisomy*, and the effect is always very severe with pronounced mental deficiency. An absence of an autosome is almost invariably lethal. Additional sex chromosomes, on the other hand, produce comparatively mild effects, and mental deficiency, though common, is by no means invariable. A single X chromosome is compatible with life and mental normality—it leads to ovarian dysgenesis. (*b*) *An alteration in structure*, i.e. deletion or translocation of part of a chromosome (see p. 31).

Both non-disjunction and loss of chromosomes may occur not only during meiosis, but also during the earliest mitotic divisions after fertilisation. The result of such post-fertilisation defects is *mosaicism*, the presence in one individual of cells which differ in their complement of chromosomes. The most important types of mosaicism are those involving the sex chromosomes, for, as already mentioned, changes implicating autosomes are usually lethal. If aberrations occur in later mitoses, a complex mosaic may result.

It should be noted that normal women are mosaics as regards the activity of their two X chromosomes, but this is not mosaicism as defined above.

SYNDROMES ASSOCIATED WITH ABNORMALITIES OF THE SEX CHROMOSOMES[24]

Since many of the X and Y chromosomal abnormalities produce sexual abnormalities, some of the features of sexual development should be noted. They may be considered under the following headings:

Anatomical Features

1. Chromosomal constitution, in respect of the sex chromosomes.
2. Structure of the gonads, as revealed by histology.
3. External genitalia.
4. Morphology of the Wolffian and Müllerian ducts.
5. Hormonal status, which is reflected in the secondary sexual characteristics, e.g. development of breast tissue and growth of beard.

Psychological Features

1. Sex of rearing, which is an indication of the sexual status of an individual as regarded by others. Usually this is based on the appearance of the external genitalia at birth.
2. Psychological sex, or the sex which the individual thinks himself or herself to have. This includes sexuality in the sense of eroticism.

In the normal person, all features correspond to one sex. When the psychological features conflict with the anatomical ones, such disturbances as homosexuality and transvestism result. These will not be considered further. When there is conflict between the anatomical features, the condition is regarded as one of intersexuality. Some of the conditions will now be considered, but for details the reader should refer to specialised texts on this complex subject.

Hermaphroditism[25]

Individuals who possess anatomical features of both sexes are termed hermaphrodites. Three groups are commonly recognised, the basis of the classification being the morphology of the gonads.

Female pseudohermaphroditism. *Congenital adrenal hyperplasia.* A defect in one of the enzymes necessary for the production of cortisol results in an oversecretion of ACTH by the pituitary, because cortisol normally inhibits the production of pituitary ACTH by its feedback effect. The excessive ACTH leads to hyperplasia of the adrenals. The common type is due to defective 21-hydroxylase, an enzyme involved in the synthesis of cortisol and aldosterone. An excess production of androgens results in the female fetus having ambiguous external genitalia at birth; later adrenal virilism develops and also a salt-losing state due in part to a failure in aldosterone secretion and in part to an overproduction of other hormones, e.g. progesterone, that antagonise aldosterone. In the male there is sexual pseudoprecosity, the testes being of normal size but the secondary sexual features being well developed.

In a less common type of adrenal hyperplasia, due to defective 11-hydroxylase, the overproduction of the mineralocorticoid deoxycorticosterone prevents a salt-losing state from developing but itself produces systemic hypertension (Fig. 3.9).

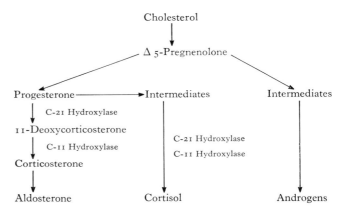

Figure 3.9
Diagram to illustrate the biosynthesis of the adrenal steroid hormones. Defective C-21 hydroxylase activity results in a failure in synthesis of aldosterone and cortisol. Overproduction of androgens causes virilism in the female, an effect also seen when there is defective C-11 hydroxylase activity. An additional effect of this defect is the overproduction of 11-deoxycorticosterone. This counters the salt-losing state, but leads to systemic hypertension.

Female pseudohermaphrodites may also be born to mothers who have an excess of androgens during pregnancy. Cases are recorded in which this was due to an arrhenoblastoma of the ovary or the administration of androgens for therapeutic purposes. All female pseudohermaphrodites have the chromosomal constitution 46,XX, and the gonads are ovaries.

True hermaphroditism. Both ovarian and testicular tissue is present, either combined as an ovotestis or in separate organs. The external genitalia are usually ambiguous. 46,XX is the usual chromosomal finding, but 46,XY and mosaics 46,XX/46,XY are known.

Male pseudohermaphroditism. The gonad or gonads present are testes, but the genital ducts and external genitalia show deviation towards female type, e.g. a small vagina is usually present with or without a uterus. At puberty masculinisation occurs, and when the patient has been brought up as a girl this leads to investigation. This type of male pseudohermaphrodite is generally 46,XY when bilateral testes are present, and a mosaic of the type 45,X/46,XY when testicular development is unilateral.

There is another type of male pseudohermaphroditism which is inherited and in which the endocrine status is fully feminine; this is the remarkable condition of *testicular feminisation*. The individual is often of above average intelligence, and has a normal, attractive, female appearance with excellent breast development. The testes are situated in the inguinal region and their tenderness may cause the patient to seek medical advice. Amenorrhoea, sterility, or dyspareunia due to a short vagina are other common complaints. The chromosomes are usually normal, 46,XY. The pathogenesis of testicular feminisation is now understood. An assay of steroid hormones reveals that they are similar to those of a normal male. The embryonic testis appears to be competent in suppressing Müllerian duct development, but although testosterone is produced, it fails to stimulate the development of the Wolffian ducts or the external genitalia. The defect lies in the unresponsiveness of these tissues to androgenic stimulation rather than to lack of hormones. The administration of androgens to the patients fails to produce masculinisation. The end-organ unresponsiveness is due to a defective gene on the X chromosome. The unopposed action of oestrogens is responsible for the breast development.

Klinefelter's Syndrome

In this syndrome, which occurs in about 1 in 500 births, there is an apparent male with gynaecomastia, small testes, poor facial hair growth, and a high-pitched voice. The limbs, especially the legs, are disproportionately long. The condition becomes apparent only at adolescence. In most cases examination of cells from skin or buccal scrapings reveals the unexpected presence of a Barr body. Chromosome counts show 47, the extra chromosome being an X. These individuals therefore have the constitution, 47,XXY. The condition usually arises by the fertilisation by a normal (Y) sperm of an XX ovum, but the fertilisation by an XY sperm of a normal (X) ovum can occur. In either event there has been nondisjunction in the abnormal gamete.

Some cases are more complicated, having a chromosomal composition of 48,XXXY, 49,XXXYY, 49,XXXXY, etc. Others exhibit mosaicism, e.g. 46,XY/47,XXY, 46,XX/47,XXY, and 46,XY/48,XXXY. 46,XX has been described (see p. 43). In general the greater the number of X chromosomes, the more likely is there to be mental retardation.

The testes in Klinefelter's syndrome are small. Early histological features are minute seminiferous tubules and a reduction in the number of germinal cells. Later there is thickening of the basement membrane, disappearance of all cellular elements apart from Sertoli cells, and ultimate hyalinisation of the tubules. The interstitial cells often show hyperplasia, but they tend to secrete an excess of oestrogen. This accounts for the gynaecomastia. Breast cancer occasionally develops. Sterility is invariable; a few patients have been claimed to be fertile, but subsequent investigations have not confirmed this.

Chromatin-negative Klinefelter's syndrome. A substantial number of cases are chromatin-negative and appear to have the make-up 46,XY. Some may be mosaics in which the cell line XXY has remained undetected, but in others there appears to be primary failure in the formation or development of the germ cells (del Castillo syndrome). Another group may be phenocopies and due to testicular atrophy caused by inflammatory disease.

Ovarian Dysgenesis

This syndrome occurs in females and is characterised by two features:

1. The presence of hypoplastic ovaries, or *streak ovaries*, which contain ovarian stroma with rete ovarii and hilus cells but no germinal follicles. The patients are therefore sterile. The term ovarian agenesis has been used previously, but is inappropriate since the organs are abnormal rather than absent.

2. *Primary amenorrhoea* and *failure to develop secondary sex characteristics*, e.g. breast development. The internal and external genitalia are infantile. Mental development is normal.

Ovarian dysgenesis may be found in females of normal stature, and the defect becomes evident with the failure to develop secondary sex characteristics at adolescence. In other cases the individual is in addition of *short stature*. *Somatic abnormalities* are striking in the remaining cases. At birth there may be redundancy of the skin of the back of the neck and lymphatic oedema of the hands and feet. Webbing of the neck, a shield-like chest with widely-spaced nipples, short fourth metacarpal bone, cubitus valgus, hypoplastic nails, multiple pigmented naevi, and coarctation of the aorta are all frequent. When two or more of these somatic anomalies are seen in a female of short stature and sexual infantilism due to streak ovaries, the eponym **Turner's syndrome** is applied.

Chromosomal abnormalities. The common defect is absence of one X chromosome giving the complement 45,X. Barr bodies are absent, and the incidence of colour blindness, a sex-linked recessive trait, is the same as in the normal male, i.e. about 8 per cent. Over 20 variants of ovarian dysgenesis have been found, and a few of these will be mentioned. Some are 46,XX*p*−, in which one of the X chromosomes has a deletion of the short arm; cells have a small Barr body. In 46,XX*qi* the abnormal isochromosome contains the two long arms of X; the Barr body is large. It therefore seems that *when an abnormal X is present, it forms the sex chromatin during the process of lyonisation.* In 46,XX*q*− the abnormal X has a deletion of its long arm. These individuals have streak ovaries but no somatic stigmata. Hence it appears that two normal X chromosomes are needed for the development of endodermal cells in the primitive ovary, so that a normal ovary with germ cells is formed. Absence of one short arm leads in addition to the somatic effects of Turner's syndrome.

Some cases of ovarian agenesis are transitional between the classical Turner's syndrome and the normal female. Some ovarian tissue may be present, and menstruation can occur. These patients are mosaics in which some cells have the normal XX, e.g. 45,X/46,XX, 46,XX/46,XX*p*−, and 45,X/46,XX/47,XXX. This emphasises the importance of examining chromosome preparations from various parts of the body in difficult cases.

Some cases of ovarian dysgenesis have male traits, e.g. 45,X/46,XY*pi*. In 46,XY*qi* the phenotype is female, but some testicular tissue may be found. It is evident that in the normal female XX, a component of the short arm of the 'inactivated' X remains active; the long arm of the Y chromosome probably also has components in common with the short arm of the X, otherwise one would except the normal XY male to have the somatic anomalies of Turner's syndrome. A normal Y is necessary for normal male development. The study of these rare but fascinating cases of ovarian dysgenesis has, therefore, led to some understanding of the functions of the sex chromosomes.

Noonan's syndrome.[26] This syndrome bears some resemblance to Turner's syndrome but it is a separate entity. It may affect either sex, and there is no known chromosomal abnormality. The main characteristics are short stature, congenital heart disease (particularly affecting the right side with pulmonary stenosis), and in many cases mild mental subnormality. Webbing of the neck may occur. Gonadal differentiation and function vary from complete absence to normal function and fertility. The condition is familial, but the exact mode of inheritance is unsettled.

Poly-X females. Many trisomy-X females, 47,XXX, have been described. The cells contain two Barr bodies. In the great majority of cases there is normal sexual development and fertility. Interestingly, the children of these women always have a normal complement of sex chromosomes; apparently XXX and XXY zygotes are either not produced or else destroyed soon after fusion. Trisomy X is associated with an increased incidence of mental subnormality, usually of mild degree. Occasional instances of 48,XXXX and 49,XXXXX are recorded; in them there is severe mental subnormality.

XYY syndrome. The chromosomal constitution 47,XYY has been noted in males with normal sexual development. Some patients have been abnormally tall, and have exhibited criminal aggressiveness or have been mentally subnormal. 49,XXXYY has been recorded.

Summary of the Mechanism of Sexual Development[27–29]

It is not possible to give a complete account of the factors which determine the normal development of sex. Abnormalities are common; indeed, aberrations of psychological sex constitute a major social problem, and one for which no adequate solution has been found. Even the factors which determine the development of the anatomical aspects of sex are not well understood, but nevertheless certain general features are evident.

The development of a normal testis is dependent on the presence of a Y chromosome. Under its influence the indifferent gonad develops into a testis. The Y chromosome determines the presence of the H-Y antigen on the cell's surface and also H-Y antigen receptor sites on the gonadal cells. Close interaction between the germ cells (with H-Y antigen) and the gonadal tissues (with H-Y antigen and H-Y receptors) results in the formation of a testis.

Once the testis has developed, further differentiation of genital tubes and external genitalia is determined by the secretion of two testicular hormones. *Factor X*, thought to be a protein, suppresses the development of the Müllerian ducts. To a considerable extent this acts locally, since if testicular tissue is absent from one side, either as a result of an experimental procedure or in some cases of true hermaphroditism, the Müllerian duct of the same side develops to produce a uterine horn. The second testicular hormone, *testosterone*, induces masculine development of the accessory glands and ducts. Feminisation occurs in the absence of these two testicular hormones regardless of the individual's sex-chromosome constitution.

Testosterone-induced masculine development is mediated by the product of a gene, itself located on the X chromosome. This product activates all the genes required for the manifestations of the male phenotype in response to circulating testosterone. The presence of a mutant gene at this site can render the tissues insensitive to testosterone, and the individual matures with a female phenotype even though testosterone-producing testes are present and the chromosomal constitution is XY. This is the condition of *testicular feminisation*, variants of which are known in mice, rats, and the human being. Specific nuclear-cytosol receptors for testosterone are absent in this condition. It should be noted that the normal female also possesses such receptors; her tissues are therefore susceptible to the effects of circulating androgens, e.g. in the condition of virilism.

The development of sexual characteristics is by no means as simple as the above account would indicate. Thus the presence of an extra X chromosome (e.g. in Klinefelter's syndrome) prevents the full maturation of the testis. There are also the 46,XX true hermaphrodite and the very rare 46,XX male. There are several explanations of the XX male. Perhaps an undetected chromosomal anomaly is present but undetected, e.g. translocation of a Y or a fragment of it to an X or other large chromosome, or XX/XY mosaics in which the XY cells are few in number or are in sites difficult to detect, such as in the testis itself. The presence of a gene for testicular development on an autosome has also been postulated.[30]

If an early embryo of either genetic sex is castrated, there is complete Müllerian duct differentiation, disappearance of the Wolffian duct, and development of female external genitalia. This state of affairs is seen in ovarian dysgenesis.

Extragonadal hormones play some part in the differentiation of the genital ducts and external genitalia. These may be derived either from the mother or from the fetus itself, as in congenital adrenal hyperplasia.

SYNDROMES ASSOCIATED WITH ABNORMALITIES OF THE AUTOSOMES[31]

The absence of one autosome (monosomy) is almost always lethal to the developing embryo, and is therefore very rarely found in post-embryonic life (monosomy 21, the converse of Down's syndrome, is described, and it too is associated with severe mental subnormality). Occasionally there is deletion of part of a chromosome, but much more frequently nondisjunction causes one pair to become trisomic: for reasons which are not apparent, this additional chromosome causes severe damage.

Trisomy 21 Syndrome (Down's Syndrome)[32]
47,XY, +21 or 47,XX, +21

This syndrome, also known as 'mongolism' because of a superficial resemblance of the face of its victims to that of members of the Mongolian race, is due to trisomy of number 21 chromosome. The condition occurs in from 1 in 600 to 700 live births. It is commoner with increasing maternal age.

Severe mental subnormality is a characteristic feature, and in individuals who live over 40 years the development of Alzheimer's disease is a constant feature. The sex chromosomes are normal, and individuals of both sexes are affected.

In Down's syndrome the palm of the hand characteristically shows a simian crease and there are abnormalities of the dermal ridges of the fingers. Indeed, the study of these fingerprints and palmar creases (dermatoglyphics) forms an important investigation in cases of chromosomal abnormality.

Occasionally an individual with Down's syndrome is found with 46 chromosomes. The constitution is: pairs (1–14), 15 alone, pairs (16–22)+XY+one odd big chromosome. This odd chromosome is thought to be a combination of 15 and 21. Thus the patient has in reality trisomy of 21, but the translocation has hidden it. In such cases one of the parents is found to have a similar translocation—45 chromosomes: pairs (1–14), 15, pairs (16–20), 21, pair 22, 15/21, XY. This is therefore called *translocation mongolism*. It is important because further children are liable to be affected also, and the parents can be advised accordingly. This type of Down's syndrome can occur in the children of young mothers, and is not related to increasing maternal age.

Trisomy 13 Syndrome (Patau's Syndrome) 47,XY,+13 or 47,XX,+13

Trisomy of number 13 chromosome is associated with a variety of congenital defects, the most common of which are mental deficiency, cleft lip and palate, microphthalmia, polydactyly, and defects of the ear, heart, and urinary and genital tracts.

Trisomy 18 Syndrome (Edwards's Syndrome) 47,XY,+18 or 47,XX,+18

Multiple abnormalities occur in this syndrome. Affected infants usually die by the third month and few survive over one year. Low-set ears, micrognathia, heart disease, mental retardation, and failure to thrive are the common findings. As with trisomy 21 and 13, mosaics and translocation cases are also described.

The Cri du Chat Syndrome 46,XY,5p− or 46,XX,5p−

The syndrome was named after the feeble mewing cry of the affected infants. Mental and growth retardation are combined with other defects. The chromosomal abnormality is a deletion of a portion of the short arm of number 5 chromosome.

Many other chromosomal abnormalities have been described in association with developmental abnormalities, and no doubt other syndromes will be recognised. Ring chromosomes have been described in most of the syndromes noted above. They arise as a result of breaks in both the long and short arms of a chromosome; this is followed by the two ends joining together. The effects vary according to the chromosome affected and the amount of lost or added chromosomal material. The most severe chromosomal aberrations are found in aborted embryos. Thus triploidy (69,XXY) and even tetraploidy (92,XXXX) are amongst the bizarre findings which have been reported. The incidence of these abnormalities has varied from 22 per cent[33] to 64 per cent[34] of spontaneous abortions in which cell cultures could be obtained. The earlier the abortion the more likely is a chromosomal abnormality to be found. About 30 per cent of zygotes are aborted spontaneously, and gross genetic errors are clearly a major cause.

CHROMOSOME ABNORMALITIES ARISING IN SOMATIC CELLS

Although mosaics are described in many of the syndromes mentioned above, the abnormality presumably occurs at an early stage of development. The possibility that a similar event could occur later in life was suggested by the findings in some cases of chronic myeloid leukaemia. Some of the haematopoietic cells show a small chromosome, which is 22 with a deleted long arm (46,XY,22q− or 46,XX,22q−). It is called the *Philadelphia* or *Ph′ chromosome*.

Other tumours have been found to exhibit a constant chromosomal abnormality. Thus in Burkitt's lymphoma the cells have an abnormally long chromosome 14. This is due to a reciprocal translocation of the end of the long arm of chromosome 14 with the long arm of chromosome 8. Retinoblastoma, multiple myeloma, meningioma, and breast cancer are amongst the tumours in which chromosomal abnormalities have been described. No doubt the list will grow as techniques of chromosomal analysis are refined.

AVOIDANCE OF GENETIC DEFECTS[35–37]

Genetic counselling will dissuade some high-risk couples from procreation, but when once conception has occurred the only course open may be the induction of abortion. Amniocentesis can be employed for the prenatal detection of fetal abnormality. Fluid can be removed from the amniotic sac from the twelfth week onwards; about the sixteenth week is the optimal time. This gives the laboratory adequate time to examine the fluid and allows abortion to be performed before the twentieth week. In some societies legal technicalities make the performance of abortion more difficult after this time. The supernatant of the fluid obtained by amniocentesis can be examined biochemically and for the presence of virus. Thus a raised level of α-fetoprotein in the amniotic fluid is associated with anencephaly and severe neural-tube defects.[38]

The cells can be examined for the presence of the X chromosome and the Y body. The sex of the fetus is sometimes of importance. In women carriers of an X-linked recessive gene the chances of a female inheriting the disease are zero; the chances for the male are 50 per cent. Amniotic cells can be cultured for full chromosomal analysis—Down's syndrome and other abnormalities can be detected readily.

In many of the inherited metabolic disorders cell culture can detect the defect.[39] In this way a prenatal diagnosis of galactosaemia, Tay-Sachs disease, the mucopolysaccharidoses, and others can be made. Amniocentesis is therefore of great value in detecting these diseases *in utero*, and the routine monitoring of a pregnancy can be carried out when the couple are at risk in as much as both are known to be carriers. This approach has been used with success in the detection of Tay-Sachs disease. Unfortunately cystic fibrosis, with a carrier rate of 1 in 25 and an incidence at birth of 1 in 1600 in Europe and North America, cannot be prevented since the biochemical defect has yet to be identified.

TREATMENT OF GENETIC DEFECTS

The treatment of patients with genetic abnormalities is often very unsatisfactory, but there are some instances where expert attention can ameliorate the condition. These can be considered under eight headings:

1. *Administration of a missing protein*—e.g. immunoglobulin in agammaglobulinaemia.

2. *Avoidance of specific substances*—e.g. lactose in galactosaemia.

3. *Administration of missing metabolites*—e.g. cytidylic and uridylic acids in orotic aciduria.

4. *Avoidance of particular drugs*—e.g. primaquine.

5. *Administration of metabolic inhibitors*—e.g. allopurinol in gout.

6. *Administration of drugs to eliminate abnormally stored material*—e.g. penicillamine in Wilson's disease.

7. *Allografts.* The grafting of normal cells into individuals lacking specific enzymes or the ability to synthesise essential substances has been hindered by the unsolved problems inherent in grafting. Thus attempts to provide thymic or lymphoid cells in cases of immunological deficiency are in the experimental stage. Allografts of spleen cells in haemophiliac subjects have not been successful.

8. *Genetic engineering.*[40] More complex means of treating genetic defects are now being investigated. Human fibroblasts from patients with galactosaemia lack the enzyme α-D-galactose 1-phosphate uridyl transferase. A λ-bacteriophage which normally infests *Escherichia coli* can carry the galactose operon. If the defective fibroblasts are infested with this phage, the enzyme activity of the cells is restored.[41,42] Whether phages or other viruses can ever be used as a vehicle for the introduction of selected genes into human cells *in vivo* is impossible to predict.

It is now possible to excise a portion of DNA using an endonuclease, and splice it into another DNA molecule. In this way hereditary material from virtually any plant or animal can be grafted into bacteria and propagated. The properties of such organisms cannot be foretold, and there is justifiable concern regarding the advisability of continuing certain types of genetic engineering.

ACQUIRED DISEASE

ENVIRONMENTAL FACTORS CAUSING DISEASE

Much of human pathology is concerned with those diseases which are acquired in post-natal life as a result of the action of external factors. The effects of physical and chemical agents, living organisms, and dietary deficiencies are the common causes of these *acquired diseases*. It must not be forgotten, however, that the developing fetus is also sensitive to environmental influences—in some instances much more so than is the adult. Intrauterine events may produce defects which are present at birth (*congenital*) but which are not inherited, since no genetic mechanism is involved. The time of onset of a disease gives no indication as to whether the cause is environmental or genetic.

The cellular and tissue responses to external agents are summarised in Fig. 3.10. It can be seen that the types of reaction which can occur are strictly limited. Any pathological process is composed of a mixture of these basic units—the nature of the mixture being largely related to the cause. The remainder of this book is devoted to a description of these basic pathological processes and the common mixtures which are found.

Figure 3.10
Diagram showing the main pathological processes of the body in response to an external agent.

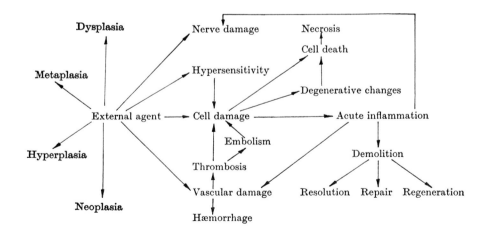

GENERAL READING

LEVINE, H. (1971) *Clinical Cytogenetics*, 572 pp. Boston: Little Brown.
NORA, J. J. & FRASER, F. C. (1974) *Medical Genetics: Principles and Practice*, 399 pp. Philadelphia: Lea and Febiger.
ROBERTS, J. A. F. (1967) *An Introduction to Medical Genetics*, 4th edn, 290 pp. London: Oxford University Press.
VALENTINE, G. H. (1975) *The Chromosome Disorders*, 3rd edn. London: Heinemann.
YUNIS, J. J. & CHANDLER, M. E. (1977) The chromosomes of man—clinical and biologic significance. *American Journal of Pathology*, **88**, 466.

REFERENCES

1. ERBE, R. W. (1976) Principles of medical genetics. *New England Journal of Medicine*, **294**, 381 and 480.
2. CARTER, C. O. (1969) An ABC of medical genetics. *Lancet*, **1**, 1014, 1041, 1087, 1139, 1203, 1252, and 1303.
3. TOWNES, P. L. (1969) Human polymorphism. *Medical Clinics of North America*, **53**, 886.
4. CARTER, C. O. (1969) Genetic counselling. *Medical Clinics of North America*, **53**, 991.
5. THOMPSON, J. S. & THOMPSON, M. W. (1973) *Genetics in Medicine*, 2nd edn. Philadelphia: Saunders.
6. HARRIS, H. (1968) Molecular basis of hereditary disease. *British Medical Journal*, **2**, 135.
7. CHILDS, B. & DER KALOUSTIAN, V. M. (1968) Genetic heterogeneity. *New England Journal of Medicine*, **279**, 1205 and 1267.
8. LA DU, B. N. (1969) Pharmacogenetics. *Medical Clinics of North America*, **53**, 839.
9. CHILDS, B. (1970) Sir Archibald Garrod's conception of chemical individuality: a modern appreciation. *New England Journal of Medicine*, **282**, 71.
10. STANBURY, J. B., WYNGAARDEN, J. B. & FREDRICKSON, D. S. (Eds.) (1972). *The Metabolic Basis of Inherited Disease*, 3rd edn. New York: McGraw-Hill.
11. O'REILLY, R. A., POOL, J. G. & AGGELER, P. M. (1968) Hereditary resistance to coumarin anticoagulant drugs in man and rat. *Annals of the New York Academy of Sciences*, **151**, 913.
12. KOLODNY, E. H. (1976) Lysosomal storage diseases. *New England Journal of Medicine*, **294**, 1217.
13. HSIA, D. Y-Y. (1969) The detection of heterozygous carriers. *Medical Clinics of North America*, **53**, 857.
14. Leading Article (1975) HL-A antigens and rheumatic diseases. *British Medical Journal*, **2**, 238.
15. BREWERTON, D. A. et al. (1973) Reiter's disease and HL-A27. *Lancet*, **2**, 996.
16. BREWERTON, D. A. et al. (1973) Acute anterior uveitis and HL-A27. *Lancet*, **2**, 994.
17. GEBHARD, R. L. *et al.* (1973) HL-A antigen type and small-intestinal disease in dermatitis herpetiformis. *Lancet*, **2**, 760.
18. The London Conference on the Normal Human Karyotype (1964) *Annals of Human Genetics*, **27**, 295.
19. Chicago Conference: Standardisation in Genetics. (1966) *Birth Defects: Original Article Series*. II: 2. New York: The National Foundation.
20. Paris Conference (1971): Standardisation in Human Cytogenetics (1972) *Birth Defects: Original Article Series* VIII: 7. New York: The National Foundation.
21. HECHT, F., WYANDT, H. E. & ERBE, R. W. (1971) Revolutionary cytogenetics. *New England Journal of Medicine*, **285**, 1482.
22. KROOTH, R. S. (1969) Genetics of cultured somatic cells. *Medical Clinics of North America*, **53**, 795.
23. EPSTEIN, C. J. (1972) Inactivation of the X-chromosome. *New England Journal of Medicine*, **286**, 318.
24. GERALD, P. S. (1976) Sex chromosome disorders. *New England Journal of Medicine*, **294**, 706.
25. NEW, M. I. (1968) Congenital adrenal hyperplasia. *Pediatric Clinics of North America*, **15**, 395.
26. GORLIN, R. J. & SEDANO, H. (1973) Noonan's syndrome (XX and XY Turner phenotype syndrome). *Modern Medicine of Canada*, **28**, 666.
27. OHNO, S. (1976) Major regulatory genes for mammalian sexual development. *Cell*, 7, 315.
28. OHNO, S. (1976) Sexual differentiation and testosterone production. *New England Journal of Medicine*, **295**, 1011.
29. WACHTEL, S. S. *et al.* (1975) Possible role for H-Y antigen in the primary determination of sex. *Nature (London)*, **257**, 235.
30. MILUNSKY, A. (1973) Sex-determining genes and the Y-chromosome. *New England Journal of Medicine*, **288**, 577.
31. Editorial (1967) Clinical chromosomology, 1967. *New England Journal of Medicine*, **277**, 825.
32. SMITH, G. F. & BERG, J. M. (1976) *Down's Anomaly*. 2nd edn. Edinburgh: Churchill Livingstone.
33. CARR, D. H. (1965) Chromosome studies in spontaneous abortions. *Obstetrics and Gynecology*, **26**, 308.
34. SZULMAN, A. E. (1965) Chromosomal aberrations in spontaneous human abortions. *New England Journal of Medicine*, **272**, 811.
35. LAURENCE, K. M. (1974) Fetal malformations and abnormalities. *Lancet*, **2**, 939.
36. MILUNSKY, A. (1973) *The Prenatal Diagnosis of Hereditary Disorders*, 253 pp. Springfield: C. C. Thomas.
37. MILUNSKY, A. (1976) Prenatal diagnosis of genetic disorders. *New England Journal of Medicine*, **295**, 377.
38. SELLER, M. J. *et al* (1974) Maternal serum-alpha-fetoprotein levels and prenatal diagnosis of neural-tube defects. *Lancet*, **1**, 428.
39. BEARN, A. G. (1972) Cell culture in inherited disease—with some notes on genetic heterogeneity. *New England Journal of Medicine*, **286**, 764.
40. COHEN, S. N. (1976) Gene manipulation. *New England Journal of Medicine*, **294**, 883.
41. Leading Article (1971) Transducing bacteriophage in genetic repair. *Lancet*, **2**, 965.
42. MERRIL, C. R., GEIER, M. R. & PETRICCIANI, J. C. (1971) Bacterial virus gene expression in human cells. *Nature (London)*, **233**, 398.

Chapter 4. Cell Response to Injury

The manner by which adverse conditions or poisons affect cells must now be examined. Most agents, it may be assumed, affect the cell by upsetting some important chemical reaction. A *biochemical lesion* is thus the first change and this in its turn may produce secondary results. Structural changes take place within the cell, and if the damage is severe the cell may die; destructive enzymes are then liberated within the cell, and the process of *self-digestion*, or *autolysis*, occurs. When this happens after the death of the whole individual, the term *post-mortem change* is used. When, however, a group of cells dies in continuity with the living, similar changes occur and it is by observing them that cell death can itself be recognised: to this process the term *necrosis* is applied—it therefore means death of cells or tissue with structural evidence of this death.

BIOCHEMICAL LESIONS[1]

The concept of a biochemical lesion was first put forward by Sir Rudolph Peters. It has been known for a long time that thiamine deficiency in pigeons leads to severe neurological complications. The birds develop opisthotonos and convulsions, but in spite of this evidence of a severe neurological lesion no abnormalities can be detected on histological examination of the brain. The situation is reminiscent of that seen in the Lesch-Nyhan syndrome.

When slices of brain tissue from thiamine-deficient birds are incubated in a Warburg apparatus, they show abnormally low oxygen consumption; if thiamine is added, the oxygen consumption rises to normal. Furthermore, if thiamine is injected intrathecally into a bird suffering from thiamine deficiency, it recovers from the neurological complications in about 30 minutes. Examination of the blood in thiamine-deficient birds reveals a raised pyruvate level, but this is not the cause of the symptoms since pyruvate itself is not toxic. The explanation of the symptoms is believed to be the hold-up in the activity of the Krebs cycle (Fig 4.1) that occurs in the absence of the co-carboxylase thiamine pyrophosphate, which is one of the factors involved in the conversion of pyruvate to acetyl-coenzyme A. Pyruvate normally enters the Krebs cycle *via* acetyl-coenzyme A. A hold-up at this point results in an accumulation of pyruvate, which is thus an effect of the lesion rather than a cause of the symptoms. The impairment of glucose metabolism in the nerve cells is presumably the cause of the symptoms.

Thiamine deficiency thus provides an excellent example of a biochemical lesion due to a deficiency: a lesion which causes severe effects and even death, but which is not detectable by the current routine histological methods. Other similar examples may be mentioned.

Lewisite poisoning. The trivalent arsenic compound lewisite was used as a poison gas in the First World War. It produces inflammation with blister formation when applied to the skin. As a systemic agent it also interferes with the action of pyruvate dehydrogenase by binding the enzyme. In this way a biochemical block is established, because pyruvate dehydrogenase plays an important part in the conversion of pyruvate to acetyl-coenzyme A.

The compound British anti-lewisite (BAL) restores the activity of the enzyme.

Fluoroacetate poisoning. This substance was shown by Peters to block the Krebs cycle by a process described as *lethal synthesis*. It enters the cycle in place of ordinary acetate and is converted to fluorocitrate. This cannot be further metabolised, and it blocks the Krebs cycle by interfering with the action of aconitase which is necessary for the conversion of citrate to *cis*-aconitate.

Diphtheria toxin. The action of diphtheria toxin has been analysed in considerable detail. The effect of its actions is to inhibit protein synthesis by inhibiting movement of the ribosomes along the mRNA.[2] It has been shown *in vitro* that

$$\text{Protein}\underset{SH}{\overset{SH}{\diagdown}} + Cl_2AsCH=CHCl \rightarrow \text{Protein}\underset{S}{\overset{S}{\diagdown}}AsCH \quad CHCl$$

Enzyme   + Lewisite   →Inactivated enzyme

$$\text{Protein}\underset{S}{\overset{S}{\diagdown}}AsCH=CHCl + \underset{\substack{CHSH \\ | \\ CH_2OH}}{CH_2SH} \rightarrow \text{Protein}\underset{SH}{\overset{SH}{\diagdown}} + \underset{\substack{CHS \\ | \\ CH_2OH}}{\overset{CH_2S}{\diagdown}}AsCH=CHCl$$

Inactivated enzyme   + BAL   →Enzyme   + BAL-Lewisite compound

Figure 4.1
The Krebs cycle. Glucose is broken
down predominantly by glycolysis, and
enters the Krebs cycle as acetylcoenzyme A. Under anaerobic conditions
pyruvic acid is converted into lactic
acid, whereby NAD is regenerated and
allows glycolysis to continue. Under
aerobic conditions the $NADH_2$ is oxidised by molecular oxygen, thus regenerating NAD, and the pyruvate is further metabolised *via* acetylcoenzyme A.
The Krebs cycle is also known as the
citric acid, or tricarboxylic acid, cycle.

Key:
1. Condensing enzyme.
2. and 3. Aconitase.
4. *Iso*-citric dehydrogenase.
5. α-Ketoglutaric dehydrogenase.
6. Succinic dehydrogenase.
7. Fumarase.
8. Malic dehydrogenase.
  CoASH—Coenzyme A.
  $CH_2COSCoA$—
  Acetylcoenzyme A.
  NAD—Nicotinamide adenine
  dinucleotide (previously called
  DPN).
  $NADH_2$—Dihydronicotinamide
  adenine dinucleotide ($DPNH_2$).
  Pi—Inorganic phosphate.

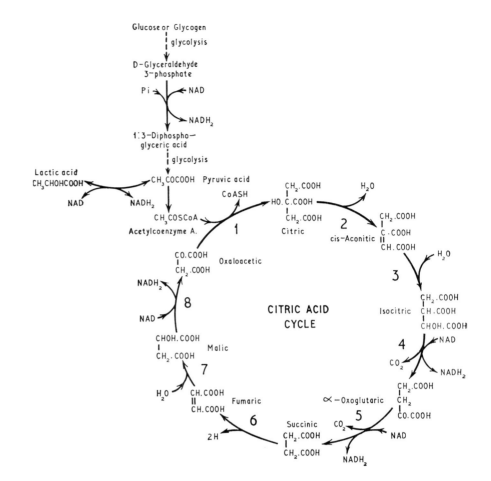

diphtheria toxin inhibits the transfer of amino acids from tRNA to the growing polypeptide chain.

Genetic Enzyme Defect

Another way in which a biochemical lesion may occur is by a specific enzyme deficiency dependent upon a genetic defect. This rare but important group of diseases is described in Chapter 3.

Some chemotherapeutic agents are used with the deliberate intention of producing a biochemical lesion in micro-organisms. This mechanism provides the basis for the action of sulphonamides and some antibiotics, e.g. rifamycin and its derivatives in bacterial and viral infections. Hopefully anti-cancer agents will also be found.

Some chemicals have a selective destructive effect, e.g. alloxan is toxic to the islets of Langerhans, and its adminis-tration to animals is followed by the development of diabetes mellitus. The drug has been used as a cytotoxic agent in cases of islet-cell tumour, but the results have been disappointing. Streptozotocin, an antibiotic, has a similar action, and pre-liminary reports indicate that it is effective in the treatment of islet-cell cancers.[3]

Finally, it has been suggested that some mental illnesses are the result of biochemical lesions. That this is possible is demonstrated by the dramatic effects of certain 5-HT anta-gonists, e.g. LSD.

Although only a few examples have been cited, this subject will certainly become increasingly important in the future. The routine methods of examining pathological material are inadequate for the detection of biochemical upsets. Other more refined methods will have to be employed for further advances to be made. For the present it may be postulated that chemical blocks or lesions may occur in the following ways:

1. The enzyme may be absent or abnormal through a genetic error.

2. The enzyme may be directly inhibited by a chemical agent.

3. There may be a deficiency of substrate for a variety of reasons—dietary deficiency, other biochemical lesions, etc.

4. Deficiency of co-enzyme.

5. Substrate competition by chemicals of similar nature to the natural substrate.

Whatever the mechanism causing the block, the effects can be brought about in three main ways:

1. The excess substrate which frequently accumulates may be toxic, or may cause some other biochemical lesion by affecting another enzyme system.

2. The inhibited reaction may be of vital importance to the cell.

3. Although the reaction itself may not be of great **impor-**

Figure 4.2
Some possible mechanisms which may be involved in the production of a biochemical lesion. The factors interfering with the basic reaction, substrate →product, are shown on the left and the effects are shown on the right.

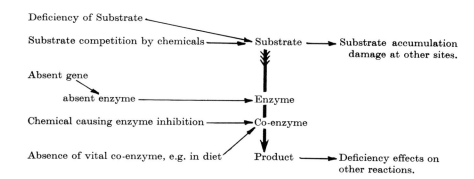

tance, the end-product may be an essential substance in some other important metabolic reaction.

The effects of a biochemical lesion vary considerably. The cell's metabolism may show gross abnormalities which may be exhibited as marked alteration in behaviour without any structural change; thus myocardium loses its capacity to contract normally within three minutes of the onset of ischaemia. This is due to a lack of energy release and an impairment of the calcium transport within the cell that is necessary for contraction. Another example is the effects of thiamine deficiency already described. The alterations in metabolism may, on the other hand, produce changes in the morphology of the cell. Such changes have been known for a long time as the *degenerations*, and great importance has been attached to them. The concepts of cellular degeneration were evolved during the last hundred years using the relatively crude methods available for cellular study. Three types of change have been described: these are firstly *cloudy swelling*, *vacuolar degeneration*, and *hydropic degeneration*. Secondly there is *fatty degeneration* and *fatty infiltration* which are related to each other. Finally there is a heterogeneous group in which eosinophilic material appears in the cell either as droplets or as ill-defined masses. This group is termed *hyaline degeneration* or *hyaline-droplet change*. These are depicted diagrammatically in Figure 4.3. It must be appreciated that these are purely descriptive terms applied to the appearance of cells when viewed in the conventional manner by light microscopy of sections from paraffin-wax embedded tissue. Before considering the impact of biochemical and electron-microscopic studies the classical changes will first be examined.

CHANGES ASSOCIATED WITH ACCUMULATION OF WATER IN THE CELL

Cloudy Swelling

The changes of cloudy swelling are frequently to be found in parenchymatous cells, e.g. liver and kidney. The cells are swollen and the cytoplasm granular. These changes closely resemble those occurring in *post-mortem* autolysis,[4] but experimentally it has been shown that they can develop in the cells of the living animal when these are subjected to such adverse conditions as ischaemia, hypoxia, and the effects of a poison.

The organ whose cells show cloudy swelling is swollen, its

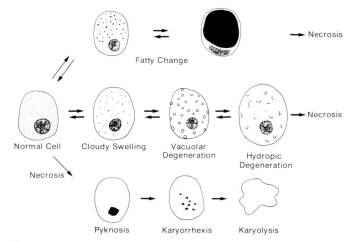

Figure 4.3
Diagram to illustrate the cellular changes which are generally described as the "degenerations". A damaged cell may exhibit progressive waterlogging, and pass through the stages of cloudy swelling, vacuolar degeneration, and hydropic degeneration. Alternatively, fat may accumulate, firstly as fine droplets, but later as the condition advances, a large globule is formed. In the bottom row the changes accompanying necrosis are depicted; these are pyknosis, karyorrhexis, and karyolysis (see p. 55). These changes become evident about 12 hours after cell death and are not reversible. (*Drawing by Margot Mackay, Department of Art as Applied to Medicine, University of Toronto.*)

cut surface bulges outwards, and it has a grey, parboiled appearance. The consistency is soft.

Vacuolar Degeneration

The naked-eye appearance described as typical of cloudy swelling is sometimes associated with swollen cells containing vacuoles rather than granules. This is vacuolar degeneration, and its causes and distribution are similar to those of cloudy swelling.

Hydropic Degeneration

The cells show great swelling due to an accumulation of fluid (water-logging). The cytoplasm is pale and homogeneous. The condition is reversible, but this is the most severe form of this group of degenerations and may terminate in death of the cell. The balloon cells seen in the early epidermal lesions of some viral infections of the skin afford a good example of this. The hydropic epidermal cells soon undergo necrosis and produce the intraepidermal vesicle so characteristic of herpes simplex, varicella-zoster, vaccinia, and smallpox infections.

CHANGES ASSOCIATED WITH THE ACCUMULATION OF FAT

An accumulation of excess stainable neutral fat is a frequent finding in parenchymal cells. It is especially common in the liver, and its causes include those which produce cloudy swelling. A fatty liver is enlarged, its cut surface bulges, and it is greasy to the touch. Its colour is pale, and in severe cases yellow. This is seen in alcoholism, cirrhosis, and in patchy distribution in the nutmeg liver of congestive heart failure. It is particularly well marked in cases of phosphorus poisoning. Fatty change is common in the convoluted tubules of the kidney, where it leads to pallor and swelling of the cortex. Accumulation of fat in the heart muscle cells is focal and may be sufficiently marked to produce yellow flecks visible on the endocardial surface (thrush-breast, or tabby-cat, heart). Severe anaemia is the usual cause.

Microscopically the cells are swollen and contain small droplets composed of neutral fat (glyceryl triesters). This is the condition at one time known as '*fatty degeneration*' (Figs 4.4 and 4.5). The fat was thought to be derived from hidden tissue fat by a process of unmasking, or *phanerosis*. In advanced cases the fat appears as one large globule pushing the nucleus to the side—an appearance described as '*fatty infiltration*', presumably because it was thought that adipose cells were infiltrating the organ (Fig. 4.4). This nomenclature

Figure 4.5

Fatty change in the liver. Electron micrograph of a rat liver cell, 4 hours following administration of ethionine. Accumulation of large lipid droplets is pronounced. The rough endoplasmic reticulum is disorganised, and the two arrows point to dilated cisterns. Lead hydroxide. × 10 500. (*Photograph by courtesy of Dr. Katsumi Miyai.*)

is misleading and has been abandoned. It is now known that 'fatty degeneration' is but an early stage in the development of 'fatty infiltration', and that in both conditions the fat is brought to the cells from the fat depots. *Fatty change* is now used to include both conditions. It should not be confused with the accumulation of true fat cells in the tissues; this is common in the heart and pancreas of obese patients. Local deposits of fat are sometimes a feature of chronic inflammation (p. 133) and following atrophy, e.g. lymph nodes and thymus. These conditions are sometimes called fatty infiltration, but confusion is most easily avoided if the term *adiposity* is used.

Hyaline degeneration and hyaline droplet change. These are described later (p. 53).

NATURE OF THE DEGENERATIVE CHANGES[5]

It is often assumed that the cellular changes of cloudy swelling or hydropic degeneration are the same regardless of the organ affected, be it liver, kidney, or islet of Langerhans. Such is not the case. Using the electron microscope, it has been possible to probe more deeply into the nature of these changes. Whereas the light microscope can give a vague impression of intracellular events and detect the changes when they are severe enough to affect the cell as a whole, electron microscopy can reveal which parts of the cell are affected and indicate the sequence of events and metabolic changes which are occurring. The structure of the cell now appears more complex than did the anatomy of the whole body a hundred years ago. Just as 'coma' ceased to be an intellectually satisfying ultimate diagnosis when specific conditions affecting the brain were recognised, so cloudy swelling is equally unsatisfactory now that organelles are known to exist. The first steps in the recognition of the cell's response to injury have been taken, and cellular pathology promises to become as complex as organ pathology. At this stage one must expect

Figure 4.4

Fatty change of liver. Many of the liver cells are distended with fat globules to the extent that their nuclei are pushed to the cell wall. In other cells the fat is present as small droplets in the cytoplasm. The material was taken at the necropsy of an elderly woman who died of septicaemia. × 80.

newly described lesions to prove as useful—and at times as misleading—as were those used initially in organ pathology.

It is not easy to give a clear generalised account of the cell's response to injury, since relatively few cell-types have been investigated to any extent. Most work has been carried out on liver and kidney subjected to a variety of chemical poisons, e.g. carbon tetrachloride, ethionine, barbiturates, ethanol, etc. Some of the changes in the cell's components will be described:

Nuclear Changes

A variety of nuclear changes have been described in poisoned cells. One of the earliest is condensation of the chromatin adjacent to the nuclear membrane and around the nucleolus. The nucleoli show loss of their granular component, and the fibrillar material is sometimes dispersed into separate fragments. Nucleoli are therefore smaller but more numerous. The loss of granular material may indicate impaired synthesis of ribosomal material and mRNA. Reduced RNA synthesis is found in damaged cells, and this is reflected in the cytoplasm as reduced protein synthesis. It should be stressed that by light microscopy nuclear changes are not obvious or characteristic in cells showing degeneration. Sometimes an increased number of nucleoli may be noted.

Cytoplasmic Changes

These may be considered under five headings:
Evidence of increased cell function. Cellular components may proliferate or reorganise in a manner which suggests a state of *hyperfunction*. In response to certain poisons the smooth endoplasmic reticulum becomes more abundant; it is produced in the rough endoplasmic reticulum and forms complex whorls and gyrations (Fig. 4.6); this is regarded as an adaptive mechanism and indicates an attempt to

Figure 4.6
Advanced proliferation of the smooth endoplasmic reticulum (ser) in the periphery of a rat hepatocyte following ethionine administration. The proliferated vesicles of the agranular reticulum are tightly packed and well demarcated from the rough endoplasmic reticulum (rer), which can be identified by the ribosomes studded on the membranes. Mitochondria (m) are elongated. cm—cell membrane; lip—lipid droplet. Lead hydroxide. × 5500. (*Photograph by courtesy of Dr. Katsumi Miyai.*)

increase the cell's ability to detoxify the substance. It may also be the morphological expression of a drug-induced enzyme induction. Thus phenobarbitone causes an increase in smooth endoplasmic reticulum as well as leading to enzyme induction. The latter has the effect of increasing the metabolism of coumarin anticoagulants, a fact that must be borne in mind if the two drugs are given simultaneously. There is also increased enzymatic glucuronidation of bilirubin, an effect of therapeutic value. However, some agents, including carcinogens, cause a proliferation of smooth endoplasmic reticulum that is accompanied by decreased enzymatic activity.

Likewise free ribosomes, rough endoplasmic reticulum, and the Golgi complex may proliferate; the number of lysosomes

Figure 4.7
Marked proliferation of mitochondria (m) in a rat hepatocyte following the administration of ethionine. The mitochondria are of uniform size and shape, and other cytoplasmic organelles are inconspicuous. Lead hydroxide. × 12 000. (*Photograph by courtesy of Dr. Katsumi Miyai.*)

may increase, and mitochondria become more abundant, enlarge, and exhibit an increase in their internal complexity (Fig. 4.7). Evidently the cell's metabolism is increased, since protein synthesis, ATP production, and catabolic activity may all be stimulated as may sometimes glycogen synthesis.

The most remarkable proliferation of mitochondria is seen in certain cells found in the salivary glands and elsewhere, which are called *oncocytes*. The cytoplasm contains little else except closely packed mitochondria, so that in paraffin sections there is an abundant eosinophilic cytoplasm. It has been suggested that the mitochondria are biochemically defective, since they do not appear to be needed for energy production.

Micropinocytotic activity may increase, and this results in the appearance of numerous vacuoles in the cytoplasm.

Evidence of decreased function. Cellular components may become less numerous and show evidence of *hypofunction*. In damaged liver cells the rough endoplasmic reticulum shows dilatation of its sacs and loss of attached ribosomes. Polysomes are reduced in number. These changes are particularly associated with hydropic degeneration, and indicate *impaired protein synthesis*. In some conditions there is disaggregation of the polysomes without degranulation of the rough endoplasmic reticulum. This also indicates decreased protein synthesis. This it is seen in normal cells during mitosis, in normoblasts as they near maturation, and in the fibroblasts of scorbutic animals.

Mitochondrial changes are frequent. These organelles may become swollen with fluid. The accumulation of fluid is nearly always in the matrix so that the cristae become shortened and reduced in number. Intramembranous fluid accumulation can also occur, in which event the cristae are swollen. Impaired function results in reduced oxidative phosphorylation, and ATP production is reduced. Since this substance forms the main immediately available source of energy for cellular metabolism, it is not surprising that many cell functions are impaired. Thus ATP is required for the operation of the mechanism, or pump, regulating the concentration of ions in the cell. The sodium pump is impeded, and sodium and water accumulate in the cell, which in this way becomes progressively enlarged and waterlogged. The electrolytes can pass freely across the cell membrane, but the proteins within the cell cannot escape. When the sodium pump breaks down, there is therefore a *tendency* for the cell to become hypertonic. This is counteracted by the entry of water into the cell which thereupon swells. The breakdown of proteins into smaller molecules may further increase this tendency to hypertonicity.

Mitochondrial swelling is commonly found in cells showing cloudy swelling. An increase in size of the intramitochondrial dense granules can precede necrosis, and is due to the deposition of divalent cations, particularly Ca^{2+} and Mg^{2+}. This change has been described in the kidney of hyperparathyroidism, as well as in cells damaged by ischaemia or poisons.

Giant mitochondria have been described in many types of damaged cells, the best known example being in the liver of alcoholics. Sometimes the giant mitochondria contain crystalline inclusions, and the phase of enlargement is merely a step towards degeneration and perhaps necrosis.

Evidence of altered function. Changes may occur which indicate that the cell has acquired a new function; thus the endothelial cells of the glomerular tuft can become actively phagocytic for fibrin, and cilia can develop in cells which are not normally ciliated, e.g. those of the olfactory mucosa.

Abnormal accumulation of substances in the cell. Lipid is an example, and is described later.

Degenerative changes. Localised areas of the cell may appear to become degenerate, and the term *focal cytoplasmic degeneration* has been applied. Sometimes cytoplasmic components, e.g. endoplasmic reticulum and mitochondria, are seen within vacuoles containing lysosomal enzymes. These are called *autophagocytic vacuoles*, *autophagosomes*, or *cytolysomes*, and an increase in their number is an indication of cell injury. Thus large numbers of autophagocytic vacuoles are seen in the cells of an organ undergoing atrophy. This may be due to progressive ischaemia or to a physiological cause, as in the breast following lactation or the secondary sex organs in old age.

Sometimes an area of cytoplasm degenerates and is actually cast off: damaged renal tubular cells can show loss of the brush border, which together with an area of the underlying cytoplasm is desquamated into the lumen. Such changes have been called necrosis of part of a cell.

Myelin figures.[6] It is not uncommon to find intracellular whorls of laminated lipid material resembling the myelin of nerves. These are called *myelin figures*, and may either be artefacts or else represent real structures. It is well known that if hydrated lipid is allowed to remain undisturbed *in vitro*, myelin figures can form. Likewise, the prolonged fixation of lipid-containing tissue with glutaraldehyde (which fixes lipid slowly) will lead to the formation of myelin figures both within cells and in the extracellular spaces. Sometimes, however, myelin figures are present in membrane-bound structures containing lysosomal enzymes. These are called *myeloid bodies*, or *myelinoid bodies*, and are present whenever the secondary lysosomes are overloaded with lipid (Fig. 2.20). Thus myelin figures are found in autophagosomes, particularly if their contents consist of much lipid-containing membranous material. Impairment of lysosomal enzyme activity, e.g. by a drug, can also lead to myelin-figure formation. Likewise genetic defects of lysosomal enzymes can impair lipid degradation, a good example being the abundant myelinoid bodies found in the affected cells in Tay-Sachs disease and Fabry's disease (Fig. 3.6).

It should be appreciated that these various changes indicating hyperfunction, hypofunction, altered function, and focal degeneration can all occur within a single cell either simultaneously or sequentially. A damaged cell is not an inactive cell, and its reaction to injury may end in recovery. Parts injured beyond recovery are lysed or extruded, and the remaining structures reform the lost components. The cell may return to normal but some alterations may persist. Thus the retention of an abnormal function is seen in metaplasia and perhaps also neoplasia. The reaction of damaged cells is a highly complex and varied affair, but so far as routine human pathology is concerned it is rarely possible to obtain tissue fresh enough to detect these intracellular events even if time and equipment were available.

Not all the changes described above occur under any single circumstance. Cells subjected to adverse conditions show a complex reaction: some changes may be regarded as degenerative, while others are adaptive. A liver cell showing cloudy swelling due to carbon tetrachloride poisoning would therefore not be expected to show the same changes as one infected with a virus, or a kidney cell damaged by hypoxia. The diversity of change is particularly well marked in cells showing hydropic change: the clarity and swelling of the β cells of the islets of Langerhans in diabetes mellitus is due to the accumulation of glycogen, while the apparent hydropic change in the kidney in hypokalaemia is due to an accumulation of fluid between the tubular cell and its basement membrane.

Nature of Fatty Change[7, 8]

Electron microscopy has revealed that many normal cells contain small droplets of lipid, but (with the obvious exception of adipose cells) these are not visible on light microscopy. The lipid is found within the endoplasmic reticulum; this is well shown in the intestinal epithelial cells during fat absorption. Excessive accumulations of fat are found in response to many adverse conditions, e.g. hypoxia and poisoning. This occurs readily in the liver, and the lipid accumulations appear in the rough endoplasmic reticulum and sacs of the

Golgi complex. Such membrane-bound lipid droplets are termed *liposomes*.[9] Later, if the adverse conditions persist, much larger, non-membrane-bound lipid droplets appear and gradually fuse together until one droplet comes to occupy much of the cytoplasm. Precisely how the liposomes evolve into these droplets is not known, but the process may be related to a defect in the synthesis of components needed to package lipid in the Golgi complex. The excess fat that appears in damaged cells is derived from the fat depots in adipose tissue.

Depot fat is composed mostly of neutral fat, and when it is mobilised it is transported in the blood as free fatty acid bound to albumin. This is removed by the tissues and utilised for metabolic purposes. If the cells are damaged by hypoxia, poisoned, etc., their metabolic activity is impaired and the fat normally brought to them is inadequately utilised; it accumulates as droplets which are at first small, but later fuse into larger globules. It might be wondered why under some circumstances damaged cells show changes described as cloudy swelling, vacuolation, etc., but at other times there is fatty change. It must be admitted that often there is no adequate explanation. Many factors affect the susceptibility of cells to exogenous poisons. Thus, certain strains of mice are excessively sensitive to chloroform and develop bilateral renal cortical necrosis. This is inherited as a sex-linked factor. Age is important; thus newborn animals are resistant to many liver-damaging compounds.

Fatty change is particularly liable to occur in the liver, and is a reflection of the key position this organ occupies in fat metabolism. In addition to being able to manufacture fatty acids themselves, the liver cells remove fatty acid from the blood stream and utilise it in the production of phospholipids. These are bound to protein, and passed back into the blood as lipoproteins by an active transport mechanism. If liver cells are damaged, protein synthesis is impaired; lipoprotein manufacture is impeded and the fat taken up by the liver is not exported. It accumulates and appears as droplets. This then is the explanation of fatty change in the liver under some circumstances.

Fatty change in the liver due to an inadequate diet. The liver is also unable to metabolise fat unless there is an adequate supply of raw materials for the manufacture of lipoprotein. Substances which are necessary for this conversion are called lipotropic factors, and in particular *choline* is important. Without it, fatty acid cannot be converted to phospholipid and therefore fatty acid in the form of neutral fat accumulates. In experimental choline deficiency in the rat fatty change readily occurs in the liver, and if this is prolonged the damage leads to a type of cirrhosis. Starvation in the human subject can also produce a fatty liver, a change most marked in the infantile protein deficiency state called kwashiorkor, but here there is no progress to cirrhosis. The fatty liver of chronic alcoholism may in part be due to malnutrition, but in addition there is the factor of a direct toxic action on the liver of large amounts of ethanol, and cirrhosis is an important complication. Paradoxically, overfed animals may also show fatty livers; this may be due to a relative deficiency of lipotropic substances.

The relationship between diet and liver disease is in fact complex. Total fasting does not lead to fat accumulation.

Ketones and fatty acids are utilised by the tissues as a source of energy, and gluconeogenesis almost ceases in the liver. Essential amino acids are therefore conserved. If small amounts of carbohydrate are given, this adaptation does not occur and the liver becomes fatty. An improper diet may be more damaging than one which simply lacks calories, a fact to be borne in mind when methods of reducing the weight of obese patients are devised. Thus the operation of small-bowel bypass effects a loss in weight, but sometimes leads to fatty liver, necrosis, and cirrhosis. It has therefore been abandoned.[10]

Although the concept of phanerosis (p. 50) has been largely discarded in relation to fatty change in the liver, it is probable that lipid droplets in other organs, e.g. in the renal tubules in glomerulonephritis, are sometimes formed by the breakdown of cytoplasmic components. Myelin figures are described on page 52.

HYALINE DEGENERATION

Hyaline is a descriptive term applied to any homogeneous eosinophilic material. Literally the term means 'glassy', and is commonly applied to changes in connective tissue (p. 67). Hyaline degeneration is also used to describe a change in cells when either the whole cell or part of it becomes eosinophilic and homogeneous. Many diverse conditions have been included. In the alcoholic patient the cells of the liver sometimes contain eosinophilic structures called *Mallory bodies*, or *alcoholic hyaline*; the material consists of a meshwork of fibrils in an area where the rough endoplasmic reticulum has broken up. The giant mitochondria which are also found in the liver cells of the alcoholic are separate structures.

The droplets which appear in the proximal convoluted tubular cells of the kidney in the nephrotic syndrome are due to the excessive reabsorption of protein which has leaked through an abnormal glomerulus (Fig. 4.8). The condition is

Figure 4.8
Hyaline droplet formation. This E.M. preparation shows part of the two adjacent proximal convoluted cells of a mouse kidney. The animal has been injected previously with egg-white. The foreign protein appears as droplets (H) which are distinct from the mitochondria (M). It is thought that the protein passes into the glomerular filtrate and then enters the tubular cells by a process of micropinocytosis. ×15 000. (*From Brewer, D. B. and Eguren, L. M. (1962), J. Path. Bact.*, **93**, 107–116)

analogous to the effects of an intravenous sucrose injection, when droplets appear in the tubular cells. Likewise, following the injection of mannitol and in diabetics with marked glycosuria these cells become greatly swollen and have a clear cytoplasm. In hyaline droplet 'degeneration' of the kidney, there may be associated degenerative changes with the formation of large cytolysomes. Nevertheless, most of the droplets seen on light microscopy consist of reabsorbed protein, and the condition is not really a degeneration.

ACCUMULATION OF ABNORMAL SUBSTANCES IN THE CELLS

The terms infiltration and degeneration have in the past been used indiscriminately in describing changes which may occur in cells. It is evident that cell function may be impaired by many agents, and the changes which ensue may be manifested either as altered function, altered appearance, or both. Sometimes the changes terminate in cell death, and at first sight it seems not unreasonable to use the term degeneration. However, the change is frequently associated with an abnormal accumulation within the cell, e.g. of water, fat, or glycogen. When this is marked the term infiltration is sometimes used. Unfortunately the same term is also used to describe a condition where an abnormal substance is deposited in a tissue which is itself normal, e.g. glycogen in the heart and kidneys in diabetes mellitus, urates in gout, and amyloid. Depositions of other substances, e.g. calcium salts, haemosiderin, bile pigments, etc., are not generally termed infiltrations in classical accounts. Attempts to apply both terms to connective tissue have further complicated the situation. It is evident that the terms infiltration and degeneration served a useful purpose in the days of descriptive pathology, but that their continued use represents an attempt to impose unity where none exists. The terms cloudy swelling, hydropic degeneration, etc., are now used much less frequently than in previous periods. This is partly because the changes are so easily confused with those of *post-mortem* autolysis, and partly because changes which appear similar on light microscopy can be due to many diverse mechanisms, as revealed by biochemical analysis and electron microscopy. It is a mistake to regard these conditions as entities in themselves. If such terms are used at all they are better referred to as granular change, fatty change, hydropic change, etc., since these are convenient and indicate a particular appearance when the light microscope is used. It must not be thought that the terms represent anything more than a morphological description, and in the future it is to be hoped that each lesion will be described more precisely relating cause, biochemical lesion, and morphological changes.

DAMAGE TO DNA[11]

Damage to DNA can occur in a variety of ways. An alteration in the sequence of nucleotides can occur as a result of a *mutation*. New nucleotides can be inserted as a result of *viral infection*. *Ultraviolet light* has the specific effect of causing damage to the bases without leading to a breakage of the polynucleotide chains. Dimers are formed between adjacent thymine molecules (50 per cent), between thymine and cytosine (40 per cent), or between adjacent cytosine molecules alone (10 per cent). This damage can be repaired by enzymatic action. First the chain is broken and the damaged segment is excised. A new section is then synthesised on the template provided by the undamaged chain. This is finally inserted into the chain by the action of a polynucleotide ligase. It follows that after the application of ultraviolet light to a tissue there is a burst of DNA synthesis which is not related to mitosis. This is termed *unscheduled DNA synthesis*. A defect in this repair mechanism occurs in xeroderma pigmentosum, and is related to the development of carcinoma (p. 373).

Ionising radiations also cause DNA damage. Both chains of the molecule can be broken and this may lead to chromosomal breaks. If only one strand of the double helix is broken, the lesion can be repaired by a process similar to that described for ultraviolet-light damage.

CHANGES FOLLOWING CELL DEATH[12]

These differ according to whether or not the dead tissue remains an integral part of a living organism.

POST-MORTEM CHANGE

In the initial stages no alteration in cellular structure is visible: in this connexion it is important to remember that no changes will be found in the myocardium of patients dying suddenly of acute coronary insufficiency.

Evidence of cell damage will be seen only when the cause of cell death has itself produced recognisable injury, e.g. disruption of cellular structures by ice-crystal formation after freezing.

In the dying cell respiration ceases, glycolysis proceeds for a while, and there results a drop in pH due to the production of lactic acid. The synthetic activities of the cell stop, but the lytic destructive enzymes continue their work. These enzymes are mostly active at a low pH and include a wide range of proteases, lipases, esterases, deoxyribonuclease, ribonuclease, etc. The cell thus undergoes a process of *self-digestion*, or *autolysis*. The enzymes may be derived from lysosomes, and it has been suggested that disruption of these bodies is an important factor in the causation of cell damage as well as in the autolysis which follows cell death. However, electron-microscopic studies of cells undergoing autolysis *in vitro* show that the changes (mitochondrial swelling, etc.) are diffuse, and not more advanced near the lysosomes.[13] Such evidence would suggest that lysosomal enzymes do not initiate the changes of necrosis.[13, 14]

Autolysis is rapid in certain tissues, and results in liquefaction, e.g. in the pancreas and gastric mucosa. In other tissues, e.g. fibrous tissue, autolysis is less rapid.

The microscopic changes that occur affect the whole cell. The cytoplasm becomes homogeneous and brightly eosinophilic; the early autolytic changes may resemble those seen in the degenerative lesions of living cells. Later on cellular and nuclear details become lost. It is important to note that these *post-mortem* changes can be distinguished from those occurring during life by the complete absence of any surrounding inflammatory response ('vital reaction'). This is particularly useful in the kidney, where it is often difficult to distinguish the changes of early necrosis from those of autolysis. The presence of oedema separating one tubule from another is good evidence that the degenerative changes existed before death.

Putrefaction in dead tissue occurs when there is invasion by protein-splitting, anaerobic, saprophytic organisms. This results in the formation of gas and a variety of foul-smelling substances which include ammonia, hydrogen sulphide, indol, skatol, and putrescent amines like putrescine and cadaverine. The tissue turns black or dark green as a result of the formation of iron sulphide from broken-down haemoglobin. The common putrefactive organisms are those clostridia normally present in the faeces, and therefore the process occurs earliest in the abdominal cavity.

CELL DEATH AND NECROSIS[12, 15]

The change in damaged cells which remain in continuity with the living varies according to the severity of the injury (Fig. 4.9). The cells may be killed suddenly by direct physical or chemical trauma, and initially these show no changes other than those directly attributable to the agent concerned, e.g. disruption in electrical injuries, effects of freezing, burning, etc. Within a few hours, however, autolysis occurs, and the cells show the morphological changes (see below) by which

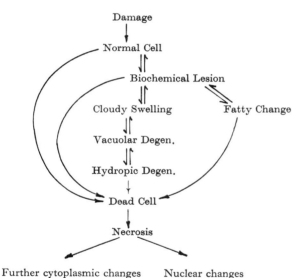

Figure 4.9
Diagram showing the stages whereby cell damage terminates in necrosis.

cell death can be recognised: this is called *necrosis*, which therefore means *circumscribed death of cells or tissues with structural evidence of this death.*

Cells less severely damaged, e.g. by poisons, may develop a biochemical lesion which may cause immediate death, or may first result in the degenerative and adaptive changes previously described. It will be recalled that these are mainly cytoplasmic, and in themselves do not indicate necrosis. Following cell death the nucleus also shows autolytic changes, and it is these which are to be regarded as pathognomonic of necrosis.

Nuclear Changes of Necrosis

The nucleus becomes smaller, while the chromatin loses its fine reticular pattern and becomes clumped. Margination of the chromatin adjacent to the nuclear envelope is an early change.

As DNA is broken down by endonucleases, short oligonucleotide fragments are formed and phosphoric-acid groups become available for binding to basic dyes such as haematoxylin. The nucleus therefore becomes acid and stains deeply. The process is termed *pyknosis*. The pyknotic nucleus either breaks up into fragments (*karyorrhexis*), or its outlines become indistinct as the nuclear material is broken down to mononucleotides, and the phosphoric-acid groups are split off; they easily leach from the cell. Hence the basophilia of the nucleic acids diminishes. This process is termed *karyolysis*.

Types of Necrosis

Coagulative necrosis. Necrotic material usually becomes firm and slightly swollen, a change well marked in 7 to 10 days old infarcts of the kidney and heart. It seems likely that the proteins are denatured. This process involves an unfolding of the three-dimensional arrangement of the molecule without necessarily changing its primary structure. This causes the tissue to become opaque, as does an egg on boiling, to fluoresce with ultraviolet light (autofluorescence), and to become more reactive. Side-chains previously saturated become exposed and available for binding. This explains why dead tissue tends to calcify. It also explains why necrotic tissue binds dyes, e.g. eosin, more avidly than does normal tissue. Increased eosinophilic staining of heart muscle fibres and neurons is a useful indication of early necrosis before an inflammatory reaction develops.

Apart from the nuclear changes, another microscopic feature is noteworthy: the preservation of the general architecture of the tissue despite the death of its constituent cells. This is *structured necrosis*. In other examples of coagulative necrosis there is no residual structure—this is *structureless necrosis*, e.g. the caseous necrosis of tuberculosis.

Caseation is a particular type of coagulative necrosis in which the dead tissue has a firm, dry, cheesy consistency and contains much lipid material. Although this type of change may occur in other conditions, the term caseation is usually restricted to the necrosis of tuberculosis.

Colliquative necrosis. Necrosis with softening (colliquative necrosis) rarely occurs as a primary event except in the central nervous system. Here necrosis (usually due to infarction) always results in softening.

Liquefaction may occur in an area of coagulative necrosis as a result of secondary changes; this is seen in:
1. Suppuration, e.g. septic infarction.
2. Liquefaction of caseous material.

Necrosis in Special Sites

Necrosis of muscle. Striated muscle occasionally undergoes necrosis during acute fevers, e.g. typhoid and smallpox. The muscle fibres lose their striations, the nuclei disappear, and the whole appears as a brightly eosinophilic, hyaline mass. The muscle, usually the rectus abdominis or the diaphragm, may rupture, and this leads to haemorrhage and pain. The condition is traditionally called 'Zenker's degeneration', but is in fact a true necrosis. A similar change has been described in cardiac muscle in severe acute infections.

Fat necrosis. Necrosis may occur in the adipose tissue of the peritoneum following the liberation of lipases from an injured or inflamed pancreas. The neutral fat is split: glycerol is removed, while the fatty acid remains and gives the damaged cells a cloudy appearance. Macroscopic areas of necrosis appear as opaque, white plaques. The lesions excite an inflammatory response, and may be removed within a week or two. Sometimes calcification ensues, and when extensive may lead to hypocalcaemia.

Traumatic fat necrosis is generally seen in the breast: the changes are similar to pancreatic fat necrosis, but the foreign-body giant-cell reaction is particularly marked (Fig. 4.10). Clinically it may resemble a scirrhous carcinoma.

glutamate-oxaloacetate transaminase and other enzymes are released from infarcted heart muscle (p. 513). Similarly, the serum level of glutamate-pyruvate transaminase is useful in detecting liver necrosis.

Creatine phosphokinase is present in high concentration in skeletal muscle, and an increased blood level occurs after muscle damage, e.g. in polymyositis, alcoholic myopathy, malignant hyperpyrexia (p. 470), after strenuous exercise, and even following intramuscular injections. The highest levels are found in the muscular dystrophies. In the Duchenne variety (p. 35) such elevation is a constant feature, and its detection may be used to diagnose the disease even before clinical manifestations appear. An elevated level is found at birth in subjects who will in due course develop the disease.[16] The level is also elevated in heterozygous carriers.

Figure 4.10
Traumatic fat necrosis of breast. The adipose tissue cells have an opaque, granular cytoplasm due to the breakdown of neutral fat and the production of fatty acid. Two large foreign-body giant cells with a foamy, fat-filled cytoplasm are present. × 180.

Figure 4.11
The lactate dehydrogenase activity of serum is shown as five component isoenzymes separated by electrophoresis. LDH 1 is the fastest component and has travelled farthest in the direction of the arrow towards the anode. In the lower part of the diagram each molecule is depicted as a tetramer made up of varying combinations of either H polypeptides (closed circles) or M polypeptides (open circles). The H and M chains are determined by separate genes. In the case of some other enzymes, the isoenzymes occur as a result of small variations in the structure of one or more polypeptides. (*After Latner, A. L.* (1970). Journal of Clinical Pathology, **24,** suppl. (Ass. Clin. Path.), **4, 8**)

'Necrosis' of collagen. Whether it is permissible to describe the degenerative changes seen in collagen as necrosis is debatable. Certainly the associated fibrocytes undergo destruction. It is, however, difficult to define necrosis in an extracellular substance like collagen. This subject, necrobiosis, and 'fibrinoid necrosis' are discussed in the next chapter.

Using column chromatography and starch-gel electrophoresis, it is possible to separate many enzymes into components called *isoenzymes* (Fig. 4.11). The pattern of concentration of the various isoenzymes differs according to the tissue of origin of the enzyme. This refinement in the study of serum enzymes has been most rewarding in the diagnosis of myocardial infarction.

DIAGNOSIS OF NECROSIS BY BIOCHEMICAL MEANS

Many soluble substances diffuse out of the cells following their death. These include potassium, protein breakdown products, and enzymes. The last are absorbed into the bloodstream, and their presence can be utilised in diagnosis. Thus

FURTHER CHANGES IN NECROTIC TISSUE

Acute inflammation. Necrotic tissue generally excites an acute inflammatory reaction in the surrounding tissue. (Fig. 4.12). This is well marked in infarction, and the infiltrating polymorphs by contributing their proteolytic enzymes to the dead tissue aid the process of autolysis. Similarly a necrotic **tumour**

Figure 4.12
Sequelae of cell death.

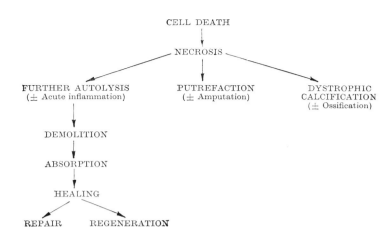

It is presumed that dead tissue releases chemicals which stimulate the inflammatory reaction, but no such substances have ever been satisfactorily identified. It a piece of liver is implanted free into the peritoneal cavity, it excites an acute inflammatory reaction and acquires the yellow-white appearance of coagulative necrosis. If it is then removed and reimplanted into another animal, very little reaction takes place. Boiled liver is similarly ignored. Presumably autolysing tissue exudes some chemical stimulus for the inflammatory reaction, but its nature remains obscure. Activation of complement is probably important.

Repair and regeneration. Following autolysis and the inflammatory reaction, there ensues invasion by macrophages and the components of granulation tissue. In this way the dead tissue is absorbed and replaced by scar tissue which may later undergo dystrophic calcification. In some instances, e.g. necrosis of skin, regeneration of specialised tissue (in this case squamous epithelium) adds its contribution to the healing process.

Calcification. Some types of necrotic tissue appear to show limited autolysis; this is particularly true of caseation. Under these circumstances healing by repair is hindered, and the necrotic tissue often undergoes dystrophic calcification (see p. 463). Sometimes bone is formed.

Gangrene. This is an old descriptive clinical term applied to any black, foul-smelling area which is in continuity with living tissue. In more precise terms it is *necrosis of tissue with superadded putrefaction*. The putrefactive organisms are usually the clostridia derived from the intestine or the soil (see Ch. 18). Necrosis of the gut is invariably followed by gangrene if the patient survives long enough. The necrosis may be ischaemic (mesenteric arterial or venous thrombosis, volvulus, etc.) or infective (acute appendicitis). Wounds infected with pathogenic saccharolytic clostridia are also contaminated by putrefactive clostridia—the result is gas-gangrene.

The putrefactive organisms that convert simple necrosis (with or without infection) to gangrene are not always clostridia. A variety of gangrenous lesions involving the skin and juxtacutaneous mucous membranes have been described: (a) noma,[17] a gangrenous lesion of the vulva or mouth (when it is alternatively called *cancrum oris*) occurring usually in malnou-

rished children after an infectious disease such as measles. It is a slowly but relentlessly spreading condition, and causes great tissue destruction. Death from inhalation pneumonia may occur. It is almost unknown in Britain, but is not uncommon in developing communities; (b) *postoperative synergistic gangrene*, which implicates the anterior abdominal wall and thighs (see p. 219); (c) *Fournier's gangrene*,[18] a fulminating lesion of the scrotum, which is usually completely destroyed, so that the testes are left exposed; (d) *puerperal gangrene*.

The organisms concerned include anaerobic streptococci, and members of the family *Bacteroidaceae*. This refers to the *Bacteroides-Fusiformis* group, currently embraced by the label *Bacteroides*. A well-known member is *Fusiformis fusiformis* (also called *Fusobacterium fusiforme*), which is often found in the company of *Borrelia vincenti*. These bacteria are anaerobic and are cultured with considerable difficulty (p. 221). They are Gram-negative bacilli, and are found as commensals in the mouth and intestine. Lesions caused by them have been called 'fusospirochaetal gangrene', but it is doubtful whether *Borr. vincenti* plays any part in the disease process.[17] These gangrenous conditions are usually due to the combined effect of the above-mentioned organisms acting in debilitated tissues in association with *Streptococcus pyogenes*, staphylococci, and coliform bacilli.

Gangrene of the lung. A putrid lung abscess is an occasional complication of dental extraction under general anaesthesia, when the root of a tooth is inhaled and lodges in a bronchus. One again organisms belonging to the family *Bacteroidaceae* are responsible for the putrefaction.

Gangrene in the limbs. All the examples of gangrene so far mentioned are 'wet'. There is progressive tissue destruction, and unless effective treatment is instituted without delay, death results. A similar type of wet gangrene occurs in the limbs. It is usually due to vascular occlusion, and is not infrequently a complication of diabetes mellitus. Generally the legs are affected rather than the arms.

There is also described another type of gangrene, 'dry gangrene'. This is usually secondary to slow occlusive vascular disease. Commencing at the tips of the phalanges the tissues become desiccated and blackened.* There is no smell and no

---

*This blackening is probably due to the slow drying and oxidation of haemoglobin and myoglobin in the tissues.

gas formation. The process is self-limiting, and the junction of dead with living tissue is sharp. Eventually the dead tissue is cast off by the process of spontaneous amputation. This lesion is in fact an infarct of a limb with minimal or no putrefactive changes. Tradition, however, dictates that it still be called gangrene. It is really an example of necrosis followed by mummification. All true gangrene is 'wet'.

Finally, it should be noted that gangrene is not massive necrosis, as is sometimes stated. Necrosis of the whole liver is not gangrene, nor is a gangrenous appendix large. It is the putrefaction of necrotic tissue, however caused, which con-stitutes the condition. It is this putrefaction which produces the smell and the blackening with iron sulphide which tog-ether are the pathognomonic features of gangrene.

It is evident from this account of cell structure and cell damage that many gaps exist in our knowledge. The advances in electron microscopy and cytochemistry are revealing wonderful details of cellular form and function. When these techniques are more widely applied to pathological material, it is to be expected that the changes occurring in damaged cells will be better understood.

GENERAL READING

GHADIALLY, F. N. (1975) *Ultrastructural Pathology of the Cell*, 543 pp. London: Butterworth. A text and atlas of physiological and pathological alterations in cell fine structure.

REFERENCES

1. PETERS, R. A. (1963) *Biochemical Lesions and Lethal Synthesis*. Oxford: Pergamon Press.
2. FARBER, E. (1972) *The Pathology of Transcription and Translation*. p. 140 *et. seq*. New York: Marcel Dekker.
3. Leading Article (1973) Streptozotocin for islet-cell carcinoma. *Lancet*, **2**, 1063.
4. TRUMP, B. F., GOLDBLATT, P. J. & STOWELL, R. E. (1965) Studies on necrosis of mouse liver *in vitro*; ultrastructural alterations in the mitochondria of hepatic parenchymal cells. *Laboratory Investigation*, **14**, 343.
5. MAGEE, P. N. (1966) Toxic liver necrosis. *Laboratory Investigation*, **15**, 111.
6. HRUBAN, Z., SLESERS, A. & HOPKINS, E. (1972) Drug-induced and naturally occurring myeloid bodies. *Laboratory Investigation*, **27**, 62.
7. LOMBARDI, B. & RECKNAGEL, R. O. (1962) Interference with secretion of triglycerides by the liver as a common factor in toxic liver injury. *American Journal of Pathology*, **40**, 571.
8. FARBER, E., LOMBARDI, B. & CASTILLO, A. E. (1963) The prevention by adenosine triphosphate of the fatty liver induced by ethionine. *Laboratory Investigation*, **12**, 873.
9. STENGER, R. J. (1970) Organelle pathology of the liver. The endoplasmic reticulum. *Gastroenterology*, **58**, 554.
10. SNODGRASS, P. J. (1970) Obesity, small-bowel bypass and liver disease. *New England Journal of Medicine*, **282**, 870.
11. BASERGA, R. (1972) In *The Pathology of Transcription and Translation*, ed. Farber, E. p. 2 (Pathology of DNA). New York: Marcel Dekker.
12. KING, D. W. *et al.* (1959) Cell death. *American Journal of Pathology*, **35**, 369, 575, 835 and 1067.
13. TRUMP, B. F., GOLDBLATT, P. J. & STOWELL, R. E. (1962) An electron microscopic study of early cytoplasmic alterations in hepatic parenchymal cells of mouse liver during necrosis *in vitro* (autolysis). *Laboratory Investigation*, **11**, 986.
14. VAN LANCKER, J. L. & HOLTZER, R. L. (1963) The fate of nuclei, deoxyribonucleic acid and deoxyribonucleases in the course of autolysis. *Laboratory Investigation*, **12**, 102.
15. DIXON, K. C. (1967) Events in dying cells. *Proceedings of the Royal Society of Medicine*, **60**, 271.
16. Leading Article (1975) Screening of the newborn for Duchenne muscular dystrophy. *British Medical Journal*, **2**, 403.
17. LINENBERG, W. B., SCHMITT, J. & HARPOLE, H. J. (1961) Noma, report of a case. *Oral Surgery, Oral Medicine and Oral Pathology*, **14**, 1138.
18. KILBY, J. O. (1962) Gangrene of scrotum and penis. *British Journal of Surgery*, **49**, 619.

Chapter 5. *Connective Tissue: Its Normal Structure and the Effects of Disease*

The non-epithelial component of the body may be regarded as a gel of ground substance in which are embedded cells and fibres. It is one of the hallmarks of connective tissue that its component cells are widely separated from each other. They are responsible for the formation and metabolism of the ground substance and the fibres, and it is these extracellular components which are largely responsible for giving each type of connective tissue its own special properties.

THE CELLS OF CONNECTIVE TISSUE

Fibroblasts. The major cellular component of the unspecialised connective tissue is the fibroblast, a cell of mesenchymal origin. The suffix 'blast' is often used to denote the young plump cell of developing connective tissue as well as the thin spindle-shaped *fibrocyte* of mature collagenous tissue. Young fibroblasts are elongated or stellate in shape, and numerous processes project from the surface. There is an abundant cytoplasm which contains much rough endoplasmic reticulum as well as a prominent Golgi complex. The structure of the fibroblast is clearly that of a cell making protein for export.

In the mature fibrocyte the rough endoplasmic reticulum is less abundant. On light microscopy the cells appear to be inactive, with a small, densely staining nucleus and sparse cytoplasm compressed between surrounding collagen bundles.

Pericytes. Around blood vessels, but not lymphatics, there are cells which somewhat resemble fibroblasts except that they are surrounded by a basement membrane, as are smooth muscle cells. The pericyte is regarded by some as a primitive cell capable of differentiating along several lines—for instance into smooth muscle, cartilage, and bone.

Histiocytes. These cells are part of the reticulo-endothelial system, and are capable of exhibiting marked phagocytic activity—in which event they are called *macrophages*. Histiocytes have a vesicular nucleus and an abundant cytoplasm. This contains many ribosomes which are free rather than attached to endoplasmic reticulum. The cell outline is irregular due to the many short processes and invaginations which the plasma membrane exhibits. Lysosomes are abundant, and their internal structure is often complex because they contain fragments of cytoplasm, organelles, phagocytosed material, etc.

Eosinophil granulocytes. These cells are characterised by possessing cytoplasmic, membrane-bound granules which contain a central structure of crystalline appearance.

Mast cells. These cells have characteristic granules which contain heparin and histamine. Their actual structure varies from one species to another. The granules are not well preserved in some species unless alcohol is used as a fixative.

In human tissue formalin is adequate, but the granules must be stained specially, e.g. with toluidine blue or Giemsa's stain, otherwise the cells may be mistaken for fibroblasts or histiocytes.

Mast cells form an important reservoir for histamine, and release this in response to certain chemical stimuli, e.g. compound 48/80, bee venom, basic peptides from polymorphs, C3a and C5a anaphylatoxins, and antigen when the cells have been sensitised by specific IgE antibody.

Plasma cells. A well-developed granular endoplasmic reticulum and Golgi complex are characteristic (p. 152). Plasma cells are particularly abundant in the lamina propria of the gastrointestinal tract, but a few are present in all loose connective tissue. A few *lymphocytes* are commonly present also.

THE GROUND SUBSTANCE

This material varies in consistency from an amorphous gel which contributes to the solid, translucent appearance of hyaline cartilage, to the glairy fluid found in the synovial joint cavities. Its name is derived from the German *grundsubstanz*, which was regarded as the material from which the formed elements of the connective tissue were derived, as indicated in the French equivalent *substance fondamentale*.

It is in the molecular meshes of the ground substance that the *extracellular interstitial fluid* is contained. This constitutes about a third of the total body water, and lies between the blood vessels and the cells. It contains various electrolytes in a concentration similar to that of the plasma (see Chapter 38) and also small uncharged solute material, such as oxygen, CO_2, glucose, and urea, which is conveyed either for cellular metabolism or for excretion.

Ground substance itself contains *glycoproteins* as well as the soluble precursors of collagen fibrils and *mucoproteins*. Many of the characteristic properties of ground substance are attributed to these mucoproteins.

Glycoproteins[1] are proteins which contain carbohydrate groups attached covalently to the polypeptide chain. Many different monosaccharides have been found in the glycoproteins. Often the terminal unit is a negatively-charged residue of *N-acetylneuraminic acid*, a sialic acid. Glycoproteins with a high content of carbohydrate are also called *proteoglycans*. Many substances normally thought of as being proteins fall into the group of glycoproteins: these include blood-group substances, fibrinogen, immunoglobulins, enzymes (such as serum cholinesterase), and hormones (such as thyroid stimulating hormone). The glycoproteins are therefore widely distributed in tissues, and since they stain red with the PAS method, their presence renders this method a useful stain for certain structures, e.g. basement membrane and fibrin.

The mucoproteins[1] are complexes of protein with acid mucopolysaccharides (also called *glucosaminoglycans*). The latter have attracted much attention: they consist of polymers of hexose sugars, some of which possess amino groups, e.g. hexosamines like D-glucosamine and D-galactosamine. The amino groups are presumably responsible in part for the mucoid properties of the polymers. Meyer[2] has subdivided the acid mucopolysaccharides as listed below. The alternative names in brackets are those proposed by Jeanloz.[3]

Non-sulphated group

Hyaluronic acid
Chondroitin

In these the acid component is the carboxyl group of a uronic acid, e.g. glucuronic acid in hyaluronic acid (which also contains *N*-acetylglucosamine, see below).

Sulphated group
Chondroitin sulphate A (chondroitin 4-sulphate)
Chondroitin sulphate B (dermatan sulphate)
Chondroitin sulphate C (chrondroitin 6-sulphate)
Heparitin sulphate (heparan sulphate)
Keratosulphate (keratan sulphate)

The physical (e.g. optical) and presumably chemical properties of each connective tissue depend to a large extent upon the nature of the ground substance as well as upon the physical arrangement and chemical composition of the fibres themselves. For example, keratan sulphate forms 50 per cent of the total acid mucopolysaccharide in the cornea, but is present only in small quantities in osteoid.

Formation of Acid Mucopolysaccharides

Metabolism of Mucoproteins

The mucoproteins are synthesised in fibroblasts and similar cells, such as osteoblasts. The protein moiety is manufactured in the rough endoplasmic reticulum, and to this acceptor protein, a polysaccharide chain of mucopolysaccharide develops by the sequential addition of individual sugars. Each sugar is donated by a uridine sugar nucleotide. Thus uridine diphosphate glucuronic acid (UDP-GlcUA) and UDP-*N*-acetylglucosamine are involved in the synthesis of hyaluronic acid. Sulphation is a separate step with the sulphate grouping being donated by 3'-phosphoadenosine 5'-phosphosulphate (PAPS).[4] The PAPS is derived from ATP and inorganic sulphate, as can be shown by using ^{35}S as a label in tracer experiments. The polymerisation of the mucopolysaccharides and their sulphation are thought to occur in the Golgi complex; granules containing mucoprotein are formed and finally discharged from the cell by the process of exocytosis.

The mucopolysaccharides show a regular metabolic turnover; thus in young animals the half-life of dermatan sulphate is 7 to 10 days. Precisely how catabolism is brought about is not known. Polysaccharidases, such as hyaluronidase*,

*The organ that contains the highest concentration of hyaluronidase is the testis. Here the enzyme's presence is related to the function of the spermatozoa rather than to connective-tissue metabolism. Nevertheless, hyaluronidase from bull's testis is a convenient source of the enzyme for use in connective-tissue studies.

have been isolated from many tissues, and may be involved in the breakdown of the mucopolysaccharides. Alternatively it may be the protein component that is broken down. That this can happen is dramatically demonstrated by injecting the proteolytic enzyme papain intravenously into a rabbit. The mucoprotein of cartilage is broken down, and the animal's ears lose their rigidity and become floppy. The released mucopolysaccharide is excreted in the urine. Toxic doses of vitamin A have a similar effect, presumably by causing damage to lysosomes and leading to the release of their proteolytic enzymes.

Abnormalities in mucoprotein metabolism. An excess or deficiency of mucoprotein in a tissue can be caused by an imbalance between synthesis and catabolism. In most pathological states the precise mechanism is not known, and they are therefore described later under the heading of changes in the ground substance.

Staining of Ground Substance

Its acidic nature renders it basophilic, i.e. blue in routine haematoxylin and eosin sections, as is seen in hyaline cartilage. The PAS method stains ground substance where it has a high glycoprotein content (p. 3). The acid mucopolysaccharides themselves are PAS negative.

Staining properties of acid mucopolysaccharides. A variety of staining techniques are in use but none can be regarded as very reliable for the identification of a particular mucopolysaccharide. Proper fixation of the tissue is important and aqueous formalin is unreliable. Basic lead acetate solution, formalin-alcohol mixtures, and cetyl pyridium chloride-formalin are commonly used.

Thiazine dyes—Azur A and *Toluidine blue*. These dyes stain the mucopolysaccharides varying shades from purple to blue. They are therefore metachromatic stains (p. 3), but the precise results depend upon the pH employed. At one time it was thought that metachromasia was exhibited only by the sulphated compounds, but this is now known to be wrong. However, if the staining is performed at pH 2 or less only the sulphated mucopolysaccharides stain metachromatically.

Alcian blue. This is not a metachromatic stain. The substances are stained blue according to the pH used. A commonly employed method stains epithelial mucin as well as that of connective tissue.

Colloidal iron (Hale, Rinehart and Abul-Haj, and others). This method depends upon the affinity of mucopolysaccharides for ferric ions in colloidal form. The addition of potassium ferrocyanide leads to the formation of Prussian blue.

Enzymatic digestion. The alteration or elimination of staining after exposure of a section to a particular enzyme may be of assistance in identifying the substance responsible for the staining. Thus testicular hyaluronidase removes hyaluronic acid, chondroitin 4-sulphate, and chondroitin 6-sulphate, whereas hyaluronidase of streptococcal origin removes only hyaluronic acid.

Changes in the Ground Substance in Disease

Remarkably little is known of the alterations that occur in ground substance under pathological conditions.

Reaction to injury. The mucopolysaccharides of ground

substance appear to undergo depolymerisation, and consequently the ground substance itself becomes more watery. Although in theory this might favour the spread of organisms, it might equally well enhance the penetrating power of the inflammatory exudate. The general loosening of the connective tissue in inflammation is well illustrated in the detachment of periosteum that occurs adjacent to a fracture (see p. 118).

The spreading factors, e.g. hyaluronidase of *Strept. pyogenes* and *Cl. welchii*, can be shown to depolymerise hyaluronic acid-containing ground substance, e.g. vitreous humour, *in vitro*. This also occurs *in vivo*, since it can be shown that dyes injected into the skin diffuse more readily when mixed with hyaluronidase. The enzyme is therefore used therapeutically for aiding the penetration of injections into the subcutaneous tissues, e.g. for parenteral fluid administration in babies. Whether hyaluronidase plays any part in the spread of infections is debatable (see p. 101).

Excessive accumulation of ground substance. The abnormal persistence of mucopolysaccharide in granulation tissue in scurvy, protein deficiency, and following glucocorticoid administration is described in Chapter 9.

The amount of ground substance in connective tissue and its state of hydration are partly under hormonal control. In *myxoedema* the increased accumulation of hyaluronic-acid containing ground substance is responsible for the puffiness of the skin which gives the patient the characteristic appearance. It is probable that the excessive secretion of pituitary thyrotrophic hormone is responsible. In the localised pretibial myxoedema of *hyperthyroidism*, LATS is incriminated (p. 455). Oestrogens and androgens also induce changes in connective tissue which are most marked in animals, e.g. the cock's comb and the sex skin of monkeys. Relaxin, secreted by the ovary, induces changes in the symphysis pubis in pregnancy.[5]

Under other less well-defined circumstances ground substance may accumulate in mature tissues, and appear as a basophilic material. The terms 'mucoid' or myxomatous 'degeneration' are generally applied to this condition, although its degenerative nature is neither always apparent nor provable. It is better to use the term *myxomatous change* to avoid this difficulty (see also p. 54).

Myxomatous change is seen in some tumours of connective tissue, such as the neurofibroma, chondroma, lipoma, and liposarcoma; myxomatous material forms the bulk of the rather uncommon myxoma. In the giant intracanalicular fibroadenoma of the breast, also called Brodie's tumour, which is a mixed tumour with a predominant connective-tissue element, the abundant myxomatous connective tissue is easily mistaken for a sarcoma.

The connective-tissue stroma of epithelial tumours may also show myxomatous change. This term should not be used for the mucoid appearance of tumour stroma when epithelial secretion has leaked into it. This is properly called 'mucoid change', and is seen in mucoid adenocarcinomata and in the pleomorphic salivary tumour.

Myxomatous change is also seen in the aorta in Erdheim's cystic medionecrosis, where it may form part of *Marfan's syndrome* (p. 66).

Myxomatous change of the heart valves.[6][7] Myxomatous change of the valves may affect the cusps, annulus, or the chordae, and this by weakening the valves leads to incompetence. The valve leaflets are thin and diaphanous and may occasionally have a blue colour in this 'floppy-valve syndrome'. It is the mitral valve which is most commonly affected, but aortic and rarely tricuspid involvement have also been reported. Intractable and progressive heart failure is the clinical manifestation of this condition, which is analogous to aortic cystic medionecrosis; moreover some cases have been associated with stigmata of Marfan's syndrome.

Genetic defects of mucopolysaccharide metabolism. There are at least six syndromes recognised in this group of diseases which may be called the *mucopolysaccharidoses*. The most common, and one of the most severe, is the *Hurler syndrome*, in which mucopolysaccharide is present in excess in connective-tissue cells as well as in certain epithelial cells, e.g. the liver. The disease becomes obvious in infancy or early childhood, and results in gross skeletal deformities with dwarfism, hepatomegaly, mental defect, and corneal opacity. Involvement of the connective tissue of the heart valves leads to aortic and mitral lesions. Coronary-artery involvement leads to myocardial ischaemia. The grotesque appearance of the head is responsible for the alternative name by which the syndrome is commonly known—*gargoylism*.

The characteristics of the other syndromes are summarised in Table 5.1. All are inherited as autosomal recessive traits except the Hunter syndrome, which is an X-linked recessive. In all of them the affected cells are distended with mucopolys-

TABLE 5.1   The mucopolysaccharidoses

Syndrome	Clinical features	Compound in urine
I Hurler	Early onset, early death, mental deficiency, dwarfism, severe skeletal defects, corneal clouding	Dermatan sulphate Heparan sulphate
II Hunter	As Hurler but less severe, skin lesions, no corneal clouding	Dermatan sulphate Heparan sulphate
III Sanfilippo	Minor skeletal changes, severe mental retardation evident by school age	Heparan sulphate
IV Morquio	Dwarfism with characteristic skeletal changes, corneal clouding, aortic regurgitation	Keratan sulphate
V Scheie	Skeletal changes mild, stiff joints, claw hands, corneal clouding is marked, aortic regurgitation, intellect little affected	Dermatan sulphate
VI Maroteaux-Lamy	Dwarfism with severe skeletal changes, hepatomegaly, corneal clouding, intellect normal	Dermatan sulphate

accharide, and present evidence suggests that in these conditions there is defective catabolism of acid mucopolysaccharide—perhaps due to a lack of a lysosomal enzyme. In each of them one or more acid mucopolysaccharides are excreted in the urine (Table 5.1); normally none is excreted. Two other laboratory tests are of value in diagnosis: (*a*) an examination of lymphocytes, neutrophils, or monocytes from the blood or marrow often reveals characteristic metachromatic granules, and (*b*) skin fibroblasts grown in culture show similar metachromatic granules; the only exception appears to be those cases of the Morquio syndrome in which the defects are restricted to the skeletal system. It is of interest that these abnormal fibroblasts can be cultured from people who are presumed to be carriers as well as from those who are clinically affected.

Diminution in amount of ground substance. With increasing age there is a diminution in the amount of ground substance in the connective tissues. There is increased sulphation of the mucoproteins and a change in the relative proportions of the various mucopolysaccharides. Thus in the nucleus pulposus the amount of keratan sulphate increases, whereas in the skin and heart there is an increase in dermatan sulphate relative to the amount of other mucopolysaccharides present.

COLLAGEN[8–10]

Collagen constitutes about one third of the body's protein: it forms a scaffold in all tissues and is the chief component of fascia, dermis, cornea, and tendon, giving these structures tensile strength. Collagen comprises almost 90 per cent of the organic matrix of bone, and its particular composition is adapted for the deposition of the bone salts.

The collagen of connective tissue is synthesised by fibroblasts or similar cells such as are found in tendon, cornea, bone, and cartilage. An exception to this is the collagen component of basement membrane which is formed by the adjacent epithelial or endothelial cells.

Light microscopic appearance of collagen. By light microscopy collagen is seen to consist of fibres, the arrangement of which varies in different tissues. In tendon the fibres are arranged in parallel bundles, whereas in skin the bundles run in different directions but are mostly parallel to the surface. The fibres have several characteristic *staining properties*:

(*a*) They stain pink with eosin.

(*b*) Picric-acid solutions combine with many dyes to form a complex that has a particular affinity for collagen. In *Van Gieson's stain* a mixture of picric acid and acid fuchsin is used, and the fibres are stained red with picrofuchsin.

(*c*) Aniline blue combined with phosphotungstic or phosphomolybdic acid stains collagen blue. This forms the basis of *Mallory's staining technique*. *Masson's trichrome stain* is similar, and collagen is stained blue if aniline blue is used or green with light green.

(*d*) The fibres are not blackened by silver impregnation methods, but are stained a brown colour.

Electron microscopic appearance of collagen. The electron microscope reveals that collagen *fibres* are made up of *fibrils*, which show a cross-banding with a periodicity of about 64 nm (Figs. 5.1a and 5.1b). It is thought that these fibrils are made up of tropocollagen molecules each of which is about 280 nm long and 1·4 nm wide. It was at first thought that the molecules were joined together end-to-end with a quarter length overlap with their lateral neighbours. It is now known that there is a gap of about 41 nm between the head of one molecule and the tail of the next as shown in Fig. 5.2. In osteoid tissue, these gaps serve as a nidus for the deposition of bone salts. The thickness of the collagen fibrils varies from tissue to tissue and with age. In cartilage they measure 15 to 25 nm while in tendon they reach 130 nm in thickness. It is evident that different lateral arrangements of the tropocollagen could form fibrils with different periodicity, and such have in fact been found to exist, for instance in the trabecular meshwork of the eye.

Solubility of collagen. Adult fully matured collagen is very insoluble, and only denaturation by strong acids or heat can render it soluble. The final product is then gelatin. In young collagen a fraction can be extracted by cold neutral buffers. This probably contains tropocollagen, and on warming the solution typical banded fibrils are reformed. An additional fraction can be extracted by dilute acid solutions and this component persists as maturation proceeds. Ultimately the collagen becomes insoluble due to the increasing number of cross-linkages which are formed (p. 64).

Chemical composition of collagen. Collagen has a characteristic X-ray diffraction pattern, and from this its structure has been surmised. The basic unit of collagen is called *tropocollagen*, a molecule 280 nm long and 1·4 nm wide, with a molecular weight of about 340 000 daltons. Tropocollagen consists of three polypeptide chains. Each of the polypeptide chains is coiled, and the three molecules are wound around a common axis like a three-stranded rope. It is thus a 'coiled coil'.

Five types of chain are known, and are designated: $\alpha1(I)$, $\alpha1(II)$, $\alpha1(III)$, $\alpha1(IV)$, and $\alpha2$. Various combinations of these polypeptide chains are known to combine to form four types of collagen:

Type I: $[\alpha1(I)]_2\alpha2$. This type of collagen is widely distributed, and is the major component of dermis, tendon, bone, and dentine. It consists of two $\alpha1(I)$ chains and one $\alpha2$ chain. Its molecular form is therefore recorded as $[\alpha1(I)]_2\alpha2$.

Type II: $[\alpha1(II)]_3$. This type of collagen consists of three $\alpha1(II)$ chains and is chiefly found in cartilage.

Type III: $[\alpha1(III)]_3$. This type of collagen comprises approximately 50 per cent of the collagen of the cardiovascular system, i.e. the heart valves and the major arteries.

Type IV: $[\alpha1(IV)]_3$. Collagen composed of three $\alpha1(IV)$ chains is found only in basement membranes.

Each polypeptide chain consists of about 1000 amino acid residues, and has a molecular weight of about 95 000. It is coiled to form a type of helix in which, unlike the usual protein α-helix, there are no hydrogen bonds between adjacent amino acids on the same chain. Each helix is stabilised by hydrogen bonds with adjacent polypeptide chains. Throughout most of the chain every third amino acid is glycine, and a common sequence is glycine-proline-hydroxyproline. Collagen indeed is characterised by its high content of glycine (33 per cent) and proline and hydroxyproline (which together constitute about 22 per cent). Hydroxyproline is an amino acid which is not found to any extent in other proteins, and an

Figure 5.1a
Section of collagen fibrils in a peripheral nerve. The fibrils show the characteristic cross-banding (arrow), which is best seen where the fibrils are cut longitudinally. Part of the cytoplasm of a Schwann cell (Sch) is also shown (×12 000). (*Photograph by courtesy of Dr. N. B. Rewcastle.*)

Figure 5.1b
Teased preparation of collagen from the *tendo achilles*. The specimen has been shadowed to accentuate the characteristic 64 nm banding. This process involves the throwing of a vaporised heavy metal such as palladium or gold on to the specimen at a small angle. Now that ultra-thin sections can be cut, this technique is not often used. ×34 000. (*Photograph by courtesy of Dr. C. I. Levene*)

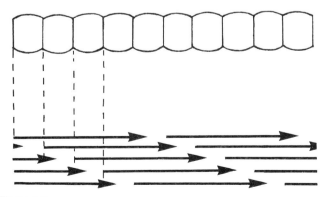

Figure 5.2
Diagram to illustrate how the lateral arrangement of tropocollagen molecules, depicted as arrows, results in the formation of a banded collagen fibril.

estimation of the amount of it in hydrolysates of tissue may therefore be used to measure the amount of collagen present. It is also noteworthy that collagen contains hydroxylysine, and it is to this amino acid that carbohydrate is attached (either galactose or glucosylgalactose).

Biosynthesis. The primary polypeptide chains are formed in the rough endoplasmic reticulum under the influence of specific mRNA. Different mRNAs exist for each type of chain; the mechanism whereby a particular gene is activated in a particular cell at a particular time is unknown. The three polypeptide chains are probably formed simultaneously, and immediately unite to form a triple helix. The molecule first formed is called *protocollagen*, and it differs from tropocollagen in that it contains no hydroxyproline, hydroxylysine, or glycosylated hydroxylysine. The next step in the formation of collagen is the hydroxylation of prolyl and lysyl residues. This step probably stabilises the molecule (Fig. 5.3).

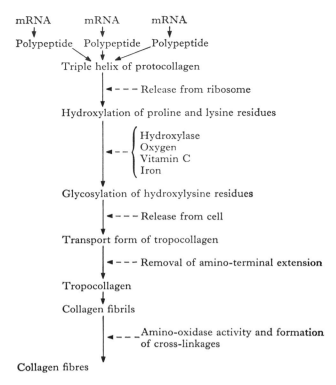

Figure 5.3
Diagram to illustrate the biosynthesis of collagen.

Requirements for hydroxylation. The two specific enzymes peptidyl proline hydroxylase (protocollagen-proline hydroxylase) and peptidyl lysine hydroxylase require the following co-factors:

(1) α-*ketoglutarate*. (2) *Ascorbic acid*. Although this can be replaced by other reducing agents *in vitro*, ascorbic acid is believed to be required *in vivo*; it may be essential for the conversion of inactive prescursors of the peptidyl hydroxylases to active enzymes. (3) *Ferrous iron*. Fibroblasts in culture fail to synthesise collagen in the presence of a metal chelating agent, such as α,α^1-dipyridyl. The cells form protocollagen, and this is released as such from the ribosomes. (5) *Oxygen*. Likewise fibroblasts in anaerobic culture synthesise protocollagen but not collagen. The oxygen of the hydroxyl group is obtained from free oxygen and not from water.

Thus the hydroxyproline and hydroxylysine in collagen are formed in the polypeptide chains by hydroxylation of the parent amino acid, and this explains the observation that, in tissue-culture experiments, radioactive-tagged proline and not hydroxyproline is the precursor of hydroxyproline in the collagen molecule. Hydroxyproline and hydroxylysine are therefore not directly encoded by specific mRNA, and this raises another problem. What factors determine which proline or lysine is hydroxylated? The particular sequence of the amino-acid residues and the position of the proline and lysine residues in relation to the length of the chain are some factors that determine where hydroxylation will take place—and where there will subsequently be glycosylation. It is not surprising that the degree of hydroxylation and glycosylation varies somewhat from one collagen to another.

Glycosylation of hydroxylysine. Glycosylation occurs at some of the hydroxylysine residues, and to some of these sites glucose in further added to the galactose. Type IV collagen in basement membrane contains the most carbohydrate, and this contributes to the positive PAS staining of this structure. It has been postulated that in diabetes mellitus excessive glycosylation could lead to the deposition of an abnormal type of collagen in the basement membrane.

Formation of tropocollagen. The manner by which the three polypeptide chains are formed simultaneously and united is not known. There is some evidence that the first-formed polypeptide chains have an extension at the NH_2-terminal end and that this contains cystine. Hence disulphide bonds could be formed and initiate the formation of the triple helix. This sulphur-containing component probably persists until the tropocollagen molecules finally polymerise into mature collagen. These findings help to explain why sulphur-containing amino acids are necessary for normal wound healing (see p. 113).

Extrusion of collagen from the cell. Tropocollagen is released from the ribosomes into the cisternae of the endoplasmic reticulum. It may then pass into the vacuoles of the Golgi complex and finally be extruded from the cell in a manner seen in typical exocrine secretion, e.g. the pancreas. This is not proven, however, and the tropocollagen may pass more directly from the ribosomes to the exterior. Whatever the route, there is some mechanism which controls the type of material which is extruded. Failure in hydroxylation or glycosylation does not immediately inhibit protein synthesis, but the defective product is not extruded and therefore extracellular collagen deposition ceases. This occurs in scurvy.

Extracellular incorporation of tropocollagen into collagen fibrils. Newly synthesised collagen consists of a molecule larger than tropocollagen because of the presence of cystine-containing extensions at the NH_2-terminal ends of the polypeptide chains. This is called *procollagen*, or *transport form*. When the extensions are removed by the action of a neutral protease, *procollagen peptidase*,* aggregation occurs. Fibres are formed by the lateral alignment of the molecules with a quarter overlap, as shown in Figure 5.2. This quarter stagger arrangement presents problems if one tries to construct a three-dimensional model with match-sticks. Perhaps four or five polymer chains are arranged so that in cross-section they form a square or pentagon. In this way there is limitation of the points of contact between the chains. Whatever the precise arrangement, the carbohydrate content of the collagen and the mucopolysaccharide composition of the ground substance seem to play a part in the determination of the size of the fibre produced.

Cross-linkage of fibrils to form fibres. The fibrils which are formed when tropocollagen aggregates have little strength. It is by the formation of firm cross-linkages that the tensile strength develops. The first step in the cross-linkage is the production of aldehyde groups on several lysyl or hydroxylysyl residues in the tropocollagen molecules:

$$R—CH_2—NH_3^+ \rightarrow R—CHO + NH_4^+.$$

*In the congenital disease dermatosparaxis of cattle this enzyme is absent or diminished in activity. The skin is abnormally fragile. No human counterpart has yet been described.

The amine oxidase catalyses this reaction, and aldehyde groups of adjacent molecules form cross-links. The process is slow, and it can be readily understood that the tensile strength of collagen in a wound steadily increases over a period of several months (p. 110).

The enzyme amine oxidase is inhibited by the nitriles that produce lathyrism. The enzyme contains copper; this explains why chronic copper deficiency in animals produces a condition which is indistinguishable from lathyrism. Penicillamine and homocysteine react with aldehyde groups so that they are unavailable for cross-linking (see p. 66). Other types of cross-linkage are known to exist at other sites of the chain, e.g. involving histidine residues.

The first formed collagen fibrils are coated with much ground substance, and it is in this that silver is deposited with suitable silver staining. Bundles of these fibrils form the *reticulin fibres* familiar to the light microscopist. As maturation proceeds the fibres increase in size and there is a diminution in the amount of surrounding ground substance. With light microscopy they are then recognised as *collagen fibres*. With silver stains the metal is deposited mainly in the region of the bands of the constituent fibrils, and the fibres therefore appear brown rather than black.

The maturation of the fibrils is usually accompanied by an increase in size due presumably to the addition of new tropocollagen units. It is only in some sites that full maturation is reached—for example, in tendon, fascia, and sclera. In organs like lymph nodes, lung, and spleen the development tends to halt at the reticulin stage.

Catabolism of Collagen

Although collagen appears to be metabolically very stable, there are indications that under some circumstances it can be formed very rapidly and equally rapidly degraded and removed. The denaturation of collagen involves the action of proteolytic enzymes, either specific collagenases or non-specific proteases. Both play a part under some circumstances.

Non-specific proteases. Proteolytic enzymes are present in the lysosomes of neutrophils and macrophages. In inflammatory lesions these enzymes may play a part in collagen degradation, but they probably play no role in the normal metabolism of collagen. There is little doubt that collagen can be phagocytosed by macrophages, but it seems that the collagen must first be damaged. Examples of this are encountered in actinically damaged skin and in the lesions of necrobiosis (p. 68).

Collagenases. The existence of normal collagenase activity was first demonstrated in 1962 by the tissue-explant technique.[11] Collagenase was found to be formed by the epidermis of the resorbing tail of the tadpole. Collagenase formed by connective-tissue cells has been shown to be important in the removal of collagen during the *post-partum* involution of the rat's uterus and in the early stages of the regeneration of the amputated newt's arm (p. 103). Another remarkable example is encountered in the carrageenin granuloma. An injection of carrageenin, a polysaccharide derived from sea-weed, produces a vigorous growth of granulation tissue with collagen formation—followed by an equally rapid catabolism of collagen so that no scarring results. Collagenases have now been described in many tissues. Thus in a healing skin wound a collagenase is produced both by epithelium and by connective tissue. Unlike the situation in the carrageenin granuloma, however, the collagenase activity is insufficient to prevent scar formation.

It seems likely that collagenases are widely distributed in the tissues and that their function is to degrade collagen. This action is balanced by collagen synthesis, so that under normal conditions the proper amount of collagen is present. Thus during development when tissues are undergoing growth or involution (physiological atrophy—see p. 300), the ratio of collagen to parenchyma remains fairly constant. When tissues are undergoing remodelling, it is probable that the tropocollagen released during collagen breakdown is used again in the formation of new fibres. When adult stature has been attained, the metabolic turnover of collagen is slow; isotope studies indicate that much of the collagen of the body is very stable. Nevertheless, there is a steady turnover, and the excretion of hydroxyproline in the urine gives some indication of its extent. Thus the excretion is increased in hyperparathyroidism, Paget's disease of bone, secondary carcinoma, and other destructive bone diseases.

Collagenase inhibitors are known to exist in the plasma α-globulins, but their role in collagen homeostasis is not known.

Reticulin

Fibres called 'reticulin' by histologists are thin (about 1 μm) and branching. They form a network in many organs, e.g. liver, lung, spleen, and lymph node, and stain an intense black with silver, but faintly with picrofuchsin (in Van Gieson's stain) and eosin. As described above, reticulin is composed of bundles of collagen fibrils which have a characteristic property of external silvering. In granulation tissue the first formed fibres are reticulin.

Whether the reticulin fibres found in the early stages of collagen formation are the same as those found in the organs mentioned above seems unlikely. A non-collagenous reticulin can be extracted from the saline insoluble residue of pig or human renal cortex or liver. The extract contains no hydroxyproline, but is 4 per cent carbohydrate and is antigenic in rabbits. The resulting antiserum gives a fluorescent staining pattern indistinguishable from that obtained with human antireticulin antibody.[12] Furthermore, this non-collagenous reticulin is capable of absorbing the characteristic staining pattern imparted by human antireticulin antibody. It has also been found that human antireticulin antibody does not stain the argyrophilic ('reticulin') fibres of the newly-formed collagen seen in healing wounds. This is probably due to the absence of a specific glycoprotein of reticulin from the young collagen fibres in this situation. The reticulin framework of the organs mentioned above thus differs chemically and antigenically as well as histologically from collagen, but as yet the chemical nature of the antigenic determinants specific for reticulin has not been elucidated.[12]

It must be understood that the name 'collagen' is used in three different connexions.

To the chemist it is a protein which may exist in solution or in insoluble form.

To the histologist using the light microscope 'collagen' exists as broad fibres with special staining properties.

To the electron microscopist it is a fibril of characteristic banded appearance; this corresponds both to the reticulin and 'collagen' of the histologist.

Microfibrils

Other fine, branching fibres called microfibrils have been described by electron microscopists. They do not show the banded appearance of collagen, but nevertheless are thought by some investigators to be the precursors of collagen fibrils. Microfibrils tend to be concentrated around elastic fibres and are present also within them. Microfibrils are closely associated with the basement membrane.

Basement Membrane[13]

Under light microscopy the basement membrane is seen as an eosinophilic, PAS-positive, hyaline, acellular sheath which is closely applied to epithelium and blood-vessel endothelium. Electron microscopy has revealed that it has two components: one is a thin band 50 to 200 nm in width which has a central dense zone, the *lamina densa*, covered on each side by a *lamina rara*. This structure is now regarded as the *basement membrane proper*, and it can be seen adjacent to epithelial cells, the endothelium of blood vessels, around pericytes, and surrounding smooth muscle cells. It is probably manufactured by these cells, and it is therefore not surprising that antigenic components of one basement membrane are different from those of another elsewhere in the body.[14]

The basement membrane proper contains glycoproteins and type IV collagen. The latter exhibits no fibrillar or banded structure, and differs in other ways from ordinary connective-tissue collagen: it contains more carbohydrate, hydroxyproline, and hydroxylysine, and also 4 to 10 cysteine molecules per 1000 amino-acid residues, so that disulphide bonds can form both between collagen molecules and with glycoproteins.

The second component of the light microscopist's 'basement membrane' is an external condensation of microfibrils, reticulin, and ground substance. It is of connective-tissue origin. See Figure 2.1, page 13.

Thickening of the basement membrane is a common pathological finding, and has been much studied in diseased glomeruli. It may be due to an increase in the amount of basement membrane material or to the addition of plasma protein components or antigen-antibody precipitates.

ABNORMALITIES OF COLLAGEN

The amount of collagen in a tissue is determined by a balance between collagen catabolism (presumably effected by collagenases) and the rate of collagen formation. Excessive catabolism, diminished synthesis, or a combination of the two lead to atrophy. The converse situation leads to fibrosis. It is unfortunate that in many human pathological conditions we are ignorant of the precise mechanisms involved and can only describe the end-results—either *atrophy* or *fibrosis*.

Collagen Atrophy

There are many conditions in which collagen degradation exceeds collagen synthesis. *Glucocorticoids* inhibit collagen synthesis, and if administered in large doses over a prolonged period lead to generalised collagen atrophy. Thus the skin becomes paper-thin, and bleeding follows mild injury.

Osteoporosis (p. 301) poses a major threat. Local injections of glucocorticoids into the skin lead to dermal atrophy: this action is utilised in the treatment of keloids (p. 113), but the results are indifferent.[15]

Excessive production of collagenase is thought to be important in the pathogenesis of several diseases. In *rheumatoid arthritis* the destruction of the joint cartilage has been ascribed to the presence of collagenase produced by the synovium. The destruction of alveolar bone that leads to loss of teeth in *chronic periodontal disease* has likewise been attributed to collagenase activity.

In old age there is a generalised atrophy of collagen and an increased cross-linkage between adjacent fibrils. Hence the amount of extractable soluble collagen decreases with age.

Fibrosis

An increase in the amount of collagen, or *fibrosis*, is a common finding in chronic inflammation (see p. 128), and is also a feature of the curious diseases called the fibromatoses (see p. 318). One of these is apparently caused by the administration of methysergide for migraine. It leads to retroperitoneal fibrosis and sometimes mitral regurgitation.[16]

In those organs where collagen fibril development is incomplete, the fibrils may mature to form histological collagen. This may explain fibrosis in organs like the spleen and lung.

There are a number of conditions in which the collagen fibres appear normal on microscopy, but are nevertheless abnormal functionally since the affected tissues are weak and can be stretched with undue ease. The defect appears to lie in the intermolecular bonds which are responsible for giving collagen its strength. This group includes three diseases which are inherited (Marfan's syndrome, homocystinuria, and the Ehlers-Danlos syndrome), and an experimentally induced condition (osteolathyrism). The precise biochemical defect is not known in any of these conditions, but they all exhibit the formation of abnormal collagen—and often elastic tissue also. Indeed, they are examples of true collagen diseases.

Marfan's syndrome. Affected individuals have long, thin limbs, spider fingers (arachnodactyly), redundant ligaments and joint capsules (resulting in double-jointedness and dislocations), hernias, and subluxation of the lens of the eye. In addition, there is weakness of the aorta which leads to aneurysmal dilatation, aortic regurgitation, and the development of dissecting aneurysm. In the aorta there is degeneration of the elastic fibres and a picture resembling Erdheim's cystic medionecrosis. However, the other lesions indicate that there is a major defect in the collagen. The disease is inherited as a Mendelian dominant trait with high penetrance.

Homocystinuria. This resembles Marfan's syndrome, but, unlike it, is inherited as a recessive trait, and there is homocystine in the urine. The skeletal changes are similar, and ectopia lentis occurs. However, the vascular lesions are characterised by thrombosis rather than dilatation; dissecting aneurysm does not occur, but there is increased platelet adhesiveness. Mental retardation is frequent.

Homocysteine probably acts by reacting with aldehydes generated by the amine oxidase reaction so that they are unavailable for cross-linkage. The drug *penicillamine* has a similar effect, and experimentally the abnormal, weak collagen contains an excess of aldehyde groups, but the formation of cross-linkages in both collagen and elastin is inhibited. Penicillamine has been used in the treatment of scleroderma, but unfortunately it is useful only in the active phase of the disease when collagen biosynthesis is taking place.[17]

Ehlers-Danlos syndrome. In this remarkable condition there is loose-jointedness and great hyperextensibility of the skin (see also p. 638).

Experimental osteolathyrism.* Young rats or chicks fed on sweet-pea (*Lathyrus odoratus*) meal develop bony deformities, weakness of tendons and ligaments, and rupture of the aorta. Although the collagen appears normal on electron microscopy, much more of the newly-formed collagen is soluble in cold saline. The collagen is deficient in aldehyde groups, and there is therefore defective cross-linkage of its fibres. The urinary output of peptides containing hydroxyproline is increased, due presumably to the fact that uncross-linked tropocollagen is more rapidly degraded than is mature collagen. The synthesis of desmosine and isodesmosine is inhibited, and since these two amino acids are important in the cross-linkages in elastic fibres, there is also a defect in the elastic tissue. The responsible agent in sweet-pea meal is β-aminoproprionitrile, and other nitriles as well as ureides and hydrazides have been found to have a similar lathryogenic activity. They inhibit the amine oxidase responsible for the formation of aldehydes and therefore cross-linkages. Chronic copper deficiency produces a disease resembling lathyrism, because copper is an essential component of the amine oxidase: in both conditions there is a tendency towards dissecting aneurysm and rupture of the aorta. The lesions of lathyrism bear some resemblance to those of Marfan's syndrome and medionecrosis of the human aorta, and this is the major reason for the current interest in the subject.

Hyalinisation

A change which occurs in abnormal deposits of collagen with the passage of time is *hyalinisation*. The individual histological collagen fibres appear to fuse together to form a glassy eosinophilic material. The intervening fibrocytes disappear, and the tissue is converted into an acellular, structureless, inert mass. Such an appearance may also be encountered in muscle fibres, and it must be understood that the term is merely descriptive of a particular microscopic appearance. Hyaline literally means glassy.

Probably several processes are included, but in the hyalinisation of collagen the material appears very uniform. It is seen in a wide array of conditions; in old scar tissue, keloids, and 'fibroid' tumours of the uterus (leiomyomata).

The glomeruli of chronic nephritis are converted into hyalinised, eosinophilic balls. These usually have two components: the remains of the glomerulus is represented by a mass of basement-membrane-like substance (which is PAS-positive), and the second component is hyalinised collagen produced by the parietal cells of Bowman's capsule. In H. and E. sections the two components cannot be distinguished (Fig. 5.4).

*Human lathyrism has been described following the ingestion of the chick pea *Lathyrus sativus*, and is characterised by spastic paralysis. The toxin responsible is not known. This neurolathyrism bears no obvious relationship to the osteolathyrism of animals described above.

Figure 5.4
Hyalinised glomerular tufts. Most of the glomeruli in this section have been converted into dense, solid balls of hyaline material, almost completely devoid of cellular structure. The patient suffered from chronic pyelonephritis with secondary hypertension. × 65.

Deposits of hyaline material may also replace epithelial cells. A good example is the hyalinisation of the islets of Langerhans that is sometimes seen in diabetes mellitus (Fig. 5.5). Apparently the substance is laid down around the sinusoids, and eventually replaces the glandular structure. This type of hyaline is probably amyloid. Indeed, amyloid may be considered as a type of hyaline material, but because of its special properties it is considered separately (Chapter 48).

Vascular hyaline. The appearance of homogeneous hyaline material in the subendothelial layer of arterioles is a common event, and in the spleen of adults may be regarded as normal. In the afferent arterioles of the renal glomeruli it is associated with benign systemic hypertension and diabetes mellitus (Fig. 5.6). The nature of this hyaline has been much debated. In the kidney it consists of granular material on electron microscopy; by some it is thought to be material, perhaps fibrin, derived from the blood. It has been claimed that fibrin, as it ages, becomes transformed into an acellular substance which has the staining properties of collagen. Other possibilities are that vascular hyaline is derived from smooth muscle or collagen, or that it consists of basement-membrane-like substance.

Necrosis of Collagen

When connective tissue is damaged, its associated fibrocytes

Figure 5.5
Hyalinisation of the islets of Langerhans. This is the pancreas of a diabetic subject. The central area is an islet largely replaced by hyaline material; the remains of epithelial cells are visible in the periphery. × 200.

Figure 5.6
Hyalinisation of renal arterioles. Two arterioles show great thickening of their wall by homogeneous hyaline material. This patient had diabetic nephropathy. × 200.

undergo necrosis and its fibres appear to degenerate. They break up, and are removed in the course of an inflammatory reaction. This necrosis of collagen differs from hyalinisation in several important respects.

(*a*) Hyaline material appears to be extremely stable; for example, the corpora albicantes seen in an old ovary have presumably been present for many years. Necrotic collagen, on the other hand, is either removed or else organised.

(*b*) Hyaline collagen retains the staining characteristics of normal collagen. Necrotic collagen, on the other hand, becomes Van Gieson negative and PAS positive. It tends to stain brightly with eosin—in fact, it takes on some of the tinctorial properties of fibrin. The term *fibrinoid necrosis* is therefore sometimes applied.

The nature of the change is a matter of much confusion due mainly to the fact that 'fibrinoid necrosis' is a morphological descriptive term of a variety of changes that occur in various tissues under very dissimilar circumstances; e.g. in the 'collagen diseases', and in tissue damaged by infective agents and ionising radiation. In blood vessels it occurs in malignant hypertension, the Shwartzman phenomenon, the Arthus phenomenon, and in polyarteritis.

In rheumatic fever and rheumatoid arthritis the fibrinoid material has been observed to be continuous with normal collagen, both on light and electron microscopy.[18] Similar degeneration of collagen with loss of cross-striations occurs in the Arthus phenomemon, but in addition antigen-antibody complexes are present. If antigen is injected into the cornea of a sensitised rabbit, a visible antigen-antibody precipitate forms as a ring around the site of injection. This area shows fibrinoid necrosis on light microscopy. On electron microscopy the precipitate is seen to be coating the collagen fibrils and filling in the ground-substance matrix. In the Shwartzman phenomenon histochemical studies indicate that the fibrinoid material contains fibrin, while in the collagen diseases there is, in addition, immunoglobulin. Another possibility is that fibrinoid is derived from the smooth-muscle coat of blood vessels. It must be concluded that although the term fibrinoid necrosis is useful in a descriptive sense, it implies no single morphological change or aetiological agent. There may be degeneration of collagen, necrosis of muscle, deposition of fibrin, precipitation of antigen-antibody complexes, or any combination of these changes.

Fibrinoid necrosis is encountered in the 'collagen diseases', but is certainly not pathognomonic of them. It is seen when connective tissue is damaged in other ways, for example, it is a prominent feature of X-ray damage to the skin. It is also found in the small arterioles in malignant hypertension, where the damage to the wall is probably caused by a sudden rise of blood pressure (Figs. 5.7 and 5.8). The necrotic walls frequently rupture, thereby giving rise to the haemorrhages in the retina and skin and the haematuria seen in malignant hypertension.

The term *necrobiosis* is commonly used to describe the fibrinoid necrosis of collagen that occurs in the lesions of certain diseases, for instance in the subcutaneous nodules of rheumatoid arthritis (Fig. 16.7). Similar lesions are seen in the skin in granuloma annulare and necrobiosis lipoidica. It is unfortunate that necrobiosis is used in this context, because the term has also been used to describe the physiological death of cells (see p. 300).

Figure 5.7
Fibrinoid necrosis of renal arteriole. This section comes from the kidney of a patient with malignant hypertension. The arteriolar wall has undergone partial disintegration and shows a blurred, deeply-staining structure. There is a surrounding acute inflammatory reaction. × 200.

Figure 5.8
Fibrinoid necrosis of glomerulus. This section comes from the same kidney as Figure 5.7. There are focal areas of necrosis of the tuft. These are blurred and darkly staining. × 200.

ELASTIC FIBRES

The elastic tissue of the aorta and its large branches, the ligamentum nuchae, lung, etc., appears very different from collagen on light microscopy. Elastic tissue appears as homogeneous, refractile fibres, or in vessels it can form an extensive, perforated, tensile sheet like a trampoline net. It stains *deep red with eosin, dark brown with orcein,* and *black with the resorcinol fuchsin stain of Weigert.* Under the electron microscope elastic tissue consists of two components. There is a central amorphous component that consists of a protein called *elastin,* and this is surrounded by microfilaments, about 10 to 12 nm in diameter, that consist of a glycoprotein. The microfibrils are obvious during the formation of elastic, but with ageing are more difficult to detect. Elastic tissue is extremely insoluble, very resistant to digestion by acids and alkalis, but readily attacked by the enzyme elastase produced by some organisms.

The formation and composition of elastin has been less extensively studied than has the biosynthesis of collagen. Elastin is probably formed from a soluble precursor called tropoelastin. Two amino acids, desmosine and isodesmosine, are thought to be important in the formation of the cross-linkages that give elastic tissue the resilience which is its characteristic property. With age there is an increase in the content of desmosine and isodesmosine, and this is accompanied by a loss of resilience. Calcification of elastic fibres is another feature of the ageing process; it also occurs in metastatic calcification (see p. 465). Agents which interfere with the formation of collagen, such as the lathyrogenic agents, also interfere with elastin formation. Hence weakness of arteries, often with the complication of dissecting aneurysm, commonly occurs.

Elastic fibres are formed by the activity of smooth muscle cells in some situations, e.g. in the aortic wall and in atheromatous plaques. In other tissues, cells which resemble fibroblasts appear to be involved. No specific 'elastoblasts' have been identified. There is little doubt that new elastic fibres can be formed in adult life. Thus degeneration of elastic tissue is sometimes accompanied by new elastic fibre formation, so as to give an appearance of fraying or reduplication.

Elastosis

Although it is sometimes stated that elastic tissue is not reformed in scar tissue in the dermis, this is probably not true. After a long time fibres do appear, and these have the staining properties of elastic. Moreover, there are certain conditions of the skin in which an excess of elastic is formed (actinic elastosis and pseudoxanthoma elasticum). It is thus evident that elastic fibres can be formed, but the situation is complicated by one uncertainty. Electronmicroscopic examination of some 'elastic fibres' has shown that they consist of typical banded collagen fibrils! It is thus sometimes difficult to distinguish between true elastic fibres and the fibres of altered collagen.

It is apparent from the above account that connective tissue is by no means the inert substance that it is often considered to be. Our knowledge of its basic structure in health and disease is still very inadequate. Changes in it are assuming an ever-increasing importance in the modern concepts of many disease processes ranging from inflammation to neoplasia. There are also a considerable number of obscure chronic inflammatory conditions which are included under the general heading of 'collagen disease'. These are considered in Chapter 16.

GENERAL READING

PEREZ-TAMAYO, R. & ROJKIND, M. (Eds) (1973) *Molecular Pathology of Connective Tissues*, 406 pp. New York: Marcel Dekkar.
McKUSICK, V. A. (1972) *Heritable Disorders of Connective Tissue*, 4th edn, 878 pp. St. Louis: Mosby.
MILLER, E. J. & MATUKAS, V. J. (1974) Biosynthesis of collagen. *Federation Proceedings*, **33**, 1197.
WEINSTOCK, M. & LEBLOND, C. P. (1974) Formation of collagen. *Federation Proceedings*, **33**, 1205.

REFERENCES

1. LEHNINGER, A. L. (1975) *Biochemistry*, 2nd edn, p. 271. New York: Worth Publishers Inc.
2. MEYER, K. (1959) In *Wound Healing and Tissue Repair*, ed. Patterson, W. B., p. 25 Chicago: University of Chicago Press.
3. JEANLOZ, R. W. (1960) The nature of mucopolysaccharides. *Arthritis and Rheumatism*, **3**, 233.
4. WINDRUM, G. M. (1958) Sulfation technics in the histologic study of granulation tissue. *Laboratory Investigation*, **7**, 9.
5. STEINETZ, B. G., BEACH, V. L. & KROC, R. L. (1959) In *Recent Progress in the Endocrinology of Reproduction*, ed. Lloyd, C. W., p. 389. New York: Academic Press.
6. Leading Article (1971) Blue-valve syndrome. *British Medical Journal*, **2**, 294.
7. TRENT, J. K. *et al.* (1970) Morphology of a prolapsed posterior mitral valve leaflet. *American Heart Journal*, **79**, 539.
8. GRANT, M. E. & PROCKOP, D. J. (1972) The biosynthesis of collagen. *New England Journal of Medicine*, **286**, 194, 242, and 291.
9. RAMACHANDRAN, G. N. (Ed.) (1967) *Treatise on Collagen*, Vol. 1, p. 556. London: Academic Press.
10. GOULD, B. S. (Ed.) (1968) *Treatise on Collagen*, Vol. 2, Part A, p. 434 and Part B, p. 488. London: Academic Press.
11. GROSS, J. & LAPIÈRE, C. M. (1962) Collagenolytic activity in amphibian tissue: a tissue culture assay. *Proceedings of the National Academy of Sciences of the United States of America*, **48**, 1014.
12. HOLBOROW, E. J. *et al.* (1977) Antibodies against reticulin and collagen. *Annals of the Rheumatic Diseases*, **36**, Supplement No.2, p. 51.
13. Various Authors (1970) In *Chemistry and Molecular Biology of the Intercellular Matrix*, ed. Balazs, E. A. Vol. 1, Chapter III, p. 471. London: Academic Press.
14. PIERCE, G. B., MIDGLEY, A. R. & RAM, J. S. (1963): The histogenesis of basement membranes. *Journal of Experimental Medicine*, **117**, 339.
15. CALNAN, J. (1977) Keloid and Dupuytren's contracture. *Annals of the Rheumatic Diseases*, **36**, Supplement No. 2, 18.
16. MUNROE, D. S., ALLEN, P. & COX, A. R. (1969) Mitral regurgitation occurring during methysergide (Sansert) therapy. *Canadian Medical Association Journal*, **101**, 536.
17. JACKSON, D. S. (1977) Nitriles, penicillamine, and substituted prolines. *Annals of the Rheumatic Diseases*, **36**, Supplement No. 2, 63.
18. LANNIGAN, R. & ZAKI, S. (1965) Electron microscope appearances of a fibrin-staining component in an Aschoff nodule from acute rheumatic fever. *Nature (London)*, **206**, 106.

Chapter 6. The Inflammatory Reaction

INTRODUCTION

One of the characteristics of living tissue is its ability to react to injury. Indeed, the survival of the individual depends upon the ability of his normal cells to respond to damage. The response in the higher animals is complex, involving not only the local cells adjacent to the area of injury, but also the body as a whole. Reaction to injury may therefore be considered under two headings.

Firstly, there is a general body response involving nervous and hormonal adjustments, and resulting in considerable metabolic alterations. At the same time the lymphoreticular system responds by proliferating to provide more phagocytes and antibody-forming cells.

Secondly, there is a local response. Initially the adjacent living tissues undergo changes which enable phagocytic cells and circulating plasma to enter the area of damage. This phase is known as acute inflammation, and continues so long as tissue damage continues. When the causative agent is withdrawn or removed, the debris of the inflammatory reaction is removed by scavenger cells. The tissue may then return to normal, but when tissue loss has been sustained, there is a final stage of healing by repair, regeneration, or both. The outline of this local reaction to injury is shown in Figure 6.1. In this chapter we shall deal with the early phase, the acute inflammatory reaction.

ACUTE INFLAMMATION

The cardinal signs of acute inflammation—*calor*, *rubor*, *dolor*, and *tumor*—have been known since the original description by Celsus in the first century A.D.: to these has been added a fifth—loss of function.* John Hunter was one of the

*The origin of this fifth sign is obscure, and to attribute it to Galen is to perpetuate a misconception which has been handed down without ·verification by many authors, including ourselves in previous editions.[1] To describe it as *functio laesa* is to give it an air of respectability which it ill deserves!

first to recognise that acute inflammation was not a disease in its own right, but rather a defence mechanism against a variety of injuries.

Definition. Although the features of acute inflammation have been known for a long time, there is no entirely satisfactory definition of the phenomenon. It is commonly defined as 'the local response of living tissue to injury', but this wrongly implies that all the succeeding events, like repair and regeneration, are included. Indeed, it also includes the cellular responses to injury, such as those described in Chapter 4, as well as neoplasia. Such a wide definition is therefore misleading and quite unhelpful.

Some definitions add the rider that the changes are beneficial and protect the tissues from further injury. This is unwarranted since not all the phenomena of acute inflammation, for instance those following the development of hypersensitivity, are necessarily of benefit. In fact, in some infections, e.g. tuberculosis, the cells of the exudate actually spread the organism through the tissues. Acute inflammation must be regarded as a mechanism which has been evolved to protect the individual from a wide range of hazards. On the whole it is a beneficial reaction, but one should not be surprised if under certain circumstances the reaction itself becomes a hazard. The formation of inflammatory oedema is probably of great importance in the limitation of bacterial infection. In the larynx, however, it may cause rapid death. Opie used the following definition: 'Inflammation is the process by means of which cells and serum accumulate about an injurious substance and tend to remove or destroy it.' While it is true that in animals which have a circulatory system the predominant features are vascular with the formation of an exudate, part fluid and part cellular, there is no doubt that a primitive type of inflammatory reaction can occur in avascular tissues. In fact, Metchnikoff did much of his work on the starfish, which has no circulatory system.

Nevertheless, it can be argued that this type of response in a lowly creature is not true inflammation comparable with that occurring in the vascular tissues of higher animals. The

Figure 6.1
Diagram to show the sequence of events which may follow local cell damage.

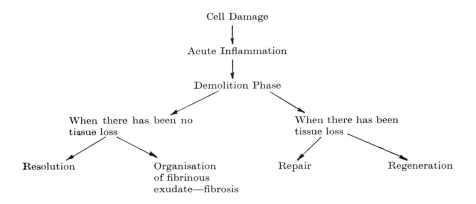

presence of a vascular system is really a prerequisite for an acceptable inflammatory response. A useful definition is the following:

Inflammation is the reaction of the vascular and supporting elements of a tissue to injury, and results in the formation of a protein-rich exudate, provided the injury has not been so severe as to destroy the area.

In avascular tissue, like the normal cornea,* no true inflammation can occur, although injury may result in changes which include the appearance of phagocytes. This response is comparable with that seen in the lower animals. An attempt to include this type of reaction under the heading of inflammation is unlikely to produce any result other than confusion.

The term *subacute inflammation* is used by some authorities: it appears to mean a mild acute inflammation, but since no exact definition is possible, there seems no good reason for retaining the term.

Causes of Acute Inflammation

Since the inflammatory reaction is a response to injury, its causes are those of cell damage. These may be briefly enumerated:

Mechanical trauma, such as cutting and crushing.

Chemical injury. There are numerous chemicals which injure cells. Many, like corrosive acids, alkalis, and phenol, are general protoplasmic poisons. Others are more selective in their action: thus mercuric chloride causes renal tubular necrosis. Some chemicals are known to act by producing a biochemical lesion, e.g. fluoroacetate. Certain body fluids, like bile and urine, cause damage when they escape into the tissues.

Radiation injury. Heat, ultraviolet light, and all forms of ionising radiations, both electromagnetic and particulate, fall into this category.

Injury due to cold and heat.

Injury associated with necrosis. A good example of this is the inflammatory reaction around an early infarct. Necrosis caused by hormonal changes is also accompanied by acute inflammation, e.g. the physiological monthly necrosis of the endometrium following the withdrawal of progesterone is associated with inflammation of the deeper part of the endometrium.

Injury due to living organisms. This includes infection with viruses, bacteria, and the larger parasites.

Injury due to an immunological mechanism. This includes the diseases mediated by antigen–antibody interaction as well as those classified as immediate and delayed-type hypersensitivity.

CHANGES IN ACUTE INFLAMMATION

Inflammation is a continuous process, the evolution of which is best studied in the living animal. The transparent web and tongue of the 'pithed' frog were originally studied, but in the higher animals the hamster cheek-pouch, the guinea-pig cochlea, the rat mesoappendix, and the rabbit ear-chamber have been used. Cohnheim (1882) gave an admirable

description to which surprisingly little has since been added. For descriptive purposes the acute inflammatory reaction may be subdivided as follows:

1. The Vascular Response.
   (i) Change in calibre of vessels.
   (ii) Changes in the vessel wall and flow of blood—stasis.
2. Swelling and Exudation.
   (i) The fluid exudate.
   (ii) The cellular exudate—phagocytosis.
3. Changes in other tissue components.

THE VASCULAR RESPONSE

Changes in the blood vessels are the most obvious manifestations of acute inflammation. They can be considered under two headings:

1. Changes in the vessel calibre.
2. Changes in the vessel wall and the flow of blood.

Changes in the Calibre of the Blood Vessels

Initial constriction. The earliest response to trauma is constriction in the small blood vessels. It can be demonstrated in the human skin: light stroking produces a white line. This vasoconstriction is apparently due to direct mechanical stimulation of the capillaries. It may also be seen when irritant chemicals are directly applied to a vascular bed. In bacterial inflammation it is questionable whether this initial constriction occurs.

Persistent vasodilatation. Vasodilatation rapidly follows the initial constriction and persists for the duration of the inflammatory process. The first result of arteriolar dilatation is that blood flows by the most direct route to the veins through the *central*, or *thoroughfare*, *channels*. Subsequent opening of the precapillary sphincters allows blood to pass into the capillary bed, and vessels which were temporarily shut down now become functional again. The inflamed part therefore appears to contain an increased number of vessels. In addition their calibre is increased.

The fact that the response of the blood vessels is so constant in acute inflammation suggests that the reaction is mediated by some common mechanism. Lewis (1924) noted that firm stroking of human skin results in a *triple response*, and his analysis of these events led to the hypothesis that histamine liberated from damaged cells was an important factor in the vascular response that follows injury (see p. 82). The features of this triple response to firm stroking of the skin are the red line, the flare, and the weal (Fig. 6.2).

The red line. After a short latent period a red line develops, at first bright red, but later tending to become cyanosed. It is sharply demarcated and is due to capillary dilatation.

The flare. After a further period of 15 to 30 seconds a flare or flush appears surrounding the red line. It is blotchy and has a crenated outline, and is due to arteriolar dilatation. If the nerve supply to the skin is sectioned, the flare can still be elicited, but if some 10 days later the test is performed again, the flare does not appear. This suggests that the flare is caused by a reflex not involving the central nervous system, but mediated *via* a local axon reflex. This is illustrated in Figure 6.3.

*The cornea may become vascularised and is then liable to true inflammation.

Figure 6.2
The triple response.
This game of naughts and crosses (tick-tack-toe) was started on the skin of the back about three minutes before the photograph was taken. Red lines developed and were soon replaced by well-marked weals. The response is more marked in this subject than in the average person, but the ability to write on the skin in this way is not uncommon and is termed *dermatographism*. It is generally asymptomatic, as in this 21-year-old nurse whose only skin complaint was that of acne vulgaris.

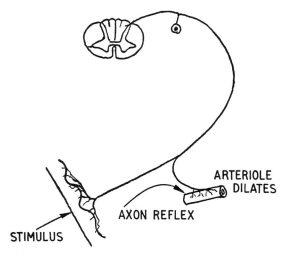

Figure 6.3
The axon reflex. Following stimulation of the skin, an impulse passing centrally also travels down the branch to the arteriole.

The weal. On the site of the red line a weal may subsequently develop due to an exudation of fluid through the vascular wall. As the oedema increases, so the weal becomes paler due to pressure on the capillaries.

It is apparent that simple mechanical injury to the skin can result in vascular changes which are typical of those seen in other types of acute inflammation. The affected part contains more blood and therefore appears red ('rubor').

The arteriolar dilatation increases the blood supply to the area. If the temperature of the part, e.g. skin, is normally below that of the blood due to its contact with the external environment, the increased blood flow that occurs during acute inflammation will be associated with a rise in temperature of the part compared with the adjacent areas. The 'calor', or heat, of acute inflammation is seen, therefore, in parts near the body surface—skin, face, ears, fingers, etc. It is not a feature of internal inflammation (Cohnheim).

Although we believe that the vasodilatation is mediated either chemically (see p. 81) or by the direct action of the agent on the blood vessels, the nervous system also plays some part.

Influence of nerve supply on the vasodilatation of acute inflammation. Inflammation can occur in completely denervated tissues, but there is no doubt that nervous influences do modify the response in the intact animal. The axon reflex is one example of this, but the autonomic nervous system can also play a part.

If the vasodilator nerve supply of a rabbit's ear is sectioned, its vessels become constricted and unresponsive. Injection of a test dose of bacteria produces a slow inflammatory reaction, and there is much more tissue destruction than when a normal ear is infected.

This effect may be correlated with the action of adrenaline. If this drug is injected together with organisms, the inflammatory response is inhibited and a spreading infection ensues. It should, however, be noted that under normal conditions the autonomic nervous system seems to play little part in the inflammatory response. When once inflammation is established, the blood vessels fail to react to sympathetic stimulation or a vasoactive drug like adrenaline.

Changes in the Vessel Wall and the Flow of Blood

Before the changes in the stream of blood in the vessels can be described, the normal flow must be understood.

The normal flow. During normal flow the blood cells tend to occupy the central, or axial, part of the stream (Fig. 6.4). This is best seen in the venules. The clear outer or plasmatic stream has great functional importance, for its viscosity is much lower than that of whole blood, and therefore the peripheral resistance is lower than it would be if the blood components were intimately mixed.

Changes in inflammation. The first change is an increase in blood velocity due to arteriolar dilatation. This phase is

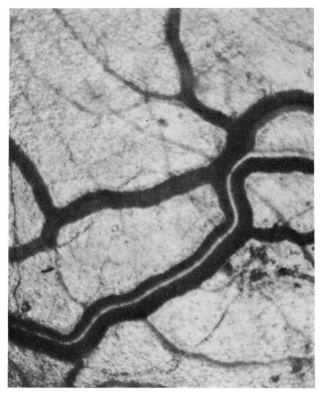

Figure 6.4
Blood flow, from right to left, in small venules seen in a rabbit ear-chamber. Note how the clear plasmatic zones in the two venules join together to produce a well-marked central clear stripe. This was a fortuitous observation which serves to illustrate the streamlining of the circulation as well as the presence of a plasmatic zone. Such a central clear stream is unusual.

short-lived, and is followed by a slowing of the stream. At the same time the white cells are seen to move into the plasmatic zone and to stick to the vessel wall; platelets also stick to the wall. The endothelial cells are swollen and appear to be covered by a gelatinous layer. This sticking of the white cells is highly characteristic of damage to blood vessels, and whereas in the normal stream the white cells cannot be distinguished, in inflammation they roll along the sticky endothelial lining in a leisurely way, quite oblivious of the red cells streaming by. These three features, *stasis*, *leucocyte adherence*, and *endothelial swelling*, must each be considered separately.

Stasis. The changes in the endothelial cells may play a small part, but the main factor in the production of stasis is an increase in the vascular permeability. Fluid is lost from the blood, which in consequence becomes more viscid. The lubricating action of the plasmatic zone is impaired or lost, and the blood stream slows down. *Thrombosis* may sometimes supervene, and is then an additional factor in causing tissue damage.

Adherence of polymorphs. With the occurrence of stasis the red cells tend to come together in the form of rouleaux, a phenomenon noted by Lister. Other factors may also play a part (see sludging, p. 421). These masses of red cells are now

the largest components in the blood stream, and the smaller white cells are pushed from the centre of the stream. They impinge more frequently on to the endothelium, which being sticky will tend to retain them. At first the white cells may escape, and either roll gently along the endothelial lining or get swept back into the blood stream. Later, however, the cells become more permanently adherent; they line the endothelium, forming great masses which may even block the lumen. This phenomenon is known as *margination* of the white cells or *pavementation* of the endothelium. It has been observed that whereas a white cell will stick to endothelium in an area of damage, it will not, if it becomes detached, stick to normal endothelium. Thus the adherence is due to the endothelial change.

Change in the endothelium. Observation of the living tissue shows swelling of the endothelial cells. They appear to be covered by a gelatinous film representing either an exudation from the surface of the injured cells, or an extracellular precipitate such as fibrin. Polymorphs adhere to this damaged area, and also adhere to each other; platelets may also be trapped. An intravenous India-ink injection demonstrates this increased adhesiveness very beautifully, for the particles stick not only to the altered endothelium, but also to the polymorphs in the vicinity. However, electron microscopy of such vessels shows carbon particles deep to the endothelial cells (see later). There can be little doubt that there is a change in the blood-vessel lining in acute inflammation, but the nature of the 'gelatinous layer' is obscure. A coating, probably of mucoprotein or mucopolysaccharide, has been reported, but most electron-microscopic studies have failed to show any extracellular material covering the endothelial cells. Whether this is due to faulty technique in the method of preparation, or whether the layer does not actually exist, is not definitely decided.

EXUDATION AND SWELLING

The most characteristic feature of acute inflammation in the higher animals is the formation of an exudate. While this usually has a cellular component, it is the exudation of fluid which is the constant feature.

The Fluid Exudate

The formation of the inflammatory exudate is dependent upon several changes. In the first place the arteriolar dilatation not only increases the flow of blood through the part, but also its pressure in the small vessels. The passage of fluid through the blood vessel walls is determined by the resultant of the hydrostatic and osmotic pressures acting upon it (Starling). These are summarised in Figure 6.5 and described in detail in Chapter 43.

In acute inflammation the pressure in the capillaries even at the venous end may exceed the osmotic pressure of the plasma proteins, and therefore fluid will tend to pass into the tissue spaces. It must not be thought that Figure 6.5 (*a*) represents the conditions in every capillary; it is known that while one group of vessels may be widely dilated and exuding fluid, another group is shut down. In this way movement of tissue fluid is increased, which may be important in the spread of infection (see p. 98). Furthermore, it must be remembered

Figure 6.5
Fluid interchanges between blood and tissue spaces:
(*a*) under normal conditions;
(*b*) in acute inflammation.

that the permeability of vessels to protein and even some smaller molecules varies considerably from one tissue to another. Thus the vessels of the brain and thymus are less permeable than those elsewhere. These differences in behaviour of capillaries are finding support from electron microscope studies, which show differences in structure. Figure 6.5 (*a*) represents a simplification of the conditions which may be expected in an average capillary in a part at heart level.

From the onset, therefore, conditions favour the formation of interstitial fluid of normal low protein content and low specific gravity. However, in inflammation the exudate differs from normal interstitial fluid; it has a very high protein content, its fibrinogen leads to clot formation, and it has a high specific gravity (over 1·020). Other important factors must therefore operate.

The crucial factor in the formation of an inflammatory exudate is an increased permeability of the vessel walls to plasma proteins. If trypan blue or pontamine sky blue is injected intravenously into an animal, the dye becomes bound to the plasma albumin and does not readily leave the circulation. When an inflammatory response is elicited, the tagged albumin can be seen to pass into the inflamed area as the exudate forms. This experimental method is often used to demonstrate an increase

in permeability to plasma protein. A similar type of labelling may be done with radioactive iodine.

The conditions in acute inflammation are shown in Figure 6.5 (*b*). The exudate has virtually the same chemical composition as plasma, with the result that the osmotic effect of the plasma proteins is largely neutralised. In addition, the breakdown of large protein molecules into several smaller ones may further increase the osmotic pressure of the interstitial fluid. Finally, there is yet another factor which plays an important part; one of the first detectable changes in experimental acute inflammation is an alteration in the ground substance, which is rendered more fluid. The effect of this increased fluidity may well be to allow exudate to diffuse more readily, thereby preventing an immediate rise in tissue tension.

To summarise, the mechanisms in the production of the fluid exudate are therefore:

1. Increased vascular permeability to proteins.
2. Increased capillary blood pressure.
3. Breakdown of large-molecule tissue proteins.
4. Increased fluidity of the tissue ground substance.

Since by far the most important of these is the increased vascular permeability, it is not surprising that this has been most extensively studied. In experimentally produced acute inflammation (thermal injury to the rat cremaster muscle) *two phases of exudation* were described by Miles. There was an *early transient phase* that was maximal at 8 to 10 minutes and was due to leakage from the venules, mediated by histamine. This was followed by a *prolonged delayed phase* which required several hours to develop and was attributed to capillary damage. The situation is more complex than this, and other patterns of reaction have been recognised. Thus three phases can be recognised:

Immediate-transient phase. This lasts about 30 minutes, affects venules, and is largely mediated by histamine.

Immediate-prolonged phase. The exudation starts immediately but persists for days. It appears to be due to direct damage to vessels.

Delayed-prolonged phase. This corresponds to Miles's delayed phase and was thought to be due to the effect of unidentified mediators on capillaries. It is now thought that both capillaries and venules are affected both by the direct injury of the agent (e.g. heat) and by chemical mediators.

Vascular permeability in normal tissues. Normally the walls of the capillaries and venules are freely permeable to water and electrolytes but not to proteins and other large molecules. Rapid exchange takes place between intravascular and extravascular water, and in fact about 70 per cent of the water in the blood crosses the vessel wall every minute and is replaced by water from the interstitial space. The mechanism whereby this exchange takes place has been much debated. In most tissues the barriers which must be considered are:

1. The endothelial cell with its attenuated extensions.
2. The basement membrane, which forms a complete sheath.
3. Pericytes, which form a discontinuous outer coat together with connective tissue fibres.

The following possibilities have been suggested:
Direct transport through the cell by simple diffusion. The lipid

(and presumably waterproof) nature of the cell membrane has led many authorities to regard this as an unlikely mechanism.

Transport across the endothelial cell by cytopempsis (p. 15). This process probably does take place, but it seems unlikely that it could explain the large volume of fluid which is known to cross the vessel walls. Furthermore, the vesicles formed by micropinocytosis would be expected to contain protein, whereas the fluid which escapes from the blood vessels has a low plasma protein content.

Passage through pores in the endothelial cells. Pores are present in the sinusoids of the liver; in certain other sites, e.g. kidney and intestine, there are fenestrations which are covered by a very thin membrane. In other areas no pores have been found, although short channels traversing the cell's cytoplasm and of the diameter of pinocytotic vesicles have been described; being tortuous, they are difficult to detect.[2]

Passage through spaces between the endothelial cells. The thick cement lines seen in silver-nitrate preparations of endothelium seem to be an artefact, for on electron microscopy the endothelial cells closely adjoin each other and the gap between them is about 15 nm wide. Junctional complexes are present.

A final consideration concerns the basement membrane, since all substances leaving or entering the vessel must cross it. The membrane appears to have no holes nor does it seem to be a barrier to the passage of water or electrolytes. Cells, large particles, and perhaps the plasma proteins are held back and their passage delayed.

Vascular permeability in inflamed tissue. Examination of the endothelial cells of capillaries in acutely inflamed tissues has revealed several changes—increase in the number and size of the micropinocytotic vesicles, blebs under the luminal cell membrane, and projections or spikes arising from the membrane. The changes are, however, inconstant and seem inadequate to explain the great increase in vascular permeability. On the other hand, it has been shown that when 5-hydroxytryptamine or histamine is applied to rat cremaster muscle important changes occur in the venules. Gaps (0·1 to 0·4 μm in diameter) appear in the endothelial lining due to the separation of adjacent endothelial cells. Histamine seems to cause contraction of the endothelial cells so that gaps appear between adjacent cells.

If the animal is first given an intravenous injection of mercuric sulphide suspension, the particles, which are 10 to 15 nm in diameter, are found to be situated between the endothelial cell and the basement membrane. It appears therefore that in acute inflammation the gap between endothelial cells widens, thereby allowing plasma to reach the basement membrane and escape to the extravascular spaces. The particles of mercuric sulphide being unable to penetrate the intact basement membrane accumulate between it and the endothelial cell (Fig. 6.6).

Similar results are obtained if India ink is used and trauma applied to produce an acute inflammation. Thus, both the early exudation of acute inflammation and the application of histamine are associated with a separation of the endothelial cells and an escape of plasma. Whether other changes occur, for instance in the basement membrane, and whether the second phase of exudation is associated with other features, are not yet clear.

Function of the fluid exudate. All the constituents of the

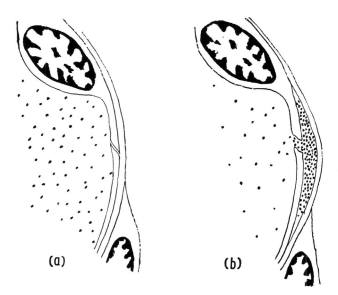

Figure 6.6
Diagrammatic representation of the changes in a venule following the intravenous injection of a suspension of mercuric sulphide (particle size 10–15 nm).

(*a*) Shows the wall of normal venule with the particles distributed in the plasma.

(*b*) After the local application of histamine. The appearances suggest that the plasma has leaked through the gap between the endothelial cells, and that the basement membrane has held back the particles but allowed the fluid exudate to pass through.

plasma are poured into the area of inflammation. These include natural antibacterial substances like opsonins and complement as well as specific immunoglobulins. Drugs and antibiotics, if present in the plasma, will also appear in the exudate. The importance of the early administration of therapeutic agents is obvious when it is remembered that they are merely carried to the inflamed area in the exudate, and are in no way concentrated. Indeed, drugs that are not bound to the plasma proteins will diffuse into the interstitial fluid at a fast rate and reach plasma concentrations in normal circumstances also. The fluid of the exudate (*inflammatory oedema*) has the effect of diluting any irritant substance irrespective of its origin. Its high fibrinogen content often results in the formation of a fibrin clot. This fibrin has three main functions:

(1) It forms a union between severed tissues, as in a cut.

(2) It may form a barrier against bacterial invasion (p. 98).

(3) It aids phagocytosis (p. 78).

The exudate accounts in part for the remaining cardinal signs of inflammation. It causes swelling ('tumor'), and the increased tissue pressure may be an important factor in the production of pain ('dolor') which itself limits activity. In fact, pain is often present before there is much swelling, and the effect of tissue tension on nerve endings cannot be the whole answer. The acid pH of the exudate, an accumulation of K^+ ions, and the presence of chemical mediators like 5-hydroxytryptamine and bradykinin have all been blamed.

Changes in the lymphatics. The small lymphatics of a tissue form a blind-ended system of vessels, which closely resemble the vascular capillaries except that a basement membrane is incomplete or absent and their walls are permeable to proteins. One of their main functions is to allow any plasma protein which has escaped from the blood vessels to drain away and ultimately reach the blood stream again. In acute inflammation the lymph vessels are held widely open and the flow of fluid, containing excess protein, is greatly increased.

The Cellular Exudate

Not only does the vascular wall allow proteins to pass through, but soon the white cells also penetrate it. It has already been described how the white cells come to adhere passively to the sticky endothelium. From there they pass actively by amoeboid motion through the vessel wall. This process is called *emigration* of the white cells into the surrounding tissues. Some authorities describe this process as diapedesis of the white cells. However, we have followed the common English practice of confining the term diapedesis to the egress of the red cells.

As previously stated, the electron microscope has failed to identify any abnormality of the endothelial surface to account for this. The white cells adhere to the endothelium and push out pseudopodia. One of these enters the gap between two endothelial cells and forces it open. Having penetrated the endothelium, it may travel laterally before bursting through the basement membrane and finally the perivascular sheath.

The first cells involved are the neutrophil polymorphs, and these take 2 to 9 minutes to penetrate the vessel wall. Several hours later the monocytes predominate, and in the tissues these large cells become phagocytic and are called macrophages; their emigration continues after the polymorphs have stopped. Lymphocytes have not yet been observed to migrate in acute inflammation. Some red cells may also escape from the vessels usually following a white cell. They merely spurt through the defect created by the white cells, being ejected as the result of the hydrostatic pressure of the blood. This passive movement is called *diapedesis*, and is to be distinguished from the active emigration of the white cells. In primates organisms may adhere to red cells by the process of immune adherence (p. 146).

The emigration does not stop when the phagocytes have penetrated the vessel wall. The cells then move towards the damaged or infected area, and form a salient histological feature of many acute inflammatory responses (Fig. 6.7).

Chemotaxis.[3] The directional movement of an organism in response to a chemical gradient is called chemotaxis and has been known for some time. A well-known example is the attraction of the spermatozoids of the male fern by malic acid, which is present in the female germ cells. The accumulation of polymorphs in acutely inflamed tissues naturally raises the possibility that they are attracted there by some chemical influence, and the movement of polymorphs has been extensively investigated. If the cells are incorporated into a film of clotted plasma placed between a slide and a coverslip, their movement can be followed by direct microscopic observation. Polymorphs exhibit *random movement*, but can also be seen to move towards certain substances; thus they exhibit this *positive chemotaxis* towards certain bacteria and starch granules. A photographic record of their movement can be obtained by means of a long exposure with the preparation illuminated using a dark-field condenser.

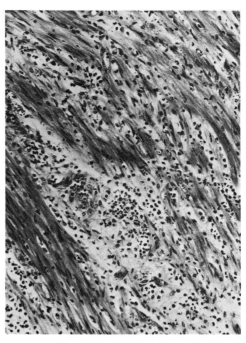

Figure 6.7
Acute inflammation in the muscular coat of the appendix. The muscle fibres are separated by the inflammatory oedema and there is a diffuse infiltration by polymorphs. × 150.

This method of investigation is time consuming, and the Boyden chamber has greatly facilitated the study of chemotaxis. The chamber consists of two tissue-culture chambers placed one on top of the other and separated by a membrane of 3 μm pore size. A suspension of polymorphs is placed in the upper chamber while the test substance is placed in the lower. The number of cells which migrate to the lower surface of the filter is a measure of the chemotactic effect (Fig. 6.8). Unless the experimental conditions are carefully controlled the Boyden chamber does not readily distinguish between chemotaxis and accelerated random movement.

Both neutrophil polymorphs and monocytes have been shown to be attracted *in vitro* to a number of agents: these include starch and certain bacteria. Antigen-antibody complexes and dead tissue are chemotactic, but only if complement is activated. Three separate components are involved. One is a soluble activated product of the trimolecular complex termed C567. The other two are small cleavage products of C3 and C5 which are designated C3a and C5a (see p. 159). Chemotactic lymphokines have been isolated (see below). The present evidence suggests that polymorphs are attracted to sites of inflammation by chemotactic agents, but the relative importance of the various factors is not known; it probably varies according to the cause of the inflammation.

With monocytes chemotaxis has also been demonstrated, and they appear to react to many of the substances which attract polymorphs. The change in the cells of the exudate from polymorphs in the early stages to monocytes later on has been the topic of frequent speculation. One explanation is that the polymorphs, which have only a short life-span, soon die and disappear. The long-lived monocytes remain, an effect

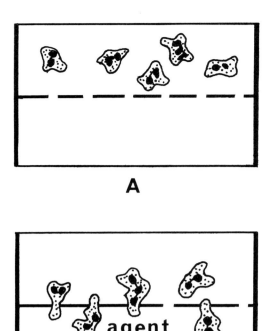

A

B

Figure 6.8
The Boyden chamber consists of two tissue-culture chambers separated by a membrane of 3 μm pore size. If the agent placed in the lower chamber is chemotactic, polymorphs present in the upper chamber migrate through the pores (B). See text.

that could be accentuated by the presence of migration inhibitory factor (p. 185). The relative number of monocytes would steadily increase. Another possibility is that the monocytes undergo division before assuming macrophage activity (p. 126).

A number of observations now suggest that some chemotactic agents are selective in their action. Thus, when sensitised lymphocytes react with antigen, factors called lymphokines are released (p. 148). Some of these are chemotactic agents, and separate agents affect polymorphs, monocytes, and eosinophils. The reaction of antigen with IgE antibody has also been shown to release a chemotactic agent for eosinophils, cells which are certainly a feature of human atopic diseases. The varied and changing population of inflammatory cells found in inflammatory disease would be more easily understood if selective chemotaxis were the mechanism. Precisely how the phagocytes sense the presence of a chemical gradient and respond to it is not known. Movement is presumed to involve the actin-myosin contractile elements in the cell.[4] The energy needed is derived from the hexose monophosphate shunt. One final point deserves consideration: so far no substance has been found to be chemotactic to lymphocytes. How they traverse the vessel wall and why, are questions which remain unanswered.

The most obvious function of the white cells in inflammation is phagocytosis. Both polymorphonuclears and mac-

rophages may be seen to ingest foreign particles, bacteria, and cell debris.

Phagocytosis. *Opsonins.*[5] The ability of polymorphonuclears to ingest organisms can be tested *in vitro*. It is found that whereas commensals are easily ingested, the presence of serum is necessary before virulent organisms may be phagocytosed. The factor in serum which is necessary is a protein called an *opsonin*. One variety appears to be non-specific and has been called a 'natural antibody'. It requires the presence of complement, and may be of importance in the recognition and subsequent phagocytosis of foreign antigenic material.

It has been found that some pathogens, usually those with capsules, e.g. pneumococci, are ingested only if specific antibodies are provided. These 'immune opsonins' are a very important type of antibacterial antibody. It is believed that opsonins coat the surface of the organism, rendering it more readily acceptable to the phagocytes. The more virulent the organism, the more noxious are its surface antigens, and one can easily understand why only 'tailor-made', or specific, antibodies are effective in promoting phagocytosis. Phagocytosis is therefore a prominent feature of inflammation occurring in an immune animal. Both polymorphs and monocytes have surface receptors for the Fc component of immunoglobulin as well as for C3. Hence these cells adhere to particles coated with antibody or complement. It will be readily appreciated therefore that activation of complement is an important process in the mediation of phagocytosis, since membrane-bound C3b is recognised by cell receptors of the phagocytes.

Opsonisation is also necessary for phagocytosis by cells of the reticulo-endothelial system, as is shown by experiments in which the liver is perfused with fluid containing organisms.

The energy for phagocytosis both by polymorphs and macrophages is derived mainly from anaerobic glycolysis. Phagocytosis of a particle is accompanied by the production of lactate (see p. 79). Following phagocytosis a series of metabolic events occur that have been called the 'respiratory burst', since they result in a dramatic increase in glucose utilisation through the hexose monophosphate shunt. This burst of oxidative metabolism, involving an increased activity of NADH oxidase and NADPH oxidase, results in the formation of powerful oxidising agents, such as H_2O_2, which are essential for the intracellular destruction of bacteria (see below).

Surface phagocytosis. Although opsonins facilitate the phagocytosis of pathogenic organisms, it has been found that, if a suitable framework is provided *in vitro*, e.g. a fibrin network, the polymorphonuclears may, by trapping an organism in a corner, be able to ingest it without its prior opsonisation. This phenomenon is known as *surface phagocytosis*, and is of importance in the immunity to infection which animals exhibit during the early (and vital) few days before antibodies are produced. When organisms gain entry to an open area like the subarachnoid space, the outcome is more serious than when they infect a compact organ like the skin or lung.

Fate of ingested particles. Ingested material is enclosed in phagocytic vacuoles, the membranes of which fuse with those of adjacent granules. The specific granules fuse first and liberate their lysozyme, lactoferrin, and alkaline phosphatase. Later the azurophil granules fuse with the vacuoles and pour in their lysosomal enzymes. In this way digestion vacuoles are

Figure 6.9
Phagocytosis.
A human peripheral blood polymorphonuclear leucocyte that has been exposed to zymosan particles (Z). At the right is a particle that has been bound to the cell but has not yet been ingested. In the lower portion of this picture are zymosan particles in phagocytic vacuoles. Lysosomes surround the particles, and have degranulated into the vacuoles (arrows). Bacteria are treated in a similar manner, and may later be destroyed ($\times 10\,000$). (*Photograph by courtesy of Dr. Sylvia Hoffstein and Dr. Gerald Weissmann, New York University Medical Center.*)

formed, and the neutrophil becomes degranulated. It is not difficult to envisage how lysosomal enzymes could escape from the cell as lysosomal membranes fuse with those of the phagosomes as they are forming (Fig. 6.9).[6] The cells also release pyrogen, and this is a major factor in the pathogenesis of the fever which accompanies acute inflammation.

Polymorphs have a short life span, 3 to 4 days at the most, and when they die, any particles which remain undigested are liberated into the intercellular spaces. Macrophages at this stage form a prominent feature of the exudate, and ingest particles, cell debris, etc. In contrast to the polymorphs they are long-lived, and those that have ingested insoluble particles remain in the tissues for long periods, possibly many years. This is well demonstrated in tattoos.

Fate of ingested bacteria. Many bacteria are destroyed in the phagosome, but the precise mechanism involved probably varies from one organism to another. The following antimicrobial agents may be involved:

1. *Lysosomal enzymes.* Although these acid-hydrolytic enzymes digest dead bacteria, it is considered unlikely that they can kill living organisms.

2. *Lysozyme* (see p. 87). This enzyme is released by both the specific and the azurophil granules of the polymorphs.

3. *Acidity.* The low pH may destroy some organisms. *Lactic acid* is produced as a consequence of the glycolysis that accompanies phagocytosis. Lactic acid is bactericidal, and its action can be reversed by certain keto compounds and carbo-

xylic acids; this may account for the fact that the leucocytes in experimentally produced diabetes mellitus can still engulf pneumococci but are unable to destroy them.

4. *Lactoferrin.* This protein inhibits bacterial growth by binding iron, which is an essential growth requirement for micro-organisms.

5. *Cationic lysosomal proteins.* At least seven different antimicrobial proteins of this type are found in neutrophils. Their importance is not known. One of these basic proteins has been called *phagocytin*.

6. *Oxidising agents.*[7] A number of oxidising agents are formed as a result of the hexose-monophosphate-shunt activity that follows phagocytosis. The superoxide anion O_2^- is thought to be an important bactericidal agent. Also important is H_2O_2, which acts on bacteria in the presence of a halide (I^-, Cl^-, or Br^-) and the enzyme myeloperoxidase that granulocytes contain. The precise mechanism of this H_2O_2-halide-myeloperoxidase bactericidal action is not settled. Singlet oxygen may be another factor. This unstable, excited state of oxygen emits light. Since activated leucocytes also emit light, it has been suggested that this is due to the continuous formation of singlet oxygen.

In summary, the neutrophil polymorph exhibits the following activities in acute inflammation: random movement, chemotaxis, adherence to bacteria and particles, phagocytosis, activation of the hexose monophosphate shunt, and bactericidal activity. A defect in any of these mechanisms is often accompanied by a decreased resistance to infection (p. 162).

CHANGES IN OTHER TISSUE COMPONENTS IN ACUTE INFLAMMATION

One of the first changes in inflammation is loss of the specific granules of the tissue mast cells. Since these contain histamine and heparin, they may be a source of chemical mediators. Another early change is an increase in the fluidity of the ground substance.

LOCAL SEQUELAE OF ACUTE INFLAMMATION

The changes which occur following the formation of an acute inflammatory exudate depend upon two major factors:

1. The amount of tissue damage sustained.

2. Whether or not the causative agent remains.

Some agents, e.g. pyogenic bacteria and turpentine, regularly produce considerable destruction of the fixed tissues of an organ. Autolysis of these elements, together with the digestion produced by the ferments of polymorphs ('pus cells'), result in the production of a cavity containing *pus* (suppurative inflammation).

In all cases of acute inflammation, unless tissue death occurs, the initial polymorph exudate is later replaced by a mononuclear one, and this appearance heralds the onset of the demolition phase.

Demolition phase. Macrophages engulf fibrin, red cells, pus cells, foreign material, bacteria, etc. They therefore contain a variety of intracellular structures including fat, haemosiderin, cholesterol, and foreign material. Sometimes the macrophages fuse together to produce giant cells.

Origin of macrophages. The macrophages which accumulate

in areas subjected to injury in lower forms of life appear to be derived from histiocytes, which are the resting tissue representatives of the reticulo-endothelial system. In mammals tissue histiocytes may also perform a similar function, but current evidence suggests that the majority of macrophages present in the stage of demolition are the progeny of monocytes that emigrated from the blood stream. Labelling experiments indicate that monocytes can divide and assume the morphology of histiocytes, macrophages, and lymphocytes. Reports that lymphocytes can change into macrophages may therefore be misleading. The cellular events in small experimental wounds in human skin have been studied by Rebuck, who placed glass cover-slips over a wound and examined the cells adhering to the glass. All stages in the transformation of small lymphocytes to macrophages have been described, but it seems unlikely that the cells described as small lymphocytes are the same as those present in the blood and thoracic-duct lymph. Lymphocytes do not readily adhere to glass, and it may well be that the small 'lymphocytes' observed in these experiments are derived from monocytes. It must be concluded that the precise origin of macrophages, histiocytes, and lymphocytes is incompletely understood at the present time.

The macrophage is the cell of prime importance during the phase of demolition. It is convenient at this stage to review its functions. See p. 392 for the functions of the reticulo-endothelial system, of which the macrophage is a member.

Functions of the Macrophage[8,9]

1. *Demolition.* This is a necessary prelude to resolution or healing, whether by regeneration or repair.

2. *Antimicrobial defence.* The monocytes are of great importance in the destruction of many invading organisms—especially those that are intracellular, such as the mycobacteria, listeria, histoplasma, and leishmania. The energy for phagocytosis is derived from glycolysis, but oxygen is required for bactericidal activity which involves the formation of intracellular hydrogen peroxide. Macrophages, unlike monocytes and polymorphs, do not contain myeloperoxidase, therefore their bactericidal mechanism must be different from that of these cells.

3. *Processing of antigen.* Macrophages phagocytose antigen and antigen-antibody complexes. They may act as a storage mechanism for antigenic determinants, or they may process the antigen and pass information on to lymphoid cells, thereby initiating an immune response (see Ch. 12).

4. *Cellular immunity.* Macrophages derived from an immunised animal are more efficient in phagocytosing and killing organisms than are the cells from a non-immunised animal. This effect appears to be non-specific (see p. 163). In addition, macrophages collaborate with immunoglobulins in killing bacteria (p. 167).

5. *Anti-tumour activity.* This role is ill defined.

6. *Control of granulopoiesis.* Human bone-marrow cells will grow in a semi-solid medium if *colony-stimulating factor* is present. The main source of this factor is the macrophage.

7. *Control of erythropoiesis.* Developing red-cell precursors often cluster around a macrophage, which is called a 'nurse cell'. It is suggested that the macrophage supplies ferritin for the synthesis of haemoglobin.

8. *Secretory activity.*[8] There is considerable evidence that macrophages, particularly when engaged in active phagocytosis, can release or secrete a number of factors, amongst which may be mentioned *lysosomal enzymes, lysozyme, plasminogen activator, collagenase, elastase, endogenous pyrogen,* and *complement* components, particularly C4 and C2. Some factors appear to act on other cells, for example there is the colony-stimulating factor noted above. Other factors act on lymphocytes, either functioning as mitogens or else stimulating them to activity, e.g. Ig production in the case of B cells, or helper function in the case of T cells. Another factor acts on fibroblasts (see pp. 106 and 135).

The importance of the secretory function of the macrophage is not known, but it is evident that this cell plays a vital role in the processes of inflammation and healing. The role of the macrophage in the defence against infection is complex and does not rest entirely on its activities as a simple scavenger cell.

Resolution

In acutely inflamed tissue in which cellular damage has been relatively slight, the cellular and tissue changes are reversible, and necrosis does not occur. The demolition phase results in removal of the exudate, and the organ returns to normal. To this process the term *resolution* is applied, and one of the best examples is found in lobar pneumonia (see p. 223). *Resolution thus means the complete return to normal of a tissue following acute inflammation.* Sometimes removal of the exudate appears to be delayed, and then the fibrin becomes invaded by granulation tissue. This is called *organisation.* It sometimes complicates bronchopneumonia, and fibrosis is the result. It often occurs in the fibrinous exudate of inflamed serous cavities; in this manner fibrous adhesions are formed. The process whereby exudate becomes organised in the absence of tissue necrosis is sometimes called 'incomplete resolution', but the term is not to be recommended.

It should be noted that while the demolition phase is proceeding, the exudate is carried by the lymphatics to the regional lymph nodes. The sinus lining cells remove cellular debris.

Suppuration

When the noxious agent produces much necrosis, resolution is impossible and the process proceeds to *suppuration.* This is typical of staphylococcal lesions, e.g. boils, but can also occur when the agent is a chemical substance, e.g. turpentine.

The first reaction is circumscribed necrosis accompanied by a profuse polymorph infiltration. The agent kills many of these leucocytes—which are called 'pus cells' by histologists. The necrotic material undergoes softening by virtue of the proteolytic enzymes released by the dead leucocytes as well as through the autolysis mediated by the tissue's own cathepsins. The resulting fluid material is called *pus* and is contained within a cavity to form an *abscess.* This is lined by a wall, or *pyogenic membrane,* which at first consists of acutely inflamed tissue heavily infiltrated with polymorphs. The copious fibrinous exudate is soon organised into granulation tissue.

The pus itself is made up of (*a*) dead and dying leucocytes, (*b*) other components of the inflammatory exudate—oedema fluid and fibrin, (*c*) organisms, many of which are living and

Figure 6.10
Sequelae of acute inflammation.

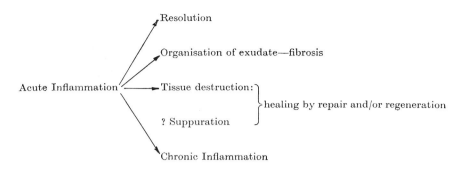

can therefore be cultured (but if the pus is chemically induced it is sterile), and (*d*) tissue debris, e.g. nucleic acids and lipids.

The pus tends to track in the line of least resistance until a free surface is reached. Then the abscess bursts and discharges its contents spontaneously—in clinical practice this is usually anticipated by surgical drainage. An abscess when drained heals by repair, but sometimes chronic inflammation ensues due to persisting infection. In this event a chronic abscess results; its wall is composed of fibrous tissue heavily in-filtrated by a pleomorphic collection of cells, including polym-orphs, macrophages, lymphocytes, and plasma cells. A large quantity of pus is produced, and is discharged through a *sinus* to the exterior or into some hollow viscus.

If, as occasionally happens, the abscess is not drained and remains sequestered in the tissues, its walls become organised into dense fibrous tissue and the pus undergoes thickening, or inspissation, as the watery part is gradually absorbed. In due course it becomes of porridge-like consistency, and may even-tually become *calcified*.

When an acute suppurative inflammation involves an epi-thelial surface, the covering is destroyed and an *ulcer* is formed. The floor is composed of necrotic tissue and acute inflammatory exudate; this layer of dead tissue forms the *slough*, and is at first adherent because the dead material has not been liquefied. Eventually, however, the slough becomes detached and the ulcer heals by the processes of repair and regeneration, as described in Chapter 9.

It should be noted that pus is also formed when an inflammatory reaction involves a surface. Necrosis of tissue need not be a marked feature, but the inflammatory exudate pours from the surface and may accumulate to form pus. In this way an empyema is formed in some cases of pneumonia even without abscess formation in the underlying lung.

Chronic Inflammation

The other sequel of acute inflammation is progression to a state of chronic inflammation, in which the inflammatory and healing processes proceed side by side. This is described in Chapter 11. It is worth noting that much chronic inflam-mation is the result of suppuration which has not been adequately drained. The slough (or sequestrum in osteo-myelitis) provides a nidus in which the causative organisms can continue to flourish. Until adequate drainage is provided, there can be no hope of terminating the infection.

Sterile chemical abscesses do not undergo this progressive course. The process is necessarily self-limiting, and apart from the effect of local tissue destruction, there are no permanent sequelae.

The sequelae of acute inflammation are summarised in Figure 6.10.

THE CHEMICAL MEDIATORS OF ACUTE INFLAMMATION[10]

Of all the changes in acute inflammation those affecting the vessels are the most striking. In addition to vasodilatation, the endothelium of the small vessels undergoes changes which not only make it sticky, but also render it more permeable both to blood cells and plasma proteins. These alterations are not dependent upon the stretching of the vessel walls consequent on dilatation, for they are not seen in the hyperaemia that accompanies increased tissue activity. Neither are they all directly related to the injury itself, as suggested by Cohnheim, for they may extend beyond the area involved (see triple response, p. 72). The most likely explanation for the vasodila-tation and the other vascular changes is that they are caused by chemical mediators. Since the vascular phenomena of acute inflammation are very similar irrespective of the cause, the most likely source of any mediators is the damaged tissue itself.

Sir Thomas Lewis, under the influence of Sir Henry Dale, suggested that *histamine* was an important chemical mediator of the inflammatory response. The first to demonstrate that other factors were also involved was Menkin. The *leukotaxine* which he isolated was later shown to be a mixture of polypep-tides and not a pure substance. Menkin also described a number of other substances (necrosin, exudin, etc.), but these have never been categorised chemically and are probably also complex mixtures. Miles described a permeability factor that could be generated by simply diluting plasma with saline. This was termed *Pf/dil* and was assumed to arise by the activation of a precursor *pro-Pf/dil*. The generation of Pf/dil was shown to be initiated by the activation of *Hageman factor* (Clotting Factor XII), but the factor itself (Pf/dil) and its precursor are not thought to be pure substances; like leukot-axine they are mixtures of other active agents. The most important of these are *plasmin*, a fibrinolytic enzyme, and *kallikrein*, which occurs in the blood in an inactive form and acts on *kininogen* to form a *kinin*. The most important kinin is *bradykinin*, a potent polypeptide previously described by Rocha e Silva. The formation of these agents and their complex inter-relationship are outlined in Figure 6.11. Other vasoactive agents are generated by activation of the comple-ment cascade; yet others are released from platelets, polym-orphs, and other cells. Thus the list of possible chemical mediators of acute inflammation seems to be never-ending, and only a brief account will be given with emphasis on those agents that seem to be of importance in human pathology. The mediators may be classified as follows:

I. Amines   (a) histamine.
                     (b) 5-hydroxytryptamine (5-HT).
II. The kinins.
III. Kinin-forming
     enzymes   (a) kallikrein.
                     (b) plasmin.
IV. Biologically active products of the complement system.
V. Biologically active components of polymorphs.
VI. Prostaglandins.
VII. Others.

The Amines

Histamine. The classical experiments of Lewis on the triple response showed that injury to the skin produced a type of inflammation which had many features in common with the effect of an injection of histamine. Lewis showed that injured skin released some substance ('H' substance) which behaved like histamine.

For a time it was accepted that histamine was the most important mediator of the vascular response in acute inflammation. Most workers have been able to identify it in inflammatory exudates, in extracts of inflamed tissues, and in the perfusate of inflamed parts. Further investigation has, however, not confirmed this belief, for tissues become refractory to continued injections of histamine and the vasodilatation of infection is long-lasting. Furthermore, work on turpentine inflammation in the pleural cavity of rats has shown that antihistamines reduce the volume of exudate during the first 30 minutes, but not thereafter. The prior administration of a histamine-depleting drug such as compound 48/80 has the same effect.

Thus, there is good evidence that histamine is liberated in acute inflammation, and that it can mimic some of the vascular events. It seems likely that it is important during the early phase, in initiating the axon reflex, and in certain hypersensitivity responses (see p. 176).

Histamine, bound to heparin, is contained in the granules of mast cells. It can be released by injury, by the action of various histamine-releasing agents (including the anaphylatoxins C3a and C5a), and by antigen if the cells have been previously sensitised by IgE (see later).

5-Hydroxytryptamine (5-HT, or serotonin). A smooth muscle contracting substance is found in the early inflammatory exudate of experimentally produced turpentine pleurisy in the rat. In this species 5-HT rather than histamine is liberated during the early phase of acute inflammation; it is liberated from mast cells or platelets.

Adrenaline and noradrenaline. These substances and their precursors dopamine and DOPA reduce the increased vascular permeability of acute inflammation. They are degraded by the enzyme monoamine oxidase, and an increase in the activity of this enzyme in acute inflammation may release the vessels from the inhibiting effect of this group of amines. This mechanism is probably not of great importance in the pathogenesis of acute inflammation.

The Kinins

The name kinin has been applied to a variety of physiologically-active polypeptides which cause contraction of smooth muscle. *Bradykinin* is the most important, and was so named because of the slow contraction which it induces in the muscle of the guinea-pig ileum; it appears to be the active agent in producing the effects of poisoning due to certain snakebites. It may also be concerned in the regulation of blood flow in the salivary glands. This same kinin is formed when human saliva acts upon blood proteins, thereby revealing an unexpected relationship between human saliva and snake venom. Similar substances have been identified from other sources—kallidin, plasma kinin, pain-producing substance, and urinary kinin. These substances are closely related chemically. Wasp venom contains another kinin.

Bradykinin, a nonapeptide, has been synthesised, and is ten times more active as a vasodilator than is histamine (on a molar basis). It produces pain when applied to tissue, and is probably identical to pain-producing substance. Bradykinin causes an increase in vascular permeability and stimulates the contraction of smooth muscle, but is not chemotactic to white cells. *Kallidin* is a decapeptide, lysyl-bradykinin, and is formed when pancreatic and other tissue kallikreins act on plasma kininogen. It is rapidly converted into bradykinin by plasma aminopeptidase.

The kinins are formed from precursor *kininogens* by the action of the enzymes *kallikrein* or *plasmin* (Fig. 6.11). Two groups of kininogens are known. The *low-molecular-weight kininogens* are acted upon by plasmin only, while the *high-molecular-weight kininogens* are the substrate for both kallikrein and plasmin. The part played by the kinins in inflammation is not yet known. Since they are capable of producing vasodilatation, increasing venular permeability, and causing pain, it has been suggested that they act as mediators during the early phases of inflammation. The suggestion that they are important during the prolonged second phase of increased permeability in inflammation seems unlikely, for, as with histamine, tissues become refractory to their actions. Kinins are degraded by the action of *kininases*, enzymes which therefore limit the duration of their action. One kininase has also been identified as an anaphylatoxin-inactivating enzyme, while another is identical to angiotensin I-converting enzyme.

Kallikrein.* Kallikrein is an enzyme that can form bradykinin from high-molecular-weight kininogen of the blood. It can also activate Hageman factor (Factor XII) to Factor XIIa, and is chemotactic to white cells. The enzyme exists as an inactive precursor (*prekallikrein*), which can itself be activated by Factor XIIf (also called prekallikrein activator before its relationship to Factor XII was known). Plasma kallikrein is one member of a group of enzymes that can form kinins from plasma. Others occur in urine, pancreas, and snake venom.

Kallikrein inhibitors. Three inhibitors are known, and presumably play a part in the regulation of kallikrein activity. These are the C1-esterase inhibitor, an α_2-macroglobulin, and α_1-antitrypsin.

The inhibitory action of these agents is not confined to

---

*Kallikrein is so called because it is found in high concentration in pancreas. *Kallikreas* is Greek for pancreas.

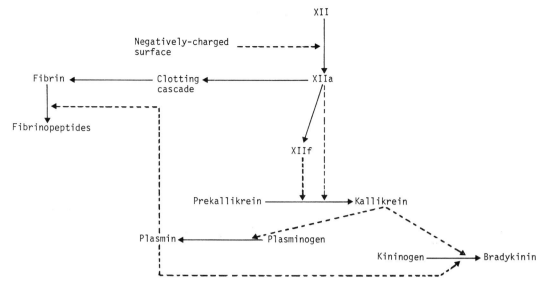

Figure 6.11

The current hypothesis for the activation of the kinin system. Note the central role of Hageman-factor (factor XII) activation which initiates clotting, fibrinolysis, and kinin formation. Factor XIIa has a major role in initiating the clotting cascade but a minor one in activating prekallikrein. Factor XIIf, on the other hand, has as its major action the activation of prekallikrein to kallikrein. The separate types of kininogen are not shown (see text). Transformations are depicted as solid lines, while enzymatic actions are shown as interrupted lines.

kallikrein. Some also inhibit plasmin, Factor XIIa, or Factor XIIf.*

Plasmin. Plasminogen is a normal component of the plasma proteins. It can be converted into plasmin by the action of kallikrein (previously called plasminogen activator). Plasmin itself is a proteolytic enzyme, and digests fibrin as well as other plasma proteins. The breakdown of fibrin leads to the formation of a variety of polypeptides (*fibrinopeptides*) that have a number of properties, including anticoagulant activity, the ability to increase vascular permeability, and being chemotactic to white cells.

Plasmin can increase vascular permeability in many ways. It can act directly on kininogen to liberate kinin; this action is slow compared with that of kallikrein. Secondly, it can activate prekallikrein to kallikrein. Finally, it can act on the third component of complement to produce C3a and on Factor XIIa to produce Factor XIIf.

Other proteolytic enzymes have been described. One is present in skin, and another, present in white blood cells, leads to the formation of leucokinin.

Biologically Active Cleavage Products of Complement

Activation of the complement system leads to the formation of two anaphylatoxins, C3a and C5a, which cause the release of histamine from mast cells. They also exert a chemotactic influence, as does C567 (p. 77). These components are impor-

tant in the pathogenesis of aggregate anaphylaxis and in the inflammation present in some lesions of immune-complex disease (p. 181). The alternate pathway of complement activation explains how vasoactive complement components can be formed following tissue damage which is not immunologically mediated. Necrotic tissue, e.g. heart muscle,[11] can release enzymes capable of activating C3, and so also can the lysosomal enzymes released from polymorphs. What part they play in inflammation in the non-immune animal and that due to trauma is not known.

Biologically Active Components of Polymorphs

Neutrophils release a variety of agents in acute inflammation. The following agents have been described:

Cationic proteins. These have various actions, including direct action on blood vessels to increase permeability, histamine-releasing factors, neutrophil-immobilising factor, and a chemotactic factor for monocytes.

Acid proteases. These act on a kininogen to produce a kinin (leucokinin).

Neutral proteases. These have been credited with many activities:— They degrade collagen, basement-membrane material, fibrin, etc., they cleave C3 and C5 to form active products, they activate kininogen to kinin, and they have a direct effect on blood vessels to increase their permeability. These actions are inhibited by α_1-antitrypsin.

The release of these various neutrophil substances may occur by a type of secretion, as the contents of granules are discharged by exocytosis—particularly during phagocytosis (Fig. 6.9). They are also released when the cell dies and undergoes autolysis. The action of *pyrogen* released by neutrophils is described in Chapter 37.

---

*The physiological role of these inhibitors is unclear. Patients deficient in C1-esterase inhibitor are subject to attacks of angio-oedema. The attacks seem to be precipitated by the action of plasmin in activating Factor XII, and thereby the kinin-forming mechanism, as well as activating complement. Subjects deficient in α_1-antitrypsin are liable to develop hepatic fibrosis in infancy or pulmonary emphysema in adult life.

It is evident that the role of polymorphs in acute inflammation is very complex. Under some circumstances they provide protection against micro-organisms, since infection introduced into animals rendered leucopenic can be spreading and lethal, while a similar infection in a normal animal would lead merely to a local acute inflammation. On the other hand, the damage seen in the lesions of the Shwartzman reaction and in the vasculitis of immune-complex disease appears to be produced by agents released by the polymorphs.

Vasoactive Acidic Lipids

The prostaglandins.[12] The name prostaglandin was given to a substance found in human seminal fluid by von Euler. Prostaglandins have been isolated from virtually every tissue of the body, and have been grouped on the basis of their chemical structure. They are derivatives of prostanoic acid, the 20-carbon parent substance. They are credited with many diverse functions—from acting as chemical transmitters in the nervous system to playing an important role in conception and parturition. Their role in thrombosis is described on page 488. They have been isolated in the tissues of human skin in allergic contact dermatitis,[13] and are released from polymorphs during phagocytosis.

Some, e.g. PGE_1 and PGE_2, produce vasodilatation, increase vascular permeability, and cause pain; others have converse effects, protecting tissues from these actions. An effect of some prostaglandins that may be of importance is their potentiation of the action of kinins in increasing vascular permeability. The prostaglandins may therefore be significant mediators of acute inflammation either by a direct action or, more likely, by regulating or *modulating* the action of other mediators.[14]

One important source of prostaglandin is the platelet, which contains prostaglandin-forming enzymes. It is significant that aspirin and indomethacin both inhibit the formation of prostaglandins from the substrate arachidonic acid;[15] this may well account for the hitherto unexplained anti-inflammatory action of aspirin. The release of prostaglandins from platelets is inhibited by glucocorticoids.

Slow-reacting substance of anaphylaxis (SRS-A). This vasoactive lipid is released from mast cells, and is described on page 176. It is not chemotactic to white cells. SRS-A is broken down by aryl sulphatase B, an enzyme found in eosinophils.

Other Possible Mediators of the Inflammatory Response

Many other possible mediators of acute inflammation have been described. *Lactic acid* is present in inflamed tissue, and may play a part in the vasodilatation and change in vascular permeability. The *lymphokines*, which are described in Chapter 12, are undoubtedly liberated in certain types of inflammation in which immune mechanisms are involved.

It is possible that some *bacterial toxins* are capable of directly initiating or modifying the inflammatory response. The gas-gangrene organisms, in particular *Cl. oedematiens*, produce toxins which appear to act directly upon blood vessels and increase their permeability. The kinases produced by some organisms, and wasp and snake venom are other examples of exogenous factors.

It is instructive to summarise the role of the mast cells and platelets at this point.

Role of the Mast Cell in Inflammation

The mast cells can release the contents of their granules when directly injured, and also in response to a number of other stimuli. C5a is a cleavage product of C5 (p. 159), and has such an action; it is the classical anaphylatoxin, so named because its formation, by causing the release of histamine, can produce a state resembling acute anaphylactic shock. C3a is another anaphylatoxin, but is less potent. Another agent is one of the cationic proteins of polymorphs. Mast-cell degranulation can be mediated immunologically; if the cells are coated with IgE, contact with antigen causes degranulation.

Mast cells release the following agents:
a. Histamine.
b. Slow-reacting substance of anaphylaxis—SRS-A.
c. Eosinophil-chemotactic factor of anaphylaxis—ECF-A.
d. Platelet-activating factor—this causes platelets to undergo the release reaction.

Role of the Platelets in Inflammation

Platelets become adherent to areas of vascular damage, and undergo a release reaction whereby the contents of their granules are liberated. The dense granules contain vasoactive amines (histamine or 5-HT according to species), while the α granules contain lysosomal enzymes.

Summary

The number of chemicals that have been suggested as mediators of acute inflammation is now so large, and their inter-relationship is so complex, that it is not possible to give any clear account of their role in acute inflammation. Indeed, as noted by Ryan and Majno, the inflammatory 'soup' is so complicated that no single individual can claim to know how the dozens of components relate to each other or how they change during the evolution of an inflammatory response.

Before any agent can be accepted as a mediator, Miles and Wilhelm have suggested that they should satisfy certain criteria:

Criteria supporting plausibility. The distribution and availability of the agent should be in keeping with its alleged actions. It should be capable of activation, and able to reproduce the change seen in inflammation. Natural antagonists should be present.

Criteria proving mediation. The agent should be isolated at the time of its proposed action; its actions should be suppressed by specific antagonists or by depleting the tissues of the mediator. With the exception of histamine, it is doubtful whether any of the proposed mediators fulfil all these criteria.

It is generally agreed that the exudation of acute inflammation involves both capillaries and venules. The capillaries are so narrow that any marked increase in their permeability would bring about their blockage; the resulting ischaemia would lead to a cessation of the inflammatory process and necrosis of the area involved. It is doubtful whether any such mechanism would be evolved. In support of this contention is the observation that capillaries do not respond to the action of vasoactive drugs. Hence it is unlikely that any mediator acts directly on the capillaries. On the other hand, capillaries do appear to respond to direct injury[16] (see the white line, p. 72, and the triple response). The present evidence suggests that the capillary changes in acute inflammation are due to a direct effect of the injuring agent— trauma or chemical or microbial toxin.

The venules, on the other hand, react to vasoactive drugs and mediators. Histamine is an accepted mediator of the early exudation of acute inflammation, and the kinins are probably important also. The prostaglandins probably modulate their actions. The mediators of the late and prolonged phases of inflammation remain enigmatic; every mediator mentioned in this chapter has at some time or another been proposed as a candidate.

The accumulation of inflammatory cells in inflammation is believed to be due to chemotaxis, and the most likely agents are the activated components of complement. The change in cell population from polymorph to macrophage, and the appearance of eosinophils in some inflammations, are related largely to the actions of different chemotactic agents that attract the particular cell in question.

Although much stress has been placed upon the uniformity of the inflammatory reaction regardless of its cause, it must not be forgotten that there is, in fact, also very considerable individual diversity, both in the amount of exudate and in the type of cell involved. This was stressed by Kettle, who recognised that the individuality of an inflammatory reaction was a reflection of the individuality of the agent causing it. It would be hard to deny the importance of many bacterial products; the leucocidins, haemolysins, kinases, permeability factors, etc., must all influence the final outcome. Products of tissue damage and mediators generated from plasma constituents are not the only agents present in the inflammation of infection. So far, much research has been done on the vasodilatation and increased vascular permeability of acute inflammation caused by trauma or chemical agents. The complex cellular changes and the intricacies of infection have been largely neglected. Until we have much more reliable information, the role of the individual chemical mediators in acute inflammation will remain ambiguous.

GENERAL READING

COHNHEIM, J. (1889) In *Lectures on General Pathology*. p. 248. London: New Sydenham Society. (This is a translation of the second edition of Cohnheim's book published in 1882.)

RYAN, G. B. & MAJNO, G. (1977) Acute inflammation. *American Journal of Pathology*, **86**, 183.

MOVAT, H. Z. (Ed.) (1971) *Inflammation, Immunity and Hypersensitivity*. New York: Harper and Row.

ZWEIFACH, B. W., GRANT, L. & McCLUSKEY, R. T. (Eds) (1974) *The Inflammatory Process*, 2nd edn, Vols 1–3. New York: Academic Press.

REFERENCES

1. RATHER, L. J. (1971) Disturbance of function (functio laesa): the legendary fifth cardinal sign of inflammation, added by Galen to the four cardinal signs of Celsus. *Bulletin of the New York Academy of Medicine*, **47**, 303.
2. SIMIONESCU, N., SIMIONESCU, M. & PALADE, G. E. (1975) Permeability of muscle capillaries to small heme-peptides. Evidence for the existence of patent transendothelial channels. *Journal of Cell Biology*, **64**, 586.
3. WARD, P. A. (1974) Leukotaxis and leukotactic disorders: a review. *American Journal of Pathology*, **77**, 520.
4. BOXER, L. A., HEDLEY-WHYTE, E. T. & STOSSEL, T. P. (1974) Neutrophil actin dysfunction and abnormal neutrophil behavior. *New England Journal of Medicine*, **291**, 1093.
5. STOSSEL, T. P. (1974) Phagocytosis. *New England Journal of Medicine*, **290**, 717, 774 and 833.
6. WEISSMANN, G. *et al.* (1971) Mechanisms of lysosomal enzyme release from leukocytes exposed to immune complexes and other particles. *Journal of Experimental Medicine*, **134**, 149S.
7. FRIDOVICH, I. (1974) Superoxide radical and the bactericidal action of phagocytes. *New England Journal of Medicine*, **290**, 624.
8. UNANUE, E. R. (1976) Secretory function of mononuclear phagocytes. *American Journal of Pathology*, **83**, 396.
9. TERRITO, M. C. & CLINE, M. J. (1975) Mononuclear phagocyte proliferation, maturation and function. *Clinics in Haematology*, **4**, 685.
10. HERSH, E. M. & BODEY, G. P. (1970) Leukocytic mechanisms in inflammation. *Annual Review of Medicine*, **21**, 105.
11. HILL, J. H. & WARD, P. A. (1971) The phlogistic role of C3 leukotactic fragments in myocardial infarcts in rats. *Journal of Experimental Medicine*, **133**, 885.
12. Leading Article: New light on inflammation (1971) *British Medical Journal*, **3**, 61.
13. GREAVES, M. W., SONDERGAARD, J. & McDONALD-GIBSON, W. (1971) Recovery of prostaglandins in human cutaneous inflammation. *British Medical Journal*, **2**, 258.
14. MARX, J. L. (1972) Prostaglandins: mediators of inflammation? *Science*, **177**, 780.
15. VANE, J. R. (1971) Inhibition of prostaglandin synthesis as a mechanism of action for aspirin-like drugs. *Nature New Biology*, **231**, 232.
16. HURLEY, J. V. (1972) *Acute Inflammation*. Edinburgh: Churchill Livingstone.

Chapter 7. The Body's Defences Against Infection

Micro-organisms can cause disease in two ways. Either they gain access to the tissues of the host, multiply and cause infection, or they manufacture powerful toxins which are subsequently introduced into the body and produce an intoxication.

Diseases caused by ingestion of preformed toxin need not be considered here in detail. Botulism and staphylococcal enterotoxic food poisoning provide typical examples; neither can be considered as bacterial infections any more than can ergotism be regarded as a fungal infection.

By far the most important method whereby micro-organisms cause disease is by their invasion of and *multiplication in the living tissues of the host*. This is the definition of *infection*, and organisms capable of producing it are termed *pathogens*. With the exception of some rare congenital conditions, all infection is derived from the external environment. The organisms may be injected directly into the host, but more usually they are first deposited on the surface of the body which is thereby contaminated. Infection may or may not follow.

Transmission of Organisms to the Body

The following modes of transmission are important:

Direct skin contact. Wound infection caused by soil or by the contact of a staphylococcal carrier is a most important example; the venereal diseases, e.g. syphilis and gonorrhoea are other examples. Contaminated air is important in causing wound infections in hospitals.

Inhalation of droplets and dust.[1] It is generally assumed that influenza, whooping-cough, the common viral diseases of childhood, meningococcal infections, diphtheria, and streptococcal sore throat are spread by droplet infection. Experimental findings have not entirely supported this belief.

Droplets are produced when air passing rapidly over a mucous membrane causes atomisation of the secretion which covers it. A few of these droplets are large (Flugge droplets), and due to the effect of gravity have a limited range. The vast majority are smaller than 100 μm in diameter, and dry up almost instantaneously to form droplet nuclei which stay suspended in the air for many hours.

Droplet formation occurs during talking, coughing, and particularly sneezing; the main source is from the *saliva in the front of the mouth*. Only during snorting is the nose an important source of droplets. The viruses of mumps, measles, smallpox, and chickenpox are found in the saliva, and these diseases may well be spread in this way. However, bacteria residing in the nose (*Staphylococcus aureus*), nasopharynx (*Streptococcus pyogenes*), or lung (tubercle bacilli) do not commonly reach the front of the mouth, and it is very unlikely that droplets are an important vehicle of their spread. Some may be expectorated as sputum, but the most important means of dissemination is by the fingers and handkerchief. Using fluorescein or test organisms as markers, it has been found that normal human beings frequently dispense nasal secretions and saliva to their hands, face, and clothing, and to every object that is touched. After desiccation the organisms are readily disseminated in the form of dust particles, and it is these which are important in the transmission of many infections.

Ingestion of contaminated food. Food may be contaminated by a human carrier, e.g. typhoid, or by flies. These insects carry many pathogenic organisms on their hairy legs. Diseases transmitted by food include typhoid fever, bacillary dysentery, and amoebiasis. Poliomyelitis and type A hepatitis are acquired by ingestion. Milk and eggs may contain bacteria because the animal itself is diseased, e.g. bovine tuberculosis, brucellosis, and *Salmonella* infections of fowls.

Inoculation. The agent may be an insect whose bite transmits pathogenic organisms, e.g. arboviruses, *Yersinia pestis*, and rickettsiae, or it may be a needle contaminated with one of the viruses of hepatitis.

Transplacental spread. This occurs in secondary syphilis, toxoplasmosis, *Listeria monocytogenes* infection, and also some viral diseases (see p. 274). Disease produced by the infection of a germ-cell before fertilisation is not recorded in human pathology.

Contamination

This is the transfer of organisms on to any object. It may be a surgical instrument, clothing, food, or a body surface.

The contamination of the body, both externally on the skin and internally in the intestinal, respiratory, and other tracts is inevitable, and many of these surfaces are habitually colonised by organisms of low-grade pathogenicity, e.g. *Staph. albus* in the skin and *Strept. viridans* in the mouth and throat. Such organisms are called *commensals*, or *resident flora*, and as will be shown later, play an important role in the decontamination of these surfaces against pathogenic organisms. Contamination with virulent organisms is certainly a common event, but infection is rare. Whether contamination with a particular pathogen is followed by infection is dependent upon:

1. *The mechanical integrity* of the body surface.

2. Its powers of removing organisms, i.e. its *powers of decontamination*.

These protective mechanisms vary greatly from one tissue to another, and each will therefore be considered separately.

THE SKIN

The skin is frequently contaminated, and its value as a protective coat ranks second only to its water-retaining properties. Its exposed position renders it liable to both major and minor physical trauma. Its protective function is carried out mainly by the epidermis, and indeed the inability of the subepithelial tissues to resist infection was one of the limiting factors in pre-Listerian surgery. Its defences are:

Mechanical Strength

The many layers of epithelial cells, the tough outer layer of keratin, and the distinct basement membrane all play a part. If this mechanical barrier is impaired, infection is almost inevitable. Excessive sweating may macerate the keratin layer; for this reason skin infections are very common in the tropics, and boils are frequently seen in moist areas like the axillae.

Intact skin appears to be completely impervious to invasion by organisms, and it is only after injury that infection can be established. Even in vaccination against smallpox minor trauma by pressure is necessary for a successful infection. Following trauma the skin becomes the portal of entry for staphylococci, streptococci, and the clostridia. In the tropics insect bites penetrate the skin barrier, and serve to introduce the causative agents of plague, typhus, yellow fever, malaria, dengue, etc.

Decontamination[2]

The powers of decontamination of the skin may be demonstrated by deliberately contaminating the hands with haemolytic streptococci, and estimating their rate of disappearance by subsequently taking swabs at regular intervals. It is found that the organism can no longer be recovered after 2 to 3 hours. The actual time taken for the skin to rid itself of organisms depends upon the organism concerned, and in some cases is as short as 10 minutes. The mechanisms involved may be considered under three headings—mechanical, biological, and chemical:

Mechanical. *Desquamation* of the surface squames removes some superficial organisms.

Desiccation is probably of some importance in destroying organisms on the surface of the skin.

Biological. Organisms normally present on the skin constitute the *resident flora*. These include *Staph. albus*, diphtheroids, sarcinae, and aerobic sporing bacilli. In addition about 25 per cent of people harbour *Staph. aureus* particularly on the hands, face, and perineum. It is impossible to remove the resident organisms from the skin; they survive in the gland ducts, and though the surface may be disinfected, the organisms are soon replaced. It is probable that the flora plays an important part in the decontaminating mechanism both by producing antibiotic substances and by competing with other organisms for essential foodstuffs.

Chemical. *Acidity of sweat.*[2] The sweat is normally acid and is unsuitable for the growth of most pathogens. The bactericidal activity is probably due to its lactic acid content. If sweating is induced, the pH is said to fall, and may at times be as low as 3. There are certain gaps in this acid coat: these are the alkaline areas where infection is quite common, e.g. axillae, groins, and interdigital clefts of the toes.

Unsaturated fatty acids. These are present in the sebaceous secretion and are bactericidal; it is interesting that some of the diphtheroids grow only in the presence of these fatty acids, so well are they adapted to their environment.

There is no doubt that the mechanical strength together with the decontaminating mechanisms are of great importance in maintaining the integrity of the skin. When one remembers how often it must be contaminated with all types of organisms, and, apart from staphylococci, how rarely it is invaded, one appreciates its efficiency as a protective coat.

THE ALIMENTARY TRACT

THE MOUTH AND THROAT

As with the skin the defence mechanism is two-fold:

Mechanical Strength

The toughness and integrity of the mucous membrane is important; this mechanical barrier is weakest at two points:

The gingival margin has only a thin epithelium, and is therefore easily traumatised. This is particularly so in the interdental region, where it is believed that a covering epithelium is present only in young healthy adults.

The tonsillar crypts. Here the epithelium is very thin; it has been shown that carmine powder dusted on to the tonsils appears in the underlying cells and connective tissue within 20 minutes. Probably the dye is transported there by phagocytes which are normally resident on the surface. Organisms may similarly reach the subepithelial tissue, and it is therefore these two sites, the tonsils and the gum margins, that are the places where infection occurs when the general body defences are impaired, e.g. in acute leukaemia and agranulocytosis. Nevertheless, it is remarkable how the tissues of the mouth, including the bone, can resist infection even after the contamination that follows dental extraction. Some form of 'tissue immunity' must be postulated, but its nature is unknown.

Decontamination

Mechanical. The continual backward flow of saliva traps organisms, which are then swallowed. Carbon particles placed on the mucosa are removed from the mouth in 15 to 30 minutes.[2]

Biological. As in the skin the resident flora is important. These organisms are α-haemolytic streptococci (*Strept. viridans*), *Neisseria pharyngis*, diphtheroids, lactobacilli*, pneumococci, *Borrelia vincenti*, actinomyces organisms, *Candida albicans*, and various *Bacteroidaceae*. Many strains of α-haemolytic streptococci produce hydrogen peroxide,[2] and this has been thought to play some part in the decontaminating mechanism.†

Chemical. The saliva inhibits many pathogens: this may be due to its *mucin*, *lysozyme*, and *antibody* content.

Lysozyme[3,4] is an acetylaminopolysaccharidase and acts on the muramic acid of the bacterial cell wall. The name *mura-*

---

*Lactobacilli are non-sporing, Gram-positive bacilli, usually microaerophilic, and conspicuously acid resistant. They are an important element in the commensal flora of the mouth, gastrointestinal tract, and vagina.

†In this connexion the rare Japanese hereditary disorder of *acatalasia* is of interest. The enzyme catalase which normally breaks down H_2O_2 is absent from the blood, and peroxide formed in the mouth produces sufficient damage to cause ulcerating, gangrenous lesions in the mouth.

midase has therefore been proposed for this agent which was first described by Fleming. By attacking the cell wall, lysozyme is able to lyse some bacteria, mostly the non-pathogens. With many organisms, however, the cell membrane must be damaged by the activation of complement or by the action of peroxides or other agents before destruction is complete. Lysozyme is present in many of the body's secretions and also in polymorphs.

Antibody. The presence of IgA antibody in many secretions (tears, colostrum, saliva, and the secretions of the respiratory, gastrointestinal, and lower urinary tracts) is important in protecting these systems from microbial infection. The antibody is produced locally and is passed into the secretion as a dimer linked to a distinct secretory peptide.

In spite of these mechanisms, potent pathogens can adapt themselves to the mouth and throat, e.g. meningococci, diphtheria bacilli, *Haemophilus influenzae*, and *Strept. pyogenes*. These may lead to infection, but if the person has considerable immunity, they may remain as 'transients' for a period of time. Such carriers are of great importance in the spread of streptococcal infections, diphtheria, and meningococcal meningitis.

SALIVARY GLANDS

The regular flow of saliva is important, for when secretion is suppressed as in conditions of shock, dehydration, and fever, or as a consequence of infective processes or neoplasia, the lips, tongue, teeth, and remainder of the mouth become coated with a mixture of food particles and dead epithelial cells. If this is not actively removed, it becomes the site of bacterial colonisation. This may result in an ascending infection of the salivary glands terminating in suppurative sialadenitis.

THE STOMACH

The stomach stands guard over the intestines, and in the human being is the first part of the alimentary tract not lined by stratified squamous epithelium. It deals not only with food, but also with the secretions of the mouth and swallowed sputum. Its defence mechanisms are:

Mechanical Strength

The continuity of the epithelium is probably not important. Acute erosions are common, and neither these nor the more serious chronic ulcers appear to provide points of entry for organisms.

Decontamination

Mechanical. Vomiting removes chemical and bacterial irritants, but is of little value in combating infection.

Biological. Under normal conditions the gastric juice is sterile.

Chemical. Without doubt the bactericidal activity of gastric juice is due to its hydrochloric acid content and not its enzymes. Proteolytic enzymes do not often kill organisms, and gastric juice loses its bactericidal activity when neutralised.

Fig 7.1 shows the levels of hydrochloric acid usually attained in the stomach following the ingestion of a meal. It is apparent that organisms such as *Strept. pyogenes*, diphtheria bacilli, pneumococci, and rhinoviruses are most unlikely to pass through the acid barrier of the stomach into the intestine. Staphylococci and *Salmonella* organisms will probably pass if ingested with food or large quantities of fluid; likewise enteroviruses can withstand moderate acidity. Milk with its potent antacid properties is a particularly favourable vehicle for organisms, e.g. *Brucella abortus*, though in fact any food is liable to have a protective action. Cholera is more likely to follow the ingestion of the organisms if the patient has

Figure 7.1
The gastric bactericidal barrier. The shaded area represents the limits of free HCl in 80 per cent of normal people following a meal. The horizontal bands are drawn at the average free acid strengths which in 20 minutes are lethal to the three bacterial groups: Group 1. *Esch. coli* and *Kl. pneumoniae*; Group 2. *S. typhi*, *Shigella* species, and *Staph. aureus*; Group 3. *Strept. pyogenes*, *Strept. viridans*, pneumococci, *N. catarrhalis*, and *C. diphtheriae*. Spore-bearing organisms are resistant to acid and cannot be shown on the chart. (*From Knott, F. A.* (1923), Guy's Hosp. Rep., **73**, 429).

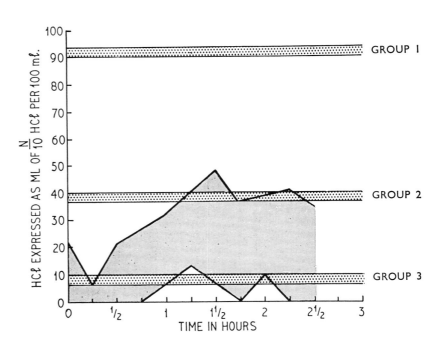

achlorhydria or has had a partial gastrectomy.[5] Coliform organisms in general are able to withstand the acidity of the stomach, as can also the cysts of *Entamoeba histolytica*. The tubercle bacillus can resist acid due to its waxy content, and therefore intestinal tuberculosis may occur when bacilli are swallowed. Gastric aspiration is carried out extensively as a diagnostic procedure in childhood tuberculosis.

The gastric contents are colonised with various organisms, and become very offensive, whenever they are dammed back as the result of pyloric stenosis. This is particularly well marked when the cause is pyloric cancer, where there is often achlorhydria.

THE INTESTINE

The intestine undoubtedly relies upon the stomach's protective action. The minor intestinal upsets of infancy may in part be related to the low gastric acidity in this age-group. Europeans living in tropical climates, especially before becoming acclimatised, usually develop hypochlorhydria, and this may be a factor in the troublesome diarrhoea that so often afflicts them. The intestine has, however, its own defence mechanism.

Mechanical Barrier

As in the stomach this is probably not important. It is interesting that some organisms, e.g. *Salmonella typhi* and the tubercle bacillus, can penetrate the mucosa without causing obvious damage. Probably phagocytes are normally present on the surface of the gut ready to ingest passing organisms. These are carried into the tissues so that infection follows. This mechanism whereby bacteria and probably also intact protein molecules gain access to the tissues may well be of great importance in the immunological development of the individual.

Decontamination

Mechanical. The development of diarrhoea is common in intestinal infection, and helps to expel the organism. If this symptom is suppressed with drugs, the disease tends to be more severe. Although in minor infections this effect may be unimportant, in typhoid fever it can be serious.

Biological. The small intestine generally contains few organisms, whereas the colon is heavily contaminated with coliforms, faecal and anaerobic streptococci, and clostridia. Spirochaetes (*Borrelia*) have been described.[6] Organisms of the genus *Bacteroides* form an important component of the intestinal flora, but are often overlooked because of the difficulties in their culture. The *Lactobacillus bifidus* occurs in breast-fed infants, and the acidity it produces is probably beneficial. Although the importance of the flora is well known, the exact mechanisms involved are not established. Some enteric bacilli release highly specific proteins called *colicines* which can kill other organisms in a variety of ways. When the flora is upset by the broad-spectrum antibiotics, superinfection with *Staph. aureus* may be a fatal complication (see p. 217).

Pseudomembranous colitis[7] is an occasional complication of broad-spectrum antibiotic therapy, particularly in postoperative patients. A characteristic, superficial, greenish-black slough of necrotic mucosa covers the colon, and there is bleeding and diarrhoea. Imbalance of the bacterial flora is one possible cause, and direct drug toxicity or a hypersensitivity reaction have also been postulated. Most cases are probably due to ischaemia of the bowel secondary to shock (p. 517).

Another indication of the importance of the bacterial flora is the experiment in which it was found possible to produce cholera regularly in adult guinea-pigs by preparing them with oral streptomycin. The animals are normally resistant to *Vibrio cholerae*.

Chemical. IgA antibodies secreted locally by plasma cells are important in providing the mucous membranes with local immunity (p. 144). It should also be noted that the lymphoid tissue of the intestine may act as the central organ responsible for the development of the peripheral lymphoid tissues destined to produce all classes of immunoglobulins (p. 151). The bile salts in the intestinal secretion destroy the infectivity of enveloped viruses (p. 267). Hence only enteroviruses, adenoviruses, reoviruses, and the viruses of hepatitis reach the intestine.

The appendix is one of the weakest links in the alimentary tract, the reason for which is not known. Possibly damage by hard concretions and the ease with which its lumen can be obstructed play a part, but it is astonishing how little we know about the cause of such a common disease as acute appendicitis.

THE CONJUNCTIVAL SAC

Although the exposed moist surface is subject to frequent contamination, infection is comparatively rare. The conjunctival sac relies partly upon the mechanical washing effect of the tears and partly upon their composition. The tears contain the highest concentration of *lysozyme* of any body fluid examined (see p. 87).

THE EAR[8]

The external auditory canal contains ear wax which is the combined product of sebaceous and ceruminous glands. Most of the Black and White races have wet, sticky, honey-coloured ear wax which contains IgA antibody and lysozyme*.[9]

THE RESPIRATORY TRACT

The respiratory tract acts as a whole, the upper part functioning as an air-conditioner for the lungs. The vibrissae filter off large particles, but the main filter is the nasal mucosa itself, covering as it does the complicated ramification of the turbinates. Not only is the inspired air warmed and humidified, but the mucus-covered surface traps organisms and particles just as flies are trapped on fly-paper. The anterior nares are distinct from the remainder of the respiratory tract, because their epithelium and bacterial flora resemble those of the skin. Their great importance lies in their frequent colonisation by *Staph. aureus*.

---

*It is of interest that among the Mongolian races over 80 per cent of people have grey, brittle, dry wax which contains IgG. Wet ear wax is determined by the presence of a dominant *W* gene.[10] Closely linked is axillary odour. Hence in a race like the Japanese, in whom the *W* gene is uncommon, the few who possess it have wet ear wax and an axillary odour.

THE NOSE AND NASOPHARYNX

Mechanical Barrier

The epithelium of the respiratory tract does not provide an adequate barrier against local infection. This is well demonstrated by the ease with which rhinoviruses and adenoviruses cause acute upper respiratory tract infection. Meningococci are apparently able to penetrate the mucosa of the nasopharynx without much difficulty (see p. 227).

Decontamination[11, 12]

Irritants are expelled by the act of sneezing. If organisms are deliberately implanted in the nose, they disappear within 15 minutes. One of the main mechanisms involved is the continuous flow of mucus backwards to the nasopharynx. The nasal secretion is both bactericidal and virucidal: antibodies have been demonstrated in it against influenza and poliomyelitis viruses (see p. 89). Lysozyme and lactoferrin are also present. Nevertheless, pathogens like meningococci and diphtheria bacilli can colonise the nose, and carriers of these constitute an important reservoir of human infection. The fact that the olfactory mucosa is non-ciliated and has beneath it much lymphoid tissue has been held to explain why some organisms gain entry through this area. Experimentally dye, proteins, and viruses can be shown to penetrate the olfactory mucosa and enter the underlying lymphoid tissue.

The nasopharynx has a resident bacterial flora similar to that of the throat (especially *Strept. viridans* and *Neisseria pharyngis*), and this has a biological decontaminating function.

THE TRACHEA AND LOWER RESPIRATORY TRACT

Mechanical Barrier

Below the larynx the respiratory tract should normally be sterile. The mucosa itself forms a poor mechanical barrier as in the nose, and is frequently infected by the influenza virus.

Decontamination[11, 12]

Mechanical. The cough reflex initiated by stimulating the larynx or upper trachea expels irritants, but may also disseminate organisms within the lung. Although the diameter of the air passages decreases steadily with each division from the trachea downwards, the total cross-sectional area increases. Thus it has been estimated that the total cross-sectional area of all the respiratory bronchioles is over 100 times that of the trachea. It follows that the velocity of the inspired air steadily decreases as it passes down the air passages, and this allows particles to fall out of the stream and adhere to the mucus-covered wall by a process of sedimentation. Most particles larger than 10 μm are removed in this way, and do not reach the alveoli. Nevertheless, some large particles, e.g. asbestos fibres, do reach the depths of the lung, presumably because of their construction as long, thin fibres.

The film of fluid which covers the mucosa is derived partly by transudation and partly from the secretions of surface goblet cells and the underlying mucous glands. By its chemical composition it protects the epithelial cells from dangerous gases, e.g. sulphur dioxide, and its proper consistency allows the cilia to move it on as a continuous sheet. The sheet of mucus ever moving upwards, at a rate of about 2 cm per minute, by ciliary activity is an important decontaminating mechanism, and any obstruction to it impairs the defences of the respiratory tract.

This frequently leads to infection, and is well seen in the bronchopneumonia which follows the obstruction caused by a foreign body or carcinoma. Ciliary action may also be impaired in bronchitis and bronchiectasis, when the normal epithelium is replaced by goblet or squamous cells. Another very important cause of breakdown of the respiratory decontaminating mechanism is the epithelial destruction caused by viral infection, e.g. influenza and measles. A similar effect is seen in whooping-cough and following the inhalation of poison gases, e.g. chlorine, phosgene, and nitrogen peroxide. Chemicals (e.g. SO_2 and tobacco smoke), drugs (e.g. atropine), cold air, and alcohol taken by mouth impair ciliary action and delay clearance from the lung. So also does the inhalation of a high concentration of oxygen; this effect, observed in the experimental animal, may be of clinical significance when giving patients with chronic chest disease oxygen therapy. Alterations in the consistency of mucus, as for example in chronic bronchitis or chronic venous congestion, when there is excessive transudation, may also impair mucociliary action.

In the respiratory bronchioles and alveoli mucociliary streams play little part in the defence of the lung, and it is here that the macrophages, or septal cells, are important. Bacteria are phagocytosed by these cells and killed in their cytoplasm. The energy for phagocytosis is provided by aerobic meta-

Figure 7.2

Macrophages in alveoli of lung. These large round cells ingest foreign particles inhaled into the lung. They phagocytose organisms, blood pigments, dust, etc. They are known as "heart-failure cells", "dust cells" etc., according to the condition that evokes their outpouring. $\times 250$.

bolism (cf. p. 78), and the hypoxia engendered by collapse or oedema might be a factor in predisposing such an area of lung to infection (Fig. 7.2)

Chemical. The bronchial mucus contains lactoferrin, lysozyme, and antibodies. Both IgG and IgM are present, but it is probable that the IgA is the most important. Nevertheless, patients with a low IgA do not seem to be particularly prone to respiratory-tract infections.[13] Cellular antibodies are also important in the defence of the lung against infection. The inhalation of vaccines has been investigated as a means of producing both cellular and humoral local immunity.

THE URINARY TRACT

Antibacterial and antiviral substances have been found in urine, but in fact the continuous flushing action of urine together with its acidity are probably of much greater importance in maintaining the sterility of the urinary tract. Obstruction always favours infection, as is seen in urethral stricture, prostatic enlargement, pregnancy, stones, and bladder diverticula. It is generally agreed that most infection arises from the lower urinary tract and reaches the ureters and kidneys by reflux from the bladder. The greater frequency of urinary infection in the female has been attributed to the shortness of the female urethra. An alternative explanation is that the male is protected by the bactericidal activity of the prostatic secretions rather than the length of the urethra.[14, 15]

Bacteria which remain on the bladder wall are believed to be killed by humoral factors or engulfed by the bladder epithelium.[16] The same probably applies to the upper urinary passages.

Some urinary-tract infection may be blood borne and attack the kidneys primarily (see p. 132).

THE FEMALE GENITAL TRACT

The vagina is protected by an acid barrier (pH 4·3–5·5) produced by the resident lactobacilli (Döderlein's bacilli), which ferment glycogen from the desquamated squamous cells to produce lactic acid. As oestrogens are responsible for the glycogen content of these cells, this acid barrier is absent in childhood and old age. Acute vulvovaginitis is therefore seen only in these two age groups.

It will be appreciated that each of the surfaces of the body is provided with a mechanism for either removing microorganisms or resisting their penetration.

Only after they have penetrated the surface epithelial barrier, either by their own efforts or as the result of trauma, can the organisms exert their influence upon the underlying tissue. If pathogenic, their continued multiplication invariably gives rise to infection.

REFERENCES

1. HARE, R. (1964) The transmission of respiratory infections. *Proceedings of the Royal Society of Medicine*, **57**, 221.
2. WILSON, G. S. & MILES, A. A. (1975) In Topley and Wilson's *Principles of Bacteriology, Virology and Immunity*, 6th edn, p. 1303. London: Arnold.
3. OSSERMAN, E. F. (1975) Lysozyme. *New England Journal of Medicine*, **292**, 424.
4. MASON, D. Y. & TAYLOR, C. R. (1975) The distribution of muramidase (lysozyme) in human tissues. *Journal of Clinical Pathology*, **28**, 124.
5. Leading article (1975) Susceptibility to cholera. *British Medical Journal*, **4**, 423.
6. LEE, F. D. *et al.* (1971) Intestinal spirochaetosis. *Gut*, **12**, 126.
7. SCOTT, A. J., NICHOLSON, G. I. & KERR, A. R. (1973) Lincomycin as a cause of pseudomembranous colitis. *Lancet*, **2**, 1232.
8. HYSLOP, N. E. (1971) Ear wax and host defense. *New England Journal of Medicine*, **284**, 1099.
9. PETRAKIS., N. L. *et al.* (1971) Demonstration and implications of lysozyme and immunoglobulins in human ear wax. *Nature (London)*, **229**, 119.
10. MATSUNAGA, E. (1962) The dimorphism in human normal cerumen. *Annals of Human Genetics*, **25**, 273.
11. NEWHOUSE, M., SANCHIS, J. & BIENENSTOCK, J. (1976) Lung defense mechanisms. *New England Journal of Medicine*, **295**, 990 and 1045.
12. Leading Article (1976) In defence of the lungs. *British Medical Journal*, **1**, 733.
13. Leading Article (1975) Selective IgA deficiency. *Lancet*, **2**, 1291.
14. STAMEY, T. A. *et al.* (1968) Antibacterial nature of prostatic fluid. *Nature (London)*, **218**, 444.
15. Leading Article (1968) Defence mechanisms of the bladder. *Lancet*, **1**, 1183.
16. Leading Article (1972) Renal localization of infection. *British Medical Journal*, **4**, 252.

Chapter 8. The Body's Response to Infection

When organisms gain access to the tissues of the body their fate depends upon the resultant of two factors: the immunity of the host and the virulence of the organism, both of which are in reality different facets of the same thing, as is explained in Chapter 13.

The possible end-results are:

1. Rapid destruction of the organisms, e.g. non-pathogens.

2. The organisms grow for a time, but are soon destroyed, e.g. minor or subclinical infection.

3. The organisms enter into a symbiotic state with the host, e.g. herpes-simplex virus.

4. There is local proliferation of organisms producing tissue damage, but little spread of infection, e.g. a boil due to staphylococcal infection.

5. Organisms may proliferate locally and produce severe damage to distant tissues by means of a soluble exotoxin. The local lesion may be insignificant, as in tetanus, or severe, as in diphtheria.

6. A local lesion is produced, but rapid spread of organisms follows, e.g. cellulitis due to *Strept. pyogenes*.

7. No local lesion forms, but the organism rapidly spreads, e.g. European typhus due to *Rickettsia prowazeki*.

8. No local lesion forms initially, but the organism spreads rapidly and later a lesion develops at the portal of entry, e.g. syphilis, typhoid fever, and scrub typhus due to *Rickettsia tsutsugamushi*.

9. The organism induces cellular proliferation, e.g. Rous's sarcoma virus. Proliferation may occur and is later followed by necrosis, e.g. smallpox virus.

This list is by no means complete. Thus, the slow viruses produce a type of infection which appears to be unique, but is not well understood. Cholera is peculiar in that the organisms multiply in the gut, and produce a toxin which increases the permeability of the blood vessels and causes oversecretion of the epithelial cells; yet the organism never penetrates beyond the basement membrane.[1] It is obvious in this example how difficult it is to separate true infection from intoxication.

Some of these possibilities will be examined in greater detail.

If organisms are non-pathogenic they are unable to multiply in the tissues; they are phagocytosed by polymorphs and macrophages and destroyed in the cytoplasm of these cells. It is often difficult to understand why some organisms cannot infect or grow in certain tissues. For example, the gonococcus is unable to grow in animal tissues, and yet is capable of causing human infection. It can grow outside the body on relatively simple media, and yet does not grow in tissues other than those of the human subject. The organisms can multiply in human polymorphonuclear leucocytes, but not in those of other animals. It seems that genetic factors are involved; this aspect of host-organism relationship is further considered in connexion with innate immunity (see p. 162).

Specific receptors are required for cells to be susceptible to certain infections. Thus the Duffy antigens Fy(a+) or Fy(b+) are necessary for the parasitisation of red cells by *Plasmodium vivax*[2] (p. 645). A further elegant demonstration of the relationship between genes and infection has come from a different quarter. Hybrid human-mouse cell lines can be prepared, and during their growth human chromosomes are eliminated preferentially. Mouse cells are not susceptible to infection with poliovirus, but the hybrid cells are susceptible only so long as human chromosome 19 is present. Hence it can be induced that this chromosome bears a gene for the poliovirus receptor.[3] It remains to be discovered whether receptors are required for other pathogens. The subject is likely to be complex: thus if the RNA of poliovirus is introduced into a mouse cell, viral replication can take place.

If an organism is capable of causing disease, it is called *pathogenic* and has the ability to grow in the tissues, and thereby cause infection. The type and severity of this infection depend on the virulence of the organism. The term *virulent* is sometimes applied to strains of an organism which have a special ability to produce severe disease. Certain strains of *Corynebacterium diphtheriae* are more virulent than others due to their greater ability to produce toxin. This implies that, while all strains of *C. diphtheriae* are pathogenic, some produce a more severe disease than others. Similar variations occur with other exotoxin-producing organisms, e.g. *Clostridium welchii*, but the term virulence is also used in connexion with an invasive organism like *Staph. aureus*. The ability of virulent strains of such an organism to produce severe disease is often not related to toxin production, but rather to some subtle alteration in the organism itself, probably in its antigenic structure. Virulence in invasive organisms can be considered under two headings:

1. *The ability of the organism to spread.*

2. *The ability of the organism to produce tissue damage.*

The ability to spread, in respect of many organisms, is inversely proportional to their tendency to produce initial local damage and a subsequent inflammatory reaction. Thus pathogenic organisms whose presence seems to excite little immediate inflammatory reaction (like *Mycobacterium leprae*, *Yersinia pestis*, and many rickettsiae and viruses), are able to spread widely without leaving any trace of their site of entry. Some organisms, although behaving essentially in the same manner, do produce diseases in which a lesion later develops at the site of entry. Syphilis is an excellent example of this; the local lesion (chancre) occurs long after the organisms have spread throughout the body, and this is presumably due to a hypersensitivity reaction. Hence, another way in which organisms may produce damage is by interacting with sensitising antibodies.[4] This is best documented with certain viral infections. Measles and respiratory syncytial virus may be more destructive in partially immunised individuals than in the non-immune (p. 274). The subject is further discussed in the section on immune complexes and disease (p. 181).

The existence of L-forms (Appendix 2) raises many possibilities. They are generally considered to be non-pathogenic, but following an overt infection they might remain in the tissues in a dormant form and provide sufficient antigen to sustain an immunological response. Rheumatic carditis and chronic post-streptococcal glomerulonephritis are obvious candidates for such a pathogenesis. L-forms might also revert to type; this could explain recurrent infections, e.g. chronic pyelonephritis and infective endocarditis.

With those organisms which do cause considerable local tissue damage, other mechanisms may enable them to spread. By producing toxins, leucocidins, fibrinolysin, hyaluronidase, etc., they may effectively counteract the body's attempt at localisation. In this way a severe local response will be followed by spread: this type of infection is seen typically with *Strept. pyogenes* and *Cl. welchii*.

Some organisms produce local damage, but have little tendency to spread. The result is a local inflammatory response which may either pass unnoticed (subclinical infection) or else be severe, e.g. a carbuncle due to *Staph. aureus*.

Finally, by not causing damage the organism may enter into a symbiotic state with the host. There are many instances of this in the lower animals. The chloroplasts of some protozoa are, for example, symbiotic algae. Many arthropods harbour rickettsiae in their cells, and indeed are infected from the ovum at the time of their conception. Sometimes the relationship is unstable; rats may carry the organism *Bartonella bacilliformis* in their red cells without harm, but if a splenectomy is performed, the animals die of acute haemolytic anaemia. Similarly, the human may harbour the virus of herpes simplex without ill effects until the development of some other infection, e.g. pneumonia, malaria, or Weil's disease, causes the characteristic lesion of herpes febrilis to appear. Adenoviruses may also lie latent in the tissues. A factor of great theoretical interest is that the host may exhibit *specific tolerance* to some organisms with which it shares common antigens (see p. 167).

Organisms which resist the decontaminating mechanisms of the body surfaces and are introduced into the tissues, may thus produce a variety of response patterns. The possibilities given on page 92 are examples of what can happen Intermediate states also exist; one type of organism may under varying circumstances produce different responses. Thus *Strept. pyogenes* may enter the body through an insignificant lesion, and rapidly kill the patient with septicaemia (pattern 7). Alternately the organism may produce a relatively minor infection such as a sore throat.

The Manner in Which Organisms Produce Damage[5]

Organisms which are capable of causing damage may do this in several ways.

Some organisms form powerful soluble *exotoxins* which produce local tissue damage. Diphtheria and gas-gangrene are diseases in which this occurs. The toxin also acts on distant tissues which it reaches *via* the blood stream. The cardiac and neurological lesions in diphtheria are produced in this way. Sometimes the toxin acts only at a distance (*Cl. tetani*). It should be noted that the lesions produced by circulating toxin are themselves sterile. The distribution of lesions depends on the sensitivity of tissues to the action of the toxin and also on their accessibility. Thus, in the guinea-pig circulating diphtheria toxin can pass the 'blood-nerve' barrier and escape into peripheral nerves, but it does not reach the spinal cord.

Exotoxins were the first toxic bacterial products to be identified. They are freely diffusible, and therefore found in the medium of a bacterial culture. They can be purified, identified, and estimated with relative ease. Their mode of action is known in many cases. On a quantitative basis they are very potent—botulinum toxin is the most poisonous substance known. Organisms whose main offensive weapon is an exotoxin are called *toxic organisms*. Examples of these are the causative organisms of diphtheria, tetanus, gas-gangrene, scarlet fever, *Shigella dysenteriae* dysentery, and botulism; the last is not an infection, but an intoxication.

With most other organisms, however, no such powerful toxins have been demonstrated. Cultures may be toxic to animals, but the responsible substances seem to be derived from the bodies of the organisms. These have been called *endotoxins*, but in reality they are the complex constituents of the bacterial body, being of protein-lipopolysaccharide constitution. The properties of exotoxins and endotoxins are summarised in Table 13.1, page 165.

Further investigations of the endotoxic group of organisms have shown that some substances do indeed diffuse out of the living cell bodies. The coagulase of *Staph. aureus* is one such substance. Some authorities call these substances exotoxins, but this is probably an error of judgement; it is even debatable whether substances like coagulase, hyaluronidase, etc. are 'toxins' at all. Therefore whatever the theoretical arguments, in practice the term exotoxins should be restricted to those substances which diffuse easily out of the organism, are highly toxic, causing some or many of the lesions of the disease, and are powerfully antigenic.

Organisms which do not produce exotoxins as defined above are called *invasive*. This term serves a useful purpose, because (with certain exceptions related to immune-complex reactions noted below) it emphasises that lesions can be produced only in the acutal presence of the organism. Generalised disease can occur only as a consequence of the systemic spread of the organisms. The clostridia of gas-gangrene, typically toxic organisms, can also spread widely in the local tissues, but except as a terminal event they do not invade the blood stream and lead to generalised colonisation of the viscera.

Strept. pyogenes provides several examples of exceptions to the above rule, for although it is an invasive organism, it can produce sterile lesions at a distance because of the development of hypersensitivity to its products. In this way acute glomerulonephritis and rheumatic fever are explained, as also the erythema nodosum and anaphylactoid purpura that occasionally follow streptococcal infection. In spite of these difficulties these two terms will be retained, because the division of organisms into 'toxic' and 'invasive' categories serves many useful purposes, especially in relationship to immunity.

Mechanisms of Damage by Invasive Organisms

The manner in which the invasive organisms produce damage is not clearly understood. Some seem to have a direct action on the tissues, and produce necrosis and acute inflammation. The pyogenic organisms fall into this group. In infection with many other organisms the situation is much more complicated. Typhoid fever and paratyphoid fever illustrate this particularly well.*

Typhoid fever. Although the evolution of the human disease is not completely known, experimental work on mice infected with *Salmonella typhimurium* (mouse typhoid) has done much to elucidate the mode of spread of the organism. During the first 24 hours following the ingestion of *S. typhimurium* the organisms can be recovered only from the contents of the gut. During the second 24 hours they are present in the mesenteric lymph nodes, and by the third day they have reached the blood, liver, and spleen. In the human disease the tempo is slower than this, but by analogy the sequence of events is probably as follows:

After being ingested, the organisms reach the contents of the small intestine; here they are taken up by phagocytes, enter the mucosa, and are carried to the local lymphoid tissue (Peyer's patches). No local damage is done, and no inflammation occurs. The organisms pass on through the lymphatics, through the mesenteric nodes, and finally reach the blood stream *via* the thoracic duct. In this way there develops a transient *bacteraemia* (see p. 100). The blood stream is rapidly cleared by the phagocytic reticulo-endothelial cells of liver, spleen, bone marrow, etc. It is at this stage that the pathogenic properties of the organisms become further manifest: they are able to live and multiply in the RE cells. By about the tenth day the parasitised cells undergo necrosis, and the blood stream is flooded with large numbers of bacilli. This is the end of the incubation period, and the patient becomes seriously ill with *septicaemia* (see p. 100). This phase lasts about one week, and is characterised clinically by a progressive rise in temperature (step-ladder pattern), a relatively slow pulse, and severe constitutional symptoms. Bronchitis is common and constipation the rule; diarrhoea is not present at this stage. The pathological diagnosis depends on obtaining a positive blood culture.

The next phase of the disease is marked by the onset of diarrhoea due to ulceration of the small intestine and the appearance of organisms in the faeces. The bacilli reach the gut *via* the bile which is heavily contaminated as a result of passage of the bacteria from the RE cells of the liver. The ulceration occurs over the inflamed Peyer's patches, and is associated with mesenteric adenitis (Fig. 8.1). In both the ulcers and the lymph nodes there is an accumulation of macrophages; polymorphs are almost completely absent (Fig. 8.2). The most likely explanation of these events is that the local lymphoid tissue of the gut has become sensitised to the

*Occasionally other salmonellae can be invasive and produce a similar septicaemic state; *S. cholera-suis*, *S. sendai*, and *S. virchow* are the most common examples.[6]

Figure 8.1
Typhoid ulceration of the bowel. There are many ulcers in the terminal ileum and ascending colon. They have retained the shape and size of the inflamed Peyer's patches and lymphoid follicles from which they arose. There is no tendency towards lateral spread. An enlarged lymph node is present in the mesentery. (A 50.2, *Reproduced by permission of the President and Council of the R.C.S. Eng.*)

organism, and that subsequent contact with it produces damage. The local production of sensitising antibodies must be postulated, because the blood level of detectable agglutinins does not rise till later in the course of the disease. During the second week diagnosis depends upon finding the organism in the faeces (and sometimes the urine). By the third week the titre of agglutinins in the serum rises (Widal reaction), and the patient gradually recovers (Fig. 8.3).

Although the nature of the *hypersensitivity* which develops in typhoid fever is not known, a type of bacterial allergy seems probable; a non-specific hypersusceptibility of the Shwartzman type is also possible. There is little doubt that the damage produced during infection is sometimes caused by the body's response to the organism. Such a mechanism should always be suspected in an infective disease that has an incubation period exceeding 7 to 10 days.

Other invasive organisms. Many *viruses*, e.g. smallpox, behave in a way similar to the typhoid bacillus: they produce no lesion on entry, but after dissemination and multiplication in the body cause extensive tissue damage.

In *syphilis* the organisms rapidly spread from the portal of entry, so that within a few hours they are widely disseminated throughout the body. Two to three weeks later an ulcerating inflammatory reaction occurs at the portal of entry. This again must be due to some alteration in tissue response to the organism. It certainly is not a primary inflammatory reaction representing an attempt by the body to localise the infection.

Figure 8.2
Typhoid ulceration of small bowel. There is considerable destruction of the mucous membrane, and an inflammatory infiltrate is present around the remaining glands. Most of the cells are macrophages, but in addition some darkly staining lymphocytes are present. Polymorphs are absent. × 200.

Some *rickettsial infections* are also characterised by a lesion at the portal of entry following their widespread dissemination.

The cause of death in septicaemia is poorly understood, and probably varies from one type of infection to another. *Anthrax* has been studied extensively because it appeared to be a typical example of an invasive organism. The pathogenesis was obscure, since neither exotoxins nor endotoxins could be demonstrated. Further research has clarified the situation.[7] A toxic factor having the properties of an exotoxin was first detected in the plasma of guinea-pigs dying of anthrax septicaemia. It has now been shown that even *in vitro* the organism produces a number of factors (termed *anthrax toxic complex*), the main action of which is to increase vascular permeability. Combined with a capsular polypeptide, which inhibits opsonisation and phagocytosis, this complex is responsible for the pathogenic action of the organism.

In *staphylococcal and streptococcal septicaemia* it is reasonable to attribute death to severe toxaemia consequent on the release of endotoxins (see p. 216 and p. 218). The cause of death in *pneumococcal septicaemia* is less easily explicable, because this organism does not appear to produce toxic substances.

A final possibility is that some invasive organisms (especially the Gram-negative ones) produce damage by means of a Shwartzman-like reaction.

The local Shwartzman phenomenon. The reaction is most easily demonstrated in rabbits. A quantity of bacterial 'endotoxin' (lipoprotein extract of certain bacteria) is injected into the skin, and 24 hours later an intravenous dose is given. The site of the skin injection then shows necrosis. The following features should be noted.

1. An effective endotoxin can be extracted from many Gram-negative organisms, especially those of the coli-typhoid group.

Figure 8.3
Chart correlating the clinical course of a typical case of typhoid fever with the principal methods of bacteriological diagnosis. (*After Harries, E. H. R. and Mitman, M.* (1947), Clinical Practice in Infectious Disease, *3rd edition, p.* 464, *Edinburgh: E. and S. Livingstone Ltd.*)

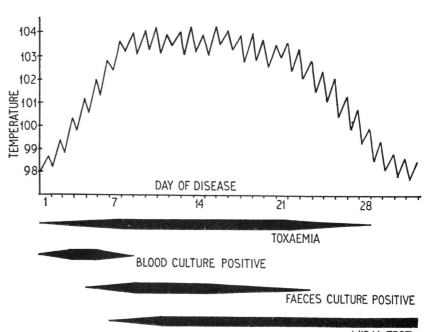

2. The interval between the first and second dose must be between 12 and 36 hours.

3. The reaction is non-specific, i.e. the two injections can be endotoxins from different organisms. The mechanism involved in this reaction is not understood, and there is little evidence that it is implicated in the lesions of bacterial infection. A similar phenomenon (Sanarelli) is considered in Chapter 32.

Variations of the Acute Inflammatory Reaction due to Infection

Although acute inflammation has been described as a common reaction to cell damage, it is only to be expected that the nature of the irritant causing the damage will influence the final picture. There will be differences depending upon the amount of irritant, and whether it is particulate, like a bacterium, or in solution, like an exotoxin. In respect of bacterial irritants there is the added factor of further growth of the organism. Finally, the presence of immunity or hypersensitivity will alter the tissue response.

In addition to considerations of the causative organism, the inflammatory response also varies according to the tissue involved. Loose tissues tend to show a greater accumulation of inflammatory oedema, and serous sacs may fill with fluid. This is called 'serous inflammation'. In a compact tissue like bone the amount of swelling is limited, but the inflammatory exudate causes a rise in tissue tension which obstructs the blood supply. Necrosis is therefore a common complication. Certain types of inflammation have been categorised, depending upon the predominance of some particular feature. The terms are useful for descriptive purposes, but are of no fundamental importance.

Suppurative inflammation (Fig. 8.4). An accumulation of neutrophil polymorphonuclear leucocytes is a feature of many types of inflammation, including that caused by traumatic injury. When tissue necrosis occurs, the disintegrating phagocytes liberate proteolytic enzymes which cause liquefaction. This fluid is pus, and the inflammation is called *suppurative* (see p. 80). Suppuration generally indicates that infection is becoming localised, and therefore in the days before chemotherapy it was regarded as a favourable sign. Hence the origin of the term 'laudable pus'. Nevertheless, diffuse suppurative lesions do occasionally occur and these are called *phlegmonous*.

Serous inflammation. As stated above, this is encountered in inflammations involving loose tissues. The fluid component exceeds the cellular one, and a large accumulation of inflammatory oedema results. Infections with *Clostridium oedematiens* are also of this type, probably because of the marked ability of the toxin to increase vascular permeability. A characteristic feature of the exudate in gas-gangrene is the absence of polymorphs. The fact that some highly virulent organisms are negatively chemotactic to polymorphs may explain this.

Fibrinous inflammation. Marked fibrin formation is a feature of inflammation in serous sacs and in the lungs. It is well marked in most forms of pericarditis, pleurisy, and peritonitis. It is also frequent in pneumococcal and staphylococcal infections. Often there is considerable serous exudate and the inflammation is then called serofibrinous.

Figure 8.4
Suppurative pyelonephritis. The structure of the kidney is almost completely destroyed except for some degenerated tubular elements at the top of the figure. There is a very heavy infiltration of polymorphs, most of which show disintegration (pus cells). × 165.

Haemorrhagic inflammation. A haemorrhagic exudate indicates that the irritant has caused severe vascular damage. It is seen in the lung in phosgene poisoning and acute influenzal pneumonia, and is typical of anthrax.

Catarrhal inflammation is seen when a mucous membrane is involved in an acute inflammatory reaction. There is some destruction of the epithelial cells and a profuse mucous secretion from the underlying glands. The common cold provides an excellent example: the running nose exudes a mixture of mucus and inflammatory exudate from the mucosa.

Membranous inflammation. A membrane covering an inflamed area of mucosa is seen in membranous bronchitis and membranous colitis. A complete 'cast' of the organ may be expelled; it consists of mucus and fibrinous exudate.

Pseudomembranous inflammation. This differs from the above in that the membrane contains necrotic epithelium as well as fibrin and inflammatory cells. It is seen in diphtheria and *Sh. dysenteriae* dysentery.

Gangrene. Gangrene occurs in inflammation whenever the dead tissue is invaded by putrefactive organisms (see p. 57).

Certain inflammations do not show the usual neutrophil polymorph response.

Inflammation characterised by mononuclear response. Typhoid and many viral infections show an inflammatory reaction virtually devoid of polymorphs. Typhoid bacilli are actively chemotactic to white cells *in vitro*, which makes this even more remarkable. A possible answer is provided by the fact that the typhoid ulcers are not produced during the primary invasion of the organism, but are secondary to a later septicaemic phase with a reinfection from bile-borne organisms. If a delayed type of hypersensitivity is involved, the monuclear response is to be expected, since this is the characteristic cell-type of that condition.

Inflammation characterised by eosinophils.[8] These cells are found instead of the usual neutrophilis in inflammation produced by helminthic parasites, e.g. ascariasis and schistosomiasis, and also in some allergic conditions (asthma, allergic rhinitis, and hay-fever). The reasons for this are as yet not understood, but there is evidence that eosinophil production is dependent on the T lymphocytes.[9] Thus, rats to whom larvae of *Trichinia spiralis* are given do not develop an eosinophilia if they have been neonatally thymectomised or treated with antilymphocytic serum, both of which procedures eliminate T lymphocytes selectively (see Ch. 12). On the other hand, such animals can develop a normal neutrophilia if suitably challenged.[9]

Eosinophils are motile, and *in vitro* are attracted by the same agents as are neutrophils. The granules of eosinophils derived from human subjects contain an arginine-rich, zinc-containing protein of molecular weight 21 000 daltons.[10] Unlike neutrophils, eosinophils are poorly phagocytic. They seem to carry receptors for complement-derived factors and histamine, and it may be that the release of the content of eosinophil granules during inflammatory reactions is mediated through surface receptors.

Eosinophilia tends to occur in diseases associated with high levels of IgE; type-1 hypersensitivity reactions are triggered off by antigen/IgE interaction on the surface of mast cells and basophils. In addition to a number of chemical mediators liberated (see p. 177), the *eosinophil chemotactic factor of anaphylaxis (ECF-A)* is also produced; it leads to the direct migration of the eosinophil from the blood stream to the site of inflammation. The eosinophil may possibly play a moderating role in allergic inflammatory process. Thus several of the granule constituents may alter the hypersensitivity reaction by inhibiting or promoting the action of mediators of inflammation, for instance aryl-sulphatase, preferentially present in eosinophils, inactivates slow-reacting substance of anaphylaxis (SRS-A). Stimulated eosinophils produce an inhibitor of histamine release which acts through the cyclic-AMP system; it seems to be a mixture of E_1 and E_2 prostaglandins.[10]

Eosinophils are conspicuous in the retest phenomenon (see p. 186) and in a number of skin diseases, e.g. pemphigus vulgaris and bullous pemphigoid.

Inflammation with no cellular exudate. This occurs typically in gas-gangrene.

The Destruction of Organisms in the Acute Inflammatory Exudate

While a wholly teleological view of the inflammatory reaction is unjustifiable, it is generally accepted that the reaction is an adaptive response having survival value for the species. It creates around the invading organisms a micro-environment unfavourable for their multiplication and survival. Inhibition of the inflammatory reaction generally decreases resistance to infection. The manner in which organisms are killed in the inflammatory exudate must now be considered.

Part Played by Phagocytes

Polymorphonuclear leucocytes. The polymorphs form the predominant cell of most acute inflammations, and play a large part in the destruction of some organisms (particularly the pyogenic group). The normal function of these cells and the manner whereby they destroy organisms is described in Chapter 6. Defects of polymorph function can lead to serious infection, a topic considered in Chapter 13.

Macrophages. These phagocytic members of the reticulo-endothelial system are particularly important in providing a defence against acid-fast bacilli, fungi, and viruses. General conditions appear to affect the RE system's ability to destroy engulfed bacteria. Experimentally, haemorrhagic shock and fasting impair the RE system's phagocytic activity. On the other hand, the administration of the endotoxin of coliform organisms and BCG vaccination produce a non-specific rise in resistance to infection. This is mediated by a greater phagocytic activity of the RE system. This topic is considered further in Chapter 13. An anamnestic rise in specific antibody may play some part (see p. 140). In the immune animal the macrophages appear better able to phagocytose and destroy bacteria.

Part Played by the Extracellular Fluids

Substances like lactic acid found in the phagocytes are liberated into the surrounding fluid during phagocytosis and following their death: the pH may fall to as low as 5·3. Reduction of the polymorph response, for example by nitrogen mustard administration which causes leucopenia, prevents this acid reaction. Glucose administration, on the other hand, increases it.

The unfavourable conditions in the area of inflammation may kill host cells as well as bacteria. The body may indeed defend itself by a type of 'scorched-earth' policy. Necrotic tissue has been shown to contain bactericidal substances. Basic peptides active against the tubercle bacillus have been isolated from caseous debris in tuberculous tissue. Humoral agents, e.g. complement and immunoglobulins, are also present in the extracellular fluids (see p. 159).

Part Played by Acquired Immunity

One way in which immunity affords protection is by speeding up the inflammatory reaction and with it the normal mechanism of destruction. This may be illustrated by the effect of diphtheria antitoxin. Virulent diphtheria bacilli inhibit the acid reaction in inflammation, but this inhibitory effect can be counteracted by administering antitoxin. Whatever the mechanism, there can be little doubt that the immune response plays an important role in the limitation of the spread of infection. This is most obvious when bacterial allergy is involved, and is considered in Chapter 14.

MECHANISMS WHEREBY ORGANISMS OVERCOME THE BODY DEFENCES

Organisms overcome the body's defences in three ways:

Neutralising action of antigens. There is evidence that organisms release their surface antigens and thereby neutralise antibody. Indeed, the detection of free antigen, by immunoelectrophoresis, in the cerebrospinal fluid has been used as a reliable diagnostic procedure in meningitis, and is comparable in accuracy with Gram's stain and culture (Fig. 8.5).[11] In meningococcal infections the presence of free meningococ-

Figure 8.5
Diagnosis of meningitis by countercurrent immunoelectrophoresis of cerebrospinal fluid. The patient was a young child with meningitis who had been admitted to hospital after having received an antibiotic; as a consequence no organisms could be cultured from the cerebrospinal fluid although it contained many polymorphs. Nevertheless, bacterial antigen was demonstrated by the technique of countercurrent immunoelectrophoresis, which is shown in the figure. The test is carried out in a sheet of agarose gel. Cerebrospinal fluid (CSF) is placed in the four wells on the right, and specific antisera are placed in separate wells on the left (Pn is antipneumococcal serum; H. i.'b' is antihaemophilus influenzae B serum; M. 'I' is antimeningococcal type-i serum; M. 'II' is antimeningococcal type-ii serum). A current is passed through the gel, and bacterial antigen, which has a strongly negative charge, is driven towards the anode (+). Under the conditions of the test, antibody moves towards the cathode (−). Hence antigen and antibody move towards each other, and a precipitate is formed where specific antibody meets antigen in optimum proportions. The well-marked precipitin line that is shown indicates that the CSF contains *Haemophilus influenzae* antigen. (*Photograph by courtesy of Dr. C. Krishnan.*)

cal antigen in the blood is associated with a very high mortality.[12] Likewise the SSS (capsular polysaccharide) is liberated in large quantities in pneumococcal infections, and is found in the lungs of fatal cases. It is capable of neutralising antibodies. In the toxic organisms, it is their exotoxins which neutralise the antibodies.

By hindering phagocytosis. Surface antigens of virulent organisms prevent phagocytosis unless specific opsonin is present. Leucocidins produced by staphylococci and streptococci destroy the white cells. Some organisms secrete substances which *in vitro* repel polymorphonuclears. In general the more pathogenic organisms exhibit this negative chemotaxis.

By spreading and countering efforts at localisation. The factors involved in the spread or localisation of infection are dealt with later (see p. 100). First the methods of spread will be considered.

SPREAD OF INFECTION

Local Spread

The natural cohesion of tissues tends to prevent the spread of organisms. The tissue fluids are, however, in constant motion under normal conditions. Particles, including organisms, will be carried in any stream of fluid which may be present. These streams are created in three ways:

1. *The functional state of the capillaries.* While the vessels in one area are dilated and exuding fluid, those in an adjacent part are at a lower pressure and absorbing fluid. This gives rise to a flow from one area to another.

2. *Pulsations of the vessels* due to the heart's action are important. If a rabbit's ear is perfused with fluid at a constant pressure, it becomes oedematous; injected dyes remain localised. Perfusion with a pulsating pressure simulating the heart's action does not result in oedema formation, and injected dyes diffuse into the tissues.

3. *Movement of muscles* both voluntary and involuntary causes considerable movement of tissue fluid. The time-honoured treatment of inflammatory lesions by rest is based upon this fact.

It should be noted that the motility of the organism appears to play no part in its spread. No correlation can be found between the two features. Of the clostridial group *Cl. tetani* is the most motile, but tetanus is a localised, non-spreading lesion. *Cl. welchii* is non-motile, yet produces a rapidly spreading gas-gangrene. Similarly *Bacillus anthracis* is non-motile, but is a very invasive organism.

Local spread may also occur in an entirely different way. Organisms ingested by phagocytes may be transported by these cells. This is an important means of spread in tuberculosis, and almost certainly occurs in many other infections, e.g. gonorrhoea.

The local defence mechanism. The acute inflammatory reaction must be regarded as a defence mechanism although, as we have seen, it is called forth only in the case of certain infections. Much stress has in the past been laid on the fibrin barrier. Certainly fibrin is laid down in localised acute inflammations, particularly in staphylococcal infections. It also forms the adhesions which appear to wall of infection in the serous sacs, e.g. around an appendix abscess. Experimentally in rabbits, when dicoumarol is given to prevent fibrin formation, staphylococcal infections are said to spread and terminate in septicaemia. Similarly urea injected locally prevents fibrin stabilisation, and staphylococcal infections tend to spread just like streptococcal ones.

Staphylococci produce coagulase, and it is tempting to postulate that this is a factor in the production of a fibrin barrier in infections with these organisms. However, it seems unlikely that it is important, because fibrin is also a prominent feature of infections with organisms which do not produce a coagulase, e.g. pneumococci. *Strept. pyogenes* produces streptokinase which activates the plasma fibrinolytic system. It might be thought that this would remove the fibrin barrier and potentiate spread. However, *Staph. aureus* produces staphylokinase, which has a similar action, and yet its infections tend to be localised. Other spreading organisms do not produce a fibrinolytic effect.

The balance of evidence favours the concepts of Menkin. Fibrin formation is evidence of a severe local reaction, and this is associated with localisation of infection. Organisms which spread produce little local reaction, and therefore no 'barrier' appears. Fibrin is therefore evidence of an attempt at localisation rather than the main cause of it. It must be admitted that the position is by no means clear. It is certain that if an acute inflammatory reaction remains localised, the exudate plays a part in this localisation. Fibrin itself aids the destruction of bacteria by surface phagocytosis. Hence experimental interference with the formation of fibrin may well upset the balance between organism and host under particular conditions. A localised lesion may thus be converted into a spreading one. On the other hand, fibrin may coat organisms and protect them from phagocytosis.

The present situation may therefore be summed up by saying that a fibrin barrier is good evidence of localisation of an infection, that it plays some part in this localisation, but is only one of the many factors involved in the inflammatory response, the sum total of which effect the destruction of the invading organisms (see also p. 216).

Spread by Natural Spaces

If local spread implicates a natural passage, infection may spread by this route. The following examples may be listed:

Peritoneum. Infection may spread rapidly throughout the peritoneal space from a localised lesion, e.g. acute appendicitis. There is rapid absorption of toxic substances from the large surface involved.

The omentum has properties which tend to limit the spread of infection. It wraps itself around inflamed parts, and walls off foci of infection. This may be correlated with the response to irritation. If a chemical irritant is injected into the peritoneal cavity of an animal, the omental and peritoneal vessels all show an inflammatory response and leak protein. The reaction in the omentum persists for longer than that of the other peritoneal vessels, and the fibrin glue which coats it may thus cause it to adhere more readily.

Pleura and pericardium. These sacs are usually infected from an adjacent lung lesion. Adhesions, at first fibrinous but later fibrous, are the usual aftermath.

Meningeal space. The subarachnoid space may be infected from adjacent structures, e.g. a nasal sinus, the middle ear, or brain. Suppurative thrombophlebitis may complicate facial infections and lead to cavernous-sinus thrombosis, and meningitis is often the result of systemic blood spread as part of a septicaemia, e.g. tuberculous, meningococcal, and pneumococcal meningitis. Under these circumstances organisms are probably filtered off in the choroid plexuses, whence they spread directly into the the cerebrospinal fluid.

Although the flow of cerebrospinal fluid is from the choroid plexus to the venous sinuses, irregular movements due to alterations in blood pressure, respiration, and posture lead to extensive mixing of the fluid. Substances artificially introduced into the spinal theca rapidly reach the ventricles. It is therefore often impossible to locate the area where infection has been introduced into the subarachnoid space.

Joint spaces. Joints may be infected from an osteomyelitis if the metaphysis of the bone is intracapsular. This is, in fact, an unusual anatomical arrangement, and most examples of suppurative arthritis are secondary to blood-borne infection or direct contamination from penetrating wounds.

Bronchi. These are a common route for the spread of invading organisms, e.g. in bronchopneumonia and tuberculosis.

Ureters. Infections of the kidney, e.g. tuberculosis, may spread down the ureters to the bladder.

Gut. This is the route for infection with parasites such as *Ascaris lumbricoides* and *Entamoeba histolytica*. Swallowed organisms from pulmonary infections may infect the intestines: a good example of this is the enteritis which occasionally complicates pulmonary tuberculosis.

Tissue planes, synovial sheaths, etc. The psoas abscess is an example of infection spreading in a potential space.

Spread by Lymphatics

The lymphatics form a capillary network almost as extensive as the vascular capillaries. None is present in spleen, brain, or bone.

In acute inflammation the vessels are held open by the increase in tissue tension. The permeability of their linings is increased, and the flow of lymph increased. Invading organisms frequently gain access to the lymphatics, and are carried to the nearest lymph node. Phagocytes that have ingested organisms but are unable to destroy them, also travel to the local nodes, e.g. in tuberculosis. The lymph nodes are thus the *second line of defence* against the spread of infection. Toxins may also be absorbed by the lymphatics. *Lymphangitis* is therefore a common event in spreading lesions, and when the vessels are near the surface, as in the forearm, they may appear as bright red streaks.

The structure of the lymph node is well adapted to its function as a filter. The afferent vessels pour lymph into the cortical sinus, whence it percolates through a spongework of reticulin fibres, around which there are numerous reticular cells and RE cells. Finally it is collected in the medullary sinuses, and passes out through the main efferent vessel. The RE cells of the node are therefore in intimate contact with the lymph fluid. When stimulated, they are actively phagocytic and capable of removing particulate matter as well as soluble toxins from the lymph.

Experimentally the efficiency of the lymph node as a filter can be tested by cannulating the efferent and afferent lymph vessels, and then perfusing the node with fluid containing organisms. Experiments of this type show:

1. The efficiency of the filter decreases as the rate of flow is increased.

2. Fatigue develops if the perfusion is continued too long.

It has been shown that exercise increases the lymph flow from a limb. This is another reason why rest is important in treating inflamed tissues.

Organisms may become arrested in the lymph nodes and yet not be destroyed. In this way *lymphadenitis* arises; the filtration will have protected the individual, but at the expense of the node. If organisms pass through the lymphatic barrier, they then enter the blood stream.

Spread by the Blood Stream

The blood stream forms the *third and last defence* against the spread of infection. It has two main defence mechanisms:

1. The circulating blood itself contains a wide array of antibacterial substances. Apart from the circulating phagocytes which probably play little part, there are natural antibacterial substances, like complement, properdin, and opsonins, as well as specific acquired antibodies.

2. The reticulo-endothelial system, especially the sinus-lining cells of the liver, bone marrow, and spleen, forms the main defence against generalised infection. Organisms injected into the blood stream experimentally are rapidly removed. In natural infections with highly invasive organisms, like the typhoid bacillus, early invasion of the blood stream occurs, and the circulating organisms are rapidly taken up by the RE system. These cells ingest foreign materials in the blood stream whether particulate or soluble. This is the first step in the afferent limb of the general immune response (see p. 152). The presence of organisms in the blood stream is not an uncommon event; it may occur under several conditions.

1. *Direct invasion of blood vessels.* A few organisms may invade blood vessels in the course of any local infection, e.g. a boil. The infection is often quite trivial, but adjacent blood vessels may be ruptured by trauma, thereby allowing organisms to enter. Periodontal infection or apical tooth abscesses are common lesions in which this is thought to occur, e.g. following dental extraction or even chewing hard food. When small numbers of organisms enter the blood stream in this way, they are readily phagocytosed by the cells of the RE system and are destroyed. This transient presence of organisms in the blood stream is called *bacteraemia*, and causes few symptoms. Rigors may occur, as in the bacteraemia that follows catheterisation. Its real importance, however, is that under certain conditions it may have serious consequences. Experimentally it has been shown that when an animal has a bacteraemia, histamine injected locally at any site will precipitate a local infection with the organism concerned. Trauma has a similar effect. Staphylococcal osteomyelitis occurs in this way. The patient, usually a child, has a transient bacteraemia usually associated with a septic skin lesion. Trauma to the limbs leads to a mild injury at the metaphysis of a long bone, and this causes localisation of the staphylococci.

In bacteraemia the kidney may filter off the organisms, and a renal infection occasionally results. In this way a large abscess of the kidney (sometimes called a carbuncle) may complicate a staphylococcal bacteraemia. The role of a coliform bacteraemia in the causation of urinary-tract infection is discussed in Chapter 11. *Strept. viridans* bacteraemia is of great importance in the pathogenesis of subacute infective endocarditis. Bacteraemia, especially with Gram-negative bacilli, has been incriminated as a cause of shock, e.g. following operations on the intestine or following the infusion of contaminated fluids (p. 418).

2. *Suppurative thrombophlebitis.* When a vein is implicated in the neighbourhood of a pyogenic infection, thrombophlebitis is liable to occur. If the thrombus is invaded by organisms, it will undergo softening, and pieces of infected thrombus will be released into the venous circulation. The resulting condition is called *pyaemia*, which is the presence in the circulation of infected thrombus which is carried to various organs where it produces metastatic abscesses or septic infarcts. Which of these develops depends on the vascular arrangements of the organ in which the emboli become lodged. The two antecedent conditions that lead to pyaemia are suppurative thrombophlebitis and acute infective endocarditis; in the latter the heart valves are the seat of the infected thrombus (vegetations), and pyaemic abscesses may be found either in the lungs or the viscera supplied by blood from the left ventricle depending on which side of the heart is involved.

If the infection involves the systemic venous circulation, pyaemic abscesses first occur in the lungs, e.g. following a carbuncle, acute osteomyelitis or suppurative arthritis (which is an important complication of rheumatoid arthritis), or puerperal infection. Pyaemic abscesses later develop in the heart, kidneys, spleen, and other organs as the pulmonary venous and systemic arterial circulation become involved.

On the other hand, suppuration occurring in the gastrointestinal tract, usually acute appendicitis or infected haemorrhoids, occasionally involves the portal vein, producing pylephlebitis suppurativa and portal pyaemia with multiple liver abscesses.

The commonest organism causing pyaemia is *Staph. aureus*, but *Strept. pyogenes*, pneumococci, and various Gram-negative intestinal bacilli may also be responsible.

3. *Spread from lymphatic system.* Organisms which are not held up in the tissues at the portal of entry or in the lymph nodes, reach the venous circulation *via* the main lymphatic ducts. Bacteraemia produced in this way is a common event with many invasive organisms, e.g. *Salmonella typhi*. The number of organisms reaching the blood is small, the condition is symptomless, and the organisms are removed from the blood by the RE cells.

If the phagocytic cells of the RE system are unable to destroy the organisms, they may proliferate in the cells. Following the death of these cells the circulation is flooded with organisms, and the patient becomes gravely ill. This is *septicaemia*. It differs from bacteraemia in the following ways:

1. It is associated with severe clinical symptoms.

2. There are more organisms in the blood.

3. It indicates that the host's resistance to the organism is very inadequate. Bacteraemia is the presence of organisms in the blood of a patient whose defence mechanisms are good. Septicaemia occurs where the defence mechanism has failed; it is therefore a much more serious condition. Septicaemia may be produced by all the pyogenic organisms (see Ch. 17), *Salmonella typhi*, *Bacillus anthracis*, *Yersinia pestis*, etc. It may sometimes lead to acute infective endocarditis, which in turn causes pyaemia.

Infection via nerves. Some viruses, e.g. rabies virus, are believed to travel up the nerves to reach the central nervous system. Whether they pass up the axoplasm or in the periaxonal spaces is uncertain. Tetanus toxin, injected or formed intramuscularly, almost certainly travels up in the tissue spaces around the axons, driven no doubt by the very high pressures (over 750 mm/water) generated in muscle by its contraction.

Factors Determining the Localisation or Spread of Infection

It is convenient at this point to summarise the factors which determine whether or not a particular organism is likely to spread from its site of primary infection.

Factors Involving the Organisms

Virulence. It should be appreciated that within each species of organism there are many strains with varying degrees of virulence. This may manifest itself both by greater infectivity during epidemics and the ability to produce a very severe spreading infection. Thus some strains of *Cl. welchii* produce a particularly spreading type of lesion, and this is related to toxin production. With *C. diphtheriae* the three strains, gravis, intermedius, and mitis, each produce the same diphtheria exotoxin, but in different amounts.

Dose. Experimentally it can be shown in calves that the lesions produced by injecting tubercle bacilli vary according to the dose. Small doses produce minor local lesions, whereas large doses result in spreading infections. A similar state of affairs probably exists with respect to many infections. In some cases it seems that there must be a minimum concentration of organisms in the tissues before an infection can be established. This concentration probably varies widely according to the organism. In some instances it has been claimed that a single organism can cause infection (*S. typhimurium* in mice), but this is probably unusual.

Portal of entry. This is a most important factor. Some organisms will cause infection only if administered by a particular route. *Vibrio cholerae* is non-pathogenic if injected subcutaneously, but causes cholera if swallowed. Experimentally the dose of tubercle bacilli necessary to cause infection of the intestine is about 100 times that needed to infect the lungs.

Synergism. The combined effect of two infecting agents may be greater than either one alone. A good example of this is seen in sheep. These animals often harbour *Cl. oedematiens* in their livers, but this is inactive and produces no disease. When, however, the animal becomes infected with the liver fluke *Fasciola hepatica*, local conditions are created which favour growth of the clostridia. The animal develops a fulminating infection of the liver known as 'black liver disease'.

The presence of two organisms, the one assisting the other, is somewhat unusual in human infection. The best-known example is Vincent's infection (*Fusobacterium fusiforme* and *Borrelia vincenti*), which is a common cause of gingivitis. Synergistic gangrene described on page 219 provides another example. *Haemophilus influenzae* provides an illustration of one organism deriving benefit from the products of another. *H. influenzae* needs for its growth a factor which is produced by staphylococci. This may be demonstrated on a culture plate where the haemophilus organisms grow as satellites around the staphylococcal colonies. Infection of the lung by these two bacteria may occur after a viral infection, e.g. epidemic influenza, and it is possible that the haemophilus organisms are aided by the staphylococci.

Products of the organisms. Spreading factor. In 1929 Duran-Reynals showed that vaccinia virus injected subcutaneously produced a widespread infection when mixed with a watery extract of testis. The action of this testicular extract was a local one, and has been shown to be due to its hyaluronidase content. A similar enzyme is produced by some bacteria.

Hyaluronidase is an enzyme which depolymerises hyaluronic acid. Hyaluronic acid forms highly viscous solutions, and is a component of the ground or intercellular substance. The enzyme converts it into a watery fluid, thereby facilitating the diffusion of injected substances.

Its relationship to the spread of infection is debatable. There is some broad correlation between hyaluronidase production and ability to spread. Thus the enzyme is produced by *Cl. welchii*, but not by *Cl. tetani*. However, the amount of hyaluronidase produced by different strains of organisms, e.g. *Cl. welchii*, does not bear any relationship to the observed virulence of the strains. Furthermore, administrations of anti-hyaluronidase do not hinder the spread of *Cl. welchii* in experimental infections. It should not be forgotten that theoretically hyaluronidase could also be a factor in the limitation of infection. If organisms and toxins are spread too widely, their concentrations at any one point might be too low to cause damage (see above). Until further proof is provided, it must be concluded that hyaluronidase production is not an important factor in the promotion of the spread of natural infection. *Streptokinase* and *staphylokinase* may play a part in the spread of infection, and so, of course, may staphylococcal *coagulase*. These have already been considered in relation to the fibrin barrier.

Factors Involving the Host

GENERAL. *The general state of health* of the host is important. Starvation and haemorrhagic shock have been shown experimentally to render animals more liable to infection. It is frequently observed that patients with chronic debilitating diseases like chronic nephritis, alcoholism, and especially diabetes mellitus are less well able to resist infection. The factors involved are complex, but probably involve both humoral factors, e.g. a low complement level, and defective action of phagocytes, both polymorphs and RE cells.

The immune state. This involves both non-specific factors like complement, and the specific antibodies of acquired immunity. Primary infections tend to spread much more than subsequent ones due to the absence of active immunity. The immunologically deficient states are described on page 170.

Low white-cell count. Infections tend to spread whenever the neutrophil (polymorphonuclear) leucocyte count is low, e.g. in agranulocytosis or acute leukaemia. Functional defects of polymorph activity are described on page 162.

LOCAL. The local blood supply is most important. *Ischaemia* from whatever cause, e.g. injection of adrenaline, nerve lesions, and peripheral vascular disease, adversely affects the inflammatory response designed to destroy the organism. Similarly *foreign bodies* and *chemicals*, by causing necrosis, are harmful. Thus silica potentiates the tubercle bacillus. The action of ionic calcium may also be mentioned in connexion with anaerobic wound infections.

It is evident from this account of the various patterns of infection that the relationship between the host and his infecting organism is extremely complex. This is well illustrated in the case of the human being and the *Brucella* organism; the infection can vary from an acute illness to a chronic disease or even to a symptomless carrier state in which a symbiotic relationship has been established. Only with the frankly exotoxin-producing organisms is the pathogenesis of the disease they cause at all clearly understood.

It is not surprising therefore that it is in this group of infections that our understanding of immunity is also most complete.

GENERAL BODY RESPONSES TO INFECTION

The last consideration concerns the general response of the body to infection. There is usually pyrexia, a raised erythrocyte sedimentation rate (ESR), and an alteration in the white-cell count depending on the organism responsible for the condition. There are various metabolic effects also, e.g. dehydration, protein breakdown with increased nitrogenous excretion in the urine, and a tendency to ketosis. All these features are discussed in later chapters. An attempt should always be made to keep the local and general responses in proper perspective.

REFERENCES

1. NORRIS, H. T. & MAJNO, G. (1968) On the role of the ileal epithelium in the pathogenesis of experimental cholera. *American Journal of Pathology*, **53**, 263.
2. GERALD, P. S. (1976) A new frontier for infectious disease research? *New England Journal of Medicine*, **295**, 337.
3. MILLER, D. A. (1974) Human chromosome 19 carries a poliovirus receptor gene. *Cell*, **1**, 167.
4. WEBB, H. E. (1968) Factors in the host-virus relationship which may affect the course of an infection. *British Medical Journal*, **4**, 684.
5. WILSON, G. S. & MILES, A. A. (1975) In Topley and Wilson's *Principles of Bacteriology, Virology, and Immunity*, 6th ed, p. 1273. London: Arnold.
6. MANI, V., BRENNAND, J. & MANDAL, B. K. (1974) Invasive illness with *Salmonella virchow* infection. *British Medical Journal*, **2**, 143.
7. GREEN, D. M. (1973) In *Medical Microbiology*, ed. Cruickshank, R., Duguid, J. P., Marmion, B. P. & Swain, R. H. A., 12th edn, Vol. 1, p. 345 *et seq*. Edinburgh: Churchill Livingstone.
8. COHEN, S. G. (1974) The eosinophil and eosinophilia. *New England Journal of Medicine*, **290**, 457.
9. BEESON, P. B. & BASS, D. A. (1977) *The Eosinophil*, 269 pp. (Vol. XIV in the series Major Problems in Internal Medicine). Philadelphia: Saunders.
10. Leading Article (1977) What eosinophils do. *Lancet*, **2**, 388.
11. GREENWOOD, B. M., WHITTLE, H. C. & DOMINIC-RAJKOVIC, O. (1971) Counter-current immunoelectrophoresis in the diagnosis of meningococcal infections. *Lancet*, **2**, 519.
12. EDWARDS, E. A. (1971) Immunologic investigations of meningococcal disease. *Journal of Immunology*, **106**, 314.

Chapter 9. Wound Healing

The word *healing*, used in a pathological context, refers to the body's replacement of destroyed tissue by living tissue. It is therefore useful, at the outset, to enumerate the causes of tissue loss or destruction:

1. Traumatic excision, whether accidental or sugical.
2. Physical, chemical, and microbial agents. These all give rise to inflammation, and in sufficient dose lead to necrosis.
3. Ischaemia, which leads to infarction.
4. The body's response to external agents can itself engender necrosis. For example, the inflammatory exudate can interfere with the blood supply of the part, as is seen in acute osteomyelitis. Hypersensitivity reactions to foreign proteins, e.g. the Arthus phenomenon, or to products of organisms, e.g. the caseation of tuberculosis, are other instances of tissue destruction brought about by the body's own vigorous responses.

In insects, amphibians, and crustaceans the ability to replace lost parts has long been known, and is truly remarkable. Thus, if the lens of the eye of a salamander is removed a new lens develops from the adjacent iris; even the complex neural part of the retina, if destroyed, can be reformed from the outer pigmented layer of the retina. Other well-known examples of regeneration are the reformation of the amputated limbs of insects and newts, and of the claws of lobsters. The process whereby whole limbs are reformed is well developed in lower forms of life; it is complex, and resembles embryonic development or asexual reproduction. The process is termed *axial regeneration* by zoologists, but the term *reconstitution* is also used by pathologists. One would think that the ability to reform a lost limb or organ was so useful to survival that it would have been retained during evolution. Such has not been the case. The higher animals—including humans—do not have the ability to replace lost limbs following their amputation. Perhaps this is because sexual reproduction has been evolved and preserved at all costs as a means of improving and remoulding the species. 'If there were no regeneration there could be no life. If everything regenerated there would be no death. All organisms exist between these two extremes. Other things being equal, they tend towards the latter end of the spectrum, never quite achieving immortality because this would be incompatible with reproduction.'*

Axial Regeneration[1]

The regeneration of the amputated arm of the newt has been extensively studied. The stump rapidly becomes covered by a layer of epidermal cells that slide in from the adjacent skin. The cells multiply to form an *apical cap*, and intimate contact of these cells with the stump, particularly its nerves, is an essential step in the regeneration process. After a brief inflammatory reaction the cells of the stump—fibroblasts, muscle cells, osteoblasts and other cell types—appear to revert from their differentiated form into a primitive cell type by a process termed *dedifferentiation*. Connective-tissue fibres—collagen, muscle, and bone—break down, and the cells of regeneration lie in an oedematous stroma that resembles the mesenchyme of the developing embryo. This mass of cells is termed the blastema. Its cells multiply rapidly in an avascular field in the first instance. Later there is vascularisation and differentiation: bone, muscle, tendon, nerves, and blood vessels are produced in a co-ordinated manner such that there is accurate replacement of the parts of the limb that were lost. No matter what the level of the original amputation, only the distal parts are replaced. Thus with a forearm amputation, a wrist and a hand are formed but never an elbow. This rule of *distal transformation* has been summed up by the trite description of 'hands from elbows, but never elbows from hands'.

The mechanism of this type of axial regeneration is presumed to be related to the genetic information residing in the cells of the stump. The presence, or formation, of a stimulating 'wound hormone' is an attractive theory to explain the onset of regeneration, but none has ever been isolated in animal tissues. In the plant world, however, stimulating wound hormones have been isolated, and have indeed been put to good use as weed-killers. In the higher animals it seems that during development as cells differentiate, there is repression of genetic expression. Following injury there is derepression, so that regeneration follows. The stimulus for derepression appears to be related to the absence of the lost part. Cells of the amputation stump dedifferentiate and then repeat the events of embryonic development; nevertheless, they are still partially repressed by the tissues that are proximal, since, as noted previously, only the distal structures are regenerated. The nature of this axial control or polarisation is not understood. Presumably tissues produce chemical repressors, and there is some evidence that these are protein in nature. The flow of these repressors is always distal and may be determined by the presence of an electric field. Thus the tip of the regenerating newt arm is negatively charged. In contrast, the stump of a non-regenerating limb, for example of a frog, does not show this negativity. Perhaps this failure to regenerate is due to the lack of a suitable electrical field—in turn this might be related to the function of nerves—for as noted previously, the contact of nerves with the epidermal epithelial cap is a vital component of amphibian regeneration. Experimental work has shown that by altering the electrical field following amputation of a limb, the regeneration that follows can be altered. Indeed, there are reports that the amputated rat limb can be induced to a limited degree of

*Quoted from Goss, R. J. (1969) *Principles of Regeneration*. New York: Academic Press.

regeneration. Amputation through the humerus can be followed by reformation of the distal half of the bone including its epiphysis.

Wound Healing in Humans

In humans the cells adjacent to the area of damage fail to dedifferentiate and no blastema comparable to that described above is formed. The healing process has two aspects:

(*a*) *Contraction*, a mechanical reduction in the size of the defect occurring in the first few weeks (see below).

(*b*) *Replacement of lost tissue*, which is brought about by migration of cells as well as division of adjacent cells to provide extra tissue to fill the gap. This can be accomplished in two ways:

Regeneration. In human pathology the term regeneration is used to describe the process whereby lost tissue is replaced by tissue similar in type. There is a proliferation of surrounding undamaged specialised cells. This process differs completely from the axial regeneration of amphibians as previously described, for it lacks the initial stage of dedifferentiation. The nearest approach to axial regeneration in humans is the regeneration of bone and cartilage that occurs in the healing of a fractured bone (p. 118).

Repair, the replacement of lost tissue by granulation tissue which matures to form scar tissue. This is inevitable when the surrounding specialised cells do not possess the capacity to proliferate, e.g. muscle and neurons.

It should be noted that the word repair is used in a rather arbitrary way be some surgeons and pathologists. Surgeons refer to the union of fractures or the closure of defects by various inert materials as examples of 'repair', but the latter is not even true healing, though it has an ameliorative effect. Some pathologists equate repair with healing and recovery, and describe 'repair by resolution', 'repair by granulation tissue', and 'repair by regeneration'. Though it is unwise to be dogmatic, there is no doubt that this variation in nomenclature is confusing; in this book the terms resolution, regeneration, and repair are used strictly in accordance with the definitions given above and on page 80.

It will readily be understood that wound healing is a complicated process involving many changes, e.g. movement of cells, division of cells, rearrangement of tissues, and biochemical changes. Depending upon the manner in which wounds are investigated, various aspects may be accentuated and various stages described.

Before describing the co-ordinated process which occurs during simple wound healing, it is convenient first to describe wound contraction, granulation-tissue formation, and changes in tensile strength.

WOUND CONTRACTION[2]

This is conveniently studied by excising a small, circular, full-thickness disc of skin from the back or flank of a rat. Figures 9.1 and 9.2 show the results of such an experiment.

New tissue formation is not included since the measurements are made from the original wound edges. It can be seen that there is an initial *lag period* of 2 to 3 days followed by a period of rapid contraction, which is largely complete by the

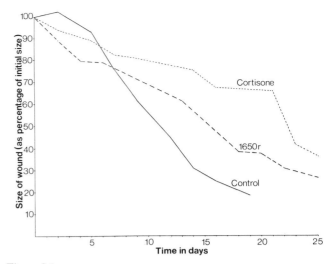

Figure 9.1
Wound contraction in the rat. Daily administration of cortisone acetate causes considerable delay in the process. Irradiation with 1650 r immediately after inflicting the wounds has a similar delaying effect.

fourteenth day. The wound is reduced by approximately 80 per cent of its original size.

The magnitude of contraction varies with the species of animal and with the shape, site, and size of the wound. In the rabbit contraction reduces large wounds to a thin linear scar, while in rats the scar occupies 20 to 30 per cent of the original wound. The importance of contraction is demonstrated in Figure 9.3.

Contraction results in much faster healing, since only one-quarter to one-third of the amount of destroyed tissue has to be replaced. If contraction is prevented, healing is slow and a large, ugly scar is formed. Not only is this cosmetically undesirable, but the large amount of fibrous tissue formed may lead to later complications following cicatrisation.

Cause of contraction. In spite of a great deal of research work neither the mechanism of contraction nor its cause is known for certainty.

Removal of fluid by drying has been suggested as a cause of the diminution in size of wound contents, but this has not been substantiated.

Contraction of collagen is the time-honoured explanation, but although collagen contracts to one-third of its original length when boiled, there is no evidence that it is capable of contracting *in vivo*.

Wound contraction is actually proceeding at a stage when little collagen is yet present in the granulation tissue. It is largely completed by the twentieth day, but collagen formation continues after this. Furthermore, in wounded scorbutic animals, although granulation tissue is formed, collagen production is inhibited. Wound contraction, however, proceeds normally, and there seems little doubt that it is not produced by direct contraction of collagen fibres of the granulation tissue.

Contraction of granulation tissue[3] The fact that contraction occurs at a time when granulation tissue is actively being formed has led most workers to regard the granulations as forming an *organ of contraction*. The observation that con-

Figure 9.2
Wound contraction in the rat and the effect of X-irradiation. The edges of the skin wounds have been tattooed with carbon so as to render them easily visible. Note how the delivery of 1650 r to the wound on the right has delayed the contraction process. (*From Blair, G. H., Slome, D. and Walter, J. B.* (1961), *Review of Experimental Investigations on Wound Healing*, British Surgical Practice: Surgical Progress, *Ed. by Ross, J. P. London: Butterworths*).

Control   Days   1650r

1

8

10

17

traction occurs normally in the scorbutic animal supports this concept.[4]

The actual location of the contracting mechanism appears to reside in the granulation tissue at the margins of the wound—the so-called 'picture-frame area'.[5] Interference with this area delays contraction, whereas careful excision of the granulation tissue of the wound centre has no such effect. The present evidence suggests that the contracting force is generated by cells of granulation tissue that closely resemble fibroblasts. These cells have several features that distinguish them from the ordinary fibroblasts of connective tissue. They have fibrillar components in their cytoplasm, and these on electron microscopy closely resemble those found in smooth-muscle cells. They contain actin, and their nuclei have infoldings of the nuclear membrane, a feature also seen in smooth-muscle cells and associated with contractility. The cells also develop a basement membrane and desmosomes: these are never found in ordinary fibroblasts.

These features all suggest that the 'fibroblasts' of granulation tissue can contract, and that they can do so has been shown *in vitro*; 5-hydroxytryptamine, angiotensin, noradrenaline, and other agents will cause contraction of a strip of granulation tissue but histamine does not have this effect. Anti-5-hydroxytryptamine agents can prevent this action, and furthermore, the local application of a smooth-muscle antagonist can inhibit wound contraction *in vivo*. These curious cells of granulation tissue have been called *myofibroblasts*, and may well be derived from pericytes. They are clearly not the same as the fibroblasts of ordinary connective tissue.

Experimental methods of inhibiting wound contrac-

Figure 9.3
Diagram showing how contraction accelerates the healing of a wound and produces a small scar. Note that in actual practice a circular wound invariably shows considerable distortion in shape by the time healing is complete. Compare this diagram with Figure 9.2. (*Drawing by Anthony J. Walter.*)

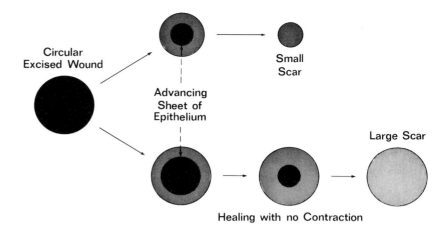

tion. *X-irradiation.* Ionising radiation applied to the wounded area at the time of wounding causes a delay in contraction (see Figs 9.1 and 9.2).

Glucocorticoids have the same effect (see Fig. 9.1).

Contraction does not proceed normally in *burns*.

Immediate skin grafting of the raw area of a wound prevents its subsequent contraction. It also halts the process if performed in an existing wound during the phase of rapid contraction. The graft must contain dermis.

GRANULATION-TISSUE FORMATION

The ingrowth of granulation tissue into a haematoma can be studied experimentally using the rabbit ear-chamber technique,[6] or by observing the changes in the interstices of an implanted plastic sponge. Three phases may be observed:

1. **Phase of traumatic inflammation.** The damaged cells set in motion the phenomenon of acute inflammation. An exudate of fibrin and polymorphs develops. Haemorrhage also occurs, and the blood clot contributes to the fibrin formation. The ground substance undergoes depolymerisation, and there is loss of granules in the mast cells. These changes have been fully described in Chapter 6.

2. **Phase of demolition.** Dead tissue cells and disintegrating polymorphs liberate their autolytic lysosomal enzymes. There is an associated macrophage infiltration. These cells ingest particulate matter, either digesting or removing it. They may fuse to form foreign-body giant cells. This demolition phase and the cells involved are described in greater detail in Chapters 6 and 30.

The initial inflammatory response seems to be essential for the subsequent proliferation of fibroblasts.[7] Recent studies suggest that the presence of platelets results in the release of a factor which stimulates fibroblast proliferation. Even more important in this respect is the macrophage. It appears to secrete a factor that is essential for fibroblast proliferation, for, if a monocytopenia is induced by pretreatment with corticosteroids and an antimacrophage serum, not only can monocytes be prevented from entering the wound, but the inflammatory response is also delayed, few fibroblasts are present, and collagen formation is delayed. By contrast, an induced neutropenia has no effect on the subsequent events in wound healing.

3. **Ingrowth of granulation tissue.** Granulation tissue is formed by the proliferation and migration of the surrounding connective tissue elements; it is composed at first of capillary loops and cells that are termed 'fibroblasts'. As noted previously, 'myofibroblast' has been suggested as a better name for this cell type, but the term has not yet come into general use and 'fibroblast' will be retained in the account that follows. Granulation tissue is thus initially highly vascular, but with the passage of time it develops into avascular scar tissue. Two stages in its formation may be recognised; firstly a stage of *vascularisation*, and subsequently a stage of *devascularisation*.

Stage of Vascularisation. The ingrowth of capillary loops and fibroblasts, so that the insoluble fibrin clot is replaced by living vascular granulation tissue, is known as *organisation*, and is conveniently studied in the rabbit ear-chamber.

Figure 9.4 shows such a chamber in position. It consists of two main transparent parts—a Perspex base and a mica coverslip. Between these parts in the central window there is a gap of between 80 μm and 100 μm (Fig. 9.5) which is first filled with blood clot and inflammatory exudate. This fibrin clot is invaded by macrophages, which advance towards the centre table, and they are followed by capillary loops and fibroblasts (Figs 9.6, 9.7, and 9.8).

Solid buds of endothelial cells grow out from existing blood vessels, undergo canalisation, and by anastomosis with their neighbours form a series of vascular arcades. At first the newly-formed vessels all appear similar, and under the electron microscope show gaps between the endothelial cells, a poorly-formed basement membrane, and long pseudopodia of the endothelial cells which reach out into the connective tissue spaces. These newly-formed vessels leak protein, and it is easy to imagine that the tissue fluid forms a very suitable medium for fibroblastic growth. Very soon differentiation occurs. Some vessels acquire a muscular coat and become arterioles, whilst others enlarge to form thin-walled venules. The remainder either disappear, or persist as part of the capillary bed. The source of the smooth muscle fibres of the arterioles is undecided, since mitosis in the existing muscle fibres is denied by many observers. Cell migration or differentiation of existing primitive mesenchymal cells are two possible though unproven suggestions. Direct arteriovenous shunts are also formed. The fibroblasts which accompany the capillary loops are at first

Figure 9.4
Two rabbit ear-chambers in position. The one in the left ear shows the clear central area in which observations are made. In the chamber on the right, the area of the central table is still filled with blood clot. (*From Blair, G. H., van den Brenk, H. A. S., Walter, J. B. and Slome, D.* (1961), 'Wound Healing', pp. 46–53, in A Symposium organised by Smith and Nephew Research Ltd. *Oxford: Pergamon Press*)

Figure 9.5
Diagrammatic representation of one type of rabbit ear-chamber; a wedge has been cut out to show its construction. The chamber is composed of a Perspex base plate which has a raised central table and three peripherally arranged pillars. The cover-slip consists of a disc of mica supported at the edge by a ring of Perspex. The cover-slip is placed upon the three pillars, and held there in position by screws which are inserted into threaded holes in the pillars. The height of the pillars is such that the gap between the top of the table and the mica is 50 to 100 μm. (*Drawing by Mr. S. P. Steward*)

large and plump, but gradually collagenous fibres form around them, and the cells become mature, elongated fibrocytes (Fig. 9.9). During this process of fibrogenesis, the pH becomes alkaline. The mode of formation of collagen is discussed in Chapter 5. The first formed fibres are described as reticulin, but these mature to form adult fibrous tissue.

Collagen is usually formed in the body by the activity of fibroblasts (or closely allied cells like osteoblasts). The cells secrete a soluble collagen which polymerises to form fibrils (see p. 64). The soluble collagen might also condense on to pre-existing fibres and thereby reinforce them. Fibroblasts are also thought to be responsible for the production of the mucopolysaccharide ground substance, because during the early phases of organisation the large fibroblasts contain granules which have similar staining reactions to those of ground substance.

The source of the fibroblasts of repair is not known for certain. Most authorities regard them as being derived from local cells of similar nature, e.g. fibrocytes. Pericytes (p. 59) or stem cells have also been suggested as the parent type. There are others who believe that they can be derived from the circulating cells of the blood—either monocytes or large lymphocytes. Part of the evidence for this is the claim that cultures of blood leucocytes may give rise to fibroblasts and collagen. Probably the cells responsible are endothelial cells or fibroblasts inadvertantly introduced during the collection of the blood. However, the matter is not finally settled.

Further changes in granulation tissue. As maturation proceeds, nerve fibres and lymphatics form. The latter develop from existing lymphatics in much the same way as do the blood vessels, only later. The two sets of vessels never communicate with each other. With the ingrowth of nerve fibres the arterioles exhibit rhythmic contraction or locomotion. Mast cells make their appearance, and are a prominent feature of vascular granulation tissue. In due course collagen fibres are produced, and their direction is determined by the stresses that are applied to the tissue. Thus, in the base of a healing ulcer the fibres are aligned parallel to the surface, whereas in a healing skin wound they are at right angles to the plane of the wound. Hence they hold the severed parts together (Fig. 9.9).

As fibroplasia proceeds, some vessels undergo atrophy whilst others show endarteritis obliterans, in which the lumen becomes obliterated due to intimal proliferation. This is the stage of *devascularisation*, and results in the formation of pale, avascular scar tissue. Mast cells disappear, and hyalinisation, calcification, and even ossification may sometimes occur. Coincident with the devascularisation there is often contracture of the scar tissue, with much local tissue distortion. This process is known as cicatrisation, and it must be clearly distinguished from contraction. *Cicatrisation* (or *contracture* as it is sometimes called) is a diminution in size of a *scar*, and is a late event; contraction is a diminution in size of a *wound*, and is an early event.

Conditions under which granulation tissue is formed (organisation). Organisation is one of the fundamental processes in pathology, and can be defined as the replacement of necrotic tissue, inflammatory exudate, thrombus, or blood clot by granulation tissue. It occurs under four conditions:

In inflammation. It is the fibrinous exudate that is organised if it is not demolished and removed expeditiously. Fibrinous exudates in serous cavities may persist and later be converted into fibrous adhesions. Granulation tissue is an important feature of all chronic inflammatory lesions and in their healing.

In wound healing. Both in open wounds and in fractures the initial haematoma between the severed ends is organised as described above. Haematomata in soft tissues (bruises) and

Figure 9.6
Granulation-tissue formation in the rabbit ear-chamber. Photographs taken at the following times after the insertion of the chamber: (*a*) 9 days, (*b*) 12 days, (*c*) 17 days, (*d*) 21 days, (*e*) 24 days, (*f*) 44 days. At 9 days vessels are seen to be invading the dark blood clot in the centre, and by the 24th day organisation is complete. The large, tortuous vessels are venules; arterioles are more difficult to see at this magnification. The arrow in (*f*) indicates an arteriole which divides almost immediately. Note how by the 44th day changes have occurred in the course of many blood vessels, although the original pattern of certain venules can still be recognized on the left-hand side of the picture. A lymphatic vessel is now visible at the top of the chamber. ×8·5.

a   b

c   d

e   f

even in serous cavities are usually completely absorbed following their demolition by macrophages, and organisation does not generally occur.

In a thrombus.

In an infarct.

Granulation tissue forms an integral part of malignant tumours where it constitutes the stroma. It is particularly prominent in scirrhous carcinoma. The manner of granulation-tissue formation under these circumstances is not altogether clear. The neoplastic cells may excite the formation of an inflammatory exudate which undergoes organisation. Alternatively, the neoplastic cells may in some way directly stimulate a proliferation of the adjacent connective tissue. The latter seems the more likely explanation, and may be likened to the formation of granulation tissue in wound healing (see Fig. 9.11).

Figure 9.7
The growing edge of granulation tissue in a rabbit ear-chamber. The rapidly moving stream of blood in the capillary loops at the top produces a streaked effect, and individual red cells cannot be distinguished; in the right-hand vessel white cells are adherent to the endothelium, and appear as transparent globules. There is no flow in the capillary buds in the lower half of the picture, and these contain plasma with few cells. Rouleaux formation is seen in one of them.

Factors Affecting Granulation-Tissue Formation and Maturation

Scurvy. Wounds in scorbutic guinea-pigs do not heal normally owing to the failure of collagen formation. Vascular granulation tissue is formed, but the fibroblasts lack orientation and show a deficiency of phosphatase. Embedded in the ground substance there are abnormal globules and thick fibres of silver-staining material. Hydroxylation of protocollagen does not take place, and since this protein cannot be extruded from the cell, collagen formation does not occur (p. 64). The ground substance itself accumulates in excessive amounts and lacks metachromasia; this is associated with its diminished sulphation, and experimentally a reduced uptake of ^{35}S-labelled sulphate can be demonstrated.

Glucocorticoid administration. With high dosage little granulation tissue is formed, fibroblasts remain small, and little collagen is formed. While this effect has been well demonstrated in the experimental animal, glucocorticoids in the dosage generally administered do not appear to influence wound healing in the human subject.

Protein starvation. This is considered later (p. 113).

Figure 9.8
Early granulation tissue. This is composed mostly of thin-walled capillaries. A few dilated vascular spaces are present, but they have not differentiated into arteries or veins. The intervening large, plump cells are fibroblasts. They have not yet started to lay down collagen fibres. × 160.

Figure 9.9
Maturing granulation tissue. The fibroblasts have started to lay down collagen fibres, and the blood vessels are better differentiated than in Figure 9.8. The section has been taken from the base of a healing ulcer; the fibroblasts and their associated collagen fibres tend to be aligned parallel to the plane of the ulcer, whereas the blood vessels tend to run at right angles to the surface. × 90.

TENSILE STRENGTH[2, 8]

The ability to resist rupture can be assessed in various ways and has been studied for centuries. Both Hunter (*circa* 1767) and Paget (*circa* 1853) used methods of measurement based on those of Leonardo da Vinci's method (*circa* 1490) for testing the tensile strength of an iron wire. By measuring the force necessary to break a wound on a tensiometer some assessment of the strength of the wound can be made. Another technique is to implant two pieces of cellulose sponge held together by a suture. When the animal is killed, the sponge is excised and the stitch removed. Part of the specimen is used for chemical estimation of the amount of hydroxyproline, while the other part is distracted on a tensiometer to measure the strength of the tissue holding the two pieces of sponge together.

Valuable as these methods may be, the results can be misleading. Other factors, such as the sectional area of the wound studied, must be taken into account. Also, the amount of tissue extension must be considered; by measuring the work done in breaking a wound it is suggested that a more meaningful measurement can be obtained. Thus a simple measurement of tensile strength indicates that taped experimental wounds heal faster than those that are sutured. However, sutured wounds are more extensible at breaking point, and if one measures the energy absorption needed to break the wounds, there is no difference detectable between the wounds that are taped and those that are sutured.

During the first few days the strength of a skin wound is only that of the clot cementing the cut surfaces together. There then follows a period of increasing tensile strength which corresponds to the increase in amount of collagen present (Fig. 9.10). If the observations are continued over a long period it is found that whereas the collagen content reaches a maximum at about 80 days, the tensile strength continues to increase for many months thereafter. The steady development of cross-linkages between collagen fibrils (see Ch. 5) is responsible for this steady increase in tensile strength. Newly-formed collagen has a high percentage of soluble collagen present, and experimental evidence suggests that collagen synthesis continues for many weeks. Since the total amount of collagen does not increase, it is evident that there must be some method of collagen breakdown and removal. Presumably this is effected by collagenases, but their nature and source are poorly documented. Nevertheless, their activity could clearly be of great importance. An over-action or unopposed action of collagenases would result in a steady diminution in the amount of collagen present in a wound: this happens in scurvy. The synthesis of collagen is blocked because hydroxylation of proline and lysine require the presence of this vitamin. The continued breakdown of collagen results in a weakening of recent scars, but it has very little effect on mature collagenous tissues.

The strength of a healing wound is of great practical importance to the surgeon because it is the main safeguard against wound dehiscence. Many factors influence the rate of healing; these are both local and general, but in the main are related to granulation-tissue and collagen formation, and are considered later. Certain additional factors should be noted:

Direction of wound. Skin wounds made in a direction parallel to the lines of Langer heal faster than those made at right angles to them. The tension lines of Langer, first described by

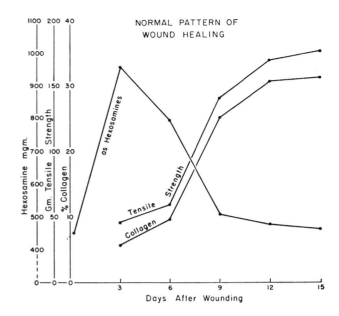

Figure 9.10
The normal pattern of healing in the rat. (*From Dunphy, J. E. and Udupa K. N. (1955), New England Journal Medicine, **253**, 847*)

Dupuytren in 1832, are due to the orientation of the collagen bundles in the dermis. The skin is less tensible in the direction of the lines than at right angles to them. In general they correspond in direction to the crease lines, although these are in fact related to the movements of the underlying muscles and joints. As skin incisions made across Langer's lines tend to gape, their healing is delayed. When planning a surgical incision the direction of pull of the underlying muscles must also be considered, and as this is related to the crease lines of flexion, the latter constitute the best guide to the placing of the incision. *Wounds parallel to or in the creases are most satisfactory and the scars least visible.* Thus it has been shown experimentally that transverse abdominal incisions produce a stronger scar than do longitudinal ones.[9]

Abdominal support. Abdominal binders reduce the rate of gain of strength of abdominal wounds.[9]

Effect of previous wounding. Pre-existing wounds at a distance do not influence the healing of a further skin wound: there is therefore no evidence of a circulating 'wound hormone'. Resutured wounds do, however, heal faster than those sutured primarily, because the reparative process has already commenced.[10] Severe trauma delays wound healing, presumably because of the adrenocortical response to the stress.

HEALING OF SKIN WOUNDS[11, 12]

Healing of a Clean Incised Wound with Edges in Apposition[13]

This process is described as *healing by primary intention*, and is the desired result in all surgical incisions.

The following changes occur:

Initial haemorrhage results in the formation of a fibrin-rich haematoma.

Figure 9.11
Diagrammatic representation of the healing of an incised wound held together by a suture, the track of which alone is shown. The wound rapidly fills with clot (A) and shortly afterwards the epithelium migrates into the wound and down the suture tracks (B). Epithelial spurs are formed, and granulation-tissue (gran) formation proceeds (C). In D the suture has been removed, and scar tissue remains to mark the site of the incision and the suture tracks. The epithelial ingrowths have degenerated.

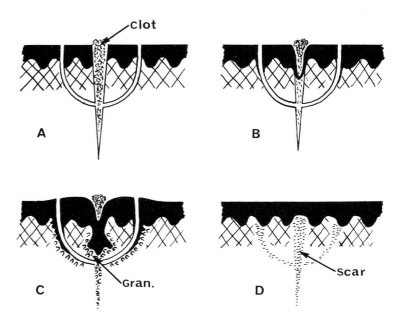

An acute inflammatory reaction occurs, and the fibrinous exudate helps to cement the cut margins of the wound together.

Epithelial Changes. Within 24 hours of injury epithelial cells from the adjacent epidermis migrate into the wound and insinuate themselves between the inert dermis and the clot (Fig. 9.11(b)). With well-approximated wounds by 24 hours a continuous layer of epidermal cells covers the surface. Overlying the area there is a crust or scab of dried clot. During the next 24 to 48 hours the epidermal cells invade the space where connective tissue will eventually develop; in this way a spur is formed (Fig. 9.11(c)). The migrating cells of the epidermis do not divide. Mitotic activity occurs in the basal cells a short distance from the edge of the wound, and in the mouse this activity is maximal at 36 hours. Epidermal cells also migrate along suture tracks, and where the suture or the incision encounters a sweat gland or other skin appendage, epithelial cells are contributed from this source (Fig. 9.11(c)). The stimulus for this epithelial growth and migration is not known. Experimentally it has been noted that cells in tissue culture continue to divide and move until they establish contact with similar cells, at which point both mitosis and movement stop. This has been called *contact inhibition* by Abercrombie, but the mechanism is obscure.

A demolition phase follows the acute inflammatory reaction in the area of the wound.

Organisation. By about the third day the wound area is invaded by fibroblasts and capillary buds growing in from the cut surfaces. This ingrowth occurs mainly from the subcutaneous tissues, with little or no contribution from the dense reticular dermis, which appears inert. There may be some contribution from the papillary dermis.

Soon after the granulation tissue appears, collagen formation commences: at first as reticulin fibres but later maturing to collagen fibres. The amount of collagen in a wound can be assessed histologically, but a more objective method is to estimate the amount of hydroxyproline in hydrosylates of the wound contents. By this technique it has been demonstrated

that the collagen content closely parallels the tensile strength of a wound during the first month. Attempts to demonstrate the amount of ground substance by chemical means have been less successful. The hexosamine content of a healing wound measures not only the hexosamine present in mucopolysaccharides but also that of the plasma glycoproteins in the inflammatory exudate. The total hexosamine level therefore measures the initial inflammatory reaction, rising to a peak at about three days and returning to normal by the ninth day (Fig. 9.10).

The granulation tissue appears to prevent excessive epithelial migration into the wound, and the epithelial cells which form the spurs and the lining of suture tracks degenerate and are replaced by granulation tissue. Only the surface epithelial cells persist, and these divide and differentiate so that a multilayered covering of epidermis is reformed. It first covers a vascular granulation tissue, but as devascularisation proceeds the scar shrinks in size and changes in colour from red to white.

Epithelial cells are thus the first cells to be stimulated, and their presence excites a connective tissue response which in its turn inhibits the epithelial growth. The early role that epithelium plays in the process of wound healing has been stressed by Gillman, and explains the formation of the epidermoid cyst from epithelial remnants (see p. 113), and also the ugly punctate scars which appear if sutures are left in position for any length of time. Punctured wounds due to injections do not form such scars, because the wound is not held open and therefore no epithelial 'invasion' occurs. The use of adhesive tapes instead of sutures for closing wounds avoids these marks and produces a better cosmetic result.[14, 15]

Healing of Wounds with Separated Edges
(*Healing by Secondary Intention*)

Although stress is sometimes laid on the difference between healing by primary intention and secondary intention, the pathological changes in both are very similar. When there is extensive tissue loss, whether by direct trauma, inflammatory

Figure 9.12

Diagram to illustrate the healing of an excised wound. The wound is rapidly filled with clot (A). Epithelium soon migrates in from the margins to undermine the clot, which dries to form a crust. Granulation tissue (gran) grows into the wounded area, and is most profuse around the circumference where it is derived from the subcutaneous tissues (B). Epithelial ingrowth continues and spurs are produced (C); these, however, do not persist, and the end-result (D) is a scar covered by epidermis which lacks rete ridges. During the healing process contraction has taken place so that the final scar is considerably smaller than the original wound.

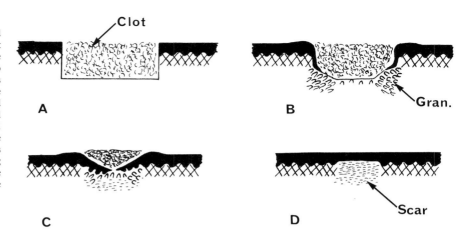

necrosis, or simply failure to approximate the wound edges, a large defect is present which must be made good. The main bulk of tissue which performs this service is granulation tissue, and this type of healing is therefore sometimes known as *healing by granulation*. The term is, however, misleading, since it wrongly implies that granulations are not formed in the simple incised wound. The differences between healing by primary and secondary intention are quantitative not qualitative.

In healing by secondary intention the wound edges are widely separated, so that healing has to progress from the base upwards as well as from the edges inwards. From the clinical point of view healing of a well-approximated incised wound (primary intention) is fast and leaves a small, neat scar. Healing by secondary intention is slow and results in a large, distorted scar. The difference lies in the type of wound and not in the type of healing.

The following account of the healing of a large uninfected wound is illustrated in Figure 9.12.

1. There is an initial inflammatory phase affecting the surrounding tissues. The wound is filled with coagulum, as described in simple incisions. This coagulum dries on its surface, and forms a scab in some wounds.

2. An important feature is *wound contraction*, which has already been fully described (see p. 104). Figure 9.3 (p. 106) shows the changes in size of full-thickness skin loss.

3. As with incised wounds, the epidermis adjacent to the wound shows hyperplasia, and epithelial cells migrate into the wound. They form a thin tongue which grows between pre-existing viable connective tissue and the surface clot with necrotic material. The epithelial cells secrete a collagenase which aids their penetration between living and dead connective tissue.

4. Demolition follows acute inflammation, and the clot in the centre of the wound is invaded and replaced by granulation tissue. This grows from the subcutaneous tissues at the wound edge, and is important in causing wound contraction. Granulation tissue is also formed from the base of the wound, the amount from this source depending upon the nature and vascularity of the bed.

When the wound is viewed with a magnifying glass, the surface (under the scab) is deep red and granular, the capillary loops forming elevated mounds. It is very fragile, and the slightest trauma causes bleeding. It was this granularity which was responsible for the name 'granulation tissue'. The covering of the wound by granulation tissue serves an important protective role. If organisms are introduced into a recent wound, infection is likely to result, but not, however, if the wound is first allowed to granulate. Thus granulation tissue forms a temporary protective layer until the surface is covered by epithelium.

5. The migrating epidermis covers the granulation tissue, and in this way a mushroom-shaped scab is formed with a central attachment, which finally becomes nipped off (Fig. 9.12(c)).

6. The regenerated epidermis becomes thicker, and sends short processes into the underlying tissue. These are transient structures and do not persist as rete ridges; neither these nor the skin appendages are reformed in humans. The epidermal incursions appear to stimulate the formation of granulation tissue, so that the scar gains thickness and is eventually level with the surface of the skin. The scar is at first pink, but the subsequent devascularisation leaves it white.

It can be seen that with full-thickness skin loss, part of the clot occupying the wound is organised but much of it is cast off. With partial-thickness skin loss, as may occur following burns or at the donor site of a Thiersch graft, the area of the wound is covered by epithelium both from the wound edges and from the cut remains of hair follicles and sweat glands. Epithelialisation is therefore very fast, and the granulation tissue which is formed is produced beneath the new epithelium. For reasons which are not known contraction does not occur.

Complications of Wound Healing

Infection. A wound may provide the portal of entry for a variety of different organisms. Infection delays healing, and if severe stops it completely. Scab formation does not occur, and often the base is composed of a slough, underlying which there is inflamed granulation tissue. Tissue destruction due to infection is common, and a simple incision then heals by secondary intention. Fibrous tissue is formed in excessive amounts, and an ugly scar remains.

Wound dehiscence.[16] Dehiscence, the bursting open of a wound, is particularly important after laparotomy, since the mortality of a burst abdomen is approximately 30 per cent. It occurs in from 0·5 to 5·0 per cent of abdominal operation, and is most common with upper abdominal incisions. Undue reliance on inappropriate suture material, such as rapidly absorbed catgut,[17] and poor surgical technique[18] are important factors, as are also those general conditions which favour poor wound healing, e.g. hypoproteinaemia, lack of vitamin C, and poor general nutrition such as may accompany malignant disease. Local factors such as infection play a part; to this must be added excessive tension due to postoperative ileus, peritonitis, or the effects of vomiting and coughing. Increased mechanical stress has been found to be a factor in over 90 per cent of cases of burst abdomen.

Implantation (or epidermoid) cysts. Epithelial cells which flow into the healing wound may sometimes persist, and they may later proliferate to form an epidermoid cyst. It should not be confused with a dermoid cyst (see p. 355).

Keloid formation.[19] Occasionally the excessive formation of collagenous tissue results in the appearance of a raised area of scar tissue called a keloid. The cause of this is unknown. Repeated trauma and irritation caused by foreign bodies, hair, keratin, etc., may play a part. They are more common in the young, especially girls, in Black people, and in tuberculous subjects. They occur most commonly in the region of the neck. They are especially frequent after burns.

Pigmentary changes. Coloured particles introduced into the wound may persist and lead to tattooing. Healed chronic ulcers sometimes have a russet colour due to staining with haemosiderin.

Painful scars. Pain, either local or referred, may be experienced if a neuroma is included in the scar tissue.

Weak scars. If scar tissue is subjected to continuous strain, stretching may result. An incisional hernia develops in this way.

Cicatrisation. This late reduction in the size of a scar is believed to differ from the early contraction of wounds. It is a frequent complication of extensive burning of the skin, and may produce great deformity. Cicatrisation is especially important in hollow viscera such as the urethra, oesophagus, and intestine. It leads to progressive stenosis with stricture formation. The heart valves may exhibit regurgitation as well as stenosis, and in a cirrhotic liver cicatrisation strangles the venous radicles and leads to portal hypertension.

Neoplasia. Trauma may under rare circumstances act as a promoting agent, and squamous-cell carcinoma occasionally develops in scars.

Factors Influencing Repair

Although it would be desirable to analyse the factors which influence repair according to whether they affect granulation-tissue formation, collagen production, contraction, etc., it must be admitted that in many instances we have insufficient information to adopt this policy. In practice the factors that cause delay in wound healing may be divided into two groups: those which act locally, and those whose influence is general.

Local factors. *Poor blood supply.* Wounds with a poor blood supply heal slowly; thus injuries heal much more slowly in the pretibial region than in parts with a good blood supply, e.g. the face. The poor circulation in the skin of the leg in patients with varicose ulcers predisposes to slow healing. Ischaemia secondary to pressure is an important factor in the

causation and poor healing of bedsores. Any condition of chronic inflammation is liable to be accompanied by endarteritis obliterans and a poor blood supply to the part; a good example of this is previous X-irradiation. Finally, the slow wound healing of old age may in part be related to coincidental atheroma.

Adhesions to bony surfaces may, by anchoring the wound edges, prevent contraction and also adequate apposition. This was noted by John Hunter and is well seen in wounds over the tibia, and also in chronic stasis ulcers.

Conditions predisposing to continued tissue breakdown and inflammation. All types of infection come under this heading. Inflammation caused by foreign bodies and irritants like disinfectants is also important. The continued trauma incurred in dressing wounds may cause much damage to the delicate regenerating epithelium.

Movement. Movement may delay wound healing in two ways.

(*a*) By subjecting the wound to persistent trauma and causing acute inflammation.

(*b*) Exercise may act in a systemic way, possibly through the adrenals. It has been shown that animals that are kept on the move show few mitoses in their epidermis.

Neoplasia.

Exposure to ionising radiation. Previous X-irradiation may affect the vascularity of the part, but apart from this X-rays inhibit wound contraction if given at the same time as the injury. The formation of granulation tissue is also delayed.

Ultraviolet light. The exposure of wounds to ultraviolet light is well known clinically to increase the rate of healing, and this has been confirmed experimentally.

General factors affecting wound healing. *Age.* Wound healing is fast in the young, but is normal in old age unless there is some associated debilitating disease or ischaemia.

Nutrition. (*a*) *Protein deficiency.* In starvation or protein depletion there is an impairment of granulation-tissue and collagen formation, resulting in a great delay in wound healing. This may be corrected by the administration of protein containing methionine or cystine. These sulphur-containing amino acids are not present in the mature collagen molecule, but cystine is a vital component of the transport form of collagen or procollagen (p. 64).

(*b*) *Vitamin-C lack.* Wound healing is notoriously slow in scurvy and even healing wounds or fractures break down again (Ch. 34).

Experimentally in guinea-pigs (scurvy does not occur in other rodents because they can synthesise vitamin C) wound contraction and epithelial regeneration proceed normally. Granulation tissue is produced, but is abnormal (see p. 109). Dead tissue, catgut sutures, etc., are poorly removed. Capillaries are unduly fragile and haemorrhages occur.

While florid scurvy is uncommon, minor degrees of vitamin-C lack are not infrequent. If guinea-pigs kept on a normal maintenance dose of the vitamin are subjected to burning, they develop a scorbutic state. Wounds then show the characteristic features of scorbutic healing.

(*c*) *The role of zinc.*[20] The addition of zinc to the diet of rats has been shown to promote the healing of thermal burns and excised wounds. The mechanism is not known, but the fact that zinc is an important component of several enzymes may be related. The oral administration of zinc sulphate has been tried in the human subject, and a beneficial effect on wound healing claimed, but the evidence is contradictory.

Hormones. (*a*) *Glucocorticoids.* Their effects on granulation-tissue formation and wound contraction have been previously noted (see pp. 106 and 109).

(*b*) *Deoxycorticosterone acetate* (DOCA) and anabolic steroids like testosterone are claimed to increase the speed of wound healing.

In general the effects of hormone administration in animals are difficult to assess. Their action may be marked, or it may be reversed by a secondary effect upon other endocrines, especially the pituitary.

Temperature. It is general experience that wounds heal much more slowly in cold weather, and experiments on cold-blooded animals (alligators) have shown that the rate of wound healing is proportional to the temperature of the environment at which they are kept. A rise of 10°C results in a two-fold increase in the speed of wound healing. In squirrels hibernating at 5°C epithelialisation of granulation tissue is completely in abeyance.[21]

Repair in the central nervous system. Repair in the central nervous system follows the same general pattern as that seen in other parts of the body. There are, however, several slight modifications due to its specialised structure. Owing to the abundance of free lipid in damaged brain tissue the macrophages in the demolition phase ingest large quantities of it. They become swollen and their cytoplasm is foamy. They are called compound granular corpuscles, because they contain lipid and haemosiderin. They are probably derived both from microglia (the histiocytes of the brain) and the blood monocytes. In the central nervous system the astrocyte is the counterpart of the fibroblast present in other connective tissues, and therefore glial tissue is found instead of fibrous tissue. Injuries involving the pia may, however, stimulate the production of a granulation tissue containing fibroblasts and collagen as well as neuroglia.

The mechanism of wound healing.[22] When one considers that in a healing wound there is cell and tissue production proceeding at a rate which exceeds that seen in most malignant tumours, it is humiliating to admit how little we know of the mechanisms involved. We understand neither the signal which starts the process, nor the mechanisms which maintain and control it.

Older workers claimed that local wound hormones, or *trephones*, were responsible for healing, but none has been isolated from animal tissue.

One explanation of cellular homeostasis is based on the proposition that there is a negative feedback mechanism whereby new cell production is inhibited by tissue-specific feedback information emanating from the mass of cells already present. An agent responsible for this inhibition is called a *chalone*,[23,24] a word derived from the Greek *chalao*, meaning I loosen or relax. Destruction of an area of tissue leads to a lack of specific chalone locally. This results in proliferation of adjacent cells so that the original bulk of tissue is restored.

Chalones are described as being water soluble and tissue specific, but not species specific. They appear to act at either the G_1 or the G_2 phase of the cell cycle and in this manner inhibit cell mitosis. There are claims that chalones which specifically inhibit the growth of epidermis, liver, kidney, circulating granulocytes, lymphocytes, and lung—amongst other tissues—have been isolated. Unfortunately no pure chalone has been demonstrated. The activity—and indeed the very existence—of a chalone must be judged by its *in-vivo* activity. Tissue extracts claimed to contain chalone can exhibit the ability to inhibit mitoses by virtue of their complement content or the presence of bacterial toxins derived from contaminants. The actual measurement of the activity of a preparation is either tedious, e.g. by counting mitoses in a tissue, or subject to possible errors, e.g. by estimating ^{3}H thymidine uptake. Hence the very existence of chalones, as at present envisaged, is in doubt.

Physical factors play an important part in tissue homeostasis; for instance epithelial cells tend to maintain contact with each other and spread over surfaces. The migration of squamous epithelium in wound healing can thus be understood. However, the subsequent division of the cells and the formation of a multi-layered epidermis cannot be so explained. Although some general factors, such as food supply, hormones, etc., affect wound healing, local factors appear to outweigh them in potency and in importance. In the control of cell division and maturation it is local factors which are most likely to be of major importance. An important component of this control appears to be related to direct cell-to-cell contact. Precisely how cells communicate information to their neighbours is unknown, but that they can do so is evident by the phenomenon of contact inhibition (p. 111), and the remarkable interaction of epidermis with dermis that takes place in wound healing.

GENERAL READING

BLAIR, G. H., SLOME, D. & WALTER, J. B. (1961) Review of experimental investigations on wound healing. In *British Surgical Practice. Surgical Progress*, pp. 462–505. Edited by E. R. Carling and J. P. Ross. London: Butterworths.

DOUGLAS, D. M. (1963) *Wound Healing and Management: A Monograph for Surgeons.* Edinburgh: Livingstone.

Leading Article (1973) To heal the wound. *Lancet*, **2**, 84.

LEVENSON, S. M., STEIN, J. M. & GROSSBLATT, N. (1966) (Eds) *Wound Healing, Proceedings of a Workshop.* Washington: National Academy of Sciences–National Research Council.

McMINN, R. M. H. (1969) *Tissue Repair*, 432 pp. New York: Academic Press.

PEACOCK, E. E. & VAN WINKLE, W. (1970) *Surgery and Biology of Wound Repair*, 630 p. Philadelphia, London and Toronto: Saunders.

SLOME, D. (1961) (Ed) *Wound Healing.* Oxford: Pergamon.

REFERENCES

1. ROSE, S. M. (1970) *Regeneration: Key to Understanding Normal and Abnormal Growth and Development.* 264 pp. New York: Appleton-Century-Crofts.
2. WALTER, J. B. (1976) Wound healing. *Journal of Otolaryngology*, **5**, 171.

3. GABBIANI, G. *et al.* (1972) Granulation tissue as a contractile organ. *Journal of Experimental Medicine*, **135**, 719.
4. GRILLO, H. C. & GROSS, J. (1959) Studies in wound healing: III. Contraction in vitamin C deficiency. *Proceedings of the Society for Experimental Biology and Medicine*, **101**, 268.
5. WATTS, G. T., GRILLO, H. C. & GROSS, J. (1958) Studies in wound healing: II. The role of granulation tissue in contraction. *Annals of Surgery*, **148**, 153.
6. CLIFF, W. T. (1963) Observations on healing tissue; a combined light and electron microscopic investigation. *Philosophical Transactions of the Royal Society, Series B*, **246**, 305.
7. JACKSON, D. S. (1977) Cell proliferation and collagen biosynthesis. *Annals of the Rheumatic Diseases*, **36**, Supplement 2, p. 2.
8. FORRESTER, J. D. (1973) Mechanical, biochemical, and architectural features of surgical repair. *Advances in Biological and Medical Physics*, **14**, 1.
9. WIANCKO, K. B., KLING, S. & MACKENZIE, W. C. (1961) Wound healing—incisions and suturing. *Canadian Medical Association Journal*, **84**, 254.
10. DOUGLAS, D. M. (1961) *In Wound Healing*, ed. Slome, D., p. 62. *loc. cit.*
11. ORDMAN, L. J. & GILLMAN, T. (1966) Studies in the healing of cutaneous wounds. *Archives of Surgery*, **93**, 857, 883 and 911.
12. GILLMAN, T. (1968) Healing of cutaneous wounds. *Glaxo Volume*, **31**, 5.
13. LINDSAY, W. K. & BIRCH, J. R. (1964) Thin skin healing. *Canadian Journal of Surgery*, **7**, 297.
14. ROTHNIE, N. G. & TAYLOR, G. W. (1963) Sutureless skin suture. *British Medical Journal*, **2**, 1027.
15. MURRAY, P. J. B. (1963) Closure of skin wounds with adhesive tape. *British Medical Journal*, **2**, 1030.
16. Leading Article (1972) Burst abdomen. *British Medical Journal*, **3**, 4.
17. Leading Article (1977) Burst abdomen—a preventable condition? *British Medical Journal*, **1**, 534.
18. Leading Article (1977) Burst abdomen. *Lancet*, **1**, 28.
19. KING, G. D. & SALZMAN, F. A. (1970) Keloid scars. *Surgical Clinics of North America*, **50**, 595.
20. Leading Article (1975) Zinc in human medicine. *Lancet*, **2**, 351.
21. BILLINGHAM, R. E. & SILVERS, W. K. (1960) A note on the fate of skin autografts and homografts and on the healing of cutaneous wounds in hibernating squirrels. *Annals of Surgery*, **152**, 975.
22. PEACOCK, E. E. (1973) Biologic frontiers in the control of healing. *American Journal of Surgery*, **126**, 708.
23. HOUCK, J. C. (Ed.) (1976) *Chalones*, 510 pp. Amsterdam: North-Holland Publishing Company.
24. RYTÖMAA, T. (1976) The chalone concept. *International Review of Experimental Pathology*, **16**, 155.

Chapter 10.   *Healing in Specialised Tissues*

The healing which follows tissue loss involves two main processes.

1. The wound undergoes contraction; this has been considered in Chapter 9.

2. The defect which remains is filled in by new cells during the processes of repair or regeneration.

Either process may predominate: for instance, repair is a salient feature of healing in excised skin wounds, and in the central nervous system. In general, tissues composed of cells that are incapable of division (i.e. permanent cells, like neurons) heal by repair. Regeneration is predominant when the cells comprising the tissue are capable of division (labile and stable cells), and is well illustrated by the healing of a damaged liver. The healing of a wound is therefore a complex process depending upon the types of cells which have been lost; these categories of labile, stable, and permanent cells are further considered on page 294.

HEALING IN CONNECTIVE TISSUE

BONE

The healing of a fracture can be appreciated only if the normal structure and formation of bone is first understood.

Structure of Bone[1-4]

Bone is composed of *calcified osteoid tissue*, which consists of collagen fibres embedded in a mucoprotein matrix (osseomucin). It is the special composition of this ground substance which imparts to bone its characteristic properties, and it is here that the bone salts are deposited. Depending upon the arrangement of the collagen fibres, two histological types may be recognised.

Woven, immature, fibrillary, or non-lamellar bone. This shows irregularity in the arrangement of the collagen bundles and in the distribution of the osteocytes. The osseomucin is usually basophilic, and is less abundant than in mature bone. It also contains less calcium. Woven bone is formed under three conditions:

(*a*) When bone forms in a sheet of differentiating mesenchyme. This occurs during embryonic development of the bones of the vault of the skull, the mandible, and the clavicle. These are therefore sometimes called *membrane bones*.

(*b*) When bone forms in the midst of differentiating granulation tissue. This is seen in fracture healing.

(*c*) In osteogenic tumours and other bone disorders.

Lamellar or adult bone. In this type of bone the collagen bundles are arranged in parallel sheets either in the form of concentric Haversian systems or flat plates (see Fig. 10.1).

In the outer dense *cortex* of a long bone Haversian systems predominate, while flat plates are seen under the periosteum and endosteum. This type of bone is called *compact*.

The central portion is hollowed out to form the medullary cavity, which contains marrow. Only a few spicules of bone remain. These are constructed of flat bundles of collagen, although in the wider trabeculae Haversian systems may be found. The central 'open' trabeculated part of the bone is called *cancellous*, but it should be noted that, like 'compact', this is a term related to the naked-eye appearance of a bone.

Lamellar bone is formed under three conditions:

(*a*) Whenever there has been a previous model of cartilage. Most of the skeleton is formed in this manner, and the process

Figure 10.1
Diagrammatic representation of a transverse section through part of the shaft of a long bone to show the arrangement of lamellar bone.

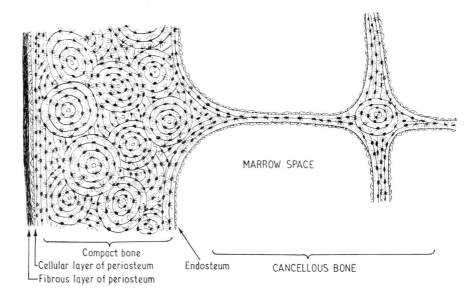

MARROW SPACE

Compact bone
Cellular layer of periosteum
Fibrous layer of periosteum
Endosteum   CANCELLOUS BONE

continues at the epiphyseal ends of long bones until adult stature is reached. The process is known as endochondral ossification. It must be understood that the cartilage is not converted into bone, but is *replaced* by bone.

The chondrocytes in the area of cartilage about to be replaced by bone enlarge and probably secrete alkaline phosphatase, since calcium salts are laid down in the intervening matrix. This interferes with the normal diffusion of nutrients to the cartilage cells (cartilage is avascular), which therefore die. The dead cartilage disintegrates, and some of it undergoes lysis to leave cavities. Into these spaces osteogenic cells and blood vessels grow; the cells differentiate into osteoblasts and lay down lamellar bone on cores of calcified cartilage. In some areas the bone remains cancellous, but on the periphery of the shaft of a long bone, successive layers of bone are laid down on the central vascular tunnel, which becomes an Haversian canal. This and the concentric lamellae of bone form an Haversian system.

The cartilage which forms during the healing of fractures is similarly replaced by bone.

(*b*) Lamellar bone is also formed whenever there has been a previous model of woven bone, whether formed during embryonic development or in fracture healing. In the normal adult the entire skeleton is composed of lamellar bone regardless of its developmental origin.

(*c*) When once lamellar bone has been formed, its progressive growth and remodelling result in further adult-bone formation.

Bone, whether woven or lamellar, is made by specialised cells called osteoblasts; microscopically these resemble fibroblasts and they manufacture collagen fibres as well as the osseomucin. They contain alkaline phosphatase, which may play a part in subsequent calcification of the osteoid. It should be noted that osteoid normally calcifies as soon as it is made. When the cells become trapped in the bone they become smaller and inactive, and are called osteocytes. These are enclosed in spaces, or *lacunae*, which intercommunicate by means of fine canaliculi. The latter are formed round the fine cytoplasmic processes of the osteocytes, but when the matrix calcifies the processes are withdrawn leaving an intercommunicating system of channels through which the osteocytes gain nourishment. These lacunae and canaliculi are seen in ground sections of bone and lie between the concentric lamellae of Haversian bone.

Bone is removed by large multinucleate *osteoclasts*, which by resorbing bone are often to be seen lying in small indentations called *Howship's lacunae*. It is generally accepted that the osteoclast is formed from a fusion of a number of macrophages.

In summary, the following classifications of bone are recognised.

Microscopic appearance:	Lamellar / Non-lamellar
Naked-eye appearance:	Compact / Cancellous
Developmental:	Membranous / Cartilaginous
Anatomical:	Long, flat, etc.

Stages in Fracture Healing (Bone Regeneration)[2, 5]

The stages in healing of a fracture are illustrated diagrammatically in Figure 10.2. It must be remembered that the entire area will not all be at the same stage of healing at the same time; thus, while the centre may be at an early stage, the changes adjacent to the bone ends will be much more advanced. However, for descriptive purposes it is convenient to divide the healing process into separate stages.

Figure 10.2

Stages in the healing of a fracture.

(*a*) Haematoma formation.

(*b*) Stages 2 and 3. Acute inflammation followed by demolition. Loose fragments of bone are removed, and the bone ends show osteoporosis.

(*c*) Stage 4. Granulation-tissue formation.

(*d*) Stage 5. The bone ends are now united by woven bone, cartilage, or a mixture of the two. This hard material is often called callus and can be divided into three parts—internal, intermediate, and external. The intermediate callus is that part which lies in line with the cortex of the bone. The internal callus occupies the original marrow cavity, while the external callus produces the fusiform swelling visible on the outside of the bone.

(*e*) Stage 6. Lamellar bone is laid down; calcified cartilage and woven bone are progressively removed.

(*f*) Stage 7. Final remodelling.

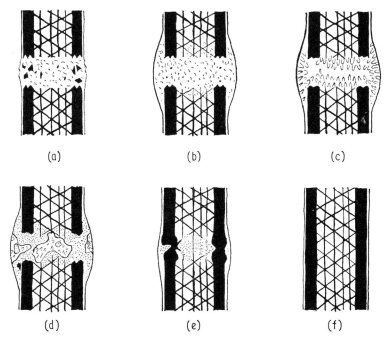

(a) (b) (c)

(d) (e) (f)

Stage 1: Haematoma formation. Immediately following the injury there is a variable amount of bleeding from torn vessels; if the periosteum is torn this blood may extend into the surrounding muscles. If it is subsequently organised and ossified, myositis ossificans results.

Stage 2: Traumatic inflammation. The tissue damage excites an inflammatory response, the exudate adding more fibrin to the clot already present. The inflammatory changes differ in no way from those seen in other inflamed tissues. There is an increased blood flow and a polymorphonuclear leucocytic infiltration. This hyperaemia has been held responsible for the decreased density of the adjacent bone ends often noted radiologically. This 'decalcification' is presumably due to osteoclastic activity, but the cause of this is not clear. The connective tissue changes accompanying the inflammatory reaction result in a loosening of the attachment of the periosteum to the bone. The haematoma therefore attains a fusiform shape.

Stage 3: Demolition. Macrophages invade the clot and remove the fibrin, red cells, inflammatory exudate, and debris. Any fragments of bone which have become detached from their blood supply undergo necrosis, and are scavenged by macrophages and osteoclasts.

Stage 4: Formation of granulation tissue. Following this phase of demolition there is an ingrowth of capillary loops and mesenchymal cells derived from the periosteum and the endosteum of the cancellous bone. The importance of the periosteum in fracture union has been much discussed in the past. The cells of its deeper layer certainly have osteogenic potentiality, and together with its blood vessels contribute to the granulation tissue. Under some circumstances this assumes great importance.

In fractures of the neck of the femur the head is dependent upon the periosteum for its blood supply. If this is damaged, there is ischaemic necrosis of the head. Thus the integrity of the periosteum is of great practical importance. The periosteum alone is capable of effecting complete regeneration of a rib following subperiosteal resection. Here its outer fibrous layer acts by forming a limiting vascular membrane around the haematoma, while its inner layer provides osteogenic cells for the formation of granulation tissue and bone.

In fractures of the long bones, however, it must not be forgotten that a very extensive area of cancellous bone is exposed. From this the endosteal osteoblasts and the medullary blood vessels grow out to form the granulation tissue. Under these circumstances the periosteum is of much less importance.

During these early phases the pH is low, and this is spoken of as the *acid tide*.

Stage 5: Woven bone and cartilage formation. The mesenchymal 'osteoblasts' next differentiate to form either woven bone or cartilage. The term 'callus', derived from the Latin and meaning hard, is often used to describe the material uniting the fracture ends regardless of its consistency. When this is granulation tissue, the 'callus' is soft, but as bone or cartilage formation occurs, it becomes hard. The word is used loosely by surgeons, radiologists, and pathologists, but exact definition of its various stages is difficult and serves no useful function. If the term is used, it is probably best to apply it to the calcified hard tissue uniting the bone ends.

Formation of woven bone. The osteoblasts form both the collagen fibres and the ground substance osseomucin in which they are embedded. The tissue produced is called *osteoid*, and is formed during maturation of the granulation tissue; as in the repair of ordinary connective tissue progressive devascularisation occurs. The collagen bundles are irregularly disposed with no attempt at lamellar structure. This osteoid undergoes calcification, and is then called woven bone.

After about ten days the pH of the uniting fracture increases. During this *alkaline tide* calcium salts are deposited in the osteoid. Osteoblasts produce an alkaline phosphatase which may play a part in the calcification by leading to a local supersaturation of phosphate following its action on hexose phosphates. However, it must be remembered that in any healing wound the fibroblasts form a similar enzyme, and yet no calcification occurs. The exact function of this enzyme is unknown. The resorption of bony spicules may play a part in causing a local supersaturation of calcium salts.

The bone ends thus become united by woven bone. It forms a fusiform mass which may arbitrarily be divided into internal, intermediate, and external callus (see Fig. 10.2 (d)).

Woven-bone formation is found whenever the bone ends are adequately immobilised. It is, therefore, predominant in human fracture healing. In experimentally-produced fractures in animals adequate immobilisation is difficult to attain, and then the granulation tissue matures not to woven bone, but to hyaline cartilage.

Formation of cartilage. The mesenchymal cells ('osteoblasts') behave as chondroblasts and form cartilage, i.e. the cells actively lead to the formation of a specialised ground substance in which the collagen fibres are embedded. The intervening matrix undergoes calcification, and the cartilage cells die. Cartilage formation occurs in fractures in which there is movement, e.g. in experimental animal fractures and human fractures where complete immobilisation is impossible, as in the ribs.

In many fractures cartilage and woven bone are formed; both are merely methods of temporarily uniting bone ends with calcified material. This acts as a scaffold on which the final adult lamellar bone can later be built. It is evident that the granulation tissue of a healing fracture bears some resemblance to the blastema of amphibian axial regeneration (p. 103), since it contains dedifferentiated cells that can subsequently form either cartilage or bone. The two embryological methods of bone formation, endochondral and intramembranous ossification, are thus faithfully repeated in the bone regeneration of later life. Indeed, under some circumstances synovial cells can be formed and a false joint produced (see later).

Stage 6: Formation of lamellar bone. The dead calcified cartilage disintegrates and is invaded by blood vessels and osteoblasts (see p. 117), whereas the woven bone is removed by osteoclasts before this vascular invasion takes place. As the initial scaffolding ('provisional callus') is removed, osteoblasts lay down osteoid which calcifies to form bone. Its collagen bundles are now arranged in orderly lamellar fashion, for the most part concentrically around the blood vessels, and in this way the Haversian systems are formed. Adjacent to the periosteum and endosteum the lamellae are parallel to the surface as in the normal bone. This phase of formation of definitive lamellar bone merges with the last stage.

Stage 7: Remodelling. The final remodelling process involving the continued osteoclastic removal and osteoblastic laying down of bone results in the formation of a bone which differs remarkably little from the original tissue. The *external callus* is slowly removed, the *intermediate callus* becomes converted into compact bone containing Haversian systems, while the *internal callus* is hollowed out into a marrow cavity in which only a few spicules of cancellous bone remain.

Abnormalities of Fracture Healing

1. **Repair, or fibrous union.** It will be recalled that the mesenchymal cells of the granulation tissue are called osteoblasts, but they are capable of differentiation along several lines. They can form bone, but if immobilisation is not complete, cartilage may develop. When movement is even more free, the cells behave as fibroblasts and the bone ends become united by simple scar tissue. Whether this can ever undergo ossification is debatable. It is claimed by some authorities that fibrous tissue can become replaced by bone, but that it is a very slow process.[5] From a practical point of view fibrous union is an unsatisfactory end-result of fracture healing because in many cases it is permanent.

Occasionally with excessive movement the cells differentiate into synovial cells, and a false joint, or pseudarthrosis, results. This is a well-recognised sequel of fractures of the tibia.

2. **Non-union.** A complete lack of union between the fracture ends results from the interposition of soft parts. Muscle or fascia separating the bone ends may prevent the formation of a uniting haematoma. Under these conditions union of any sort is impossible.

3. **Delayed union.** In the presence of a persisting haematoma any of the causes of delayed healing (see p. 113) will retard bone regeneration. If the adverse conditions are severe there may be fibrous union rather than delayed union with bone.

In practice the following are the most important:

Movement. Movement of any sort is harmful, because it causes damage to the delicate granulation tissue and thereby excites an inflammatory reaction. In surgical practice every attempt is made to reduce movement to a minimum. In impacted fractures this is usually easy, but where the bone ends are mobile, pins, plates, or other forms of internal splinting may have to be used. The damage caused by overdistraction is an important cause of delayed union or non-union. By contrast, if the bone ends are brought together under high compression, there is rigid immobilisation and healing is accelerated.[6]

Infection. By prolonging the acute inflammatory phase infection is an important cause of delayed union or non-union. Since the tension engendered by the formation of exudate in a bone is particularly liable to lead to extensive ischaemic necrosis, it is especially important to avoid contaminating previously closed fractures during open reduction. Rigorous asepsis must be maintained by employing a no-touch technique.

Poor blood supply. While complete loss of blood supply results in necrosis of bone, poor blood supply leads to slow granulation-tissue formation and therefore delayed union.

Certain sites are notorious for this complication, e.g. fractures of neck of femur, shaft of tibia, and the carpal scaphoid. In these situations the avoidance of other causes of delayed healing e.g. movement, is particularly important. The slow healing of fractures in old age is probably due to ischaemia.

Spontaneous fractures. Sudden unexpected strains may cause fractures in normal bones. The violent convulsive movements of tetanus and strychnine poisoning or electroconvulsive therapy (ECT) without prior anaesthesia not uncommonly result in the collapse of a vertebral body, causing wedging. Avulsion of the spinous process of the seventh cervical vertebra ('clay-shoveller's disease') and march fracture of the metatarsal are other examples of spontaneous fractures due to muscular stress.

Pathological fracture. This term is applied to fractures occurring in diseased bones subjected to a normal strain. Any lesion that weakens the bones is liable to cause fracture. Generalised conditions, e.g. osteitis fibrosa cystica of von Recklinghausen and osteogenesis imperfecta, are well-known but uncommon examples. Solitary and aneurysmal bone cysts, hydatid cysts, giant-cell tumours, and angiomatous hamartomata are other examples. Secondary tumours must always be borne in mind, and indeed a fracture is often the first symptom of such a tumour. Somewhat surprisingly, most pathological fractures heal well, even when due to metastatic carcinoma.

Cartilage

Regeneration in cartilage is generally poor. In the hyaline cartilage of joint surfaces small defects are made good by regeneration. With larger injuries which damage the underlying vascular bone, a haematoma is formed which becomes vascularised and converted either into fibrous tissue or bone.

Tendon[7]

Regeneration in tendon is good, but the process is slow. It is said that the tendon ends should be accurately united and under some tension, otherwise union is by fibrous scar tissue.

Muscle[8]

Smooth muscle.[9] Smooth muscle has limited regenerative capacity. In large destructive lesions of unstriped muscle a permanent scar remains to mark the site of the original injury, and this is well illustrated in a healed chronic peptic ulcer. Nevertheless, it is not uncommon to find no trace of an ulcer at necropsy despite convincing radiographic evidence that one existed previously.

That smooth muscle cells have definite powers of regeneration has been shown in an experimental crush injury of the taenia of the guinea-pig caecum. Although about 10 000 cells are destroyed, they are so rapidly replaced that by 14 days there is little microscopic evidence of injury. Furthermore, the proliferating cells that fill in the gap show the electron-microscopic features of smooth muscle.[10]

The arterioles of granulation tissue acquire a muscular coat; the origin of these fibres is debated: perhaps they arise by differentiation of adjacent connective tissue cells that migrate with the endothelial cells.

Cardiac muscle. The heart muscle in human beings appears to show no regenerative capacity, and once necrosis has occurred, as in infarction, a permanent scar remains. Under special circumstances cardiac muscle cells may form giant cells similar to those seen in voluntary muscle. It has been suggested that the Aschoff giant cell of rheumatic fever is of this nature.

Skeletal muscle. The capacity of skeletal muscle to regenerate has usually been underestimated by pathologists. When part of an individual fibre is damaged, regeneration follows. Cells of the original syncytium appear to dedifferentiate, separate as individual cells, and undergo division. The regenerating cells fuse and differentiate into a new muscle fibre that is continuous with the old. Thus, in a surgical wound of voluntary muscle the regenerating cells on either side of the incision may unite, so that in time the continuity of the muscle is restored.[11] Similarly, when part of a muscle fibre has been damaged, as in Zenker's necrosis, full restoration of structure and function is possible. When muscle damage is extensive, and particularly if accompanied by ischaemia as with infarction, healing is mainly by scar tissue.

The considerable regenerative capacity of striated skeletal muscle can be demonstrated experimentally.[12] If a rat's gastrocnemius is removed, minced into 1 mm cubes with scissors, and replaced into the animal's leg, a new muscle is formed. The restoration is not perfect; the muscle is smaller than the original, and there is some scarring. Nevertheless, the muscle fibres are correctly aligned with the long axis of the limb, and function returns. The original muscle cells dedifferentiate, multiply, and then differentiate again into muscle fibres. Whether human muscle can regenerate in this manner is not known; restoration of a blood supply would seem to pose a major problem.

Bone Marrow

Bone marrow provides an excellent example of tissue in which regeneration is complete.

Fat

Although fat cells may appear in fully mature granulation tissue, as sometimes seen in the rabbit ear-chamber, defects in fatty tissue are usually made good by fibrous tissue. The process of repair shows a characteristic feature during the demolition phase: the macrophages ingest large quantities of fat, becoming greatly swollen in the process. These 'foam cells' form a prominent feature of traumatic fat necrosis. Fatty acid and cholesterol crystals may also be laid down and excite a giant-cell reaction.

Mesothelial Lining of Peritoneum and Other Serious Cavities[13]

Denuded areas are healed by metaplasia of the underlying connective tissue cells, which take on the form and function of flattened mesothelium. Hence following abdominal surgery raw areas are rapidly covered by newly-formed mesothelium. Adhesions do not develop unless healing is complicated by inflammation caused either by infection or the presence of irritant chemicals, such as talc or starch in glove powder. Likewise sutures can cause inflammation and adhesion formation: raw areas are best left to heal unaided by the surgeon's attempts at covering them with peritoneum.

Synovial lining cells are also replaced from underlying connective tissue. The adjacent uninjured synovial cells are inert and play no part in the process of healing.[14]

Vascular endothelium.[15] The regeneration of vascular endothelium has been extensively investigated in the hope that it might provide a clue to the pathogenesis of atheroma. Following the mechanical removal of an area of endothelium from the rabbit's aorta, new endothelial cells arise by mitotic division from pre-existing lining cells, and slowly spread over the denuded area covering it in about one year. When a section of baboon aorta is replaced by a knitted fabric prosthesis, a new endothelial lining forms within ten weeks. New endothelial cells are derived from vessels penetrating the fabric as well as from the aorta itself. A similar re-endothelialisation occurs following endarterectomy. The vasa vasorum here contribute to the process.

It has been suggested that endothelial cells can also evolve from deposited circulating mononuclear cells. This view is not supported by the observation that the new endothelial cells can initiate fibrinolysis; it has been found that only endothelial cells in a vessel wall have this property. Flattened monocytes forming a pseudo-endothelium do not have this ability, and they differ also in their electron microscopic appearances.

Nervous Tissue

Adult nerve cells are unable to divide and therefore are incapable of taking part in any regenerative process. In lower animals, e.g. some amphibians, following the loss of the tail, ependymal cells proliferate and later mature into neurons. Thus the spinal cord can be regenerated in these animals; no such phenomenon occurs in the human subject.

When the axon of a nerve cell is severed, changes take place which may result in the reformation of the severed end. The process has been studied most frequently in the peripheral nerves, where the axons are enclosed in the Schwann cells and are myelinated when they exceed 2 μm in diameter.

Peripheral nervous system.[16,17] Following section of the axis cylinder, the nerve cell shows changes described as *chromatolysis.* The cell swells and its Nissl granules disappear. These bodies are zones of endoplasmic reticulum studded plentifully with ribosomes, and their disappearance reflects dysfunction in the protein-synthesising system of the nerve cell. The axis cylinder becomes irregular and varicose, and by 48 hours has become broken up. The myelin degenerates and becomes broken up into segments called ovoids. These are engulfed by the Schwann cell to form autophagosomes, for the cell that once formed the myelin now engulfs it and breaks it down into small vacuoles. The broken-down material derived from the axons and the myelin is finally engulfed and removed by macrophages. These cells are derived from the blood monocytes, as they are during a demolition phase in other parts of the body. Precisely how the lipid droplets pass from the Schwann cells to the macrophages is not known. These changes were originally described as *Wallerian degeneration,* and affect the nerve fibre distal to the point of section and also, in myelinated fibres, a short area proximally up to the first node of Ranvier.

In addition to their phagocytic activity the Schwann cells proliferate; those from the segment distal to the cut join with those proliferating from the proximal stump. In this way continuity is established across the gap by a mass of Schwann cells. Next, from the proximal portion of the cut axon numerous neurofibrils sprout out, and are seen to lie invaginated into the cytoplasm of the Schwann cells. They push their way distally through the Schwann cells at the rate of about 1 mm per day. Many of the fibrils lose their way and degenerate, but some reach an appropriate end-organ and persist to form the definitive replacement axon. It is evident that accurate apposition of the cut ends of the nerve is of great importance in facilitating this process. The final stage involves the reformation of the myelin sheath as the regenerating axon matures and increases in diameter.

The functional end-result of nerve damage depends on various factors: if the axons are damaged but the nerve trunk itself is not severed, an excellent result may be expected. When the nerve is severed, careful suturing and the exclusion of infection are important for good recovery. Functional recovery is more complete when a pure motor or sensory nerve is cut. Recovery from a lesion of a mixed nerve, like the median nerve, is often poor.

Central nervous system.[18, 19] Here oligodendroglia take the place of the Schwann cells in relation to nerve fibres. It is often taught that regeneration of central nerve fibres does not occur: the affected nerve cells show chromatolysis often followed by necrosis, and the destroyed tissue is replaced by proliferating neuroglia to form a dense glial scar. Nevertheless, there is considerable evidence that some regeneration is possible. In the clinical field it is noticeable that in patients with partial spinal-cord lesions, voluntary muscle strength seems to increase steadily for 9 to 12 months. This is generally attributed to improved utilisation of residual undamaged pathways, but in addition new fibres may be formed; sometimes these appear to originate from cells in the posterior root ganglia. Certainly in the lower animals regeneration of the long-tract axons in the spinal cord and in the optic nerve is a usual feature, and there is good reason to believe that this can also occur in the higher animals, including the human. How important these fibres are from a functional point of view, and whether means could be found to improve regeneration, are subjects which are being studied at the present time. The isolation of a nerve-growth factor in certain tumours, snake venom, and salivary gland has aroused much interest, but the role of this protein, hormone-like substance is at present not known.[20]

HEALING IN EPITHELIAL TISSUES

It is often stated that the greater the degree of specialisation of a tissue, the less well developed are its powers of regeneration. Certainly nerve cells are highly specialised and incapable of division, but degrees of specialisation in cells are as difficult to define as they are amongst human beings. Is a liver cell more or less specialised than a simple unstriped muscle fibre? Liver cells show remarkable powers of proliferation, yet perform functions of which they alone are capable. Similarly, it is impossible to compare the degrees of specialisation of the different types of epithelium, each of which has its own peculiar characteristics. It seems more likely that the power of regeneration is best developed in those organs and tissues which are most liable to injury, and the replacement of which has survival value for the individual.

All covering epithelia show good regenerative power. This is hardly surprising since they are being continuously subjected to trauma, and their integrity depends upon their ability to replace the lost cells.

Skin and Other Squamous Epithelia

These show good regeneration, although specialised structures like the rete ridges, hair follicles, sweat glands, and sebaceous glands are not replaced in humans. The details of the epithelial changes in skin wounds, involving both movement and division of cells, have already been described (Ch. 9). Wounds of the oesophagus behave similarly. In both it should be noted that the actively migrating cells do not undergo mitosis; this occurs only when they gain attachment to the underlying connective tissue.

OTHER LINING EPITHELIA[21]

Intestinal Epithelium

Complete regeneration results in perfect replacement of lost epithelium, including in the small intestine the crypts and villi. It is interesting that because there is normally a very high rate of mitotic activity in the epithelium of the small intestine, no further increase occurs at the wound margins.

Stomach

Here regeneration is good, and in contrast to stratified squamous epithelium the migrating cells show mitosis. Acute ulceration of the mucosa of the stomach is a common event, but healing occurs rapidly without any scarring because the underlying connective tissue and muscle is not destroyed. In chronic peptic ulcers epithelial regeneration is inhibited, the reason for which is not known. When healing does occur, the newly-formed epithelium may be of intestinal type, showing well-marked villi.

Bladder

In experimental wounds of the bladder mucosa there is active migration and mitosis of cells. As in the intestine and gall-bladder mitosis occurs in the migrating cells. After one month the wound shows characteristic crypt-like downgrowths of epithelium, such as are described in the condition of cystitis glandularis.

Transitional epithelium shows a remarkable regenerative capacity after complete removal of the bladder mucosa. In the dog, within 16 weeks the organ is completely relined by epithelium which has grown from the ureters and the urethra.[22] Complete resection of the bladder mucosa has therefore been suggested as a treatment for multiple papillomatous tumours, but whether the new mucosa is any less liable to neoplasia is not known. Another surgical application is the use of vein grafts to replace the ureter, for they are soon lined by transitional epithelium.[23]

Gallbladder

Regeneration is good, resembling that of the bladder.

Respiratory Tract

Loss of epithelium, such as occurs in acute influenzal

tracheobronchitis, is quickly followed by the division of basal cells leading to a reformation of ciliated pseudostratified columnar epithelium. Sometimes after repeated damage the new epithelium may change to a simple columnar or squamous type (see metaplasia, p. 303).

GLANDULAR EPITHELIA

Liver[24-26]

The liver has remarkable powers of regeneration. Within 15 hours of resecting 70 per cent of the liver of a rat, many of the hepatocytes previously in the G_0 phase of the cell cycle resume DNA synthesis. By 24 hours 30 per cent of the cells are in the S phase, and this is followed by a wave of mitoses. By two weeks the liver has been restored to its original weight.[26]

In the human being regeneration of liver cells is seen after any type of necrosis, provided the patient survives. The end-results of this regeneration vary so widely, depending upon the type of necrosis, that this important subject will be considered in some detail. The clinical manifestations of liver disease are considered in Chapter 47.

Three categories of hepatic necrosis are recognised:

Focal necrosis, in which there are small foci of necrosis scattered throughout the liver. This occurs in many acute infections, e.g. typhoid fever and pneumonia, and may be related to the parasitisation of Kupffer cells during the incubation period. When these are destroyed, the adjacent liver cells undergo necrosis. Healing presumably occurs by regeneration, because old foci of scarring are not found *post mortem* in such patients when they die of other diseases. Focal necrosis is typical of viral hepatitis.

Zonal necrosis, in which a zone of each lobule throughout the liver undergoes necrosis. Central zonal necrosis is the characteristic lesion of many liver poisons, e.g. chloroform, carbon tetrachloride, muscarine, cinchophen, monoamine-oxidase inhibitors, and paracetamol (when taken in large overdoses).[27] Midzonal necrosis is characteristic of yellow fever. Peripheral zonal necrosis is seen typically in phosphorus poisoning, where there is also severe fatty change, and in eclampsia, where there is gross haemorrhage around the portal tracts. Recovery with regeneration is the usual sequel, and during this phase the remaining liver cells undergo division and replace those which have been destroyed. Since the reticulin framework of each lobule is undamaged, the resulting healing leaves a perfectly normal architecture. After repeated attacks of zonal necrosis, however, some distortion of the liver pattern may occur (see cirrhosis).

A slowly developing destruction of cells, more akin to atrophy than frank necrosis, affects the central zones of the lobules in chronic venous congestion (see cardiac cirrhosis).

Massive necrosis, in which there are extensive areas of necrosis involving the whole liver indiscriminately. It is either idiopathic or the result of severe viral hepatitis or the poisons mentioned above. Death in cholaemia usually ensues within a few days. At necropsy the liver is shrunken, its capsule wrinkled, and the cut surface soft and yellow ('acute yellow atrophy') or dark reddish-brown due to congestion. Sometimes the clinical course is more protracted and there is sufficient time for regeneration to occur. The liver is then small but contains numerous irregular nodules of regenerated parenchyma, many of which also show necrosis. This condition has been called subacute yellow atrophy, but subacute hepatic necrosis is a better name. Sometimes the regeneration of liver is adequate to sustain life, and further necrosis does not occur. However, large areas of liver have been destroyed and the reticulin framework of the lobules has collapsed. Regeneration from surviving islets of liver cells occurs, but the irregular nodules so produced are not normal lobules. Although this is an excellent example of regeneration, the anatomical and functional end-result is not as satisfactory as that occurring after zonal necrosis.

In addition to the regenerative nodules described above, areas of liver where the lobular structure is preserved also show regeneration. A considerable amount of scar tissue is formed. The bile ducts exhibit hyperplasia, and numerous tubules are present amid the fibrous tissue surrounding the liver nodules. The end-result is a coarsely scarred liver with numerous nodules of parenchyma separated from each other by broad bands of fibrous tissue. The larger nodules show a recognisable lobular pattern. The condition has been called postnecrotic scarring and macronodular cirrhosis.

Cirrhosis of the liver. The term cirrhosis was introduced by Laennec who was impressed by the tawny colour of the liver in this condition, but this is due merely to fatty change of the liver cells. The essential feature is diffuse destruction of the parenchyma and its replacement by fibrous tissue which disrupts the normal lobular architecture of the liver. There is usually active regeneration of liver cells occurring at the same time as this fibrous reparative process.

Cirrhosis is best regarded as an *end-stage condition*, as it can be the end-result of liver damage due to many causes— poisons, alcohol, hepatitis, infection, genetic error, etc. Classifications are very unsatisfactory since in most cases the cause is unknown. A descriptive classification is the most useful[28]:

Macronodular cirrhosis. This has been described above.

Micronodular cirrhosis (portal or Laennec's cirrhosis). The liver shows numerous regenerative nodules which are small and fairly uniform in size, and are separated by strands of fibrous tissue (Figs. 10.3 and 10.4). The condition may be idiopathic but is often found in alcoholics. It is often preceded by fatty change which, by leading to necrosis, appears to be responsible for the progressive fibrosis which disrupts the liver lobules.

It must be emphasised that there is no sharp line of division between these two types of cirrhosis, and that mixed types occur. At the present time it is wisest to describe cirrhosis in morphological terms, and accept that any type may follow any cause. Cirrhosis of the liver is an important complication of the metabolic abnormalities that lead to haemochromatosis, Wilson's disease, and galactosaemia.

CARDIAC CIRRHOSIS. In prolonged cardiac failure, especially in young people, there may be a fibrous replacement of the destroyed central zones of the lobules. A fine 'reversed' type of cirrhosis, i.e. starting from the centres of the lobules instead of the portal tracts, may follow.

BILIARY CIRRHOSIS. In persistent obstructive jaundice due either to intrahepatic or extrahepatic factors, e.g. obstruction to the common bile duct, there is an inspissation of bile in

Figure 10.3
Cirrhosis of the liver. A section through the liver shows the regular pattern of small, uniform nodules typical of micronodular cirrhosis. At the top of the specimen there is a large rounded tumour which, in the fresh state, was white in colour and partly bile stained. Histologically it was a well-differentiated hepatoma. The patient was an elderly man who had no history of liver disease, but died with a haemoperitoneum consequent on rupture of the hepatoma. (A108.1, *Reproduced by permission of the President and Council of the R.C.S. Eng.*).

Figure 10.4
Micronodular cirrhosis. A thick strand of cellular fibrous tissue intersects two nodules, the cells of which show severe fatty change. × 32.

many lobules, and this produces an inflammatory reaction, necrosis of neighbouring cells, and progressive fibrosis. The deeply jaundiced liver is finely granular.

It is evident that although the liver and bile-duct epithelial cells possess remarkable powers of regeneration, destructive liver disease is not always attended by a satisfactory end-result. Some of the factors governing the regeneration of liver are:

Age. Experimentally-induced regeneration is better in young animals.

Blood supply. Interference with the blood supply impairs regeneration; this may be a factor in the production of cardiac cirrhosis.

Maintenance of lobular architecture. The marked difference between the regeneration following zonal necrosis compared with that of massive necrosis has already been mentioned.

Cirrhotic livers have limited powers of regeneration. This may, however, be merely a question of poor blood supply.

Bile-duct obstruction appears to impair healing.

Stimulus for liver regeneration.[24] Small wounds of the liver produced surgically, e.g. when performing a biopsy, heal by granulation tissue and scarring. It is evident that the stimulus for liver regeneration is a metabolic one, but its precise nature remains unknown.

The stimulus for liver regeneration acts on the organ as a whole and comes into play when a mass of liver is *resected*, undergoes *necrosis*, or is induced to *atrophy* as by tying off a branch of the portal vein. It has been postulated that an excessive accumulation of some substance in the blood is the stimulus, but none has been identified. No known hormone plays a significant part. Alternatively, it might be that the liver normally produces some inhibiting substance, or chalone, the depletion of which allows regeneration to occur. In spite of much experimental work with much conflicting evidence, the stimulus for liver regeneration is obscure.

Thyroid

Experimentally the thyroid has good powers of regeneration. This may be impaired by the administration of thyroxine, presumably because of pituitary inhibition.

Kidney

The renal tubular epithelium has considerable powers of regeneration; thus in acute tubular necrosis, in spite of extensive damage, complete return to normal may occur. This type of lesion is therefore most eligible for treatment with haemodialysis since recovery is possible. When damage to the kidney results in the destruction of a complete nephron, regeneration does not occur. Glomeruli once destroyed cannot be replaced.

Following unilateral nephrectomy the remaining kidney increases in size. No new nephrons are formed, even in the newborn, and the enlargement is due to an increase in size and number of the cells in the glomeruli and proximal convoluted tubules. The enlargement is greater in young animals than in the old and in well-nourished ones than in the starved. The stimulus for compensatory enlargement is unknown, but is assumed to be humoral.[29]

HYPERPLASIA AND REGENERATION COMPARED

In both conditions there is a division of cells that is kept strictly under control, in contrast with the type of cell division seen in neoplasia. In regeneration there is replacement of lost cells, whilst in hyperplasia there is excessive multiplication of cells, resulting in a larger amount of tissue than normal. The stimulus for cell division is probably the same in both conditions and varies from organ to organ; possibly the withdrawal of an inhibiting influence, such as a chalone, is involved (p. 114). In the case of the endocrine glands hormonal factors are important. In most instances we are quite ignorant of the exact mechanism.

While the distinction between hyperplasia and regeneration is quite clear, the terms are frequently confused. The designation of hepatic cirrhosis as an example of a 'hyperplastic regenerative' condition is a reflection of this confusion. In point of fact the liver cells clearly show regeneration, since the bulk of the liver is not greater than normal in the majority of cases. The bile ducts do show hyperplasia, but nevertheless the use of the term 'hyperplastic regeneration' can only serve to cause confusion and render each word meaningless.

It must be admitted that regeneration and hyperplasia may exist side by side. In a healing skin wound the lost epidermis is regenerated, but the edges of the wound show marked epithelial hyperplasia (see Fig. 9.12). This further stresses the point that the stimulus for both conditions is probably the same. Nevertheless, as long as both pathological terms are used it is desirable that they be used in their correct connotation.

REFERENCES

1. BLOOM, W. & FAWCETT, D. W. (1975) In *A Textbook of Histology*, 10th edn, p. 244. Philadelphia: Saunders.
2. HAM, A. W. (1974) *Histology*, 7th edn, p. 378. Philadelphia: Lippincott.
3. GOLDHABER, P. (1962) Some current concepts of bone physiology. *New England Journal of Medicine*, **266**, 870 and 924.
4. BAKER, S. L. (1959) In *A Textbook of X-Ray Diagnosis*, ed. Shanks, S. C. & Kerley, P., 3rd edn, Vol. 4, p. 55. London: Lewis.
5. PRITCHARD, J. J. (1963) In *The Scientific Basis of Medicine Annual Reviews*, p. 286. London: Athlone Press.
6. MÜLLER, M. E. (1969) Compression as an aid in orthopaedic surgery. In *Recent Advances in Orthopaedics*, ed. Apley, A. G., p. 79. London: Churchill.
7. BUCK, R. C. (1953) Regeneration of tendon. *Journal of Pathology and Bacteriology*, **66**, 1.
8. HAY, E. D. (1971) Skeletal-muscle regeneration. *New England Journal of Medicine*, **284**, 1033.
9. McGEACHIE, J. K. (1971) Ultra-structural specificity in regenerating smooth muscle. *Experimentia*, **27**, 436.
10. McGEACHIE, J. K. (1975) *Smooth muscle regeneration, Monographs in Developmental Biology*, Vol. 9, 90 pp. Basel: Karger.
11. GAY, A. J. & HUNT, T. E. (1954) Reuniting of skeletal muscle fibres after transection. *Anatomical Record*, **120**, 853.
12. CARLSON, B. M. (1972) *The Regeneration of Minced Muscles, Monographs in Developmental Biology*, Vol. 4, 128 pp. Basel: Karger.
13. HUBBARD, T. B. *et al.* (1967) The pathology of peritoneal repair. *Annals of Surgery*, **165**, 908.
14. LEVENE, A. (1957) The response to injury of rat synovial membrane. *Journal of Pathology and Bacteriology*, **73**, 87.
15. Leading Article (1967) Endothelium and atherosclerosis. *Lancet*, **2**, 1239.
16. DYCK, P. J., THOMAS, P. K. & LAMBERT, E. H. (1975). *Peripheral Neuropathy*, Vol. i, pp. 179–181 and 205–208. Philadelphia: Saunders.
17. WALTON, J. N. (Ed.) (1974) *Disorders of Voluntary Muscle*, 3rd edn, see Wallerian Degeneration, pp. 239–244. Edinburgh: Churchill Livingstone.
18. WINDLE, W. F. (Ed.) (1955) *Regeneration in the Central Nervous System*. Springfield: Thomas.
19. Leading Article (1976) Any hope for the cut central axon? *Lancet*, **1**, 1224.
20. Leading Article (1972) Nerve growth factor. *Lancet*, **1**, 1375.
21. McMINN, R. M. H. (1960) The cellular anatomy of experimental wound healing. *Annals of the Royal College of Surgeons of England*, **26**, 245.
22. SANDERS, A. R., SCHEIN, C. J. & ORKIN, L. A. (1958) Total mucosal denudation of the canine bladder; experimental observations and clinical implications. Final report. *Journal of Urology*, **79**, 63.
23. BOHNE, A. W., OSBORN, R. W. & HETTLE, P. J. (1955) Regeneration of the urinary bladder in the dog, following total cystectomy. *Surgery, Gynecology and Obstetrics*, **100**, 259.
24. WEINBREN, K. (1966) Problems in restoration of the liver. In *Wound Healing*, ed. Illingworth, C., p. 69. London: Churchill.
25. BUCHER, N. L. R. (1967) Experimental aspects of hepatic regeneration. *New England Journal of Medicine*, **277**, pp. 686 and 738.
26. VERLY, W. G. (1976) The control of liver growth. In *Chalones*, ed. Houck, J. C., p. 401. Amsterdam: North-Holland Publishing Company.
27. Leading Article (1975) Paracetamol hepatotoxicity. *Lancet*, **2**, 1189.
28. ANTHONY, P. P. *et al.* (1978) The morphology of cirrhosis. *Journal of Clinical Pathology*, **31**, 395.
29. MALT, R. A. (1969) Compensatory growth of the kidney. *New England Journal of Medicine*, **280**, 1446.

Chapter 11. Chronic Inflammation

The tissue response to injury has been divided into three phases. The initial vascular and exudative phenomena of acute inflammation are followed by a second phase of demolition. This is accomplished by macrophage activity. The third and final phase is one of healing, by which lost tissue is replaced by the processes of repair and regeneration.

It is evident that complete healing can occur only when the acute inflammatory and demolition phases are themselves completed. Since these are the consequences of the initial damage, it follows that healing results only when the cause of the inflammation is removed. If the body is unable to remove the irritant, a disease process develops in which there is present a mixture of the phenomena of acute inflammation, demolition, repair, and regeneration. To such a lesion the term 'chronic inflammation' is applied. *Chronic inflammation may therefore be defined as a prolonged process in which destruction and inflammation are proceeding at the same time as attempts at healing.*

Causes of Chronic Inflammation

Since all agents which cause cell damage initiate an acute inflammatory response, they may, if they persist, also lead to chronic inflammation. In this way insoluble particles such as silica, asbestos, and other foreign bodies very readily cause chronic inflammation. Organisms such as the tubercle bacillus and actinomyces, against which the body has only a limited resistance, are another important cause. Moreover, if local or general conditions impair the body's defences, an organism which usually produces a self-limiting acute inflammation may persist to cause a chronic one. Any of the causes of delayed healing (p. 113) may so turn the scales against the host that there develops the 'frustrated healing' which chronic inflammation has so aptly been called. Finally, a state of hypersensitivity, if persistent, may lead to exuberant chronic inflammatory reactions. This is seen in many chronic infective diseases, of which tuberculosis is the prototype, and is also important in non-infective conditions such as allergic contact dermatitis and hypersensitivity angiitis. The collagen diseases afford excellent examples of chronic inflammation associated with progressive destruction of collagen. It is possible that they too are related to hypersensitivity or autoimmunity (see Ch. 16).

Classification of the Types of Chronic Inflammation

Clinical. Although chronic inflammation may follow obvious acute inflammation (e.g. osteomyelitis), some irritants (e.g. the tubercle bacillus) usually cause only a mild or fleeting acute reaction, but nevertheless persist and lead to the development of a chronic disease.

The initial acute phase is often inconspicuous, and clinically it may be completely missed. It can therefore be induced that two types of chronic inflammation occur: (*a*) following acute inflammation, and (*b*) starting *de novo*.

Specific and non-specific. It is customary to subdivide chronic inflammation in another way: certain irritants cause a tissue reaction which is histologically characteristic. By examining such a lesion, one can infer its origin without either seeing or isolating the causative agent. Such a lesion is said to be *specific*. Tuberculosis, leprosy, and syphilis are included under this heading. In fact, many lesions encountered in these diseases are not histologically characteristic, and therefore, strictly speaking, the term 'specific' should not be used. Thus, while the histological appearances of a gumma are fairly typical, the lesions of secondary syphilis are by no means diagnostic. The reaction is 'non-specific'.

With increasing knowledge it has been realised that tissue reactions that were once regarded as diagnostic of a particular disease are by no means as specific as was at one time thought. Thus, a 'typical tuberculous' lesion may be found in leprosy, sarcoidosis, or even in a reaction to a foreign body like talc.

The use of the terms 'specific' and 'non-specific' are, however, retained, even though it is not really justified in terms of the original conception. Since this convention is so time-honoured, it is unlikely to be altered, but it should be remembered that the distinction between specific and non-specific is quite artificial.

Histological. The histological features of a chronic inflammatory lesion may be used in descriptive classification. Where polymorphs abound and abscess formation is present, the lesion may justly be called a *chronic suppurative inflammation*. In some examples of chronic inflammation the lesions contain numerous macrophages, which either infiltrate the tissues diffusely (diffuse granulomatous reaction) or form groups or follicles and develop into epithelioid cells. This maturation commonly occurs in tuberculosis, and the term *tuberculoid* is frequently applied for this reason. Three variants occur:

Non-caseating tuberculoid reaction, as seen in sarcoidosis (Fig. 21.4), lupus vulgaris, and tuberculoid leprosy.

Caseating tuberculoid reaction, as commonly seen in tuberculosis (Fig. 20.2).

Suppurative tuberculoid reaction, in which small abscesses filled with polymorphs are formed and are surrounded by a mantle of epithelioid cells. This occurs in lymphogranuloma venereum, tularaemia, coccidioidomycosis, and cat-scratch disease (Fig. 21.3).

Granulomatous inflammation.[1] Some chronic inflammations are characterised by the formation of tumour-like masses, and the term granuloma has been applied to them. In some instances the mass is composed of inflammatory granulation tissue, and Virchow included this type of lesion amongst the granulomata. Most contemporary workers, however, use the term in a descriptive sense restricted to a microscopic appearance rather than related to the formation of a tumour-like mass. In this sense a granuloma is defined as a chronic inflammatory reaction containing a predominance of cells of the macrophage series. This includes both a diffuse infiltration of macrophages as well as the follicular type of lesion in which epithelioid cells are formed (tuberculoid reaction). Some pathologists restrict the term granuloma to a lesion characterised by the formation of epithelioid cells and giant cells arranged in follicular groups; in this case the terms granulomatous and tuberculoid are synonymous. Actinomycosis and sporotrichosis are often included in the group of granulomatous inflammations, even though their lesions are typically suppurative. It is evident that granulomatous inflammation is a term without a precise meaning, and it is wise not to use it without qualification. The concept of granuloma is further discussed on page 129.

General Features of Chronic Inflammation

Although there are wide differences between various types of chronic inflammation, depending partly upon the tissues involved and partly upon the causative agent, there are, nevertheless, certain basic similarities. These are best considered under the heading of the three component reactions which together constitute chronic inflammation.

Acute inflammation. Evidence of acute inflammation is frequently seen in chronic inflammation. Exudation is particularly well marked in chronic suppurative disease. Pus, rich in polymorphonuclear leucocytes, is very evident in chronic suppurative conditions such as chronic brain abscess, osteomyelitis, empyema, pyosalpinx, and pyonephrosis, to mention only a few examples. It is also typical of actinomycosis. Fibrin may be seen microscopically, and on occasions forms large masses easily visible to the naked eye. This is prominent in chronic empyema thoracis due to pneumococcal or staphylococcal infection.

Eosinophils are sometimes present in large numbers in the exudate in chronic inflammation. This is sometimes mediated by an immune reaction, but whether it is always a manifestation of hypersensitivity is not known.

Fluid exudation is a feature of draining chronic suppurative lesions, and the continued protein loss may lead to hypoproteinaemia. Accumulations of a protein-rich fluid are frequent in chronic inflammation of the serous sacs, e.g. tuberculous peritonitis, and in some forms of serositis, including that due to tuberculosis, abundant fibrin formation is evident (see Fig. 11.1). The spider-web clot seen in the cerebrospinal fluid of tuberculous meningitis will also be recalled. Usually, however, overt acute inflammation is not an outstanding feature of tuberculosis.

Demolition. This is accomplished by macrophages. These cells are derived from emigrating monocytes of bone-marrow origin, and they constitute the bulk of 'granulomatous' lesions. By transfusing monocytes labelled *in vitro* with tritiated thymidine to animals bearing granulomata of various types and ages, it has been found that some lesions, notably those due to the local injection of *B. pertussis* vaccine or heat-killed tubercle bacilli in mineral oil, show a high turnover of monocytes[2,3]. Probably these high-turnover lesions are associated with toxic destruction of monocytes. By contrast a carrageenan

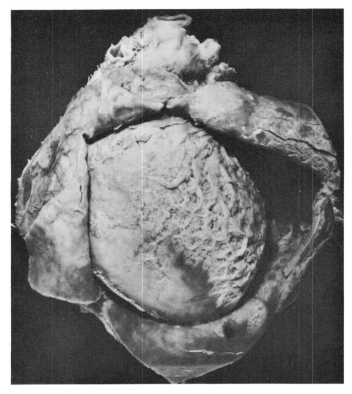

Figure 11.1
Tuberculous pericarditis. The patient was a man aged 22 years, who had had pulmonary tuberculosis for 5 years. The specimen shows the opened pericardial sac, in which the heart is seen to be covered by a thick fibrinous exudate. Over the apex there is a layer of blood clot due to recent haemorrhage. The parietal pericardium is greatly thickened, and is also covered by fibrinous exudate and blood clot. (EC 12.1, *Reproduced by permission of the President and Council of the R.C.S. Eng.*)

(polysaccharide derived from seaweed) granuloma is a low-turnover lesion, and the monocytes remain for many weeks. Monocytes from the blood appear to undergo mitosis soon after leaving the circulation, and then enter a resting phase for several days before further division. The long-lived monocytes neither die nor divide for long periods of time, and are replaced by a local macrophage population (derived from histiocytes) irrespective of the bone marrow. Thus low-turnover granulomata are not affected by bone-marrow X-irradiation, but local X-irradiation reduces DNA synthesis almost completely. The converse occurs in high-turnover lesions, which need constant replenishment of cells from the marrow.

Chronic inflammatory lesions with a heavy macrophage infiltration are traditionally called 'proliferative'; as can be induced from this recent experimental work, the macrophages arise both from an exudation of blood monocytes and their subsequent local proliferation. Nevertheless, an 'exudative' lesion is traditionally defined as one showing an exudate of plasma with fibrin and polymorphs (see also pp. 184 and 240).

Under certain circumstances macrophages become large and polygonal with pale, oval nuclei and abundant, cloudy, eosinophilic cytoplasm. These cells are called *epithelioid* cells[4] from a resemblance in appearance to the epithelial cells of epidermis. The apposing cell membranes of epithelioid cells exhibit a high degree of interdigitation, so that on light microscopy the cell outlines appear to be indistinct. The cytoplasm of the cells contains many organelles including mitochondria, lysosomes, endoplasmic reticulum, and Golgi complex. No phagosomes are present, and it is evident that epithelioid cells lack the ability to phagocytose material (such as staphylococci). These cells can, however, avidly take up small particles (such as colloidal gold) by the process of pinocytosis. Material taken up in this way can later be extruded either piecemeal or as a vacuole together with lysosomal enzymes.

Precisely why macrophages differentiate into epithelioid cells is not clear, but they do so under a number of circumstances. It has been found experimentally that macrophages become epithelioid cells when they have not undertaken phagocytosis, or have completely digested phagocytosed material, or have successfully extruded phagocytosed material by exocytosis. Epithelioid-cell formation is inhibited if phagocytosed material cannot either be digested or extruded. Thus, the lepra cells of lepomatous leprosy and the foam cells found in xanthomata do not become epithelioid cells. In a tuberculous granuloma, however, epithelioid cells are typical.

It would appear therefore, that epithelioid cells develop when the influx of macrophages exceeds the number required to ingest a non-digestible substance, or when the substance is digestible and not very toxic to the macrophages, but is constantly available so that new macrophages are involved in the process and do not die before they can develop epithelioid features. It may be that epithelioid cells form a barrier between macrophages containing organisms and the host, and that they ingest subparticulate material which is digested, detoxified, or excreted. Their life-span is short, being one to four weeks. The cell either dies or else undergoes mitosis to form small round cells (easily mistaken for lymphocytes) which mature to young macrophages. These may become epithelioid if the circumstances are right.[4]

When macrophages encounter insoluble material, they frequently coalesce to form *giant cells*. It has been found that non-proliferating macrophages may fuse in this way,[5] but despite the darkly-staining, rather inactive appearance of the nuclei of the chronic inflammatory giant cell, DNA synthesis does occur, but only when the cells are 2 to 4 weeks old.[2,3]. This is associated with a burst of mitotic activity, the nuclei all often entering the mitotic cycle synchronously. Thus it appears that, in an experimental situation, giant cells can renew themselves. Nevertheless, in human tissue one does not see mitotic figures in typical giant cells.

Giant cells are frequently seen around exogenous foreign bodies, e.g. catgut, silk, talc, plastic sponges like Ivalon, etc., and they are also present around such endogenous debris as sequestra, cholesterol crystals, and uric-acid crystals (in gout). They are formed in response to the tubercle bacillus and many other organisms causing chronic inflammation.

Various types of giant cells are described. In some the nuclei are disposed around the periphery of the cell in the form of a horseshoe or a ring, and these are called *Langhans giant cells*; they are particularly frequent in tuberculous lesions. Another type is the *Touton giant cell* found in xanthomata. (Figs. 11.2a and 11.2b). Its peripheral cytoplasm has a

TABLE 11.1 Giant cells formed by fusion of macrophages

(1) Reaction to exogenous insoluble material, e.g. talc, silica, and ligatures (*foreign-body giant cells*).
(2) Reaction to insoluble material formed in the body, e.g. sodium urate crystals, cholesterol, keratin, and fat.
(3) Touton giant cells.
(4) Reactions to certain organisms, e.g. tuberculosis (*Langhans giant cell*) fungal infections, and syphilis.

Figure 11.2a
Xanthoma showing Touton giant cell. The lesion consists of many foam cells some of which have fused to form giant cells. The cell in the centre is a typical Touton giant cell. The nuclei are arranged in a circular manner to form a wreath. The peripheral part of the cytoplasm is vacuolated due to its lipid content. The central part of the cytoplasm, enclosed by the nuclei, has a homogeneous, eosinophilic appearance. × 215.

Figure 11.2b
Touton giant cell. This Touton giant cell differs from that shown in Figure 11.2a in that the peripheral cytoplasm is less vacuolated. The section is from a naevoxanthoendothelioma (juvenile xanthogranuloma). This curious lesion appears during the neonatal period as a rapidly-growing, red skin nodule which almost invariably involutes spontaneously. × 320.

foamy appearance, and the nuclei surround a central area of clear eosinophilic cytoplasm. In the *foreign-body giant cell* the nuclei are scattered haphazardly throughout the cell, and some are present centrally. In many lesions giant cells of both Langhans and foreign-body type are present. The two types should not be regarded as distinct.

It is evident that monocytes can be regarded as undifferentiated cells that are released from the bone marrow, circulate in the blood stream, and subsequently invade areas of damage and inflammation; here they differentiate into macrophages which are characterised by their phagocytic activity. Under some circumstances macrophages tend to aggregate to form follicles, and the cells differentiate into epithelioid cells and giant cells. Although these derivatives of the monocyte have obvious phagocytic or pinocytotic activity, other roles, noted on page 80, have been attributed to them. They may process antigen as part of the efferent limb of an immune response. They are credited with secreting a considerable number of substances including interferon, pyrogen, complement components, lysozyme, acid hydrolases, neutral proteases, cytotoxic factors, and ill-defined proteins that regulate the function and proliferation of other cells (for instance fibroblasts and the granulocyte precursors in bone marrow).

As noted previously, macrophages may be derived from local tissue histiocytes.[6] This is probably an unimportant source under most circumstances; nevertheless, some pathologists use the term 'histiocytic infiltrate' as synonymous with a macrophage infiltrate as seen in a diffuse granulomatous reaction.

Features of healing. *Repair.* The granulation tissue of repair contains a variety of cells, chief amongst which are:

1. Endothelial cells forming blood and lymphatic vessels.
2. Fibroblasts forming collagen (astrocytes forming a glial scar in the central nervous system).
3. Small round cells—lymphocytes and plasma cells.

These features are all seen in chronic inflammation. In chronic suppuration the pus-filled cavity is lined by acutely inflamed granulation tissue. This is the *pyogenic membrane.* The vascularity of the granulations predisposes to haemorrhage from the delicate thin-walled capillaries. Repeated haemorrhage is a frequent accompaniment of chronic peptic ulcer, and one of the commonest causes of haemoptysis is the chronic infection invariable in bronchiectasis. It is probable that haemoptysis in cancer of the lung is more frequently due to the associated bronchiectasis than from the tumour itself.

Fibroblasts are prominent in most chronic inflammations. They lay down collagen, which is the product of the repair process that is an integral part of chronic inflammation. The proliferation of fibroblasts and their synthesis of collagen appears to be stimulated by a humoral factor released from macrophages.[7] This also occurs in the early stages of wound healing (p. 106).

Repair is seen in fibroid tuberculosis, chronic peptic ulcer, chronic cholecystitis, in the walls of chronic abcesses, etc. If fibrin is characteristic of acute inflammation, fibrosis can be considered the salient feature of chronic inflammation. The *cicatrisation* that results leads to many of the important complications of chronic inflammation. Thus chronic rheumatic valvulitis leads to valvular stenosis and regurgitation, chronic gastric ulcers may proceed to pyloric stenosis or hour-

Figure 11.3
Endarteritis obliterans. This is a section through a gumma. The periphery shows fibrous tissue heavily infiltrated by small round cells, but the central area is defined by the internal elastic lamina of a medium-sized artery. Inside this lamina there is a considerable proliferation of the more palely-staining tunica intima, which shows a moderate cellular infiltration. The lumen of the vessel is reduced to a small channel near the middle of the field. × 70.

glass stomach, while fibrous ankylosis with severe limitation of movement is a frequent end-result of rheumatoid arthritis.

A very common feature of chronic inflammation is *endarteritis obliterans*, in which the lumen of the small arteries is gradually occluded as the result of a progressive proliferation of the tunica intima. (Fig. 11.3). It is seen in the bed of chronic peptic ulcers, following radiation damage, around gummata, etc.

A feature of chronic inflammation which is worthy of special note is the accumulation of lymphocytes and plasma cells. These are the 'cells of chronic inflammation' or 'small round cells' (Fig. 11.4), and their presence is related to an immune reaction. Present in the granulation tissue of a healing wound, they are much more numerous in chronic inflammatory granulation tissue. Frequently they assume a perivascular distribution, e.g. in syphilitic aortitis, and are presumably derived from the blood rather than from local lymphoid tissue or stem cells.

There is little doubt that plasma cells are concerned with the production of immunoglobulins. Heavy plasma-cell infiltrations are common in chronic inflammatory lesions of juxtacutaneous mucous membranes. In ageing plasma cells there are sometimes intracytoplasmic accumulations of strongly eosinophilic, PAS-positive material called *Russell bodies* (Fig. 11.5). Despite their prominent appearance they are of no great importance.

Regeneration. When the tissue destroyed in chronic inflammation is of a type capable of division, regeneration rather than repair takes place. This is particularly obvious in surface epithelia. Indeed, regeneration may become so exuberant that the line of demarcation between it, hyperplasia, and neoplasia may be difficult to define. For this reason malignancy has frequently been ascribed to 'chronic irritation'. A well-known

Figure 11.4
Plasma cells. This is the section of a chronic inflammatory response in which plasma cells are predominating. The round and pear-shaped contour of the cells is well marked. Their nuclei are eccentric, and have a conspicuous cart-wheel disposition of clumped chromatin. The cytoplasm is comparatively darkly-staining due to its high content of RNA. The clear area adjacent to the nucleus is the Golgi complex × 400.

Figure 11.5
Russell bodies. (*a*) Nasal biopsy from patient with rhinoscleroma showing many plasma cells and one Russell body. (*b*) Chronic inflammatory granulation tissue showing one Russell body in the cytoplasm of a plasma cell. The nucleus of the cell is compressed to one side. (*c*) Russell body lying free in tissue; same case as (*a*). (*d*) Russell bodies stained with Giemsa's stain. These structures are stained strongly with the PAS method and must not be mistaken for fungi. × 600.

example of this is the regeneration of the epithelium which occurs in ulcerative colitis, and which may progress to polypoid overgrowth and malignancy.

In the gallbladder chronic inflammation may cause the epithelium to 'invade' the wall, giving rise in extreme cases to cholecystitis glandularis proliferans which may easily be mistaken for cancer* (Fig. 11.6). The 'tumourlets' seen in the lung in bronchiectasis are also regenerative and hyperplastic rather than neoplastic (Fig. 24.2, p. 296).

The epithelial overgrowth at the edge of a chronic gastric ulcer is another pitfall for the unwary. The greatly divergent views expressed in the past on the frequency of malignant change in chronic gastric ulcer are largely due to the difficulties in interpreting the microscopic appearances.

The Granuloma[1]

The contemporary definition of a granuloma is a lesion consisting predominantly of macrophages. It need not ne-

*The normal gallbladder often shows epithelial-lined diverticula (Rokitansky-Aschoff sinuses) beneath the muscular coat. The possibility that some examples of cholecystitis glandularis proliferans are, in fact, congenital abnormalities (ectopias) cannot be excluded.

Figure 11.6
Chronic cholecystitis with epithelial hyperplasia (cholecystitis glandularis proliferans). The gallbladder wall is thickened, and there is a wide zone of chronic inflammatory tissue deep to the attenuated muscle layer. There are many glandular spaces in this inflammatory zone, and one is connected with the overlying epithelium by a narrow duct which penetrates the muscle coat. It is called a Rokitansky-Aschoff sinus. × 25.

cessarily show necrosis, fibrosis, or giant cells. Three types can be distinguished.

(*a*) *Reactive granuloma.* In this there is simply a collection of macrophages without any other cells. Good examples are afforded by the reactions that develop around colloids, such as aluminium hydroxide, and bland mineral oils.

(*b*) *Toxic granuloma.* Good examples are seen in association with silica and probably beryllium.*

(*c*) *Immunological granuloma.* This occurs in certain infections, such as tuberculosis, leprosy, and schistosomiasis, in sarcoidosis, in the vicinity of some malignant tumours, and as a reaction to metal haptens. A good example of the last is the zirconium granuloma mentioned on page 137. In the toxic and immunological granulomata the macrophages may develop into epithelioid cells and giant cells, and lymphocytes, plasma cells, polymorphs, and eosinophils may also be present. The lymphocytes may be stimulated to form organised lymphoid tissue with B and T cells. There may be necrosis, often the result of ischaemia or the liberation of lysosomal enzymes, and there may also be a later fibroblastic proliferation with the laying down of collagen.

The two factors that seem to lead to the development of an immunological granuloma are a deposition of antigen-antibody complexes with a predominance of antibody (a predominance of antigen leads to immune-complex disease, see p. 181) or a delayed-type hypersensitivity reaction.

It is interesting to compare the two types of granulomata seen in leprosy.[8] In the *lepromatous* type there is a massive collection of undifferentiated macrophages full of bacilli (lepra cells) with virtually no lymphocytes. Delayed-type hypersensitivity is in abeyance, but there is hypergammaglobulinaemia and there are many immune-complex reactions in the tissues where they produce erythema nodosum leprosum. In the *tuberculoid* type, on the other hand, there is a typical epithelioid-cell granuloma with many lymphocytes, bacilli are

very scanty, and there is an accentuated delayed-type hypersensitivity as evidenced by a strongly positive lepromin reaction (see p. 183). The plasma globulins are usually normal, and there are no immune-complex reactions in the tissues.

The tuberculoid type of leprosy is the high-resistance form, and the lepromatous type the low-resistance form. Furthermore, there is a spectrum of clinical points between these two poles clustering around a central *borderline* position. The full spectrum is as follows[8]:

TT – tuberculoid polar (high resistance)
BT – borderline tuberculoid
BB – borderline
BL – borderline lepromatous
LI – indefinite lepromatous
LL – lepromatous polar (low resistance).

Between LI and BT patients may move across the spectrum in one direction or another according to the level of cellular immunity which may vary as the antigenic load increases or decreases in relation to chemotherapeutic treatment. Progress from LI to BT is associated with an increase in lymphocytic infiltration and a progressive differentiation of macrophages into epithelioid cells. At the same time there is a progressive decrease in the number of organisms in the lesions, so that in BT they may be difficult to demonstrate by conventional staining techniques. At the lepromatous pole, despite low host resistance, there is a high level of circulating antimycobacterial antibody present in the plasma in the great majority of patients. Immune-complex disease and amyloidosis are important complications.[9]

General Effects of Chronic Inflammation

The general effects of chronic inflammation depend upon the nature and extent of the responsible agent. In a localised foreign-body reaction or a chronic varicose ulcer there is no noteworthy general response at all. On the other hand, in chronic infective diseases like tuberculosis or actinomycosis there may be widespread changes in the reticulo-endothelial system and in the blood stream.

---

*It is still undecided whether the mechanism of the beryllium granuloma is toxic or immunological.

Changes in the reticulo-endothelial system (see also Ch. 30). Most chronic inflammatory conditions lead to hyperplasia of the RE system. The presence of large mononuclear cells derived from monocytes in the local response has already been described. The lymph nodes draining a chronic infective lesion show hyperplasia affecting the sinus-lining cells and sometimes the germinal centres and medullary cords.

If organisms gain access to the blood stream, they are taken up by the other members of the RE system, namely the sinus-lining cells of spleen, liver, marrow, etc. Generalised parasitisation of the system is seen in kala-azar, miliary tuberculosis, and histoplasmosis. These hyperplastic changes are undoubtedly related to the phagocytic functions of the cells; in addition they also play some part in the immune response. Hyperplasia indeed occurs without obvious widespread dissemination of the organisms, and this may be due to the formation of antigen-antibody complexes in the bloodstream which are subsequently removed by the RE system.

The immune response. Antibody production is a feature of most chronic inflammatory diseases, and the demonstration of specific immunoglobulins is a useful diagnostic procedure. Antibody production may be so marked that the γ-globulin blood level is raised. Kala-azar affords a good example of this.

The antibodies may, on the other hand, be of the lymphocyte or cell-bound type, and be associated with delayed hypersensitivity. Tests like the tuberculin, lepromin, and Frei are based upon this. This cell-mediated hypersensitivity itself results in tissue damage, and is a major factor in the pathogenesis of chronic inflammation. Tuberculosis would not be a chronic destructive disease were it not for the development of this type of hypersensitivity.

The immune response may be reflected in definite morphological changes. Hyperplasia of the splenic cells may be sufficient to render the spleen clinically palpable, hence splenomegaly is seen in chronic malaria, subacute infective endocarditis, Felty's syndrome, etc.

Finally, the long-continued stress on the antibody producing mechanism may be associated with *amyloid disease* (Ch. 48).

Changes in the blood. The white cells frequently show changes which are related to the causative agent and to the extent of the infection: these are considered in Chapter 53. Anaemia is frequent and usually of the normochromic, normocytic type, but it may become hypochromic and microcytic as a result of repeated haemorrhage, e.g. in peptic ulcer.

The reduction in plasma albumin, the rise in γ-globulin, and other changes that occur in the plasma proteins are described elsewhere (see Ch. 49). A rise in the ESR occurs in many chronic inflammatory diseases, and is commonly used as an aid both to diagnosis and prognosis, e.g. in tuberculosis and rheumatoid arthritis.

Other changes. Although 'toxaemia' is put forward as the explanation of many of the general symptoms, it cannot be regarded as anything more than a cloak for our ignorance. The following signs and symptoms are frequent and attributed to this state: tiredness, malaise, headache, anorexia, loss of weight, anaemia, loss of libido, and pyrexia.

Toxaemia is often assumed to be due to the liberation of endotoxins, but although such substances have been identified in some organisms, e.g. staphylococci and *Escherichia coli*, there are others, such as *Treponema pallidum*, in which no such endotoxins are known. Possibly toxic substances are formed when tissue is damaged either as a result of direct bacterial action or hypersensitivity. However, there is no direct evidence as to the nature of the endotoxins or products of tissue damage which are responsible for the 'toxaemia' of infection.

EXAMPLES OF CHRONIC INFLAMMATION

Examples of chronic inflammation can be considered in the following groups:

(*a*) Those due to 'non-specific', pyogenic, bacterial agents (*Staph. aureus* and *Esch. coli*).

(*b*) Those due to inanimate foreign bodies, e.g. catgut.

(*c*) Those due to 'specific' organisms, e.g. tubercle bacillus and *Tr. pallidum*. This third group is so important that it is dealt with separately in Chapters 20 and 21.

(*d*) Those associated with hypersensitivity or autoimmunity. These are discussed in Chapter 16. The collagen diseases can be conveniently included in this group.

The first group includes a wide collection of conditions that are very commonly encountered in clinical practice. For the purposes of this discussion a few important examples have been selected.

Osteomyelitis. Acute osteomyelitis occurs most often in children at the metaphysis of one of the long bones of the lower limbs. This is the area which is most easily traumatised, and should this occur during the course of a *Staph. aureus* bacteraemia, the organisms may become lodged and produce a metastatic lesion. A typical acute inflammatory reaction occurs, and owing to the rigidity of the bone the increased tension produced by the exudation causes compression of the blood vessels and subsequent ischaemia. Necrosis of bone therefore follows; pus is then formed, and it tracks under the periosteum, thereby further imperilling the blood supply to the cortex. In this way extensive necrosis may occur, sometimes involving the whole shaft. This dead bone acts as a foreign body; it cannot be easily removed, and it not only provides a focus for organismal growth but also prevents adequate drainage of pus. Conditions are ideal for the development of chronic infection.

Pus ruptures through the periosteum into the muscular and subcutaneous compartments. Usually it is discharged on to the skin surface through sinuses. The vascular periosteum attempts to reform the shaft of the bone; in this way the sequestered shaft becomes encased in a thick bony *involucrum* (Fig. 11.7). The shaft is bathed in pus which escapes through holes, or *cloacae*, in the involucrum, and is then discharged to the surface. Osteoclasts slowly erode the sequestrum, detaching it at each end from living bone and slowly destroying it. This must be completed before healing can be accomplished. In practice this is seldom possible without surgical intervention. If nothing is done, the condition may lead to death as the result of pyaemia, 'toxaemia', or amyloid disease.

This chronic infection is fortunately uncommon nowadays since the advent of antibiotic therapy, which is used in combination with early surgical drainage in the acute stage. Once chronicity develops, the outlook for the limb is still very poor.

Figure 11.7
Osteomyelitis of tibia. The limb was amputated 6 months after the presence of necrosis was established. In this specimen the extensive central sequestrum is largely concealed by an exuberant involucrum formed from the detached periosteum. There is a cloaca at the base of the shaft (it has been enlarged artificially), and through it the pitted sequestrum is plainly recognisable. (HS 44.1, *Reproduced by permission of the President and Council of the R.C.S. Eng.*)

From a pathological point of view the disease illustrates many points. It shows how an acute infection can become chronic due to the inadequate drainage of pus as well as to the presence of a foreign body, in this case the sequestrum. Moreover, all the features of chronic inflammation are present. Acute inflammation is evidenced by the polymorphonuclear and fluid exudate, demolition by macrophage and osteoclastic activity, regeneration by bone formation, and repair by surrounding scarring.

Chronic pyelonephritis. Chronic pyelonephritis is now recognised as a common cause of chronic renal failure and an important aetiological factor in systemic hypertension.

The organisms usually implicated are the Gram-negative intestinal bacilli, but the exact mode of infection is debated. Certainly urinary obstruction plays an important part. It has

been shown in the rabbit that if one ureter is tied, an intravenous injection of *Esch. coli* results in acute pyelonephritis in that kidney.

On the other hand, there is no doubt that organisms can be introduced into the bladder during catheterisation, and that this manipulation is a potent cause of acute cystitis. From the bladder urine may reflux up the ureters; it is generally agreed that this ascending spread of infection is the cause of most cases of acute pyelonephritis.

Chronic pyelonephritis may commence either as an overt acute disease or may appear insidiously. During the acute phase the cortex contains multiple minute abscesses, and the congested medulla shows streaking due to pus cells in the tubules. Why this condition becomes chronic is not altogether clear. Urinary obstruction is liable to perpetuate the infection, and in some cases evidence of this in the form of hydroureter or hydronephrosis may be found. Often, however, there is no obvious obstructive element.

The importance of scars in predisposing to recurrent attacks of pyelonephritis has been stressed by a number of workers. Thus, it has been shown that rabbits whose kidneys have been scarred by electrical burning are very liable to subsequent infection. In another experiment it was found that the intravenous injection of Gram-negative intestinal bacilli produced acute pyelonephritis only in those rabbits whose kidneys already bore the scars of a previous staphylococcal infection. It has been suggested that in the human subject also the presence of old scars predisposes to acute pyelonephritis, and that many such scars are due to congenital abnormalities of the parenchyma. Be this as it may, it seems very probable that one attack of acute pyelonephritis predisposes the patient to repeated ones because of the damage it produces.

In the chronic stage the kidney shows focal scarring and infiltration with chronic inflammatory cells (Fig. 11.8). In the affected areas many glomeruli are hyalinised, and others show typical periglomerular fibrosis. The surviving tubules are often dilated and contain eosinophilic material, producing a picture which resembles normal thyroid tissue. The vessels may show the changes of either benign or malignant hypertension.

Hypertension often occurs, and since this may occasionally be due to unilateral renal disease, and therefore amenable to surgical treatment, it has attained considerable prominence. The exact incidence is, however, disputed as is its pathogenesis; probably from 15 to 20 per cent of all cases of malignant hypertension are due to pyelonephritis.

Chronic inflammation in the alimentary tract. *The stomach.* The factors which determine whether the frequently occurring acute gastric ulcers will heal or persist as chronic ulcers are not known. In chronic ulceration the destructive process penetrates the muscle and destroys it. The ulcer base is then composed of scar tissue, superficial to which there is a layer of vascular granulation tissue heavily infiltrated with pus cells, macrophages, plasma cells, and lymphocytes. Overlying this there is a slough.

Since the smooth muscle undergoes incomplete regeneration, it is replaced to greater or lesser extent by scar tissue. The epithelium attempts to grow over the ulcer bed; its invaginations at the ulcer edge may simulate neoplastic invasion, and in occasional cases cancer does develop at this site.

Figure 11.8
Chronic pyelonephritis. Most of the renal parenchyma has been replaced by fibrous tissue heavily infiltrated by lymphocytes in some parts. The glomerular buds are partly fibrosed, and there i• well-marked periglomerular fibrosis. The tubules are atrophic. ×90.

The incidence is probably low (less than 4 per cent) in gastric ulcers, and never in duodenal ulcers. If healing does occur, the regenerated epithelium may be of intestinal type with villi, Paneth cells, etc.

The colon. Chronic inflammatory lesions of the colon may follow specific infections by the *Shigella* species or *Entamoeba histolytica*, but in Britain the commonest colonic lesion is *idiopathic ulcerative colitis*. This disease can commence as a fulminating acute condition which either leads to rapid death or else follows a more chronic course. Usually the onset is insidious and the disease is chronic from the beginning.

The rectum and distal part of the colon are generally worst affected, and in the acute phase the mucosa is intensely hyperaemic. On proctoscopy the muscosa bleeds very easily. Occasionally the colon undergoes acute dilatation, and may perforate, a condition called acute toxic megacolon and one that is frequently fatal.

In the common type of ulcerative colitis small mucosal abscesses form as a result of blockage of the openings of the crypts of Lieberkühn (crypt abscesses); the mucosa undergoes ulceration and chronic inflammatory changes. The changes are largely confined to the mucosa, in contrast to the transmural involvement that is characteristic of Crohn's disease (p. 261).

The colon becomes rigid and shortened due mainly to hypertrophy of the muscle coat, the cause of which is not known; fibrosis is not marked, and does not affect the muscle. An increase in fat occurs in the subserosal layer. Fat accumulation of this type is a feature of many chronic inflammatory conditions, e.g. chronic pyelonephritis, but the reason for this is not known.

As the disease progresses the outstanding feature is generalised hyperaemia and oedema of the mucosa together with infiltration by lymphocytes. Polymorphs are relatively scanty and are confined to the areas of ulceration which are usually arranged longitudinally over the taeniae coli. The ulceration tends to surround and undermine areas of swollen mucosa which then constitute *pseudopolypi*. This is an example of catarrhal inflammation, for in addition to the pus there is an abundant secretion of mucus; pus, blood, and mucus are

Figure 11.9
Chronic ulcerative colitis with pseudopolyposis. The appearance of these multiple foci of polypoid overgrowth of epithelium is to be distinguished from true polyposis coli. In pseudopolyposis the bowel itself is chronically inflamed, and in this specimen the wall is considerably contracted. Furthermore, the intervening mucosa is roughened and inflamed. In polyposis coli there is no evidence of inflammation. (EA 70.1, *Reproduced by permission of the President and Council of the R.C.S. Eng.*)

therefore all present in the stools. In only the very chronic stages of the disease does epithelial overgrowth occur and lead to polypoid excrescences. Although the hyperplastic condition superficially resembles true polyposis coli, the intervening mucosa is normal in polyposis coli, whereas it is inflamed in ulcerative colitis (Fig. 11.9). Ulcerative colitis is sometimes complicated by cancer (see p. 374).

TISSUE RESPONSE TO INSOLUBLE INANIMATE FOREIGN MATERIALS

The tissue response to these substances is very complex, and with the increasing use of metals and plastics in reconstructive surgery is a matter of considerable importance. It is probably true to state that all foreign materials are capable of producing an inflammatory response under certain circumstances. Nothing is truly 'inert'. The factors which determine the severity of the inflammatory response are not completely understood, but the following are important.

The chemical nature of the material. The chemical stability and solubility are of great importance: thus stainless steel is more inert than ordinary steel.

Physical state of the substance. Smooth, highly-polished surfaces provoke much less reaction than do rough, irregular surfaces. It is important to bear this in mind when inserting metallic prostheses or pins. Finely-divided or colloidal substances, e.g. silica, are particularly irritating.

Electro-chemical potentials set up by the close proximity of dissimilar metals cause tissue damage. It should not be forgotten that there are many different types of 'stainless steel'. This is particularly important in orthopaedic surgery. Plate and screws must be of exactly the same composition. Otherwise there is sufficient reaction to cause loosening of the screws. Even the metal scraped off the screwdriver may be sufficient to produce this effect.

The relatively insoluble foreign materials cannot be removed by the inflammatory reaction which they excite, and it follows that the lesions induced are typically chronic in character. Giant cells abound (Fig. 11.10). Most of these are of the foreign-body type, but sometimes Langhans giant cells are also prominent. As already indicated, it is unwise to distinguish categorically between them.

A few important examples of reaction to foreign materials will be cited.

Carbon. Tattooing consists of introducing carbon into the dermis; it excites little inflammatory reaction, and is soon taken up by macrophages; when these cells die it remains free in the tissues indefinitely. Inhaled carbon is transported by macrophages to the lymphoid tissues in the lung, where it remains throughout life. Usually there is some dilatation of the respiratory bronchioles ('focal dust emphysema'), which should be distinguished from destructive centrilobular emphysema. Coalminer's pneumoconiosis due to carbon alone produces little disability by itself; it is the associated chronic bronchitis or silicosis that is crippling.

Metals. Vitallium and stainless steel cause little reaction when used in the form of polished plates, Smith-Petersen pins, and arthroplasty cups. Tantalum, titanium, and zirconium are also used because of their inertness. Other metallic objects, e.g. bullets, excite more reaction, and eventually

Figure 11.10
Foreign-body reaction. This is a section through an old operation scar at the site of an unabsorbed nylon suture, which is not recognisable in the figure. There is a heavy accumulation of foreign-body giant cells, around which there are empty spaces. The whole is enclosed in dense fibrous tissue in which there is a moderate lymphocytic infiltration. × 100.

become encapsulated in fibrous tissue. Steel or iron fragments lodged in the eye after penetrating injuries can cause a severe reaction resulting in blindness.

Plastic sponges (e.g. Ivalon, Etheron, and Polyfoam). In surgical practice these materials have been inserted as a means of inducing fibrosis as well as for mammoplasty. There is an initial acute inflammatory reaction with polymorphs, but this is rapidly followed by a macrophage response. Giant cells are formed in abundance, and the interstices of the sponge are invaded by granulation tissue. This matures until eventually dense, contracted scar tissue results. For this reason the materials are not uniformly successful for breast reconstruction. Futhermore, there is experimental evidence that in animals they may induce the formation of sarcoma.

Silicones and silastics.[10] Silicones are oily liquids of the basic formula:

$$CH_3 \quad CH_3$$
$$| \qquad |$$
$$CH_3 - Si - O - Si \text{ etc.}$$
$$| \qquad |$$
$$CH_3 \quad CH_3$$

They are heat stable, chemically non-reactive, and non-toxic, and excite little or no inflammatory or immunological response. Oxygen is ten times more soluble in them than in water, and fish and even small mammals can survive when immersed in them. They have been used in the human for many purposes. Injected into arthritic joints, they relieve pain and increase the range of movement. Subcutaneous injections have been used to recontour the face and breasts, but drifting of the fluid is a disadvantage.

Rubbers of varying degrees of hardness and known as *silastics* are formed from silicone by the addition of ferric or aluminium chloride followed by oxidation. They too are inert and can withstand bending without fatigue almost indefinitely. They have been used to form a variety of prostheses—the lens of the eye, the ear drum, breasts, joints, etc.

Suture materials. Catgut excites a brisk acute pyogenic inflammatory reaction which is soon followed by the appearance of macrophages and giant cells. The strength of plain catgut is reduced to half within two days, whereas for chromic gut the time is ten days.

The tissue reaction to linen, nylon, etc., does not succeed in removing the material, which is therefore retained for a long time.

Silica.[11] Colloidal silica solutions are very toxic to cells, and produce extensive necrosis if injected into the tissues. When silica is inhaled in the form of particles 2 to 5 μm in diameter, it is taken up by macrophages, which are usually destroyed by the effect the silica has on the cell membrane in increasing its permeability.[7] The silica is taken up by further macrophages, and the effect may be repeated; if sufficient quartz is present to overwhelm the macrophages, it is then taken up by the type II alveolar epithelial cells, also called granular pneumocytes (see p. 537), which discharge their lamellar bodies and associated lipids from the lysosomes, leading to a localised alveolar proteinosis (in which the alveolar space is full of proteinaceous material), which may in severe cases be quite widespread.

The alveolar fluid is carried by the lymphatics to small lymphoid aggregations in the connective tissue where the silica crystals are taken up by the local histiocytes, which are destroyed in a similar manner to the alveolar macrophages. Other histiocytes are less severely damaged, and suffer only an increased permeability of their lysosomal membranes, so that enzymes are released into the connective tissue; enzyme secretion from intact cells follows the induced fusion of lysosomal with cell membranes. These enzymes and lipids appear to attract more macrophages to the area, and a factor from the macrophages also stimulates fibrogenesis and possibly also fibroblast multiplication. Thus there develops a focus of perivascular dust reticulation in which fibroblasts, macrophages, and other cells of inflammation become enmeshed in proliferating reticulin fibres surrounding the blood vessel. Many of the macrophages appear to be destroyed, and their content of quartz and other dust lies free in the fibrous connective tissue. The fibroblasts produce exuberant collagen fibres which replace the reticulin.

If the process continues, the quartz is conveyed by the larger lymphatics to the hilar lymph nodes, which similarly contain dense whorls of fibrous tissue containing crystals of silica. Likewise fibrous nodules may develop under the visceral pleura as subpleural lymphoid follicles become involved. The silicotic islets occur in the apical segments of the upper and lower lobes, and are initially discrete but later coalesce to form conglomerate nodules. The fully matured silicotic islet consists of whorled, concentric hyaline fibres. This glassy appearance of the collagen fibres is due to a coating consisting of blood proteins, mainly γ-globulins, that remain *in situ* for a long time.

Silicosis is seen in miners, stone-workers, and sand-blasters, and can produce great disability due to progressive lung destruction. The condition predisposes to tuberculosis but not to lung cancer. It used to be taught that necrosis within a silicotic islet indicated tuberculous infection, but it is now known that small areas of necrosis are often due merely to ischaemia in the centre of an acellular nodule.

Silicosis can be more severe in patients who have autoantibodies in the serum.[12] One good example is the exuberant silicotic nodule found in patients who suffer from rheumatoid disease, which is analagous to Caplan's syndrome occurring in coalminers (p. 208). Antinuclear antibodies are often found in patients with severe progressive disease, but it is not certain whether they precede or follow the lung condition.

It should be noted that silica introduced into small cuts, e.g. of the fingers, produces a non-caseating tuberculoid granulomatous reaction resembling sarcoidosis.

Asbestos.[11] Another important disease produced by the inhalation of a dust (pneumoconiosis) is asbestosis. Asbestos belongs to a group of silicate minerals called amphiboles, in which only 2 oxygen atoms of the SiO_4 tetrahedra are shared with adjacent tetrahedra. The asbestiform minerals comprise chrysotile ('white asbestos'), which is a magnesium silicate, and the amphibole group consisting of crocidolite ('blue asbestos'), amosite ('brown asbestos'), anthophyllite, tremolite, and actinolite. Crocidolite, amosite, and actinolite all contain iron silicate.[13] Chrysotile accounts for 95 per cent of the exploited fibres, whereas crocidolite and amosite together account for about 4 per cent of the commercially-used asbestos.

When fibres are inhaled and retained in the lung parenchyma, some become coated with an iron-protein complex which is smooth, golden-brown in colour, and with bulbous ends resembling a drum-stick. These *asbestos bodies* (Fig. 11.11) are striking when viewed under light microscopy, but electron microscopy shows that in fact they are in the minority, being grossly outnumbered by uncoated fibres. These are so fine as to escape detection by the light microscope. The fibres vary greatly in length from less than 5 μm to over 200 μm. Short fibres are readily phagocytosed by macrophages, but those over 30 μm are not completely ingested. Fibres that are not ingested can react with the cell membranes of macrophages over a long period, and this may be relevant to their biological effects.[7] Compared with silicosis, cell death is delayed in asbestosis, but it may often be observed after exposure to moderate amounts of chrysotile. More usually asbestos fibres induce the selective release of lysosomal enzymes from cultured macrophages. These hydrolases have a fibrogenic activity.[7]

Lesions from the inhalation of asbestos dust consist initially of fibres, some in macrophages and other free, asbestos bodies, and cell debris accumulating in the alveoli arising directly from the respiratory bronchioles. These deposits become organised; the initial reticulin web is soon replaced by collagen fibres which spread into the wall of the respiratory bron-

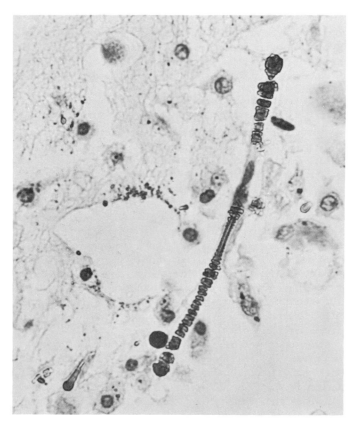

Figure 11.11
Asbestos body in lung. Note the dumb-bell shape of the elongated fibre and its segmented structure. Surrounding it there is organising proteinaceous material in an alveolus. The head of a second, broken asbestos body is also present. × 320.

chioles. At first only a few scattered respiratory bronchioles are affected, but later the fibrosis spreads both upwards into the walls of the terminal bronchioles and peripherally into the whole of the acinus, eventually reaching the terminal air-sacs. If sufficient fibres are retained in the lung, most of the parenchyma is replaced by a fibrous-tissue network surrounding distorted, collapsed air-spaces and containing clumps of asbestos bodies and fibres. There is also an infiltration of lymphocytes and plasma cells.

The lesions in asbestosis appear first at the bases of the lower lobes of the lungs, and the interstitial fibrosis gradually spreads upwards as the disease progresses. The visceral and parietal pleura is often involved with the formation of plaques of varying size, some quite large. These often calcify later on. Asbestosis is a very important precancerous condition, but predisposes less to tuberculosis than does silicosis.

Talc. Talc (magnesium silicate) causes a typical foreign-body reaction which terminates in fibrosis (Fig. 11.12). Its use as a glove-powder is liable to lead to postoperative adhesions following abdominal surgery.[14] Starch powder, although safer, may have a similar effect.

A few patients have developed fever, ascites, and other signs of peritonitis 2 to 3 weeks after abdominal surgery. At laparotomy the numerous peritoneal granulomata that are encountered may mimic seedling deposits of cancer or tubercle follicles. The symptoms subside on steroid therapy, and the condition is probably mediated by a hypersensitivity reaction, since the patient's lymphocytes have been found to undergo blast transformation when mixed with corn starch *in vitro*. It is evident that surgeon's gloves should be thoroughly washed before use in the peritoneal cavity.[15]

Beryllium.[16] This excites an acute inflammatory response which progresses to chronic inflammation with fibrosis and sometimes a non-caseating tuberculoid reaction. It is seen in

Figure 11.12
Starch granuloma. This granuloma was found in the appendix. A central area of necrosis is bounded by a layer of radially disposed macrophages and giant cells. The starch granules, represented as clear oval spaces, are seen within the necrosis and the giant cells. × 150. (*From Neely, J. and Davies, J. D. (1971), British Medical Journal, 3, 625.*)

the lungs of workers whose occupation entails inhalation of beryllium compounds.

Zirconium. Though metallic zirconium is inert, salts of this metal in deodorant sticks have been reported (mostly from the USA) to produce non-caseating tuberculoid lesions in the skin (see p. 261). The tuberculoid reaction to zirconium is an immunological granuloma related to delayed-type hypersensitivity.[1]

REFERENCES

1. ADAMS, D. O. (1976) The granulomatous inflammatory response. *American Journal of Pathology*, **84**, 164.
2. RYAN, G. B. & SPECTOR, W. G. (1970) Macrophage turnover in inflamed connective tissue. *Proceedings of the Royal Society*, B, **175**, 269.
3. SPECTOR, W. G. (1971) The cellular dynamics of granulomas. *Proceedings of the Royal Society of Medicine*, **64**, 941.
4. PAPADIMITRIOU, J. M. & SPECTOR, W. G. (1971) The origin, properties and fate of epithelioid cells. *Journal of Pathology*, **105**, 187.
5. CARTER, R. L. & ROBERTS, J. D. B. (1971) Macrophages and multinucleate giant cells in nitrosoquinoline-induced granulomata in rats: an autoradiographic study. *Journal of Pathology*, **105**, 285.
6. DAEMS, W. T., KOERTEN, H. K. SORANZO, M. R. (1976) In *The Reticuloendothelial System in Health and Disease* (Differences between monocyte-derived and tissue macrophages), ed. Reichard, S. M., Escobar, M. R. & Friedman, H. p. 27. New York: Plenium Press.
7. ALLISON, A. C., CLARK, I. A. & DAVIES, P. (1977) Cellular interactions in fibrogenesis. *Annals of the Rheumatic Diseases*, **36**, Supplement p. 8.
8. TURK, J. L. (1975) *Delayed Hypersensitivity*, 2nd edn, p. 275. Amsterdam: North Holland.
9. Leading Article (1975) Amyloidosis and leprosy. *Lancet*, **2**, 589.
10. HELAL, B. (1969) In *Recent Advances in Orthopaedics*, p. 91, ed. Apley, A. G. London: Churchill.
11. WAGNER, J. C. (1977) Pulmonary fibrosis and mineral dusts. *Annals of the Rheumatic Diseases*, **36**, Supplement p. 42.
12. TURNER-WARWICK, M. *et al.* (1977) Chemical fibrosis: the model of silica. *Annals of the Rheumatic Diseases*, **36**, Supplement p. 47
13. SPENCER, H. (1977) *Pathology of the Lung*, 3rd edn, vol. 1, p. 423. Oxford: Pergamon Press.
14. SAXÉN, L. & MYLLÄRNIEMI, H. (1968) Foreign material and postoperative adhesions. *New England Journal of Medicine*, **279**, 200.
15. Leading Article (1973) Glove powder: a surgical hazard. *British Medical Journal*, **2**, 502.
16. FREIMAN, D. G. & HARDY, H. L. (1970) Beryllium disease; the relation of pulmonary pathology to clinical course and prognosis based on a study of 130 cases from US Beryllium Case Registry. *Human Pathology*, **1**, 25.

Chapter 12. The Immune Response

One of the characteristic features of the adult vertebrate is its ability to distinguish between its own normal constituents ('self') and those of external or foreign origin ('non-self'). Damaged or degenerating tissue components are included in this group of non-self substances. The reaction to foreign substances involves the elimination of the foreign material, and is an important homeostatic mechanism.[1] It has been adapted during evolution as a protective mechanism against infection, and for this reason the response has been called the *immune response*.*

In the first description of antibody formation by von Behring and Kitasato in 1890, it was shown that animals injected with tetanus or diphtheria toxin produced substances which were capable of neutralising the toxins. The antibodies gave protection against these diseases, and the subject of immunology naturally grew around the central theme of immunity to bacterial infection.

Soon, however, with the description of the tuberculin reaction by Koch and anaphylaxis by Richet, it was realised that the body's reaction to foreign protein was also responsible for the phenomena of hypersensitivity.

More recently it has been recognised that under certain conditions the body is capable of reacting against its own constituents, thereby revealing diseases whose pathogenesis can be explained on an 'autoimmune reaction'. Great interest is now centred on this aspect, which affords a new pathogenesis to many well-established diseases, and also shows how the body can react against whole living tissues as well as simple protein antigens. The grafting of tissues from one animal to another is a further exploitation of the science of immunology.

Inevitably the highly specific and sensitive methods which have been developed in immunology have been applied to other fields, e.g. in the analysis of protein structure, blood group antigens, etc.

The immune response is therefore a reaction to foreign material which results in the formation of antibodies. These may be either immunoglobulins or cell-bound. Two separate systems are involved. *The lymphoid tissue associated developmentally with the thymus is responsible for the production of cell-bound antibodies, while the immunoglobulins are synthesised in cells which are dependent developmentally on lymphoid tissue associated with the gut: in birds this is the bursa of Fabricius.*

ANTIGENS

An *antigen* is usually defined as a substance which when introduced parenterally into the tissues stimulates the *production* of an antibody, and when mixed with that antibody *reacts specifically* with it in some detectable way. An *antibody* is a substance produced as a result of the stimulus provided by the introduction of an antigen with which it reacts in a specific way. Advances in immunology have demanded some modification of these definitions.

An *antigen* may be defined as a substance that when introduced parenterally into the tissues evokes an immune response which results in the production of *antibodies*, the development of *immunological memory*, and under some circumstances the induction of *specific immunological tolerance*. The antibodies produced may be immunoglobulins or cellular, and react *specifically* with the antigen in some detectable way. Immunological memory or tolerance are evident when the antigen is introduced on a subsequent occasion, for there is a response differing from that seen on the first encounter. Indeed, an antigen may be directly defined in these terms: it is *a substance which when introduced into the body of a susceptible animal leads to an immune response which results in a specific change such that when the antigen is introduced on a subsequent occasion there is a response differing from that seen when the substance was first introduced.*† The difference observed may be local or general depending on the route of administration; the reaction leads to the more rapid elimination from the body, except perhaps in certain cells, and in such a form as to provide for immunological memory.

Two classes of antigen may be considered: (*a*) *haptens*, which show little or no antigenic properties until first combined with protein; this may occur spontaneously *in vivo* when the substance is introduced into the body, or be performed *in vitro* by chemical manipulations, and (*b*) *true antigens*, which are nearly always proteins. In fact there is no hard and fast line of division between these two classes.

Characteristics of Antigens

Most true antigens are high-molecular-weight substances of protein nature, but even proteins of low molecular weight can be antigenic; a good example is insulin with a molecular weight of 6000 daltons. Lipids are not antigenic, but polysaccharides have antigenic properties provided they have a high enough molecular weight. Thus dextran of molecular weight

---

*It is of interest to note that there is no immune response in non-vertebrates, and presumably their defences against infection must rely on other mechanisms. The Californian and Atlantic hagfish are primitive vertebrates which occupy a similar position. The sea lamprey can form cellular antibodies but few immunoglobulins. Higher vertebrates produce both types of antibody.

†It is of historical interest that von Pirquet coined the term *allergy* to describe this altered response. It included those changes which led both to immunity and to hypersensitivity. However, by common usage the original meaning has been changed, and allergy is now equated with hypersensitivity (p. 174).

100 000 daltons is not antigenic, whereas dextrans of molecular weight 600 000 daltons are antigenic.

Haemoglobin is an example of a poor antigen, whereas those proteins found in skin are highly antigenic. It must be appreciated that antigenicity, like pathogenicity with micro-organisms, is not an absolute quality. A substance can be considered antigenic only in relation to a specific host. The skin antigens of an individual are not antigenic to himself, but are highly antigenic to all other individuals (except an identical twin).

The antigenic specificity of each protein is due to specific areas of the molecule called *determinant sites*, or *epitopes*. One protein molecule can have several epitopes, and these may differ from each other not only in specificity but also in antigenic potency. It is therefore an oversimplification to think of a protein like serum albumin as exhibiting a single specificity (see p. 145). The precise nature of the epitopic sites is poorly understood, but the shape of the molecule due to its secondary and tertiary structure is believed to be involved (see footnote, p. 15). It is of interest that even a slight difference in the chemical composition of a protein can greatly affect the antigenic properties of a protein. Thus in the ABO blood-group substances a single sugar molecule in a side chain can determine antigenic specificity (see Ch. 55).

Denaturation of protein involves changes in its secondary structure and changes in antigenicity. New epitopes may be uncovered and old ones lost. A similar phenomenon may occur *in vivo*; antibodies may appear against fragments of an injected antigen due to the exposure of new determinants which were not on the surface of the original molecule.

Haptens.[2] It has been found that even slight changes in the chemical composition of a protein are capable of altering its antigenic properties. One of the ways in which this may be done is by its conjugation with a second small molecule known as a *hapten*. This is a non-protein substance which has little or no antigenic properties itself, but which combines with a protein to form a new antigen. The latter is capable of stimulating the production of specific immunoglobulins, the specificity of which depends upon the hapten fraction rather than the carrier protein.

A secondary response can be obtained by a subsequent challenge by the same carrier-hapten complex, but *not by the hapten combined with a different carrier*. This is because the carrier is recognised by T cells, while the hapten is recognised by B cells. Hence the immune response to a protein-hapten complex involves T cell recognition and T cell help (by T helper cells) to enable B cells to produce immunoglobulin. In the immune response to a carrier-hapten complex the specificity is largely dominated by the hapten, and the response to the carrier is suppressed. This suppression is not necessarily complete, for antibodies specific for the carrier protein may also appear (p. 184). This applies particularly to the cell-bound type.

Haptens on their own have the property of combining with their specific immunoglobulin, although usually no precipitate is formed. However, the treated antibody is no longer capable of forming a precipitate when added to the antigen–hapten complex. Therefore, while haptens must be combined with protein to elicit their specific antibody response, they do not require the protein to react with the antibody so produced.

The more complex haptens, e.g. pneumococcal polysaccharide, do react with their specific antibodies to produce a precipitate.

Lipids and simple carbohydrates, which are not antigenic, and the more complex polysaccharides, which are poorly antigenic (see above), produce powerful antigens when they are combined with protein.

The importance of haptens may be illustrated by three examples.

(1) Pneumococci contain an important polysaccharide in their capsules which determines their pathogenicity and antigenicity (see p. 221). Similarity β-haemolytic streptococci contain polysaccharide haptens (see Lancefield grouping, p. 218).

(2) Simple chemicals may combine with body proteins, thereby producing an antigenic complex. This is the basis of allergic contact dermatitis and many types of drug hypersensitivity.

(3) Several important tissue antigens are either haptens or haptens combined with protein. Thus, the blood-group substances (ABO system) are glycoproteins, and transplantation, Forssman, and Wassermann antigens are lipid in nature.

Heterophile antigens. This name is applied to antigens which are identical (or very closely related), and which are found in the tissues of different and unrelated species of animals. Antibodies to them thus appear to be non-specific. The best known is *Forssman antigen*, a lipopolysaccharide-protein complex, which is widely distributed in nature, being found in certain bacteria, e.g. *Sh. dysenteriae*, and the tissues and red cells of many animals. Guinea-pig kidney is a convenient laboratory source. Other important examples are the antigen shared between (a) *Proteus* organisms and certain rickettsiae (see Weil-Felix reaction, p. 169), and (b) the virus of infectious mononucleosis and sheep red cells (Paul-Bunnell test, Ch. 53).

Alloantigens. Substances which are present in one individual and are antigenic to some (but not all) individuals of the *same species* are termed alloantigens. Good examples are the blood-group and transplantation antigens, and those associated with the genetically determined variants of the immunoglobulins and other plasma proteins. Alloantigens were previously called isoantigens, but this terminology has now been changed to bring it into line with the terms used in transplantation immunology. Likewise the term alloantibody replaces isoantibody.

TYPES OF ANTIBODY

The immunoglobulins were for long regarded as the most important products of the immune response, but it is now well established that other types of antibody are produced. One type is confined to the cells, and therefore regarded as *cell-bound*, or *cellular, antibody*. The cells involved in this type of immunity are the lymphocytes. These play an important part in *homograft rejection*, in *delayed-type hypersensitivity*, and in *immunity to microbial infection*.

Interferon may be regarded as yet another mechanism involved in immunity to infection.

The following important types of antibodies may therefore be recognised.

IMMUNOGLOBULINS

Detectable in vitro

Agglutinins
Precipitins
Amboceptors, e.g. lysins
Opsonins
Blocking antibodies
Neutralising antibodies, e.g. antitoxins and anti-enzymes

Detectable in vivo

Antibodies causing immunity (see Ch. 13)
Antibodies causing hypersensitivity (see Ch. 14)

CELLULAR ANTIBODIES

Cell-bound antibody (see p. 147 and p. 184)

Factors Influencing Antibody Production

A large number of factors affect the response of an animal to the introduction of an antigen. The following account includes the important generalisations, but as with all generalisations many exceptions will be found.

Genetic factors. The response to a particular antigen is probably determined by the animal's genetic constitution. Alleles at the Ir locus are of great importance in the mouse; this recently recognised aspect of the immune response is described further on page 162.

Previous contact with antigen. When an antigen is introduced into an animal for the first time, there is an interval varying from about 4 days to 4 weeks before any immunoglobulin can be detected in the serum. Then follows a rise in antibody titre which reaches a maximum at a time which may vary from 6 days to 3 months. Even then the level reached is comparatively low (*primary response*).

When the same antigen is injected on a second occasion, there is an immediate drop in circulating antibody level due to its neutralisation by the injected antigen. However, after 2 to 3 days a rapid exponential rise in titre is noted, which reaches a peak after 7 to 14 days and again falls off, rapidly at first and later more slowly. The final level of antibody is usually above the previous one. The features of the *secondary response* are that a smaller dose of antigen is needed to produce it, the lag period is shorter, and there is a greater production of antibody which is mostly of the IgG class. Thus the prior introduction of antigen has led to a state in which, although the antibody titre is low, the animal is in a particularly favourable position should it ever in the future need to make the same antibody again. This state, known as *potential immunity*, is of great importance when considering active artificial immunisation. Potential immunity is dependent upon *immunological memory*, and this appears to reside in small lymphocytes. Thus if small lymphocytes from the thoracic duct of an immunised animal are injected into a syngeneic host, the latter will respond to a first injection of antigen by a typical secondary response. Figure 12.1 contrasts the two responses.

Repeated injections of antigen lead to variable responses depending upon the type of substance used, the frequency of injection, etc. Usually the antibody response is less marked with each injection, and under some circumstances the antibody level may even fall. This may be due to a type of

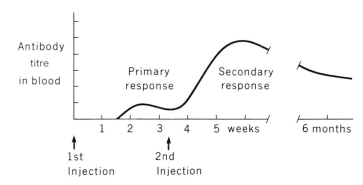

Figure 12.1
Diagram showing the differences between a primary and a secondary response to an antigenic stimulus. (*Drawn by Margot Mackay, Department of Art as Applied to Medicine, University of Toronto.*)

tolerance or immunological paralysis (see p. 141). The unreactive state is not permanent.

Anamnestic reaction. During the stage of potential immunity the production of specific antibodies may also occur in response to the stimulus of an unrelated antigen. The introduction of an antigen may therefore give rise not only to its own specific antibodies but also to others which are specific to the many antigens which the individual has met previously. This 'recall' phenomenon is known as the *anamnestic reaction*;* it may also be seen in infection, but fortunately, from a diagnostic point of view, the general rise in titre thereby induced is small.

It is important to remember this phenomenon when interpreting the results of the Widal, Weil-Felix, or other agglutination tests. Any infection is liable to cause an increased production of agglutinins; this affects the anti-H agglutinins especially, and in the Widal test is most marked in those who have been inoculated previously with TAB (p. 169).

The anamnestic reaction has been used to investigate the epidemiology of past influenza epidemics. A persons who has suffered from influenza due to one strain of virus will produce antibodies to that strain many years later when infected with an influenza virus of different strain.

Type of antigen. Antigens vary considerably in their ability to elicit antibody production. As a general rule particulate antigen produces a better response than does soluble material. For this reason an antigen precipitated with alum is used for diphtheria immunisation. Another method of improving antibody response is to mix the antigen with Freund's adjuvant† (dead mycobacteria in a liquid oil-in-water emulsion). These methods probably act by delaying the absorption of antigen from the site of injection and from the regional lymph nodes which the adjuvant reaches in 1 hour, but it has also been suggested that the local inflammatory reaction (particularly macrophage activity) may play some part

---

* Some authorities use this term in a different sense and apply it to the secondary response (see above).

† In the complete 'Freund's adjuvant', the acid-fast bacilli are included and a delayed-type hypersensitivity is also induced. The adjuvant is too irritating for human use. The 'incomplete' antigen does not contain bacilli, and its use merely augments the immunoglobulin response. Arachis oil is commonly used in Freund's adjuvant.

in the heightened response. In addition, the inflammatory response may be a factor in stimulating the production of cell-bound antibodies. *Bordetella pertussis* also acts as a potent adjuvant, and is included with diphtheria and tetanus toxoid in triple vaccine. The administration of several antigens together does not always enhance the immune response—sometimes there is inhibition, the explanation for which competition is unknown.

Quantity of antigen given. Within wide limits the antibody response is not closely related to the quantity of antigen injected. When very large doses are given there may be a complete failure of antibody production; moreover, the animal may for many months be incapable of reacting to further smaller doses of the same antigen. This phenomenon, known as *immunological paralysis*, is a type of immunological tolerance (p. 155) and has been most studied in mice injected with pneumococcal polysaccharides, substances which are not metabolised and remain in the body for a long period. Immunological paralysis is produced by soluble antigens much more easily than with particulate material. Very small doses of antigen may also induce a state of tolerance.

Route of administration. With some antigens, e.g. bacteria, an intravenous injection gives rise to immunoglobulin production, whereas subcutaneous or intraperitoneal administration causes, in addition, an immune response associated with the production of cell-bound antibodies. Chemicals applied to the skin are particularly liable to induce delayed-type hypersensitivity as a result of this T cell response.

Duration of antigenic stimulation. The first-formed immunoglobulins are of the IgM class (see Rhesus sensitisation, p. 648). The more usual IgG antibodies appear later, and their presence inhibits IgM production. The IgM antibodies are produced when there is antigen excess as occurs during the early phase of an immune response. If IgG is administered, IgM production is inhibited. The production of IgM antibodies appears to be a primitive response, since this type of antibody is the only one produced in some primitive vertebrates, e.g. sharks. It is the first type of antibody produced by the human fetus whilst *in utero*.

The antibody titre already present. The presence of circulating immunoglobulin may depress or completely abolish the response to injected antigen as expressed by immunoglobulin or cell-bound antibody formation (see also tumour enhancement, p. 372). The implications of this should be remembered when artificial immunisation is being attempted. Thus, the response to diphtheria toxoid is poor in infants who have a high titre of passively transferred maternal antibody (see also tetanus prophylaxis, p. 232). The phenomenon can be used to advantage to prevent sensitisation of Rh-negative mothers who have recently given birth to Rh-positive children. If anti-Rh globulin is administered within 48 hours after delivery, sensitisation is inhibited. The explanation for this is not definitely known, but the rapid binding of the antigen by antibody and its subsequent elimination probably play an important part.

Age of animal. During early fetal life animals will accept foreign protein without antibody production. Furthermore, they may be rendered incapable of reacting to the same antigen on a subsequent occasion. This is *immunological toler-*

ance and is described in detail later (p. 193). As fetal development proceeds, the ability to produce immunoglobulin appears. At this stage small doses of antigen excite an immune response, while *large* or *very small* doses produce tolerance. The human fetus has the ability to produce antibodies from about the age of 3 months. Nevertheless, it produces little antibody, and the immunoglobulins present in the blood at birth consist almost entirely of IgG of maternal origin. As this is catabolised, endogenous antibody is produced. Adult levels of IgM are attained by one year, IgG by the age of 5 or 6 years, and IgA by 10 years. Infection of the fetus, e.g. with syphilis, leads to IgM antibody production and not tolerance. Indeed, the presence of a high IgM at birth may be used as an indication of intra-uterine infection, since this type of antibody, being unable to cross the placental barrier, cannot be of maternal origin.[3]

Mice are relatively immature at birth, and can be rendered tolerant with small doses of antigen.

Nutrition. Starvation has little or no effect on antibody production. An exception to this is the immunological deficiency exhibited by pyridoxine-deficient rats; the explanation for this is not known.

Anergy. A loss of the ability to express a cell-mediated immune response is called anergy. Thus a person previously sensitive to tuberculin, trichophytin, and mumps antigen becomes negative. Anergy is not uncommon in terminal states due to many causes, e.g. infections and malignancy. In cancer it is associated with a bad prognosis.[4] It is also a well-known feature of sarcoidosis, lepromatous leprosy, and measles. The pathogenesis is not known, and indeed may not be the same in all instances. Destruction of normal lymphoid tissue may be postulated as the mechanism in extensive malignant disease, Hodgkin's disease, and widespread sarcoidosis. However, this cannot be the explanation in early sarcoidosis or measles.

The action of blocking antibodies or of suppressor T cells may be involved, but non-immunological agents may also play a part. Thus a factor has been found in the serum of patients with Hodgkin's disease that inhibits the patient's T cells.[5]

Immunologically deficient diseases. See page 170.

Artificial Methods Designed to Reduce the Immune Response

Immunological unresponsiveness can be induced in one of two ways. The induction of *tolerance* is described on page 155. *Immunosuppression* refers to the diminution of the immune response in an otherwise normal animal. The following have been used:

Glucocorticoid administration. The continuous administration of a glucocorticoid, usually prednisone, impairs the antibody response to a primary antigenic stimulation. The secondary response is not appreciably affected unless large doses are given.

Antilymphocytic serum.[6, 7] The production of antilymphocytic serum by the injection of lymphocytes of one species into an animal of another species was described by Metchnikoff in 1899. Administration of the serum blocks T cell function, but does not suppress antibody responses that do not require the participation of T lymphocytes, nor those that are fully established at the time of its administration. It prolongs the life of allografts, and has been used in patients for suppressing the graft reaction and in treating autoimmune disease. The active factor is a γ-globulin, but serum for human use is difficult to standardise and its administration has many unwanted effects, e.g. local pain, anaphylactic shock, thrombocytopenia, and renal damage; this last is due to a contaminating anti-basement membrane component. Although antilymphocytic serum may produce lymphopenia, this is not invariable, and the degree of suppression of graft rejection does not parallel this effect. It has been suggested that the serum coats the lymphocytes or in some way renders them less active, thus impeding the afferent limb of the immune response. The serum appears to block immunological memory for some previously encountered antigens. Thus if an animal previously sensitised to bovine serum albumin is treated with the serum and subsequently challenged with the antigen, it reacts with a typical primary response. This effect might prove to be of immense value in the treatment of some diseases, but the danger on the other side of the coin is quite considerable: the immunological memory for past infection would also be blocked, and the organisms would promote a primary response.

The lack of standardisation of antilymphocytic serum—there is no satisfactory way of assessing its immunosuppressive activity *in vitro*—and the cost of its production have limited the use of this potentially useful agent.

Total body exposure to ionising radiation.[8] Following exposure to X-rays, animals show a poor response to primary antigenic stimulation. The antibody response to a secondary stimulation is much less inhibited, indicating that it is the development of potential immunity which is affected by the action of ionising radiation. This again stresses the fact that two distinct steps are involved in the immune response. The primary stimulus produces a 'conditioning' effect which results in the state of potential immunity. Subsequent stimulation triggers off a different mechanism which leads to the rapid production of antibodies. There is evidence that ionising radiation reduces macrophage activity and that it is this effect which is responsible for inhibiting the primary response (p. 153).

If ionising radiation is given after the injection of antigen, the peak of antibody production may actually be increased.[9] Alkylating agents, such as nitrogen mustard, produce effects similar to those of ionising radiation.

Administration of antimetabolites. The administration of 6-mercaptopurine, or its more potent and less toxic derivative *azathioprine (Imuran)*, inhibits the primary response; indeed, a state of tolerance may be induced. These agents are most effective if given about one day *after* the administration of antigen, in contrast to ionising radiation which must be given beforehand for a maximal inhibiting effect. Large doses of 6-mercaptopurine also inhibit the secondary response. Actinomycin D has an effect similar to that of 6-mercaptopurine.

Depletion of the body's lymphocytes. This experimental procedure also inhibits the development of a primary response. It depletes the body of T cells, and may be performed by establishing a thoracic-duct fistula or by the extracorporeal irradiation of blood.

Nature and Properties of Immunoglobulins

Antibody activity in the plasma is due to a group of globulins which, on electrophoretic separation, form a broad band in the γ fraction together with some activity in the α and β regions. They are highly specific and react with their corresponding antigens in various ways, although this action may not always be demonstrable *in vitro*. The in-vitro reactions between antigens and antibodies are considered later in this chapter, but it may be noted at this stage that in general the antibodies tend to neutralise their antigens and lead to their elimination.

The antibody produced in an animal after the injection of an antigen is not a single distinct protein, for one antigenic compound may have several epitopes, and therefore antibodies of different specificities are produced. Furthermore, even the antibody possessing a single specificity is heterogeneous and consists of a group of proteins differing somewhat in molecular composition and size, and in electrophoretic mobility.

Nomenclature and Chemical Structure

The estimation of the molecular size led to the recognition of two major groups. The antibodies with a molecular weight of about 150 000 daltons form the 7S group, while the macroglobulins of molecular weight 10^6 daltons form the 19S component. Electrophoresis further subdivided the antibodies into γ_1, γ_2, β_1, β_2, etc., and this led to a complex terminology—thus the macroglobulins were variously called the $\beta_2 M$, $\gamma_1 M$, or 19S fraction. It is now agreed that all antibodies be termed *immunoglobulins* with the designation Ig regardless of their electrophoretic mobility.

The work of Porter has shown that each immunoglobulin molecule is composed of four polypeptide chains, one pair half the length of the other—these are called the *light chains* and consist of about 217 amino acids, and their molecular weight is about 25 000 daltons. The longer pair are called *heavy chains* and their molecular weight is about 50 000 daltons. It follows that the molecular weight of a typical immunoglobulin is about 150 000 daltons.

As Figure 12.2 indicates, the light chains are united to the heavy chains by a single disulphide bond at the carboxy-terminal end of the chain* (here the terminal amino acid has a free carboxyl group, whereas at the amino-terminal end of the chain there is a free amino group). The heavy chains are united together by from 1 to 5 disulphide bonds (in the diagram two have been depicted). If the molecule is digested with papain, three fragments are produced. Two are identical and have one antibody-combining site each; they are called the *Fab fragments*, and, as can be seen in Figure 12.2, they consist of the light chains and the amino-terminal portions of the heavy chains. The third fragment is crystallisable (which indicates the homogeneity of the amino-acid sequences in that part of the molecule), and is therefore called the *Fc fragment*. Although it has no antibody activity and consists only of part of the heavy chains, it contains many of the antigenic determinants of the molecule as a whole, and is also responsible for the properties of skin fixation, complement fixation, and placental transfer. If the molecule is digested with pepsin, there is a splitting of the heavy chains on the carboxy-terminal

---

*The carboxy-terminal part of a polypeptide is the first portion to be released from the ribosome, while the amino-terminal portion is released last.

Figure 12.2

Diagrammatic representation of the structure of IgG. The molecule is composed of two light polypeptide chains and two heavy chains joined together by disulphide bonds. Digestion with the enzyme papain splits the molecule into three fragments, as indicated by the dotted lines. The two Fab fragments have one antibody-combining site each, whilst the Fc fragment has none. The sites for the antigenic determinants governed by the *Inv* and *Gm* genes are shown.

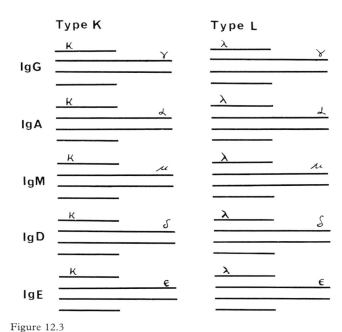

Figure 12.3

Structure of the immunoglobulins. The classes resemble each other in that the molecules are composed of two identical light polypeptide chains and two identical heavy chains. The difference lies in their heavy chains. In any one class there are two types. In the K type there are two κ light chains while in the L type there are two λ light chains.

side of the disulphide bonds; the remainder of the heavy chains fall apart, and a residue composed of two Fab fragments combined together is left. This acts as a bivalent antibody.

It is evident that the antibody-binding properties of the molecule reside in the Fab fragments at the amino-terminal end. The amino-terminal halves of the light chains and the associated halves of the heavy chains (called the Fd fragments) are described as *variable*, because the amino acids that constitute them vary both in type and sequence in each molecule. Some areas of the variable regions display much more variation than others. These are the *hypervariable* regions. It is in this way that so many different antibodies can be derived from any class of immunoglobulin. The carboxy-terminal halves of the light chains and the Fd fragments are much more constant, and are spoken of as *invariable* or *constant*. The Fc parts of the heavy chains are the most invariable, hence their tendency to crystallise.

Electron microscopy indicates that immunoglobulins are Y shaped, with the two arms of the Y joining at a *hinge area*. Movement at this point can result in a change of shape from a narrow Y to a T.

The immunoglobulins are themselves antigenic when injected into other species, and immunoelectrophoretic studies have revealed that the light and heavy chains are not homogeneous. Human antibodies can be divided into classes depending upon specific antigenic determinants on the light and heavy chains. There are five types of heavy chains, which are named: γ, α, μ, δ, and ε. Each antibody molecule has a pair of identical heavy chains and therefore five *classes* are recognised: IgG, IgA, IgM, IgD, and IgE respectively. Each class has been further subdivided into two types: K, for Korngold, and L, for Lipari, after the two workers who first recognised them. The difference lies in the light chains which are termed κ (kappa) and λ (lambda). Each molecule, whether IgG, IgA, IgM, IgD, or IgE, has either two κ or two λ chains, *but never one of each*. In a normal individual within each class of immunoglobulin, e.g. IgG, IgA, etc., about 70 per cent of the molecules have κ light chains and the remainder have the λ.

The five classes of immunoglobulins are depicted in Figure 12.3.

Variants of the heavy chains have now been detected. Thus there are four subtypes of the γ chains, called γ_1, γ_2, γ_3, and γ_4. Four subclasses of IgG are therefore recognised. Likewise there are two subclasses of IgA and of IgM to add to the remarkable heterogeneity of the immunoglobulins.

IgA, which exists mainly as a dimer, and IgM, which exists as a pentamer, both contain an additional small polypeptide chain that joins the monomers together. This is the J chain, and it is manufactured by the same cell that makes the immunoglobulin.

Inherited variation. Inherited antigenic differences have been found in both the light and heavy chains. The first two to be identified were the Gm antigens on the heavy chains, and the InV on the light κ chains. These alloantigens are comparable with the alloantigens of the red cells, but naturally occurring alloantibodies are uncommon. They are occasionally produced when immunoglobulin from one individual is transfused into another of different genotype. Alloantibodies also occur in rheumatoid arthritis, and are termed collectively the *rheumatoid factor* (p. 208). A third independent group of genetic markers, called the Am factors, has been described in the IgA molecule. Antibodies occur after transfusion with blood of a different Am type.

Properties of the Immunoglobulin Groups[10]

IgG immunoglobulin. This is the slowest component on electrophoresis, forms about 15 per cent of the total plasma proteins (6 to 15 g per litre), and contains about 3 per cent of

Figure 12.4
Diagrammatic representation of IgM and IgA.
IgM is shown as a pentamer. IgA is a dimer with its
two subunits united by a secretory component
represented by a triangle. Disulphide bonds are
depicted as solid circles.

carbohydrate. It is the only immunoglobulin capable of crossing the placenta and is found in all extracellular fluids. It has the longest half life of all the immunoglobulins: about 5 days.

IgA immunoglobulin[11] is present in the plasma (2 to 4 g per litre), but its highest concentration is found in secretions (mucus, colostrum, etc.) and it is an important factor in preventing infection of mucous membranes. It contains about 7·5 per cent of carbohydrate. Dimers and trimers and higher multimers of the 7S monomers are found in the blood, so that 9S and 11S components are present. Some IgA is made locally in the lymphoid tissue of the intestinal wall and secreted as a dimer bound to a third polypeptide called the secretory, or transport, piece, which may serve to stabilise the IgA against proteolysis or to facilitate secretion of this immunoglobulin (Fig. 12.4). The secreted IgA is an 11S component with a molecular weight of 385 000 daltons. It does not fix complement by the classical pathway, and it has been suggested that its function is to react with antigens absorbed from the gut and neutralise them without the damaging activation of complement.[12–14]

IgD immunoglobulin. This has been identified on immunoelectrophoresis of plasma and as an M protein in occasional cases of multiple myeloma. IgD molecules have been identified on the surface of lymphocytes, and are believed to act as antigen receptors in that situation. No other function has yet been attributed to this immunoglobulin.

IgE immunoglobulin is a 7S fraction with a molecular weight of 200 000 daltons, which is responsible for human anaphylaxis (p. 177) as well as for hypersensitivity states such as hay-fever and asthma. IgE binds to specific receptors on mast cells, and its subsequent interaction with antigen leads to the degranulation of the cells and the release of histamine, 5-HT, ECF-A, and SRS-A (p. 176). While this is the mechanism involved in type-1 hypersensitivity reactions, it may also increase vascular permeability such that other antibodies, e.g. IgG, can enter the area and destroy an infecting agent. Thus IgE may be of importance in defence against infection.[15] IgE will not fix complement even when aggregated.

IgM immunoglobulin. This is a 19S globulin containing about 10 per cent carbohydrate, and has a molecular weight of 900 000 daltons. It can be dissociated into five 7S subunits, each of which has a similar structure to that of IgG except that the heavy μ chains are present instead of γ (Fig. 12.4). It is largely restricted to the intravascular compartment (0·5 to 2 g per litre), and appears in the plasma at the age of 2 to 3 months.

Although it might be expected that IgM would have ten combining sites, the antibody is in fact sometimes pentavalent. The explanation for this is not known.

Specificity of Antibodies

The differences between the various chains of the immunoglobulins lie in their amino-acid sequence. Furthermore, the actual specificity of an antibody also lies in its exact chemical composition. Patients with multiple myeloma provide a ready source of homogeneous immunoglobulin whose amino-acid sequence can be analysed. It has been found that there are areas of constant sequence and areas that are variable on both light and heavy chains (p. 143). It is the differences in these variable areas that determine specificity. However, it is not yet possible to identify antibody specifically by chemical analysis; the only method of identification and estimation is by a reaction involving union with the appropriate antigen, either *in vitro* or *in vivo*.

Antigen-Antibody Union

The forces which unite antigen to antibody are not known for certain, but it is generally agreed that non-covalent bonds are involved. The union can certainly be broken; thus potent toxin can be recovered from toxin-antitoxin combinations.

The ability of an antibody to form stable complexes with antigen is termed its *avidity*. Antibodies of high avidity are usually formed in the later stages of an immune response or during a secondary response.

Following the primary union of antibody with antigen secondary phenomena occur; these are of great practical importance and are described below:

Types of Antibodies

Agglutinins. When a particulate antigen is added to its antibody, the particles may adhere together to produce large visible clumps. This clumping is called agglutination, and the antibody is called an agglutinin. The particles may consist of whole organisms, in which case it is a *surface antigen* that is involved. Alternatively, tanned red cells or collodion or polystyrene particles may be coated artificially with antigen, and then used for detecting agglutinating antibodies. This type of haemagglutination technique is very sensitive, being about ten times as effective in detecting antibody as the most sensitive gel-diffusion technique (see p. 145). Coated particles are in

Figure 12.5
Agglutination test. The titre of the antibody is 1 in 64. The failure of the first tube (1 in 2 dilution) to show agglutination is known as the prozone phenomenon and is not uncommonly seen in *Brucella* agglutination tests and in the standard serological tests for syphilis, such as the VDRL.

FINAL DILUTION OF SERUM

common use to detect antibodies in rheumatoid arthritis, infectious mononucleosis, thyroid disease, and systemic lupus erythematosus. Commercial tests are also available for the detection of C-reactive protein and fibrinogen (as a test for hypofibrinogenaemia) in blood, and chorionic gonadotrophin in urine (as a test for pregnancy).

Agglutination is dependent on the pH of the medium, its electrolyte content, and also on the temperature at which it takes place. It may take an appreciable time. It fails to occur if there is great excess of antigen, and also in some cases in the presence of excess antibody (see below). In performing agglutination tests these factors must be taken into account. Estimation of the strength, or titre, of these antibodies is frequently of value, and is performed as follows:

A series of tubes is prepared, the first containing neat serum (left-hand tube, Fig. 12.5), while each subsequent tube contains serum diluted with saline in proportions 1 in 2, 1 in 4, 1 in 8, etc. (doubling dilutions). To each is added an equal volume of a suspension of particles, after which the tubes are incubated at 37°C for a suitable period. The dilution of the serum in the last tube which shows definite agglutination is described as the titre of the antibody. Sometimes the left-hand tubes containing the highest concentrations of antibody fail to show agglutination. This is termed the 'prozone' phenomenon.

Precipitins. Precipitation is the formation of an insoluble product when two soluble substances are mixed together. In this type of reaction the antigen must therefore be in solution. To demonstrate antibacterial precipitins a soluble extract of the organism is first prepared, and then added to the antibody. This may be done by simple mixing, but precipitation does not occur in the presence of excess antibody. A better technique is to layer the one fluid carefully on the other, in which case a precipitate forms at or near the interface. Using this method Lancefield was able to sub-divide the β-haemolytic streptococci into many groups.

Probably the most sensitive method, however, is to perform the reaction in an agar gel (Oudin). If an antigen is placed in a cup cut in an agar plate in which there is incorporated the corresponding antibody, there develops a zone of precipitation which steadily advances with a sharp leading edge. Precipitation occurs where antigen and antibody are in optimal proportions. Another method is to allow antigen and antibody to diffuse towards each other from separate cups (see Fig. 12.6). This technique, developed by Ouchterlony, can be used to identify unknown antigens or antibodies. Thus, if a mixture of antibodies is allowed to diffuse towards different antigens each in a separate cup, lines of precipitation will be formed (see Fig. 12.6). If the lines fuse it may be assumed that they

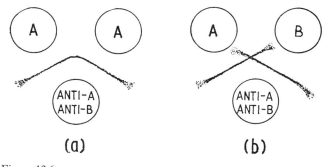

Figure 12.6
Ouchterlony plates showing precipitin reactions. In (a) the precipitin lines join together, as they are both due to the same A-anti-A reaction. In (b) the lines cross, as they are formed by different antigen–antibody reactions.

are caused by the same antigen-antibody precipitation, while if they intersect they are due to different reactions.

As with agglutination, electrolyte concentration and pH are important. Precipitation may not occur in the absence of electrolytes, and reactions are usually performed with physiological concentrations of saline.

The investigation of the composition of the precipitate has shown that the ratio of antigen to antibody varies according to the manner in which the precipitate is formed. A plausible hypothesis of the mode of formation of the precipitate is the lattice theory. There is considerable evidence to show that many antibodies are bivalent, while antigens are multivalent. By valency is meant the number of combining units, or arms, attached to each molecule. Thus, when a precipitate is formed with antigen and antibody in optimal proportions, the compound formed has the structure as shown in Figure 12.7 (A). Less compact precipitates are formed if either antigen or antibody is in excess (Fig. 12.7 (B) and (C)), while soluble products can be explained when either component is present in great excess (Fig. 12.7 (D) and (E)). It should be remembered that one antigen may contain several epitopes, and its introduction into an animal can lead to the formation of separate antibodies each with different specificities. The cooperative action of these may be involved in an antigen-antibody reaction (Fig. 12.8).

Precipitin reactions are used in streptococcal grouping (Lancefield), the medico-legal identification of human blood or semen, and in the diagnosis of syphilis (e.g. the VDRL and Kahn tests). In the Kahn test the precipitate is so soft and flocculent that it is usually called a 'flocculation test'.

Figure 12.7
Diagrammatic representation of the composition of various antigen-antibody combinations (see text). Antibody, assumed to be bivalent, is depicted as hollow rods. The solid circles are antigen molecules and have six combining units. (*After Pauling, L.* (1940), *Journal of the American Chemical Society,* **62**, 2643.)

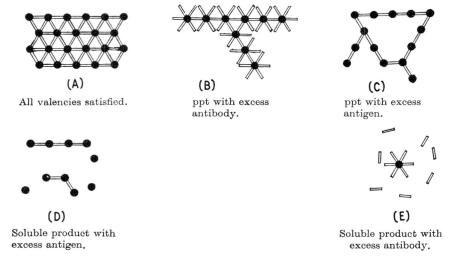

(A)
All valencies satisfied.

(B)
ppt with excess antibody.

(C)
ppt with excess antigen.

(D)
Soluble product with excess antigen.

(E)
Soluble product with excess antibody.

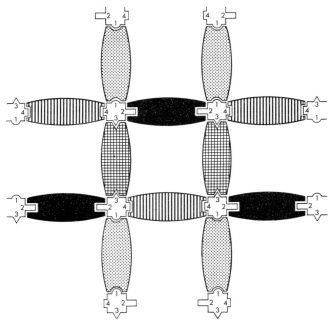

Figure 12.8
Schematic illustration of the diversity of antibodies formed against a pure antigen and their cooperative effects in the precipitin reaction with the antigen. The antigenic determinants (epitopes) are arbitrarily labelled 1, 2, 3, and 4. The diagram is based on Fig. 13.14 in Davis, B. D., Dulbecco, R., Eisen, H. N., Ginsberg, H. S. and Wood, W. B. (1967), "Microbiology", p. 386. New York: Harper and Row-Hoeber.

Amboceptor. This type of antibody, when combined with its corresponding antigen, can sequentially activate a group of proteins which collectively are called *complement* (see p. 159). The activation of complement may produce some visible effect, for instance the lysis of a bacterium or red cell, or it may be invisible. In such instances the reaction can be detected by using a second 'haemolytic system', as in the complement fixation test.

The Wassermann reaction is a good example of this. The test is explained diagrammatically in Table 12.1, in which it will be seen that serum, which has been heated to 56°C for half an hour, is mixed with a standard quantity of complement and antigen. The antigen is in fact a cholesterolised extract of heart muscle. The object of heating the serum is to inactivate the unknown quantity of complement which is normally present, so that a known, measured amount can be added for the reaction. The serum-antigen-complement mixture is allowed to incubate for a standard length of time, e.g. 2 hours at 37°C. If the relevant antibody is present in the patient's serum, the antigen will combine with it, and at the same time 'fix', or combine with, the added complement.

The detector system is then added. It is also of an antigen-amboceptor type, and utilises red cells with a corresponding haemolysin. If complement is not used up in the first reaction, it is available for the second system. Therefore, haemolysis of the red cells denotes the absence of syphilitic antibody, and the Wassermann reaction is said to be negative. On the other hand, the absence of haemolysis indicates a positive reaction. The question of false positive reactions is considered on page 248.

Amboceptors are either IgM or IgG (IgM is the stronger amboceptor of the two), and the commonly encountered examples are bacteriolysins and haemolysins. Complement fixation tests are employed in the diagnosis of syphilis, gonorrhoea, hydatid disease, and nearly all the viral infections. They are also of diagnostic use in Hashimoto's disease.

Antibodies causing the immune adherence phenomenon. Antigens (e.g. trypanosomes, spirochaetes, bacteria, viruses, or proteins) when combined with antibody are found to adhere to human red cells, thereby causing them to agglutinate. This is due to the activation of complement and the formation of a C3 cleavage component (p. 161). Only primate red cells behave in this manner. In non-primates antigen-antibody-complement complexes adhere to platelets. This adherence can be used *in vitro* as a sensitive means of testing for antibodies, and may also play some part in immunity to infection (see p. 167).

Opsonins. Opsonins are substances which render organisms more readily susceptible to phagocytosis. Polymorphs are in

TABLE 12.1

	Wassermann reaction	
First reaction	*Second or detector reaction (haemolytic system)*
Patient's serum with ? antibody heated to 56°C for 30 minutes (to inactivate any complement which is present)	Red cells (sheep)
	Haemolysin (serum of rabbit immunised against sheep red cells). This is inactivated commercially to remove its complement.
Antigen (standard quantity)	
	? complement unused
Complement (carefully measured amount)	

general able to phagocytose virulent organisms only if the latter are first coated with a specific opsonin. This type of opsonin and also the non-specific type are considered in the sections of acute inflammation (see p. 78) and immunity (see p. 161). Opsonisation also aids the clearance of organisms from the blood by the reticulo-endothelial system.

Cytotoxic antibodies. Antibodies destructive to cells grown in tissue culture can be demonstrated in the serum of patients with Hashimoto's disease. Bacteriolysins and haemolysins are other examples of this type of antibody.

Antibody-dependent cell-mediated cytotoxicity.[16–18] B lymphocytes, null lymphocytes, monocytes, and polymorphs have Fc receptors on their cell surfaces by which they can attach to IgG-coated cells. In the case of monocytes and neutrophils this is an opsonic effect, and is a prelude to phagocytosis. With lymphocytes the attachment results in cell death by some ill-defined mechanism that depends on close cell-to-cell interaction. The phenomenon of antibody-dependent cell-mediated cytotoxicity is yet another example of the co-operation between humoral and cellular components in the immune response. It is one mechanism whereby cancer cells and allografts can be destroyed by an immune response.

Blocking (or incomplete) antibodies. These combine with their corresponding antigens without visible effect, and prevent the action of some other antibody added subsequently. The best-known antibody of this type is found in cases of Rhesus incompatibility (see Ch. 55); its action may be illustrated as follows:

D cells + Anti-D = agglutination (D-Anti-D combination)
D cells + Anti-D blocking antibody = no agglutination (D-blocking-anti-D combination)
D-blocking-anti-D + Anti-D = no union, no agglutination

The agglutinating action of anti-D is thus blocked by the prior union of blocking anti-D with the red cells. The presence of such an incomplete antibody on the surface of red cells can be detected by the Coombs test (p. 648). In this an anti-human globulin serum is added to the coated red cells and causes their agglutination.

Blocking antibodies are often erroneously assumed to be univalent. A bivalent antibody can combine with its antigen under conditions which are unfavourable for agglutination. Under other conditions agglutination may occur. Thus blocking anti-D antibody causes red-cell agglutination if the test is carried out in a strong albumin solution or if the red cells are first trypsinised.

Precipitin reactions may be blocked by incomplete antibodies. The prozone phenomenon (p. 145) can be due to their action.

Blocking antibodies are formed during the desensitisation therapy of patients with atopic disease (p. 179). They also play a part in the enhancement of tumour growth by immunoglobulins (p. 372), as well as in the acceptance of allogeneic grafts (p. 192).

Antibodies which neutralise the antigen. *Antienzymes and antitoxins.* Many organisms produce toxins or enzymes which are antigenic. The exotoxins, lecithinases, coagulases, haemolysins, leucocidins, hyaluronidases, etc., are examples of these; corresponding antibodies are formed in bacterial infection, and are considered in Chapter 13.

Virus neutralising antibodies probably coat the virus particles and prevent their attachment to cells (see p. 274).

Antibacterial antibodies may have effects not already described, e.g. bactericidal antibodies kill organisms, and these are closely related to the bacteriolysins. Syphilitic antibody causes immobilisation of the organism, a fact utilised in the *Treponema pallidum* immobilisation test.

It cannot be stressed too strongly that the globulin antibodies have been named according to the nature of the test used to detect them. At one time it was thought that each type was distinct, but it is now known that in many cases a single antibody can perform several functions depending upon the conditions under which it is examined. For instance, a substance may be capable of neutralising toxin, e.g. diphtheria toxin, in an *in vivo* experiment. It is therefore rightly called an antitoxin. However, *in vitro* it can produce a precipitate with its antigen, and may therefore be labelled a precipitin. Some agglutinins, e.g. to red cells, produce agglutination only in the absence of complement. When this is present there is lysis and the complement is fixed.

Nevertheless, such a unitarian theory is too simple, for it is known that a single antigen can lead to the formation of a heterogeneous group of immunoglobulins, each with the same specificity but differing in chemical composition (IgG, IgA, etc.). This is reflected in their avidity and their ability to sensitise, cross the placenta, and engage in the many *in vitro* activities by which antibodies are detected. Furthermore, antibodies with different specificities may be produced (p. 143).

Cell-bound Antibodies[19]

Cell-mediated immunity and hypersensitivity are related to antibodies residing in lymphocytes. The manner by which such sensitised or immune lymphocytes produce their effect is incompletely understood; when the cells come into contact with the appropriate antigen, they release a number of effector proteins which can be recognised by their specific actions and are called *lymphokines*. Many such actions have been described, and it is not certain how many agents are involved. One agent may produce several effects, and conversely several agents may produce the same effect. The present situation is very similar to that encountered with the immunoglobulins in the early days of immunology. The following factors may be listed; they are released when specifically sensitised lymphocytes are incubated with the specific antigen, and can be measured by *in vitro* methods as well as by their effects *in vivo*.

1. **Migration inhibition factor.** This substance has a molecular weight of 25 000 to 55 000 daltons. It acts on macrophages and prevents their migration (see Fig. 14.3, p. 185). The agent also seems to activate the macrophages, increase phagocytic activity, and make the cells better able to kill organisms. It may be postulated that this factor causes macrophages to accumulate at a site of infection and overcome it.

2. **Transfer factor.** This has a molecular weight of less than 10 000 daltons, and has the property of acting upon uncommitted lymphocytes and rendering them sensitised (see p. 184). The agent may well recruit more immune cells, which are then available to react with further antigen.

3. **Lymphotoxin.** This protein of molecular weight 80 000 to 150 000 daltons causes a cytopathic effect on cells such as fibroblasts grown in culture as monolayers. *Growth inhibiting factor* is closely related if not identical. Sensitised T cells may kill their target cells (e.g. a graft) by the liberation of a lymphotoxin. Nevertheless, such *killer T cells* may produce their effect by some other mechanism—one that involves close cell-to-cell contact.[20]

4. **Skin reactive factor.** On injection into the skin, this produces a picture similar to that of a delayed-type hypersensitivity reaction.

5. **Chemotactic factors.** At least 3 have been described. One affects monocytes while the other attracts polymorphs. Yet another may affect eosinophils.

6. **Mitogenic factor.** This causes lymphocyes to transfer into blast cells and divide. Enhanced incorporation of ^{3}H thymidine can be used to measure this.

7. **Interferon.** See page 275.

Other lymphokines have been isolated: one acts on neutrophils and causes the release of endogenous pyrogen. Another is the colony-stimulating factor in granulopoiesis (p. 80). Yet another is the macrophage arming factor (p. 190).

The subject of cell-mediated immune responses is considered in greater detail in the sections on delayed-type hypersensitivity and cell-mediated immunity.

THE ANTIBODY-FORMING TISSUES

Before describing the cellular features of the immune response it is essential to understand the structure and development of the lymphoid tissues of the body.

The Lymphoid Tissues[21-24]

The thymus.[25] The first lymphoid tissue to develop in mammals is the thymus. It contains an epithelial element in the form of reticular cells and Hassall's corpuscles. In addition there are many thymocytes which morphologically resemble lymphocytes. It is taught that germinal centres are not normally present, but this has been disputed.

The bursa of Fabricius. In birds the next lymphoid organ to develop is the *bursa of Fabricius*. This is situated near the cloaca, and, like the thymus, has an epithelial as well as a lymphoid element. It is suspected that mammals have an equivalent tissue, perhaps more widely distributed, and forming the lymphoid tissue of the appendix and colon, and the Peyer's patches of the small intestine.

Lymph nodes. Lymph comes into the lymph node through the peripheral sinus, traverses the cortex, enters the sinusoids of the medulla, and finally leaves through the efferent duct (Fig. 12.9). The sinuses are lined by plump, *littoral*, or *sinus-lining cells*, which have eosinophilic cytoplasm and are phagocytic. Reticular cells are present and appear to be concerned with the formation of reticulin, which constitutes the connective tissue framework of the node. In the outer part, or *cortex*, of the node there are densely packed lymphocytes which are focally aggregated into *follicles*. In the centre of each follicle there is often a well-defined *germinal*

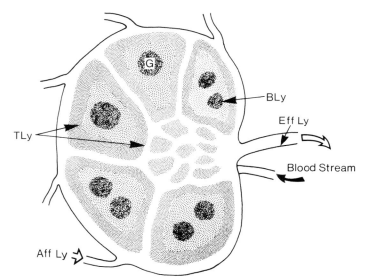

Figure 12.9
Diagram of a lymph node. Lymph enters the node through several afferent lymphatic vessels (Aff Ly), and percolates through a meshwork formed by reticular cells and their reticulin fibres. In the medulla the fluid is collected into sinuses that are lined by phagocytic sinus-lining cells, which are members of the reticulo-endothelial system. The cortex contains collections of B lymphocytes (B Ly), some of which have one or more germinal centres (G). Surrounding these areas there is a mantle of T lymphocytes (T Ly); this is designated the *paracortical zone*. In the medulla there are groups, or cords, of B cells—both lymphocytes and cells that have differentiated into plasma cells—The B cells tend to remain in the node, and are therefore described as sessile. T cells, on the other hand, leave the node *via* the solitary efferent lymphatic vessel (Eff Ly), enter the blood stream *via* the thoracic duct, and finally return to a lymph node. They leave the blood stream by passing through the walls of the postcapillary venules in the paracortical zone. Lymph containing lymphocytes from tissues or other lymph nodes also enters the lymph node through the afferent lymphatics (Aff Ly). (*Drawn by Margot Mackay, Department of Art as Applied to Medicine, University of Toronto.*)

Figure 12.10
Part of a reactive lymph node. At the edge of the section there is a lymphoid follicle with a central germinal centre. Interior to it there is an extensive paracortical zone of lymphocytes. Inward from this there is the looser medullary area with cords of lymphocytes. × 30.

Figure 12.11
A lymphoid follicle. This is a magnified view of the lymphoid follicle shown in Figure 12.10.

centre of Flemming[24] (Figs. 12.10 and 12.11). This contains large cells which are generally called lymphoblasts. They show a high turn-over rate and therefore mitoses are abundant.

In addition, the centres have large macrophages which usually contain nuclear debris in their clear, abundant cytoplasm. On microscopy the macrophages produce clear spaces which have been likened to the stars in a starry sky. The purpose of this macrophage activity is probably related to the recycling of DNA. The germinal centres are sites of rapid production of cells which have a short life. Components of DNA such as thymidine are used again, and it follows that measurements of cell proliferation using tritiated thymidine as a marker show a deceptively low uptake because of the existing pool of unlabelled thymidine.

The *medulla* of the node shows prominent sinuses and medullary cords of cells between them. These cells are mainly small lymphocytes together with a variable number of plasma cells and granulocytes.

Between the cortex with its germinal centres and the medulla there is a third zone which is packed with lymphocytes but less densely so than the cortex. There are no follicles in this *paracortical zone*.

T lymphocytes (see below) from the blood normally enter the lymph node by moving through gaps between the endothelial cells of the post-capillary sinusoids in the paracortical zone; they subsequently leave the node in the efferent lymph. The lymphocytes therefore re-enter the blood stream through the thoracic duct. It follows that if this duct is exteriorised and drained, the body is steadily depleted of T lymphocytes.

The lymphocytes.[26-31] The lymphocytes in the blood range from the large to the small variety. The latter have a dense spherical nucleus and little cytoplasm. Lymphocytes are motile cells, and in culture can sometimes be seen to send processes into other cells and even enter their cytoplasm, a process called *emperiopolesis*. Although lymphocytes appear to form a relatively homogeneous group on morphological grounds, it is now appreciated that the population is heterogeneous. Two distinct types have been identified:

T lymphocytes. These cells are thymus dependent and are long lived—in the human being they live for many months and certainly over 1 year. The cells continuously recirculate through the paracortical zone of the lymph nodes as described above. T lymphocytes cannot be identified morphologically in the human being, although scanning electron microscopy has shown that they have fewer microvilli on their surface than do B cells.[32] They also behave differently when placed in an electrical field on electrophoresis.[33] A number of specific antigens have been identified on the T cell membrane, e.g. an antigen shared with brain tissue; in mice the θ antigen is characteristic. The cells also carry a number of specific receptors by which they may be identified. The most characteristic is a receptor for sheep red cells. The erythrocytes adhere to T cells and form rosettes (termed E rosettes) when the two types of cell are mixed at 0°C. This is a useful way of identifying T cells: thus it has been found that 70 to 80 per cent of the blood lymphocytes form E rosettes, and are therefore T cells.

Committed T cells have specific surface receptors for antigen. The nature of this receptor is uncertain, but it is probable that it consists of part of an IgM molecule. Nevertheless, specific anti-IgM does not block the attachment of antigen to sensitised cells, and much of the IgM molecule must be buried in the plasma membrane. For this reason also fluorescent techniques have generally failed to detect the presence of immunoglobulin on the surface of T lymphocytes. It is believed that when antigen binds to several adjacent receptors, the cell is stimulated to activity (see blast transformation and lymphokine formation).

B lymphocytes. B lymphocytes are so named because they are dependent on the bursa, or bursal-equivalent tissue. This type of cell can be found in the blood, but their numbers are small as they tend to remain sessile in the lymphoid tissues. They occupy the primary germinal follicles and are short-lived cells, their life-span being measured in days.

On scanning electron microscopy B cells are found to have numerous microvilli on their surface, but this may be an artefact produced by the method of preparation and of no fundamental importance. B cells have many surface markers that aid in their identification. They have readily demonstrable (by immunofluorescence) immunoglobulin on their surface membranes. The cells develop in three stages; the first of these is independent of antigen and involves the appearance of surface IgM and later IgD. The IgM is monomeric (8S), and both the IgM and IgD share the same variable regions and presumably have the same specificity.

Other markers on B cells are receptors for EB virus, C3 (the third component of complement), and the Fc portion of IgG.* These Fc receptors can be detected by the formation of rosettes by red cells coated with IgG antibody (EA rosettes). If complement is also present, the C3 receptors also take part (EAC rosettes). These must be distinguished from the E rosettes formed by washed sheep red cells around T lymphocytes.

The Fc receptors take part in many reactions. Thus B lymphocytes, even uncommitted ones, adhere to antibody-coated cells, e.g. tumour cells, and perhaps kill them. Immune complexes also adhere to the B cell's Fc receptors, and this adherence may stimulate the cells to further development into immunoblasts (plasmablasts) and finally into plasma cells. These are the second and third phases in the development of B cells.

Null lymphocytes. Some lymphocytes lack both B and T markers and are termed null cells. Some, however, have Fc

receptors and can take part in antibody-dependent cell-mediated cytotoxicity (p. 147). These are called *K*, or *killer*, *cells*.

Yet another group of lymphocytes lack both T and B-cell markers and Fc receptors. They appear to be capable of killing cells without the co-operation of immunoglobulins, and since their action is non-specific, have been called *NK cells*.

Some workers are not convinced of the lymphocytic origin of these two groups of cells and believe them to be of monocyte-macrophage lineage.

Spleen. In the spleen the blood passes through the central (malpighian) arterioles to enter the sinusoids which are, as in the lymph nodes, lined by phagocytic cells. In the red pulp there are reticular cells, lymphocytes, and plasma cells as well as occasional granulocytes and megakaryocytes. The lymphoid cuffs are situated around the malpighian arterioles, and the T lymphocytes are derived from the blood as part of the recirculation of cells as in the paracortical zones of the lymph nodes. Germinal centres may be prominent.

Development of the peripheral lymphoid tissues. The thymus, and in birds the bursa, are well developed and large before the peripheral lymphoid tissue matures. The thymus is

Figure 12.12
Diagram showing the postulated development of the peripheral lymphoid tissue of the lymph nodes.

the central organ responsible for the formation of the paracortical zone of the lymph nodes and for the sheath of lymphocytes around the central arterioles in the spleen. These are the *thymus-dependent areas*. The bursa is necessary for the formation of the germinal centres in the spleen and in the cortex of the nodes, and also for cells which develop into plasma cells in the splenic red pulp and the medullary cords of the nodes. It is believed that the earliest immunological cell is to be found in the bone marrow (*reticular anlage*). This *stem cell* may differentiate to a blood-cell precursor (see p. 600) or develop into a lymphoid cell (Fig. 12.12).

It is not known whether the marrow cells migrate to the peripheral tissues and there develop under the influence of a thymic or bursal hormone, or whether the cells migrate first to the thymus or bursa, develop for a while, and then are released to populate the peripheral lymphoid tissue. There is good evidence that in the mouse, marrow cells migrate to the thymus and develop into lymphoid tissue. It seems likely that in this species there is a continuous replacement of stem cells in the thymus from the marrow.

The Thymus in Relation to the Immune Response

If antigen is given intravenously, the thymus does not take part in the immune response unless it is first inflamed: thus

---

*It should be noted that macrophages also have C3 and Fc receptors. An attachment of these cells to antibody or complement-coated particles aids phagocytosis (see opsonins, p. 78). Another possible function for the Fc receptors of macrophages (and also B lymphocytes) is to trap circulating immune complexes, so that antigen is retained in many parts of the body and there plays a part in immunological memory.

there appears to be a blood-thymus barrier which under normal conditions keeps the organ isolated. The thymus undergoes atrophy in the adult animal, and its removal is not associated with any immediate, significant depression of the immune response. However, reduced immunological responsiveness is seen after about 1 year and also following total body irradiation. Recovery from irradiation is impaired as compared with normal animals.

Thymectomy performed shortly after birth can produce dramatic effects in some species. Mice, for example, appear normal for 3 to 4 weeks, and then a wasting syndrome usually develops which closely resembles runt disease (p. 194). This is probably a result of microbial infection, since it does not occur in germ-free animals.* Significantly there is a deficiency of small lymphocytes in the splenic white pulp, the paracortical zones of lymph nodes, and in the circulating blood. The animals exhibit an impaired ability to develop delayed-type hypersensitivity, and are tolerant of allografts and sometimes even of xenografts. The production of immunoglobulins to some antigens is normal, but to others, e.g. sheep red cells, it is impaired.

The implantation of syngeneic thymus tissue will restore the immunological competence of the thymectomised animal, and the graft becomes repopulated by lymphoid cells derived from the *bone marrow of the host*. Even if the thymic implant is enclosed in a Millipore chamber which will not allow the egress of cells, it is reported that it will restore to some extent the immunological competence of the recipient. Presumably the graft cells secrete some substance which allows the animal's lymphoid tissue to develop; the nature of this factor is controversial. A substance called *thymin* (and later *thymopoietin*[34]) has been isolated by some workers, but as yet the hormonal nature of this is not widely accepted. Its action is weak in relation to its concentration, a property not at all like that of the high potency of a hormone.

Alternative to this humoral theory there is the possibility that the thymus produces lymphocytes which migrate to populate the lymphoid tissues. Experiments using ³H-labelled thymidine indicate that there is very active cell proliferation in the thymus, but that many of the cells die and relatively few leave the organ. A massive overproduction of cells which have a very short life-span is also a feature of lymphoid tissue in the bone marrow and germinal centres.[23] It may be postulated that this apparently wasteful lymphopoiesis serves a purpose in that it provides a constant supply of undifferentiated, uncommitted cells—either marrow stem cells, T cells, or B cells. It is possible that somatic mutation could provide many cell types, as proposed by the selective theory of antibody production (see p. 154). It is also conceivable that abnormal cells could arise and lead to an autoimmune process. Indeed, the thymus has been regarded as an organ commonly involved in the pathogenesis of autoimmune disease.

The Bursa of Fabricius in Relation to the Immune Response

Removal of the bursa, especially if combined with non-lethal total body irradiation, results in an immunologically

*A germ-free animal is one that has been specially reared under sterile conditions. Caesarian section is generally employed in the initiation of such a colony.

deficient state characterised by a failure to produce immunoglobulins when suitably challenged by an antigen. It is possible that in mammals the intestinal lymphoid tissue corresponds to the bursa, since its removal in rabbits produces a similar failure in immunoglobulin production. This may be regarded as the *gut-associated central lymphoid tissue*. It is presumed to be responsible for the development of that part of the peripheral lymphoid tissue which is responsible for the production of immunoglobulins, namely germinal centres, B lymphocytes, and plasma cells. The lymphoid aggregates should not be confused with the more diffuse lymphoid tissue and plasma cells which are responsible for the production of IgA.

Lymphocyte Transformation

One of the most remarkable observations of recent times is that the small lymphocytes of the blood and the lymph can be stimulated *in vitro* to become large cells with basophilic, pyroninophilic cytoplasm containing many free ribosomes and nuclei with nucleoli. These cells have been called *immunoblasts*, pyroninophilic cells, and blast cells. They exhibit DNA synthesis and mitotic activity, a feature which has led to them being intensively used in studies of human chromosomes.

Agents which lead to lymphocyte transformation and mitosis are termed *mitogens*, and include:

Lectins. These are proteins or glycoproteins derived from plant tissue, and have affinity for certain cell-surface carbohydrates. They include:

Phytohaemagglutinin, derived from red kidney beans; this substance was used originally to produce agglutination of red cells in experiments designed to facilitate the isolation of white cells from the blood.

Concanavalin A, derived from jack beans.

Pokeweed mitogen.

Some lectins, e.g. from wheat germ or mushrooms, inhibit lymphocyte transformation.

Streptolysin S

Antilymphocytic serum

Antigen-antibody complexes

Other allogeneic lymphocytes. If small lymphocytes from another individual are mixed with test lymphocytes, both groups of cells undergo blast transformation.

Antigen, if added to the lymphocytes from a sensitised individual. This occurs regardless of whether the sensitisation is of the immediate or delayed type.

If a sample of lymphocytes is exposed to a mitogen, the number of cells that undergo transformation varies; so also does the speed at which they respond. This is because some mitogens (phytohaemagglutinin and concanavalin A) stimulate T cells only, others (bacterial endotoxin) B cells only, while others (antilymphocytic serum and pokeweed mitogen) affect both types of cells. T cell transformation occurs faster than does B cell transformation; hence the number of cells that transform, and the speed at which they do so, is related to the number of B or T cells that are involved.

The precise role of the blast transformation phenomenon in the intact animal is not known, but various suggestions have been made:

Proliferating B cells can form the germinal centres of lymphoid tissue. Each centre may indeed be a clone derived from one cell. In other situations, e.g. the medulla of lymph nodes, the cells may differentiate into plasma cells. Others may revert to small lymphocytes and remain as memory cells.

Proliferating T cells can revert to small lymphocytes and act as effector cells in a cell-mediated immune response; others remain as memory cells.

Functional Steps in the Immune Response

The following steps may be postulated as occurring after the introduction of an antigen:

The recognition system. A mechanism must exist for recognising an antigen as foreign. Furthermore, the system must have a *memory* so that the same antigen can be recognised again.

The processing system. Once having been recognised as an antigen, its determinants must be processed in such a way that specific antibody can be produced.

The production system. The final outcome of the immune response is the manufacture of antibody. This often involves synthesis of a range of specific proteins as well as the formation of immune cells. The production system must be *regulated* in some way, so that the immune response can be turned off when the antigenic stimulus is withdrawn.

Anatomical Site of Antibody Production

Antibodies are not produced in any one organ or site. With intravenously administered antigens they are produced in the spleen, liver, and lymph nodes, whereas locally introduced antigen stimulates antibody production at the local site and in the regional lymph nodes.

Since all antibodies are either cellular or else proteins produced by cells, a complete understanding of the immune response entails an understanding of the cellular events involved. It is generally agreed that the lymphoreticular tissues are of prime importance and that two morphological cell types are concerned. There are the large mononuclear, potentially phagocytic cells grouped together as the RE system, and the lymphocytes. Detailed knowledge about the origin, morphology, and function of these cells is unfortunately lacking, and much confusion has been caused in the past by making wholly unwarranted assumptions. Cells which look alike, e.g. small lymphocytes, do not necessarily have the same origin or function.

The Recognition System

A cell which is capable of recognising antigen and of initiating an immune response, although not necessarily producing antibody itself, is termed an *immunologically competent cell*. There is considerable evidence that such a cell is morphologically a small lymphocyte, and that both B and T cell variants exist. The evidence may be summarised as follows: 1. Procedures which deplete the population of small lymphocytes also inhibit the development of a primary response to antigenic stimulation. The following may be mentioned: total body irradiation, administration of drugs (p. 142), thoracic-duct drainage (p. 142), bursectomy, and thymectomy in the neonate (p.151). 2. Animals rendered tolerant to an antigen (p. 155) can have their immunological responsiveness restored by the injection of lymphocytes from a non-tolerant adult syngeneic animal.

Precisely how the appropriate cells recognise the antigen is not known. One possibility is that the cells have specific immunoglobulin on their surface, and that the stimulus is an antigen-antibody complex. There is evidence that both the T and B lymphocytes have immunoglobulin on their surfaces, but this in itself does not prove that the mechanism outlined above is operative.

Prior to contact with antigen, the B and T cells are regarded as uncommitted. Contact with antigen stimulates the cells to divide, and the cellular products of this proliferation may either participate directly in an immune response by producing immunoglobulins or effector T cells, or they may persist as *memory cells*. These cells are therefore regarded as committed, because they have specific receptors for the antigen concerned.

The process of recognising antigen is sometimes known as the *afferent limb* of the immune response. Actual production of immunoglobulins, or effector cells in cell-mediated immune responses, constitutes the *efferent limb*.

Cells Involved in Immunoglobulin Synthesis

There is abundant evidence that immunoglobulins are synthesised in B cells. When stimulated by antigenic contact, they develop rough endoplasmic reticulum, pass through a stage that has been termed an immunoblast or plasmablast, and finally evolve into a plasma cell. Fluorescein or ferritin-labelled anti-immunoglobulin readily demonstrates abundant antibody in the cytoplasm of these cells.

The plaque technique. A technique developed by Jerne has shed some light on the morphology of antibody-producing cells. Lymphoid cells from an animal immunised with foreign red cells are mixed with the same type of red cells in heated agar; a thin layer of this is poured into a Petri dish, allowed to set, and incubated for one hour or more, during which period the cells produce antibody. A more sensitive modification of this technique has been described in which lymphoid cells, red cells, and complement are incubated in a shallow chamber under a coverslip. A clear halo, or plaque of haemolysis, is seen to surround single cells. The technique has been modified to detect antibody formation against bacteria and other antigens. The antibody forming cells (*plaque-forming cells*) have been examined by light and electron microscopy. Some resemble lymphocytes, others blast cells, immature plasma cells, or typical mature plasma cells. Thus the plasma cell is regarded as the end-stage in the development of a B lymphocyte whose function is directed to immunoglobulin production. It has a short life-span—probably 2 to 3 days—and is found in conditions in which antibody production is occurring and in sites which are actively engaged in making antibodies, such as splenic pulp, medullary cords of lymph nodes, and chronic inflammatory granulation tissue. Indeed, the plasma cell is the characteristic cell of chronic inflammation.

The plaque technique has been used to study the type of antibody produced by single cells.[35] When an animal is stimulated by two dissimilar antigens, an individual cell from that animal produces antibody against either one antigen or the other, but probably never against both. Furthermore, only one class of antibody is produced at any one time, although there is some evidence that a cell can switch from one class, e.g. IgM, to another, e.g. IgG.

Morphological Aspects of Immunoglobulin Production

When an antigen such as pneumococcal polysaccharide, which is known to stimulate immunoglobulin production and not delayed-type hypersensitivity, is injected into the skin, some is carried to the regional lymph nodes and is taken up by the sinus-lining cells. There is a dramatic fall in the number of lymphocytes leaving the node, but shortly afterwards the cell count in the efferent lymph rises and reaches a maximum at about 2 days. Many of the cells are large pyroninophilic cells. The lymph also contains specific antibodies. The medullary cords contain pyroninophilic cells, and these appear to mature to adult plasma cells which contain specific immunoglobulin antibody. The germinal centres enlarge and new ones form, but this is a late event in the primary response.

The secondary response has certain distinctive features. Germinal centre formation is a marked feature and occurs early. Antigen can be demonstrated in them, and later on so also can antibody. Antibody formation also occurs in distant sites, e.g. the spleen, and it is possible that the cells responsible for this are derived from the large pyroninophilic cells that migrated from the node during the primary response. A sensitised animal drained of small lymphocytes by thoracic-duct drainage will still give a secondary response to injected antigen. The cells which form antibody in the secondary response are therefore derived from *sessile cells*: these are the B lymphocytes and cells derived from them.

It is evident that immunoglobulin production is related to the formation of germinal centres, and the greatest amount of antibody is formed in the cells of the medulla which finally appear as plasma cells. These are the bursal, or bursal-equivalent, dependent areas. It is not clear whether cells from the germinal centres migrate into the medulla and differentiate into antibody-producing cells.

Number of Cell Types Involved in the Immune Response[36]

There is considerable evidence that both immunoglobulin production and cell-mediated immune responses involve the co-operative action of more than one cell type.

Immunoglobulin production to many antigens is greatly enhanced by the activity of T cells.[37, 38] These *helper T cells* appear to release soluble substances (which may be included amongst the lymphokines) that, combined with the stimulus provided by the antigen, provide a signal for the B cells to produce specific antibody. Various soluble factors can provide this second signal; they may be either non-specific or else specific for the particular antigen. Antigens that do not require T-cell co-operation in order to provoke the formation of antibodies appear to act as B cell mitogens (p. 151). The interrelationship between B and T cells is very complex, for T cells can also act as *suppressors* to some antibody responses.[39] Thus in some T cell-deficient animals there is an exaggerated immunoglobulin response to some antigens. The human counterpart of this situation is lepromatous leprosy, in which abeyance of T cell function is combined with an excessive immunoglobulin response. Indeed, the polyclonal hypergammaglobulinaemia that results is responsible for one of the serious complications of leprosy: the combination of specific immunoglobulin with lepra-bacillus antigen produces complexes that cause a vasculitis. Erythema nodosum leprosum is the result, and its pathogenesis parallels that of the Arthus reaction (p. 179).

There is considerable evidence that *macrophages* are required for T cell activation—not only the activation of sensitised cells by antigen *in vivo*, but also the non-specific stimulus provided by a mitogen *in vitro* (p. 80). It is probable that B cell activation also requires macrophage co-operation, particularly those B cell functions that require the aid of helper T cells. Research in this area is hindered by the fact that it is difficult to separate B cells from macrophages. Hence experiments in which B cells appear to have been directly stimulated by antigen are sometimes invalidated by the presence of small numbers of macrophages.

Macrophages readily take up antigen, the bulk of which is catabolised. Some antigen, however, is retained and presented to the lymphocytes in such a form that it stimulates antibody production. This antigen probably remains on the cell membrane of the macrophage before presentation to the lymphocytes. Nevertheless, there is some evidence that antigen may enter the cell by endocytosis and be processed in some way. The transfer of antigen, or processed antigen, appears to be related to direct cell-to-cell contact, and lymphocytes can be observed to form clusters around macrophages. Nevertheless, macrophages appear also to release a soluble *lymphocyte-activating factor* that can, under some circumstances, replace direct cell-to-cell contact. The situation is further complicated by the fact that macrophages can also act as suppressor cells; hence both macrophages and T lymphocytes are involved in the complex regulation of the immune response.

Cell-bound Antibody Production

This has been studied in experimentally induced allergic contact dermatitis. Oxazolone (p. 184) applied to the skin readily causes allergic contact dermatitis due to the formation of sensitising cell-bound antibodies. The changes in the lymph nodes are instructive.[40] In the paracortical, or thymus-dependent, areas, large pyroninophilic cells appear. DNA-synthesis can be demonstrated in them by the usual technique of ^{3}H-thymidine labelling, and they probably arise from small lymphocytes. The number of these pyroninophilic cells reaches a maximum by about the fourth day. Subsequently they disappear, and are replaced by small lymphocyes which are derived from them. At the same time hypersensitivity develops. Excision of the area of skin within 16 hours of application of the sensitising agent, or excision of the regional lymph nodes before 3 days, prevents sensitisation of the animal. An intact lymphatic drainage is therefore necessary for the development of cell-bound sensitising antibodies under these circumstances. With skin allografts the same conditions apply, but a lymphatic connexion is not necessary for sensitisation to occur when grafts are connected by vascular anastomosis, e.g. kidney and heart.

THEORIES OF IMMUNOGLOBULIN ANTIBODY PRODUCTION

Immunoglobulins are proteins, and it is reasonable to believe that their formation in the rough endoplasmic reticulum of plasma cells is largely determined by genetic information residing in the nucleus. The problem which has taxed immunologists is the mechanism whereby the body can be induced to produce new specific protein following external stimulation by an antigen. Two main theories have emerged.

The Instructive Theory

This classical but improbable theory postulated that an antigen acts as a mould, or template, and that its presence leads to a slight alteration in the chemical composition of immunoglobulin, thereby rendering it highly specific and able to react with that particular antigen. Even a slight difference in the spatial arrangement of the molecule of an antigen leads to the production of a different specific antibody. The template theory assumes that the antigen is present throughout the period of potential immunity, which in many cases lasts for years and possibly the whole life of the animal. Some antigens, e.g. pneumococcal polysaccharides, are known to persist for long periods in an unchanged state, but with others the situation is less clear.

An estimation of the rate of elimination from the blood of injected ^{131}I-labelled antigen (bovine γ-globulin) shows that it is metabolised fastest in the immune animal with circulating antibodies present prior to the injection. In the non-immune, antigen can be detected for 7 days and irradiation prolongs the period considerably (see Fig. 12.13 and legend).

It is evident that the development of the immune response leads to the disappearance of circulating antigen. Antigen-antibody complexes in the blood are rapidly taken up and catabolised by the reticulo-endothelial system. Nevertheless, there is evidence that small quantities of antigen, or antigen fragments containing the determinant groups, are retained in cells for a long period in the immune animal. It is possible to envisage that, by becoming attached to RNA, they might modify protein synthesis, i.e. lead to antibody production.

An alternative explanation, one not requiring the continued presence of the antigen, is that there occurs a permanent modification of some self-duplicating mechanism in the cell. The nature of this change has, however, never been described in exact terms.

The Selective Theory

An alternative hypothesis is that formulated by Jerne and elaborated by Burnet. It differs from the classical approach in postulating that antigen does not itself determine the pattern or the specificity of the antibody, but is only responsible for the amount produced. The chief supposition of this approach is that during the early stages of embryonic development there occur many somatic mutations in the immunologically competent cells (p. 152). This results in the formation of a whole range of cells which between them is capable of mounting an immune response specific for any antigen which the body may subsequently meet. It is postulated that the effect of contact with antigen in the adult is to stimulate the growth of the cells which are capable of making the appropriate immune response. In this way a body of cells, or clone, develops, and as its size increases so does antibody production appear. A feature of the immune response which is not readily explicable by the selective theory is the interference of the response to one antigen when another unrelated antigen is administered. This suggests that both antigens act on the same cell type, and therefore compete (p. 141).

It is obvious that if somatic mutation occurs so frequently that cells are produced which can form antibodies against all possible antigens, then inevitably some mutations will produce cells capable of forming antibodies against the host's own tissues. It must therefore be postulated that there exists some mechanism during embryonic life for the destruction of these harmful, or *forbidden*, *clones*: contact with antigen has to destroy the clone rather than stimulate it. This is one explanation of the phenomenon of immunological tolerance.

Figure 12.13

Showing the blood levels of antigen (^{131}I-labelled bovine γ-globulin) and antibody in the rabbit following one intravenous injection of antigen. The initial rapid fall in antigen level is due to equilibration between the blood and the tissues. In the group of animals already possessing antibodies due to previous immunisation, the antigen is rapidly eliminated, and antibody appears by the 2nd day. In immunised animals with no circulating antibodies (potential immunity) antigen is eliminated by the 4th day, and antibody production is correspondingly delayed. The control animals show the development of an immune response on the 4th day as evidenced by the rapid elimination of antigen during the next 2 to 3 days. By the 7th day antibodies appear in the circulation. 200 r delays the immune response till the 7th day, and after 500 r the response is completely suppressed. The slow, steady elimination of antigen in the heavily irradiated group is due to its gradual metabolism, and corresponds to the fall seen in the other groups prior to the development of an immune response. Other experiments show that it also corresponds to the elimination of injected ^{131}I-labelled homologous γ-globulin (this is not antigenic). These results show that the first indication of immune response is the disappearance of antigen from the circulation, and that this precedes the liberation of γ-globulin antibodies. (*From Talmage, D. W., Dixon, F. J., Bukantz, S. C., and Dammin, G. J.* (1951), Journal of Immunology, **67**, 243.)

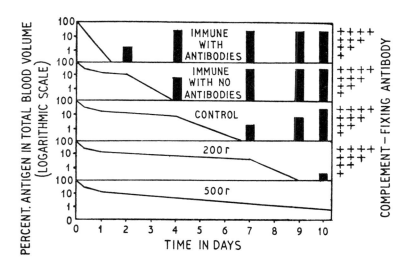

Specific Immunological Tolerance

The administration of an antigen to an embryo results not in the formation of antibodies but in the acceptance of the foreign substance as 'self'. The phenomenon was first noticed when embryos were grafted with allogeneic cells, i.e. from an animal of the same species but of a different genetic constitution. So long as the grafted cells survived in the host the animals were tolerant of further grafts from the same donor, but not from those of any other donor. The tolerance was therefore specific and not due to a generalised depression of the immune response. This subject is considered further in Chapter 15.

Specific immunological tolerance to non-living antigens can also be induced, but it persists only for so long as the antigen remains. Repeated injections are therefore usually required.

The theory of Burnet explains how early contact with antigen could destroy the appropriate clone, but in order to explain why tolerance is lost when the antigen is dissipated, it must be assumed that the capacity to relearn 'self' from 'non-self' is also present during adult life. It could be that new immunologically competent cells are being formed throughout life, and that at an early stage in their development they learn to recognise as 'self' those antigens which are present at that time. Thus, during embryonic life when antibody-forming cells are few and many immunologically competent cells are being formed, tolerance is easy to establish with relatively small doses of antigen. In the adult, on the other hand, there are many antibody-forming cells and few developing immunologically competent cells; therefore tolerance is difficult to establish.

Induction of tolerance. There are various ways in which tolerance may be induced.
(1) Administration of antigen to a fetus or immature animal.
(2) Administration of massive doses of antigen to a mature animal.
(3) Administration of very small, often repeated, doses of antigen to young animals.
(4) Administration of antigen following extensive damage to the lymphoreticular system by ionising radiations or cytotoxic drugs. Antibody formation is temporarily in abeyance, and regeneration of the immunologically competent cells occurs in the presence of antigen.
(5) Administration of antigen to an immunologically defective animal such as one subjected to a neonatal thymectomy.
(6) Administration of certain antigens, e.g. picryl chloride, by mouth.

Tolerance to an antigen can be broken by administering a related antigen or the original one combined with Freund's adjuvent. Guinea-pigs can be rendered so tolerant to bovine serum albumin that they cannot make immunoglobulin or exhibit delayed hypersensitivity. If bovine serum albumin is given with Freund's adjuvant, the animals are then capable of responding to a further injection of antigen by immunoglobulin production, and yet many remain tolerant in respect of delayed hypersensitivity. This dissociation of tolerance has been called *immune deviation*, and again indicates that the two aspects of the immune response, cellular and humoral, are independent of each other.

Maintenance of tolerance. To maintain the state of tolerance the antigen must usually persist in the body, and this can be ensured either by injecting living cells as antigen or by the repeated injection of non-living antigens.

Explanation of tolerance. Two major theories have been put forward.

Production of tolerant cells. Under some circumstances antigen can act on immunologically competent cells to render them unresponsive. It has been suggested that if antigen acts directly on the cells they are rendered tolerant. If antigen is taken up by macrophages first, the immunologically competent cells are stimulated to initiate an immune response. This concept explains how *very large doses* of antigen can produce paralysis, for antigen can act directly on the cells. Likewise *very small doses* of antigen may fail to initiate antibody production and yet can act on the immunologically competent cells to render them tolerant. Another possibility is that antigen-antibody complexes stimulate the immunologically competent cells to divide and lead to further antibody production. Tolerance is easier to produce if specific antibodies are absent and if the animal's capability of producing them is impaired, e.g. in fetal life and following X-irradiation and administration of cytotoxic drugs.

Elimination of potentially reactive cells. It is possible that there is no such thing as a tolerant cell, but rather that the appropriate cell has been eliminated as suggested by Burnet's theory.

The theory implies that one cell can produce one type of antibody only. The plaque technique has produced evidence that most B cells produce antibody with one specificity and of one class. However, the possibility that a few cells can produce antibodies of different specificities has not been completely excluded. Nevertheless, these observations tend to support the theory that tolerance is due to an absence of cells capable of initiating or completing an immune response to a specific antigen.

The postulation that tolerance is due to the elimination of the appropriate reactive cells has run into some difficulties. Thus thyroglobulin normally circulates in the bloodstream, and the body is presumably tolerant to it. Yet injections of thyroglobulin *combined with adjuvant* lead to the production of antibodies. An explanation suggested independently by Weigle and Allison is that the formation of antibodies under these circumstances requires the co-operation of T and B lymphocytes. When antigen is present in the circulation in low concentration, T cells are presumed not to respond and no antibody is formed, even though B cells with specific receptors are present. The addition of adjuvant could by-pass the T cells. In support of this hypothesis is the finding of B cells with specific binding sites for labelled human thyroglobulin. The phenomenon of immune deviation (see above) provides further evidence that T cells can be rendered inactive while B cells are still capable of responding.

Tolerance can be produced in various ways, and it is probable that the mechanisms involved differ from one circumstance to another. The elimination of potentially reactive cells, as suggested by Burnet, is one possibility. More likely the cells are still present but are tolerant because they are incapable of reacting. This could be because they have lost their specific receptors (e.g. by capping and subsequent endocytosis, p. 16); they could be blocked by specific antibody or inhibited by the action of suppressor T cells or macrophages. The antigen may not be processed (perhaps by macrophages) correctly and thereby fail to provide the correct stimulus. Which of these explanations is the correct one under a particular circumstance remains to be discovered by further research.

It must be concluded that we are very ignorant about the manner in which antigens bring about a lifelong change in immunoglobulin synthesis. Probably the processing of antigen by macrophages or some other helper cell is important in producing a primary response, but the stimulation for a secondary response is a direct action of the antigen on sensitised cells, possibly with the formation of an antigen-antibody complex. Tolerance is a state in which a particular antibody mechanism is in abeyance, but whether this is due to chemical repression or to physical elimination of the appropriate mechanism is undecided.

The concept that the immune response plays a major role in destroying malignant cells has attained great popularity and stimulated much research. The immunological surveillance function of lymphocytes is described on page 372. Tumours, mostly lymphomata, are more common in immunologically deficient individuals than in the normal, but the concept that the major cause of cancer is a breakdown of the immune response cannot be accepted.[41] As at present conceived, the immune response has evolved as a mechanism for the removal of unwanted material from the body. The material may be derived from degenerate tissue that forms as a result of development or disease: this includes some tumour cells or their products. It includes also extraneous material, whether inanimate antigens or microbial agents.

Although it is convenient, and currently popular, to subdivide the immune response in the human being into two distinct parts, there are indications that the division is by no means complete. Subpopulations of B and T cells have been recognised, and together with macrophages they frequently interact with each other and with immunoglobulins. Furthermore, no definite bursal-equivalent tissue has been recognised in human beings. It is evident that the cellular and the humoral aspects of the immune response are no more separated than they were in the days of Metchnikoff.

GENERAL READING

GELL, P. G. H., COOMBS, R. R. A. & LACHMANN, P. J. (Eds.) (1975) *Clinical Aspects of Immunology*, 3rd edn, 1754 pp. Oxford: Blackwell.
THALER, M. S., KLAUSNER, R. D. & COHEN, H. J. (1977) *Medical Immunology*. Philadelphia: Lippincott.
TURK, J. L. (1978) *Immunology in Clinical Medicine*, 3rd edn. London: Heinemann.

REFERENCES

1. BELLANTI, J. A. & GREEN, R. E. (1971) Immunological reactivity: expression of efficiency in elimination of foreignness. *Lancet*, **2**, 526.
2. BULLOCK, W. W. & MÖLLER, E. (1974) The continuing carrier problem. *Transplantation Reviews*, **18**, 3.
3. Annotation (1966) Intrauterine infections. *Lancet*, **2**, 1403.
4. EILBER, F. R. & MORTON, D. L. (1970) Impaired immunologic reactivity and recurrence following cancer surgery. *Cancer (Philadelphia)*, **25**, 362.
5. SIEGAL, F. P. (1976) Inhibition of T-cell rosette formation by Hodgkin-disease serum. *New England Journal of Medicine*, **295**, 1314.
6. Leading Article (1975) Current status of antilymphocyte globulin. *British Medical Journal*, **1**, 644.
7. Leading Article (1976) A.L.G. and transplantation. *Lancet*, **1**, 521.
8. TALIAFERRO, W. H., TALIAFERRO, L. G. & JAROSLOW, B. N. (1964) *Radiation and Immune Mechanisms*. New York: Academic Press.
9. DIXON, F. J. & McCONAHEY, P. J. (1963) Enhancement of antibody formation by whole body x-radiation. *Journal of Experimental Medicine*, **117**, 833.
10. COHEN, S. & MILSTEIN, C. (1967) Structure and biological properties of immunoglobulin. *Advances in Immunology*, 7, 1.
11. TOMASI, T. B. (1972) Secretory immunoglobulins. *New England Journal of Medicine*, **287**, 500.
12. BUCKLEY, R. H. & DEES, S. C. (1969) Correlation of milk precipitins with IgA deficiency. *New England Journal of Medicine*, **281**, 465.
13. TOMASI, T. B. (1970) Structure and function of mucosal antibodies. *Annual Review of Medicine*, **21**, 281.
14. GOOD, R. A. & CHOI, Y. S. (1971) Relation of IgA and IgE to bodily defenses. *New England Journal of Medicine*, **284**, 552.
15. FRANKLIN, E. C. (1976) Some impacts of clinical investigation on immunology. *New England Journal of Medicine*, **294**, 531.
16. TRINCHIERI, G. & de MARCHI, M. (1975) Antibody-dependent cell-mediated cytotoxicity in humans. *Jounal of Immunology*, **115**, 256.
17. SCORNIK, J. C. (1974) Antibody-dependent cell-mediated cytotoxicity. *Journal of Immunology*, **113**, 1519.
18. GALE, R. P. & ZIGHELBOIM, J. (1975) Polymorphonuclear leukocytes in antibody-dependent cellular cytotoxicity. *Journal of Immunology*, **114**, 1047.
19. DAVID, J. R. (1973) Lymphocytic mediators and cellular hypersensitivity. *New England Journal of Medicine*, **288**, 143.
20. HENNEY, C. S. (1974) Killer T cells. *New England Journal of Medicine*, **291**, 1357.
21. ELVES, W. M. (1972) *The Lymphocytes*, 2nd edn. London: Lloyd-Luke.
22. SMITH, R. T. & MIESCHER, P. A. (1966) *Phylogeny of Immunity*. University of Florida Press.
23. YOFFEY, J. M. (1967) *The Lymphocyte in Immunology and Haemopoiesis*. London: Arnold.
24. COTTIER, H. *et al.* (1967) *Germinal Centers in Immune Responses*. New York: Springer Verlag.
25. CANTOR, H. & WEISSMAN, I. (1976) Development and function of subpopulations of thymocytes and T lymphocytes. *Progress in Allergy*, **20**, 1.
26. CRADDOCK, C. G., LONGMIRE, R. & McMILLAN, R. (1971) Lymphocytes and the immune response. *New England Journal of Medicine*, **285**, 324 and 378.
27. ROWLANDS, D. T. & DANIELE, R. P. (1975) Surface receptors in the immune response. *New England Journal of Medicine*, **293**, 26.
28. PARKER, C. W. (1976) Control of lymphocytic function. *New England Journal of Medicine*, **295**, 1180.
29. SELIGMANN, M., PREUD'HOMME, J. L. & KOURILSKY, F. M. (1973) *Membrane Receptors of Lymphocytes*. Amsterdam: North Holland Publishing Co.
30. FU, S. M., WINCHESTER, R. J. & KUNKEL, H. G. (1974) Occurrence of surface IgM, IgD and free light chains on human lymphocytes. *Journal of Experimental Medicine*, **139**, 451.
31. ZUCKERMAN, S. H. & DOUGLAS, S. D. (1976) The lymphocyte plasma membrane: markers, receptors, and determinants. *Pathobiology Annual*, **6**, 119.

32. LIN, P. S., COOPER, A. G. & WORTIS, H. H. (1973) Scanning electron microscopy of human T-cell and B-cell rosettes. *New England Journal of Medicine*, **289**, 548.
33. MEHRISHI, J. N. & ZEILLER, K. (1974) T and B lymphocytes: striking differences in surface membranes. *British Medical Journal*, **1**, 360.
34. MILLER, J. F. A. P. (1974) Endocrine function of the thymus. *New England Journal of Medicine*, **290**, 1255.
35. CUNNINGHAM, A. J. (1973) Antibody formation studied at the single-cell level. *Progress in Allergy*, **17**, 5.
36. MILLER, J. F. A. P. (1975) T-cell regulation of immune responsiveness. *Annals of the New York Academy of Sciences*, **249**, 9.
37. MILLER, J. F. A. P. *et al.* (1971) Cell-to-cell interaction in the immune response. VII Requirement for differentiation of thymus-derived cells. *Journal of Experimental Medicine*, **134**, 1266.
38. OPPENHEIM, J. J. & ROSENSTREICH, D. L. (1976) Signals regulating *in vitro* activation of lymphocytes. *Progress in Allergy*, **20**, 65.
39. GERSHON, R. K. *et al.* (1972) Suppressor T cells. *Journal of Immunology*, **108**, 586.
40. TURK, J. L. (1975) *Delayed Hypersensitivity*, 2nd edn. Amsterdam: North Holland.
41. Leading Article (1977) Immunological deficiency and the risk of cancer. *British Medical Journal*, **2**, 654.

Chapter 13. *Immunity to Infection*

The ability to resist infection (immunity) is a property common to all living creatures. It is due in part to the immune response which follows a previous exposure to micro-organisms or their products. This type of immunity is specific, and has been known for a long time. It was well recognised that second attacks of many acute infections were very uncommon, and this observation led to the deliberate infection of the skin with smallpox virus (variolation) as a means of preventing this disease. Although used widely with success its dangers were considerable; the practice fell into disrepute and was made illegal by an Act of Parliament in 1840. Jenner's introduction of 'vaccination' in 1796 using the less virulent cow-pox virus proved to be much more satisfactory.

Before describing the various types of immunity, it must be appreciated that the resistance of an animal and the virulence of an organism are merely alternative ways of describing the relationship between host and parasite. The Lancefield Group-B streptococcus is virulent to cows, but not usually to the human being. This may be considered from the host's point of view—the human is immune, while cows are susceptible. Furthermore, some organisms produce disease only if introduced into a particular tissue. As an example of this, cholera vibrios are harmless when injected subcutaneously, but highly virulent if ingested. Not only is the portal of entry important, but so also is the number of organisms. A dose of tubercle bacilli capable of causing infection in the lung may be insufficient to produce intestinal disease. Some organisms are normally either 'avirulent' or produce minor infections, but when the body's defences are weakened can lead to severe disease. This event is called *opportunistic infection*, and good examples are the deep-seated mycoses occurring in patients with one of the immunologically deficient diseases. Immunity, pathogenicity, and virulence are relative terms, which are meaningless unless not only the host and organism are specified, but also the conditions under which the two interact are defined.

Immunity may be divided into two main classes depending on whether or not it is related to previous contact with the organism or its antigens. These types are summarised below.

Non-Specific Immunity

This type of immunity is not dependent on previous contact with the organism or its products. Three factors are involved:

Cellular factors

Humoral factors

Genetic factors — Species / Racial / Individual

Specific Immunity

This type of immunity is related to a specific immune response to the organism or its products, and can be considered under two headings:

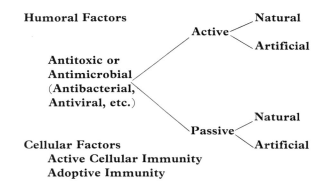

Humoral Factors

Antitoxic or Antimicrobial (Antibacterial, Antiviral, etc.)

Active — Natural / Artificial

Passive — Natural / Artificial

Cellular Factors
Active Cellular Immunity
Adoptive Immunity

NON-SPECIFIC IMMUNITY

All individuals possess an inherent ability to destroy invading micro-organisms which is not dependent on either the presence of antibodies or previous contact with the organism. Both cellular and humoral mechanisms are involved, and in the past there has been much discussion as to which is the more important. These arguments are now largely of historical interest, for it is believed that both phagocytes and humoral bactericidal substances are involved, and indeed often work hand in hand.

In addition other factors are involved. An organism may be capable of causing severe infection in one species, and yet incapable of causing disease in others. We are quite ignorant of the reasons for this difference, because neither known humoral nor cellular factors are involved. The tissues of an immune animal appear to be unsuitable for bacterial growth, even though by our present methods of investigation they do not differ from those of a susceptible animal. This type of immunity is probably dependent on subtle biochemical differences, which are generally assumed to be governed by genetic factors. To this type of immunity the terms 'innate' or 'inborn' are applied.

CELLULAR FACTORS

Foreign particles and organisms are ingested by phagocytes both in the blood and tissues. Polymorphonuclear leucocytes and the large mononuclear cells of the reticulo-endothelial system are involved. These cells accumulate as a result of an inflammatory response; this has been described in Chapter 6. The manner whereby polymorphs destroy organisms is described on page 78, and defects in this function are described later.

HUMORAL FACTORS

It has been known for a long time that blood and serum possess bactericidal power. For this reason blood is always well diluted with broth when it is cultured bacteriologically. Of the substances involved, those that belong to the complement system are the best defined.

Complement[1,2]

Complement was originally conceived by Bordet as a plasma component which aided or complemented the union of antigen to antibody. It is now known to consist of at least eleven components which can be sequentially activated in a cascade manner similar to that described in the clotting of blood. The components of complement are designated C1, C2, to C9. C1 has three components. The activation of the early components of complement involves the formation of enzymes which cleave the next component by limited proteolysis. Cleavage products are suffixed by a lower-case letter, e.g. C3a and C5a are small cleavage products of C3 and C5. Components in an active state are symbolised by a bar over the component numbers, e.g. $\overline{C42}$. The component of complement that is most plentiful is C3, and indeed the activation of C3 by cleavage into C3a and C3b is the central feature of the complement pathway.* Enzymes that act on C3 (C3 convertases) can be generated in three ways.

1. *The classical pathway*, by the formation of the C3 convertase $\overline{C42}$.

2. *The alternate pathway*, by the formation of the alternate C3 convertase $\overline{C3bBb}$.

3. *Cobra venom factor*, with the formation of the convertase $\overline{CVF,Bb}$.

*C3 is also called β_1C, and an antibody to it is commonly used to detect complement deposits (see Coombs's test, p. 648). The antibody is mainly directed against determinants of C3b. C3d, which is the degradation product of C3b, is liable to be missed.

The Classical Pathway of Complement Activation

The most intensively studied complement reaction is that of immune haemolysis initiated by the interaction of a site on the membrane of an erythrocyte E with a specific antibody A. The antigenic determinant may either by a natural constituent of the red-cell membrane or an antigen or hapten artificially attached to it. In either event interaction with specific antibody results in the formation of a complex EA (Fig. 13.1). This so aligns the heavy chains of the antibody molecule that the first component of complement (C1) is bound to the cell membrane. Actually C1 has three components C1q, C1r, and C1s, but these are held together in the presence of Ca^{++} ions. C1q is a collagen-like protein with binding sites for IgG and IgM. The addition of the immunoglobulin molecules causes a change such that the altered C1q activates C1r to $\overline{C1r}$, which in turn activates C1s to form a serine esterase $\overline{C1s}$. This acts on C4 and cleaves it into C4a and C4b. The major component C4b remains attached to the red-cell membrane. $\overline{C1s}$ also cleaves C2 into two fragments; the major fragment C2a combines with C4b, and is added to the complex on the red-cell membrane. The complex is now depicted as $\overline{C4b2a}$, and during its formation a polypeptide fragment, termed C kinin or C2 kinin, is released.† The complex $\overline{C4b2a}$ is unstable, and may revert to EAC4b by loss of the C2 component. However, under favourable conditions the active complex $\overline{C4b2a}$, also called *C3 convertase*, acts on C3 and cleaves it into C3a and C3b. C3a (anaphylatoxin) is released into the fluid phase, while C3b remains bound to the cell membrane. C1 probably plays no part in this or any subsequent reaction. The amplification effect of the C3b feedback mechanism is described later, and it results in the generation of more C3b. The complex $\overline{C4b,2a,3b}$ cleaves C5 into C5a (the classical anaphylatoxin) and C5b. This is the last enzymatic action in the pathway. C5b binds C6 and C7, and the resulting trimolecular complex binds C8 and C9. The details of these two remaining steps have yet to be clarified.

†C2 kinin is thought to be an important mediator in familial angiooedema due to C1 esterase deficiency (p. 525).

Figure 13.1
Diagram to illustrate the stages in the activation of complement, the components of which are designated C1, C2, etc. E represents a receptor site on a red cell, while A is a specific antibody. The complete reaction results in lysis of the red cell, but intermediate products are formed which result in opsonisation, immune adherence, chemotaxis, and the formation of anaphylatoxin. For the sake of clarity the activated fragment of each component which is added to the reaction chain is not identified. See text for details.

The end-result is that the receptor site on the cell is so altered that lysis is inevitable. Electron microscopy has revealed the appearance of holes in the cell membrane, 10nm in diameter; these are too small to allow the cell's contents to escape, but appear to enable fluid to enter and thereby destroy the cell by osmotic distension and rupture. It should be noted that all the components of complement must be activated for this haemolytic effect, and also for bacteriolysis.

One molecule of IgM antibody is necessary to initiate the complement mediated damage at one site on the red cell. Two molecules of IgG1, IgG2, or IgG3 are needed. Thus with IgM antibody, however much diluted, a particular number of red cells is lysed. With IgG the chances of two molecules becoming attached to one receptor site are much less likely as dilution proceeds. IgM antibodies are therefore much more efficient than IgG in sensitising cells. IgG$_4$, IgA, IgE, and IgD do not activate complement in this way.

Although haemolysis is the important *in-vitro* mechanism of complement mediated red-cell destruction, *in vivo* there is another important mechanism that involves the reticuloendothelial system. Macrophages have a surface C3b receptor, and by this means attach themselves to red cells coated with C3b. The red cells may be released unharmed, or may be first changed and converted into spherocytes. Alternatively they may be phagocytosed and destroyed. This type of red-cell destruction is typical of Rh incompatibility and the type of autoimmune haemolytic anaemia due to warm autoantibodies.

The Alternate Pathway of Complement Activation

It is known that C3 and the terminal components of the complement pathway can be activated by a number of agents without the involvement of C1, C4, or C2. Zymosan (a polysaccharide derived from yeast), bacterial lipopolysaccharide endotoxin, and cobra snake venom are amongst the agents that can lead to the generation of a C3 convertase from constituents of blood other than C1, C4, or C2. Pillemer in 1954 was the first person to describe *properdin* as a plasma protein which, in the presence of zymosan, can generate a C3 convertase and thereby activate C3 in the absence of an antibody. Additional factors (called Factor A, Factor B, and others) are required but C1, C4, and C2 are not consumed. *Magnesium* ions are necessary, but not Ca^{++}. Hence Pillemer had demonstrated an alternative pathway for the activation of complement, but its significance was not appreciated for many years. Other workers have investigated the generation of C3 convertase by the action on blood of endotoxin lipopolysaccharide, cobra snake venom, and aggregated immunoglobulins. Many names have been employed to describe the factors that are involved, but it now seems that many of them are identical with the factors in the properdin system—this is the alternate pathway.*

The initial steps in the activation of the pathway are incompletely understood, and no clear account can be given at

*The nomenclature of these various factors is very confusing, since one substance may be given different names by different authors. Note the following: *factor A* is identical with C3; *activated factor A* is C3b; *factor B* is also called C3 proactivator, C3PA, glycine-rich betaglobulin, or GBG; *factor C* is the same as C3bina, an inactivator of C3b also called conglutinogen activating factor, or KAF; *factor D* is C3 proactivator convertase, C3PA convertase, C3PAse, or GBGase.

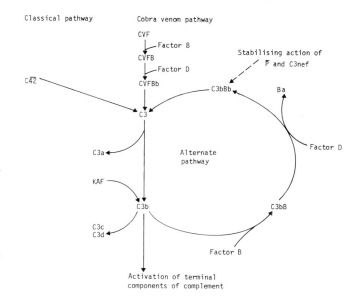

Figure 13.2
The alternate pathway to the activation of complement. The activation of properdin by zymosan, aggregated immunoglobulin, or bacterial endotoxin, in conjunction with factor B, factor D, and other factors is thought to cleave C3 to C3a and C3b. This step is poorly documented and is not shown in the diagram. C3b combines with factor B (also called C3 proactivator) in the presence of magnesium ions to form a loose complex C3bB. Factor D, which is a serine esterase, also called C3 proactivator convertase, cleaves factor B into Ba (which enters the fluid phase) and Bb which remains attached to C3b. The complex C3bBb is the C3 convertase of the alternate pathway, and can cleave C3 to form C3a and C3b. The latter can bind to cell membranes, cleave C5, and initiate the activation of the remaining components of the complement pathway. Note that C3 can be cleaved by two other factors: C$\overline{42}$ is the convertase of the classical pathway of activation. Cobra venom factor (CVF) is an analogue of C3b, and in conjunction with factor B and factor D forms the convertase CVFBb. Activated properdin ($\bar{P}$) and the C3 nephritic factor (C3nef stabilises the labile C3bBb) help to give the feedback cycle of the alternate pathway another turn. Conglutinogen activator factor (KAF), by inactivating C3b to C3c and C3d, acts as a brake on the complement-activating mechanism.

this time. Under the influence of the initiating factor (e.g. zymosan), properdin is activated, and native C3 together with factor B and factor D can form a convertase that is capable of acting on C3 to generate C3b. Next there is an interaction of C3b with activated properdin (P) and factors B and D to form a C3 convertase, which will cleave C3 to form more C3b and also activate C5. An important aspect of this mechanism is the positive feedback of C3b as shown in Figure 13.2. This mechanism clearly demands some homeostatic control, or else the formation of a little C3b would lead to massive complement activation. The enzyme KAF (p. 161) plays a part in this by inactivating C3b.

C3bBb (the alternate pathway convertase) is labile and decays rapidly. It can be stabilised by activated properdin; this is probably one of the main functions of properdin in the activation of the alternate pathway.†

†Another substance that stabilises C3bBb is C3nef, or C3 nephritic factor; this is a serum protein that is found in some patients with hypocomplementaemic membranoproliferative glomerulonephritis.

Summary. The complement components C3 to C9 can be activated via the alternate pathway by a number of factors including aggregated IgA, IgE, and IgG4, immunoglobulins which previously were thought not to activate complement. The precise role of this pathway has yet to be determined, but abnormalities in it are known to affect immunity to infection (see below), and its activation can explain how defects in the classical pathway may be circumvented. Thus C4-deficient guinea-pigs can exhibit the Arthus phenomenon. Furthermore, the positive C3b feedback cycle can act as an amplification mechanism regardless of whether the classical or alternate system is activated. One disease in which the alternate pathway appears to play a major role is paroxysmal nocturnal haemoglobinuria.

Cobra Venom Activation of Complement

It has been known since the beginning of this century that a factor in cobra venom can activate complement without the consumption of C1, C4, or C2. The cobra venom factor CVF is an analogue of C3b and combines with factor B. The complex is acted upon by factor D to form the stable active complex CVFBb. This mechanism is clearly not of any physiological importance.

Inhibitors of Complement Activation

Apart from the rapid decay of some complexes, e.g. $C\overline{42}$, there are three enzymes whose actions tend to prevent complement activation:

1. **C1 esterase inhibitor.** This forms a stable complex with C1s, and inhibits the enzymatic action of C1. Absence of this enzyme is associated with familial angio-oedema (p. 525).

2. **C3b inactivator, also called conglutinogen activating factor, or KAF.** This enzyme degrades C3b by splitting off a peptide and thereby exposing a carbohydrate determinant in C3 that reacts with conglutinin (see below).

3. **Serum carboxypeptidase B.** This enzyme inactivates both C3a and C5a.

During the process of complement activation various components are formed which have important actions. These components are formed not only when the complement is activated at cell receptor sites as in immune haemolysis but also when the reaction takes place in solution. This can be initiated not only by antigen-antibody complexes but also by other mechanisms, for instance by the enzyme plasmin and other proteolytic enzymes such as those from lysosomes. Furthermore, the process need not proceed to completion. The components of complement which are released during activation are responsible for:

Opsonisation. Bound C3b is a powerful opsonin and therefore aids *phagocytosis*.

Immune adherence. C3b is also responsible for this phenomenon (p. 146). This is closely related to the opsonic effect, for bacteria adherent to cells are more easily phagocytosed.

Chemotaxis. $C\overline{567}$ is chemotactic for polymorphs. This is an important mediator in the Arthus phenomenon (p. 179), aggregate anaphylaxis (p. 177), some types of vasculitis, and probably in acute inflammation in general (p. 83). C3a and C5a are also important chemotactic agents.

Anaphylatoxin production. Anaphylatoxin is an agent which will act on mast cells and lead to the liberation of histamine. At least two types are known; one is a small cleavage product of C3 labelled C3a and the other is C5a derived from C5. Anaphylatoxin can be formed not only by the interaction of antigen with antibody, but also *via* the alternate pathway by incubating serum with agar, kaolin, barium sulphate, and inulin. They are also generated when the serum proteases are activated. Thus both plasmin and bacterial proteases can cleave C3 and C5 to produce the anaphylatoxins C3a and C5a (see aggregate anaphylaxis, p. 177 and anaphylactoid reactions, p. 177).

Complement is therefore an important component of plasma; after its activation it can directly effect the lysis of bacteria; indirectly it can mediate an acute inflammatory reaction by increasing vascular permeability, attracting white cells, and promoting phagocytosis. It might therefore be deduced that complement is a vital factor in the immune mechanism. Nevertheless, a deficiency of various factors has been noted in apparently normal animals. Thus hereditary deficiency of C2 in the human, C5 in mice, C4 in guinea-pigs, and C6 in rabbits is not associated with undue liability to infection. Further examples have now been discovered in which the converse is true. In one family, a girl with a dysfunction of C5 activity was found to be unduly susceptible to *Staphylococcus aureus* and Gram-negative bacilli.[3] Another case is recorded of a young man with a lifelong susceptibility to infection in whom there was a lack of C3. The defect was due to KAF deficiency. This enzyme normally inactivates C3b and impedes the positive feedback mechanism whereby C3b activates the alternate pathway (Fig. 13.2). Hence in this patient all his C3 was consumed (and converted into C3b), as also was factor B.[4] It is evident that with such a complex system as complement, subtle errors at critical points can have serious effects, while relatively gross errors at other points can be by-passed or corrected.

Conglutination. This is mentioned here because of its relationship to complement. Red cell-complement-antibody complexes are agglutinated by a protein, *conglutinin*, present normally in the sera of cattle. It is not an antibody, and appears to be specific against C3.

A similar substance, termed *immune conglutinin*, appears in the blood in man following many infections and immunisation procedures. It is an antibody directed against epitopic sites on C3 and C4 which are normally hidden, but which become exposed when complement is activated. It is therefore a type of autoantibody.

OTHER FACTORS

Bactericidal substances have been extracted from tissue and serum, but in no case has identification been successful. The basic peptides extracted from tuberculous tissue may be cited as an example.

Natural Opsonin

Normal serum contains a protein which can coat relatively avirulent organisms, rendering them more easily phagocytosed by polymorphs. It is said to be heat-labile, and to require the presence of complement. A deficient natural opsonin for pneumococcal phagocytosis is found in patients with sickle-cell anaemia, and these patients are unduly susceptible to infection.[5] The nature of the missing factor is not known. It has been found with *S. typhimurium* infection in animals that serum from a naturally resistant species (the rat) contains an opsonin which will protect a susceptible species (the mouse) from a dose of bacteria that would normally be lethal. How frequently innate immunity is mediated by humoral factors is not decided.

GENETIC FACTORS—INNATE IMMUNITY

Species. Species immunity is the most absolute immunity known. The human species has almost complete immunity to many animal diseases; distemper and foot-and-mouth disease do not normally affect it, while certain typically human diseases like poliomyelitis, syphilis, and leprosy do not easily affect animals. Adult humans are immune to Lancefield Group-B streptococci; these organisms are, however, capable of producing mastitis in cattle. On the other hand, Group-A streptococci cause serious human infection, thus illustrating the high degree of specificity of innate immunity. In other words, virulence is sometimes dependent upon quite small changes in antigenic structure. Nevertheless, some organisms do produce disease in several species, a fact utilised by Koch in the formulation of his famous postulates (see Appendix 2).

Racial. The selective breeding of disease-resistant plants is well known in agriculture, where it is of great practical importance. Selective breeding in animals is more difficult; the work of Lurie, who succeeded in breeding rabbits of varying degrees of susceptibility to tuberculosis, is a noteworthy achievement in this field. Another instance often cited is that of Algerian sheep, which are said to be immune to anthrax.

In the human the position is more difficult to assess. There is considerable evidence to show that individuals with the sickle-cell trait are resistant to *Plasmodium falciparum* malaria. The trait is due to a genetic error, which lends some weight to the thesis that innate immunity is dependent upon inherited characteristics. Likewise individuals who are Duffy negative are resistant to infection by *Plasmodium vivax*. (p. 645). Other examples are on less firm ground. The European races are said to be more susceptible to yellow fever than are the native races of West Africa. The Irish and the Welsh are generally held to be more susceptible to tuberculosis than are the English. However, the possibility of immunity acquired in early childhood, as well as the question of widely differing social and economic levels in different peoples, make it difficult to prove that these are true examples of innate immunity. Nevertheless, the work with plants and animals would lead us to suppose by analogy that racial differences do exist in human beings.

Individual. The existence of individual immunity is difficult to prove either in humans or animals. The study of tuberculosis in twins has shed some light on this problem. In the case of uniovular twins it is found that when one twin has tuberculosis, the chances of the other twin also having it are over 85 per cent. When, however, one of binovular twins has tuberculosis, the chances of the other twin also having it are only 25 per cent. This percentage corresponds to that which is usually encountered in siblings who are not twins.

Other examples of an individual's genetic make-up affecting his response to an infection may be cited.[6] Susceptibility to *Haemophilus influenzae* epiglottitis and meningitis has been shown to be related to a major histocompatibility gene in the human. In animals it is well known that the immune response to a particular antigen is linked to hereditary factors. A cross-reaction between the bacterial antigen and a tissue antigen, such as a blood-group substance, is sometimes the cause of this.

These examples of innate immunity—species, racial, and individual—are dependent upon genetic make-up. In some instances the ability to mount an immune response is invoked, and sometimes the presence of a specific receptor for an organism or its toxin on a cell membrane is involved (p. 92), but until recently we have been ignorant of the mechanisms involved in the genetic control of the immune response.

Recent work, mainly in the mouse, has clarified the position to some extent. The ability to mount an immune response against a particular antigen (*immune responsiveness*) is inherited as an autosomal dominant trait.[7, 8] The genes responsible are the *immune response* (*Ir*) *genes*, and are part of the major histocompatibility complex (see Appendix 4). The presence of an *Ir* gene can determine an animal's ability to respond to a given antigen at all (responders and non-responders), or it may control the *level* of the response—i.e. the amount of antibody produced and whether it be IgM, IgG, etc. The gene product has not been identified, but it appears to affect T cell function primarily. The *Ir* gene has its human counterpart in the *HLA-DR* locus.

DEFECTS IN NON-SPECIFIC IMMUNITY[9]

Defects in the Polymorphs[10]

These may be considered under two main headings:

Quantitative polymorph defects. The causes and effects of neutropenia (agranulocytosis) are described in Chapter 53. An unusual example is *cyclic neutropenia*, in which polymorphs virtually disappear from the circulation for a few days every 21 days. It is characterised by recurrent skin infections, otitis media, and oral ulceration, together with arthritis. The cause is not known, nor is there effective treatment.

Qualitative polymorph defects.[11] The behaviour and functions of the polymorphs have been considered in Chapter 6: abnormalities can be considered under the following headings: abnormality of

1. random movement
2. chemotaxis
3. adherence to bacteria
4. phagocytosis
5. intracellular bactericidal activity.

Each of these functions can be investigated, and many defects have been described. Unfortunately reports in the literature are contradictory, and often several defects have been found in one clinical entity. Hence at the present time it is best to consider the subject under the headings of the various clinical syndromes that have been identified.

The lazy leucocyte syndrome.[12] Two children have been found with recurrent respiratory and gingival infection, in whom neutropenia was associated with defective polymorph random movement and chemotaxis. Other polymorph functions have been reported as normal.

Familial chemotactic defect. This has been described in three children with ichthyosis vulgaris and recurrent *Trichophyton rubrum* infection.

Chediak-Higashi syndrome. This rare condition is inherited as an autosomal recessive trait, and is characterised by repeated pyogenic infections, a type of partial oculocutaneous albinism, and the presence of large, abnormal, membrane-bound granules in various cells of the body. Thus there are giant melanosomes in the melanocytes of the skin and giant azurophil granules in the neutrophil polymorphs. The polymorphs exhibit defective random movement, defective chemotaxis, and impaired degranulation on phagocytosing particles. Death is usually due to infection or the development of lymphoma.

Chronic granulomatous disease.[13] This disease affects only boys, as it is inherited as an X-linked recessive trait. It is characterised by repeated infection, often staphylococcal, of the skin, lymph nodes, lungs, and other internal organs. The patients' polymorphs can phagocytose bacteria, but the characteristic 'respiratory burst' does not occur (p. 78); hence H_2O_2 and superoxide are not formed due to this defect in the hexose monophosphate shunt. The precise defect is not known, but a defective NADH oxidase activity is probably at fault. In the absence of H_2O_2, the H_2O_2-halide-myeloperoxidase mechanism, which plays a key role in microbial killing, is in abeyance, and the polymorphs fail to kill phagocytosed bacteria. This applies particularly to those organisms, e.g. *Staph. aureus*, that produce a catalase. Bacteria which form H_2O_2 are killed by their own product.

The nitroblue tetrazolium (NBT) test is useful in the diagnosis of chronic granulomatous disease. This dye is taken up by polymorphs and converted into the pigment formazan.[14] Fewer than 10 per cent of patient's neutrophils reduce the dye even when stimulated by phagocytosis. In normal individuals 70 to 90 per cent of neutrophils are positive. The test is dependent on the production of hydrogen peroxide and superoxide in the cells, and as noted previously, the basic defect in chronic granulomatous disease is a failure of neutrophils to produce these agents on phagocytosing bacteria.*

Other defects associated with impaired bacterial killing. *Job's syndrome*† resembles chronic granulomatous disease clinically except that it affects girls with red hair. No defect in the neutrophils was found in some cases, but in others the NBT was negative and phagocytosed staphylococci were not killed. Chronic granulomatous disease and Job's syndrome probably cover a group of conditions each with different defects and modes of inheritance. Patients with *glucose-6 phosphate dehydrogenase deficiency* show an increased susceptibility to infection, as do some individuals with *myeloperoxidase deficiency*. Recurrent staphylococcal infections have also been reported in a patient with *pyruvate kinase deficiency*; it is evident that the bactericidal activity of neutrophils is a complex affair and can be upset by many metabolic defects. In addition to the enzyme defects described above, many other factors are known to affect neutrophil function. Amongst these

*Early hopes that the NBT test would distinguish between bacterial and viral infections have not been fulfilled.[15]

†'So went Satan forth from the presence of the Lord, and smote Job with sore boils from the sole of his foot unto his crown.' JOB 2:7.

are: diabetes mellitus,[16] cirrhosis of the liver,[17] severe infections, Hodgkin's disease, the administration of drugs (e.g. phenylbutazone, alcohol,[18] and glucocorticoids), and deficiency of complement components such that anaphylatoxins and chemotactic factors are deficient.

Defects in the Monocytes and RE System

Defects in the monocytes are less well documented than the neutrophil abnormalities. Defective monocyte chemotaxis has been reported in neoplastic disease, the Wiskott-Aldrich syndrome (p. 171), and in some cases of mucocutaneous candidiasis. The spleen plays an important role in phagocytosing agents which are not opsonised.[19, 20] Individuals with *congenital splenic hypoplasia* are particularly susceptible to infections with organisms against which they lack antibodies.[21] Splenic infarction and atrophy in *sickle-cell anaemia* may in part explain the susceptibility to pneumococcal infections (septicaemia and meningitis) that these patients display. They also lack specific opsonin. *Splenectomy* is sometimes followed by overwhelming infection, particularly if performed in children and for a severe disease, e.g. thalassaemia.

A non-specific *increase* in immunity occurs after BCG vaccination. It also follows injections of certain colloids and the endotoxins of Gram-negative bacilli. This appears to be due to an enhanced phagocytic activity of the reticulo-endothelial system which follows an initial period of depression ('RE blockade').

Defects in Complement

Subjects have been found who lack a particular component of complement. Deficiencies of C1, C4, C2, C3, C5, C6, and C7 have been reported. Some patients have shown no apparent clinical effects, but others have exhibited an increased susceptibility to infection: thus the patient described on page 161 with low C3 due to C3b inactivator deficiency suffered from repeated infections. Some patients (e.g. C1, C4, and C2 deficiency) have developed lupus erythematosus, glomerulonephritis, or Henoch-Schönlein purpura. This relationship between immune deficiency and autoimmune disease is not understood, but is also seen in patients with specific immunological defects (p. 171).

Conclusion. The existence of these rare syndromes indicates the complexity of the mechanisms on which immunity to infection depends. Indeed, it seems likely that the ability to overcome infections varies from one organism to another. It is to be expected that many more cases will be recognised in which individuals are unable to combat particular organisms or groups of organisms.

SPECIFIC IMMUNITY

This type of immunity is always associated with the presence of antibodies which may be of either humoral or cellular nature. When the host produces its own antibodies, the immunity is called 'active'. This may occur naturally or artificially. When the antibodies are donated to the host from another source, e.g. the serum of a convalescent patient or an immunised horse, the immunity is described as 'passive'. The antibodies are both immunoglobulins and cell bound.

Active Immunity

Natural active immunity follows an overt attack of the disease. Not infrequently people who deny ever having suffered from the infection are found to be immune, and their blood contains specific antibodies. In these cases it is likely that the infection has occurred, but in so mild a form as to escape notice. Subclinical attacks of this type are common in many diseases, e.g. tuberculosis and poliomyelitis, and probably play an important part in preventing epidemics. When an infection is introduced into a virgin population, a widespread, severe outbreak may ensue. This was seen when measles was first introduced into the Fiji Islands (1875),[22] and is also well known with myxomatosis in rabbits: first described in Montevideo by Sanarelli in 1898, devastating outbreaks have since occurred in Australia (by government initiative) and Europe (by private enterprise).[23] Natural selection of individuals having innate immunity is another factor which may operate.

Artificial active immunity follows the injection of toxoids or vaccines. These are considered in detail later.

Passive Immunity by Transference of Immunoglobulins

Immunoglobulins may be passively transferred either naturally or artificially.

Natural passive immunity: although at birth the body is poorly equipped for making its own antibodies, it nevertheless has immunoglobulins in considerable quantity, and these confer immunity. They are of maternal origin, and gain access to the child in one of two ways depending upon the species:

In utero, either *via* the placental or the vitelline circulation.

By *absorption through the gut* of antibodies contained in the colostrum and milk.

In humans and other primates humoral antibodies are transferred across the placenta, but in guinea-pigs and rabbits absorption is from the uterine lumen through the vitelline circulation. In horses, pigs, and cattle the transfer occurs after birth from the colostrum and milk. Dogs, rats, and mice occupy an intermediate position; some transfer occurs before birth, but most antibodies are received afterwards.

The value of passively acquired antibodies in human breast milk has been much debated. The milk contains IgA as well as non-immunoglobulin agents, such as lysozyme and lactoferrin, that neutralise or inhibit the growth of viruses and bacteria. Breast feeding is currently regarded as being far superior to the use of cow's milk preparations.[24]

Transmission across fetal membranes is a highly selective affair. IgG tends to be easily transferable, while IgA, IgM, and IgE are held back. Some antibodies (e.g. diphtheria antitoxin) are found in higher concentration in the offspring than in the mother. There is no adequate explanation for this. Transmission of *antigen* across the placenta is also a possibility, and might lead to the development of potential immunity.[25]

Relationship of immunoglobulins to immunity. Although some antibodies give good protection to the newborn child, e.g. to diphtheria, others do not. Thus, staphylococcal infection is common, although the staphylococcal antihaemolysin titre of the baby is higher than that of its mother. Whooping-cough is another disease for which no protection is afforded.

Artificial passive immunity is deliberately induced by injecting immunoglobulins for prophylactic or therapeutic purposes. The protection afforded is short-lived, because the antibodies are metabolised. It has been shown that in neonatal life the antibodies are destroyed at a slower rate than in the adult. Infants therefore retain their passive immunity for several months, whereas the effect of a serum injection in adults is measured in days rather than weeks.

Passive Immunity by Transference of Cells

If lymph-node cells from an immunised animal are transferred to another animal which is either syngeneic, tolerant, or non-reactive, e.g. due to X-irradiation, the grafted cells lead to the production of immunoglobulins in the new host. This is called *adoptive immunity*. Whether passive cellular immunity, e.g. to tuberculosis, can be transferred by lymphocytes (or in humans, transfer factor—see p. 184) is not known.

Before considering the mechanism of acquired immunity, it is important to remember that bacteria produce their harmful effects in two main ways: (1) by elaborating powerful exotoxins; (2) by invading tissues. Although both methods are used by a few bacteria, it is convenient to divide pathogenic organisms into two groups. Those which produce their main effect by means of a soluble exotoxin are called the *toxic organisms*; those which produce their main effect by means of endotoxins are termed *invasive*. As these two types of organism produce their effects in different ways, it is not surprising that the immunity which the body develops is different in the two instances (see Table 13.2). The main differences between exotoxins and endotoxins are shown in Table 13.1.

There are therefore two main subdivisions of this acquired type of immunity:

(1) Antitoxic, against the toxic organisms.
(2) Antibacterial, against the invasive organisms.

ANTITOXIC IMMUNITY

Toxic organisms produce their effects by means of powerful, diffusible exotoxins which are highly antigenic. The antibodies (antitoxins) are capable of neutralising the toxin, and act in the body by intercepting the toxin before it reaches susceptible tissues. They are commonly of IgG type.

Diphtheria bacilli alighting on a mucous membrane produce their effect, and indeed the disease, by elaborating an exotoxin, which acts upon the local tissues as well as being absorbed by the blood stream and causing damage at distant sites. If the host has a high antitoxin level in the circulation, and therefore in the tissues and mucus, the toxin is rapidly neutralised, thereby leaving the organism without its main offensive weapon. It then becomes in effect avirulent, and is removed by the normal decontaminating mechanism of the part. A virulent organism attacking a host with a high antitoxin level is in the same position as an avirulent organism attacking a normal host.

Virulent organisms may sometimes persist in the nose or throat in spite of a high level of circulating antitoxin. This constitutes the *carrier state*, and the individual, although not suffering any ill-effects from this colonisation, is nevertheless a source of danger to non-immune contacts.

TABLE 13.1   Showing the main differences between exotoxins and endotoxins

Property of toxin	Exotoxin	Endotoxin
Liberation	Large amounts liberated in broth culture: easily diffuses out of bacterium	Small amounts liberated with living organisms: liberated when organisms are destroyed.
Composition	Protein (relatively simple)	Complex protein-lipopolysaccharide.
Lethal dose	Small. Action specific	Larger. Action not specific.
Action of heat	Heat-labile in general*	Heat-stable in general.
Number of strains producing one toxin	Often all strains*	Often only one.
Ability to stimulate the production of demonstrable antibodies	Strong tendency	Some factors are antigenic (e.g. the surface antigens). Others are poor antigens.
Corresponding antibody	Antitoxin	Many types; some are antibacterial, others (e.g. antihaemolysins) are not.
Value of antibody in infection	Good protection	Variable—some antibodies protective, others are not.
Union with antibody	Simple direct relationship, often precipitation	Complex relationship. Agglutination, complement fixation, etc.

*Botulinum toxin is an exception to these generalisations.

TABLE 13.2   Types of immunity

Type	Due to	Mode of action
Antitoxic	Immunoglobulins (antitoxins)	Neutralises toxin and speeds its elimination. No direct effect on organism.
Antibacterial (and Antiviral)	*Humoral antibodies* Antibacterial Antiviral	Aids phagocytes and activates complement. Prevents attachment.
	Local Tissue Immunity due to IgA	Prevents infection.
	Cellular antibody Immune lymphocytes	Lymphokines: Cytotoxic action or lymphotoxin. Chemotaxis. Macrophage immobilisation. Interferon.

Evidently some type of antibacterial immunity is also involved in diphtheria.

It will be seen that the level of antitoxin in the circulating blood is a good measure of the degree of immunity, and this information is of great value in the assessment of immunity to toxic organisms. The degree of immunity as assessed in terms of an antibody titre is in fact an underestimate, because more antibodies are rapidly formed as a result of the stimulus of the infection.

Examples of Antitoxic Immunity

Diphtheria. The exotoxin produced by the diphtheria bacillus is mainly responsible for the organism's ability to survive and multiply at the site of infection. A reasonable level of circulating antibody will therefore confer immunity. This forms the basis of the *Schick test*.

A small quantity of toxin* is injected intradermally into the forearm, and the reaction observed after 48 hours. If the individual's blood contains no antitoxin, the introduced toxin causes tissue damage which is manifested by an acute inflammatory reaction (Schick-positive). If, however, the blood contains a fair level of antitoxin, then the introduced toxin is immediately neutralised, and no reaction occurs (Schick-negative).

*The amount used is generally that which is just neutralised by 1/1000 unit of antitoxin. In the skin of the other forearm a control of heated exotoxin is injected.

This type of biological test is found to be most useful in diphtheria; the actual measurement of the antitoxin titre in the blood would be more efficient, though more tedious to perform. The Schick test is usually negative after an attack of diphtheria. Subclinical attacks frequently occur, as evidenced by the fact that many adults are Schick-negative without ever having suffered from a clinical infection. The significance of Schick testing is shown in Table 13.3.

Table 13.3

Schick	Throat swab for diphtheria bacilli	Condition
+	−	Susceptible
+	+	Diphtheria
−	−	Immune
−	+	Carrier

Diphtheria can occur in a Schick-negative child, but the infection is not accompanied by generalised toxaemia. This again indicates that there is an antibacterial component to the immunity of diphtheria. However, it cannot be measured, and for practical purposes the antitoxin titre as gauged by the Schick test is of value. It has three uses: (*a*) to assess the general state of immunity to diphtheria in a large community; (*b*) to assess the necessity for active immunisation; (*c*) as a retrospective diagnostic aid in cases suspected of being diphtheria.

Active immunity of the artificial type is produced by the introduction into the body of *toxoid*. If APT (Alum Precipitated Toxoid) is used two doses are given, but with TAF (Toxoid Antitoxin Floccules) three injections are necessary. In practice the toxoid is often given in conjunction with tetanus toxoid, pertussis vaccine, and Salk vaccine.

Antitoxin administration is an essential part of the treatment of diphtheria. It is derived from horses that have been immunised against toxoid (and toxin). By producing a high blood level of antitoxin the toxin liberated at the site of infection is neutralised, and is therefore unable to reach distant organs, e.g. heart, adrenals, and nerves. Toxin which has already reached these tissues is firmly bound to them, and cannot be dislodged by the antibody. Treatment at an early stage of the disease is therefore essential if the full benefits of antitoxin therapy are to be obtained. The organisms themselves are not directly affected, but are destroyed by the acute inflammatory exudate. A carrier state may persist after the attack, and it is therefore advisable to insist on negative throat-swab cultures before discharging the patient.

Scarlet fever. The skin manifestations of this disease are caused by the erythrogenic exotoxin of *Strept. pyogenes*. Immunity may be detected by the *Dick test*, which involves exactly the same principle as the Schick test. A small quantity of erythrogenic toxin is injected intracutaneously. A positive reaction denotes susceptibility to the effects of the toxin.

The ability of antitoxin to neutralise erythrogenic toxin is used in the *Schultz-Charlton reaction*. In this test some antitoxin* is injected into the skin of a patient who has a

* From animals immunised with erythrogenic toxin

scarlatiniform eruption. If the patient has scarlet fever, the toxin is neutralised, and blanching occurs in the region where the antitoxin was injected. Although this reaction has great theoretical diagnostic value, it is not found to be very useful in practice, being positive only in those cases which are fairly obvious clinically.

Many of the different Griffith types of *Strept. pyogenes* produce the erythrogenic exotoxin, which consists of three antigenic types only (see p. 218, but in fact a single attack of scarlet fever is the rule). Therefore a scarlet-fever patient infected with any one of these types of streptococcus produces an antitoxin against one of the erythrogenic exotoxins, and is thereafter immune to it. There is, however, no immunity to streptococcal infection in general, because this depends on separate antibacterial antibodies against each Griffith type, of which there are about 50. As in diphtheria, the antitoxin merely neutralises the toxin and does not kill the organisms. On the other hand, whereas the neutralisation of the diphtheria toxin automatically allows the organism to be destroyed by the acute inflammatory exudate, the same does not apply after the neutralisation of the erythrogenic exotoxin of streptococci. The invasiveness of this organism depends on surface antigens, which have to be neutralised by specific antibacterial antibodies (see p. 167).

Tetanus. The tetanus bacillus has limited powers of invasion, and produces a severe disease by liberating a powerful exotoxin. This neurotoxin affects the anterior horn cells; once inside the cells it cannot be neutralised by its antitoxin. As with diphtheria early treatment of the disease is essential. Both horse and human antitetanic sera (ATS) are available, and can be given in large doses to intercept any further toxin which may be liberated. The horse protein is liable to produce hypersensitivity reactions, and its routine use is frowned on by many authorities.

Formaldehyde converts the toxin into toxoid (TT), which is extensively used as an active immunising agent. The prophylaxis and treatment of tetanus are further considered in Chapter 18.

Gas-gangrene. The clostridia causing this infection produce powerful exotoxins, the α-toxin of *Cl. welchii* being the most important. It is a powerful necrotoxin, and prepares ideal conditions for the invasion of the organisms. Antitoxin prevents this local necrotising action, thereby checking further spread of the bacilli. The antitoxins have no direct effect on the organism.

Botulism. The various strains of *Cl. botulinum* produce toxins which are antigenically distinct. Unless the particular strain involved is known, a polyvalent antiserum must be given. Botulinum toxin is very heat stable, unlike most exotoxins (staphylococcal enterotoxin is also relatively thermostable).

Summary of Antitoxic Immunity

(1) Immunity is conferred by circulating immunoglobulins, which are called antitoxins.

(2) The circulating antibody titre is a good measure of the degree of immunity.

(3) Reaction between toxin and antitoxin is a relatively simple, quantitative affair, about which much is known.

(4) Active immunisation with toxoid is reliable.

(5) Passive immunisation is effective in the treatment of the disease, if given early enough.

ANTIBACTERIAL IMMUNITY

Antibacterial immunity is much more complex than antitoxic immunity. The reason for this is the antigenic complexity of organisms, for although they are said to contain 'endotoxins', these are in effect the contents of the bacterial cell and many of them are not related to the pathogenic action of the organism. The globulin antibodies which are formed against the invasive organisms are therefore described as antibacterial rather than anti-endotoxic. They are IgM and IgG immunoglobulins.

Antigenic Structure of Invasive Organisms

Bacteria are living unicellular organisms, and as such are composed of a complex mixture of proteins, carbohydrates, and lipids. Many of these substances are antigenic, and one may well regard bacteria as made up of a mosaic of antigens. The virulent or invasive properties are often dependent upon a single substance, which is usually on the cell surface. The polysaccharide hapten capsule of the pneumococcus is a good example of this. Sometimes more than one surface antigen is present, the external one covering those beneath it to a greater or lesser extent. This phenomenon is well shown by the typhoid bacillus. Organisms containing the O surface antigen are virulent, and are agglutinated by anti-O serum. Some virulent strains have an additional Vi antigen coat. They are agglutinated by anti-Vi but not by anti-O. Although it is convenient to consider the Vi antigen as an additional coat which covers the O antigen, it is quite possible that one surface antigenic site can, by its presence, inhibit other antigenic determinants from reacting with their respective antibodies.

Organisms can acquire additional antigens from their surrounding media. Electron microscopy of virus particles escaping from a cell has shown how this can occur with viruses (see Fig. 22.5). If infective agents acquire antigens from their hosts, this might be a factor in promoting their virulence. Thus a future host, by exhibiting tolerance to these antigens, might show a reduced or delayed antibody response to the whole organism. As against this, it must be remembered that with some infections much of the tissue destruction might be caused by the immune response. Thus tolerance would cause immunity. An example of this is seen in mice infected with the virus of lymphocytic choriomeningitis. Infection *in utero* leads to little antibody formation, and the mice develop a chronic carrier state.[26] Ultimately immunoglobulin is produced, and the animals develop immune-complex glomerulonephritis. Thus their tolerance to the organism is split—affecting T-cell function more than B-cell mechanisms. Mice first infected as adults succumb to a severe disease (see p. 274).

It will be seen that there may be considerable variation in the structure of a single bacterial species. Not only does this affect the virulence, but also the colonial appearance of the organisms on a solid medium. For instance, pneumococci whose virulence has been enhanced by animal passage frequently produce *smooth* colonies on plate culture. Continued growth on the artificial media, however, often results in loss of virulence due to a loss of the surface antigen. These colonies appear *rough*. Such attenuated strains may be produced in other ways, e.g. passage through mice in the case of viruses. This change which affects an organism's virulence, colonial appearance, antigenic structure, etc., is known collectively as *microbial variation*.

This multiplicity of antigens leads to the formation of a large number of different antibodies when an animal is infected with the whole organism. As only a few of the bacterial antigens are responsible for invasiveness or virulence, it is only the corresponding antibodies that are of protective value. Many other antibodies may also be present, but in all probability they play no part in immunity. On the other hand, their presence may be of great diagnostic help, e.g. the Widal reaction of typhoid fever.

Organisms in the body are dealt with by two methods: they are destroyed either by phagocytosis or by complement activation. Both have already been described with regard to innate immunity, and it seems likely that antibacterial antibodies protect merely by aiding or activating these existing mechanisms.

Phagocytosis by polymorphs and macrophages is aided by the action of specific opsonins. Moreover, organisms adherent to red cells (see p. 146) are more easily phagocytosed *in vitro*, an effect which may also occur in the blood stream or in a local area of inflammation. The reticulo-endothelial system clears the blood stream of organisms more quickly in the immune animal.

Examples of Antibacterial Immunity

Pneumococcal infections. Pneumococci produce no powerful toxin, and their virulence depends upon the polysaccharide capsular hapten called the *specific soluble substance* (SSS), which by repelling phagocytes enables the organism to invade the tissues. Pneumococci without capsules are 'rough' and avirulent.

Immunity to pneumococcal infection is due to a type-specific antibody, which may be produced both by infection and the administration of the capsular substance. The antibody acts as an *opsonin* both *in vitro* and *in vivo*. It can also act as a precipitin and agglutinin, but is incapable of killing the organism even in the presence of complement. A specific reaction on the capsule can be demonstrated. This is generally described as the 'capsular swelling reaction', but in fact there is little or no actual swelling, the appearance being due to an increased opacity of the capsular substance, when it is acted upon by the type-specific antibody. Organisms so treated are still viable, and it seems certain that polymorphs must be present for their destruction.

Immune serum was once used in treating pneumococcal infection, but it has been rendered obsolete by the introduction of sulphonamides and the antibiotics.

Streptococcal infections. The virulence of *Streptococcus pyogenes* is dependent upon its type-specific M protein content, which too is present on the surface of the organism, and like the SSS hinders phagocytosis. Antibodies to it confer good immunity in experimental animals. The organisms produce many toxic and enzymatic products, e.g. haemolysin, hyaluronidase, streptokinase, and sometimes the erythrogenic exotoxin. Antibodies to these are produced, but confer no immunity against streptococcal infection. Although theoretically useful, the large number of different types of streptococcal antigens makes artificial immunisation by vaccines or sera an impracticable proposition. In any case the organism responds well to chemotherapeutic agents, although early treatment with these agents reduces the immune response.

Staphylococcal infection. Staphylococci are readily phagocytosed by polymorphs, but these may then be killed by the organism, presumably by its leucocidins. The α-toxin, coagulase, and leucocidins are all antigenic; however, their antibodies provide little or no protection. Unfortunately we are ignorant about the antigenic components which are responsible for the virulence of staphylococci, and it is therefore impossible to make effective vaccines. Many preparations have been used, but their value is doubtful.

Typhoid. Typhoid bacilli may be killed by phagocytosis or by humoral mechanisms. Antibodies confer immunity by their opsonic and complement-activating effects. The important antigens are not yet clearly defined. Phenolised preparations preserving the O and H antigens are effective. But an acetone killed and dried (AKD) vaccine was superior in a trial conducted in Guyana, and has been adopted by the US Armed Forces. An alcoholised vaccine, high in O and Vi antigens, was introduced for a period during the Second World War, and was of little value.[27] H antibodies do not confer immunity, but nevertheless find great use in the laboratory for the identification of *Salmonella* organisms. Presumably the important antigens in a vaccine are the O and others as yet undetermined.

Whooping-cough. The situation is the same as with typhoid, in that the antigen responsible for virulence has not been identified. Vaccines prepared from freshly isolated smooth strains have, however, proved of great value in prophylaxis.

Tuberculosis. The mechanism of immunity to tuberculosis is poorly understood; precipitins, agglutinins, and complement-fixing antibodies have been identified, but these do not confer immunity. The Mantoux test is used to detect hypersensitivity to tubercle-bacillus protein, and it is generally assumed that where hypersensitivity exists, so also does immunity. Active immunisation with a living attenuated bovine strain of bacillus (BCG) is widely used, apparently with good effect, although the degree of protection afforded cannot be directly measured. It is probable that acquired immunity to tuberculosis is due to cellular antibodies. The subject is discussed in Chapter 20.

Viral infections. The immunity to viral infection is considered in detail in Chapter 22. IgA antibodies in the secretions covering mucous membranes prevent initial infection, while IgG neutralising antibodies in the plasma limit dissemination should infection occur. Cell-mediated immunity is also important, since patients with a defect in the thymus-dependent immune response are particularly liable to viral infections. Interferon appears to be a major factor in the recovery from established infection.

Action of the Humoral Antibacterial Antibodies in the Body

Although the action of some antibodies appears to be beneficial, e.g. the opsonins, with others, like the agglutinins and precipitins, the effect is much less clear. Thus, it is possible that agglutinins by causing the organisms to remain localised to one site may so raise their local concentration that infection is favoured. On the other hand, it is possible that agglutination may prevent spread, and help to localise infection and facilitate phagocytosis.

It has already been stressed (p. 147) that antibodies have been named according to the nature of the tests employed to detect them. Furthermore, a single antibody may be detected as a precipitin, agglutinin, or lysin. To attempt to explain antibacterial immunity on the basis of *in-vitro* antibody reactions is not rewarding. It seems certain that the only way in which they can kill bacteria is by aiding one of the normal body defences; thus some antibodies activate complement, and others collaborate with phagocytes in the actual destruction of the organisms. In general, it may be said that the antibacterial antibodies produce their beneficial effect by localising infection.

It has been shown that in an animal rendered leucopenic, although there may be a high titre of antibacterial antibodies present, injected pneumococci tend to remain localised for only a limited time, and then spread and kill the animal. Therefore, without the intervention of the phagocytes antibacterial immunity is impotent. With other organisms phagocytosis may not be so vital, because humoral bactericidal mechanisms are also effective.

The antigenic structure of most organisms is highly complex, and there are many slight variations which affect their virulence; for instance, antibacterial antibodies to one particular strain of organisms may not protect against other strains. Serum therapy is on this account extremely difficult and rarely efficacious.

In-vitro tests, e.g. agglutination, are dependent on the occurrence of certain specific antigens within the organism. It does not follow, however, that these antigens are the ones that confer the property of virulence on the organism. It is very apparent that the titre of antibodies in a patient's serum, as demonstrated *in vitro*, often bears no relationship to the degree of immunity possessed against that particular organism. It often happens that the antigens responsible for an organism's virulence are not the ones investigated in the common *in-vitro* tests. Antibacterial antibodies probably afford as complete a protection against invasive organisms as do antitoxins against toxic organisms. It is unfortunate that the common serological tests investigate the antibody response to antigens that do not concern the organism's virulence. This does not, however, detract from their great value in diagnosis.

Immunity due to IgA in secretions. IgA is the principal antibody found in the secretions of the nose, salivary glands, and the alimentary tract. Its presence appears to be responsible for the local immunity which follows ingestion of live poliomyelitis vaccine. Antibodies to other viruses have also been detected in the IgA fraction, and it remains to be discovered whether the same mechanism applies to bacterial infection.

Value of Estimating Antibodies in Diagnosis

The Wassermann complement fixation test and Kahn flocculation test are well-known methods of detecting the syphilitic antibody. In typhoid fever agglutinins can be detected against both flagellar H antigens and the somatic O and Vi antigens (Widal test). The titre rises towards the end of the second week of the disease, and particular significance should be attached to a rising titre of anti-O agglutinins. An anamnestic rise following other infections is less liable to affect these than the anti-H agglutinins. In patients previously vaccinated with TAB the Widal test is of much less value in diagnosing typhoid fever, because high titres of antibody may be present even before the onset of the infection, and the subsequent anamnestic rise confuses the picture even more.

In the Weil-Felix test advantage is taken of the fact that certain *Proteus* organisms share a common antigen with the rickettsiae; antibodies which agglutinate *Proteus* OX19 are found in European louse-born typhus, while in mite-borne scrub typhus the antibodies react with *Proteus* OXK.*

Cell-mediated Immunity in Bacterial Disease

Although in the past great stress has been laid on the part played by humoral antibacterial antibodies, it is evident that cell-mediated responses are also important. Sensitised lymphocytes in contact with antigen release lymphokines which augment the inflammatory response and immobilise macrophages. Thus lymphocytes play an important role in immunity; passive immunity to an intracellular parasite such as *Listeria monocytogenes* may be accomplished by the transfer of lymphoid cells to a syngeneic, recipient animal, but not by the administration of immunoglobulin.

The increased phagocytic power of macrophages in Mantoux-positive individuals indicates that a change in them may play a part in the antibacterial immunity to the tubercle bacillus. Curiously enough, although the delayed-type hypersensitivity which develops during an infection with the tubercle bacillus is specific, the increased phagocytic activity of the macrophages which accompanies it is non-specific. Indeed, this is the basis for giving BCG in an attempt to control malignant disease.

Anergy, indicating a lack of cell-mediated responses, can lead to an increased susceptibility to infection: measles has a reputation for reactivating a tuberculous infection (p. 172).

It is evident that the interrelationship between delayed-type hypersensitivity, cell-bound antibodies, and immunity is poorly understood. Individuals who display defective cell-mediated immunity show particular susceptibility to certain infections, e.g. to viruses, fungi, and some bacteria (p. 170).

Artificial Antibacterial and Antiviral Immunity

The artificial production of immunity to the invasive organisms is much more difficult that to those of the toxic group. The reasons for this are twofold.

(1) The antigens responsible for the virulence of the organisms are in many cases unknown. Preparations of vaccine may therefore be deficient in vital antigens, and the antibodies which they provoke are then not protective.

(2) Immunity is in part cell mediated, and this is difficult to stimulate other than by infection with living organisms.

The injection of toxins or toxoids is quite unsatisfactory, and it is found that the whole organism, i.e. a *vaccine*,† must be used. Attention has to be paid to the relevant surface antigen of the organism which is used in the preparation of the vaccine. Furthermore, if the strain of organism selected does not happen to be the one which is prevalent at the time, vaccination is unlikely to produce satisfactory immunity, e.g. influenza.

In many diseases dead vaccines are not effective, and a vaccine containing live, attenuated organisms is much more efficient.

The artificial induction of local immunity has so far been utilised only in poliomyelitis.

Summary of Antibacterial Immunity

1. Many strains of bacteria exist, and they may differ widely in their antigenic structure and virulence.

2. It is difficult to prepare effective vaccines, because it is not always possible to include all the possible antigenic variants in the preparation.

3. Antibacterial immunity is only partly dependent upon the production of immunoglobulin antibacterial antibodies.

4. It is difficult to measure the immunity because of the wide bacterial variation.

5. Many *in-vitro* actions of humoral antibodies can be demonstrated, but their activity *in vivo* is not necessarily related to their *in-vitro* properties.

6. The effect of the antibodies is to aid localisation of the infection.

7. Local immunity due to local IgA plays a part in some infections.

8. Antibacterial immunity is also related to cellular antibodies.

Artificial Immunisation[29]

Specific immunity to infections may be increased artificially by giving antisera (passive) or by the administration of vaccines or toxoids (active).

A toxoid is a preparation of an exotoxin which has been so treated (usually with formaldehyde) that its toxicity is abolished without impairing its essential antigenic determinants. Satisfactory preparations of diphtheria and tetanus toxoid are in current use (see pp. 166 and 231).

Vaccines are suspensions of whole organisms either alive or dead. They may be administered orally, but the common route is by parenteral injection. BCG, smallpox, yellow fever, and poliomyelitis (Sabin) are examples of live vaccines; TAB, pertussis vaccine, and Salk poliomyelitis vaccine are dead.

Although there is general agreement that active immunisation of the population is desirable, there is no unanimity on the schedule to be adopted. With living vaccines one dose is generally sufficient, since the organism multiplies during the

---

*It is of interest that a high titre of antibodies against *Proteus* OX19 can be produced by injecting a vaccine of *Proteus* OX19 organisms. This method is reported to have been used by Polish patriot doctors during the Second World War as a means of deceiving the Nazis into believing that individuals had typhus fever. 'Epidemics' of typhus could thereby be created, and the individuals and the area in which they lived were thereby left relatively free of oppression.[28]

†The term is derived from the Latin *vacca*, a cow, and was coined by Pasteur in honour of Jenner's observation that an infection with cow-pox protected against smallpox.

course of the subclinical infection which follows, and this provides a sufficient antigenic stimulus (but see p. 278). A cellular type of immunity also ensues. With dead vaccines and toxoids a two or three-dose procedure is adopted for primary immunisation. In order to avoid multiple injections, there has been a trend to combine several antigens into one preparation e.g. combined diphtheria, tetanus, poliomyelitis, and pertussis. The pertussis organisms have been found to exercise an adjuvant effect and improve the response to the toxoids.

Maintenance of immunity. Regular booster doses are usually recommended, but there is a tendency to regard these as unnecessary, and indeed, if repeated too frequently, as harmful. Following a satisfactory primary course, immunity to diphtheria and tetanus persists for many years, and booster doses can be given in the event of an exposure to infection.

It is apparent that the immunisation procedures that are adopted are based upon factors determined by administrative convenience, finance, and the patient's comfort as well as on the results obtained from previous experience. The best plan for the individual practitioner is to adopt the procedure which is generally accepted in his own area, and to modify it as the results of well-planned field trials become available.

COMPLICATIONS OF ARTIFICIAL IMMUNISATION[29]

Although serious complications are very uncommon, their occurrence has been a serious handicap to the public's acceptance of widespread immunisation. In some instances particular preparations, e.g. horse ATS, have fallen into disfavour because of their complications. The hazards of artificial immunisation will be summarised here, since many aspects are described in greater detail elsewhere in this book.

Reactions Following the Use of Any Agent:

Infection. With carefully controlled methods of preparation and adequate aseptic technique this is an infrequent complication.

Local acute inflammation due to the irritant properties of the preparation. In severe cases there is also a general reaction with pyrexia, malaise, etc. Such reactions are usually seen after the use of dead vaccines, e.g. TAB, and to a lesser extent alum-containing toxoids.

Provocation poliomyelitis, especially with alum-containing toxoids.

Reactions Following the Use of Specific Agents:

Animal Sera.

Hypersensitivity reactions: local reactions, serum sickness, anaphylaxis, and death.

Neurological complications. Encephalitis, myelitis, polyneuritis (of Landry or Guillain-Barré type), neuritis affecting a group of nerves, e.g. 'radiculitis' of the brachial plexus, and lesions of individual nerves have all been described. The pathogenesis is obscure; a hypersensitivity reaction may be involved, as neurological complications may also occur with serum sickness.

Human Serum.

Infection: viral hepatitis is the most important.

Passive transfer of immediate-type hypersensitivity is a minor hazard.

Hypersensitivity reactions to minor geneticaly-determined protein variants is a possibility.

Live Vaccine.

Excessive local spread of the agent, e.g. BCG and vaccinia.

Widespread dissemination of the organism to produce severe disease, e.g. vaccinia.

Neurological complications, e.g. postvaccinal encephalitis.

Toxoids and Dead Vaccines.[30]

Hypersensitivity. Local reactions due to immediate and delayed-type hypersensitivity. Anaphylaxis is rare. Encephalitis following antirabies injections is probably a reaction to foreign nervous tissue.

Neurological complications resemble those seen following the use of serum. Thus, pertussis vaccine is occasionally followed by encephalitis or blindness.

IMMUNOLOGICALLY DEFICIENT DISEASES[9, 31, 32]

In 1952 Bruton described the case of a young boy whose sequence of repeated pneumococcal infections was shown to be related to a very low plasma γ-globulin level. Since that time numerous instances of immunological deficiency disease have been described, and attempts to understand the mechanism in each case have served to test our understanding of the mechanisms involved in the defences of the body against infection.

On the hypothesis that the thymus is necessary for the proper development of cell-mediated immune reactions, while the gut-associated lymphoid tissue is essential for the immunoglobulin responses, attempts have been made to separate the syndromes into groups according to which system is presumed to be at fault. In some cases this has been eminently successful, but there are others in which the defect is such that our knowledge of the immune response is inadequate to explain them. A feature which can cause confusion is a patient with a specific immunological deficiency developing other immunological defects as a secondary event, as the disease and its complications progress.

The term *agammaglobulinaemia* is generally used to describe cases in which the γ-globulin level is very low (under 1 g per litre). *Hypogammaglobulinaemia* would be more accurate, but is usually reserved for cases in which the level of γ-globulins, although low, is over 1 g per litre. Although no hard and fast rules can be made, this group of diseases is characterised by repeated pyogenic bacterial infections and also viral hepatitis. When there is a defect in the formation of cellular antibodies, infections with *Mycobacterium tuberculosis*, viruses, and fungi (especially *Candida*) often dominate the picture.

Stem-cell Deficiency

Reticular dysgenesis. This is described in infants who possess no white cells or lymphoid tissue. Presumably the primitive marrow reticular cells failed to develop. The longest period of survival has been 90 days.

Pure Thymic Deficiency Syndromes

In *thymic alymphoplasia* of Nezelof, sometimes called thymic dysplasia, the thymus is absent or rudimentary and there is a complete absence of all the cell-mediated responses of delayed hypersensitivity. Germinal centres, plasma cells, and the production of γ-globulins are, however, normal. In *thymic aplasia*, described by Di George, there is in addition absence of the parathyroid glands, which causes the disease to present in infancy with hypocalcaemic tetany.

Pure Immunoglobulin Deficiency Syndromes

Bruton's congenital sex-linked agammaglobulinaemia. This is restricted to males, and usually appears at about the age of six months when maternally derived immunoglobulins are exhausted. There is a striking absence of plasma cells everywhere and atrophy of the lymphoid tissue of the tonsils, appendix, and Peyer's patches. The thymus is normal and cell-mediated responses are normal. There is, however, a virtual absence of the three main classes of immunoglobulins, and this is associated with a liability to repeated, serious, pyogenic, bacterial infections which invariably lead to death. In addition, fulminating hepatitis may occur. Curiously enough, if these patients are given human γ-globulin they sometimes manufacture antibodies to it.[33] Polyarteritis and rheumatoid arthritis are more frequent in these patients, indicating perhaps that this is not simply a disease in which there is a failure of immunoglobulin synthesis.

Late-onset agammaglobulinaemia and hypogammaglobulinaemia.[34] A variety of syndromes, including a polyarthritis affecting the large joints,[35] and malabsorption accompanied by infection with *Giardia lamblia*, have been described in which a low immunoglobulin level is first detected in childhood or adult life. The conditions are sometimes called acquired, but probably inherited factors are involved in many cases. Plasma cells are not formed in response to antigenic stimulation, but germinal centres are seen and may even be hyperplastic, particularly in the tonsil and bowel.

Dysgammaglobulinaemia. This term is used to describe the condition in which there is a low level or absence of one or more, but not all, of the immunoglobulin classes. So far as the three main classes of immunoglobulins are concerned, there are six possible combinations. Thus in one type found in male infants with recurrent infections, IgG and IgA are low or absent, while IgM is elevated (the *hyper-IgM syndrome*). In the *hyper-IgE syndrome* patients are also plagued with recurrent pyogenic infections. *Isolated IgA deficiency* is the most common immunodeficiency state.[36]

Some cases suffer from sinusitis and pulmonary infections with intestinal malabsorption and a sprue-like syndrome, and also show a tendency to develop rheumatoid arthritis or other autoimmune disease; most individuals, however, appear normal, and there is no apparent increase in the incidence of respiratory infection. Several other types of dysgammaglobulinaemia are known, and some exhibit a malabsorption syndrome—steatorrhoea with nodular hyperplasia of the intestinal lymphoid tissue or lymphadenopathy and hepatomegaly. Liability to infection is common.

This group of immunoglobulin deficiency syndromes may be regarded as disorders of the B cells. In some cases all classes of antibody are reduced, while in others the defect spares one or more classes of antibody. In many instances the defect appears to be inherited, but some are probably acquired; viral infection, e.g. rubella, has been implicated. An interesting but unexplained feature of this group of conditions is that the patients or their families exhibit a high incidence of rheumatoid arthritis, systemic lupus erythematosus, Crohn's disease, lymphoma, and thymoma.

Deficiency Syndromes of Mixed Type

In this group, in addition to thymic hypoplasia and defective cell-bound antibody production, there is also depression of some or all of the immunoglobulins.

Severe combined immunodeficiency syndrome. This form of deficiency shows a total lack of both cell-mediated and humoral immunity, and is the most severe immunological defect known. It is inherited as an autosomal recessive trait and is also known as *Swiss-type lymphopenic agammaglobulinaemia*.

The disease is noticed during the first few weeks of life. There is a failure to thrive, infection particularly by viruses, *Candida albicans*, and *Pneumocystis carinii* (see p. 259), and diarrhoea. The infants seldom survive more than two years. The thymus and all the lymphoid tissue are hypoplastic, and both cell-mediated and humoral immune responses are absent. Allografts are not rejected. Administration of fresh blood to these patients often leads to a fatal *graft-versus-host* reaction beginning in 7 to 10 days with a high fever, morbilliform rash, hepatosplenomegaly, and diarrhoea. Pancytopenia develops and death occurs within 15 days. In some patients who have not been transfused, a skin rash similar to that of the GVH rash has been seen, and it is suggested that it is due to a GVH reaction by maternal lymphocytes.

Other types of combined immunodeficiency syndrome have been described, and may be inherited as X-linked traits or occur sporadically.

Some patients with severe combined immunodeficiency syndrome lack the enzyme adenosine deaminase. This enzyme catalyses the conversion of adenosine to inosine, and plays a part in the re-utilisation of purines; the relationship of the defect to the immunodeficiency is not known.

Ataxia telangiectasia. This is inherited as an autosomal recessive character and is characterised by progressive cerebellar ataxia, oculocutaneous telangiectasia, and recurrent sinus and pulmonary infections by viruses and bacteria. The onset is in early childhood and death usually occurs by adolescence. The thymus is absent or hypoplastic, and delayed-type reactions are markedly depressed. In addition there is a low level of plasma IgA and often IgE. Unexpectedly, plasma cells are present in the alimentary tract, but they contain IgM rather than the normal IgA immunoglobulins. A considerable number of patients develop a malignant lymphoma or other tumour.

Wiskott-Aldrich syndrome. This is characterised by atopic *eczema*, bleeding due to *thrombocytopenia*, and an increased susceptibility to *infection*. It is inherited as a sex-linked recessive characteristic, and death usually occurs in infancy. The major defect appears to be in the afferent limb of the immune response such that the individual fails to react to polysaccharide or lipopolysaccharide antigens. This leads to a low IgM level. As the disease progresses, there is a failure in T-lymphocyte development. Infection with a wide range of viruses, fungi, and bacteria occurs, and patients rarely survive over 10 years of age.

Treatment of immunological-deficiency diseases. Patients who lack particular immunoglobulins can be treated by the administration of suitable antibody concentrates. When cell-mediated function is defective, marrow and thymic grafts have been used. The administration of transfer factor has also been tried both in some primary immunological deficiency states and in acquired ones such as lepromatous leprosy.[37] Results are being assessed, and such treatment is at present the task of specialised centres.

Acquired Immunological Deficiency

Antibody levels are low in a number of naturally occurring diseases.

Secondary to infection. During measles, German measles, and following measles vaccination there is depression of cell-mediated hypersensitivity. There is a similar anergy in lepromatous leprosy (p. 130).

Hodgkin's disease. The major defect is suppression of the reactions dependent upon cell-bound antibodies. There is an increased liability to infection with tubercle bacilli, viruses, and fungi, a liability aggravated by the treatment.

Sarcoidosis. The defect is as in Hodgkin's disease, but there is no increased liability to infection.

Multiple myeloma and *Waldenström's macroglobulinaemia.* Both exhibit impairment of normal immunoglobulin production.

Lymphocytic lymphoma and *chronic lymphatic leukaemia.* There is depression of both immunoglobulin and cell-bound antibody production.

Intestinal lymphangiectasia. The dilated, abnormal lymphatic vessels leak fat, plasma proteins, and lymphocytes into the intestine. Cell-mediated responses are particularly affected. Since the long-chain fatty acids are absorbed into the lymphatics and increase the lymph flow, their administration worsens the disease. A low-fat diet, or one containing medium-chain triglycerides which are absorbed into the portal venous system, has a beneficial effect.

Iatrogenic immunological deficiency. In the treatment of patients with grafts or 'autoimmune' diseases, deliberate suppression of the immune response is often attempted by the administration of glucocorticoids, cytotoxic drugs, antilymphocytic serum, and ionising radiation. The results of this are often disappointing in relation to the aims of the treatment and devastating in terms of the infections that result.

REFERENCES

1. VOGT, W. (1974) Activation, activities and pharmacologically active products of complement. *Pharmacological Reviews*, **26, 125.**
2. RUDDY, S., GIGLI, I. & AUSTEN, K. F. (1972) The complement system of man. *New England Journal of Medicine*, **287,** 489, 545, 592 and 642.
3. MILLER, M. E. & NILSSON, U. R. (1970) A familial deficiency of the phagocytosis-enhancing activity of serum related to a dysfunction of the fifth component of complement (C5). *New England Journal of Medicine*, **282,** 354.
4. ALPER, C. A., ROSEN, F. S. & LACHMANN, P. J. (1972) Inactivator of the third component of complement as an inhibitor of the properdin pathway. *Proceedings of the National Academy of Sciences*, **69,** 2910.
5. Editorial (1968) On the preparation of victuals for phagocytes. *New England Journal of Medicine*, **279,** 489.
6. Leading Article (1971) Haemophilus disease and cell-surface antigens. *Lancet*, **2,** 914.
7. GREEN, I. (1974) Genetic control of immune responses. *Immunogenetics*, **1,** 4.
8. BENACERRAF, B. & KATZ, D. H. (1975) The histocompatibility-linked immune response genes. *Advances in Cancer Research*, **21,** 121.
9. HAYWARD, A. R. (1977) *Immunodeficiency.* p. 125. London: Arnold.
10. BELLANTI, J. A. & DAYTON, D. H. (Edrs) (1975) *The Phagocytic Cell in Host Resistance.* New York: Raven Press.
11. GALLIN, J. I. & WOLFF, S. M. (1975) Leucocyte chemotaxis: physiological considerations and abnormalities. *Clinics in Haematology*, **4,** 567
12. MILLER, M. E., OSKI, F. A. & HARRIS, M. B. (1971) Lazy-leucocyte syndrome. *Lancet*, **1,** 665.
13. Leading Article (1976) Microbial killing by neutrophils. *Lancet*, **1,** 1393.
14. SEGAL, A. W. (1974) Nitroblue-tetrazolium tests. *Lancet*, **2,** 1248.
15. Leading Article (1974) Another look at the N.B.T. test. *Lancet*, **1,** 664.
16. MOWAT, A. G. & BAUM, J. (1971) Chemotaxis of polymorphonuclear leukocytes from patients with diabetes mellitus. *New England Journal of Medicine*, **284,** 621.
17. DEMEO, A. N. & ANDERSEN, B. R. (1972) Defective chemotaxis associated with a serum inhibitor in cirrhotic patients. *New England Journal of Medicine*, **286,** 735.
18. BRAYTON, R. G. et al. (1970) Effect of alcohol and various diseases on leukocyte mobilization, phagocytosis and intracellular bacterial killing. *New England Journal of Medicine*, **282,** 123.
19. ERAKLIS, A. J. et al. (1967) Hazard of overwhelming infection after splenectomy in childhood. *New England Journal of Medicine*, **276,** 1225.
20. Leading Article (1976) Infective hazards of splenectomy. *Lancet*, **1,** 1167.
21. MILLER, M. E. (1970) Enhanced susceptibility to infection. *Medical Clinics of North America*, **54,** 713.
22. BURNET, F. M. (1962) *Natural History of Infectious Disease*, 3rd edn, p. 205. Cambridge University Press.
23. FENNER, F. (1959) Myxomatosis. *British Medical Bulletin*, **15,** 240.
24. Leading Article (1976) Breast-feeding: the immunological argument. *British Medical Journal*, **1,** 1167.
25. GILL, T. J. (1973) Maternal/fetal interactions and the immune response. *Lancet*, **1,** 133.
26. SILVERSTEIN, A. M. (1972) Fetal immune responses in congenital infection. *New England Journal of Medicine*, **286,** 1413.
27. Leading Article (1967) Typhoid vaccines. *Lancet*, **2,** 1075.
28. Leading Article (1977) Deception by immunisation. *British Medical Journal*, **2,** 716.
29. WILSON, G. S. (1967) *The Hazards of Immunisation.* London: Athlone Press.
30. Leading Article (1974) Reactions to tetanus toxoid. *British Medical Journal*, **1,** 48.

31. SELL, S. (1968) Immunological deficiency diseases. *Archives of Pathology*, **86**, 95.
32. HITZIG, W. H. (1976) Congenital immunodeficiency diseases, clinical appearance and treatment. *Pathobiology Annual*, **6**, 163.
33. Editorial (1968) Immunologic paradox. *New England Journal of Medicine*, **278**, 1174.
34. Leading Article (1976) Idiopathic late-onset immunoglobulin deficiency. *Lancet*, **2**, 838.
35. WEBSTER, A. D. B. *et al.* (1976) Polyarthritis in adults with hypogammaglobulinaemia and its rapid response to immunoglobulin treatment. *British Medical Journal*, **1**, 1314.
36. Leading Article (1975) IgA deficiency. *Lancet*, **2**, 1291.
37. BLOOM, B. R. (1973) Does transfer factor act specifically or as an immunologic adjuvant? *New England Journal of Medicine*, **288**, 908.

Chapter 14. *Hypersensitivity*

Hypersensitivity is a state in which an animal exhibits an excessive reactivity to the introduction of an antigen or hapten. Strictly speaking, *hypersensitivity* means excessive reaction, e.g. anaphylaxis, whereas *allergy* implies an altered reaction as exemplified by the Mantoux test. It is debatable whether such a distinction can be justified, and for practical purposes the two words are best regarded as synonymous. The excessive or altered reaction to bacteria as seen in the Koch phenomenon is conventionally called *bacterial allergy*. However, diseases like asthma and hay-fever are also called 'allergic', although in fact they differ markedly from the bacterial allergies. It is obvious that the two terms mean different things to different people, and therefore no useful purpose is served by trying to distinguish between them, even if this were desirable on theoretical grounds.

Two distinct types of hypersensitivity can be recognised. In one the reaction to administration of antigen is immediate (within minutes), while in the other it is delayed for 24 to 48 hours. The distinction between these two types is of fundamental importance. The *immediate-type* hypersensitivities are related to the formation of sensitising immunoglobulins. In *delayed-type* hypersensitivity, the reaction is cell mediated.

It is now realised that immunoglobulins can cause hypersensitivity in various ways and that in only one of these is the reaction immediate in the sense that this term is usually used. Indeed, injury due to immunoglobulins can be caused in three distinct ways, and these have been classified by Gell and Coombs thus:

Type I, immediate hypersensitivity. This is commonly mediated by IgE and is typified by acute anaphylaxis in humans.

Type II, or cytotoxic reaction. Antibodies, IgG or IgM, are directed against cellular or tissue antigens, e.g. as in haemolytic anaemia.

Type III, due to antigen-antibody complexes. IgG is mainly involved.

In the *delayed-type* hypersensitivities no such sensitising antibodies can be demonstrated, and the hypersensitivity is cell-mediated. This type of hypersensitivity is classified as *Type IV*.

Other types of hypersensitivity responses probably exist, and some examples are mentioned at the end of this chapter.

TYPE I IMMEDIATE HYPERSENSITIVITY

Many examples of this type of hypersensitivity occur in the human subject; the offending antigen is usually a dust, food, or drug. The features of immediate-type hypersensitivity have been the subject of intensive experimental study in animals. Anaphylaxis, which represents the most severe manifestation, will be described in some detail, because it illustrates the main features of this group.

ANAPHYLAXIS[1]

The term 'anaphylaxis' was first used to describe the severe reaction classically described by Richet and Portier in 1902. Since that time a localised, usually cutaneous manifestation of hypersensitivity has been labelled *cutaneous anaphylaxis*, and it is therefore advisable to describe the generalised form as *generalised*, or *systemic*, *anaphylaxis*.

Systemic Anaphylaxis

Richet and Portier were attempting to immunise dogs against the toxins of the sea-anemone, and noted that animals that had survived a sublethal injection of toxin were unduly sensitive to a second injection—so sensitive indeed that quite small doses produced a severe reaction, often resulting in death. At first the phenomenon was explained on the basis of the toxic nature of the extract, but subsequent work showed that other antigenic proteins could produce the same effect, even though they were not in themselves toxic. Richet called the reaction anaphylaxis because it seemed to represent the antithesis of immunity (Gr. *ana*—against, *phylaxis*—protection).

Anaphylaxis may be elicited by giving a single large, *shocking* dose of antigen at a suitable interval after one or more *sensitising* doses.

Active sensitisation. The first dose of antigen must reach the tissues in an unaltered state. It may be injected, but as the dose need only be small, a sufficient amount may be absorbed by inhalation or ingestion, provided the antigen is not denatured during absorption. Haptens may induce anaphylactic sensitisation if injected into the skin, because they combine with body proteins to produce complete antigens; in some instances, e.g. neoarsphenamine, intravenous injection leads to sensitisation. Presumably the drug combines with a body protein, thereby becoming antigenic.

Although some animals, e.g. guinea-pig, are easily sensitised by one small injection, others like the rabbit respond less readily, and may require several sensitising doses combined with an adjuvant.

Development of hypersensitivity. Anaphylactic shock can be demonstrated only if the shocking dose is given some time after the sensitising dose. The period is usually 8 to 10 days. The existence of this latent interval strongly suggests that an immune mechanism is involved. Once established, the state of hypersensitivity remains unaltered for a long time.

Production of shock. Following the injection of the second or 'shocking dose' of antigen, the animal develops a state which closely resembles acute histamine poisoning. The following features of the shocking dose should be noted:

Specificity. The same antigen must be used, a fact which indicates that the sensitisation is specific.

Dosage and rate of administration. The shocking dose must be administered quickly so that the damaging antigen-antibody reaction can produce systemic effects. In experimental work the intravenous route is used. The dose of antigen to be given varies with the type of anaphylaxis. It is often large when compared with the sensitising dose (in aggregate anaphylaxis), but enormous doses must not be given because antigen-antibody union is less damaging when there is great antigen excess, and shock may not occur.

Action of haptens. Haptens will induce shock provided they are capable of causing precipitation when mixed with their corresponding antibodies. Haptens that do not precipitate in this manner will not produce shock; instead they induce a refractory state to the subsequent injection of whole antigen. This state lasts only a few hours.

The shock. The manifestations of anaphylactic shock resemble those of histamine poisoning. They vary considerably in different species, but in any one species the reaction is fairly constant.

Guinea-pig. A few seconds after the injection of the shocking dose, the animal begins to twitch its nose. It rapidly develops respiratory distress, having great difficulty in expiration. Cyanosis appears, and death from asphyxia usually occurs within 5 to 10 minutes. The symptoms are due to severe bronchospasm, and over-distension of the lungs can be demonstrated at necropsy.

Rabbit. The onset of shock is slower than in the guinea-pig. The animal becomes unsteady, rests on the ground, and frequently urinates and defaecates. Cyanosis develops, consciousness is lost, and in well-sensitised animals death follows. There is generalised arteriolar constriction which affects the pulmonary vessels in particular. Measurements of pulmonary blood pressure reveal hypertension, and death is usually ascribed to acute cor pulmonale.

Dog. The dog shows a fall in systemic blood pressure. It is believed that the hepatic veins undergo constriction, leading to acute venous congestion of the liver and organs drained by the portal system. Vomiting of blood and diarrhoea occur before death. There is an increase in the clotting time due to the release of heparin.

Rat. The animal exhibits prostration, rapid and laboured breathing, cyanosis, hypotension, hypothermia, and marked haemoconcentration.

Human being.[2] The symptoms of anaphylaxis in the human closely resemble those of the guinea-pig, being characterised by acute respiratory distress of an asthmatic type. Generalised oedema develops, causing obvious swelling of the eyelids and dependent parts. Oedema of the larynx may add to the respiratory distress caused by bronchospasm. Itching and diffuse erythema of the skin may occur. Urticaria is characteristic.

Anaphylaxis is rare in the human, and usually follows the injection of horse serum, e.g. ATS, either intravenously or intramuscularly. It may also follow bee stings and the administration of drugs, e.g. penicillin and neoarsphenamine. In two cases it has been reported to follow sexual intercourse, being due to antibody directed against mucoprotein present in seminal fluid.[3] Occasionally the shock resembles that seen in the dog, rabbit, or rat.

It has been suggested that sudden death in infancy ('cot death') is due to hypersensitivity to milk. The sensitised child is presumed to inhale regurgitated milk during sleep and to die of acute anaphylaxis. But this hypothesis has received little direct support, and the cause of cot death still awaits solution. Infection may be important in some cases.[4]

Although the manifestations of anaphylaxis vary in different species, the disturbance is fundamentally the same in all of them. The two main effects are:

(1) *Spasm of smooth muscle*—either blood vessel or bronchial.

(2) *Damage to small blood vessels and an increase in their permeability.* Generalised oedema, although not obvious in animals, may nevertheless be demonstrated.

Systemic anaphylaxis is a generalised reaction affecting all parts of the body, though not with equal intensity. Some organs appear to be particularly sensitive, and the disturbances produced in them not only dominate the clinical picture but may also cause death. This is well illustrated by anaphylaxis in the dog. The liver is the organ most affected; obstruction to the hepatic venous outflow causes circulatory failure followed by death. In hepatectomised dogs anaphylaxis can still be demonstrated, but with much greater difficulty.

Cutaneous Anaphylaxis

If a small quantity of antigen is injected into the skin of a sensitised animal, an immediate local reaction occurs which is characterised by erythema and increased vascular permeability. A weal forms in the human but not in animals, and intravenous trypan blue is given to detect the increase in vascular permeability (p. 75).

This type of reaction may be used clinically to detect sensitisation before giving a large therapeutic dose of foreign serum, thereby avoiding acute anaphylactic shock and possibly death.

Unfortunately, the results of such skin tests are not a reliable indication of a possible sensitisation to anaphylaxis. The antibodies that cause skin sensitisation are not necessarily the same as those responsible for anaphylaxis. It is suggested that the safest procedure when administering foreign sera is to give a small test dose subcutaneously and watch for any mild general reaction. Adrenaline and a syringe should, of course, be at hand (see p. 232).

Pathogenesis of Anaphylaxis[1]

There is abundant evidence that anaphylaxis is initiated by the interaction of antigen with antibody; this leads to the release of pharmacologically active compounds that are directly responsible for the characteristic features of the syndrome. There has been much speculation in the past concerning the type of antibody involved, the site of the interaction, and the nature of the chemicals released. *It is now evident that at least two groups of antibodies are concerned and that there are at least two distinct mechanisms whereby the shock is produced.* Much of the experimental work performed in the past was on actively sensitised animals in which both mechanisms were involved, either separately or in combination. The anaphylactic shock produced under one set of circumstances was not identical with that produced under different experimental conditions; thus many apparently conflicting findings were published. Sometimes complement was shown to be involved in anaphylaxis and sometimes not. Likewise, antihistamine drugs may or may not protect. The use of passively sensitised animals has clarified the situation, because relatively pure antibody can be administered in known quantity and its role in sensitisation to anaphylaxis can be assessed.

Cytotropic anaphylaxis. Anaphylaxis is described as *cytotropic* when it is the result of antigen reacting with immunoglobulin (IgE in the human) fixed to cells—usually mast cells. When the antibody is manufactured by the test animal itself, or in passive anaphylaxis by an animal of the same species, the antibody is termed *homocytotropic*. When the antibody is derived from a different species it is called *heterocytotropic*. Cytotropic anaphylaxis is the classical type of reaction as exemplified by anaphylaxis in the actively sensitised guinea-pig.

Aggregate anaphylaxis. This type of anaphylaxis occurs in the actively sensitised rabbit, and is due to the formation of antibody-antigen aggregates in the circulation. Fixation of antibody to cells plays no part in the pathogenesis of aggregate anaphylaxis, but activation of complement is vital and polymorphs are essential.

Both types of anaphylaxis must be examined in more detail.

Cytotropic Anaphylaxis

This type of anaphylaxis is dependent upon immunoglobulin in the circulating blood becoming attached to certain target cells and thereby sensitising them.

Evidence that circulating antibodies are involved.

(1) The blood of a sensitised animal contains antibodies which precipitate with the corresponding antigen or hapten.

(2) That these antibodies are related to the sensitisation is indicated by the evidence derived from passive sensitisation.

Passive sensitisation. Serum from one sensitised animal will, if injected intravenously, sensitise another animal to anaphylaxis. The passive sensitisation is made manifest only after a time-interval of several hours. It appears therefore that the mere presence of circulating antibody is not sufficient, and that some other conditions have to be fulfilled before sensitisation can occur. The present evidence suggests that antibody has first to be fixed to cells. The Schultz-Dale phenomenon and passive skin sensitisation provide more conclusive evidence.

Schultz-Dale phenomenon. If a piece of the uterine muscle is removed from a sensitised guinea-pig, it is found to contract vigorously when placed in contact with the antigen. The muscle is first thoroughly washed in Tyrode solution to remove blood and serum, and then suspended in a bath containing Tyrode solution at 37°C. The addition of antigen to the bath results in contraction, which can be recorded by means of a suitable system of levers. The Schultz-Dale reaction can also be carried out on uterine muscle sensitised *in vitro* by immersing it in sensitising antibody, and also by using the uterus removed from a passively sensitised animal. Isolated intestinal muscle behaves in the same way as myometrium. As under the conditions of these tests no blood or plasma is present, it seems certain that the antibody is firmly fixed to the cells.

Passive cutaneous anaphylaxis. A small amount of serum

from a sensitised animal* is injected into the skin of a guinea-pig, and this is followed a few hours later by an intravenous injection of antigen mixed with Evans blue. Within a few minutes an exudative reaction is detectable by the leakage of the dye into the skin site.

Reversed passive cutaneous anaphylaxis. If *antigen* is injected into the skin of an animal it will sensitise the skin provided it is itself an immunoglobulin that will fix on to the tissues, e.g. rabbit serum injected into guinea-pig skin. When a specific antibody is injected intravenously some hours later, a local reaction is seen at the site of the injected skin. This is termed reversed passive cutaneous anaphylaxis. *Reversed systemic anaphylaxis* may similarly be produced by injecting antigen intravenously followed some time later by a specific antibody.

Guinea-pigs sensitised to anaphylactic shock can be desensitised by repeated small injections of antigen. In this way a very high titre of circulating antibody is produced. Administration of antigen to such an animal does not produce anaphylaxis, because the circulating antibody is sufficient to neutralise all the injected antigen, none being left over to react with fixed antibody.

Target cells involved in cytotropic anaphylaxis. Although anaphylaxis is produced by an antigen-antibody interaction in close association with cells, precisely which cells are involved is by no means certain. Mast cells are important in the guinea-pig, rat, dog, and mouse; these show degranulation and are presumed to release histamine. In the rat 5-hydroxytryptamine is released, whereas in the dog sufficient heparin enters the circulation to cause prolongation of the clotting time. In the human the polymorphs are thought to be involved, and in the rabbit both polymorphs and platelets. Whether fixation occurs in other cells, e.g. the liver macrophages, argentaffin cells, or the parenchymal cells of skin and muscle, is not known. It is evident that very considerable species differences exist, and that if human disease is to be elucidated, people themselves must be investigated.

Mediators of cytotropic anaphylaxis.[5] The action of specific antigen on mast cells coated with specific IgE is to cause the release of the following agents: *histamine, 5HT, SRS-A, ECF-A, platelet activating factor*, and *prostaglandins*. These are described below. In addition, the platelets release vasoactive amines as part of the platelet release reaction.

Histamine. Histamine can be detected in the blood in acute systemic anaphylaxis, and is released if antigen is applied to sensitised tissue *in vitro*. Antihistamine drugs inhibit the production of acute anaphylactic shock, and likewise if a sensitised animal is depleted of histamine by the administration of a histamine-releasing agent like compound 48/80, it is protected temporarily.

5-Hydroxytryptamine (serotonin). This is present in the platelets of all species and in the mast cells of rats and mice. Its release may be important in anaphylaxis of these rodents.

Slow-reacting substance of anaphylaxis (SRS-A). If the lungs of a sensitised guinea-pig are perfused with a fluid containing antigen, histamine can be demonstrated in the fluid issuing at the beginning of the experiment. Alternatively, antigen can be added to lung chopped into small pieces. Later, another

---

*This test will not detect the IgE responsible for human anaphylaxis.

substance appears, which, when applied to isolated uterine muscle, causes a slow sustained contraction, unlike the more rapid 'kick' produced by histamine. This substance is a lipid of unknown composition, and might be responsible for the bronchospasm seen in the human subject. Histamine is not so important in this connexion; histamine-releasing compounds given to humans cause pruritus, oedema of the face, and hypotension, but not bronchospasm.

Eosinophil chemotactic factor of anaphylaxis (ECF-A). This is probably responsible for the local accumulation of eosinophils that is such a prominent feature of some local type-I hypersensitivity reactions in the human subject.

Platelet activating factor. This triggers the platelet release phenomenon and leads to the liberation of vasoactive amines from the platelets.

Kinins. There is evidence that kinin-forming enzymes are activated in anaphylactic shock.

If one compares the mediators of cytotropic anaphylaxis with those of acute inflammation, one is struck by the similarity of the factors involved. Indeed, the main reactions are very similar in both phenomena, for both are characterised by an increased vascular permeability. However, in our present state of knowledge it would be unwise to pursue the analogy too far.

Species variation. In addition to the species variation as regards the target cells and the nature of the mediator released, there is very considerable difference in the type of response and sensitivity of different species to these agents. Thus the human being and guinea-pig are highly sensitive to histamine, whereas the mouse and rat are very insensitive. The reverse is true of serotonin. It is hardly surprising that the manifestations of anaphylaxis vary so greatly from one species to another (p. 175).

Protracted anaphylaxis. Although the manifestations of anaphylactic shock in the guinea-pig are very similar to those of histamine poisoning, antihistamine drugs do not completely counteract the shock. Indeed, when death in the acute phase is prevented, the animal sometimes dies of protracted shock some hours later. The cause of this syndrome of *protracted anaphylaxis* is not known, but it has been suggested that a continuing production of kinin is responsible. The animals show hypotension and hypothermia. At necropsy there is congestion of and haemorrhage into the abdominal viscera but no overinflation of the lungs. A similar prolonged anaphylaxis has been demonstrated when antigen is given to a sensitised animal by the intraperitoneal or subcutaneous route so that its absorption is delayed.

Aggregate Anaphylaxis[1]

The recognition of this type of anaphylaxis was based on various observations which were contrary to what would be expected in the classical anaphylaxis of the guinea-pig. In the rabbit the sensitivity to anaphylactic shock is proportional to the level of plasma antibody; a high level does not confer immunity. Passive transfer in this species is best accomplished by injecting a large dose of antibody, and the sensitisation is immediate, indicating that cell fixation is not a prerequisite. Furthermore, complement is required, and sensitisation to shock can be abolished by depleting the animal of complement, e.g. by injecting zymosan.

Aggregate anaphylaxis is a type III reaction, and the damaging antigen-antibody complexes are produced in the circulating blood. Precipitates are formed, and the complement system is activated. The anaphylatoxins (C3a and C5a) are produced, and they lead to the release of histamine from mast cells. C567 component causes polymorphs to join the aggregates, and these can be seen in the circulation. They plug the capillaries in many organs, but more important than the mechanical interference with the circulation is the liberation of their damaging lysosomal contents.

Antibodies Concerned in Anaphylaxis[1]

The sensitising immunoglobulins may be divided into two groups: the *cytotropic antibodies*, which are responsible for cytotropic anaphylaxis, and a second group responsible for *aggregate anaphylaxis*.

Cytotropic anaphylaxis antibodies. In the guinea-pig and the mouse the important antibody is a 7S, γ_1 or fast γ-globulin. It is thermostable and will sensitise animals of the same species to cytotropic anaphylaxis. This type of antibody is therefore called a *homocytotropic antibody*, and a similar type of immunoglobulin is produced in other species. In the human the important antibody concerned in anaphylaxis is thermolabile, and is an IgE immunoglobulin. It was originally called a *reagin*, and is non-precipitating. It has the unusual property of *firm, long-lasting fixation to skin*, and on this property the Praunitz-Küstner reaction is based (p. 178). It is difficult to detect it in serum by the commonly used *in-vitro* tests, but it can be recognised and measured by highly sensitive methods such as the radio-immuno-inhibition technique and by the use of living cells (p. 178).

Aggregate anaphylaxis antibody. This is a γ_2 or slow γ-globulin which acts as a precipitin and can *fix complement*. It can passively sensitise an animal of the same species to aggregate anaphylaxis. A confusing facet of this subject is that this antibody, when injected into an animal of a *different species*, will sometimes sensitise it to cytotropic anaphylaxis. The latter type of anaphylaxis is therefore called *heterocytotropic anaphylaxis*.

Conclusion

The precise manifestation of anaphylaxis exhibited by an actively sensitised individual depends upon the relative proportions of the various sensitising antibodies which are produced. It is probable that all commonly used laboratory animals can manufacture antibodies for both cytotropic and aggregate anaphylaxis, but that preference is often shown for one of them. Thus, γ_1-globulin predominates in the guinea-pig, γ_2-globulin in the rabbit, and IgE immunoglobulin in the human.

Anaphylactoid shock. A condition very like anaphylactic shock can be produced by the intravenous injection of the following substances:

1. Antigen-antibody mixtures—especially those with moderate antigen excess. This in fact is a type of aggregate anaphylaxis.

2. Serum which has been incubated with kaolin, starch, and other polysaccharides—this procedure leads to the formation of kinins and anaphylatoxin by the activation of complement *via* the alternate pathway.

3. Forssman antibody. Some writers refer to this as an example of 'cytotoxic anaphylaxis'. It is a type II reaction.

4. Trypsin. This leads to the formation of kinin.

5. Peptone.

6. Salts of heavy metals.

DUST AND FOOD HYPERSENSITIVITY AND ATOPY[6]

This group of hypersensitivity reactions occurs after the ingestion of certain foods and the inhalation of antigens like pollen and dust. The symptoms differ according to the route of absorption, and there is considerable variation from one person to the next. The offending chemical may be a complete antigen or a hapten: the latter presumably combines with tissue or plasma proteins to produce a complete antigen.

Types. *Inhalation* of antigens like pollen, horse dander, and dust usually produces symptoms referable to the respiratory tract, e.g. allergic rhinitis (hay-fever), and asthma of the extrinsic type.

Ingested substances produce either gastrointestinal symptoms or skin eruptions of an urticarial type. Shellfish, mushrooms, strawberries, and milk are among the numerous foods to which some people are sensitive.

Nature of the lesions. The lesions are exudative, and frequently contain eosinophils. The appearance of these cells in the secretions in hay-fever and asthma is of diagnostic value, and is presumably due to the formation of ECF-A (p. 177). Blood eosinophilia may also be conspicuous. It will be recalled that eosinophils are also present in many parasitic diseases, in which allergic manifestations are often prominent. Eosinophils are not, however, a feature of atopic dermatitis.

Characteristics. *Genetic influence.* Patients with this type of hypersensitivity frequently give a family history of similar complaints. The pattern of reaction differs in members of the same family; one may have hay-fever, another asthma, and another atopic dermatitis. What is inherited is the capacity to react to antigens in this peculiar way. The antigens involved may vary, because they are determined by environmental factors. Nevertheless, families are on record in which there has been a constantly recurring response, e.g. hypersensitivity to a particular food.

Hypersensitivity in which there is a strong hereditary element and expressed in hay-fever, asthma, and atopic dermatitis, is called *atopy*. The basis for this may be an overproduction of sensitising IgE, perhaps accompanied by a deficiency of IgA, IgG, or IgM.[7] Thus atopy is often a feature of immunological deficiency states, e.g. the Wiskott-Aldrich syndrome, IgA deficiency, and Bruton's agammaglobulinaemia.

Sensitisation. Previous contact with either antigen or hapten is necessary, but as only small quantities are needed, the event may be forgotten. Nurses who spill streptomycin on their fingers may react with skin eruptions to subsequent injections of the drug; they would, however, deny any previous streptomycin treatment.

Detection. A scratch test or intradermal injection with the antigen produces an immediate-type reaction with a weal appearing in a minute or two. This occurs whether the hypersensitivity is of respiratory, alimentary, or cutaneous type. Haptens may not produce a positive test until they are first conjugated with protein. Some, e.g. aspirin, produce a reaction if applied to the buccal mucous membrane or the tongue.

Skin testing is of limited value in atopic patients. Such individuals tend to make sensitising IgE against many antigens, and it is often impossible to decide which of the positive results is of significance in relation to the current illness.

The sensitivity shown by some individuals is extreme. Thus the active antigens in the grass pollens are polypeptide or protein carbohydrate substances of low molecular weight, and doses of the order of $10^{-7}\gamma$ to $10^{-8}\gamma$ are sufficient to elicit an intradermal reaction in a sensitive person; 10 000 times this dose given intravenously can be fatal.

Passive transfer. Although for a long time antibodies could not be detected in the serum by the ordinary *in-vitro* techniques, serum will passively sensitise a normal person. This was first demonstrated by Prausnitz and Küstner.

Prausnitz-Küstner (P-K) reaction. Küstner was hypersensitive to cooked fish. Some of his serum was injected into Prausnitz's skin, and after 24 hours this area responded to the local injection of an extract of cooked fish by the immediate formation of a weal. The ingestion of fish was also capable of eliciting an urticarial reaction in the local area. This passive hypersensitivity remained for weeks, but was dissipated after eliciting the P-K reaction. The P-K test is still performed, but is inconvenient and exposes the test subject to the danger of viral hepatitis. Monkeys may be used, but they are now more scarce than humans!

Antibodies. The IgE antibodies detected by the P-K reaction were originally called reagins. They have a strong affinity for human and monkey skin but not that of other species. A reliable *in-vitro* method of detecting them would be of great value in the investigation and treatment of patients with hypersensitivity, and many techniques, none of them very satisfactory, have been devised. Thus in ragweed-sensitive people it is found that the addition of antigen to the patient's white cells leads to the release of histamine. Chopped human lung can be sensitised passively *in vitro* so that, on addition of antigen, histamine and SRS-A are released. This release can be inhibited by β-adrenergic drugs such as adrenaline, and the action has been ascribed to an increase in the cell's content of cyclic AMP. α-Adrenergic stimulation has the converse effect.[8] A rather similar observation is that the basophils of penicillin-sensitive patients show degranulation when mixed with the drug. Monkey ileum can be sensitised with human IgE and used in a Schultz-Dale reaction.

Another method is the exposure of the patient's serum to red cells to which antigen has been attached. IgE coats the cells but, being an incomplete antibody, causes no agglutination. The addition of anti-human IgE globulin causes agglutination. In this way the IgE levels in the blood may be measured, and the results in one group of patients (exposed to castorbean extract) with asthma correlated well with the clinical state and with the level of IgE as measured by passive cutaneous anaphylaxis using the baboon.[9] IgE protein obtained from a patient with myeloma will specifically inhibit the P-K reaction, presumably by competing with the other IgE antibody. Indeed, there seems little doubt that human reaginic antibody is an IgE immunoglobulin, the level of which is raised in asthma, hay-fever, and atopic eczema.

Desensitisation in the human. Very small doses of antigen administered at 30-minute intervals may be given without the occurrence of anaphylactic shock. Fixed antibody is steadily neutralised, but the desensitisation is of temporary duration and the method is not recommended since it may be followed by accelerated serum sickness (see also p. 180).

Antigen administered in weekly doses of increasing size confers some degree of desensitisation. This method is used in hay-fever and asthma, but the results are not uniformly satisfactory. The mechanism involves the production of excess antibody, some of which is of the blocking type. This type of antibody, when injected into a P-K prepared site, will desensitise the skin so that the antigen no longer provokes the response, i.e. it 'blocks' the reaction. This it does by competition for antigen. The degree of hypersensitivity which an individual exhibits may thus be related to the relative proportions of heat-labile sensitising IgE and heat-stable blocking antibody.

Desensitisation is of no value in the prevention or treatment of the skin manifestations of atopy (infantile eczema and atopic dermatitis). Indeed, there is no obvious relationship between the dermatitis and the presence of sensitising IgE. Exacerbations of the dermatitis are not apparently related to contact with, or ingestion of, the antigens to which the patient is sensitive, as demonstrable by skin tests.

As previously pointed out, the hypersensitivity under consideration is of the immediate type. Histamine and SRS-A are the important mediators that are released. Antihistamines counteract the vascular effects, but, as would be expected, not the bronchial-muscle spasm (see p. 177). Glucocorticoids, however, have the converse effect, and find an important place in the treatment of asthma.

Infection

Immediate-type hypersensitivity to microbial products may develop during the course of an infection. Thus, during convalescence from lobar pneumonia, an injection of the capsular polysaccharide (SSS) of the causative pneumococcus into the skin produces an immediate-type reaction (weal). The Casoni test is a similar reaction, and is used in the diagnosis of hydatid disease. Whether this type of sensitisation plays any part in the pathogenesis of lobar pneumonia is not known (see p. 222).

TYPE II HYPERSENSITIVITY

This type of hypersensitivity is mediated by antibodies which react with tissue components and are usually cytotoxic. The following are examples of this, and are considered in greater detail elsewhere:

Autoantibodies against blood cells. Autoimmune haemolytic anaemia and idiopathic thrombocytopenic purpura are examples.

Drug-induced lesions. For example Sedormid purpura (p. 639) and the anaemia caused by α-methyldopa (p. 614).

Cytotoxic alloantibodies. See haemolytic disease of the newborn (p. 613).

Autoantibodies against tissue components. Antibodies against glomerular basement membrane in Goodpasture's syndrome is an example of this type. The production of LATS in Graves's disease may be included under this heading.

TYPE III HYPERSENSITIVITY

This type of hypersensitivity is dependent on the formation of damaging antibody-antigen complexes: hence the alternative name *immune-complex disease.*

THE ARTHUS PHENOMENON

This can be demonstrated both in humans and animals. Repeated weekly subcutaneous injections of antigen even into different areas lead to progressively more severe local reactions. Oedema and erythema appear within 1 hour, and over the next few hours haemorrhage and necrosis develop. Microscopically, there is an acute inflammatory reaction with a massive accumulation of polymorphs both within the vessels and in their walls. Necrosis of the vessel wall leads to haemorrhage, and completes the picture of an acute vasculitis (Fig. 14.1).

Pathogenesis. The interaction of antigen with antibody in the vessel walls leads to the formation of complexes which activate complement. The formation of anaphylatoxins and chemotactic factors leads to an acute inflammatory reaction and the accumulation of many polymorphs. Antigen, antibody, and complement can be detected in the vessel walls by immunofluorescent techniques and electron microscopy. The polymorphs release their lysosomal enzymes, and the damage produced contributes to the increase in vascular permeability and the tissue necrosis. There is no evidence that histamine is a mediator, nor do antihistamine drugs inhibit the reaction. The Arthus reaction cannot be elicited in an animal depleted of polymorphs, nor in one depleted of complement by the prior administration of zymosan or the venom of the cobra *Naja naja.*

The antibody concerned in the Arthus reaction is of the precipitating IgG type. Passive transfer (passive Arthus reaction) can be demonstrated by the intravenous injection of antibody, e.g. 10 mg in the rabbit. This large dose contrasts with the much smaller quantities required to transfer sensitivity to anaphylaxis of either the cytotropic or the aggregate type. No latent period is required, and there is no cell fixation.

This explanation is supported by the phenomenon of the *reversed passive Arthus reaction.* This is demonstrated when a local injection of antibody (obtained from a sensitised animal) is introduced into the skin of a normal animal, which is then given a large intravenous dose of corresponding antigen. Thus, an Arthus-type reaction can be produced whenever antigen and appropriate complement-fixing antibody meet in the vessel wall.

SERUM SICKNESS

Serum sickness differs from most other forms of hypersensitivity response in that only one dose of antigen is

Figure 14.1
The Arthus reaction. This section is taken from a rabbit, and it includes the subcutaneous tissues and the underlying muscle (Musc). The blood vessel in the centre is sectioned obliquely and shows occlusion of its lumen by thrombus. Its walls are heavily infiltratedaby polymorphs (Poly), many of which are degenerating. Free red cells (RBC) in the tissues bear witness to the severity of the vascular damage. ×470.

necessary to produce it. It usually appears between the 7th and 14th day after the administration of a foreign protein, e.g. therapeutic serum of horse origin. The reaction may be accelerated, appearing after 3 or 4 days, in patients who have had serum previously; occasionally it may occur immediately. The main features are fever and a skin eruption, which is sometimes first apparent at the site of injection. A generalised urticarial or morbilliform eruption is frequently seen. The skin lesions often cause intense irritation. Other features are generalised lymphadenopathy, joint pains, oedema of the eyelids and dependent parts, proteinuria, and early leucopenia followed by leucocytosis. Increased vascular permeability accounts for many of the signs of the disease. Polymorphonuclear leucocytes leave the circulation, and can be found in the oedema fluid.

Experimental production. A single large injection of foreign protein in a rabbit produces a disease with lesions similar to those described in the few fatal cases of human serum sickness. By using ^{131}I-labelled antigen the following sequence of events may be observed (Fig. 14.2):

1. There is an immediate drop in the blood level of antigen due to equilibration with extravascular, extracellular fluids.

Figure 14.2
Time relations between fall of circulating antigen, formation of antigen-antibody complexes, lesions of serum sickness, and rise of circulating antibody in rabbits injected with large doses of ^{131}I-labelled bovine serum albumin. (*From Gladstone, G. P. (1961), in Florey, H. W. General Pathology, 3rd edn., after Dixon, F. J. et al. (1959), in Lawrence, H. S. Cellular and Humoral Aspects of the Hypersensitive States, p.354 New York: Harper and Row.*)

2. During the first 10 days the blood level of antigen is high, but shows a slow progressive fall because of its catabolism.

3. From the 10th to 13th day antigen is rapidly catabolised, and by the 13th day none is present in the circulation. This rapid disappearance of antigen is called *immune catabolism*. During this period even the antigen which is still present in the blood is bound to antibody, and fluorescent techniques have demonstrated that soluble antigen-antibody complex is also found in the affected inflamed arteries.

4. From the 13th to 14th day the disease abates, all antigen is eliminated, and precipitating antibodies appear in the blood.

On the basis of these observations the following mechanism is postulated: the disease is caused by persistence of circulating antigen which reacts with newly-formed antibody. As only one exposure to antigen is given, the delay of 7 to 14 days is easily explicable in that this is the usual time-interval for antibody production after a primary injection. The damaging antigen-antibody reaction occurs in certain tissues, but when once the antigen is combined with antibody, it is rapidly catabolised. The disease is therefore self-limiting. Finally excess antibody is produced, and appears in the circulation.

Antigen-antibody complexes are formed in the circulation and are deposited in the vessel walls. As in the Arthus reaction, complement is activated, polymorphs accumulate and release their enzymes, and tissue damage results. An acute vasculitis is the characteristic lesion and is seen in many organs, for instance the skin and heart. The development of these lesions can be prevented by the prior depletion of complement or polymorphs. Another characteristic lesion of experimental serum sickness is glomerulonephritis; immune complexes are deposited in the glomerular basement membrane as granular deposits. There is a proliferation of glomerular cells but, unlike the other vascular lesions, polymorphs do not accumulate. Increased vascular permeability accounts for the proteinuria.

The deposition of antigen-antibody complexes in the vessel wall is probably due to a local increase in vascular permeability mediated by histamine. Antihistamine drugs therefore inhibit the development of the lesions of acute serum sickness. In the rabbit it is believed that the histamine is derived from platelets which adhere to the complexes by the process of immune adherence (p. 146). An alternative explanation is that leucocytes sensitised by specific IgE release soluble factors when acted upon by antigen. The factors cause the clumping of platelets and the release of histamine and serotonin.[10] Whatever the mechanism, a local increase in vascular permeability appears to be the important event which localises the lesions of serum sickness.

The pathogenesis of the Arthus reaction and acute serum sickness both involve the formation of immune complexes which initiate complement activation and result in vascular damage. They are conveniently grouped together under the term *immune-complex disease*, and it is instructive to consider some other examples at this point.

Chronic immune-complex disease. If daily injections of antigen are given to animals in doses such that antigen-antibody complexes with antigen excess are formed in the blood, a chronic glomerulonephritis develops. Histologically there is thickening of the basement membrane (membranous change), and fluorescent studies reveal a coarsely granular deposit containing antigen, antibody, and complement. This 'lumpy-bumpy' deposit can be located electromicroscopically on the epithelial side of the basement membrane. The pathogenesis is similar to that of acute serum sickness, but the dominant lesion is renal—a localisation which is not explained. It appears that the kidneys are readily damaged by circulating immune complexes; this mechanism may be the explanation of the renal component of many diseases, particularly those associated with a chronic infection (often viral) and in individuals with a defective immune response, e.g. the *glomerulonephritis* of lupus erythematosus, post-streptococcal nephritis, NZB and NZB/NZW mice, Aleutian mink disease, and lymphocytic choriomeningitis[11] of mice.

Other organs may be affected. After the use of killed measles vaccine, a natural infection with measles virus can cause an excessive *lung lesion* due to immune complexes;[12] a similar response can be seen with respiratory-syncytial-virus infection.[13] *Immune-complex arthritis*[14] and *urticaria* may occur with viral hepatitis, especially in the virus B type. Polyarthritis, urticaria, and angio-oedema are the main features of this syndrome, which has also been noted with other viral diseases, e.g. rubella, mumps, vaccinia, and variola.

Detection of immune complexes in serum.[15] The detection of immune complexes in the circulation now constitutes an important means of investigating immune-complex disease. Many methods are available, but none is easy. Some methods depend on the physical or chemical properties of the large complexes. In one of them the property of forming a precipitate with Clq is utilised by an agarose gel technique.[16] Another promising method utilises the peculiar properties of the Raji cell,[17] a neoplastic B-type lymphocyte derived from a patient with Burkitt's lymphoma. The cells have various surface receptors for IgG and complement components. In particular the receptors for C3b are of importance, because it is to them that immune complexes adhere. Hence Raji cells incubated with test serum can be shown to have adherent immune complexes by the use of tagged anti-human immunoglobulin; the tagging may be done by either a fluorescent or a radioactive-isotope method. These methods can detect immune complexes, but they are not specific. In the investigation of a specific condition it is often desirable to detect complexes containing a particular antigen. Such methods are available, but are not in routine use.

Some Clinical Examples of Hypersensitivity Mediated by Immunoglobulins

In clinical practice it sometimes happens that hypersensitivity reactions are mediated by several mechanisms, commonly a combination of type I and type III responses. Three subjects will be described: acute allergic vasculitis, drug hypersensitivity, and allergic lung disease.

Acute Allergic Vasculitis

Many forms of acute vasculitis are believed to be examples of immune-complex disease. Vasculitis of the vessels in the subcutis is a feature of erythema nodosum leprosum (p. 153), in which immune complexes and complement can be demonstrated in the inflamed vessel walls. In the common type of erythema nodosum affecting the subcutaneous tissues of the shins in young women, drugs (often the birth-control pill) or a streptococcal infection often provide the antigen component of the complexes that are presumed to be deposited. Vasculitis of the dermis is a feature of the skin lesions of *Streptococcus viridans* endocarditis, meningococcal septicaemia, and gonococcal septicaemia (p. 510). Histologically the lesions closely resemble those of the Arthus reaction.

Drug Hypersensitivity[18, 19]

Hypersensitivity to drugs is a common clinical event and is due to the drug, or one of its degradation products, acting as a hapten and stimulating the formation of sensitising antibodies. Virtually any drug can produce a reaction, but common offenders are penicillin,[20] sulphonamides, aspirin, para-aminosalicylic acid (PAS), barbiturates, and quinine. Relatively few people given a drug manifest hypersensitivity, and the tendency to do so is probably inherited. Thus atopic individuals are particularly at risk especially in respect of IgE-mediated effects.

Types of drug reaction. The reaction may be *immediate*: if the drug is given by injection it can occur within a few minutes. Urticaria is common and in more severe cases laryngeal oedema, asthma, hypotension, and death complete the features of acute anaphylaxis. Immediate reactions are due to the presence of sensitising IgE antibodies.

Later drug reactions begin several days after the administration of the drug and have the features of immune-complex disease. Urticarial, morbilliform,* petechial, and other types of skin eruptions are common, and the addition of arthralgia, renal damage, and fever produce a disease resembling serum sickness. In other cases individual features may occur alone, e.g. renal damage, drug fever, or acute vasculitis of the skin. Antibodies concerned in these reactions are either IgG or IgM.

Late drug effects are thrombocytopenia (p. 639), haemolytic anaemia (p. 614), erythema multiforme (which if severe and affecting the mucous membranes is called the Stevens-Johnson syndrome), cholestatic jaundice, and a syndrome resembling systemic lupus erythematosus. Methicillin appears to be responsible for some cases of interstitial nephritis, and is accompanied by anti-renal-tubule basement-membrane antibodies.[22] The pathogenesis of many of these effects is obscure. In some instances, e.g. haemolytic anaemia, cytotoxic antibodies are present (type II reaction); they may be directed against the drug as in penicillin-induced haemolytic anaemia, or against the red-cell surface antigens, an effect induced by α-methyldopa (p. 614).

Detection of drug sensitisation. With most drugs it is not possible to detect sensitisation other than by giving a test dose. The sensitivity to penicillin has been the most studied. Benzylpenicillin is broken down to several products. The major component forms a benzylpenicilloyl haptenic group which appears to be unimportant, because not only does it induce the formation of IgE antibodies but also IgG blocking ones. A minor breakdown product is benzyl penamaldic acid mixed disulphide group which acts as a hapten for the

*The morbilliform rash that commonly occurs when ampicillin is administered to patients with infectious mononucleosis is not a hypersensitivity reaction, and does not indicate future hypersensitivity to penicillin.[21] Possibly it is a type of Jarisch-Herxheimer reaction.

formation of sensitising IgE only. It is possible to perform skin tests using these components, but the test itself can lead to sensitisation. This may be avoided by using a reagent composed of the haptenic group attached to a small synthetic polypeptide. Nevertheless, skin tests detect only IgE sensitising antibody, and do not eliminate the possibility of the presence of IgG or IgM, which can lead to immune-complex effects. Skin testing is therefore not a routine clinical procedure. *In-vitro* tests are described on page 178.

Allergic Lung Disease [23-25]

Lung tissue is constantly confronted with airborne antigens, and it is not surprising that allergic disease is common. Several patterns of reaction can be found:

The extrinsic type of bronchial asthma. This is a component of atopy and is a type I reaction mediated by IgE. It has been described above.

Extrinsic allergic alveolitis.[26] This disease is due to the inhalation of fine particles of organic material and the subsequent development of precipitin, IgG, sensitising antibodies. The later exposure to the same dust results in an immune-complex reaction in the alveoli (type III reaction). Clinically there is a sudden onset of fever, headache, dyspnoea, and cough coming on 4 to 6 hours after exposure. The lung compliance is decreased and the pulmonary defect is restrictive in contrast to the airways obstruction of bronchial asthma. The best known example of extrinsic allergic alveolitis is *farmer's lung*; the antigen is derived from fungal spores in mouldy hay. Many other examples are known and are related to occupation, habit, or hobby. The antigen can be fungal (baggassosis and malt-worker's lung) or of insect or animal origin (bird fancier's lung, pituitary-snuff taker's lung, etc.).

Asthma with pulmonary infiltrates and eosinophilia. This is a mixed group and is mediated by a combination of types I and III hypersensitivity. The term Loeffler's syndrome has been applied but this is not a defined entity. Some cases are due to parasites. *Broncho-pulmonary aspergillosis* is due to the colonisation of cavities or bronchi by *Aspergillus fumigatus* and the development of sensitising IgE and IgG. Skin tests reveal an immediate reaction followed later by an Arthus-type response. The condition should not be confused with an aspergilloma,[27] in which a fungus-ball forms in a pre-existing cavity or area of necrosis.

There are other types of lung disease in which an allergic basis has been postulated with varying degrees of conviction. Thus there is Goodpasture's syndrome (type II reaction) and the various forms of pulmonary vasculitis (see p. 211).

TYPE IV (DELAYED-TYPE) HYPERSENSITIVITY[28]

As the main features and pathogenesis of anaphylactic and immune-complex hypersensitivity were clarified, it became evident that there also existed a separate, completely distinct type of hypersensitivity. Its recognition stemmed from the early observations of Robert Koch on the effects of tuberculous infection in guinea-pigs. Since similar reactions were noted in other infections the term *bacterial allergy* was applied. However, the term is not appropriate because immediate-type hypersensitivity may also be induced by bacteria. **Delayed-type** is a more acceptable term, and it can occur not only as the result of infection but also as a response to antigens of non-bacterial origin. **Cell-mediated hypersensitivity** is another term which is commonly used to describe these reactions, since it is currently believed that they are mediated by the activity of cellular antibodies. The term is useful in that certain immune-complex reactions which are related to humoral antibodies may take many hours to develop, and are therefore difficult to distinguish if the classification is based strictly on the time taken for the reaction to appear. In this book the terms delayed-type, cell-mediated, and type IV reactions are used synonymously. The subject is most easily understood by first considering Koch's observations.

The Koch Phenomenon

If tubercle bacilli are injected into a normal guinea-pig, there is an incubation period of 10 to 14 days followed by the appearance of a nodule at the site of injection. Ulceration follows and persists till the death of the animal. The bacilli spread to the local lymph nodes, finally reach the blood stream, and produce generalised miliary tuberculosis and death. The injection of tubercle bacilli into an animal infected 4 to 6 weeks previously evokes a different type of response. A nodule appears in 1 to 2 days, ulcerates, and then heals. There is little tendency to spread to the local lymph nodes. This second type of response was described by Koch, and it should be noted that the reaction of a tuberculous animal to tubercle bacilli differs from that of a normal one in three important respects:

1. The incubation period is greatly shortened—this may be described as hypersensitivity.
2. The lesion heals quickly.
3. There is no spread. These are the features of immunity.

The heightened tissue response of the tuberculous animal can be demonstrated not only to the living tubercle bacillus, but also to dead organisms and extracts of organism. Koch originally used 'old tuberculin', but more recently a Purified Protein Derivative (PPD) has been introduced.

The intradermal injection of a small quantity of PPD into a normal animal results in a negligible inflammatory response. In the tuberculous animal, however, there develops a raised erythematous lesion **appearing within 24 hours and reaching a peak by 72 hours.** This is the *Mantoux*, or *tuberculin*, *test*, and a positive result indicates the existence of hypersensitivity to tuberculoprotein. The delay in the appearance of the reaction is noteworthy, and contrasts with the rapid appearance of anaphylactic reactions. The injection of a larger quantity of PPD into a tuberculous animal may result in a flare-up of the local tuberculous lesion. Attempts to 'immunise' patients may therefore do more harm than good.

Tuberculin shock. The injection of a relatively large dose of PPD into a highly sensitised animal will produce a systemic reaction characterised by prostration, hypothermia, and death within 30 hours. Inhalation of an aerosol can have the same effect.

Although tuberculoprotein is capable of eliciting the Mantoux reaction in a sensitised subject, it does not induce this delayed type of hypersensitivity. It is antigenic, but its use as a sensitising agent results in the development of immediate-type hypersensitivity.

Under natural conditions bacterial allergy occurs only as a result of infection with the organism. A conversion from Mantoux-negative to positive during the course of an undiagnosed illness is therefore good evidence of its tuberculous aetiology. If the infection is completely eradicated the test may, over a period of years, revert to negative. Nevertheless, the Mantoux test is of great importance clinically since a positive reaction indicates a past or present tuberculous infection.

Delayed-Type Hypersensitivity in Other Infections

Hypersensitivity reactions akin to the Mantoux test are of diagnostic value in other infections, and indicate the existence of sensitisation. The following tests may be cited: Frei (lymphogranuloma venereum), coccidioidin (coccidioidomycosis), histoplasmin (histoplasmosis), and blastomycin (blastomycosis).

The intradermal injection of lepromin elicits a tuberculin-like reaction at 24 to 48 hours, which is called the *Fernandez reaction*, but even more significant is a much more slowly developing papular lesion which develops in about 4 weeks, and is diagnosed by biopsy when epithelioid-cell granulomata are sought. This is called the *Mitsuda reaction*; a similar type of test is done in sarcoidosis (Kveim test, see p. 261) and to diagnose hypersensitivity to zirconium salts (p. 137). The lepromin test is negative in lepromatous leprosy and positive in the tuberculoid type* as well as in many non-lepers. Hypersensitivity to Candida antigen, mumps antigen, streptokinase, streptodornase, and trichophytin is very common in normal people. A negative response to these, and to tuberculin and coccidioidin in California, indicates an abnormal state (see anergy, p. 141).

It seems certain that this type of hypersensitivity develops in many chronic infections, and indeed plays an important part in the production of the lesions. Even in acute infections delayed-type hypersensitivity may occur. Thus, following lobar pneumonia a delayed-type skin reaction can be demonstrated by injecting the specific pneumococcal protein. Delayed-type hypersensitivity to antigens of infective agents is seen after recovery from many, if not all, viral infections. This aspect is further discussed in other parts of this book (see lobar pneumonia, p. 222, syphilis, p. 249, typhoid, p. 94, and smallpox, p. 274).

Features of Delayed-Type Hypersensitivity

Active induction. Delayed-type hypersensitivity may be induced in humans or animals by the following methods:

Infection. This has been described above.

Injection of antigen with adjuvants. Delayed-type hypersensitivity develops if antigen is injected together with Freund's complete adjuvant (p. 140). The essential component of the tubercle bacillus appears to be a high-molecular-weight mycoside, termed Wax D. The explanation of this observation is not known, but there is some evidence to suggest that the local tissue response to the injection is of some importance. If a simple antigen, e.g. egg albumin, is injected into a tuberculous focus in an animal, both immediate and delayed-type hypersensitivities develop to the egg protein.

*The Mantoux test may also be positive, and the two mycobacteria concerned appear to have antigens in common. BCG vaccination has been advocated in leprosy prophylaxis.

Application of simple chemicals to skin. Hydrophobic compounds are most effective since they penetrate the skin more readily than do hydrophilic substances. Detergents aid absorption and, therefore, sensitisation. Sensitisation by skin application, e.g. of picryl chloride, dinitrochlorobenzene, and 2-ethoxymethylene-5-oxazolone (oxazolone),[29] have been used extensively in animal experimental work (p. 153). In the human subject many agents lead to allergic contact dermatitis (p. 185).

Tissue grafting. See Chapter 15.

Time of appearance of reaction. The reaction is not visible before 12 hours and is maximal at 24 to 72 hours. Injected antigen finds no antibody with which to interact and there is no immediate reaction. The reaction is dependent upon an intact blood supply to the part, and presumably sensitised lymphocytes and macrophages are brought to the site. The stimulus for this emigration is not known, but one may suppose that the cells accumulate slowly and that this is the explanation of the delay which is typical of all cell-mediated hypersensitivity responses.

Type of tissue response.[28] An early acute inflammatory response with oedema and polymorph infiltration is soon followed by an accumulation of macrophages, lymphocytes, sometimes eosinophils and mast cells, and later epithelioid cells and giant cells. The predominant reaction is mononuclear in contrast to the exudative response of anaphylaxis and the polymorph accumulation of the immune-complex reaction. In severe reactions necrosis is prominent.

Inhibition of reaction. Glucocorticoid administration inhibits delayed-type responses, but the effect is non-specific since many inflammatory responses are also affected. The effect is temporary, and reactivity returns on withdrawing the drug. Antihistamine drugs produce no inhibition.

Specificity. With few exceptions, the delayed-type hypersensitivity responses are even more specific than the usual serological and immediate-type reactions. When hapten-protein conjugates are used, the sensitisation is directed against both the hapten and the carrier protein.

Tolerance. Delayed-type hypersensitivity cannot be induced in animals rendered tolerant by the procedures listed on page 141. A curious feature noted in guinea-pigs is that animals given picryl chloride by gastric tube, to avoid contact with skin, are permanently tolerant to this chemical, so that subsequent application to the skin does not produce sensitisation. The mechanism is not understood.

Passive transfer. Although antibodies of precipitating, agglutinating, and complement-fixing types can be found in the serum, they are not causally related to the hypersensitivity. An injection of these immunoglobulins into a normal animal does not passively transfer the state of hypersensitivity. This contrasts markedly with the immediate-type sensitisation which is transferable by serum. It seems certain that immunoglobulins are not concerned, and this is supported by the observation that patients with agammaglobulinaemia can become Mantoux-positive, although they are virtually incapable of forming immunoglobulin antibodies.

Delayed-type hypersensitivity can be transferred to another animal by transferring living cells. Intraperitoneal injections of splenic or lymph-gland cells from a tuberculous animal will confer passive hypersensitivity. There is no appreciable latent period, and the hypersensitivity lasts for as long as the grafted cells survive, e.g. months if syngeneic cells are used. Passive transfer has been reported in guinea-pigs using serum from irradiated sensitised donors.[30] It is postulated that a cell-bound factor can be released into the circulation by the irradiation.

The mechanism whereby transferred lymphocytes render the host hypersensitive is poorly understood. One possibility is that the specific sensitised lymphocytes accumulate selectively at the site of antigen administration, and are therefore responsible for the positive reaction. By labelling lymphocytes with tritiated thymidine in the donor the fate of injected cells can be followed. Results are contradictory—some workers claim that donor cells accumulate specifically at the site of a skin test, while others maintain that the majority of cells are of host origin. The latter is almost certainly correct and supported by the following experimental observation: if lymphocytes from an immunised host are injected into an X-irradiated animal, immunoglobulin antibody formation can be detected (see adoptive immunity, p. 164). The transferred cells do not, however, support the transfer of delayed-type hypersensitivity, indicating that host cells are necessary. These results apply to animals; in the human host cells are certainly involved, for the injection of small numbers of white cells from the blood of a sensitised person (e.g. 0·1 to 0·5 ml of a concentrate) will transfer hypersensitivity of bacterial, fungal, viral, and contact-dermatitis types. This passively induced, delayed-type hypersensitivity is generalised, appears within 24 hours, and lasts for many months. Furthermore, in contrast to the findings in animals, transfer can be effected by extracts of white cells. The active agent is called transfer factor.

Transfer factor.[31,32] This is a stable substance that has the property of transferring sensitivity to previously uncommitted lymphocytes. It has a molecular weight of under 10 000 daltons, and consists of a short polypeptide chain joined to three or four RNA bases. The precise mode of action of this remarkable substance is not known.

Antibody involved. There are two theories:

Serum antibody. It has been suggested that delayed-type hypersensitivity is, like other immune phenomena, mediated by serum antibodies, and that since passive transfer by serum cannot be demonstrated, the antibodies must be in very low concentration and of high avidity. Alternatively the antibodies might be of a special class (*cytophilic antibody*) such that they have a high affinity for lymphocytes and macrophages. Another variant of this theory is that antibody is produced locally by lymphocytes when stimulated by antigen. The antibody reacts locally, and does not appear in detectable amounts in the serum. It seems unlikely that any of these explanations is true.

Cellular antibody. The alternative and currently accepted hypothesis is that the antibody concerned in delayed-type hypersensitivity is entirely *cell-bound*. This theory is attractive in that it explains the failure of serum transfer, and also that it presupposes the existence of a completely separate type of antibody. The unsolved mystery of the transfer factor certainly indicates that the mechanisms involved in delayed-type hypersensitivity are separate from those related to immunoglobulin production. So also do the effects of thymectomy and bursectomy (p. 151).

Figure 14.3
Specific inhibition by antigen of the migration of cells from sensitised animals. The cells, mostly macrophages and lymphocytes from a peritoneal exudate, are placed in capillary tubes and incubated in a microchamber. Normally the macrophages migrate from the open end and produce a tufted appearance. The cells derived from animals with delayed-type hypersensitivity show no migration in the presence of the specific antigen. (*From David, J. R., Al-Askari, S., Lawrence, H. S., and Thomas, L. (1964), Journal of Immunology,* **93,** 264.)

In spite of the potent effects exhibited by sensitised lymphocytes *in vivo,* the manner by which they produce tissue damage is poorly understood. As described on page 148, when T-lymphocytes come into contact with specific antigen, a number of potent low-molecular-weight factors called *lymphokines* are liberated.[33,34] Insofar as cell-mediated hypersensitivity is concerned, lymphotoxin is probably the most important, but the other factors may recruit cells and augment the inflammatory reaction. In practice, the most useful *in-vitro* test has been one that measures the migratory inhibitory factor.

This can be demonstrated by packing the lymphocytes and macrophages from the peritoneal exudate of a sensitised guinea-pig into a capillary tube and incubating it in a suitable chamber containing culture fluid. Normally the cells migrate from the free ends of the tube to form tufts. These tufts do not appear if the cells from a guinea-pig showing delayed-type hypersensitivity are incubated in the presence of antigen (Fig. 14.3). If cells from a normal animal, mixed with about 10 per cent of cells from a sensitised one, are placed in a tube and cultured in the presence of antigen, *none* of the cells migrate. Hence a few sensitised cells can transfer information to other cells *in vitro,* just as they can *in vivo.* It should be noted that lymphocytes from an animal sensitised towards immunoglobulin production and not delayed hypersensitivity do not show this phenomenon.

The effect of antigen on sensitised human cells can be assessed by using white blood cells from the buffy coat. If these are packed into capillary tubes as described above, their migration is inhibited by antigen to which the patient is sensitive.

Allergic Contact Dermatitis[35]

The occurrence of a localised dermatitis following the repeated exposure of the skin to a chemical is a frequent event. Sensitisation may occur to a wide variety of substances; tulips, primulas, poison ivy, wool, iodine, atropine, paraphenylenediamine (used as a hair dye), and nickel are common examples. The last is usually seen in women; costume jewellery and the nickel-plated buckles of watch-straps and brassières cause dermatitis where they come into contact with the skin. Sensitivity to chromium compounds is an important cause of industrial dermatitis, since chromium is present in cement, paint, and other products used in the building trade.[36] It is also a cause of shoe dermatitis, because chromium is used in the tanning process of leather.

Heredity is sometimes involved, but the liability to become hypersensitive is not related to atopy. The reaction is essentially local, and consists of intra-epidermal oedema with vesiculation and a dermal inflammatory reaction. The lesions are therefore dermatitic. The offending substance taken by mouth is harmless. Only direct application to the skin is effective.

Sensitisation can be detected by a *patch test*: the suspected agent is kept in contact with the skin for 24 hours, and a positive reaction is indicated by the appearance of swelling and redness about 24 hours later.

Performing a patch test is not without its disadvantages, for the test may itself induce hypersensitivity in persons not previously sensitive. Sometimes following a negative response a *flare reaction* occurs at the site of the test 10 to 20 days later. This is due to persistence of the antigen at the test site, and the mechanism is therefore analogous to that of serum sickness. The ability to develop hypersensitivity to dinitrochlorobenzene is used clinically to test the cell-mediated immune response.

The patch test can be demonstrated on any part of the body surface, and has the characteristics of delayed-type hypersensitivity. Passive transfer can be obtained only by injecting sensitised cells or transfer factor. The condition therefore closely resembles other cell-mediated reactions, except that the skin is the only tissue where this hypersensitivity is normally manifested.

The offending chemical probably acts as a hapten, and by combining with skin protein produces a potent antigen. A plausible explanation of the delayed-type hypersensitivity which develops is that this new antigen is in fact a living skin cell, and is therefore treated like a foreign graft. Once sensitisation has occurred, further application of the chemical to the skin results in the reformation of the abnormal cells, and therefore a 'graft rejection' phenomenon occurs. An alternative, but less satisfactory explanation is that lipids of the skin act as adjuvants in much the same way as perhaps the wax of the tubercle bacillus.

It is interesting that atopic eczema, although generally linked with asthma, appears to be due to a delayed-type hypersensitivity. Indeed, it has been reported that lymphocytes from atopic patients sensitive to grass pollen, when cultured in the presence of specific antigen, show blast transformation and the formation of IgE antibody.[37,38] The atopic diseases, although classified as examples of immediate hypersensitivity, are clearly complex and poorly understood. Since they are so common they are deserving of careful study.

Experimentally-Produced Autoimmune Disease

There is considerable evidence that autoimmune encephalomyelitis is cell mediated (see Ch. 16).

Allograft Rejection

The hypersensitivity which develops during the rejection of an allograft is of the cell-mediated type. This is considered in Chapter 15.

The Retest Phenomenon[39]

If a positive tuberculin test is performed on a hypersensitive person, and the same site is retested with tuberculin at a later date, an accelerated reaction is observed. It appears at 2 hours and is maximal at 8 hours. The lesion is characterised by an exudation of fluid and a massive accumulation of eosinophils. Immediate-type hypersensitivity is not involved, but the mechanism concerned in the retest reaction is not known. Perhaps a specific chemotactic lymphokine for eosinophils is liberated[40] (p. 148). This phenomenon deserves further study, for eosinophils develop in response to repeated injections of antigen or antigen-antibody complexes, and many human diseases of an 'allergic' nature are also characterised by exudation and eosinophil infiltration. These are curiously unresponsive to antihistamine drugs (e.g. asthma, allergic rhinitis, nasal polyps, etc.).

The Jones-Mote Reaction

If repeated small doses of protein antigen are injected into the skin of guinea-pigs or human beings, a state of delayed-type hypersensitivity develops. This phase is usually transient and is soon replaced by Arthus-type hypersensitivity as immunoglobulins appear in the blood. It seems unlikely that this Jones-Mote type of delayed hypersensitivity is the same as the classical delayed type; the skin reactions tend to develop rather more quickly and to fade earlier. Histologically they are characterised by the accumulation of basophils, and the term *cutaneous basophil hypersensitivity* has been proposed.[41,42] Its role in human pathology remains undetermined, but it may be related to the presence of basophils in some inflammatory lesions, e.g. in the lesions of allergic contact dermatitis.[43]

OTHER TYPES OF HYPERSENSITIVITY[44]

Other types of hypersensitivity reactions are known that do not readily fit into the four categories previously described. Thus the stimulating effect of antibody (LATS) on thryoid cells has been cited as an example of 'type V' hypersensitivity. The retest phenomenon and the Jones-Mote reaction have been described above.

Another example is *antibody-dependent cellular cytotoxicity*, in which target cells coated with immunoglobulin are killed by non-immune effector cells, whether lymphocytes, macrophages, or polymorphs.

SUMMARY

It is evident that in response to antigenic stimulation the body is capable of reacting in a variety of ways. Antibodies are produced which have the effect of altering the individual's response to the same antigen should this substance be introduced on a subsequent occasion. The best-known antibodies are the immunoglobulins found in the plasma. These may neutralise toxins or aid in destroying micro-organisms and thereby confer immunity on the individual. Alternatively the immunoglobulins may lead to sensitisation of the immediate type. The difference between those antibodies which confer immunity and those which cause hypersensitivity appears to be qualitative rather than quantitative. The liability of an individual to produce sensitising antibodies is, to some extent at least, determined by genetic factors.

The role of the cell-bound type of antibody is more difficult to understand. The sensitised lymphocytes release factors which can kill cells and induce an inflammatory reaction. In particular the macrophages are affected, and they become more phagocytic to bacteria, and by remaining localised may be an important factor in the localisation of infection. Sensitised lymphocytes are responsible for the features of delayed-type hypersensitivity. It is not known whether immunity and delayed-type hypersensitivity are two aspects of a single process or whether they are distinct and separable components of the cell-mediated immune response. At first sight the tissue destruction of allergic contact dermatitis or at the site of a positive Mantoux reaction may seem to be of no advantage to the individual. The process may be seen in a different light when it is remembered that cellular antibodies are usually produced against living cells (see p. 199). These cells may be foreign, as with bacteria and grafts, or they may be host cells altered by contact with chemicals or following degenerative or neoplastic changes. Destruction of these cells would be of great survival value to the individual. The value of immediate-type hypersensitivity is more difficult to see, but it is possible that the inflammatory reaction which results is of advantage in that cells and plasma are brought rapidly to the site of bacterial invasion. Nevertheless, of the two types of hypersensitivity the delayed type appears to be more closely related to immunity than does the immediate type.

REFERENCES

1. MIESCHER, P. A. & MUELLER-EBERHARD, H. J. (1976) *Textbook of Immunopathology*, 2nd edn, Vols 1 and 2. New York: Grune and Stratton.
2. AUSTEN, K. F. (1974) Systemic anaphylaxis in the human being. *New England Journal of Medicine*, **291**, 661.
3. LEVINE, B. B., SIRAGANIAN, R. P. & SCHENKEIN, I. (1973) Allergy to human seminal plasma. *New England Journal of Medicine*, **288**, 894.
4. Leading Article (1970) Sudden death in infancy. *Lancet*, **2**, 1021.
5. BROCKLEHURST, W. E. (1975) In *Clinical Aspects of Immunology*, ed. Gell, P. G. H., Coombs, R. R. A. & Lachmann, P. J., 3rd edn, p. 821. Oxford: Blackwell.
6. PEPYS, J. (1975) In *Clinical Aspects of Immunology*, 3rd edn, p. 877, *loc. cit.*
7. KAUFMAN, H. S. & HOBBS, J. R. (1970) Immunoglobulin deficiencies in an atopic population. *Lancet*, **2**, 1061.
8. ORANGE, R. P., AUSTIN, W. G. & AUSTEN, K. F. (1971) Immunological release of histamine and slow-reacting substance of anaphylaxis from human lung. I. Modulation by agents influencing cellular levels of cyclic $3',5'$-adenosine monophosphate. *Journal of Experimental Medicine*, **134**, 136S.
9. COOMBS, R. R. A. *et al.* (1968) Detection of IgE (IgND) specific antibody (probably reagin) to castor-bean allergen by the red-cell-linked antigen-antiglobulin method. *Lancet*, **1**, 1115.
10. COCHRANE, C. G. (1971) Mechanisms involved in the deposition of immune complexes in tissues. *Journal of Experimental Medicine*, **134**, 75S.
11. OLDSTONE, M. B. A. & DIXON, F. J. (1971) Immune complex disease in chronic viral infections. *Journal of Experimental Medicine*, **134**, 32S.
12. FULGINITI, V. A. *et al.* (1967) Altered reactivity to measles virus. Atypical measles in children previously immunized with inactivated measles virus vaccines. *Journal of the American Medical Association*, **202**, 1075.
13. CHANOCK, R. M. *et al.* (1968) Possible role of immunological factors in pathogenesis of RS virus lower respiratory tract disease. *Perspectives in Virology*, **6**, 125.
14. KOFF, R. S. (1971) Immune-complex arthritis in viral hepatitis? *New England Journal of Medicine*, **285**, 229.
15. ZUBLER, R. H. & LAMBERT, P. H. (1977) In *Recent Advances in Clinical Immunology*, ed. Thompson, R. A. number one, p. 125. Edinburgh: Churchill Livingstone.
16. AGNELLO, V., WINCHESTER, R. J. & KUNKEL, H. G. (1970) Precipitin reactions of the Clq component of complement with aggregated γ-globulin and immune complexes in gel diffusion. *Immunology*, **19**, 909.
17. THEOFILOPOULOS, A. N., WILSON, C. B. & DIXON, F. J. (1976). The Raji cell radioimmune assay for detecting immune complexes in human sera. *Journal of Clinical Investigation*, **57**, 169.
18. DASH, C. H. & JONES, H. E. H. (1972) *Mechanisms in Drug Allergy*. Edinburgh: Churchill Livingstone.
19. PARKER, C. W. (1975) Drug allergy. *New England Journal of Medicine*, **292**, 511, 732 and 957.
20. LEVINE, B. B. (1972) Skin rashes with penicillin therapy: current management. *New England Journal of Medicine*, **286**, 42.
21. Annotation (1969) Ampicillin rashes. *Lancet*, **2**, 993.
22. FLAX, M. H. (1974) Drug-induced autoimmunity. *New England Journal of Medicine*, **291**, 414.
23. MCCOMBS, R. P. (1972) Diseases due to immunologic reactions in the lungs. *New England Journal of Medicine*, **286**, 1186 and 1245.
24. Leading Article (1969) Organic dusts and allergic lung diseases. *Lancet*, **1**, 1195.
25. Leading Article (1970) Allergic alveolitis. *British Medical Journal*, **1**, 708.
26. KATZ, R. M. & KNIKER, W. T. (1973) Infantile hypersensitivity pneumonitis as a reaction to organic antigens. *New England Journal of Medicine*, **288**, 233.
27. Leading Article (1977) Aspergilloma. *Lancet*, **1**, 637.
28. TURK, J. L. (1975) *Delayed Hypersensitivity*, 2nd edn. Amsterdam: North Holland.
29. OORT, J. & TURK, J. L. (1965) A histological and autoradiographic study of lymph nodes during the development of contact sensitivity in the guinea-pig. *British Journal of Experimental Pathology*, **46**, 147.
30. DUPUY, J.-M., PEREY, D. Y. E. & GOOD, R. A. (1969) Passive transfer, with plasma, of delayed allergy in guineapigs. *Lancet*, **1**, 551.
31. LAWRENCE, H. S. (1970) Transfer factor and cellular immune deficiency disease. *New England Journal of Medicine*, **283**, 411.
32. Leading Article (1974) Transfer factor. *British Medical Journal*, **2**, 397.
33. Leading Article (1973) Lymphokines. *Lancet*, **1**, 1490.
34. Leading Article (1978) Lymphokines: an increasing repertoire. *British Medical Journal*, **1**, 62.
35. CALNAN, C. D. & TURK, J. L. (1975) In *Clinical Aspects of Immunology*, 3rd edn, p. 1019, *loc. cit.*
36. POLAK, L., TURK, J. L. & FREY, J. R. (1973) Studies on contact hypersensitivity to chromium compounds. *Progress in Allergy*, **17**, 145.
37. BROSTOFF, J., GREAVES, M. F. & ROITT, I. M. (1969) IgE in lymphoid cells from pollen-stimulated cultures. *Lancet*, **1**, 803.
38. WARD, P. A. (1971) Complement-derived leukotactic factors in pathological fluids. *Journal of Experimental Medicine*, **134**, 109S.
39. ARNASON, B. G. & WAKSMAN, B. H. (1963) The retest reaction in delayed sensitivity. *Laboratory Investigation*, **12**, 737.
40. COHEN, S. & WARD, P. A. (1971) *In vitro* and *in vivo* activity of a lymphocyte and immune complex-dependent chemotactic factor for eosinophils. *Journal of Experimental Medicine*, **133**, 133.
41. RICHERSON, H. B., DVORAK, H. F. & LESKOWITZ, S. (1969) Cutaneous basophilic hypersensitivity: a new interpretation of the Jones-Mote reaction. *Journal of Immunology*, **103**, 1431.
42. RICHERSON, H. B. (1971) Cutaneous basophil (Jones-Mote) hypersensitivity after 'tolerogenic' doses of intravenous ovalbumin in the guinea-pig. *Journal of Experimental Medicine*, **134**, 630.
43. DVORAK, H. F. & MIHM, M. C. (1972) Basophilic leukocytes in allergic contact dermatitis. *Journal of Experimental Medicine*, **135**, 235.
44. PATTERSON, R., ZEISS, C. R. & KELLY, J. F. (1976) Classification of hypersensitivity reactions. *New England Journal of Medicine*, **295**, 277.

Chapter 15.   The Graft Reaction

Having described the immunological response to bacteria and simple antigens, no study of immunity would be complete without including the body's response to complex living cells. This includes the allied subjects of graft immunity and autoimmunity.

TRANSPLANTATION OF TISSUES[1,2]

Although it is usually assumed that the art of grafting is a modern one, it is interesting to note that it has been performed for over two thousand years. Local skin flaps were used by Indian surgeons for the operation of rhinoplasty, and the techniques were described by Celsus. During the fifteenth century the use of pedicle flaps was devised in Italy, but the practice fell into disrepute because of the opposition of surgeons and the Church. For nearly 300 years no further advance was made, until in 1794 two Army doctors stationed in India witnessed the operation of rhinoplasty performed by an Indian surgeon, and reintroduced the art into England. With the development of anaesthesia in the nineteenth century and the advent of two world wars in the twentieth century plastic surgery came into its own, and with it extensive transplantation of tissue. In addition to the practical value in surgery of transplantation of tissue, recent work on grafting has done much to extend our knowledge of the body's response to foreign tissues.

Classification of Transplants

The terms transplant and graft are used synonymously. They may be conveniently classified in the following ways:

Species of origin. Grafts may be classified as autologous, homologous, or heterologous.

An autograft is a transplant made from one site to another site in the same individual.

A homograft is a transplant made from one individual to another of the same species. If the two individuals are syngeneic (isogeneic), i.e. of identical or nearly identical genetic structure, then the terms *syngeneic homograft* or *isograft* are used. In the human being this applies only to grafts from one identical twin to another. In all other instances, when the two individuals are of different genetic make-up, the terms *allogeneic homograft* or *allograft* are used. In practice the unqualified term homograft is taken to refer to the latter type of graft.

A xenograft, or *heterograft*, is a transplant from one animal to another of a different species.

Nature of the tissue transplanted. Tissue may be fetal, normal mature, or neoplastic. It may be transplanted directly from the donor, or there may be some intermediate period of storage or growth *in vitro*.

Viability of the graft. Those grafts whose function is

Figure 15.1
The Chimera, a mythical monster who dwelt in Lycia, was the terror of the neighbourhood, until she was killed by Bellerophon mounted on his winged steed, Pegasus.

> A mingled monster of no mortal kind:
> Behind, a dragon's fiery tail was spread,
> A goat's rough body bore a lion's head,
> Her pitchy nostrils flaky flames expire,
> Her gaping throat emits infernal fire.
> Iliad, VI, 180.

Quoted in Precope, J. (1954), *Medicine, Magic and Mythology*, p. 160. London: Heinemann.
The term *chimera* is now used in medicine to describe an animal which for long periods contains living cells belonging to another individual who is genetically different. The condition may arise naturally, as in the case of binovular twins sharing a common placenta, or artificially by the immunological tolerance technique of Medawar or by the induction of irradiation chimerism. (*Photograph of an Etruscan bronze by courtesy of the director of The Archaeological Museum, Florence*)

dependent upon the continued survival of their cells are called *vital*. This contrasts with a *static* graft in which the cells die, but the matrix performs an important function, e.g. many bone grafts. Thus, one may have homovital and homostatic grafts if the material is derived from a member of the same species.

Method of grafting. Grafts are called free, when they are completely disconnected from the donor before subsequently being implanted in the host site. They may be grafted by means of pedicle transplants, in which case they remain partially attached to the donor's site for a while. In general such grafts are autologous, although homologous pedicle transplants have been tried, and are called parabiotic transplants.

A third manner of transplantation is by vascular anastomosis: the major blood vessels of the transplant are connected with those of the host at the time of operation. This method is used for transplanting kidney, liver, and heart.

Site of grafting. An *isotopic* graft is one which is placed in an anatomical position similar to that from which it came, e.g. the cornea to cornea. An *orthotopic* graft is one which is surrounded in the host by the same kind of tissue as that previously present in the donor, e.g. skin grafted from the leg to the arm. A *heterotopic* graft is one which is placed in a situation which differs from that of the donor site. An example of this is the transplantation of cornea to a sub-cutaneous situation.

For practical purposes the most important feature of any graft is its origin. Therefore it is convenient to subdivide grafts into the three main groups—autografts, homografts, and xenografts.

AUTOGRAFTS[1]

Autotransplantation, the transplantation of tissues from one site to another in the same individual, occurs spontaneously in a variety of conditions. It is a familiar feature of malignant tumours when they metastasise, but also occasionally occurs with some normal tissues. It is believed, for instance, that the cells of the haematopoietic tissues are capable of circulating in the blood and settling down in abnormal sites. Rupture of the spleen is occasionally followed by the implantation and growth of splenic tissue in the peritoneal cavity (*splenosis*).

Deliberate autotransplantation is frequently carried out surgically, and such grafts survive provided they once become established; the conditions necessary for this may be classified as follows:

Tissue must be healthy. Transplants do not survive if the tissue is subjected to undue mechanical or chemical trauma.

Freedom from infection. Sepsis effectively prevents vascularisation, and leads to rapid necrosis of the graft.

Adequate nutrition. In tissues which have a reasonably high oxygen requirement, large free transplants undergo central necrosis because vascularisation does not occur sufficiently fast to prevent death of tissue.

Hormonal stimulation. Free transplants of endocrine glands are more likely to be successful if the animal is deficient in that type of tissue. This is sometimes known as *Halsted's law*, but it is not strictly true and was not first described by him; it was noted in 1905 by Cristiani. It is not the deficiency of the endocrine secretion itself which stimulates the growth of the graft, but rather the excess of pituitary hormone which is attendant upon the deficiency.

Nervous stimulation. Muscle grafts, even when embryonic, atrophy unless left attached to their nerve supply.

Mechanical stimulation. Bone grafts persist only if subjected to a mechanical stimulation. Heterotopic grafts in soft tissue tend to disappear.

Temperature. Free testicular grafts take only if placed in sites where the temperature is lower than that of the remainder of the body; thus in the rabbit testicular grafts can grow in the ears.

Other factors. Free autografts of pieces of kidney, liver, and pancreas may survive for a while, but always die later. The whole organs can be transplanted successfully if connected by vascular anastomosis.

FATE OF AUTOGRAFTS[1]

The body does not respond by any immunological mechanism, and provided the local conditions are satisfactory, most autografts survive. Avascular tissue, like cartilage and cornea, can live without vascularisation, but with all other grafts survival is dependent upon the acquisition of an adequate blood supply.

Vascularisation. It has long been debated whether the vessels which supply autografts are those of the original transplant, or whether they are new ones derived from the local site. It appears that vascularisation occurs in two phases. During the first 3 days new host capillaries develop and anastomose with the existing vessels of the graft. In this way rapid vascularisation is accomplished. During the second phase which occurs from the fourth day onwards, the graft is invaded by new host vessels. Some of these grow along the lumina of the original vessels of the graft. It seems fairly certain that the small capillaries of the graft persist, but that larger vessels, although they may develop a circulation during the first phase, do not long persist.

Tissue induction. The term *induction* is used to describe the changes which occur in one tissue as a result of the juxtaposition of other tissues. The best-known example is the ossification which is induced in connective tissue by heterotopic autotransplants of urinary-tract epithelium. It is also found that fascia used to suture bladder injuries may undergo ossification; gall-bladder epithelium has similar 'osteogenic' properties.

Creeping substitution. This process, although not the same as induction, has many features in common with it. It is applied to the process whereby a graft is gradually replaced by host tissue. It is, for instance, believed that grafts of bone are steadily replaced by host bone. Similarly, nerves are invaded by axons from the host, and transplanted blood vessels appear to be steadily replaced by host tissue.

FUNCTIONS OF GRAFTS

Autografts usually function in exactly the same way as do normal tissues. However, skin and bone function only if transplanted orthotopically. The endocrine glands present certain special problems. If ovarian, testicular, and possibly thyroid tissue is transplanted into an area which is drained by the portal vein, its secretion is carried to the liver and inactivated. Although the graft may function normally, it fails to produce the expected, generalised hormonal effect. Although the anterior pituitary may survive if transplanted heterotopically, its function is retained only when it is placed under the median eminence of the tuber cinereum; only in this situation does it receive the necessary hypothalamic hormonal stimulation.

HOMOGRAFTS[1, 3]

There are two types of homograft, the *syngeneic*, in which there is genetic identity between donor and recipient and the *allogeneic*, in which there is genetic disidentity. It is the latter, usually called an *allograft*, that evokes a rejection reaction, and is the subject of this discussion. Indeed, it is around the fate of the allograft that great interest continues to be centred, firstly because of the potentialities of grafting tissue from one individual to another, and secondly because of the fundamental biological properties that the homograft reaction has revealed. These have far-reaching effects in many branches of medicine.

FATE OF HOMOGRAFTS

Allografts are usually rejected, and three patterns of this *homograft rejection phenomenon* may be recognised: 1. *Hyperacute rejection*, 2. *Acute rejection*, and 3. *Chronic rejection*.

Hyperacute rejection. Free grafts are not vascularised, and the graft dies—see white graft reaction, page 191. With transplants attached by vascular anastomosis, the graft vessels become obstructed by polymorphs and fibrin until the circulation through them ceases—see hyperacute renal rejection. Humoral antibodies are mainly responsible for hyperacute rejection.

Acute rejection. Free allografts become vascularised in much the same way as autografts. The graft, however, remains viable for only a limited period. This varies from about 8 days in mice to 13 to 14 days in rats and 2 to 3 weeks in the human: rarely this period may extend to 6 weeks in the human subject. The first sign of rejection of a homograft is infiltration with lymphocytes and pyroninophilic cells, so called because their cytoplasm stains with pyronin due to the presence of many free ribosomes. These cells are of host origin, and are derived from small lymphocytes by transformation (p. 151). Monocytes are also present in the infiltrate, making up about 30 per cent of the population. It has been suggested that sensitised T cells elaborate a lymphokine called *macrophage-arming factor* that can stimulate macrophages to destroy graft cells.[4]

The cellular infiltrate is followed by stasis in the vessels of the graft, thrombosis both in the graft and the bed, haemorrhage, and oedema. Finally the whole graft becomes necrotic, and there follows an acute inflammatory response with an infiltration of polymorphs, which may include a large number of eosinophils. The graft is cast off if on the surface, while in the deeper parts of the body it is invaded by macrophages and granulation tissue.

The survival time of allografts is related to the size of the graft. Thus in rats small grafts may remain viable for 22 days, whereas large grafts survive only for 8 days. It is also worthy of note that where two grafts are applied to the same animal from the same donor, even though the grafts are of a different size, they are both rejected at the same time. These features all point to graft rejection involving an immunological mechanism. The cell-mediated response is the most important.

When the transplant is attached by a vascular anastomosis, the changes are similar. These have been studied most extensively by transplanting kidneys in dogs. It is found that the homotransplanted kidney begins to function within an hour or even less. During the next 3 or 4 days, although the organ functions, it increases in weight and becomes swollen. The cortex is wider than normal and is somewhat nodular.

By the second to third day the cortex shows cellular infiltration with lymphocytes and pyroninophilic cells; later

cells of the plasma-cell series appear. The kidney becomes oedematous, and vascular damage leads to a reduction in blood flow, tubular necrosis, and haemorrhage. In the terminal stages there is an inflammatory response with polymorph infiltration. The glomeruli tend to remain intact until quite late in the process.

The route by which graft antigen reaches the host immune mechanism varies. With skin grafts the presence of intact lymphatics at the host site is important—if these are blocked sensitisation is impeded. With kidney grafts the lymphatics are not important, and activation of the immune response depends either on host cells passing through the kidney or on the release of antigen into the plasma leaving the graft.

Chronic rejection. The graft appears to be accepted, but its vessels gradually become obstructed by intimal thickening. This type of rejection has been most studied in patients with renal and heart transplants.

Factors Which May Determine Long Survival of Homotransplants

Although allografts are usually rejected as described above, there are conditions under which the graft may survive for a long period. These are best divided into three groups.

1. Factors which affect the graft itself. Certain tissues are found to behave differently and to be capable of long survival.
2. Grafts in certain situations behave differently.
3. The condition of the recipient may alter the fate of the graft.

SPECIAL PROPERTIES OF CERTAIN TISSUES

Normal tissues. *Cartilage.* Allografts of cartilage may remain intact with viable cells for months or even years. It is found also that grafts of dead cartilage may remain intact for very long periods. The reason for this long survival is not known, but is presumed to be related to its peculiar composition. It is suggested that its avascularity may play a part, but this explanation is hardly convincing when it is remembered that epidermis is also avascular and yet rapidly rejected.

Cornea. Allografts of cornea remain intact only if grafted isotopically—that is to say, into the eye. Heterotopic transplants are rapidly destroyed. Isotopic grafts of cornea may go cloudy prior to their rejection. Those, however, that do not behave in this way may remain clear and functional for a long time. It is found that when a successful corneal graft is applied to an animal, and some 2 to 6 weeks later a skin graft is applied from the same donor, not only is the skin graft rejected, but at the same time the cornea becomes opaque and is rejected. It therefore appears that the cornea grafted isotopically is nevertheless vulnerable to the rejection mechanism that can be evoked by skin grafting.

It is, however, found that if the skin graft from the same donor as that from which the cornea is obtained is applied 6 weeks or more after the corneal graft, it has no effect on that graft. It would therefore seem that in the rabbit the corneal graft is in danger only during the first 6 weeks, but thereafter is protected from any immunological mechanism which may subsequently be elicited. The explanations offered are:

(*a*) the graft becomes walled off by fibrous tissue;

(*b*) the graft is steadily replaced by host cells or at least its epithelial and endothelial components are replaced;

(*c*) the graft undergoes a change known as *adaptation*, in which it is presumed that the foreign cells are gradually modified to become more acceptable to the mechanisms of the host. An alternative explanation is that immunoglobulins are formed which act as *blocking antibodies*. In this way lymphocytes and macrophages are prevented from attacking the graft cells.

Ovary. There is a vast literature on the results of allografting ovarian tissue; it appears that occasional grafts may survive permanently, or more probably that occasional grafts may survive for a long time. It seems certain that ovarian grafts remain viable longer than do skin grafts.

Tissues from embryos and immature individuals. It is generally stated that fetal tissues grow better and survive longer than do normal mature tissues, but there is much conflicting evidence. There seems little doubt that in the anterior chamber of the eye fetal tissue does grow better. Such a transplant may increase in size 1000 times, while a normal adult tissue increases only three times.

Neoplastic tissue. Under some circumstances there is no doubt that allografts of tumours can grow quite easily. A good example of this is the Brown-Pearce carcinoma of rabbits.

TRANSPLANTATION TO SPECIAL SITES

Anterior chamber of the eye. It is well known that transplants grow particularly well in the anterior chamber of the eye. Medawar has shown that in the rabbit allografts survive indefinitely in this situation, so long as they are not vascularised. Woodruff,[1] on the other hand, has demonstrated survival and vascularisation of allografts of thyroid tissue in the guinea-pig. Fetal tissue may also grow well in the anterior chamber and become vascularised. The actual results of transplanting tissue into the anterior chamber of the eye therefore depend largely upon the species involved and the tissue which is transplanted.

In general it appears that grafts in the anterior chamber excite a slow immune response, that is, slow as compared with grafts placed in other situations. Any immunity already present as the result of previous grafting is made manifest also in the anterior chamber. In addition, it seems likely that the first few weeks in the anterior chamber are critical for the graft. If it survives this period, it is capable of withstanding any immune response. It can even be removed from the anterior chamber and placed in another site, and still grow. This is another good example of a graft showing adaptation.

Brain. Brain, and to a lesser extent testis, kidney, and uterus, are sites where homotransplants seem to survive longer than elsewhere.

FACTORS CONCERNING THE HOST

The antigenic compatibility between graft and host is the single most important factor in determining the fate of a graft. The antigens concerned are the *transplantation antigens*, and are considered on page 673. Since the antigens are determined by *histocompatibility genes*, it follows that the genetic compatibility between graft and host is important. Thus a graft from one identical twin to another (syngeneic homograft, or isograft) excites no immune response and is

treated as an autograft. It is also found that with highly inbred strains of animals, tissues may be freely interchanged between individuals. An exception to this is that in certain strains of mice, grafts donated from males to females die. This is sometimes known as the *Eichwald and Silmser effect*, and is due to a histocompatibility gene on the Y chromosome (p. 43).

Constitutional abnormalities of the host. A variety of conditions may cause prolonged survival of homografts.

Immunological deficiency syndromes. The graft rejection mechanism is impaired in the syndromes described on pages 170 to 172, in which the thymus-dependent system is affected; of the acquired conditions, Hodgkin's disease is the best documented.

Uraemia. It is well known that kidney and skin transplants last longer in uraemic patients.

Pregnancy. Pregnant animals seem more tolerant to allografts (see also p. 194).

Experimental procedures. Experimental procedures including specific immunological tolerance are described later (see pp. 193–194).

HOMOGRAFT IMMUNITY

If following the rejection of an allograft another graft is applied to the same animal from the same donor, this second graft is rejected even more rapidly. This is known as the *second set phenomenon*.

The application of a second skin graft within a short time (about 12 days) of the rejection of the first results in the *white graft reaction*: the graft is not vascularised, but becomes pale, undergoes necrosis, and is cast off. If the second graft is applied after a longer interval, it shows early vascularisation, but suddenly by the fourth to fifth day it becomes cyanosed and the surrounding skin shows marked erythema and oedema. The vessels thrombose and the graft undergoes necrosis. This is termed the *accelerated graft rejection phenomenon*. At the same time the site of the original graft becomes inflamed (*recall flare*) due, it is thought, to persistence of graft antigen.

The same type of rapid rejection has been shown to occur with kidney transplants. If a second kidney from the same donor is grafted into a dog, it begins to secrete urine like the first kidney, but the flow diminishes after 12 hours and stops completely after 24 hours. Histologically there is severe tubular damage with haemorrhage, oedema, and fibrinoid material in the glomeruli. It should be noted that skin grafts will immunise an animal against kidney and *vice versa*.

The leucocytes of the blood are also capable of causing immunisation against skin, and appear to act much more rapidly than do skin grafts. Thus, if white cells are given intraperitoneally, a state of immunity rapidly develops. If white cells are injected intraperitoneally at the same time as skin is grafted, it is found that the skin graft is rejected much more rapidly than a first graft ought to be. This is easily explained by the fact that the injection of leucocytes causes the rapid development of a state of immunity.

It is not difficult to show that the second set rejection phenomenon is dependent upon the development of an immunological reaction. Both humoral and cellular factors have been implicated, and it is instructive to examine the evidence on which the various hypotheses have been based.

Humoral Factors

Following the rejection of a first skin graft there appear in the blood stream a variety of immunoglobulins. Some are capable of agglutinating the red cells of the donor and are therefore called *haemagglutinins*. Haemolysins, leucocytic agglutinins, complement-fixing antibodies, and precipitins have all been described. Factors have also been found in the plasma which are toxic to donor cells grown in tissue culture.

Attempts to transfer the state of immunity to another animal by the injection of serum have not generally been successful, and confirmatory evidence that immunoglobulins were not important in causing graft rejection came from diffusion-chamber experiments. These chambers are composed of a Millipore membrane of a porosity chosen to allow the inward diffusion of soluble substances but to prevent the entry of host cells. Allografts enclosed in such a chamber and placed in the peritoneal cavity of an incompatible host were found to survive even in animals previously immunised. These results have been challenged on the grounds that the pores of the chamber do not allow antibodies and complement to penetrate easily. Furthermore, it has been found that some grafts, usually of tumour tissue, can be destroyed within a diffusion chamber.

It is evident that the immunoglobulins play some role in the rejection of certain grafts under certain circumstances. The following factors are concerned:

1. The amount of transplantation antigen on the cell surface. Cells with a large amount combine with a large amount of antibody, activate complement, and are thereby lysed. Cells with little antigen are protected against complement lysis.

2. The complement-fixing properties of the antibody involved.

3. Physical factors; thus the injection of antibodies in and around a graft can lead to its rejection. Likewise dissociated cells are more readily killed than are solid grafts. The hyperacute rejection in both skin and kidney is mediated by humoral antibodies, and they may also play some part in chronic rejection.

Immunoglobulins sometimes have a second and quite opposite effect on a graft: the life of the graft is sometimes prolonged in an animal which has been passively immunised. This phenomenon is known as *enhancement*. Two mechanisms at least are involved.

1. The antibody may combine with antigenic sites without harming the graft by activating complement. By covering the sites, the immune response is inhibited by blocking the *afferent* pathway so that complement-fixing and cellular antibodies are not produced.

2. The immunoglobulin may compete with immune lymphocytes for the receptor sites on the graft cells. Since immunoglobulin formation will continue, the state of enhancement can be self-perpetuating.

The phenomenon of graft enhancement has a parallel in infection by the tubercle bacillus. The preliminary immunisation of an animal with tuberculoprotein interferes with the development of delayed tuberculin reactivity induced by the administration of BCG.

Cellular Factors

As the relationship between immunity and humoral antibodies is complex, it was not unnatural that cellular factors should be considered. There is much evidence to show that the type of immunity is cell mediated, and indeed the state of immunity to grafts can be passively transferred by the conveyance of lymphoid tissue from an immune animal to a normal one which is syngeneic (*adoptive immunity*). If animals sensitised to a graft are injected intradermally with cells or extracts of cells from the donor strain, an inflammatory reaction akin to the tuberculin reaction ensues. A similar reaction is seen if lymphocytes from the sensitised host are injected into an animal of the donor strain. This is called the *transfer reaction*, and may be regarded as a local graft-versus-host reaction. This occurs only if the animal's own lymphocytes are active, and it can be abolished by prior irradiation.

Passive transfer of homograft immunity can be performed by an intravenous injection of lymphocytes prepared from the regional lymph nodes and spleen of an animal which has rejected a graft. If the transferred cells are suitably labelled, they can be found in the lymph nodes and spleen of the recipient. They do not, however, appear preferentially in a graft when the animal is challenged even though the graft is rapidly rejected. Adoptive immunity of this type cannot be induced in an animal if it has been irradiated previously. Host cells are essential, and it seems that the injected sensitised lymphocytes alter the host's own lymphocytes. Such a transfer of information from sensitised to non-sensitised lymphocyte can also be demonstrated *in vitro* as with the transfer factor of delayed-type hypersensitivity.

There seems little doubt that small lymphocytes are capable of causing the rejection of a graft. Thus, if a tolerant animal with an established graft is injected with syngeneic small lymphocytes from either a normal or a previously immunised animal, the graft is promptly rejected. If the antibodies which cause the accelerated graft rejection are closely associated with the lymphoid series of cells, it is curious that these cells are not always in evidence histologically. The accelerated reaction is characterised by vascular damage and necrosis. The explanation of this is not at all clear.

Antigens concerned.[3] The antigens in tissue grafts which are responsible for the development of homograft immunity are termed the transplantation antigens. They are associated almost entirely with the cell membrane and are of glycoprotein nature, and they have now been isolated with some degree of purity. The transplantation antigens are determined genetically, and are described in Appendix 4.

Distribution of antigens.[5] Transplantation antigens are present in all nucleated cells of the body, but the quantity varies from one tissue to the next. Thus some tissues, e.g. skin and spleen, are rich in antigens, while others are poor, e.g. aorta, muscle, brain, and fat. Liver and lung occupy an intermediate position.

Conclusions. The pathogenesis of homograft rejection is still poorly understood. As with bacterial immunity both humoral and cellular factors have been implicated, but their relative importance differs according to the particular circumstances. It may well transpire that, as in bacterial immunity, cellular and humoral factors work hand in hand. It has, for instance, been found in tumour transplantation work that normal macrophages can be so changed by the addition of specific immunoglobulins that they are enabled to phagocytose tumour cells. They thus behave in the same manner as do the macrophages of an immune animal. It is evident that much careful work has yet to be done before the problems of transplantation immunity can be solved.

Experimental Procedures Which Affect Behaviour in Allografts

Procedures affecting primarily the host. *Total body irradiation.* Although total body irradiation impairs the body's capacity to form antibodies to bacterial toxins and red cells, its effects on grafts are more complex. Total body irradiation does indeed prolong the life of a primary allograft. It does not, however, seem to affect the survival time of second set grafts even though the lymphocyte count is much reduced.

Cytotoxic chemicals. Nitrogen mustards and aminopterin are said to be without effect on the life of allografts. But, other drugs, e.g. azathioprine, are being used clinically for their effect on the survival of kidney and other transplants (see pp. 142 and 196).

Lymphocyte depletion by chronic thoracic-duct drainage impairs the rejection of first set homografts in rats.

Antilymphocytic serum, see page 141.

Reticulo-endothelial blockade. The results obtained by RE blockade are somewhat conflicting, but most workers claim that blockade does prolong graft survival. Most of this work has, however, been done on transplantable tumours, e.g. Brown-Pearce carcinoma in rabbits.

Glucocorticoids. While these can prolong the life of allografts in some animals, there is much species variation. Prednisone is used in the human subject in transplant work (pp. 196–197).

Enhancement. This has been described on page 192.

Procedures affecting the transplant. Procedures designed to alter the antigenicity of the transplant with a view to prolonging its life have been largely unsuccessful.

Specific Immunological Tolerance of Allografts

The acceptance of foreign tissue by immature animals has been known to experimental embryologists for many years. The grafting of parts of one embryo on to another was carried out without realising its more general biological significance. In 1948–49 Burnet and Fenner predicted that immature animals would be capable of accepting foreign tissues. They postulated that the tissues of an animal and their breakdown products possessed 'self-markers', which were recognisable to its immunological system. In this way animals did not make antibodies against their own tissue components. These workers further postulated that the capacity to learn to recognise these 'self-markers' is present only during embryonic and early post-natal life. The presentation of foreign antigens to a developing embryo could therefore be expected to lead to their being recognised as 'self' throughout the rest of the life of the individual. Owen, in 1945, described red-cell chimerism in cattle. This condition results when binovular twins share a common placenta. The blood cells from each twin are shared, and each is born with two sets of red cells. It has since been

shown that the state may exist throughout life, due to the fact that each twin has accepted and become tolerant to the erythrocyte-forming tissue of its fellow. This type of chimerism has been described in cattle, lambs, and chickens, and several instances are on record of its occurrence in the human.

However, the fundamental significance of these facts was not fully realised until 1952, when Medawar showed that red-cell chimeras could also exchange skin grafts. It was later shown that they also exchanged kidney grafts. Then Medawar and his colleagues, Billingham and Brent, undertook a series of experiments upon which our understanding of immune tolerance is based. In their early experiments they injected mouse embryos of CBA strain with cells of the testis, kidney, and spleen from mice of strain A. The injection of this mixture of cells was given with a fine needle inserted through the abdominal wall, after an incision had been made through the skin of the pregnant CBA mice. Many of the embryos survived this injection, and were subsequently born as normal mice which were then allowed to grow up. When 8 weeks old they were challenged with skin grafts from strain A mice, and it was found that these grafts behaved like autotransplants, i.e. they survived. This experiment clearly demonstrated the existence of a specific immune tolerance, which developed in response to intra-uterine contact with foreign cells.

Further experiments have shown that the injection of foreign cells into young animals, e.g. the rat, at birth may also induce tolerance. Glucocorticoid treatment does not interfere with the development of tolerance; in fact it permits tolerance to be induced for up to 2 weeks when given from the time of birth onwards. A direct proof that tolerance is acquired during early life has been provided by an ingenious experiment performed on the tree frog *Hyla regilla*.[6] The buccal part of the pituitary was removed from an embryo, maintained in culture, and later replaced in the same animal when it had attained maturity. There was a typical allograft reaction to the implant, which was not seen when only a part of the buccal pituitary was removed beforehand.

It should be noted that immunological tolerance is not an all-or-nothing affair. There are varying degrees of tolerance, and these are manifested as gradations of prolongation of graft survival. When fully developed, tolerance is attended by the permanent survival of allografts.

Maternally-induced tolerance. It has been suggested that maternal cells enter the fetal circulation, and the fetus should therefore be tolerant to maternal tissue. Although it is known that this may occasionally happen, it does not seem likely that it is a common event. It may, however, explain the occasional case in which grafts from a mother have been accepted by her child.

Induction of Tolerance after the Development of Immunological Maturity

Enhancement. The growth of tumour allografts may be enhanced by the prior injection of killed cells of the prospective donor. This effect is probably due to the formation of haemagglutinins. The effect is much less marked when normal tissue is used as a graft.

The survival of skin grafts in rabbits may be prolonged by a previous intravenous injection of a suspension of dissociated epidermal cells of the donor (Billingham-Sparrow phenomenon).[1] A second graft may survive even longer than the first. The explanation of these findings is not clear; it is probably related to enhancement.

Induction of tolerance after irradiation. It is known that total body irradiation of lethal dose will inhibit the immune response. Under these circumstances the injection of foreign bone-marrow cells, either allografts or xenografts, results in the repopulation of the bone marrow with foreign cells. The animal may survive in this state for some time, and can accept grafts, e.g. skin grafts, from the same donor as the marrow cells. Frequently, however, these *x-ray chimeras*, as they are called, die of *secondary disease*, a condition which closely resembles runt disease and is due to a GVH reaction (see below).

The administration of cytotoxic drugs, see page 193.

Pregnancy.[7-9] It is a remarkable fact that pregnancy, even repeated, rarely causes the mother to react immunologically against her developing fetus. There is some degree of maternal immunosuppression during pregnancy, an effect that can be correlated with the presence of four immunosuppressive agents in the maternal plasma: glucocorticoids; placental chorionic gonadotrophin; human somatomammotrophin (also known as human placental lactogen); and α-fetoprotein. All these compounds are secreted by the placenta, and it is therefore possible that the local concentration at the junction of fetal and uterine tissues is considerably higher than might be expected from the maternal plasma levels. Oestrogens are also excreted by the placenta, and they too have a mild, general, immunosuppressive effect.

However, the maternal uterus is capable of mounting an immune response. Thus a lymphocytic infiltration develops around the blastocyst that implants in the uterine decidua, and there is marked enlargement of the aortic lymph nodes in pregnant rats and mice following the mating of genetically disparate animals, but not with genetically identical animals. In the human the most familiar example of an immune response against fetal antigens is the development of Rhesus antibodies by Rh-negative women (p. 613). Many women also develop antibodies against HLA antigens which can be detected on their husbands' leucocytes. These antibodies in all probability have developed against the same antigens present on the cells of the fetus. Some women develop such antibodies in high titre and with high specificity, and their sera are of value in tissue typing (p. 674).

Thus there is the paradox of maternal immune response against fetal antigens without the rejection of the fetus, a phenomenon not adequately explained by the moderate degree of immunosuppression that occurs in pregnancy. Both the fetus and the placenta are sufficiently antigenic to stimulate an immune response, but the trophoblast seems to be the one tissue that is very feebly antigenic. Indeed, large numbers of trophoblastic cells are swept into the maternal circulation (about 100 000 a day) and masses of them lodge in the lung capillaries, but there is no evidence that they ever stimulate an immune response. As a poorly antigenic layer of fetal tissue lying directly in contact with maternal lymphocytes would be very effective as an immunological barrier and protect the underlying placental tissue from immune attack, much investigation has been directed towards establishing the degree of antigenicity of the trophoblast. It seems that the trophoblast does contain some HLA antigens that are of importance in initiating graft rejection, but these appear to be masked.

A layer of 'fibrinoid' material on the maternal surface of the syncytial trophoblast has been described, which may be sialomucin, a proteoglycan which has the property of masking HLA antigens on the cell surface. But this claim awaits confirmation by other investigators.

It is evident that, considering the intimate contact that exists between the fetal placenta and the maternal lymphocytes, the immunosuppressive mechanisms are remarkably effective in preventing rejection. However, there is also evidence that immunological mechanisms are involved in the selection of gametes at fertilisation and at implantation of the blastocyst. Animal studies have shown that genetic disparity of the parents results in placentas that are larger than those developing when the parents are genetically identical through inbreeding. Labour itself is not an immunological event; its onset is possibly hormonally induced by the fetus, but the matter is not decided.

The ease with which tolerance can be induced is therefore related to many factors. The antigenic differences between graft and host are very important. Thus, it is relatively easy to produce tolerance in mice when they differ at the H-1 or H-3 locus, but difficult when the difference lies at the H-2 locus. Tolerance is easier to induce in immature animals than in adults unless the immune response has been depressed. Large doses of antigen tend to produce tolerance, although the curious fact that very small quantities can do the same has been noted on page 155. Finally, the route of administration plays a part; the intravenous route sometimes leading to tolerance when an intraperitoneal injection results in immunity.

Graft-Versus-Host Reaction[10,11]

It was soon found that the injection of foreign cells into young or embryonic animals was not free from danger. Some died, and the percentage mortality varied considerably according to the exact circumstances of the experiment. In some instances the injected animals developed a disease which was characterised by wasting, atrophy of the lymphoid tissue, and a liability to intercurrent infection. The condition has come to be known as *runt disease*, and is due to the graft cells reacting immunologically against the host. It is an example of a graft-versus-host (GVH) reaction, and occurs when the following conditions are fulfilled:

(1) If the host is tolerant of the grafted cells.

(2) If the graft cells are immunologically competent. Indeed, the ability to produce a GVH reaction can be used to assess immunological competence. Thus, adult small lymphocytes from the thoracic duct are effective.

(3) If the host contains antigens which are not present in the grafted cells and to which the grafted cells are not tolerant.

When the antigenic difference between the host and the graft is great, as when there is a difference at the H-2 locus in mice, there is a severe GVH reaction and the animals die. When the difference is slight the grafted animals may survive.

A local method of demonstrating a GVH reaction in guinea-pigs is to inject lymphocytes into the skin of an allogeneic host. After 24 to 36 hours a reaction develops which resembles a positive Mantoux test. This test has been used as a means of selecting suitable donors for renal transplantation in the human. Thus, if lymphocytes from the proposed recipient are injected into the skin of a panel of willing donors, the intensity of the reactions is a measure of the future reaction to the transplanted kidney. Although of great theoretical interest, this test, sometimes called the *normal lymphocyte transfer test*, presents obvious difficulties and dangers. Its value in predicting the fate of a graft in the human has not been established, and tissue typing is more commonly used.

Pathogenesis of runt disease. It can be shown that the injected cells populate the host. If small lymphocytes from the thoracic duct of a rat are injected into lethally irradiated mice, it can be shown that the mouse spleens contain many pyroninophilic cells of rat chromosomal type. By administering tritiated thymidine 12 hours before examination it is evident that most of these cells are synthesising DNA. Furthermore, 12 hours later the labelled cells are all small lymphocytes. This and other experiments indicate that the small lymphocytes can change into pyroninophilic cells, divide, and produce small lymphocytes again. Nevertheless, the splenic enlargement which is a characteristic feature of runt disease is due not only to this effect, for there is considerable evidence that many of the proliferating cells are of host origin. How the cells, whether of host or donor origin, produce the lesions of runt disease is not known.

GVH reactions in the human. A GVH reaction is seen when allogeneic marrow is given after the heroic treatment of leukaemia with total body irradiation or with cytotoxic drugs. It can also follow the administration of fresh whole blood to cases of immunological deficiency (see p. 171), and has been described in infants following intrauterine and exchange transfusions for haemolytic disease of the newborn.[12] The reaction occurs even when the recipient and donor are siblings and compatible insofar as the HLA antigens are concerned.[13] Salient features of the syndrome are wasting, anorexia, diarrhoea with malabsorption, exfoliative dermatitis, liver damage with jaundice, and an increased susceptibility to fungal and viral infections.

XENOGRAFTS (HETEROGRAFTS)[1]

Xenografts are destroyed even more rapidly than are allografts; they are indeed treated like 'second-set' allografts. There is no vascularisation, and the graft undergoes necrosis which stimulates an acute inflammatory reaction. The rejection certainly involves an immunological mechanism, but there is no reason to assume that this is the only mechanism involved. The ultimate consequences of bringing together tissues of very dissimilar genetic constitution are not known and cannot be foreseen.

Xenografts of living skin usually die within a few days, whereas cartilage may last for up to three weeks. Xenografts of cartilage serving a static function may remain in the body much longer, and, as with arteries, dead material is usually more satisfactory than a fresh, living graft.

Special sites. Tumour xenografts may grow in the anterior chamber of the eye, brain (Fig. 15.2), testis, hamster cheekpouch, and in the yolk-sac. Xenografts of embryonic tissue

Figure 15.2
Coronal section through the head of a mouse which 66 days previously had been given an intracerebral inoculation of human oat-cell carcinoma of the lung. The xenografted tumour showed active growth, and produced the large, circular, tumour mass which is here seen in section × 9. (*From Chesterman, F. C.* (1955), *Intracranial heterotransplantation of human tumours*, British Journal of Cancer, **9**, 51)

may also survive in these sites, but normal adult tissue does not usually do so.

Second set phenomena. Second grafts are probably destroyed even more quickly than are the first, but this is difficult to assess in view of the rapidity with which even first grafts are eliminated.

Antibodies concerned. Many antibodies have been identified in animals that have rejected xenografts. These include haemolysins and cytotoxic factors. They may be species-specific and sometimes even organ-specific. Immunoglobulins can in fact be present even in normal animals, and are perhaps induced by previous contact with heterophile antigens. Thus, many human sera contain lymphocytotoxic and haemagglutinating activity against sheep's cells and pig's cells.[14] It is worth noting that xenografts in diffusion chambers are killed in immunised animals. It is therefore probable that xenograft immunity is effected by humoral antibodies, but the role of cellular antibodies has not been excluded.

Glucocorticoids have been administered in the study of the heterotransplantability of tumours; human tumours may be grown in animals treated with these agents. Total body X-irradiation has similarly been used. Animals subjected to total body irradiation of lethal dose may be made into red-cell chimeras as described in connexion with allografts. These xenograft chimeras will accept other grafts from the same donor, so long as the state of chimerism persists.

CLINICAL USE OF GRAFTS IN SPECIAL SITUATIONS[1, 2, 15]

Grafting has now become an established procedure. With some tissues, e.g. heart valves and cornea, immediate rejection is not a problem, while with skin no practical means have been found to prevent it. With renal transplants a fair degree of success has been obtained; tissue matching and immunosuppressive therapy have played an important part in this, and no doubt the methods evolved will be applicable to the grafting of other organs, e.g. liver, lung, and heart, which is at present in an experimental stage. Renal grafts will therefore be considered in some detail.

RENAL TRANSPLANTATION[16, 17]

Renal transplantation is now a common procedure, and a one-year survival time can be expected in over 50 per cent of cases if the donor is a living relative (and in 65 to 75 per cent of cases when the donor is a parent or sibling). With unrelated donors the figure is lower—about one third. With sibling grafts the results are much better when there is compatibility for the HLA locus. How important compatibility is when the donor is not related is debated.[18] The risk of rejection is greatest during the first year, and few grafts fail after the second year; indeed, sepsis is then the problem. Grafted kidneys appear to exhibit adaptation, for when one is accepted, a subsequent kidney graft or skin graft from the same donor can be rejected and yet the original graft remains unaffected.

Renal Complications of Grafting

Acute tubular necrosis. This is liable to occur regardless of the origin of the kidney. It is due to the hypoxia sustained during the transfer of the organ from the donor to the patient.

Recurrence of the original renal disease. In patients with chronic glomerulonephritis the grafted kidney may develop the same disease. This is seen more frequently with isografts, when no immunosuppressive drugs are given, than with allografts. Presumably the additional therapy prevents the development of the disease. The recurrence of other renal disease varies according to the disease. Thus it is very common with oxalosis, rare in amyloidosis, and has not yet been encountered in diabetes mellitus or Fabry's disease.

Rejection. *Hyperacute rejection.* This occurs immediately, and the kidney becomes swollen and congested. The vessels in the graft become blocked by fibrin and polymorphs. The reaction is due to major ABO incompatibility or the presence of immunoglobulin antibodies to the graft, e.g. following the rejection of a previous graft. The reaction is complement dependent. Antigen-antibody-complement complexes are deposited and lead to polymorph and platelet deposition in the vessels, as in the Arthus reaction.

Acute rejection. This may occur at any time from days to months after the operation. The lesion is brought about by infiltrations of host lymphocytes reacting against the endothelium of the capillaries and venules situated around the tubules in the cortex. The capillary walls are disrupted with extravasations of blood in the interstitial tissue. The kidney shows infiltration by mononuclear cells (p. 190) and severe tubular damage. Fibrinoid necrosis may occur in the arterioles. The role of immunoglobulins is generally considered to be unimportant in this type of rejection. Nevertheless, deposits of immunoglobulin and complement can be found in the kidney undergoing acute reversible rejection. As in other areas of immunology the distinction between the cell-mediated and the humoral response is less clear-cut than was considered previously (see also antibody-dependent cell-mediated cytotoxicity, p. 147).

Clinically the onset of acute rejection is sudden, with fever, swelling of the graft, oliguria, and a decrease in renal function. There is a marked diminution in urinary sodium excretion, proteinuria, and an increase in the plasma creatinine. These clinical manifestations are best defined if the rejection episode occurs within the first few weeks of transplantation. In delayed episodes the onset is less acute and the manifestations are less clear-cut.

Chronic rejection. This occurs at any time after one year. One type of chronic rejection is due to platelet thrombi in the capillaries of the glomeruli; this can be rapidly reversed by glucocorticoids. A later type of chronic rejection is due to a lesion resembling membranous glomerulonephritis, and is caused by a deposit of IgM in the capillary walls. This is of linear deposition, as in Goodpasture's syndrome. It may be that the IgM forms against components of the basement membrane. Clinically there is proteinuria and progressively decreased renal function.

Non-Renal Complications

Infection is a constant danger in patients on immunosuppressive therapy, and may be due to a wide variety of opportunistic organisms.

Various late syndromes have been described in patients with renal grafts—the symptoms include splenomegaly, fever, synovitis, and muscle pains. Pulmonary changes may occur ('transplantation lung'). It is not clear whether these syndromes are caused by an immunological reaction and comparable to Goodpasture's syndrome, or by an undetected infection, such as with *Pneumocystis carinii*.

Immunosuppressive Therapy

The early attempts at immunosuppression utilised total body irradiation, but although some long-term survivors appeared, the risk of marrow aplasia was great, and the balance between survival of the patient and acceptance of the graft was too precarious. The method is therefore no longer used. 6-Mercaptopurine was introduced in 1959, and later replaced by the less toxic azathioprine ('Imuran'). This, together with glucocorticoids, is now the mainstay of therapy. Antilymphocytic serum is under study at some centres. In the experimental animal it greatly prolongs the life of allografts and xenografts. Its action seems to be directed against the mobile long-lived lymphocytes which recirculate through the lymph nodes.[19] Anti-thymus serum is reported as being superior in that it also abolishes the second set rejection.

The administration of prednisone and actinomycin C, and the local irradiation of the graft are additional measures which are often instituted if signs of acute rejection occur.

An unfortunate effect of immunosuppressive therapy is an increased susceptibility to infection, e.g. cytomegalovirus and herpes simplex. Nearly half the patients treated for over 1 year develop recurrent crops of warts.[20]

Another problem which accompanies immunosuppressive therapy is the development of malignant tumours. A number of patients have developed a lymphoma within 1 year of grafting. There are several reports of malignancy present in the graft which has spread and killed the recipient of a renal transplant.[21] In one case where the kidney contained a secondary carcinoma of the lung, withdrawal of immunosuppressive therapy resulted in rejection of both the kidney and the carcinoma.[22] It seems possible that immunosuppression encourages the growth of tumour cells and that organ replacement with homografts is unlikely to be of value in the treatment of cancer.

Enhancement. This has been used experimentally as a means of preventing graft rejection. The animal may be given tissue antigen, or antibody can be administered passively.[23]

Tests of Tissue Compatibility

The following tests have been employed to assess the antigenic compatibility between graft and host.

ABO blood grouping. Success is impossible if the donor blood group is not compatible with that of the host.

Normal lymphocyte transfer test (p. 195). One drawback of this test is that the lymphocytes of uraemic patients react poorly.

Mixed leucocyte culture. If donor and recipient lymphocytes are cultured together, both undergo transformation and division (p. 151). This may be measured by the uptake of tritiated thymidine. The test can be made one-way and more specific if the donor cells are treated with mitomycin C prior to mixing, so that only the recipient's reaction to the donor is measured. The test detects antigens determined by the HLA locus, and about 25 per cent of siblings are compatible. Unrelated individuals are rarely compatible.

Detection of preformed serum antibodies in the recipient which are cytotoxic to the lymphocytes of the donor.

Tissue matching. Tissue typing is described in Appendix 4. An attempt is made to match the donor and recipient as closely as possible. In general, it has been found that the best matches are obtained between siblings and that these give the best clinical results. Antigenic matching of graft with host appears to be the most promising development in recent years. The techniques are, however, complex, and the supply of donor material erratic; there is no satisfactory way of preserving tissue. The organisation of a transplantation unit is now beyond the resources of a single hospital, and regional cooperation is essential.[24]

Bone[25]

Bone grafts have in the past been used to provide internal fixation, but advances in metallurgy have largely obviated this function. Grafts are now commonly used to provide a temporary scaffold to fill a cavity, to bridge the gap between an ununited fracture, or to fuse a joint in the operation of arthrodesis. Free grafts are unable to acquire a blood supply sufficiently fast to prevent necrosis of most of the bone cells. With fresh autografts some of the superficial osteocytes and the endosteal and periosteal osteoblasts may survive, but their contribution to the subsequent healing process is probably small. Blood vessels grow into the Haversian canals, and the bony matrix is slowly eroded by osteoclasts and subsequently replaced by living lamellar bone. With solid, cortical bone grafts this process may take many months, but with cancellous bone the process is quicker; cancellous bone is therefore preferred. In addition to the slow replacement of the graft by this process of creeping substitution, the presence of the graft excites the formation of granulation tissue around it. This is derived from the vascular medullary cavity and to a lesser extent from the periosteum. The granulation tissue matures to form woven bone, and this is replaced by lamellar bone. Coincidentally, there is a general remodelling process as the area adapts to the local stresses to which it is exposed. It will be seen that a bone graft has an inductive effect on local tissues and can lead to the formation of new bone. This can occur even if the bone graft is embedded heterotopically in an extraskeletal site.

In clinical practice *fresh autografts* are most satisfactory, and some of the osteogenic cells which take part in the incorporation process may be of graft origin. *Fresh allografts* excite an inflammatory reaction due to rejection and this delays healing. Allografts preserved by various means, e.g. freezing, freeze-drying, and X-irradiation, can be stored in bone banks. In some hands their use has been satisfactory. *Xenografts*, usually calf, are less useful. Preserved bone grafts of any origin serve as a temporary scaffold on which host bone can be formed, but there is no agreement as to the best method of preservation. In clinical work there are so many variables, such as the age of the patient, the site of insertion of the graft, the technique and skill of the surgeon, etc., that evaluation of the results obtained is virtually impossible. There is, however, general agreement that fresh autografts of cancellous bone are better than any other type.

Blood Vessels

Both autografts and allografts have been used in the replacement of blood vessels in the human subject, and it seems likely that in all cases the cells of the graft die. They therefore behave as static grafts. For obvious reasons autografts of large arteries are not practicable in the human, and allografts are therefore the only material available. There is considerable evidence to show that freeze-dried material is superior to both frozen and fresh grafts. This is possibly due to its lack of antigenicity.

The tissue of the graft remains in an unaltered state for a long period, but is eventually replaced by the host tissue. It appears therefore that arterial grafts act merely as mechanical dead tissues, and recent workers have favoured their substitution by synthetic plastic material.

The main problems involved in both types of grafts are mechanical, i.e. fitting the graft or prosthesis, and subsequently preventing rupture or thrombosis.

Heart[26, 27]

The recent heart transplants have been attended by more publicity than success. Of over 100 cases very few long-term survivors are recorded. The graft may fail within the first month, and the microscopic signs of rejection comprise infiltration of the myocardial interstitial tissue by lymphocytes, macrophages, and polymorphs. Late rejection is characterised by intimal thickening and fibrosis of the coronary vessels, and an infiltration by lymphocytes, plasma cells, and macrophages. Somewhat unexpectedly, the heart appears to be more vulnerable than the kidney to rejection, and histocompatibility is the critical factor in the survival of the patient. With our present immunosuppressive agents there seems to be no reliable method of preventing rejection of a heart that is a poor antigenic match—10 years is the longest survival to date.

Heart-valve grafts,[28, 29] mostly aortic, have been in use since 1955, but the best technique is difficult to assess because of the many variables that have been introduced. The aortic valve may be inserted isotopically or be placed in the descending aorta. It may be fresh or freeze-dried and sterilised by β-propiolactone, ethylene oxide, formaldehyde, or γ-rays. The major complications are incompetence, endocarditis (often an infection by an organism not generally encountered), and thrombosis with subsequent embolism. In spite of these hazards many valves have remained functional for several years. It appears that there is little or no homograft reaction, for the valve is virtually avascular and it remains acellular. This being so, it is probable that xenografts will also be satisfactory; indeed pig valves have been used.

Nerves

Much work has been done on the replacement of a resected portion of nerve employing autografts, allografts, or xenografts of nerve tissue.

Autografts. A living autograft shows classical Wallerian degeneration with proliferation of Schwann cells, into which regenerating nerve fibres of the host nerve subsequently penetrate. When large nerve grafts are used, there is some danger of necrosis of the central portion, and for this reason several smaller strands or cables are used to bridge the defect. The good results obtained with experimental autografts are reflected in equally good results obtained in human beings, although many early reports were extremely pessimistic. There is little doubt that, provided the segment of nerve is not too long, fresh autografts can be invaded by regenerating nerve fibres, and the results can be at least as good as those obtained after suture of a severed nerve.

Allografts. An allograft also shows Wallerian degeneration, but the process is much slower than with autografts. The Schwann cells proliferate, but subsequently die as the graft becomes infiltrated with lymphoid cells. The dying graft is invaded by host Schwann cells and axons; with small segments there may be sufficient invasion to bridge the gap. Allografts have been of some use experimentally where small defects have to be bridged, but are valueless where the segment to be replaced is long.

In clinical work allografts have produced extremely disappointing results. It seems probable that attempts at allografting with suppression of the homograft reaction might produce better clinical results, but no reports are as yet available.

Xenografts. These show Wallerian degeneration with some degree of proliferation of Schwann cells in certain species. There is little tendency for the graft to be invaded by host axons, and in general xenografts fail. Their use is therefore not to be recommended in human beings.

Skin

Autografts take readily, the only limiting factor being the readiness with which the graft acquires a blood supply. Split skin grafts have been extensively used, and readily take on a suitable bed. Free whole-thickness, or Wolfe grafts, if stripped of subcutaneous fat, take well on fresh, clean surfaces, but survive much less readily on granulation tissue. Pedicle grafts are extensively used in plastic surgery.

Human isografts take as readily as autografts. Allografts are almost invariably rejected except in non-identical twins showing blood chimerism. In about 25 per cent of allografts from mother to child, and less commonly in allografts from child to mother, survival has been reported for periods up to 1 year. Allografts between other individuals, however, are usually rejected in from 1 to 4 weeks, and rarely survive longer than 10 weeks.

Various attempts have been made to prolong the life of allografts. The most valuable appears to be the use of grafts from multiple donors. This work is based upon the fact that the immune response is to some extent related to the size of the graft. Several small grafts from a number of donors therefore excite less response than does a large graft from a single donor. The use of fetal tissue or skin from infants has been tried, but no convincing evidence has been forthcoming that it is of any value. This also applies to pure epidermal grafts. At the present time the value of human allografts is to provide temporary cover when this is needed, e.g. for patients with extensive burns. Xenografts are invariably rejected, but in recent years the use of embryo calf skin has been advocated for severely burned patients. The graft persists for periods ranging from 12 to 17 days, and may therefore provide a temporary cover, much the same as an allograft.

The Cornea[30]

The privileged position which isotopic corneal grafts enjoy is an important factor in their clinical use. Under normal conditions host lymphocytes are unable to reach the graft, but should iritis occur, inflammatory cells enter the anterior chamber, and this is followed by oedema of the graft.

The fate of the grafted cells has been the subject of much speculation. It is generally agreed that the surface epithelial cells are soon replaced by those of the host. With full-thickness grafts the endothelial cells remain viable for many months, but it is likely that they too are replaced. Since the integrity of the graft is dependent on the presence of a healthy layer of endothelial cells, it is evident that this component of the graft must be viable. At present only the use of fresh material can ensure this; freeze-dried grafts are of no value. They may, however, be successful as lamellar, or partial-thickness, grafts.

Bone Marrow[31]

Marrow grafts, administered by intravenous injection, have been used in an attempt to treat aplastic anaemia and various immunological deficiency states. They have also been used in malignant conditions, particularly leukaemia; 1000 rad total body irradiation and cyclophosphamide therapy is used to destroy the malignant cells prior to the grafting. The initial results of these attempts were not very encouraging, for not only is there a possibility of graft rejection, but should the graft survive the patient is at risk from a GVH reaction. Hence close tissue and ABO matching are essential. In spite of the difficulties, stable chimerism can be obtained in some patients, and grafted cells appear to become tolerant of the host. The mechanism is not understood, but blocking antibodies and the action of suppressor cells are possible factors.

Other Organs

Other organs which have been transplanted include liver [32-34] and lung.[35] The number of cases is small, and although some long-term survivors are recorded, the procedures are still experimental. Thymus and spleen grafts have been employed in some cases of immunological deficiency, e.g. Di George's syndrome, and have been found useful.[36] Another potential value of grafting is to supply enzyme-forming tissue to patients with inborn errors of metabolism. Renal transplantation has been carried out in patients with Fabry's disease and cystinosis. Advanced Wilson's disease has been treated by liver transplantation. Very few cases have been treated in this manner, and the value has yet to be proven.[37]

It is evident from this brief account that the fate of an allograft is dependent upon a large number of factors. The genetic difference between host and graft is most important. The content of antigen varies from one tissue to another, and the graft may show adaptation. The site of grafting is sometimes important, and also whether the graft establishes lymphatic or vascular connexion with the host. Finally, there is the host response, humoral and cellular, both of which can be modified by therapy. Tolerance may develop to graft antigens. It is hardly surprising that in human transplantation there is enormous variation in the end-result, so that some grafts function for years while others are rejected immediately. The complexity of the allograft reaction is to be regarded as a challenge, for as its intricacies are being unravelled, so is allotransplantation finding a valuable place in clinical medicine.

One final point deserves consideration. Why do the vertebrates possess such an efficient mechanism for the rejection of grafts, bearing in mind that such a function could have had no obvious survival value in the past? Various suggestions have been made, but none is satisfactory. The invasion by organisms which characteristically multiply in the host macrophages may have prompted the development of a cellular immune response. Another suggestion is that the mechanisms of cellular immunity have been evolved in mammals (and other viviparous animals) to prevent invasion of the mother by fetal cells during gestation. Yet another possibility is that the graft rejection phenomenon is a manifestation of a homeostatic mechanism whereby damaged or abnormal cells, such as those of neoplasia, are destroyed and eliminated. Although there has been no dramatic increase in the incidence of malignancy in patients on immunosuppressive therapy, lymphomata have been reported,[38] and there is one case of a histiocytic lymphoma (reticulum-cell sarcoma) developing at the site of injection of antilymphocytic serum.[39] The long-term effects of powerful immunosuppressive therapy may well provide an answer to this problem.

REFERENCES

1. WOODRUFF, M. F. A. (1960) *The Transplantation of Tissues and Organs*. Springfield, Ill.: Thomas.
2. RAPAPORT, F. T. & DAUSSET, J. (1968) *Human Transplantation*, 278 pp. New York: Grune and Stratton.
3. RUSSELL, P. S. & WINN, H. J. (1970) Transplantation. *New England Journal of Medicine*, **282**, 786, 848 and 896.
4. DIMITRIU, A. *et al.* (1974) Macrophage cytotoxicity in the mouse immune response against a skin graft. *Journal of Immunology*, **114**, 195.
5. BERAH, M., HORS, J. & DAUSSET, J. (1968) Concentration of transplantation antigens in human organs. *Lancet*, **2**, 106.
6. TRIPLETT, E. L. (1962) On the mechanism of immunologic self recognition. *Journal of Immunology*, **89**, 505.
7. MUIR, V. Y. (1977) Concept of the fetus as a transplant. *Hospital Update*, **3**, 621.
8. BEER, A. E. & BILLINGHAM, R. E. (1976) *The Immunobiology of Mammalian Reproduction*. Englewood Cliffs, New Jersey: Prentice-Hall.
9. BORLAND, R., LOKE, Y. W. & WILSON, D. (1975) Immunological privilege resulting from endocrine activity of trophoblast *in vivo*. In *Immunobiology of the Trophoblast*, ed. Edwards, R. G., Howe, C. W. S. & Johnson, M. H., p. 157. Cambridge: Cambridge University Press.
10. SLAVIN, R. E. & SANTOS, G. W. (1973) The graft versus host reaction in man after bone marrow transplantation: pathology, pathogenesis, clinical features, and implication. *Clinical Immunology and Immunopathology*, **1**, 472.
11. ELKINS, W. L. (1971) Cellular immunology and the pathogenesis of graft versus host reactions. *Progress in Allergy*, **15**, 78.
12. SCHWARTZ, R. S. (1974) Trojan-horse lymphocytes. *New England Journal of Medicine*, **290**, 397.
13. GRAW, R. G. *et al.* (1970) Graft-versus-host reaction complicating HLA matched bone-marrow transplantation. *Lancet*, **2**, 1053.
14. McKENZIE, I. F. C. *et al.* (1968) Human lymphocytotoxic and haemagglutinating activity against sheep and pig cells. *Lancet*, **2**, 386.
15. HAMBURGER, J., CROSNIER, J. & DESCAMPS, B. (1978) The transplanted kidney. *Advances in Internal Medicine*, **23**, 195.
16. CALNE, R. Y. (1967) *Renal Transplantation*, 2nd edn. London: Arnold.
17. PORTER, K. A. (1974) In *Pathology of the Kidney*, ed. Heptinstall, R. H., 2nd edn. Edinburgh: Churchill Livingstone.
18. Leading Article (1971) Tissue-typing in organ transplantation. *Lancet*, **1**, 639.
19. Leading Article (1968) A.L.S. and the heterograft. *Lancet*, **1**, 1238.
20. SPENCER, E. S. & ANDERSEN, H. K. (1970) Clinically evident, non-terminal infections with herpesviruses and the wart virus in immunosuppressed renal allograft recipients. *British Medical Journal*, **3**, 251.
21. HUME, D. M. (1966) Progress in clinical renal homotransplantation. *Advances in Surgery*, **2**, 419.
22. WILSON, R. E. *et al.* (1968) Immunologic rejection of human cancer transplanted with a renal allograft. *New England Journal of Medicine*, **278**, 479.
23. STUART, F. P., SAITOH, T. & FITCH, F. W. (1968) Rejection of renal allografts: specific immunologic suppression. *Science*, **160**, 1463.
24. TERASAKI, P. I., WILKINSON, G. & McCLELLAND, J. (1971) National transplant communication network. *Journal of the American Medical Association*, **218**, 1674.
25. BURWELL, R. G. (1969) In *Recent Advances in Orthopaedics*, ed. Apley, A. G., p. 115. London: Churchill.
26. Ellis, B. *et al.* (1971). Clinical and pathological findings in human cardiac rejection. *Archives of Pathology*, **92**, 58.
27. NORA, J. J. *et al.* (1969) Rejection of the transplanted human heart. *New England Journal of Medicine*, **280**, 1079.
28. BARRATT-BOYES, B. G. (1967) Homograft replacement for aortic valve disease. *Modern Concepts in Cardiovascular Disease*, **36**, 1.
29. Ross, D. (1967) Homograft replacement of the aortic valve. *British Journal of Surgery*, **54**, 842.

30. Rycroft, B. W. (1955) *Corneal Grafts.* London: Butterworth.
31. Thomas, E. D. *et al.* (1975) Bone-marrow transplantation. *New England Journal of Medicine,* **292**, 832 and 895.
32. Leading Article (1969) Liver transplantation. *Lancet,* **1**, 868.
33. Williams, R. *et al.* (1969) Liver transplantation in man—III, Studies of liver function, histology, and immunosuppressive therapy. *British Medical Journal,* **3**, 12.
34. Williams, R. (1970) Transplantation of the liver in man. *British Medical Journal,* **1**, 585.
35. Leading Article (1970) Lung transplantation reviewed. *British Medical Journal,* **3**, 600.
36. Leading Article (1969) Graft treatment of immunity deficiency. *Lancet,* **1**, 243.
37. Leading Article (1972) Enzyme transplants. *Lancet,* **2**, 1235.
38. Leading Article (1972) Immunosuppression and malignancy. *British Medical Journal,* **3**, 713.
39. Deodhar, S. D. *et al.* (1969) Development of reticulum-cell sarcoma at the site of antilymphocyte globulin injection in a patient with renal transplant. *New England Journal of Medicine,* **280**, 1104.

Chapter 16. Diseases Mediated by Immunological Mechanisms

Although it is evident that under normal conditions the body does not make antibodies against the antigens of its own tissues, the mechanisms which prevent their formation may on occasion break down.

It is assumed that an individual's proteins have 'self' markers, which are recognised by the immunologically competent cells. If the theory of Burnet is true, the ability to recognise these 'self' markers is learned by the contact of immunologically competent cells with the antigens during embryonic development and is maintained during life by continued contact.

It may be postulated that antibodies against the individual's own tissues (*autoantibodies*) may be manufactured under three circumstances.

Alteration in antigenicity of tissue proteins. This may be due to:

Degenerative lesions, e.g. lens protein in cataracts and skin in burns.

Attachment of hapten, e.g. allergic contact dermatitis.

Specific antibodies should be formed against the affected tissue or the hapten.

Release of an antigen which has always been 'isolated' from the immunologically competent cells or which has become 'sequestered' during development, e.g. lens protein. Such a protein will be labelled 'non-self', and the antibody produced should be specific for it.

Loss of tolerance. Tolerance of self proteins might be expected to be lost in a variety of ways.

Forbidden clones might be formed as a result of some disease of the lymphoreticular system, e.g. lymphoma. Alternatively the defect might be a failure to eliminate a forbidden clone due to a disorder of the regulating mechanism. Whether tolerance to self proteins is complete or not is undecided. For some antigens it is thought that only T cells are tolerant and that B cells are fully capable of reacting if given a suitable stimulus. Hence tolerance can be broken; one way in which this can occur is by the appearance of a closely related, cross-reacting antigen. In this manner animals made tolerant to bovine serum albumin (BSA) can manufacture anti-BSA when injected with human serum albumin. Loss of tolerance can therefore occur as a result of some degenerative process, the attachment of a hapten, or by infection with an organism which has an antigen in common with its host.

Another type of tolerance may be due to the activity of T suppressor cells. Loss of these cells, e.g. in old age, may explain the autoimmune phenomena of elderly people and in immunologically deficient states.

If it is assumed that the continued presence of antigen in reasonable quantity is necessary for the maintenance of tolerance, then the atrophy of any tissue (e.g. adrenal or thyroid) might cause the level of relevant antigen to fall below the critical point, and tolerance would be lost.

Types of antibody. It may be postulated that the autoantibodies will either be immunoglobulins or cell-bound. The immunoglobulins may be of any class and fall into two types:

1. *Organ-specific* immunoglobulins, whose specificity is directed against a determinant present in one organ, e.g. haemolysins and antithyroid antibodies.

2. *Non-organ-specific.* Immunoglobulins directed against DNA, mitochondria, smooth muscle, and immunoglobulin determinants (rheumatoid factor) fall into this group.

ROLE OF AUTOANTIBODIES IN DISEASE PROCESSES

Antibodies may directly attack a tissue and cause damage. The immunoglobulins acquire destructive properties in two ways; they may collaborate with lymphocytes, monocytes, or polymorphs (see antibody-dependent cellular cytotoxicity, p. 147) or they may activate complement by either the classical or the alternate pathway. An example of complement activation is seen in the haemolytic anaemia due to autohaemolysins. Cell-bound antibodies can also destroy cells; experimental allergic encephalomyelitis is the most clear-cut example. Diseases in which the major lesions are caused by an immune mechanism may with justification be called autoimmune diseases. However, it must be stressed that the autoimmunity merely provides a mechanism in the pathogenesis of a disease. It does not provide the cause, which as noted later may be inherited or acquired.

Autoimmune mechanisms may cause lesions which are minor manifestations of the disease, e.g. the vasculitis of lepromatous leprosy. Clearly, there is no sharp line of distinction between this group and those described above. Sometimes the autoantibodies appear to play no part in the disease process. The Wassermann antibody in syphilis may provide an example of this.

An important mechanism whereby antibodies produce pathological lesions is by forming damaging immune complexes with antigen. This has been described under immune-complex disease (p. 181).

AETIOLOGY OF IMMUNOLOGICALLY MEDIATED DISEASES

1. **Genetic factors.** Antigen-antibody complexes are damaging when in antigen excess. An inherited defect in antibody production may favour this,[1] and indeed some autoimmune diseases tend to be familial, e.g. lupus erythematosus and rheumatoid arthritis. Furthermore, these diseases are common in patients with immunological deficiency, e.g. agammaglobulinaemia (p. 171).

2. **Acquired factors.** Any of the extrinsic causes of disease can precipitate an autoimmune process. Thus, drugs (e.g. hydralazine) and sunlight can precipitate the onset of lupus erythematosus. Infection, particularly with viruses, can lead to the formation of autoimmune haemolytic anaemia (e.g. in mycoplasmal pneumonia) or renal damage of immune-complex

type, e.g. NZB mice. Tissue damage however caused can presumably so alter the tissue's antigenicity that antibodies are formed. These may aid the elimination of the dead tissue and provide the basis for useful diagnostic tests. Sometimes they may themselves cause further lesions, e.g. the post-cardiotomy syndrome following heart-muscle damage.

When the aetiology of a disease is clearly established, as in smallpox, the immunologically mediated manifestations of the disease, such as the skin eruption, are readily accepted as part of the whole condition. It is when the cause of a disease is not known, e.g. rheumatoid arthritis, that stress is laid on the autoimmune component of the illness. The label 'autoimmune disease' should not, however, delude one into thinking that one knows the cause of the disease—one has only described part of its pathogenesis.

It is instructive to describe some diseases in which there is a prominent autoimmune component.

RENAL DISEASE[2, 3]

Nephrotoxic nephritis (Masugi type). The injection of heterologous antibody against glomerular basement membrane produces a glomerulonephritis; rats have generally been used and injected with duck anti-rat serum. The antibody becomes attached to the basement membrane and appears as a linear ribbon on immunofluorescence. A similar effect can be induced in animals if they are given basement-membrane substance with Freund's adjuvant. In the Masugi type of nephrotoxic nephritis the initial glomerulonephritis due to heterologous antibody is soon followed by a second phase—the autogenous phase—as antibody to the foreign immunoglobulin is produced and deposited in the basement membrane.

The linear pattern of immunoglobulin deposition in the glomeruli is seen in some types of human glomerulonephritis. The best known is *Goodpasture's syndrome.* This is an acute disease which generally attacks males of the age-group 25 to 35 years and is characterised by extensive pulmonary haemorrhage (resembling idiopathic pulmonary haemosiderosis, p. 589) combined with a rapidly progressing glomerulonephritis. Immunoglobulin is desposited in the basement membrane of lung and glomeruli; presumably the damage caused by this explains the lesions, but the aetiology of the disease is unknown; a respiratory viral infection has been suggested. Apart from Goodpasture's syndrome, a linear pattern of immunofluorescence is uncommon in human glomerulonephritis.

Immune complex disease. Glomerulonephritis due to the glomerular deposition of non-glomerular antigen-antibody complexes is a characteristic finding in serum sickness. The localisation of the complexes is related to their nature. Large complexes formed with antibody excess tend to accumulate in the subendothelial space or in the mesangium. Small complexes formed with antigen excess tend to pass through the basement membrane and come to lie under the epithelial cells. These subepithelial deposits are the most damaging, and give a 'lumpy-bumpy' appearance on immunofluorescence.

Glucocorticoids tend to hold up the passage of the complexes through the membrane, and the mesangial cells are able to phagocytose and eliminate them. Steroid administration therefore tends to prevent renal damage. Immune-complex glomerulonephritis can be produced most easily in animals

which have a poor immune response to the given antigen. This underlines the fact that immune complexes are most damaging when in antigen excess. The administration of steroids can indeed increase the incidence of nephritis by inhibiting the immune response.

Immune-complex glomerulonephritis can be produced in animals in many ways, e.g. after injection of brush-border antigen, or indeed many other antigens such as thyroglobulin, when combined with Freund's adjuvant. It occurs spontaneously in NZB/NZW hybrid mice and in NZB mice infected with murine leukaemia virus. In the human it is seen in serum sickness itself, in secondary syphilis, quartan malaria, and in allergic drug reactions, as in penicillamine therapy.[4] Clinically there is usually a nephrotic syndrome. Immune-complex deposition is probably the explanation of the nephrotic syndrome that is sometimes encountered in patients with cancer (p. 339). DNA-antiDNA complexes are of major importance in the pathogenesis of the nephritis of systemic lupus erythematosus (see later). The most important example, however, is post-streptococcal glomerulonephritis.

Post-streptococcal glomerulonephritis. Like acute rheumatic fever, *acute glomerulonephritis* usually occurs after an obvious *Strept. pyogenes* infection. After pharyngitis the mean period is about 10 days, whereas after impetigo it is generally 3 weeks or longer.[5] The glomeruli exhibit 'lumpy-bumpy' immunoglobulin deposits situated between the epithelial cells and the basement membrane. The glomerular damage appears to be caused by the deposition of immune complexes followed by the activation of complement, probably by the alternate pathway. An impaired immune response by the patient may favour the formation of immune complexes with antigen excess. Nevertheless, streptococcal antigen cannot always be demonstrated in the deposits, and the precise pathogenesis of the disease is not known. Some streptococci have antigens in common with kidney, and the formation of anti-kidney antibodies may be an additional factor in the pathogenesis of the disease.[6]

However the damage is produced, there is an infiltration of the glomeruli with polymorphs and a proliferation of mesangial cells. The glomeruli are enlarged, relatively bloodless, and hypercellular (Fig. 16.1). Resolution usually ensues, but sometimes the disease progresses. With severe glomerular damage the parietal epithelial cells of Bowman's capsule proliferate to produce characteristic crescents (Fig. 16.2). This is *rapidly progressive chronic glomerulonephritis,* and death occurs within 2 years. More usually the disease progresses slowly over a period of many years until the glomeruli are converted into hyaline, functionless masses. Uraemia, hypertension, and heart failure are the clinical accompaniments. Before reaching this stage the glomeruli may take on a lobular appearance (*lobular nephritis*), and the patients often exhibit a nephrotic syndrome.

Acute nephritis most often follows a type-12 streptococcal infection. Rabbits given a culture filtrate of type-12 streptococci intravenously develop a nephritis-like condition, but the interpretation of these findings is complicated, for they may all be examples of non-specific immune-complex damage.

Other types of glomerulonephritis. Other types of nephritis are not post-streptococcal in type and their aetiology is unknown. Glomerulonephritis occurs in *anaphylactoid purpura*

Figure 16.1
Acute glomerulonephritis. The two glomeruli included in the section are considerably enlarged. They are hypercellular due to an infiltration of polymorphs and a proliferation of mesangial cells. The vascular lumina have been occluded, with the result that few red cells are present in the tuft. × 200.

Figure 16.2
Chronic glomerulonephritis. The glomerular tuft is severely deformed and shows a somewhat lobular appearance. There are adhesions between the tuft and the cells of the parietal layer of Bowman's capsule. In one segment these cells have proliferated sufficiently to form an early crescent. The proximal convoluted tubules are atrophic and there is some increase in the amount of interstitial tissue. × 200.

(p. 640), and deposits of IgG and complement are found in the glomeruli. The pattern is neither linear nor 'lumpy bumpy', since the deposits are seen in the mesangium and are not related to the basement membrane. As already noted, the nephrotic syndrome may be a feature of immune-complex disease.

In chronic active hepatitis and some cases of cirrhosis of the liver, cellular and immunoglobulin antibodies to liver-cell components are formed, and these cross-react with a protein component of the distal renal tubules called Tamm-Horsfall glycoprotein. This may be of significance in the pathogenesis of the renal tubular acidosis that is common in these patients.[7]

Liver disease. There is little doubt that an immune mechanism is responsible for the liver-cell necrosis in acute viral hepatitis, for the virus itself is not cytotoxic. Whether the antibodies responsible are directed against viral antigens (e.g. HBsAg) or against liver-specific antigens is undecided. Nor is it known why some cases proceed to chronic hepatitis and cirrhosis. Nevertheless, there is considerable evidence to show that chronic liver disease is accompanied by autoimmune phenomena even if they are not caused by them.[8]

Non-organ-specific autoantibodies are found in chronic active hepatitis, primary biliary cirrhosis, and some cases (cryptogenic) of cirrhosis. These have been grouped as 'autoimmune liver disease', but the relationship between the antibodies and the pathogenesis of the diseases in unknown.

Rheumatoid factor and antinuclear antibodies may be found, but the most frequent are anti-smooth muscle (in chronic active hepatitis) and anti-mitochondrial antibody (in primary biliary cirrhosis).

Skin diseases.[9] Antibodies to skin components have been reported in burns and a number of skin diseases. The best documented examples are to be found in the bullous diseases. In bullous pemphigoid antibody is present in the basement membrane of the skin in the lesions (Fig. 16.3), and it can also be detected in the serum. Likewise in pemphigus vulgaris there is antibody directed against the intercellular substance of the epidermal cells. Dermatitis herpetiformis is the latest disease to join this group, for IgA has been detected in the early, characteristic, papillary lesions of this condition. The antibodies in lupus erythematosus are noted on page 209.

Haemolytic anaemias. There is no doubt that some haemolytic anaemias are caused by autoantibodies. Some are frank autoagglutinins, whereas others act *in vitro* as incomplete antibodies. Both types of antibody cause red-cell destruction *in vivo*. The Donath-Landsteiner antibody is a true haemolysin. Viral, mycoplasmal, and rarely spirochaetal infections may lead to autoimmune haemolytic anaemia.

Autoimmune haemolytic anaemia may be due to an abnormality in the recognition system, as in histiocytic lymphoma or

Figure 16.3
Deposition of IgG antibody in the basement membrane of skin in bullous pemphigoid. A frozen section of skin taken adjacent to a recent vesicle was stained with fluorescein-labelled anti-IgG and examined microscopically under ultraviolet light. The linear staining of the basement membrane is characteristic of this disease. The ill-defined fluorescence on the surface of the skin is nonspecific staining of the stratum corneum.

Figure 16.4
Hashimoto's disease. There is a heavy infiltration of the thyroid gland by a mass of lymphocytes among which there are some plasma cells also. The remaining acini are atrophic and contain small amounts of colloid. × 80.

chronic lymphatic leukaemia, or there may be some obscure defect in the red cells themselves. Alternatively, a foreign factor may act as a hapten and render the cells antigenic, e.g. penicillin (p. 614).

Agranulocytosis and thrombocytopenia may also be associated with autoantibodies (see Chs 53 and 54).

Thyroid disease. *Hashimoto's disease.*[10] The finding of antithyroglobulin antibodies in this condition has led to the hypothesis that it is an autoimmune disease. It is argued that the thyroglobulin is normally sequestered from the body as a whole, and therefore not recognised as 'self'. Damage to the gland (possibly due to a viral infection like mumps) might cause a release of thyroglobulin, and the body then responds by making antibodies. It has been suggested, that, whereas the T cells are tolerant of thyroglobulin, the B cells are fully reactive; the release of thyroglobulin, possibly altered by disease, could by-pass the T cell block. If the antibodies cause further damage to the gland, a vicious circle is established. Histologically the gland shows atrophy of its epithelial elements, together with a dense infiltration of lymphoid cells often with germinal centres. There are also many plasma cells (Fig. 16.4). These findings are very suggestive of local antibody production by B cells.

Antithyroglobulin antibodies are found in about 90 per cent of cases of Hashimoto's disease, and appear to be produced by the lymphoid tissue in the thyroid gland itself. In addition other factors are also present. Antibodies to microsomal fractions occur, but these may be found in some cases of *primary myxoedema*, *thyrotoxicosis*, and even in normal people. Other antibodies are present which are cytotoxic to thyroid cells grown in tissue culture. An agglutination test using coated latex particles or red cells is used extensively as a diagnostic procedure. On the other hand, the injection of serum from patients cannot reproduce the disease in animals.

The possibility of cellular antibodies has been investigated, and lymphocytes from cases of Hashimoto's disease are said to behave abnormally in tissue cultures of thyroid cells. It seemed for a time that T cell-mediated cytotoxicity was the likely pathogenesis of Hashimoto's disease, and that immunoglobulin formation was an incidental phenomenon useful in diagnosis but not directly related to the cause of the disease. Present evidence has reversed this concept, and it now seems likely that the thyroid damage is caused by the immunoglobulin-mediated cytotoxic activity of killer lymphocytes. T cells merely play a part as suppressor cells.

Two experimental models support this concept. Thus Wistar rats (which do not normally develop thyroiditis) depleted of T cells by thymectomy and exposed to total-body, sublethal X-irradiation, develop a chronic thyroiditis. Suppressor T cells are radiosensitive whereas helper T cells are relatively radioresistant; hence under the conditions of the experiment enough helper T cells remain to assist immunoglobulin synthesis by B cells, while the suppressor T cells are eliminated. Experiments with obese chickens support this concept. These chickens have a high spontaneous incidence of thyroiditis. Bursectomy (either surgical or hormonal by injecting androgens) markedly decreases the incidence of thyroiditis. On the other hand, thymectomy or whole-body X-irradiation both increase the incidence and severity of the disease. Thus present evidence suggests that thyroiditis can be mediated by immunoglobulins and the activity of killer lymphocytes. The same may well apply to Hashimoto's disease.

LATS and other autoantibodies involved in the pathogenesis of Graves's disease are discussed in Chapter 35.

Eye diseases. *Sympathetic ophthalmia.*[11] This condition follows perforating injuries of the eye involving the uveal tract. A chronic inflammatory granulomatous lesion commences in the injured eye, and is followed 1 to 2 months later by a similar reaction in the other eye. The second eye is usually more severely damaged than the first, and blindness often results. The 'sympathetic' inflammation can be prevented by removal of the injured eye within 1 to 2 weeks of injury. The condition is rare, and occurs in less than 2 per cent of penetrating injuries.

The lesions are caseating tuberculoid granulomata, but no causative organism has been isolated. There is evidence to suggest that the lesions might be due to the development of type-IV hypersensitivity to uveal antigen, possibly the pigment or the matrix of the pigment granules.[12] This would explain the bilateral nature of the disease and its favourable response to glucocorticoids. If uveal pigment is regarded as sequestered and 'non-self', it is easy to see how an injury could result in the formation of antibodies. What is less easy to explain is why the other eye is subsequently involved, because if it is postulated that the pigment is sequestered from the immunologically competent cells, it is difficult to imagine how the antibodies, which are probably effector T cells, could gain access to the normal uveal pigment.

Phako-anaphylactic endophthalmitis[11] (lens-induced endophthalmitis). This name is applied to an inflammatory reaction in the region of the lens capsule which occasionally occurs following the extracapsular extraction of a cataract, or sometimes after an injury involving the lens. It is thought to be due to the development of antibodies to lens protein, which by becoming sequestered from the immune mechanism during development, is treated as 'non-self'. However, an alteration in the antigenicity of the lens protein itself may also be an important factor.

Other conditions. Autoantibodies have been described in many other conditions, although their relationship to the diseases is ill-defined. Thus antibodies are found against the microsomal fraction of gastric parietal cells and against intrinsic factor in pernicious anaemia.[13] Autoimmune adrenalitis is thought to be a major cause of Addison's disease, and antimicrosomal antibodies are found in the blood. Primary hypoparathyroidism is yet another disease in which autoantibodies are found.

Experimentally-produced autoimmune diseases. Injections of emulsions of normal tissues, usually mixed with Freund's adjuvant, into animals sometimes produce characteristic lesions. If brain is used, a demyelinating *allergic encephalomyelitis* is produced. Nerve tissue produces an *allergic neuritis.* With thyroid a condition somewhat resembling Hashimoto's disease results. Damage can be produced against other tissues, e.g. testis and uveal tissue, by this type of experiment. Passive transfer experiments indicate that the antibodies involved are cell bound and not immunoglobulins.

What relationship these experimental lesions have to any human disease is not known. Certainly the encephalitis following immunisation against rabies (due to its rabbit spinal-cord content) may fall into this group, but there is no evidence that other demyelinating conditions, e.g. multiple sclerosis, can also be included. The typically relapsing course of the human disease is not seen in experimental autoimmune encephalitis.

Post-vaccinal encephalitis is also characterised by perivascular demyelination, and although an autoimmune mechanism is postulated, direct evidence is lacking.

Conclusions

It is obvious that under a wide range of conditions the body can produce antibodies to its own normal or slightly altered tissue antigens. The immunoglobulins that appear in the circulation are of interest in diagnosis, and sometimes play an important role in the pathogenesis of the disease.

The association of cell-mediated antibody with disease is much less clear. In the experimentally-produced autoimmune conditions they appear to be of great importance. Unfortunately methods of detecting this type of antibody are not reliable and have only recently been applied to human disease; for the present no categorical statement can be made about the role of cellular autoantibodies in human disease.

THE COLLAGEN DISEASES

In 1933 Klinge first drew attention to the damage to the fine collagen framework of the myocardium that occurs in *acute rheumatic fever*, and suggested that this condition was fundamentally a disease of collagen. In 1942 Klemperer and his colleagues were struck by the many morphological features that were common to diseases as distinct as acute rheumatic fever, *rheumatoid arthritis*, *systemic lupus erythematosus*, and *polyarteritis nodosa*. They felt that this group could be classified under the heading of the 'collagen diseases'. Indeed, the feature common to all these diseases is extensive fibrinoid necrosis involving collagen, though this is also invariable in malignant hypertension, which is never classified in the group. A fifth member, *scleroderma*, was subsequently added, but here proliferation with later condensation of collagen is much more typical than fibrinoid necrosis, which is present only in certain uncommon lesions of the disease.

The term 'collagen disease' (or 'connective-tissue disease'), also sometimes called 'collagen-vascular disease' to emphasise the vascular damage that is often a predominant feature, has been a convenient repository for a number of conditions of obscure aetiology in which there is a chronic inflammatory reaction and widespread parenchymatous destruction. The presence of autoantibodies in some of these conditions has confused the issue still further, so that the collagen diseases have been regarded as important examples of autoimmune processes. There is little evidence that any of the five diseases mentioned above, in which there is damage to collagen, are caused by autoantibodies, nor does the collagenous lesion appear to be primary. The present consensus of opinion favours an immune-complex type of allergy as the basis of most of these conditions, and it seems that the concept of collagen disease will pass into disuse. It has been retained here because of its past association and its value in linking the five conditions closely together.

Acute Rheumatic Fever

This is typically a disease of childhood, and it is closely related to a *Strept. pyogenes pharyngitis* which usually occurs about 3 weeks before the onset of the disease. It almost never follows streptococcal impetigo or pyoderma.[5] The present view is that there is an immune-complex reaction between large amounts of streptococcal antigen and small amounts of antibody in the patient's serum. The formation of soluble antigen-antibody complexes, and their localisation on the walls of small blood vessels in the heart and joints predominantly, leads to the activation of complement and tissue damage (see p. 181). The peculiar localisation of these complexes is not understood; in the other streptococcal immune-complex disease, acute glomerulonephritis, the localisation is entirely glomerular. The tissue reactions of this group of diseases usually start as acute inflammation which persists and enters a chronic stage. Instead of an organismal agent being the cause of the reaction, the precipitating factor is a focus of damaged connective tissue.

The basic lesion of rheumatic fever is the *Aschoff body*, which is typically situated in the interstitial tissue of the myocardium close to a coronary arteriole (Fig. 16.5). It is fusiform in shape and microscopical in size, and consists of a small area of necrotic connective tissue. Around this there is a pleomorphic cellular infiltration, of which the most characteristic elements are large cells with basophilic cytoplasm and vesicular nuclei having prominent nucleoli (Anitschkow cells). These nuclei are sometimes multiple, in which case the cell is called an 'Aschoff giant cell'. The origin of these cells has given rise to much debate. They are generally regarded as myocardial histiocytes, though a rival school of thought believes that they are derived from damaged heart muscle.[14] The other cells present are lymphocytes, macrophages, and occasional polymorphs and eosinophils. These foci are also present under the pericardium and the endocardium. Furthermore, there is extensive oedema of the entire heart muscle in the acute stage. Indeed, in those uncommon cases of death from fulminating rheumatic fever, the oedema is the most prominent feature, the cellular infiltration is diffuse, and there are no true Aschoff bodies.

The cause of heart failure in acute rheumatic fever is unknown. The muscle fibres themselves look normal; perhaps there is a more subtle biochemical type of lesion. Mitral regurgitation is the common valvular defect in the acute disease and is due to dilatation of the valve ring.

As recovery occurs, so these foci heal to form scars. This is of great importance in the endocardium and valves. Even in

Figure 16.5

Aschoff nodule in myocardium. In the connective tissue between two muscle bundles there is a fusiform lesion arranged near to a small blood vessel. It consists of a minute focus of damaged connective tissue surrounded by typical Aschoff giant cells and a non-specific small round cell infiltration. × 180.

the acute stage the inflammatory oedema leads to endocardial damage, which is most severe around the mitral and aortic valves. The formation of rheumatic vegetations is the result of this. As healing occurs, so there is progressive scarring and shrinkage of the valve cusps and the chordae tendineae. In due course valvular stenosis or regurgitation ensues. The mitral valve is most commonly attacked in acute theumatic fever, and then the aortic valve. The right side of the heart is only occasionally affected.

There may be an acute sero-fibrinous pericarditis which is organised to form pericardial adhesions. These are of little functional importance and should not be confused with constrictive pericarditis, which is never due to acute rheumatic fever; it is usually tuberculous or pyogenic in origin or else due to rheumatoid disease.

Essentially similar lesions may occur in the joints, producing a characteristically flitting *arthritis*. Rheumatic *pleurisy* is an occasional feature, and from time to time lesions in the *aorta* and the *medium-sized arteries* have been reported. Cerebral involvement gives rise to *Sydenham's chorea*; vague lesions have been described in the basal ganglia and the cortex.

A more typical lesion is the *rheumatic nodule* (Fig. 16.6). Crops tend to erupt subcutaneously along tendons and over bony pressure points. Histologically they are merely florid Aschoff bodies with little central necrosis. The lesions merge

Figure 16.6
Rheumatic nodule. The section shows a small central lattice of degenerating collagen, surrounded by a zone of small round cells. There are no Aschoff giant cells; these are found only in cardiac lesions. × 200 approx. (*From Bywaters, E. G. L. and Scott, F. E. T.* (1960), '*Rheumatism and the connective tissue diseases*', *in* Recent Advances in Clinical Pathology, *Series III, edited by Dyke, S. C. p.* 301, *Fig. 6. London: Churchill*)

into the surrounding tissue. Rheumatic nodules are typically transient, usually disappearing after a few days.

On the whole, the lesions of acute rheumatic fever do not leave significant residual foci of damage; for instance the arthritis resolves spontaneously. Very rarely, however, it progresses and produces severe deformities, especially of the hands, which resemble those of rheumatoid arthritis. This is called *Jaccoud's syndrome*, and has also been seen after the joint involvement of systemic lupus erythematosus.[15] But it is the cardiac lesions that proceed to chronic disability, and the importance of acute rheumatic fever depends on this fact.

Nevertheless, the disease is mild nowadays, a tendency noticeable in streptococcal lesions generally. Some cases of rheumatic heart disease survive to extreme old age.

Rheumatoid Arthritis

This disease has its maximal incidence during early adult life, and it afflicts women much more frequently than men. The lesions are characteristically polyarticular, and the smaller joints tend to bear the brunt of the disease. Clinically it starts as an acute arthritis, and this is reflected histologically in an acutely inflamed synovial membrane. There is proliferation of the synovial lining cells and a heavy infiltration of lymphocytes, plasma cells, macrophages, and numbers of polym-

orphs. The synovial fluid contains many pus cells. As the disease progresses, so the synovial membrane becomes crowded with lymphocytes. Sometimes lymphoid follicles develop in their midst.

There is later an ingrowth of granulation tissue from the perichondral margins. This spreads over the articular surfaces in the form of a pannus, and eventually destroys them completely. Progressive deformity and ankylosis follow. Associated with this there is atrophy of the neighbouring bones and muscles, and the overlying skin becomes smooth and shiny.

In the articular lesions there is little evidence of necrosis, but a very characteristic feature of the disease is the appearance over bony prominences of large *rheumatoid nodules*. These are composed of an extensive central area of necrotic connective tissue which is surrounded by a zone of erectly-orientated histiocytes which are later replaced by fibroblasts. These cells form a 'palisade' around the necrotic collagen, and for this reason the lesion is classified as a palisading granuloma. In the periphery there is an infiltration of lymphocytes, plasma cells, and macrophages. Rheumatoid nodules persist for years. The large amount of necrotic material is probably the cause of this (Fig. 16.7). Similar nodules may sometimes be found in the internal viscera.

Figure 16.7
Rheumatoid nodule. There is an extensive central area of necrotic connective tissue surrounded by a palisade layer of fibroblasts. In the periphery there is reparative fibrosis and a moderate small round cell infiltration. × 200 approx. (*From Bywaters, E. G. L. and Scott, F. E. T.* (1960), '*Rheumatism and the connective tissue diseases*', *in* Recent Advances in Clinical Pathology, *Series III, edited by Dyke, S.C. p.* 301, *Fig. 6. London: Churchill*)

Rheumatoid arthritis is often associated with visceral lesions, so that the composite condition is generally referred to as *rheumatoid disease*. The *heart* is not uncommonly involved, the most frequent lesion being pericarditis which may occasionally be constrictive.[16] Myocardial lesions are rarer, and may take the form of diffuse small round-cell infiltrations, fusiform foci reminiscent of Aschoff bodies, and even discrete rheumatoid granulomata.

Necrotising arteritis, rather similar to that of polyarteritis nodosa, occasionally affects the vessels of the heart, bowel, nerves, and muscles; infarction may thus complicate rheumatoid arthritis.

The pulmonary lesions of rheumatoid disease are important. The commonest is pleurisy, with or without an effusion.[17] A type of diffuse fibrosis (or fibrosing alveolitis) may occur, and also the more typical rheumatoid pneumoconiosis (Caplan's syndrome). This occurs in coalminers who are afflicted with rheumatoid arthritis. In the lungs there are nodular foci composed of a large area of central necrosis, which is surrounded by inflammatory cells and fibrous tissue. It seems that the pneumoconiosis acts as a local precipitating factor for the development of rheumatoid nodules in the lungs. Much more rarely nodules develop in previously normal lungs.

There is often *regional lymphadenitis* in rheumatoid disease. Sometimes this is generalised, and there may be moderate enlargement of the liver and spleen also. The histological changes are those of non-specific reactive hyperplasia. This may occur at any age, but is most prominent in the juvenile condition (Still's disease). If it is accompanied by leucopenia and melanotic pigmentation of the skin, it is called Felty's syndrome.[18]

Ocular lesions are sometimes present. The commonest is keratoconjunctivitis sicca; another is scleromalacia perforans, in which rheumatoid nodules form in the sclera where they break down and often destroy the use of the eye. Iridocyclitis is not a feature of rheumatoid disease. While it is found in some cases of Still's disease, these cases are probably instances of juvenile ankylosing spondylitis rather than rheumatoid disease.

The triad of dry eyes (keratoconjunctivitis sicca), dry mouth (xerostoma), and rheumatoid arthritis constitutes *Sjøgren's syndrome*.[19] The ocular and buccal lesion occurring together is called the *sicca syndrome*,[20] and is common in many diseases in which non-organ-specific autoantibodies are found, e.g. Hashimoto's thyroiditis, liver disease, and renal disease.

Generalised amyloidosis is an important complication of rheumatoid disease.

The nature of rheumatoid disease is unknown. It has been placed in the autoimmune group because there may be autoantibodies present, though there is no evidence that these play a causative part in the disease process. About 80 per cent of patients with active disease have the *rheumatoid factor* in their sera. This is an IgM antibody which reacts against human IgG containing the corresponding Inv or Gm specificity (see p. 143). In practice the globulin is adsorbed on to red cells or latex particles; these are then agglutinated by the rheumatoid factor. Antinuclear antibodies are found in about 20 per cent of cases, but the LE-cell phenomenon is seldom present.

In rheumatoid arthritis IgG, IgM, complement, and rheumatoid factor have all been detected in the synovium of affected joints, and the synovial fluid may contain immune complexes. Furthermore, there is also an increase of T lymphocytes in the synovium of affected joints. The nature of the antigenic stimulus remains obscure; attempts at isolating an organism, e.g. mycoplasma or rubella virus, have been inconclusive.[21,22]

Ankylosing spondylitis. This is mentioned to contrast it with rheumatoid arthritis. It occurs chiefly in young men, and affects the vertebral and sacro-iliac joints predominantly. Although the early histological changes closely resemble those of rheumatoid disease, there is later bony ankylosis and calcification of the ligamentous attachments to the spine. The end-result is a rigid 'bamboo spine'. In about a quarter of cases the peripheral joints are also affected, especially the hip joints.

Ankylosing spondylitis is seronegative. On the other hand, there is a very strong association with transplantation antigen HLA-B27 (see p. 675). Its complications also differ from those of rheumatoid disease: iridocyclitis, aortitis, and a rare apical fibrosis with cavitation of the lungs simulating tuberculosis. Both diseases may lead to amyloidosis.

Systemic Lupus Erythematosus (SLE)

For a long time the skin disease *chronic discoid lupus erythematosus* has been known to dermatologists. It consists of plaques of scaling erythema on the skin of the exposed parts, notably the face and hands. These lesions persist for long periods and heal by scarring. Histologically there is atrophy of the epidermis, hydropic degeneration of the basal cells, a tendency to plugging of the hair follicles with horny material, and an infiltration of small round cells (mostly lymphocytes) in the dermis. It is particularly dense around hair follicles and sweat glands. Foci of altered collagen may be present in the dermis, but this is inconstant.

It was known that occasionally this chronic disease could spread rapidly, especially after prolonged exposure to sunlight. Then a 'sub-acute' or even an 'acute' type of lupus erythematosus could supervene, in which there were severe constitutional disturbances. Death frequently ensued.

More recently the incidence of the acute disseminated or 'systemic' type of disease has increased considerably. It almost always arises *de novo*, though there is no doubt that the chronic discoid type of the disease is related to the systemic variety, for there are subtle gradations in severity between these two extremes. The question arises whether this great increase in incidence of systemic lupus erythematosus is a true indication of the establishment of a new disease, or whether it was always present but remained unrecognised. The disease is much commoner in women than in men, and the age group 20 to 40 years is most often affected.

The manifestations of this disease are very protean. There may be widespread *erythematous eruptions* (involving especially the sun-exposed areas) but on the whole it is the visceral manifestations which predominate. Of these the most important are *arthritis, pericarditis, pleurisy, endocarditis*, and *nephritis*. Fever is present during active phases, and there is usually leucopenia. The disease runs an erratic course, and over 40 per cent of cases survive 15 years. Nephritis is the commonest lethal lesion, and glucocorticoids also contribute to the mortality figures.[23]

Figure 16.8
Systemic lupus erythematosus. This glomerulus shows the typical 'wire-loop' lesion. The thickened capillary wall stains brightly with eosin, because there is widening of the basement-membrane zone. Not all the basement membrane is affected. Thus accounts for the patchy appearance of the lesion in the glomerulus. ×240. (*From Heptinstall, R. H. (1960), 'Diseases of the kidney', in Recent Advances in Pathology, 7th edition, edited by Harrison, C. V. p 103, Fig. 4.11. London: Churchill*)

The characteristic histological lesion of the systemic disease is fibrinoid necrosis of the connective tissue under the endothelium of the serous sacs (e.g. pleura and pericardium), beneath the synovial lining cells of joints, and under the endocardium. The disease also attacks the walls of small arterioles. In the kidney a characteristic appearance is produced in the glomeruli because of a thickening of the basement membrane of the capillaries. The process is focal, and the affected vessels have a brightly eosinophilic, thickened wall thereby resembling the bacteriologist's wire loop: this is called the *wire-loop lesion* (Fig. 16.8). Many glomeruli show foci of mesangial proliferation, and ultimately undergo necrosis. Another characteristic, but distinctly uncommon, lesion may be seen in the splenic arterioles situated in the centre of the lymphoid follicles: a concentric laying-down of collagen fibres without much necrosis, producing an onion-skin appearance.

In the heart the necrotic connective tissue under the endocardium may erupt through on to the surface and lead to the formation of vegetations. These may be mural or valvular, and unlike rheumatic disease, both sides of the heart are equally affected, the brunt being borne by the mitral and tricuspid valves. This lesion is called *Libman–Sacks endocarditis*, and is a characteristic, though uncommon, manifestation of SLE. The myocardium is not primarily affected, but foci of necrotic connective tissue may be found in it.

Around the areas of fibrinoid necrosis there is an inflammatory reaction in which lymphocytes and plasma cells are present. A very important diagnostic feature of the disease is the presence of lilac-staining *haematoxyphil bodies* amid the necrotic debris. They are foci of degraded nuclear material, and are the histological counterpart of the 'LE cell'. These bodies are small, round, and homogeneous.

A prominent feature of the condition is the presence of many autoantibodies in the serum. Acute haemolytic anaemia may occur, and the Coombs test is sometimes positive. Circulating anticoagulants may be present, and there may also be thrombocytopenic purpura due to platelet antibodies. These patients are also prone to develop alloantibodies against transfused red cells, and if they require a transfusion expert selection of blood and cross-matching are essential. The serological tests for syphilis may be falsely positive, and the rheumatoid factor is present in about a third of the cases.

The most important antibodies from a diagnostic point of view are those that are active against nuclear components. These may be detected by immunofluorescence. Suitable cells are incubated with patient's serum, thoroughly washed, and then incubated with fluorescein-labelled anti-IgG. Many patterns have been described but four are commonly recognised:

1. *Homogeneous pattern.* The entire nucleus is seen to fluoresce evenly. This is associated with antibody against nucleoprotein—the same antibody that is responsible for the LE test (see below).

2. *Peripheral, or rim, pattern.* This pattern is associated with antibodies to DNA and nucleoprotein. Renal involvement is most common with this pattern.

3. *Nucleolar pattern.*

4. *Speckled pattern.* This is characteristic of the mixed connective-tissue disease.

The presence of autoantibodies against native double-stranded DNA is virtually pathognomonic of systemic lupus erythematosus, particularly if there is renal involvement. Antibodies to single-stranded DNA or denatured DNA are less specific, and are found also in other diseases.

The *LE-cell phenomenon* was the first specific laboratory test described for the diagnosis of SLE. It is found that when normal leucocytes are incubated with the serum of a patient for about 2 hours at 37°C, some of the neutrophils contain a homogeneous mass of uniformly purplish material (using a Romanowsky stain) in their cytoplasm. The mass consists of altered nuclear material. The neutrophil is called an 'LE cell', and it must be distinguished from a 'tart cell', which is a monocyte which has phagocytosed a nuclear fragment, the basic structure of which is still recognisable. It is the homogeneous, structureless nature of the inclusion that is typical of the LE cell. The exact nature of the phenomenon is ill-understood. The current view is that the patient's serum contains an antibody against a component of nucleoprotein—probably a nucleohistone. When the leucocytes die, e.g. after prolonged incubation, the antibody reacts with this component. The nucleus is then ingested by a polymorph. Apparently the process of ingestion causes the alteration in the nuclear appearance.

With the exception of chronic active hepatitis the LE test is not positive in diseases other than SLE. It is not, however, as sensitive as the fluorescent-antibody tests.

Patients with SLE also have an antibody that kills lymphocytes in the presence of complement and at a low temperature. Similar cold-reactive lymphocytotoxins are also found in patients with Crohn's disease, and are presumed to be a manifestation of an altered immune reaction.[24]

The wide range of antibodies present in SLE react with widely distributed antigen, and are non-organ specific. There is no evidence that the antibodies against intracellular fractions are active against living cells. It is interesting that the relatives of patients with SLE show an increased incidence of autoantibodies and related diseases (see also pp. 171 and 213).

There is good evidence that lupus nephritis is an immune-complex disorder due to the localisation of soluble complexes of nuclear antigen and antinuclear antibody in the glomeruli.[25,26] The nuclear antigen is DNA, and it may be autologous or foreign, e.g. from a bacterium or virus. Patients with active lupus nephritis almost invariably have a reduced serum level of complement.[25] It seems probable that many of the manifestations of SLE are attributable to damaging immune complexes in the small blood vessels of the viscera, e.g. heart, joints, and serous cavities. The agent is thought to be a drug or an organism which acts on autologous DNA or contributes its own DNA. The antihypertensive agent hydralazine stimulates antibodies to native DNA when it produces a lupus syndrome.

In a number of cases of lupus nephritis filamentous, tubular structures, variously called undulating tubules (p. 26) and tubuloreticular inclusions, were seen in the glomerular endothelial cells, and these have been interpreted as being viral, e.g. orthomyxovirus or paramyxovirus. It seems more likely that they are modified endoplasmic reticulum,[27] and neither these structures nor others that have been described can be regarded as being proven virus particles. In one case haemobartonella-like organisms were found in the red cells.[28] In other cases high titres of antibodies to various viruses, especially EB virus, have been reported.[29]

A C-type RNA virus appears to be involved in the pathogenesis of murine SLE in New Zealand black (NZB) mice,[30] and a similar virus may well occur in human tissues. The distinction between viral and host DNA is not easy, and both can be transmitted from parent to offspring; this again emphasises the close connexion between inherited disease and viral infection. In the disease of NZB/NZW hybrid mice, the glomerulonephritis that occurs closely resembles that found in human SLE. The development of the glomerular lesions is greatly enhanced and intensified by incidental viral infection (e.g. lymphocytic choriomeningitis virus). The glomerular deposits contain lymphocytic choriomeningitis virus antigen and Gross virus antigen as well as native DNA.

Systemic lupus erythematosus therefore appears to be caused by the deposition of antigen-antibody complexes with the subsequent activation of complement. The antibodies may be directed against native DNA or viral DNA. The reason why only certain individuals are affected by the disease may be related to genetic constitution or *in-utero* viral infection analagous to the Gross virus infection in mice.

Polyarteritis Nodosa

Polyarteritis nodosa of the classical, or Kussmaul-Maier, type is a *necrotising arteritis* affecting the *medium-sized muscular vessels* of the heart, kidneys, bowel, liver, spleen, pancreas, and also the nutrient arteries of the peripheral nerves. The usual victims are middle-aged men, and the clinical manifestations are a febrile, wasting illness to which the effects of regional vascular occlusion are added. Multiple asymmetrical neuritis (*mononeuritis multiplex*) due to ischaemia of peripheral nerve trunks is a common finding. The effects of polyarteritis nodosa are extremely widespread; recovery is exceptional.

Histologically there is an extensive zone of fibrinoid necrosis involving a segment of the artery. The whole thickness of the wall is affected (i.e. it is a panarteritis), and there is a profuse inflammatory response with infiltrations of lymphocytes, plasma cells, macrophages, polymorphs, and often many eosinophils as well. The weakened wall tends to yield to the intra-arterial pressure, and small nodular aneurysms may form (hence the name polyarteritis nodosa) and subsequently rupture. An even commoner complication is thrombosis and infarction. At necropsy there are often large extravasations of blood, e.g. around the kidneys and in the wall of the bowel, as well as extensive areas of infarction of the kidneys, spleen, and other organs. The lesions may heal, especially under the influence of glucocorticoids, and then the arterial wall is invaded by granulation tissue. This in no way lessens the danger of infarction; indeed, the worst ischaemic effects may be seen in the healing stage.

The renal lesions of polyarteritis are particularly severe; not only is there often necrosis of the arcuate and interlobular arteries, but there is also much fibrinoid necrosis of individual glomeruli. Systemic hypertension is commonly present, especially as the renal lesions heal.

The aetiology of polyarteritis nodosa is unknown in most cases, but sometimes hypersensitivity to drugs, e.g. sulphonamides, phenylbutazone, tetracyclines, and thiazides, appears to be the precipitating factor.

Variants of polyarteritis nodosa. A type of polyarteritis occurs which affects small vessels and spares those of larger calibre. This *microscopical polyarteritis* is characterised by vascular necrosis and an accompanying acute inflammatory reaction (Fig. 16.9). This is often marked, and the initial polymorph exudate is followed by a mononuclear one sometimes with epithelioid-cell and giant-cell formation. Vascular obstruction leads to tissue necrosis, and later there is granulation-tissue formation. The lesions may therefore show extensive necrosis and chronic inflammation, and resemble those produced by bacteria and fungi. These granulomatous variants generally are examples of Wegener's granulomatosis or allergic granulomatous vasculitis (Churg and Strauss), as described below.

A variety of names has been attached to this group of conditions, e.g. necrotising arteritis (or vasculitis, if small veins are also involved) and hypersensitivity angiitis. In the latter, described by Zeek, the lesions all tend to be at the same stage. The distribution of the lesions varies from case to case and a large number of clinical syndromes are recognised. In some, e.g. Wegener's granulomatosis, the lesions are severe and, if untreated, the disease is invariably fatal. In others the arteritis is confined to one area and the disease is benign and self-limiting, e.g. erythema nodosum and Henoch-Schönlein purpura (p. 640). In the syndromes which affect the kidney

Figure 16.9
Polyarteritis nodosa with pulmonary involvement. This small pulmonary artery shows severe fibrinoid necrosis. It is surrounded by a heavy cellular infiltration. ×198. (*From Harrison, C. V.* (1960), (*Diseases of arteries', in* Recent Advances in Pathology, *7th edition, edited by Harrison, C. V. p.* 172, *Fig.* 5.8. *London: Churchill*)

the characteristic lesion is glomerulonecrosis and capsular crescent formation, very much like that seen in rapidly progressive glomerulonephritis.

Recognised syndromes. A few only of these will be outlined.

Lethal midline granuloma, or *malignant granuloma.* This affects males rather more frequently than females, and usually in the 20 to 50 age group. It often commences with epistaxis, and is characterised by inflammatory granulation-tissue formation in the nose and nasopharynx. This is combined with necrosis and gangrene, so that eventually the palate and nasal structures are destroyed. This terrible disease usually kills by local infection or haemorrhage.

Progressive allergic granulomatosis. This variant often starts with the development of asthmatic attacks. Nodular, necrotic lesions are present in the lungs, and these are accompanied by chronic inflammation with epithelioid cells and giant cells (Fig. 16.10). The lesions therefore resemble those of tuberculosis.

Wegener's granulomatosis.[31,32] This is usually defined as a polyarteritis affecting amongst other organs the *kidneys, lungs,* and *upper respiratory tract.* In the last site the lesions resemble those described in lethal midline granuloma. Death is usually due to renal failure. Treatment with cytotoxic drugs has greatly improved the prognosis of this otherwise uniformly fatal disease.[33]

Figure 16.10
Two allergic granulomata in the portal area of the liver. Note the central necrosis and the surrounding zone of macrophages and giant cells. The small cells at the periphery of the lesions are eosinophils, plasma cells, and macrophages. ×120. (*From Abell, M. R. et al.* (1970), New England Journal of Medicine, **282,** 665)

Although many separate syndromes are described, the validity of regarding them as separate entities must be questioned. On the one hand, it is common to encounter cases in which the features, although clearly those of a vasculitis, do not fit readily into any one of the described syndromes. On the other hand, it is also doubtful whether the custom of including these many syndromes under the heading of polyarteritis is a valid basis for classification. In some instances the disease appears to be a manifestation of hypersensitivity to drugs, food, or infection. The only feature which is common to all members of this group is a morphological one—namely the presence of an arteritis.

Although the precipitating agent is usually not discovered, the morphology of the lesion and its not infrequent association with hypersensitivity make an immune-complex mechanism the most probable. Lesions of experimental serum sickness in animals closely resemble human polyarteritis nodosa. Of great interest is the occasional association of hepatitis-B surface antigen (HBsAg) with polyarteritis nodosa.[34] In the incubation period of hepatitis B the following immune-complex lesions have been described: polyarteritis, glomerulonephritis, urticaria, and arthritis.[35]

Another example of vasculitis due to the deposition of immune complexes is erythema nodosum leprosum;[36] this is seen in lepromatous leprosy when treated with dapsone. There is a cutaneous vasculitis manifest as erythematous indurated areas which may ulcerate. Fever, lymphadenopathy, proteinuria, and arthritis are present, as in serum sickness.

On the other hand, Wegener's granulomatosis does not seem to be related to circulating immune complexes, but there is not infrequently evidence of partial impairment of cell-mediated immunity.[37]

Polyarteritis nodosa and its variants are not usually associated with autoantibodies, although from time to time non-organ-specific ones are found in the serum. The diagnosis is histological from a skin or muscle biopsy, or from a deep-seated lesion.

Scleroderma

As with LE, scleroderma was first described as a skin disease. Two types are recognised: circumscribed scleroderma, or morphoea, and systemic scleroderma, or progressive systemic sclerosis.

Morphoea. The disease is usually restricted to the skin. Well-demarcated plaques are formed which are stiff and firm. These lesions are of little significance unless they are extensive, when they are associated with atrophy of the underlying subcutaneous tissue and skeletal muscles. If the face is affected there may be hemiatrophy. Morphoea rarely, if ever, progresses to the systemic form.

Progressive systemic sclerosis. The skin lesions may start centrally on the trunk and spread peripherally, or they may start on the face and hands. The latter type is usually associated with Raynaud's phenomenon, and calcification may occur particularly in the pulps of the fingers. The affected skin becomes indurated, stiff, and tight so that if the area involved is great, considerable impairment of movement ensues. This is accentuated by atrophy of the subcutaneous tissues, so that the skin is bound to underlying muscles. Muscle weakness due to *myositis* is common and often severe. In contrast to morphoea, the skin lesions are poorly defined. Nevertheless, the changes which occur are very similar in both types of disease.

In the skin lesion of scleroderma the collagen fibres are at first swollen and oedematous, and there is a small round cell infiltration which is most heavy around the blood vessels. Later on the collagen fibres become condensed into compact masses in which the normal spaces between individual bundles are greatly reduced in extent. New collagen is formed, and this results in the thickening of the dermis. In due course the fibroblasts become very scanty and the cellular infiltration disappears. The hair follicles and sebaceous glands atrophy. The elastic tissue may also disappear, but more usually it persists. Hyperelastosis is occasionally reported. There is also a tendency towards increased melanin pigmentation over the affected areas of skin, and Addison's disease may be simulated.

Visceral lesions. *Skeletal muscle* is nearly always affected. There is degeneration of muscle fibres with an associated inflammatory response, and ultimately replacement by fibrous tissue occurs. Similar changes are often seen in the smooth muscle of the *gastrointestinal tract*. The oesophagus is the most common site, and dysphagia and regurgitation of food

result. *Cardiac muscle* may be affected and heart failure occurs. The *lungs* often suffer, not only as the result of the oesophageal lesion, but also primarily. Diffuse fibrosis leads to contraction of the lung substance, and there may be the formation of cysts lined by bronchiolar epithelium surrounded by dense fibrous tissue (honeycomb lung). This fibro-cystic change is usually most pronounced at the periphery of the lung, and the cysts may rupture into the pleural cavity to produce a pneumothorax. The exuberant proliferation of epithelium in these cysts may sometimes proceed to neoplasia, and adenocarcinoma is a well-recognised complication of scleroderma lung.

The smaller *arteries* in sclerodermatous lesions show intimal proliferation (endarteritis) with medial hypertrophy and a mild inflammatory reaction around them. In the extremities this may lead to Raynaud's syndrome, which sometimes precedes overt disease.

A similar type of lesion is occasionally found in the interlobular arteries of the *kidney*, and the thickened tunica intima contains large amounts of an acid mucopolysaccharide (Fig. 16.11). Distal to this there may be fibrinoid necrosis of the arteries which can extend to the afferent glomerular arterioles and the glomeruli. The appearance is identical to

Figure 16.11
Progressive systemic sclerosis involving a renal artery. This interlobular artery shows great intimal proliferation; the thickened tunica intima contains a large amount of mucoid material in which the cellular element is splayed out. The lumen is almost occluded. The smaller arteries and arterioles showed severe fibrinoid necrosis. × 250.

that of severe malignant hypertension, but in scleroderma the blood pressure is usually normal. This renal lesion is rare, and when present is rapidly fatal.

Of all the 'collagen diseases' scleroderma is the most chronic. Inflammatory change is seldom conspicuous, and apart from the renal lesion, the process is a very prolonged one. Non-organ-specific autoantibodies may be found in the serum, e.g. low titres of antinuclear factor. Rheumatoid factor may also be present in those cases with a higher titre of antinuclear factor. The titre of these factors bears no relationship to the severity or extent of the disease. Antibodies to RNA may also be present.[38]

The nature of the condition is obscure, but some authorities consider the vascular lesion to be the primary one. On electron microscopy similarities have been noted in the small vessels of cases of SLE, dermatomyositis, and scleroderma.[39] The last shows more advanced changes than those of the first two. In one case of scleroderma that progressed to a fatal polyarteritis nodosa, immunoglobulin and complement were found free within the acutely inflamed small arteries,[40] but there is no evidence that scleroderma itself is an immune-complex disease.

Polymyositis[41]

Polymyositis is frequently included among the collagen diseases. Histologically there is a diffuse inflammatory infiltration affecting many skeletal muscles, accompanied by destruction of muscle fibres. There may also be cutaneous lesions, in which case the condition is called *dermatomyositis*. The skin changes can take many forms. Periorbital oedema and heliotrope erythema are characteristic, but other lesions may resemble those of systemic lupus erythematosus or progressive systemic sclerosis. There is a well-recognised association between dermatomyositis and deep-seated malignant disease.

Mixed Connective-Tissue Disease[42–44]

This term has been applied by Sharp and associates to a syndrome having features of systemic lupus erythematosus, progressive systemic sclerosis, and dermatomyositis. Raynaud's syndrome is common, and the condition has a good prognosis since renal complications are uncommon and the response to prednisone is good. Specific antinuclear antibody is present and gives a speckled pattern on immunofluorescence. This is due to the presence of an antibody to a ribonuclease-insensitive component of an extractable nuclear antigen (ENA), which itself is a complex of nuclear RNA and protein.

Conclusions

The 'collagen diseases' comprise a group of conditions that have the following features in common:

There is widespread degeneration of collagen, and fibrinoid necrosis is present in all of them. The necrosis is greatest in polyarteritis and SLE, and is least conspicuous in scleroderma. Nevertheless, degeneration of collagen can occur following many types of injury, and it is difficult to accept that these conditions are primarily diseases of collagen. They do, however, involve the connective tissues of many organs in addition to being associated with parenchymal damage, e.g. epidermis in SLE.

Collagen, like its denatured derivative gelatin, is antigenic, and antibodies to both substances have been demonstrated in human sera. Human autoantibodies against gelatin may be found in normal sera, but their titre is raised in rheumatoid arthritis, SLE, and scleroderma, as well as in some other chronic conditions associated with collagen breakdown. Native collagen is less antigenic than its denatured derivative, but antibodies against it are also reported in the conditions mentioned above. Their true incidence in health and disease awaits further investigation.[45]

Whether these two collagen antibodies play any part in the collagen diseases is unknown, but tissue-culture experiments suggest that the antigelatin autoantibodies may stimulate fibroblasts to synthesise and secrete more cell product.

They all respond well to glucocorticoids and ACTH. Their action is presumably not only anti-inflammatory but also inhibitory to autoantibody formation. More recently *immunosuppressive agents* have been used, e.g. cyclophosphamide and azathioprine, and good results have been reported, especially in polyarteritis nodosa and its more lethal variants.[33] Once again the effect is anti-inflammatory as well as immunosuppressive.

There is a marked constitutional effect typified by a greatly raised red-cell sedimentation rate. This is useful prognostically in gauging the progress of the condition. In scleroderma the ESR may be normal, as it is the most torpid of all these conditions. There is a general tendency to hypergammaglobulinaemia, which is most pronounced in rheumatoid arthritis and SLE.

There is an inter-relationship between the disorders. Some cases of rheumatoid arthritis develop features of SLE, and polyarteritis nodosa may complicate SLE or rheumatoid arthritis. Scleroderma occasionally merges into rheumatoid arthritis and SLE. Furthermore there is sometimes an increased familial incidence of this group of diseases. The increased incidence in patients with certain congenital immunological deficiency syndromes has been noted on page 171. The explanation of this is not known, for while it might be taken to support the thesis that an altered immune response is of prime importance, an increased liability to infection with an unidentified agent is equally possible.

The initial enthusiasm for including the collagen diseases under the heading of autoimmunity has now waned. Certainly autoantibodies are present, especially in SLE and rheumatoid arthritis, and hypersensitivity is important in some types of polyarteritis. An alteration in the immune response is a feature of this group of diseases, but its relationship to their pathogenesis is obscure.

It is of interest to conclude with a brief account of certain animal diseases which closely mimic the human collagen diseases.[46] *Aleutian mink disease* resembles SLE and is due to a viral infection. The *autoimmune haemolytic anaemia* that develops in New Zealand black (NZB) mice is suspected of being a viral infection, perhaps acquired *in utero*, because the disease still develops if the animals are reared under germ-free conditions.[47] The NZB mice occasionally, and the hybrids NZB/NZW frequently, develop an immune-complex nephritis which closely resembles human lupus nephritis. Genetic, viral, and immunological factors are therefore involved. Swine develop a polyarthritis due to an infection with *Erysipelothrix insidiosa*, while *equine viral arteritis* resembles human polyarteritis. An arteritis is also a feature of equine infectious anaemia (a viral disease) and Aleutian mink disease. Now that an autoimmune aetiology for this group of diseases is no longer favoured, there is a search for similar infective agents in the human subject.

REFERENCES

1. PETERS, D. K. & LACHMANN, P. J. (1974) Immunity deficiency in pathogenesis of glomerulonephritis. *Lancet*, 1, 58.
2. GERMUTH, F. G. & RODRIGUEZ, E. (1973) *Immune Complex Deposits and Antibasement Membrane Disease*. Boston: Little Brown.
3. McCLUSKEY, R. T. & KLASSEN, J. (1973) Immunologically mediated glomerular, tubular and interstitial renal disease. *New England Journal of Medicine*, 288, 564.
4. ROY, L. P. *et al.* (1972) Etiologic agents of immune deposit disease. *Progress in Clinical Immunology*, 1, 1.
5. WANNAMAKER, L. W. (1970) Differences between streptococcal infections of the throat and of the skin. *New England Journal of Medicine*, 282, 23 and 78.
6. REED, R. W. & MATHESON, B. H. (1960) Experimental nephritis due to type specific streptococci. IV. The effect of type 12 nephrotoxin in monkeys. *Journal of Infectious Diseases*, 106, 245.
7. TSANTOULAS, D. C. *et al.* (1974) Cell-mediated immunity to human Tamm-Horsfall glycoprotein in autoimmune liver disease with renal tubular acidosis. *British Medical Journal*, 4, 491.
8. PARONETTO, F. & POPPER, H. (1976) Two immunologic reactions in the pathogenesis of hepatitis? *New England Journal of Medicine*, 294, 606.
9. BEUTNER, E. H., CHORZELSKI, T. P. & JORDAN, R. E. (1970) *Autosensitisation in Pemphigus and Bullous Pemphigoid*. Springfield, Illinois: Thomas.
10. ALLISON, A. C. (1976) Self-tolerance and autoimmunity in the thyroid. *New England Journal of Medicine*, 295, 821.
11. HOGAN, M. J. & ZIMMERMAN, L. E. (1962) *Ophthalmic Pathology*, 2nd edn, pp. 367 and 153. Philadelphia: Saunders.
12. MANSKI, W. *et al.* (1976) In *Textbook of Immunopathology*, 2nd edn, Vol. 2, p. 877, ed. Miescher, P. A. and Müller-Eberhard, H. J. New York: Grune and Stratton.
13. JAMES, D. *et al.* (1974) Cell-mediated immunity to intrinsic factor in autoimmune disorders. *British Medical Journal*, 4, 494.
14. MURPHY, G. E. (1960) Nature of rheumatic heart disease with special reference to myocardial disease and heart failure. *Medicine (Baltimore)*, 39, 289.
15. BYWATERS, E. G. L. (1975) Jaccoud's syndrome. A sequel to the joint involvement of systemic lupus erythematosus. *Clinics in Rheumatic Diseases*, 1, 125
16. HARROLD, B. P. (1968) Non-tuberculous constrictive pericarditis. *British Medical Journal*, 1, 290.
17. Leading Article (1972) Pleural effusion in rheumatoid arthritis. *Lancet*, 1, 480.
18. Leading Article (1971) Felty's syndrome. *British Medical Journal*, 4, 379.
19. Leading Article (1973) Sjøgren's syndrome. *British Medical Journal*, 4, 62.
20. GOLDING, P. L. *et al.* (1970) 'Sicca complex' in liver disease. *British Medical Journal*, 4, 340.
21. HIRSCHHORN, R. (1975) The blind man and the rheumatoid elephant. *New England Journal of Medicine*, 293, 554.
22. Leading Article (1976) Immune complexes in rheumatic disease. *Lancet*, 2, 79.
23. Leading Article (1971) Systemic lupus: history and natural history. *Lancet*, 1, 1283.
24. Leading Article (1976) Lymphocytotoxic antibodies. *Lancet*, 1, 785.
25. Leading Article (1971) Treatment of lupus nephritis. *Lancet*, 2, 964.
26. CHRISTIAN, C. L. (1969) Immune-complex disease. *New England Journal of Medicine*, 280, 878.
27. GRIMLEY, P. M. & SCHAFF, Z. (1976) Significance of tuburoreticular inclusions in the pathology of human disease. *Pathology Annual*, 6, 221.
28. KALLICK, C. A. *et al.* (1972) Systemic lupus erythematosus associated with haemobartonella-like organisms. *Nature New Biology*, 236, 145.
29. EVANS, A. S., ROTHFIELD, N. F. & NIEDERMAN, J. C. (1971) Raised antibody titres to E.B. virus in systemic lupus erythematosus. *Lancet*, 1, 167.
30. CHRISTIAN, C. L. (1976) Systemic lupus erythematosus and type C RNA viruses. *New England Journal of Medicine*, 295, 501.
31. Leading Article (1971) Wegener's granulomatosis. *British Medical Journal*, 3, 446.
32. HARRISON, D. F. N. (1974) Non-healing granulomata of the upper respiratory tract. *British Medical Journal*, 4, 205.
33. Leading Article (1972) Wegener's granulomatosis. *Lancet*, 2, 519.
34. GOCKE, D. J. *et al.* (1970) Association between polyarteritis and Australia antigen. *Lancet*, 2, 1149.
35. Leading Article (1971) Extrahepatic manifestations of serum hepatitis. *Lancet*, 2, 805.
36. WEMAMBU, S. N. C. *et al.* (1969) Erythema nodosum leprosum: a clinical manifestation of the Arthus phenomenon. *Lancet*, 2, 933.
37. SHILLITOE, E. J. *et al.* (1974) Immunological features of Wegener's granulomatosis. *Lancet*, 1, 281.
38. JAYSON, M. I. V. (1977) Collagen changes in the pathogenesis of systemic sclerosis. *Annals of the Rheumatic Diseases*, 36, Supplement p. 26.
39. NORTON, W. L. (1970) Comparison of the microangiopathy of systemic lupus erythematosus, dermatomyositis, scleroderma, and diabetes mellitus. *Laboratory Investigation*, 22, 301.
40. TOTH, A. & ALPERT, L. I. (1971) Progressive systemic sclerosis terminating as periarteritis nodosa. *Archives of Pathology*, 92, 31.
41. TALBOTT, J. H. (1974) *Collagen-Vascular Diseases*. New York: Grune and Stratton.
42. SHARP, G. C. *et al.* (1972) Mixed connective tissue disease—an apparently distinct rheumatic disease syndrome associated with a specific antibody to an extractable nuclear antigen (ENA). *American Journal of Medicine*, 52, 148.
43. KITCHINER, D. *et al.* (1975) Mixed connective tissue disease with digital gangrene. *British Medical Journal*, 1, 249.
44. MINKIN, W. & RABHAN, N. (1977) Mixed connective tissue disease. *Archives of Dermatology*, 112, 1535.
45. HOLBOROW, E. J. *et al.* (1977) Antibodies against reticulin and collagen. *Annals of the Rheumatic Diseases*, 36, Supplement p. 51.
46. LEADER, R. W., GORHAM, J. R. & WAGNER, B. M. (1967) In *The Connective Tissue*, ed. Wagner, B. M. & Smith, D. E. pp. 95–131. Baltimore: Williams and Wilkins.
47. EAST, J. *et al.* (1967) Autoimmune reactions and virus-like particles in germ-free NZB mice. *Lancet*, 1, 755.

Chapter 17. Acute Pyogenic Infections

The organisms responsible for suppuration account for some of the most important lesions seen clinically. Although most of these bacteria respond to antibiotic therapy, surgical drainage of abscesses caused by them is still often necessary. The most important members of this group are:

The pyogenic cocci, viz. *Staphylococcus aureus*, *Streptococcus pyogenes*, pneumococcus, meningococcus, and gonococcus.

The Gram-negative intestinal bacilli, viz. *Escherichia coli*, *Proteus* species, *Pseudomonas aeruginosa* (*Ps. pyocyanea*), and organisms of the genus *Bacteroides*.

Of these it is the staphylococcus, streptococcus, and Gram-negative bacilli that produce the most widespread lesions. Not only do they infect wounds, burns, and chronic ulcerative skin lesions secondarily, but they can also spread to any organ of the body. No tissue is exempt from these non-specific bacterial infections.

By contrast, the pneumococcus nearly always affects the lungs. Though an initial septicaemia is characteristic of lobar pneumonia, the organism produces metastatic lesions only exceptionally. Likewise, the meningococcus and gonococcus usually confine themselves to the meninges and genital tract respectively.

The local tissue response to each of these bacteria is similar: acute inflammation with a copious outpouring of neutrophil polymorphs. The process and its possible sequelae have been described in Chapter 6. If the organisms are destroyed early by the inflammatory response, there is resolution; otherwise the condition proceeds to suppuration with abscess formation. If the pus is successfully drained healing follows; otherwise the lesion becomes chronic. Many of the common chronic inflammatory lesions due to non-specific bacterial infections come into this category, e.g. chronic pyelonephritis, chronic diverticulitis, chronic cholecystitis, and chronic osteomyelitis. It should be remembered, as stressed in Chapter 11, that a neutrophil infiltrate is not pathognomonic of a simple acute inflammatory reaction; it occurs also in chronic abscesses and in other chronic infections such as actinomycosis and sporotrichosis. When a pyogenic lesion becomes chronic there is an admixture of other cells, e.g. lymphocytes, plasma cells, macrophages, and eosinophils, as well as a proliferation of connective tissue and specialised cells.

In generalised pyogenic infections there is a severe constitutional reaction with fever and a neutrophil leucocytosis. The ESR is raised, and immunoglobulins are produced which are important in the defence against the organisms (see Ch. 13). The diagnosis is generally made by isolating the organism either from a local lesion or by blood culture. Nevertheless, in some instances serological methods are of value. Thus the gonococcal complement fixation test may be indicative of the aetiology of an obscure arthritis and the anti-staphylococcal haemolysin titre rises in patients with deep-seated staphylococcal abscesses. A rise in anti-DNAse and antistreptococcal haemolysin O (commonly shortened to ASO) is seen following streptococcal pharyngitis and tonsillitis, and this may help to confirm the diagnosis of acute glomerulonephritis and rheumatic fever. With streptococcal skin infections no such rise in ASO titre is seen[1] (see also p. 202 and 206).

GENERAL BACTERIOLOGY OF PYOGENIC ORGANISMS

It is important to note the salient bacteriological features of these organisms because of the frequency with which they cause infection. By examining the properties of each organism an attempt can be made to understand the type of disease it causes.

STAPHYLOCOCCI

Morphology. They are Gram-positive, spherical organisms about 1 μm in diameter, which are arranged in grape-like clusters. They are non-motile, non-sporing, and non-capsulate.

Cultural characteristics. They grow easily on most media. They are aerobic organisms, but can tolerate an anaerobic atmosphere quite well, i.e. they are facultative anaerobes. They grow best at 37°C. On blood agar, shiny, convex colonies about 3 mm in diameter appear within 24 hours, and these are pigmented. Most have a creamy white or dull yellow colour, but some species are golden, lemon yellow, and even red. Though pigmentation is no longer regarded as important, the organisms are still called *Staphylococcus albus* when non-pathogenic (whatever the actual colour of the colony) and *Staphylococcus aureus* when pathogenic. *Staph. aureus* is sometimes called *Staph. pyogenes*, and *Staph. albus* is occasionally called *Staph. epidermidis*. Staphylococci are divided into these two groups according to their production of coagulase in the laboratory. The term non-pathogenic is not strictly true, for *Staph. albus* can produce infection (p. 218).

Coagulase production. Coagulase is an enzyme that converts the fibrinogen of citrated human or rabbit plasma into fibrin. *Staph. albus* does not produce it but *Staph. aureus* does. It can be demonstrated by a slide test, in which a suspension of staphylococci in water is mixed with a drop of plasma. The organisms clump together at once if coagulase is present, because fibrin sticks to the surfaces of the cocci and makes them adhere to one another.

Typing of staphylococci. Not all varieties of *Staph. aureus* are equally virulent. Some are associated with superficial skin lesions only, while others may lead to disastrous ward epidemics. In such an epidemic of hospital infection it is necessary to type the staphylococcus to see whether all the patients are infected with a single strain or with a number of strains, as explained in Chapter 19. Staphylococci are typed with a bacteriophage (which is a virus that parasitises bacteria) that acts specifically against staphylococci. Some bacteriophages, however, lyse more than one strain of staphylococcus, and some strains of staphylococci are lysed by a number of bacteriophages. However, the number of bacteriophages lysing a particular strain of staphylococci is constant, and the organism is typed according to the *pattern* of lysis by a set of 24 different anti-*Staph. aureus* bacteriophages. For example, a well-known epidemic strain of staphylococcus is lysed by phages 47, 53, 75, and 77, and is therefore typed 47/53/75/77. One of the most notorious epidemic strains is the phage type 80 staphylococcus. This was first recognised in Australia in 1953, and has since then wreaked havoc in many hospitals throughout the world.

The various phage types can be allocated to one of three groups: Group I contains many hospital epidemic strains. Group II strains cause minor sepsis and impetigo. Group III includes strains of animal origin, most of the enterotoxin-producing strains, and many of the antibiotic-resistant hospital strains.

Toxin production. The staphylococcus is an invasive organism, but the factors responsible for its virulence are not clearly defined. Nevertheless, some toxins are known, and these mainly have the properties of endotoxins. Many microbiologists, however, prefer to group these toxic products under the heading of exotoxins. Be this as it may, there is no doubt that their action is less potent than that of the enterotoxin, which is noted below.

The most important of these toxic products is the *α-toxin*, which produces local tissue necrosis, and is lethal when injected intravenously. It is also haemolytic to red cells, and destroys white cells, i.e. it is a haemolysin and a leucocidin.

Another staphylococcal toxin acts only on white cells, and is called the *Panton-Valentine leucocidin*. Two other endotoxins are also described, and these have haemolytic and necrotising actions. An erythrogenic factor has also been described on a few occasions (see footnote, p. 219).

In addition three enzymes are produced by staphylococci:
Coagulase.
Staphylokinase, which lyses fibrin by activating the plasmin system.
Hyaluronidase. These last two enzymes are produced by most strains, but do not play a notable part in the pathogenesis of the lesions.

Some strains also produce an exotoxin called *enterotoxin*, which produces symptoms of food-poisoning when ingested. It is the only exotoxin produced by the staphylococcus, and unlike most exotoxins it is thermostable.

Lesions produced by staphylococci. The typical staphylococcal lesion is a *circumscribed abscess*. It contains thick creamy pus which is odourless. Coagulase production has been suggested as an important factor in the localisation of the infection by virtue of the copious fibrin formation that it induces (see fibrin barrier, p. 98). On the other hand, some authorities regard coagulase as a factor aiding the spread of infection, because the deposition of fibrin acts as a protective covering for the organism. It is evident that our ideas on the importance of coagulase in staphylococcal infection are still purely speculative. It seems likely that the local damage inflicted by the α-toxin leads to a marked inflammatory reaction, which in its turn successfully localises and overcomes the infection.

The most important surgical staphylococcal lesion is *wound infection*, which is often acquired while the patient is in hospital.

Staphylococcal skin lesions are very frequent and include boils, carbuncles, paronychia, impetigo, and its bullous variant in the newborn (Fig. 17.1).

In *impetigo* the organism invades the superficial layers of the skin and produces characteristic superficial, intraepidermal bullae and pustules.

A deeper infection is the common *boil*, or *furuncle*, in which

Figure 17.1
Diagram illustrating some staphylococcal infections of the skin. (A) *Impetigo*. The infection is very superficial, and a pustule forms beneath the stratum corneum of the epidermis. (B) *Superficial folliculitis*. The suppurative inflammation involves the superficial part of a hair follicle. Clinically this appears as a small pustule; the condition is also called impetigo of Bockhart. (C) *Furuncle or Boil*. The infection involves an entire hair follicle, and the inflammatory oedema produces a considerable swelling, which can be 1 cm or more in diameter. Nevertheless, a boil has one head only. (D) *Carbuncle*. The infection involves the subcutaneous tissues, and loculated pockets of pus are present. These pockets are formed between fibrous septa, which are not shown in the diagram. Note the multiple heads through which pus can be discharged. (*Drawing by Margot Mackay, Department of Art as Applied to Medicine, University of Toronto.*)

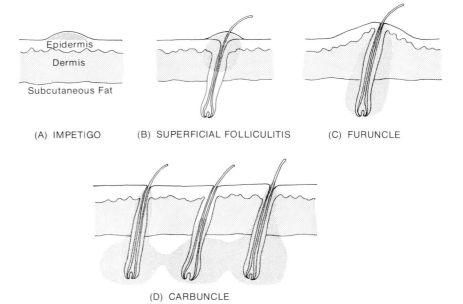

(A) IMPETIGO   (B) SUPERFICIAL FOLLICULITIS   (C) FURUNCLE

(D) CARBUNCLE

a hair follicle is involved. Suppuration is the usual result, and pus is discharged from a single opening. A well-known regional boil is the stye, or hordeolum, in which an eye-lash is implicated. Boils are particularly common in the axillae and the back of the neck, and they are often multiple in these sites due to the regional concentration of hair follicles and sebaceous glands. Nevertheless, each boil has its own 'head', through which pus is discharged.

In a *carbuncle* the infection extends to the underlying fatty subcutaneous tissue. The anatomical arrangement of the superficial fascia is such that it is divided into compartments by dense fibrous septa which extend from the deep fascia up to the dermis above. This is particularly well marked in the back of the neck. It therefore follows that when infection spreads to the subcutaneous tissue, many separate loculated abscesses form, and each bursts on to the surface through its own 'head', or sinus. In this way a single carbuncle has multiple heads, one for each loculus.

Two other examples of subcutaneous staphylococcal lesions are *abscesses of the pulp spaces* of the fingers and the *palmar spaces* of the hand.

*Bullous impetigo of the newborn** is the result of similar cross-infection in maternity wards. Many infants become carriers and may transmit the staphylococci to their mothers during breast feeding. A *breast abscess* may result if the nipple is cracked.

Two other important examples of cross-infection are pneumonia and enterocolitis. *Staphylococcal pneumonia* is due to the inhalation of virulent organisms, and is characterised by the development of lung abscesses which may spread to the pleural cavities and lead to empyema. *Staphylococcal enterocolitis* is an occasional complication of gastrointestinal surgery, especially in patients who have been given antibiotics. There is an acute, patchy inflammation of the intestinal mucosa, which causes severe diarrhoea. The shock engendered by this in a patient in the early postoperative period is an important cause of the very serious *pseudomembranous enterocolitis,*† in which long strips of mucosa undergo necrosis and remain attached to the wall to form a membrane. Most cases die rapidly of the combined effects of diarrhoea and intestinal haemorrhage, and microscopically there is often thrombosis of the mucosal and submucosal vessels.[2]

Staphylococci are the most important causal agents in *acute osteomyelitis*, a disease commonest in growing children (see p. 131). It is believed that a few organisms, probably derived from the skin, during the course of a bacteraemia infect the metaphysis of a long bone that may have been injured during play. Sometimes the lesion becomes circumscribed and chronic leading to a *Brodie's abscess*.

In similar fashion staphylococci may produce a spreading cortical abscess of the kidney. This is sometimes called a *renal*

---

*The alternative name pemphigus neonatorum is best abandoned, since the condition is not related to the pemphigus group of diseases.

†The term pseudomembranous enterocolitis is best used to describe a morphological entity. It occurs under several circumstances. Some cases are of staphylococcal origin, whereas others are due to *Candida* infection (usually in immunologically-compromised patients). Many cases are due to ischaemia (p. 517). It has also been described in patients on clindamycin therapy, and in these no specific infection or other cause has been identified.

Figure 17.2
'Carbuncle of kidney'. The kidney is the seat of a large, loculated, cortical abscess which has extended as far as the hilum. (U 13.6, *Reproduced by permission of the President and Council of the R.C.S. Eng.*)

carbuncle; it spreads outwards to produce a perinephric abscess rather than inwards to the calyceal system. Intravenous-drug users are prone to develop this disease which has otherwise become very uncommon (Fig. 17.2). On the other hand, Gram-negative organisms, possibly from ascending urinary-tract infections, are being found increasingly often in renal carbuncles.[3]

Staphylococci may spread *via* the lymphatics to produce a *lymphadenitis* that may undergo suppuration. If the infection is not arrested, there will be massive blood-stream invasion to produce a fatal *septicaemia*.

Staphylococcal *pyaemia* is not uncommon, and usually follows the involvement of a large vein in the course of a local infection (suppurative thrombophlebitis). Pyaemia is also a complication of *acute infective endocarditis* which occasionally complicates staphylococcal septicaemia.

Staphylococcal food-poisoning is the only condition due entirely to the exotoxin, enterotoxin. It follows the ingestion of food products contaminated by toxin-producing strains. The resulting gastroenteritis is severe, but is seldom fatal. The condition is a true intoxication (see p. 86), and is to be contrasted with enterocolitis, in which there is an invasion of the bowel wall by staphylococci.

Occurrence. The reservoir of pathogenic staphylococci is the anterior nares. About 40 per cent of healthy adults are nasal carriers, and in a hospital population the figure may rise to over 70 per cent. From the nares they are transferred to the skin, particularly of the hands and perineum. Staphylococci are also present in the faeces, but this is probably not an important source of infection except in patients with enterocolitis.

Staphylococcus albus. This organism is coagulase negative and a universal commensal of the skin. It has become important as a cause of opportunistic infection especially following surgery when foreign material is inserted. Thus it causes endocarditis following open-heart surgery, and may colonise the artificial shunts (Spitz-Holter valves) inserted into the brain to relieve congenital hydrocephalus. It causes urinary-tract infection especially in association with stones. Occasionally it produces septicaemia.

STREPTOCOCCI

Morphology. These too are Gram-positive, spherical organisms, slightly smaller than staphylococci. They tend to be arranged in chains, but this is conspicuous only when the organisms are cultured in fluid media. These chains vary in length, and some are very short indeed. Sometimes the organisms are disposed simply in pairs. They are non-motile and non-sporing. Some strains possess very thin capsules called microcapsules.

Cultural characteristics. They grow less easily than staphylococci, but are also aerobes and facultative anaerobes. A few strains are obligatory anaerobes.

They can be cultured on blood agar at 37°C, and within 24 hours, transparent colonies 0·5 to 1 mm in diameter develop. Around these there may be a zone of haemolysis, and according to this the organisms are classified into three main groups:

α-haemolytic streptococci, which produce a narrow zone of partial haemolysis often with a greenish pigmentation. These organisms are often reported as *Strept. viridans*.

β-haemolytic streptococci, which produce a sharply demarcated, clear zone of complete haemolysis.

Non-haemolytic streptococci. These are also called 'anhaemolytic' or *γ-type* streptococci.

Although both the first two varieties produce a haemolytic effect on blood agar, it is only the β-haemolytic group that possesses a soluble haemolysin capable of completely lysing horse red cells in suspension. β-haemolytic streptococci are particularly important in producing serious pyogenic infections. Not all, however, are human pathogens; some produce disease only in cattle and other animals. It is therefore important to distinguish between the different groups of β-haemolytic streptococci. One point of difference is the greater sensitivity of the human pathogen to *bacitracin*, but of more importance is serological grouping.

Lancefield grouping of streptococci. Beta-haemolytic streptococci can be divided into 18 groups by a precipitation test, first described by Lancefield, according to the presence

of a specific carbohydrate hapten, called the C antigen, in the wall of the organism. The great majority of human pathogens fall into Lancefield's group A, and a group-A organism is called *Strept. pyogenes*.

Griffith typing. *Strept. pyogenes*, like its staphylococcal counterpart, may give rise to epidemics of hospital infection and also acute nephritis in army camps, schools, and similar institutions. Typing is carried out, not by bacteriophage lysis, but by serological methods. Griffith discovered that group-A streptococci could be subdivided into over 50 different types depending on the presence of protein antigens, called M and T antigens, on the surface of the organism. The M antigen is particularly important because its presence is related to virulence (see p. 167). Typing is carried out by agglutination and precipitation tests using type-specific rabbit antisera. There seems to be little variation in the virulence of the different types, except that a few, especially type 12, are related to acute glomerulonephritis.

Toxin production. Like the staphylococcus, *Strept. pyogenes* is an invasive organism that produces powerful toxic products, most of which are intermediate between endotoxins and exotoxins, and also a potent exotoxin.

There are two haemolysins designated *streptolysin O* and *streptolysin S*. Streptolysin O is also cardiotoxic and leucocidic, whereas streptolysin S is a pure haemolysin. As the chemical nature of endotoxins is generally so poorly understood, it is right to include the M protein among them. This is powerfully antigenic. It acts by interfering with phagocytosis, and the antibody formed against it is an opsonin.

The organism produces the following enzymes:

Hyaluronidase.

Streptokinase, which induces fibrinolysis by activating the plasmin system.

Streptodornase, which depolymerises DNA. The name streptodornase is derived from the first letters of the syllables **deoxyribonuclease**.

The exotoxin referred to is the *erythrogenic toxin* responsible for the punctate erythema characteristic of scarlet fever. There are three antigenic types of erythrogenic toxin. The toxin is produced by some strains only, and those that do so are lysogenic.* Virulent strains of *C. diphtheriae* are also lysogenic, and it seems that the production of exotoxin is related to the presence of prophage in the organism's DNA.

Lesions of Strept. pyogenes. The typical streptococcal lesion is a *spreading cellulitis*. The poor localising tendency has been associated with the hyaluronidase and streptokinase produced by most strains, often in large amounts (but see p. 101). Abscesses occur much later than in staphylococcal infections, and the pus is thin, pinkish-grey in colour, odourless, and sometimes blood-stained. It is probable that the streptodornase and streptokinase are responsible for this watery consistency, because the viscosity of pus is due to DNA and fibrin.

*A bacterium is *lysogenic* when it harbours a bacteriophage which lies latent in its DNA. Such a bacteriophage is said to be *temperate*, and it lies latent in the bacterium as *prophage*. Some external circumstances, e.g. exposure to ultraviolet light, may cause the bacteriophage to become *virulent*, whereupon it promptly lyses the organism. Although prophage causes no obvious damage to the bacterium, it may alter or modify some of its functional characteristics. Lysogeny is an example of a latent virus infection (see p. 272).

In recent years the virulence of *Strept. pyogenes* has declined so markedly that many of its classical lesions which produced so much damage in the past are now rarely seen. By contrast, staphylococcal lesions are commoner and more severe than ever.

Streptococci are occasional causes of *wound infection* and are also responsible for some cases of *impetigo*. *Erysipelas*, a cellulitis of the dermis, is a classical streptococcal lesion.

Necrotising fasciitis[4] is usually caused by *Strept. pyogenes*, but occasional staphylococcal cases have been described. The condition was first described by Meleney as haemolytic streptococcal gangrene. It is an uncommon fulminating infection which follows trauma, sometimes quite trivial. There is a rapidly spreading infection of the subcutaneous fatty tissues. Thrombosis of the dermal vessels causes a red discoloration of the skin with bulla formation and necrosis. The skin lesions are ill defined in contradistinction to erysipelas, and if the patient survives there is extensive sloughing. Although the infection is due to an organism which is sensitive to antibiotics, surgical relief is also necessary.

Streptococci are important causes of tonsillitis and pharyngitis (*streptococcal sore throat*), and these may be complicated by *otitis media* and *sinusitis*. In the 1918 influenza pandemic many people died of a complicating *streptococcal pneumonia*. *Streptococcal puerperal infection* killed thousands of women before the introduction of the sulphonamides, but today it is very uncommon.

The invasiveness of streptococci is evidenced by their tendency to spread by the lymphatics with the production of streaks of red, linear *lymphangitis* under the skin and *lymphadenitis*. This is followed rapidly by *septicaemia*.

If an infecting streptococcus produces the erythrogenic exotoxin, and if the patient has no circulating antitoxin, the local lesion will be complicated by the effects of this toxin. A punctate erythema appears, and the condition is called *scarlet fever*.*

There is a more indirect relationship between streptococcal infections on the one hand and *acute rheumatic fever* and *acute glomerulonephritis* on the other. These two conditions may occur about 3 weeks after the initial infection, and it is generally held that they are manifestations of immune-complex allergy to the streptococcal antigen. Some cases of *erythema nodosum* are similarly related to streptococcal infection, but here delayed-type hypersensitivity is probably involved.

Occurrence. *Streptococcus pyogenes* is found in the throats of about 10 per cent of people, and in from 2 to 5 per cent it is present also in the anterior nares.

Other β-haemolytic streptococci.[6-8] These are occasionally incriminated as human pathogens. *Group-B streptococci* (*Strept. agalactiae*) are not infrequently found in the female genital tract, and are recognised as a common cause of serious perinatal infection. An infection during the first 24 hours of life (early onset) is manifest as respiratory distress with shock, septicaemia, and meningitis. Infection is probably acquired during labour from the vaginal flora. Later infection (after 7 days of age) commonly presents as meningitis.

Group-C streptococci may be involved in puerperal infection, wound infection, cellulitis, and scarlet fever.

Group-G streptococci may also be associated with puerperal infection.

Infections Due to α-haemolytic Streptococci

Strept. viridans is not a single-defined species, but is the collective name given to α-haemolytic streptococci. These organisms are invariable commensals of the mouth and throat, and a number of strains, e.g. *Strept. mitis*, *Strept. mutans*, and *Strept. sanguis*, have been incriminated in *dental caries* and *periodontal disease*. Of greater importance, however, is the association of *Strept. viridans* with *subacute infective endocarditis*, described on page 501.

It should be noted that the pneumococcus is often included among the α-haemolytic streptococci, but it is such a distinctive organism that it is described separately on page 221.

Infections Due to Non-haemolytic Streptococci

The non-haemolytic streptococcus is always present in the colon, hence its alternative names *Strept. faecalis* and *enterococcus*. If it leaves its normal habitat, this organism has a range of pathogenicity similar to the Gram-negative intestinal organisms. It is also an uncommon cause of *subacute infective endocarditis*, and may be found in association with *dental caries* and *periodontal disease*.

Occasionally *Strept. faecalis* produces a true β-haemolysis on blood agar, but it does not possess a soluble haemolysin. It belongs to Lancefield's group D.

Anaerobic Streptococcal Infections

The strictly anaerobic streptococci have different biological characteristics from the above-mentioned aerobic streptococci. They are often much smaller, and exhibit pleomorphism (variation in size and shape) on artificial culture. They do not produce haemolysis in blood agar. *Peptostreptococcus putridus* is the best documented species.

Anaerobic streptococci are normal inhabitants of the bowel and vagina. They are occasionally associated with *infected wounds*, and in civilised countries used to be an important cause of *puerperal infection*. *Suppurative myositis* is an unusual condition caused by these organisms.

Meleney's postoperative synergistic gangrene[9] usually follows the drainage of a deep abscess, either peritoneal or in the chest. There is a slowly spreading infection of the skin; the margin of the area is bright red and as the lesion expands this becomes purple, then black and gangrenous, and finally the necrotic skin is sloughed off leaving a granulating surface (Fig. 17.3). The infection is caused classically by a microaerophilic non-haemolytic streptococcus acting synergistically with *Staph. aureus*, but other synergistic pairs have also been incriminated.

Meleney's chronic undermining, or burrowing, ulcer is a different condition. It usually follows an operation on the intestinal or genital tract, and is caused by an infection with a haemolytic microaerophilic streptococcus. It involves the subcutaneous tissues and burrows deeply into the pelvis. The condition is very painful.

---

*A scarlet-fever-like illness due to staphylococci has also been described. A filtrate of the *Staph. aureus* contained on erythrogenic factor, which was antigenically distinct from the streptococcal erythrogenic toxin.[5]

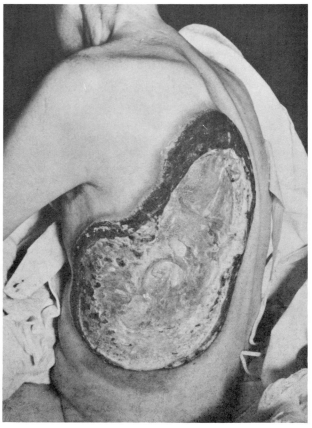

Figure 17.3
Meleney's postoperative synergistic gangrene. This patient developed an empyema as a complication of bronchopneumonia with abscess formation. Attempts to drain this resulted in a spreading gangrene which finally involved a large area of the chest wall.

THE GRAM-NEGATIVE INTESTINAL BACILLI

In the account that follows no attempt has been made to delineate the features of each genus, for this is the task of the bacteriologist. For the present the clinician must be prepared to accept a nomenclature which varies from one centre to another depending on the classification adopted and the effort which the laboratory is prepared to put into the typing of each isolated 'coliform organism'.

Most of the members of this group belong to the family *Enterobacteriaceae*. The important pus-forming genera are *Escherichia*, *Klebsiella* and *Enterobacter* (sometimes grouped together as *Aerobacter*), *Citrobacter*, *Hafnia*, and *Proteus*. Other important members of the family *Enterobacteriaceae* are *Salmonella*, responsible for typhoid fever and food poisoning, and *Shigella*, responsible for bacillary dysentery; these two groups of organisms are not distinguished by suppuration and are not described further. Another important Gram-negative intestinal genus that causes suppuration is *Pseudomonas*. It does not belong to the *Enterobacteriaceae*, for although it may occur in the human intestine, this is not its natural habitat. It is found widely distributed in nature. Of the many *Pseudomonas* species only one, *Ps. aeruginosa* (commonly called *Ps. pyocyanea*) is pathogenic to the human.

There are a number of *Proteus* species, e.g. *Pr. mirabilis*, *Pr. vulgaris*, *Pr. morganii*, and *Pr. rettgeri*, and they can be distinguished by biochemical reactions.

Morphology.* They are all Gram-negative rods 1 to 4 µm long, with a tendency to considerable variation in size. With a few exceptions, e.g. *Klebsiella*, they are vigorously motile. *Klebsiella* also differs from the others in having a capsule. None of these organisms forms spores.

Cultural characteristics. These organisms grow well at 37°C, being aerobic and facultatively anaerobic. On blood agar most members of this group produce greyish, shiny colonies, 3 to 5 mm in diameter, within 24 hours. Some *Proteus* species are distinctive in spreading over the surface of the agar in a confluent layer and submerging other colonies that may be present. This is called *swarming*. *Ps. aeruginosa* produces a bluish-green pigmentation due to the formation of the pigments fluorescin and pyocyanin. These are best seen on nutrient agar, because the haemoglobin in blood agar obscures them. In addition, colonies of *Ps. aeruginosa* have a characteristic fresh odour resembling fruit.

Biochemical reactions.* The most important ones are the sugar fermentation tests. Nearly all ferment some sugars, e.g. glucose, often with the production of gas (see p. 667). But it is the fermentation of lactose which is most distinctive. *Esch. coli* ferments lactose vigorously with the production of acid and gas, and most of the related coliform group do likewise, but in some instances without gas formation.

The distinctive property of lactose fermentation by some organisms is made use of in MacConkey's selective medium, the composition of which is described in Appendix 2. The lactose in this medium is fermented by *Esch. coli* and most coliform organisms, and the lactic acid produced turns the neutral-red indicator a pink colour. Therefore these colonies are pink, while those of *Salmonella*, *Shigella*, *Proteus*, and *Pseudomonas* are colourless.

Occurrence. Unlike the pyogenic streptococci and staphylococci, these organisms may be regarded as normal inhabitants of the body, causing disease only when they leave their normal habitat.

Esch. coli is always present in the bowel, and about a third of all human faeces harbour *Proteus* species. *Ps. aeruginosa* is less commonly present, being found in from 3 to 16 per cent of faeces.[10]

Pathogenicity. The pathogenic action of these organisms is believed to be due to an endotoxin, which as yet has been poorly defined. When they escape from the lumen of the bowel and invade the tissues, they produce suppurative lesions. *Ps. aeruginosa* produces an elastase, which may explain the organism's tendency to invade blood vessels.

Esch. coli and the **coliform organisms** always predominate in infective lesions associated with the bowel, e.g. *appendix abscess*, *acute sigmoid diverticulitis*, *ischioerectal abscess*, and *generalised peritonitis following perforation of a hollow viscus*. They frequently infect *penetrating wounds of the abdomen* and furthermore are the commonest agents in *urinary-*

Salmonella and *Shigella* are not considered here. Both genera are characterised by a failure to ferment lactose (except *Sh. sonnei*). The *Salmonellae* are motile, while the *Shigellae* are non-motile (see p. 667).

tract infections (see p. 234). They are also commonly associated with *acute cholecystitis*, presumably reaching the gall-bladder from the liver to which they are conveyed by the portal vein. The alternative route of infection *via* the bile duct seems unlikely.

Esch. coli is often cultured from sputum and is a cause of *bronchopneumonia*.

Esch. coli and the other Gram-negative intestinal bacilli can easily invade the blood stream, and produce a *septicaemia*. A typical feature of this is a state of profound shock (*Gram-negative shock*, see p. 418).

Klebsiella organisms share the general pathogenicity of *Esch. coli*, but one species, *Kl. pneumoniae* (also called Friedländer's bacillus) causes an uncommon, but very dangerous type of *bronchopneumonia* characterised by a slimy exudate. Two diseases of the upper respiratory tract caused by *Klebsiella* organisms are *rhinoscleroma*, a chronic granulomatous inflammation of the nose and nasopharynx, and *ozaena*, an atrophic rhinitis associated with offensive crusts in the nasal passages.

Proteus organisms and **Ps. aeruginosa** have a similar range of pathogenicity, but they are less frequently commensals of the bowel, and are much more often transmitted by cross-infection. This is particularly true of *Ps. aeruginosa*, which is the commonest cross-infecting organism after *Staph. aureus*. Serological and bacteriophage typing has been used in investigating hospital epidemics.

Proteus organisms are a very important cause of *urinary-tract infection*. They decompose urea readily and produce ammonia. The urine therefore becomes alkaline, a factor favouring the formation of phosphate calculi in the bladder (see Ch. 51). *Proteus* organisms are important agents in *wound infection*, and secondary invaders of chronic ulcerative skin lesions.

Ps. aeruginosa is even more widespread in its infecting tendencies, and is easily recognisable clinically by the bluish-green pus it produces. It frequently *infects the urinary tract*, and it can spread through a urological ward very rapidly. It is of importance in *wound infection* and *eye infection* (see p. 234), and is frequently the cause of *chronic otitis media* and *otitis externa*. Like the *Klebsiella* and *Proteus* organisms, it is an important cause of *respiratory infections*. It is very invasive, and the *septicaemia*[11,12] it produces is characterised by an acute necrotising angiitis due to the invasion of the vessel walls by the organisms. There are large areas of haemorrhagic infarction in the skin and internal organs, particularly the lungs and kidneys. On the skin the haemorrhagic lesions rapidly break down to form necrotic ulcers (*ecthyma gangrenosum*).[13] Microscopically these are seen to be teeming with organisms, and show destruction of vessels with little inflammatory reaction.

It should be noted that although *Esch. coli* is an inevitable and harmless inhabitant of the bowel, there are a few well-recognised enteropathogenic strains. These are of no special importance as causes of suppuration, but they may produce epidemics of *gastroenteritis amongst infants*. Only a few enteropathogenic types are described, e.g. 026, 055, 0111, 0119, and 0128, and they are typed serologically by agglutination tests. The condition is most common in artificially-fed babies, and is probably spread by fomites and contaminated food.

Enteropathogenic strains are also responsible for many cases of traveller's diarrhoea.

Gram-Negative Anaerobic Intestinal Bacilli

The Gram-negative intestinal organisms of the genus *Bacteroides* are an important group, because they form the bulk of organisms in the intestine as well as being present as part of the normal flora of the vagina. They are non-sporing, strict anaerobes, and are very sensitive to the toxic effect of oxygen. They cause infection of wounds, the peritoneal cavity, and the uterus following labour or abortion (see p. 57). Localised *Bacteroides* infections are characterised by a particularly foul odour. They may invade the blood stream, and are a cause of Gram-negative shock. Infections by *Bacteroides* are probably missed quite frequently because of the extreme oxygen sensitivity of this group of organisms. Not only must culture be performed under anaerobic conditions, but oxygen must also be excluded from the specimen during its transit to the laboratory. The ordinary type of swab is therefore quite inadequate for isolating this organism.

THE PNEUMOCOCCUS

Diplococcus pneumoniae is closely related to the streptococci, and is often called *Strept. pneumoniae*, but it is better to regard it as a separate genus.

Morphology. It is oval or lance-shaped, and is arranged in pairs with the long axes in line with each other. It is the same size as the streptococcus, and like it is Gram-positive, non-motile, and non-sporing. An important feature is the presence of a prominent capsule.

Cultural characteristics. It resembles the α-haemolytic streptococcus very closely, and produces a diffuse greenish pigmentation into the surrounding blood agar. Its colonies are somewhat larger than those of *Strept. viridans*, and have raised margins. They resemble in shape the chequers used in a game of draughts.

Unlike the streptococcus, the pneumococcus is lysed by bile salts very rapidly. Another point of difference is the great sensitivity of the pneumococcus to *optochin* (ethyl hydrocuprein hydrochloride).

Typing of pneumococci. Type-specificity depends on the polysaccharide hapten (the specific soluble substance, or SSS) present in the capsule of the organism, and it is this that determines its virulence (see p. 167). When a type-specific rabbit antiserum is mixed with a suspension of pneumococci, their capsules become clearly delineated and give an appearance of swelling if the SSS corresponds to the antibody in the serum. Over 70 different types of pneumococci have been recognised, but pneumococcal typing is seldom carried out nowadays because serum therapy is obsolete in lobar pneumonia. Types 1, 2, and 3 are the most virulent, and are responsible for most cases of lobar pneumonia. The remainder used to be called 'Type 4', but nowadays each type is given a number of its own. Types 5, 7, and 14 are also quite virulent, but the others appear to be commensals of the nose and throat, and cause little harm in healthy people.

Pathogenic lesions. The most important pneumococcal lesion is *lobar pneumonia*, which will be described in detail.

Figure 17.4
Pneumococcal meningitis. The patient was an
infant of 8 months who had had recurrent attacks
of pneumonia, the last of which was complicated
by meningitis. The specimen is the left cerebral
hemisphere, and the sulci of the frontal portion
are filled with a thick, opaque layer of inflammatory exudate. N 6.2, *Reproduced by permission
of the President and Council of the R.C.S. Eng.)*

Other primary pneumococcal conditions are *otitis media* and *suppurative sinusitis*, both of which may lead to *meningitis* (Fig. 17.4). Pneumococci may cause *purulent conjunctivitis*. Another interesting condition is the *primary pneumococcal peritonitis* which is described in young girls. Whether it is really primary, the organism gaining entrance to the peritoneal cavity by way of the uterine tubes, or whether it is blood-borne from an undetected lesion in the respiratory tract, is undecided.

Lobar Pneumonia

This is a disease especially of healthy young adults. The organism is a pneumococcus of high virulence, usually type 1, 2, or 3, and it is acquired from another victim or a convalescent carrier. 'Contact' carriers, i.e. those who have never had clinical infection, may also transmit the organisms. The infection is exogenous, and the contending parties are a virulent organism and a healthy, though unimmunised host.

The infection is acquired by inhalation, but it is probable that the organism first establishes itself in the nasopharynx. Then after some days or weeks, if the person is particularly susceptible, say because of a common cold or after chilling or an alcoholic spree, the organism may spread to the lung, middle ear, nasal sinus, or meninges. If the lung is involved there is an acute inflammatory reaction. If immunity is good, the condition may never pass beyond this stage, but otherwise a rapidly-spreading inflammatory oedema soon implicates a whole lobe, and sometimes several lobes (Fig. 17.5).

The rapid spread of the infection to the periphery in a gigantic wave of oedematous exudate suggests that allergy is involved in the process. The earlier nasopharyngeal infection may have been enough to initiate an immune response. Alternatively, the organisms may have passed through the lungs symptomlessly, proliferated in the RE system, and then returned to the blood, thereby causing septicaemia. When they reach the lungs again, an allergic episode follows the recently acquired immune response. This mechanism would be anal-

ogous to that described in typhoid fever (p. 94) and syphilis (p.249).

Whatever the mechanism there is no doubt that during this acute stage there is septicaemia, and sometimes the pneumococci may become localised and produce *meningitis, acute infective endocarditis, peritonitis,* and *suppurative arthritis.* For the first week the organism has the upper hand, and if death occurs, it is due to overwhelming 'toxaemia' (though the nature of the toxic principle is unknown) sometimes accompanied by the metastatic lesions already named. After a week the titre of antibodies (opsonins) in the circulation rapidly rises, and with their aid the polymorphs are able to phagocytose the organisms (see Ch. 13). The disease resolves dramatically, and the fever abates precipitously by 'crisis'.

Corresponding with this general effect, the local lesion in the lungs passes through four stages:

(1) **Inflammatory oedema.** There is engorgement of the alveolar capillaries which show margination of leucocytes. In the alveoli there is an oedematous exudate containing macrophages ('septal cells') and a few polymorphs. The oedema fluid spreads rapidly through the entire lobe *via* minute openings in the alveolar walls (the pores of Kohn) and through the lumina of the alveolar ducts. At this stage it is teeming with pneumococci.

(2) **Red hepatisation.** The capillary engorgement persists, while the oedema in the alveoli coagulates into fine skeins of fibrin. The alveoli are crowded with polymorphs, and there are also considerable numbers of red cells present (Fig. 17.6). These enter by diapedesis, and their products of haemolysis are responsible for the rusty colour of the sputum that is coughed up. It is very tenacious due to the large amount of fibrin present.

The lobe itself is firm (consolidated), airless, and red in colour. In consistency it resembles liver (red hepatisation).

(3) **Grey hepatisation.** This follows on the red stage. The alveolar capillaries are now closed down, partly because the

Figure 17.6
Lobar pneumonia. The two adjacent alveoli are filled with a loose fibrinous exudate containing pus cells and macrophages. The alveolar capillaries are dilated and contain many red cells. This corresponds to the stage of red hepatisation. × 320.

Figure 17.5
Lobar pneumonia. The left lower lobe is completely consolidated while the upper lobe is unaffected. (R 30.2, *Reproduced by permission of the President and Council of the R.C.S. Eng.*)

acute inflammatory reaction has to an extent spent itself, and partly because of pressure exerted on the capillaries by the distended, solid alveoli. These are full of dense inspissated fibrin, around which there are numerous degenerating and dead polymorphs (Fig. 17.7). At this stage bacteria and red cells are scanty. The fibrin tends to retract from the alveolar walls, and then the capillary circulation becomes active again.

The lobe is even firmer now than before, and it has a grey colour due to the relative bloodlessness. It is so voluminous that the ribs indent the lateral surfaces.

(4) **Resolution.** This is carried out by macrophages as part of the process of demolition. The inspissated fibrin is removed with great rapidity, and all remaining debris is cleared away. The fluid exudate and macrophages leave the alveoli mainly *via* the lymphatics, and they are intercepted at the hilar lymph nodes which show the features of reactive hyperplasia (see p. 393). Some of the exudate leaves *via* the alveolar capillaries, and so re-enters the blood stream.

During the process there is an acute fibrinous pleurisy over the

affected lobe. Because the fibrinous exudate is so extensive it is unusual for it to be completely 'demolished' by macrophages during resolution. Remnants of it persist long enough to undergo organisation into permanent pleural adhesions. These are of little functional significance.

Though the stages of lobar pneumonia have been described sequentially, it must be remembered that pathological processes rarely proceed as methodically as this. While one part of a lobe shows red hepatisation, an adjacent area will be grey and solid, while elsewhere resolution may be progressing. Nevertheless, in contradistinction to bronchopneumonia, it is usual for all the alveoli in one low-power microscope field to be at one stage. The stages described above are seldom seen nowadays, because the infection is curtailed by chemotherapy.

Local sequelae of lobar pneumonia. (*a*) The commonest sequel is *resolution*, which is usually so complete that only the residual pleural adhesions remain as a testimony to the attack of pneumonia.

(*b*) Rarely the fibrinous exudate in the alveoli does not undergo demolition, but persists and is organised into fibrous tissue, a process called *carnification*. Fibrosis of the lung results.

(*c*) *Suppuration* with the production of a lung abscess is also

Figure 17.7
Lobar pneumonia. The alveoli are crowded with pus cells, and the fibrinous exudate has condensed into thick strands. The alveolar capillaries are inconspicuous, and appear to have shut down. This corresponds to the stage of grey hepatisation. × 320.

very uncommon in lobar pneumonia, but it may be encountered in individuals with a poor resistance to infection, e.g. alcoholics and diabetics. There is usually an associated pneumococcal empyema, and the pericardial sac may be involved by direct contact.

Bronchopneumonia

In bronchopneumonia, unlike lobar pneumonia, there are numerous discrete foci of inflammation around terminal bronchioles (Fig. 17.8). As the disease progresses these tend to become confluent, and occasionally the process becomes so extensive that a whole lobe is consolidated. However, the wildfire spread of lobar pneumonia is not present.

There are many varieties of bronchopneumonia. They are best considered as follows:

Endogenous bronchopneumonia due to commensal organisms of the upper respiratory passages. Of these the pneumococci of low-grade virulence are by far the most important. The host is invariably in a poor state of health. The antagonists are therefore a poorly virulent endogenous organism and an enfeebled host (cf. lobar pneumonia). The following conditions in the host predispose to endogenous bronchopneumonia:

Extremes of age. It is commonest in infancy and old age.

General debilitating illness. It is a common terminal event in cancer, cerebral vascular accidents, and uraemia.

Pre-existing respiratory disease, e.g. chronic bronchitis, influenza, measles, whooping-cough, and mycoplasmal pneumonia.

Local obstruction to the upward flow of mucus which is wafted along by ciliary action (see Ch. 7). The dammed-up secretion forms an admirable medium for bacterial growth. Examples of such conditions are foreign bodies and tumours of the bronchi.

Figure 17.8
Bronchopneumonia. Part of a terminal bronchiole (Term Br) is shown with its lining of ciliated columnar epithelium. The bronchiole is crowded with inflammatory cells, the majority of which are polymorphs. Alveoli (Alv) adjacent to the bronchiole also contain inflammatory exudate with polymorphs and fibrin. An alveolus further away from the bronchiole merely contains oedema fluid. × 80.

Pulmonary oedema, e.g. after chest injuries, ether anaesthesia (which also damages the cilia), heart failure, and in any terminal condition ('hypostatic pneumonia').

The untreated disease lasts much longer than does lobar pneumonia. If the primary condition is fatal and the pneumonia merely a terminal event, there will be little attempt at cure, but even in the childhood bronchopneumonia that follows measles and pertussis, a prolonged course is the rule and is often punctuated by relapses and remissions, depending on whether the organism or the host is gaining the upper hand. The fever gradually subsides in step-like fashion, a process described as 'lysis'.

The general pathological process is, of course, similar to that of lobar pneumonia, but there is no attempt at the orderly sequence described in that condition. The disease is usually basal and bilateral in distribution.

If an area of bronchopneumonia is examined microscopically, it is found to consist of acutely inflamed bronchioles full of pus (Fig. 17.8). Some of the surrounding alveoli contain oedema fluid in which there are macrophages and polymorphs, while others are filled with a dense fibrinous exudate in which there are innumerable polymorphs. Some are collapsed as the result of the absorption of air distal to the blocked bronchioles ('absorption collapse'), whereas neighbouring alveoli are empty and distended due to compensatory dilatation. As the process proceeds, some of the alveoli show evidence of demolition of exudate by macrophages, but in others there is progressive organisation.

SEQUELAE OF BRONCHOPNEUMONIA

(*a*) *Resolution.* This is less frequent than in lobar pneumonia.

(*b*) *Progressive Fibrosis of the Lung.* This is correspondingly more frequent, and is due to the organisation of fibrinous exudate. In addition there is often a continuance of the inflammatory process, so that the lung is progressively destroyed and converted into fibrous tissue. This is, of course,

chronic inflammation, and bronchopneumonia often becomes chronic. In due course the infection spreads, and the muscle and elastic tissue of the adjacent bronchi are destroyed and replaced by granulation tissue. In consequence the lumina widen, and eventually the dilatation becomes so extensive that secretion accumulates, forming the nidus for further infection and inflammatory destruction. This is the pathogenesis of *bronchiectasis*, which is both a sequel of bronchopneumonia and a predisposing cause of further attacks of it.

(*c*) *Suppuration.* This is also not uncommon, particularly when the host's resistance is exceptionally poor.

Table 17.1 contrasts untreated pneumococcal lobar pneumonia and endogenous bronchopneumonia.

Another type of endogenous bronchopneumonia follows the inhalation of material from the mouth. The root of a tooth inhaled during extraction under general anaesthesia is a classical example of this. It lodges in a bronchus, and the *Bacteroides* organisms present in it lead to a putrid type of pneumonia which terminates in abscess formation (see p. 57).

Exogenous bronchopneumonia. A large variety of virulent organisms, when inhaled, can lead to severe bronchopneumonia. The host may be a healthy adult, or else be enfeebled as the result of a previous disease.

Examples of virulent organisms causing exogenous bronchopneumonia are:

Staph. aureus, as a result of hospital cross-infection (Fig. 17.9).

Strept. pyogenes, e.g. during the 1918 influenza pandemic.

Kl. pneumoniae; and also *Esch. coli*, *Proteus* organisms, and *Ps. aeruginosa*.

Yersinia pestis ('pneumonic plague').

Bacillus anthracis ('woolsorter's disease').

Myco. tuberculosis (see Ch. 20) and the deep-seated fungal diseases (see Ch. 21). This type of disease is quite distinct, as the lesion produced is always chronic. Furthermore, the cellular response is not pyogenic.

Most of these organisms are very virulent, and suppuration

TABLE 17.1 A comparison of lobar and endogenous bronchopneumonia

	Lobar Pneumonia	*Bronchopneumonia*
Host	Healthy young adult	Enfeebled patient at extremes of life or chronically ill; after viral infections or with bronchial obstruction
Organism	Highly virulent exogenous pneumococcus	Poorly virulent endogenous pneumococcus and other organisms
Type of lesion	Rapid spread throughout an entire lobe	Discrete foci, usually basal, around bronchioles. Affects several lobes. Bilateral.
Progress	Wildfire spread with resolution after a week. Fever falls by crisis	Prolonged course with slow convalescence. Fever falls by lysis
Sequelae	Resolution and organised pleural exudate. Fibrosis of lung and suppuration exceptional.	Complete resolution uncommon. Residual fibrosis and bronchiectasis frequent. Suppuration is not uncommon
Mode of death	Toxaemia. Metastatic pneumococcal lesions, e.g. meningitis, peritonitis, and acute infective endocarditis	Precipitating condition, e.g. cancer. Progressive lung damage

Figure 17.9
Staphylococcal bronchopneumonia. There are discrete foci of consolidation scattered throughout the lung. (R 29.3, *Reproduced by permission of the President and Council of the R.C.S. Eng.*)

or necrosis is usual. There is generally an accompanying septicaemia, and only the most vigorous treatment will prevent death. Apart from the extremely destructive potentialities of these agents, the pneumonia they produce is basically similar to that of endogenous pneumococci. Streptococcal and *Klebsiella* pneumonia may be so extensive as to simulate lobar pneumonia.

Legionnaires' disease.[14] This is a newly-described pneumonia that derives its name from its first occasion of dramatic manifestation: among the delegates at the Pennsylvania State American Legion at Philadelphia in July, 1976. The incubation period was about a week, and there was a mortality rate of 16 per cent. The main pathological feature was a severe pyogenic type of bronchopneumonia of almost lobar distribution. The fascinating feature of this outbreak, which was probably airborne, was the extreme difficulty in isolating a causative organism. Eventually a bacillus of varying length and thickness was found. It is Gram negative inasmuch as it does not take up Gram's stain, but it is demonstrated by silver impregnation. It grows freely in the yolk-sac of the chick embryo, and can be cultured on a special agar medium.

Yolk-sac suspensions can be used for fluorescent antibody tests on the sera of suspected patients. By this method it has been discovered that this type of pneumonia has occurred in small epidemics in the USA at least since 1965, but in them the disease was sometimes milder with a smaller mortality rate. Cases have also been reported in Spain and Britain.

The bacterium has not yet been assigned to a genus or even classified more broadly. The antibiotics tetracycline and erythromycin seem to be the most effective in treatment.

Primary atypical pneumonia. This term may be used to include those pneumonias that are not pyogenic. Some are mycoplasmal, rickettsial (Q fever), or chlamydial (psittacosis and ornithosis), and others again are of viral origin due to adenoviruses, myxoviruses, and others that are noted in Chapter 23. Histologically these pneumonias are characterised by moderately heavy macrophage and lymphocyte infiltrations in the alveolar walls, and to a lesser extent in the alveoli. Polymorphs are scanty, unless there is a secondary bacterial pneumonia. A hyaline membrane lining the alveoli is a common finding.

THE NEISSERIAL ORGANISMS

The genus *Neisseria* includes a large number of Gram-negative cocci. Many of these are commensals of the mouth, nose, and throat, and are named collectively *N. pharyngis*. There are in addition two highly pathogenic members of the group, *N. meningitidis* (meningococcus) and *N. gonorrhoeae* (gonococcus), which merit a brief consideration.

Morphology. These two organisms are kidney shaped and arranged in pairs with their concave surfaces opposed. They are non-motile and non-sporing. The meningococcus has a very fine capsule. Both organisms are encountered most typically within the cytoplasm of polymorphs (Gram-negative intracellular diplococci), and it is impossible to distinguish between them morphologically.

Cultural characteristics. Many *Neisseria* organisms grow quite easily on blood agar at 37°C under aerobic conditions, but the two pathogens are much more demanding in their requirements than the others. An atmosphere of 5 per cent CO_2 is essential for the gonococcus and helpful for the meningococcus, which is the more easily cultured of the two. Both grow quite well on blood agar, chocolate agar, and serum agar (see Appendix 2). The colonies are small, translucent, circular discs rather like those of the streptococcus. They do not produce haemolysis.

It is evident that there is great similarity between the meningococcus and the gonococcus; one point of difference is that whereas the meningococcus ferments both glucose and maltose, the gonococcus ferments only glucose.

Typing. As with the pneumococcus typing plays very little part in the study of these organisms. The meningococcus can be divided into four types (nowadays designated A, B, C, and D) using special agglutinating antisera.

Pathogenicity. In human beings both are invasive organisms, and both produce an ill-defined endotoxin. Neither organism is found naturally in any other host, but a typical meningitis follows the injection of the meningococcus into the cerebrospinal fluid of rabbits and monkeys. It has recently been claimed that urethritis can be produced in the chimpanzee by the local inoculation of gonococcal pus.[15]

Meningococcal Infections[16]

From 5 to 30 per cent of healthy individuals carry the meningococcus in the nasopharyngeal area. Epidemics of meningococcal infection are prone to occur when a large number of people are herded together in cramped quarters, e.g. barracks. Under these conditions the carrier rate may rise to over 50 per cent, and then the danger of infection becomes great. This state of affairs also occurs in pneumococcal lobar pneumonia.

It is possible that there is first an insignificant infection in the nasopharynx, but it must be admitted that the factors involved in the invasiveness of the organism are ill-understood. It may be that the meningococcus invades the cranial cavity directly through the cribriform plate, because the olfactory area of the nasal mucosa appears to be specifically vulnerable in that it does not possess cilia.

More usually, however, there is a stage of *septicaemia*, during which the patient develops severe constitutional symptoms and a profuse petechial eruption. Occasionally the septicaemia may be so fulminating that death occurs before there is evidence of meningeal infection. Under such conditions there is an extensive bleeding tendency with bilateral adrenal haemorrhages (Waterhouse-Friderichsen syndrome).

The septicaemia is rapidly succeeded by meningeal involvement. The reason for this specific localisation is unknown. There is a generalised fibrinous *meningitis* which rapidly becomes purulent. The pia mater acts as an efficient barrier against the invasion of the brain by organisms; the cerebral substance is merely congested and oedematous. In untreated cases death rapidly occurs. Pyogenic meningitis, unlike the tuberculous variety, tends to affect the vertex of the brain rather than the base. Hence there is seldom any organisation of adhesions in the area of the cisterna magna with subsequent hydrocephalus, such as was often seen in fatal cases of tuberculour meningitis in the pre-antibiotic era.

More rarely the meningococcus also becomes localised in other tissues, in which case such complications as *arthritis* (in which immune-complex allergy is important),[17] *endocarditis*, and *otitis media* occur. *Primary meningococcal conjunctivitis* is a rare, though well-recognised, condition. *Chronic meningococcal septicaemia* is a rare variant; there is a remittent fever resembling malaria, a maculopapular skin eruption that fades and recurs, and migratory arthralgias.

Gonococcal Infections

The usual manifestation of gonococcal infection is the venereal disease *gonorrhoea*. In the male it commences as an acute suppurative urethritis, which if untreated may spread to the prostate, seminal vesicles, and epididymes. The destruction of tissue and the subsequent scarring lead to such permanent sequelae as urethral stricture and sterility.

In the female the disease is often less acute, and it affects the urethra, vestibular glands, and cervix uteri. The vagina is characteristically immune because of its acidity (see Ch. 7), except in prepubertal girls. The disease may spread and lead to salpingitis and pelvic peritonitis (pelvic inflammatory disease, or PID). The subsequent occlusion of the uterine tubes is an important cause of sterility.

Other venereal presentations of gonorrhoea are *proctitis* in those, commonly male, homosexuals who practise sodomy, and *pharyngitis* and *tonsillitis* in those who practise oral methods of intercourse. Such manifestations are not rare nowadays, and should always be remembered when a throat lesion is accompanied by a marked systemic reaction which does not respond promptly to chemotherapy.[18]

The gonococcus is much more invasive locally but much less so systemically than is the meningococcus. Nevertheless, gonococcal *septicaemia* is becoming more common nowadays. A conspicuous feature of this is a rather scanty maculopapular and pustular skin eruption found especially on the extremities.[19] Fever and polyarthralgia are invariably present (see Figs. 42.1 and 42.2, p. 510). *Acute infective endocarditis* is a rare complication.

Another important gonococcal lesion is *purulent conjunctivitis*. This often used to occur in the newborn, whose eyes were contaminated during passage through the birth canal. A patient with gonorrhoea may also develop conjunctivitis by contaminating his eyes with his hands. The invasive character of the organism is obvious in gonococcal ophthalmia; the infection starts as a superficial conjunctivitis, but it soon implicates the cornea, the substance of which is rapidly destroyed and converted into scar tissue. Blindness was almost invariable, but the prognosis has completely changed since the introduction of penicillin.

An important later complication of gonorrhoea is *arthritis*. It is typically monarticular, and is said to be commoner in women and in Black people. It must be distinguished from the joint lesions of *Reiter's disease*,[20] which comprises a diagnostic triad of non-gonococcal urethritis, conjunctivitis, and arthritis, and may manifest iridocyclitis and a horny thickening of the skin of the palms and soles called keratoderma blenorrhagica. This condition is of unknown aetiology, and may be acquired non-venereally—sometimes there is a history of dysentery beforehand. The arthritis is polyarticular, and men are much more commonly affected than are women. The sacro-iliac joints are often affected, and in chronic cases the changes of ankylosing spondylitis may be seen in the spine.[21] It is noteworthy that there is a very strong association with transplantation antigen HLA-B27 in Reiter's disease.

As gonorrhoea and Reiter's disease can both occur at the same time, it is wiser not to diagnose gonococcal arthritis until the organisms are isolated from the synovial fluid. It is probable that in both types of arthritis there is an immune-complex type of allergic reaction in addition to the possible presence of an infective agent in the joint.

TREATMENT OF THE PYOGENIC INFECTIONS

It is in the treatment of the pyogenic group of infections that chemotherapy has had its greatest triumph. The sulphonamides have been extremely valuable (especially in meningococcal infections), but they are now largely superseded by the vast range of newly-discovered antibiotics.

Against the pyococcal infections generally penicillin is the drug of choice. Tetracyclines are also very useful. The Gram-negative intestinal bacilli are penicillin resistant, but respond well to the tetracyclines and the streptomycin group, especially kanamycin and gentamicin. *Ps. aeruginosa* is a very resistant organism, but responds to polymyxin and gentamicin.

An advance of great importance has been the development of new penicillins which have extended properties over the generally employed penicillin G. Some of the broad-spectrum penicillins, e.g. ampicillin, are effective against many Gram-negative intestinal bacilli, and one, carbenicillin, can be used in *Ps. aeruginosa* infections.

GENERAL REFERENCES FOR CHAPTERS 17 *to* 20

CRUICKSHANK, R., DUGUID, J. P., MARMION, B. P. & SWAIN, R. H. A. (1973) *Medical Microbiology*, 12th edn, Vol. 1. Edinburgh: Churchill Livingstone. An excellent account of medical microbiolgy, with the accent on laboratory findings and the properties of bacteria and viruses.

WILSON, G. S. & MILES, A. A. (1975) *Topley and Wilson's Principles of Bacteriology, Virology and Immunity*, 6th edn, Vols. 1 and 2. An authoritative account of the whole subject.

YOUMANS, G. P., PATERSON, P. Y. & SOMMERS, H. M. (1975) *The Biological and Clinical Basis of Infectious Diseases*. Philadelphia: Saunders. An excellent account of medical microbiology and infectious disease, with particular emphasis on the clinical features.

REFERENCES

1. WANNAMAKER, L. W. (1970) Differences between streptococcal infections of the throat and of the skin. *New England Journal of Medicine*, **282**, 23 and 78.
2. Leading Article (1971) Haemorrhagic ulceration of gut. *British Medical Journal*, **3**, 132.
3. Leading Article (1978) Renal carbuncles. *British Medical Journal*, **1**, 1166.
4. STRASBERG, S. M. & SILVER, M. D. (1968) Hemolytic streptococcus gangrene. *American Journal of Surgery*, **115**, 763.
5. DUNNET, W. N. & SCHALLIBAUM, E. M. (1960) Scarlet-fever-like illness due to staphylococcal infection. *Lancet*, **2**, 1227.
6. FEIGIN, R. D. (1976) The perinatal group B streptococcal problem: more questions than answers. *New England Journal of Medicine*, **294**, 106.
7. Leading Article (1977) Group-B streptococci in the newborn. *Lancet*, **1**, 520.
8. FINCH, R. G., FRENCH, G. L. & PHILLIPS, I. (1976) Group B streptococci in the female genital tract. *British Medical Journal*, **1**, 1245.
9. Leading Article (1975) Acute dermal gangrene. *British Medical Journal*, **3**, 607.
10. WILLIAMS, R. E. O., BLOWERS, R., GARROD, L. P. & SHOOTER, R. A. (1966) In *Hospital Infection*, 2nd edn, p. 43. London: Lloyd-Luke.
11. CURTIN, J. A., PETERSDORF, R. G. & BENNETT, I. L. (1961) Pseudomonas bacteremia: review of ninety-one cases. *Annals of Internal Medicine*, **54**, 1077.
12. RABIN, E. R. *et al.* (1961) Fatal pseudomonas infection in burned patients. *New England Journal of Medicine*, **265**, 1225.
13. FORKNER, C. E. *et al.* (1958) Pseudomonas septicemia: observations on twenty-three cases. *American Journal of Medicine*, **25**, 877.
14. Leading Article (1978) Legionnaires' disease. *British Medical Journal*, **1**, 2.
15. LUCAS, C. T. *et al.* (1971) Transfer of gonococcal urethritis from man to chimpanzee. *Journal of the American Medical Association*, **216**, 1612.
16. Leading Article (1974) Meningococcal infections. *British Medical Journal*, **3**, 295.
17. DAVIS, J. A. S. *et al.* (1976) Circulating immune complexes in a patient with meningococcal disease. *British Medical Journal*, **1**, 1445.
18. BRO-JØRGENSEN, A. & JENSEN, T. (1971) Gonococcal tonsillar infections. *British Medical Journal*, **4**, 660.
19. SHAPIRO, L., TEISCH, J. A. & BROWNSTEIN, M. H. (1973) Dermatohistopathology of chronic gonococcal sepsis. *Archives of Dermatology*, **107**, 403.
20. Leading Article (1971) Reiter's disease. *British Medical Journal*, **3**, 386.
21. MOLL, J. M. H. *et al.* (1974) Associations between ankylosing spondylitis, psoriatic arthritis, Reiter's disease, the intestinal arthropathies, and Behçet's syndrome. *Medicine (Baltimore)*, **53**, 343.

Chapter 18. Wound Infections: The Clostridia

THE SOURCE OF WOUND INFECTION

The most important organisms responsible for wound infection are (a) *Staph. aureus*; (b) *Strept. pyogenes*; (c) Gram-negative intestinal bacilli; and (d) clostridia. Certain uncommon wound infections should be noted. *Anaerobic streptococci* and *Bacteroides* are described in Chapter 17. *Fusospirochaetal* infections have been noted following human bites, as has also *actinomycosis*. In tropical countries wounds are occasionally infected with *Corynebacterium diphtheriae*, producing cutaneous diphtheria. Other tropical oddities are *mycetoma* (see p. 253) and *myiasis*, the infestation of a cutaneous wound with fly larvae.

Wounds may be infected primarily at the time of injury or else secondarily at a later date; either infection may be derived from the patient himself or from an outside source. The types of wounds most liable to primary infection are those that follow battle or agricultural accidents, when gross soiling is almost inevitable. Likewise wounds implicating the bowel are contaminated by the patient's faeces. The organisms found in such wounds include clostridia and Gram-negative intestinal bacilli. On the other hand, wounds following industrial accidents may be only lightly contaminated with staphylococci, and clean surgical wounds should, at least theoretically, be free of pathogens.

It is regrettable that wounds that were primarily sterile, or else rendered sterile by appropriate antibiotic therapy, often become infected during convalescence. The source of such infection may be the patient himself, as a result of touching his injuries, but more commonly the infection of a wound is from an extrinsic source following cross-infection. The most prevalent wound infections nowadays are the result of cross-infection in hospital wards, and the organisms usually responsible are *Staph. aureus* and *Ps. aeruginosa*. These are considered in Chapter 19. The remainder of this chapter is devoted to anaerobic wound infections due to the clostridial group of organisms.

ANAEROBIC WOUND INFECTIONS

These infections are of great clinical importance, and with few exceptions, e.g. those due to anaerobic streptococci, actinomyces, and bacteroides, all are due to the clostridial group of anaerobic spore-bearers. The clostridial organisms are responsible for two extremely serious conditions, *gas-gangrene* and *tetanus*. Gas-gangrene is produced by the combined action of a number of clostridia, the most important of which are *Cl. welchii* (also called *Cl. perfringens*), *Cl. oedematiens*, and *Cl. septicum*, whereas tetanus is caused by a single organism, *Cl. tetani*. The rare, lethal form of food-poisoning, botulism, is produced by another clostridium, *Cl. botulinum*.

BACTERIOLOGY OF THE CLOSTRIDIAL ORGANISMS

Morphology. They are large, Gram-positive bacilli approximately 5 μm long and 0·5 to 1 μm broad. The most characteristic feature is the spore, which is produced whenever the organism is placed in adverse conditions. It is usually central or subterminal, but in *Cl. tetani* it is situated terminally producing a characteristic drum-stick appearance. These organisms are all motile and non-capsulate with the exception of *Cl. welchii*, which is non-motile and capsulate.

Cultural characteristics. They all grow easily but demand absolute anaerobiosis, i.e. they are obligatory anaerobes. They are most conveniently cultured at 37°C on blood agar in the anaerobic atmosphere afforded by a McIntosh and Fildes jar. There appear flat, rather irregular colonies, and these may be surrounded by a zone of complete haemolysis, depending on the species.

Robertson's meat medium, which consists of cooked meat suspended in infusion broth, is useful in that it allows the growth of both anaerobes and aerobes (see Appendix 2). The anaerobes can then be subcultured anaerobically on to blood agar to obtain pure colonies.

Biochemical reactions. These are of considerable importance in relation to the pathogenesis of gas-gangrene. Clostridia are divided into two categories, saccharolytic and proteolytic.

Saccharolytic clostridia ferment many sugars, e.g. lactose and glucose. They do not break down proteins, and they merely turn the meat in Robertson's medium a pink colour due to the production of acid. The principal pathogens of gas-gangrene, viz. *Cl. welchii*, *Cl. septicum*, and *Cl. oedematiens*, come into this category.

Proteolytic clostridia. These break down protein and produce foul-smelling gases like hydrogen sulphide and ammonia. The meat in Robertson's medium becomes black due to the formation of iron sulphide. The putrefactive organisms of gas-gangrene, e.g. *Cl. sporogenes* and *Cl. histolyticum*, come into this category.

It is a fair generalisation that the saccharolytic clostridia are the important pathogens in gas-gangrene and the proteolytic clostridia mostly saprophytes. However, the demarcation is not clear cut, since the proteolytic clostridia have some saccharolytic capacity. In addition, *Cl. histolyticum* is moderately pathogenic despite its predominantly proteolytic activity. *Cl. welchii* has slight proteolytic activity.

Cl. tetani does not ferment sugars, but is moderately proteolytic.

Toxin production. The clostridia are typical toxic organisms, the lesions they produce being due entirely to exotoxins. The infection is localised, but the systemic effects are far-reaching.

Of the gas-gangrene group *Cl. welchii* is the most important. Five types are described, and type A is the human pathogen, causing gas-gangrene and food-poisoning. The other four types affect sheep and cattle. The toxin of type A is called α-*toxin*. It is lethal for laboratory animals and is necrotising. It is a lecithinase, and attacks the phospholipid constituents of red cells thereby causing severe haemolytic anaemia. This lecithinase is used in detecting *Cl. welchii*: if egg-yolk, which is rich in lipoprotein, is incorporated into nutrient agar, it is rendered opalescent by *Cl. welchii* by virtue of its lecithinase. This effect is prevented if the agar plate is first treated with an antitoxin to the α-toxin. This is called *Nagler's reaction*.

In addition, some strains of type-A *Cl. welchii* produce variable amounts of haemolysin (θ-toxin), collagenase (κ-toxin), hyaluronidase (μ-toxin), and deoxyribonuclease (ν-toxin).

Cl. septicum produces various toxins: one that is lethal and haemolytic, a haemolysin, a deoxyribonuclease, and a hyaluronidase. *Cl. oedematiens* produces a toxin that is haemolytic and has a lecithinase activity and is also necrotising and lethal.

By contrast, *Cl. tetani* produces only two exotoxins. The important one is a neurotoxin called *tetanospasmin*, which is responsible for the convulsions of tetanus. Tetanospasmin has been separated in a pure crystalline form. It is an immensely potent poison, being second only to the exotoxin of *Cl. botulinum* in this respect. The other exotoxin is haemolytic, and is known as *tetanolysin*.

Occurrence. The spores of these organisms are widely dispersed in nature, and are especially plentiful in soil. These organisms are contaminants of the human and animal intestine, and their spores are excreted in the faeces and returned to the soil in the form of manure. *Cl. welchii* is an invariable inhabitant of the human bowel, but *Cl. tetani* is somewhat more sporadic. Clostridial organisms must be expected in all environments, including the air and furniture of wards and even operating theatres. As regards the latter, plenum filtration systems (see p. 235) are important in preventing the entry of spores from the atmosphere.

By virtue of their ability to form spores in adverse circumstances, these organisms are resistant to heat and desiccation. Only well-devised sterilising methods can destroy them.

Apart from the role played by *Cl. welchii* in gas-gangrene, certain specific strains are an important cause of *food-poisoning* when they contaminate meat in heavy culture. The symptoms, which may be quite severe and occasionally fatal, are dysenteric in type. The causal organisms are isolated with ease from the meat and the patient's faeces.

GAS-GANGRENE

Gas-gangrene may follow the contamination of a wound with the spores of the pathogenic clostridia. Considering the very widespread distribution of these spores and the rarity of gas-gangrene in civilian practice, it is evident that the contamination of a healthy incised wound is not followed by infection. The factor essential for spore germination is a reduced oxygen tension. This is present in severely contused or lacerated wounds containing much dead tissue, which has been devitalised as a result of compression or impaired blood supply. Deep punctured wounds are particularly dangerous. Foreign bodies like shrapnel or pieces of clothing exert local pressure, and also favour pyogenic infection. Soil is particularly dangerous, because its ionisable calcium salts and silicic acid lead to tissue necrosis. Finally, any coincidental infection by aerobic organisms serves to augment the anaerobiosis. The local injection of adrenaline has a similar effect by causing vasoconstriction, and this drug should not be injected into the buttocks where the skin is liable to be contaminated with clostridial spores.[1]

It therefore follows that most gas-gangrene is exogenous in origin, and is due to the contamination of large wounds. It is seen typically in battle casualties or in agricultural accidents. An appreciable amount of gas-gangrene is, however, endogenous from the bowel. Examples of this are the clostridial puerperal sepsis that follows criminal abortion, and the gas-gangrene of the high thigh stump after amputation of the lower limb for peripheral vascular disease. The stump is often soiled with faeces, especially in an elderly, incontinent patient.[2]

Spores of clostridia have been known to remain dormant in healed wounds, and to have germinated following surgical intervention. This is particularly important with regard to tetanus, and immunisation is always advisable before surgery is performed on old war and agricultural wounds.

Pathogenesis. Gas-gangrene is not due to infection by a single clostridial organism; it is the consequence of a combined assault by numerous saccharolytic and proteolytic organisms. The true pathogens, *Cl. welchii*, *Cl. septicum*, and *Cl. oedematiens*, germinate, and the powerful exotoxins which they liberate produce local tissue necrosis. At this stage the proteolytic saprophytes, such as *Cl. sporogenes* and *Cl. histolyticum*, flourish on the dead material, and break it down into putrid products.

If the wound is merely superficial, it will discharge foul-smelling fluid in which there are bubbles of gas (*anaerobic cellulitis*), but if it is extensive enough to implicate the underlying muscles, the *anaerobic myositis* typical of gas-gangrene develops.

(*a*) There is a rapidly progressive necrosis of muscle fibres due to the necrotising exotoxins of the saccharolytic clostridia.

(*b*) The muscle carbohydrate is fermented by these organisms. Lactic acid and gas (mostly hydrogen and carbon dioxide) are formed. This is the origin of the 'gas' in gas-gangrene. At this stage it is odourless.

(*c*) There is rapid spread of infection due to the breaking down of intercellular ground substance and local tissue barriers (e.g. endomysium and perimysium) by the hyaluronidase and collagenase produced by the organisms. A whole muscle bundle may be affected with great rapidity. Indeed, gas-gangrene resembles an invasive infection in the extent of its local spread, but the organisms show no tendency towards blood-stream invasion, except perhaps at the time of death. This accounts for the gas bubbles in the liver (*foamy liver*) and other organs sometimes found at necropsy. Moreover, this appearance is not confined to gas-gangrene; clostridial organisms may also enter the blood stream from the bowel as an agonal phenomenon during the course of any fatal disease.

(*d*) As the infection spreads, so the necrosis increases both by toxic action and the ischaemia following pressure by the gas and exudate on the surrounding blood vessels. The area is tense, oedematous, and crepitant, and the muscle is odourless and brick-red in colour.

(*e*) Following the extensive necrosis there is progressive putrefaction, which is brought about by the proteolytic clostridia. These thrive on and decompose the dead muscle, which becomes greenish-black in colour. Necrosis with superadded putrefaction is called gangrene (see 'p. 57), and these saprophytes complete the evolution of 'gas-gangrene'. It is at this stage that the characteristically foul odour appears.

(*f*) During this local process there is severe toxaemia due to circulating exotoxins. It is manifested by profound shock and a rapidly-developing haemolytic anaemia (see p. 230). It is this toxaemia which brings about the death of the patient.

The local pathological effects of gas-gangrene are acute inflammation with much muscle necrosis and spreading oedema. Polymorph infiltration is not conspicuous while the process is advancing, a point of difference between clostridial and streptococcal myositis. In the oedema fluid there are large numbers of organisms. The severe oedema may be related to the permeability factor produced by some clostridia, especially *Cl. oedematiens*. The absence of polymorphs is strange; perhaps the powerful exotoxins exert a negative chemotactic influence.

Treatment of gas-gangrene. It is usual to give a polyvalent antiserum against the exotoxins of the three main pathogens, as well as penicillin or a tetracycline.

The use of hyperbaric oxygen also has its place in treatment. The patient is placed in a special pressurised chamber in which he breathes oxygen at 2 to 3 atmospheres pressure absolute for periods of 1 to 2 hours twice daily on several successive days. This treatment requires special experience as well as apparatus, and oxygen is potentially dangerous to the lungs when in high concentration (see p. 526).

For prophylaxis in cases of grossly contaminated wounds penicillin has replaced antiserum therapy. There is no doubt, however, that a proper wound toilet is the most important aspect of prevention and treatment.

TETANUS

The spores of *Cl. tetani* not infrequently contaminate wounds, but as with the gas-gangrene organisms a reduced oxygen tension is essential for their germination. The conditions conducive to tetanus infection are therefore similar to those already described. Quite often the degree of trauma is very mild, because an insignificant punctured wound like the prick of a contaminated thorn can be the site of origin of a fatal tetanus infection.

Exogenous infection has also resulted in *surgical tetanus*, i.e. the introduction of spores into a wound during the course of a surgical operation. For such spores to germinate they must be presented with a nidus where conditions are relatively anaerobic. Contaminated foreign materials embedded in the tissues, e.g. catgut, talc, or cotton-wool, provide the necessary nidus, and are the causes of surgical tetanus, which nowadays is very rare. Catgut, which is made from the intestine of sheep, is almost inevitably contaminated, but fortunately modern processes of sterilisation during its manufacture are so effective that it has ceased to be a hazard in most countries.

Although tetanus is now uncommon in the Western world, the situation in the poorer countries is quite different. It has been estimated that over one million people die each year from tetanus, and that this disease is a leading cause of death among hospital admissions in many of the developing countries. Among the ways by which the spores may be introduced into the tissues of the unprotected population are injecting quinine (for malaria), ear piercing, and applying soil (or even dung) to the umbilicus of the newborn.

Endogenous tetanus infection is rare, but it has been reported after septic abortions.

Pathogenesis

Tetanus is clinically a disease of the central nervous system. The local lesion may be so mild that only very careful search will reveal it, yet the exotoxin produced may be sufficient to cause death.

After peripheral absorption, the toxin reaches the central nervous system probably by passing along the motor trunks; it spreads up the spaces between the nerve fibres. It acts by interfering with the inhibition processes at the motor neurons. This accounts for the generalised increase in tone, and also explains *local tetanus*. This is the early tendency to spasms of those muscles controlled by the same spinal segment as that supplying the area infected.

The incubation period varies from a few days to several weeks, and the shorter it is, the worse the prognosis. Tetanus developing from wounds of the upper extremities, neck, and face is said to be more frequently fatal than that arising after injuries to the lower parts of the body.

The condition usually commences with stiffness and spasm confined to the area of infection (local tetanus). This is soon followed by severe trismus due to masseteric spasm (lock-jaw), dysphagia, spasm of the facial muscles producing the characteristic *risus sardonicus*, and finally generalised tetanic convulsions, in which there may be opisthotonos. The picture resembles strychnine poisoning quite closely, but unlike it there is residual muscle stiffness between periods of convulsion. Death is due to asphyxia following involvement of the respiratory muscles. There are no characteristic *post-mortem* findings.

Prophylaxis of Tetanus[3]

Since tetanus may occur following quite trivial wounds, by far the best method of prophylaxis is active immunisation. This is carried out by a course of three injections of tetanus toxoid, a formolised preparation of the exotoxin adsorbed on to aluminium hydroxide or phosphate. The second injection is given about 6 weeks after the first, and the third from 6 to 12 months after the second. Routine booster doses are recommended at 10-year intervals unless during this period the patient has received a booster dose at a time of wounding. Hypersensitivity reactions, usually pain at the site of injection, may occur, particularly when tetanus toxoid is given frequently to boost immunity.[4] Therefore unnecessary booster doses of toxoid are to be avoided.

When a person is severely wounded, tetanus prophylaxis is

essential. If the patient has had a complete basic course of toxoid or a booster within the past 5 years, he is adequately immune, and nothing further should be done apart from the local treatment of the wound. If the period since the last dose of toxoid exceeds 5 years but is less than 10 years, a booster dose should be given. If, however, the period exceeds 10 years, immediate passive immunisation must also be performed, since any residual immunity may not be adequate to protect the patient even under the stimulus of a booster dose. If there is no history of active immunisation, the need for passive immunisation is even stronger, since the first dose of toxoid cannot produce an adequate active immunity to shield the patient in time from the possible development of tetanus. Nowadays in many countries passive immunisation is carried out with *human tenanus immunoglobulin*, also called *tetanus immune globulin (human)*, 250 units of which are given intramuscularly. This will produce a serum concentration of antitoxin greater than 0·01 unit per ml for about four weeks, a level which is adequate to prevent the development of tetanus. If the wound is still unhealed after 4 weeks, a second dose should be given. Human immunoglobulin only rarely causes adverse allergic reactions in healthy patients who receive it only for the prevention of tetanus (it is more dangerous when used repeatedly in the treatment of hypogammaglobulinaemia, when anaphylactic reactions may occasionally occur). Nevertheless, adrenaline solution should always be available when it is given (0·5 to 1 ml of Adrenaline Injection (B.P.), which is 1 in 1000 aqueous solution, intramuscularly in adults).

At the same time a dose of adsorbed toxoid is given, but into a different limb. In the case of a patient who has never been immunised actively before, this constitutes the first of the three immunising doses; in those who have allowed their active immunity to lapse for more than 10 years, this is a booster dose. Since the toxoid is of the adsorbed type and

adminstered at a distance from the immunoglobulin, its action is not interfered with by the initially high level of passive immunity.

In those areas where human immune globulin is still unavailable, the much less satisfactory and more dangerous *horse antitetanic serum (ATS)* must be used in a dose of 1500 to 10 000 units. There is such a great danger of anaphylactic reactions occurring that a small subcutaneous test dose has first to be given. If symptoms such as a drop in blood pressure, tachycardia, or dyspnoea develop, adrenaline must be administered immediately. In any case, the treatment will have to be abandoned, since these manifestations indicate that antibodies are already present in the patient's serum, and these will neutralise the horse ATS. Even if there are no adverse reactions and the remainder of the ATS can be given in safety, its immunising effect is soon vitiated, since the foreign serum is cleared from the patient's blood much more rapidly than the homologous human serum. It is seldom detectable immunologically after 16 days. It therefore follows that human immunoglobulin is by far the better agent for the passive immunisation against tetanus, and it is to be hoped that it will soon be available in all countries.

Treatment of Tetanus

The treatment of established tetanus is still unsatisfactory. Large doses of antitoxin (even up to 100 000 units) are recommended, sometimes even intravenously after preliminary subcutaneous and intramuscular test doses, but by the time the disease is clinically manifest much of the exotoxin is firmly bound to the affected cells, and is therefore invulnerable to the action of circulating immunoglobulins. The therapeutic value of antiserum is, however, not accepted by all workers. Penicillin and a tetracycline should also be given. The most important factor is undoubtedly the maintenance of respiratory function; on this especially does recovery depend.

GENERAL REFERENCES

See Chapter 17, page 228.

REFERENCES

1. Harvey, P. W. & Purnell, G. V. (1968) Fatal case of gas gangrene associated with intramuscular injections. *British Medical Journal*, 1, 744.
2. Leading Article (1969) Postoperative gas gangrene. *British Medical Journal*, 2, 328.
3. Smith, J. W. G., Laurence, D. R. & Evans, D. G. (1975) Prevention of tetanus in the wounded. *British Medical Journal*, 3, 453.
4. Leading Article (1974) Reactions to tetanus toxoid. *British Medical Journal*, 1, 48.

Chapter 19. Hospital Infection

The present pre-eminence of surgery can be attributed to advances in the two ancillary fields of anaesthesia and microbiology. The advisability of analgesia on the grounds of humanity and cleanliness on the grounds of necessity was recognised by surgeons at least as early as the third millennium B.C., yet even in the nineteenth century these were blatantly ignored. A change was precipitated by Ignaz Semmelweiss in Vienna and Oliver Wendell Holmes in Boston. Independently they revived the idea of the contagious nature of wound infection by showing that puerperal sepsis was related to the unclean hands and clothing of the obstetrician rather than to an act of God. The idea was unacceptable to the medical establishment of the day: Holmes was ignored but did at least live to see his ideas vindicated; Semmelweiss, on the other hand, was derided and dismissed from his post, and he subsequently died insane.[1] A century later we fully appreciate the dangers of hospital infection.

Hospital infection is the result of the transmission of pathogenic organisms to a previously uninfected patient from a source in the environment of a hospital. If the organisms are derived from some external source the infection is called *cross-infection*; if they are derived from the patient himself, it is called *auto-infection*. In *maternity wards* epidemics of staphylococcal bullous impetigo of the newborn (and subsequent maternal breast abscess) may be encountered, while amongst the older infants explosive epidemics of gastro-enteritis due to enteropathogenic species of *Esch. coli* and to *Salmonella* and *Shigella* organisms are not uncommon. In a *children's ward* the common viral diseases like chickenpox and measles, when once introduced, will spread like wildfire, and epidemics of hepatitis A may also occur. In *mental hospitals*, *Shigella* diarrhoea is often a great nuisance. Even in *general medical wards* the menace of cross-infection is always present. A patient with open pulmonary tuberculosis is an obvious source of danger, and should be isolated as soon as possible. It is quite common for patients admitted with cerebral vascular accidents to succumb to staphylococcal pneumonia, and for patients with neurological disorders like multiple sclerosis and cauda equina lesions, who require repeated catheterisation, to develop intractable *Ps. aeruginosa* infections of the urinary tract.

It is, however, in *surgical and maternity wards* that the incidence of cross-infection reaches its peak, because the patients often have large areas of denuded integument as a result of wounds and extensive burns, or following delivery. These provide an admirable avenue for bacterial invasion. The most common infecting organisms are *Staph. aureus* and the Gram-negative intestinal bacilli. *Strept. pyogenes* has had an evil reputation for producing wound infections and puerperal sepsis, but nowadays streptococcal lesions of this type are uncommon. When present, streptococci are usually found in association with staphylococci.

Staphylococcal cross-infection manifests itself as (*a*) wound infection; (*b*) skin infections, e.g. boils and bullous impetigo of the newborn; (*c*) enterocolitis; (*d*) pneumonia; (*e*) breast abscesses in lactating women; (*f*) acute conjunctivitis in the newborn. The Gram-negative bacilli are the usual causes of urinary-tract cross-infection, and they are also responsible for much wound infection. Herpesvirus infection has been described as a complication of burns.[2]

The incidence of hospital wound infection varies from 2 to 20 per cent, and it depends on such variable factors as the patient's age, the size of wound, the duration of operation, the presence of drainage tubes, the normal bacterial flora of the part, and the hospital in which the patient is treated.

SOURCE OF AND TRANSMISSION OF ORGANISMS

Staph. aureus. The reservoir is the anterior nares, from where the organisms are conveyed to the skin of the hands. The hands and perineum are areas on which staphylococci tend to multiply with greatest readiness. The organisms are excreted either from overt lesions like boils and pustules, or else they may be discharged from the skin of symptomless carriers. The nose is the ultimate reservoir, but is of less importance in the actual transmission of the organism, except perhaps during heavy breathing and snorting.

The staphylococci are transferred either by direct contact on to a patient, or else to objects that may come into contact with patients (*fomites*). A perineal carrier is very liable to contaminate his bedding. A carrier may likewise contaminate a communal bath or bowl.

It is important to realise that not all carriers are equally efficient excretors, nor does it necessarily follow that carriers who suffer from recurrent overt lesions are more dangerous than those who are symptomless. Some of the most virulent staphylococcal cross-infections have been transmitted by carriers who have not even exhibited evidence of local nasal infection. These dispensers of staphylococci are particularly dangerous. The nature of local immunity to staphylococcal infection and the relationship between carriage and excretion are ill-understood.

Finally, excretors of staphylococci may contaminate the air around them both directly and indirectly from their sheets and blankets. It is well recognised that movement in bed increases the number of organisms in the surrounding air.

There are two good methods of assessing the bacterial content of the air, the *settling* or *sedimentation plate* and the *slit-sampler*. The former consists of a culture plate of standard diameter, on which the organisms in the air are allowed to settle. This is a time-consuming procedure but is particularly valuable in operating theatres, where the danger is most liable to arise from particles settling on the area of incision. The exposed plate is comparable with the exposed wound. The slit-sampler consists of a narrow slit through which air is sucked on to a rotating culture plate beneath it. This is a very efficient method of collecting most of the organisms in the sampled volume of air, and is speedy as compared with the settling plate.

Air-borne staphylococci are particularly liable to contaminate wounds in the operating theatre, where the area of incision must of necessity be exposed for some time; even in a ward these bacteria can contaminate wounds while they are being dressed. Furthermore, staphylococci will almost certainly be inspired by other patients and attendants, whose anterior nares may then be colonised. In this respect it is most important to note that a considerable amount of staphylococcal auto-infection from the nose is really the result of cross-infection at a slightly earlier period. Many patients become nasal carriers during the pre-operative period, and subsequently contaminate their wounds. Air-borne organisms may be inspired or swallowed and lead to staphylococcal pneumonia or enterocolitis.

Some types of staphylococci spread much more rapidly than others. The type-80 staphylococcus is notorious for the severity of its lesions as well as for its speed of spread. Most epidemic strains are resistant to the commonly-used antibiotics, but it does not follow that sensitive organisms are necessarily less virulent than resistant ones. With the constant use of antibiotics over the years most of the sensitive strains have been eliminated, so that a predominantly resistant population has been left behind. This is one of the results of the abuse of antibiotics. Once a resistant population has developed, it is perpetuated by infecting new victims. In this way cross-infection plays a major part in maintaining resistant strains.

The two cardinal hazards of hospital practice, the abuse of antibiotics and the presence of cross-infection, tend to reinforce each other and set up a vicious circle.

Strept. pyogenes. The reservoir is the throat, but it is particularly those people who harbour streptococci in their noses who are likely to transmit infection. The important mode of transmission is by close direct contact. Unlike staphylococci, these organisms do not survive long on the skin, nor is the transmission of infection by fomites of much importance. There is good experimental evidence that blankets heavily contaminated with streptococci do not infect people who sleep in them. The part played by airborne transmission in streptococcal cross-infection is also not of great moment, except perhaps in extensive burns.

Gram-negative intestinal bacilli. *Esch. coli* is a universal commensal of the bowel, and *Proteus* organisms are present in about a third of all specimens of faeces. It is probable that a considerable amount of wound infection caused by these organisms is the result of true auto-infection, but until the established methods of typing come into general use, the actual amount of cross-infection produced by them will remain unknown. It is also important to note that the anterior urethra is frequently colonised by *Esch. coli*, *Proteus* organisms, and *Strept. faecalis*, and that these organisms can be forced into the bladder during catheterisation. Cystitis may then ensue.

Faecal carriage of *Ps. aeruginosa* is uncommon enough to make it unlikely that auto-infection is the explanation of the majority of infections it causes. The reservoirs are the infected wounds and urinary tracts of individual patients. Most urinary cross-infection is carried by the hands of attendants from urine bottles to bladder drainage apparatus connected to indwelling catheters. The role played by inadequately-sterilised cystoscopes has also been demonstrated.

The Gram-negative intestinal bacilli can be shed quite easily into the air, but they are much less resistant to drying than are the staphylococci and streptococci. Therefore airborne spread is not so important as with these cocci. On the other hand, stagnant water affords a suitable environment for the Gram-negative organisms, especially *Ps. aeruginosa*, which has been known to contaminate the humidifiers of operating theatres and infant's incubators. It can survive in certain disinfectants, notably cetrimide, and has caused suppurative panophthalmitis (with the loss of the eye) when contaminated eye-lotions have been used to irrigate eyes on which surgery had been recently performed. Similar ocular infection has been described in a special-care nursery among neonates, and the source was contaminated resuscitation apparatus.[3]

MODE OF CROSS-INFECTION

In surgical cases cross-infection may occur either in the operating theatre or else later in the ward. Infections acquired during the period of operation usually manifest themselves within the next seven days, whereas later manifestations are more likely to be due to subsequent ward infection. Both ward and operating-theatre infections may be superficial in nature, but if the infection is obviously deepseated, it is almost certain to have been acquired during the operation.

Cross-Infection in Operating Theatres

The three methods of theatre cross-infection are (a) *by direct contact from the surgeon or attendants*, (b) *from the air*, and (c) *from contaminated instruments*.

The surgeon may have overt infection on the hands or some other part of the body, or more likely be a nasal carrier with contaminated hands. The most dangerous areas for transmitting staphylococcal infection are the hands and wrists. Even the most scrupulous 'scrubbing up' cannot sterilise the skin, for some organisms are bound to find shelter in its pores. Impermeable gloves are therefore essential for all surgical procedures, and they must be changed at once if they are perforated during the operation. The sweat that accumulates under the glove is bound to contain many organisms. The area of the wrist just above the rim of the glove is also dangerous to the patient. The sleeve of the theatre gown soon becomes sodden with blood, and organisms can penetrate it with ease, and so be introduced into the wound. By contrast, the nose is less dangerous as an immediate source of infection, but should be masked in order to obviate the danger of violent expulsion of droplets during sneezing or coughing.

Much interest has been centred around the problem of the *air-borne transmission of infection*, which is particularly important in operating theatres. In poorly ventilated rooms there is a progressive accumulation of pathogenic organisms derived in part from the patient and bedclothes and in part from the attendants and spectators who have gathered around to watch the operation. All movements of the spectators cause settled organisms to rise in the air, from where they may alight on to the wound.

Efficient ventilation is obviously necessary to remove these organisms, but unless intelligently devised, it may cause more harm than good. In the past there have been epidemics of theatre infection due to suction of air from an adjacent contaminated source by means of a reduced pressure exhaust system of fans. In fact the air that was drawn in came from near-by wards, and was heavily contaminated with staphylococci. Clostridia are the commonest pathogens found in the outside air. The inlet for fresh air to the air-conditioning plant should be as high as possible.

Inadequately sterilised instruments are of the greatest danger in transmitting infection. The role played by cystoscopes has already been mentioned.

Prevention of Theatre Cross-Infection

Architecture and design of theatre. In theory it is best either to have the theatres completely separate from the wards, or else in one composite block. In practice the most that can be hoped for is that a single floor may be reserved entirely for a suite of theatres, adequate in number for the size of the hospital. It is better situated in a cul-de-sac than near a main thoroughfare.

The *accessory compartments*, e.g. the scrub, sterilising, and sink rooms, should be separate from, though connected to, the theatre. In this way the splashes produced during 'scrubbing up' will not contaminate the theatre, nor will the contaminated instruments washed up in the sink room come in contact with the theatre environment. The heat engendered by autoclaving, and the steam subsequently produced, make a separate sterilising room desirable, and furthermore the dirty atmosphere of the theatre may contaminate sterilised instruments. In fact, sterilisation is best done in a central sterile supply department away from the theatre. The anaesthetic room is useful for preparing the patient for reception on to the operating table prior to entering into the theatre. It should have close access to the theatre.

The *walls* and fittings of a theatre should be smooth and easy to wash down. There should be no ledges to collect dust. The *floors* should have a smooth finish, and slope gently towards a gully so that they can be swilled down with ease. The *temperature* most suitable for work varies according to the country; in temperate climates 18 to 21°C (65 to 70°F) is a good air temperature for a theatre, and the *relative humidity* should be about 55 per cent.

Ventilation is of paramount importance. Not only is it essential for the comfort of the staff, but it also serves to remove anaesthetic gases. The air admitted must be free of pathogenic organisms, so that it does not endanger the area of operation or the sterile equipment.

A positive pressure (plenum) system is essential, and the air should be filtered before admission. Positive pressurisation serves to prevent contaminated air infiltrating into the theatre. It is also necessary to direct the air flow, so that any organisms released in the theatre may be removed as expeditiously as possible. There are two methods of distributing the incoming air. In one, turbulent ventilation, the air is rapidly mixed with that already present in the theatre, while in the other method, displacement ventilation, the air is introduced gently, and merely displaces that in the theatre by quiet downward movement. In both types of ventilation the air is introduced at ceiling-level. It is customary to extract some of it by exhaust fans situated near the floor. It is said that displacement ventilation is better in a room which is generally contaminated, whereas turbulent ventiliation is preferable if the source of contamination is confined to the area of the operating table, for it will produce less contamination of the incision. In practice either is acceptable.

The *filter* itself should have pores of about 5 μm in diameter. At first sight this seems very large in relation to the size of the organisms, but in fact bacteria seldom occur singly as unattached particles in the air. They are usually attached to particles of dust which are considerably larger than 5 μm. Filters made of disposable fabric and oiled mesh are very effective; they must be adequately maintained, otherwise there may be heavy contamination of air entering the theatre, or else the pores may become so blocked that no air can enter at all.

The surgeon and attendants.[4-6] Nobody with overt staphylococcal infection, whether a boil or a superficial skin lesion anywhere on the body, should be allowed into the theatre. Streptococcal sore throat is another contraindication, and so also are infections of the respiratory tract, which could be transmitted to the patient in a most vulnerable state. It is impractical to exclude staphylococcal carriers unless they bear epidemic strains. The use of a cream containing chlorhexidine and neomycin or gentamicin in the nose can reduce the staphylococcal population there. The ritual of a shower bath before operating is useless, and indeed increases the dispersal of bacteria, particularly staphylococci, in the air for some hours. Even washing with a hexachlorophane soap is not helpful. The removal of underclothes is another ritual; it does not decrease the infectivity of the surgeon because the underlying skin is the source of the organisms. The surgeon should be gowned and masked to prevent direct contact between the incised area and his own skin. Theatre gowns are unfortunately inefficient in preventing the escape of organisms, which penetrate between the pores of the fabric and at the trouser openings at the ankles. The use of an operating suit made of a woven fabric with pore size of 7 to 10 μm, and the securing of trousers around the ankles greatly reduces the dispersal of bacteria, and should certainly be considered in operations on patients who are at high risk of infection.

The method of washing up, no matter how painstaking and prolonged, will remove only those 'transient' organisms which are picked up adventitiously; it will reduce but cannot eliminate the 'resident' flora. A six-minute scrub with soap and water reduces the bacterial flora by about 50 per cent, while a two-minute handwashing in one of the liquid preparations containing hexachlorophane or iodophors can reduce the population to as little as 1 per cent. Rinsing in a 0.5 per cent solution of chlorhexidine is equally effective. Liquid soap or detergent preparations are more effective than are antiseptic bar soaps. Prolonged washing is not only unnecessary but is indeed harmful to the skin if frequently carried out. It has been recommended that two or three minutes' scrubbing, with careful attention to the nails, before the first operation, and two or three minutes' washing without a brush before the subsequent operations of a list should be an adequate routine for a surgeon.[4] Rings should be removed from the fingers before washing up.

Caps are important as the hair often harbours staphylococci, and a mask should be worn to protect the wound from salivary droplets and mucus emitted during talking or sneezing. Cotton masks with impervious material inserted between the two layers are simple and adequate. Some paper masks are also suitable. Shoes should be removed, and theatre boots or shoes worn. Finally, intact gloves must be worn; the pretested ones are best. A waterproof fabric is useful for protecting the sleeve area.

The spectators. These should wear masks and caps and be gowned and properly shod. Above all there should be as little movement as possible, and this means limiting the number of spectators and assistants. The surgical team should be as small as possible, and the equipment so well placed that extraneous movements are unnecessary.

The patient. The patient's bedclothes and blankets should not be allowed into the theatre.

The ritual of shaving the skin of the operation site increases the risk of wound sepsis in proportion to the time elapsing before operation.[5] Bacterial colonisation of the slightly damaged skin is probably responsible. Therefore shaving should be avoided where possible, and in very hairy sites it should be deferred until the day of the operation. The disinfection of the skin can be carried out for some days in advance with hexachlorophane soap to cut down the staphylococcal flora. This is done particularly in orthopaedic cases, but could be applied to other types of surgery. Skin disinfection at operation is discussed on page 661.

Surgical equipment. The amount of theatre equipment present should be limited, since all objects accumulate organisms. Sterile packs should have a double wrapping and must be kept dry, as organisms move by capillary action through moist, porous material. All equipment should be disinfected, or sterilised if it comes into contact with the incision. This is described in Appendix 1.

Systemic chemoprophylaxis.[5] The value of systemic antibiotics in preventing wound infection is limited. Broad-spectrum antibiotics, e.g. tetracyclines and ampicillin, may actually lead to an increased incidence of postoperative sepsis.[7,8] Antibiotics with a narrow spectrum are preferable, e.g. penicillin where vascular disease or trauma predisposes to gasgangrene, or with dental operations on patients with endocardial disease of the heart valves. In patients undergoing operations for the insertion of a heart-valve prosthesis, the combined use of penicillin and streptomycin (or else a penicillinase-tolerant penicillin) should be continued for as long as three months (until the valve cuff becomes endothelialised). Patients with an infected urine should have prophylaxis with an antibiotic selected on the basis of sensitivity tests before operation or instrumentation of the urinary tract. The drug metronidazole is useful in preventing *Bacteroides* infection after abdominal and gynaecological surgery.[9]

The surgical isolator.[5] This consists of a transparent plastic tent distended with filtered air under moderate pressure and completely enclosing the patient, except for the head. It provides a radical means of preventing the spread of organisms to the wound from the staff and the environment. Access is through glove sleeves and entry ports incorporating air locks.

Cross-Infection in Surgical Wards

The modes of staphylococcal cross-infection in a ward are not very different from those in a theatre, except that many other patients are also present. They are potential sources of infection.

Patients with obvious septic lesions, e.g. extensive skin infections with a copious purulent exudate or chronic osteomyelitis with pus seeping through the plaster, are particularly dangerous. The organisms soon contaminate the bedding, and are shed into the air. The same applies to patients suffering from staphylococcal pneumonia or enterocolitis. Others may merely be carriers, but of these a few may harbour virulent strains, which can lead to a ward epidemic.

The *air* may be sufficiently contaminated to endanger wounds during dressing, especially such complicated lesions as extensive burns. In this respect it is important that sterilised dressings which have been exposed to the air should be discarded if not used at the time of exposure. It is bad practice to keep a large supply of dressings in metal drums, using some as required and keeping the remainder. If small packages are used, there will be less temptation to retain any dressings that are left over.

Another source of mischief is contaminated bedclothes, especially blankets. Apart from the possible danger of direct contat with patients, contaminated blankets are of even greater importance in shedding staphylococci into the air. An experiment in which woollen and cotton blankets were heavily contaminated with *Staph. citreus* demonstrated the great speed with which the organisms were dispersed throughout the ward. When the blankets were covered by a counterpane, the dispersion was even greater; this was attributed to friction on the surface of the blankets.[10]

It must finally be reiterated that much postoperative infection due to organisms in the patient's nose or on his skin is really the result of initial cross-infection and subsequent autoinfection.

Quite apart from direct implantation into the wound, it is possible that nasal carriers are subjected to a period of bacteraemia during the inexpert insertion of endotracheal tubes. The tissue damage in the wound could be sufficient to localise infection there.

Prevention of Cross-Infection in Surgical Wards

Isolation policy. Under ideal circumstances all patients harbouring staphylococci should be isolated from the remainder of the hospital community, but in practice this is impossible. There is no doubt, however, that patients suffering from extensive, discharging, staphylococcal lesions should be separated from uninfected patients. Carriers of virulent strains, e.g. the type-80 staphylococcus, should be treated likewise.

On the other hand, there are patients who are particularly susceptible to infection, and they too should be isolated in their own interests. This is called *reverse isolation*. Patients who have undergone extensive skin grafting or organ transplantation, or who are suffering from agranulocytosis or immunological deficiency disease fall into this category.

The type of isolation recommended is again subject to the

criterion of practicability. *Complete isolation* in an air-conditioned cubicle in a special hospital is an ideal but is rarely practical, and it may have the additional disadvantage of necessitating a break in the continuity of the medical attendants responsible for the patient's treatment. *Ward side-rooms*, on the other hand, are convenient and practical, but it is important to ensure that the flow of air is in the right direction. If the patient is excreting large numbers of staphylococci, the ventilation must be adjusted so that the air is discharged without contaminating the main ward. Care must also be taken to prevent the nursing staff from contracting infection from the patient. The use of protective clothing is advisable.

Communal segregation of infected patients in 'septic wards' is another possibility. It protects the uninfected, but entails the risk of the infected patients acquiring each other's infection. In practice it is very useful in times of emergency. Barrier nursing, so useful in an intestinal infection like typhoid fever, is of very limited value in preventing staphylococcal cross-infection, because it cannot reduce the air-borne transmission of organisms. In an epidemic of staphylococcal infection the whole ward may have to be evacuated and then disinfected.

Dressing technique. The danger of doctors and attendants who have overt infection, or who carry virulent staphylococci on their skin, has already been discussed. People who have infected lesions should not dress wounds. All dressers should be properly clothed and masked, and a *rigorous no-touch technique* should be employed by the use of sterile forceps. Alternatively gloves should be worn.

It is bad practice to dress wounds in general wards even if there is no evidence of overt infection among the patients. It is far better to use separate, well-equipped, properly ventilated *dressing rooms*. The question of ventilation is particularly important if infected wounds are being dressed in the room. In a short time there will be an accumulation of pathogenic organisms in it, and they must be discharged to the outside atmosphere and not into the general ward. Likewise it is foolish to allow ward air to contaminate the dressing room.

Urinary drainage. Catheterisation should be avoided whenever possible because of the danger of cystitis (see p. 234), but when the use of the catheter is necessary the operator should be gloved. Where continuous bladder drainage is necessary, the weight of evidence incriminates open systems for cross-infection. The use of *closed drainage systems*, especially those which do not need to be disconnected periodically during bladder irrigation, has reduced the amount of urinary cross-infection very considerably.[11]

Disposal of contaminated articles. Wound dressings should be placed in paper bags and burnt. They should not be left lying around the wards. Used instruments should be sterilised without delay, and dirty bedclothes should be sent to the laundry as soon as possible.

General cleaning and disinfection of the ward. This includes the disinfection of bedding and the cleaning of the ward furniture, walls, and floors.

It is recommended that cotton *blankets* should be used and changed on the patient's discharge, after two weeks, or when contaminated with infected material. *Sheets* should be changed every two days (or more frequently if contaminated) and on the patient's discharge. *Bed-covers* should be changed weekly (or more often if contaminated) and when the patient is discharged.

The laundering process itself will sufficiently disinfect the bedding, but if the patient is suffering from particularly dangerous diseases like tuberculosis or staphylococcal enterocolitis, the bedding must be disinfected before it is sent to the laundry. In the case of smallpox, anthrax, or plague the bedding must be burnt.

Screens should be disinfected at monthly intervals. *Curtains* reach their maximum of contamination within a few days. Since frequent changing is impractical, they should be changed when they are dirty or for obvious aesthetic reasons, and at least every three to six months. *Communal baths* should be disinfected after use. The *walls, floors*, and *furniture* of wards should be cleaned so frequently that there is no visible dirt on them. This entails the daily washing of floors and dusting of furniture. Walls and ceilings should be cleaned at least once a year.

It is easy to adopt a sanctimonious attitude towards ward hygiene. A state of mind may result in which the staff are more concerned about preventing infection than about treating patients under their care. A sense of proportion is always essential. The scope of hygiene depends on the size and position of the hospital, and the nature of the surgery that is performed in it. Hospital infection will be overcome only when aseptic methods are used by every member of the staff as part of an unwritten, instinctive routine in the treatment of each patient that is admitted.

Investigation of an Epidemic of Surgical Cross-Infection

First of all, the infecting organism must be isolated, and it should then be typed.

Secondly, it should be decided by clinical assessment whether the infections occurred during the time of operation or later on in the ward. The time of first appearance of the lesions and their depth are good indications.

If all the organisms are of one type, it is strong presumptive evidence that the infection has originated from a single source. It is therefore important to swab the anterior nares of the relevant theatre and ward staff, and also to examine any overt or healing infected lesions that may be present on their skin. In ward infections all the patients should be similarly investigated.

If a carrier is found, that person should be isolated and treated. Sometimes there may be several carriers, or else the source of infection may not be discovered. All the infected individuals may have to be isolated, and the ward closed and disinfected. When it is re-opened, it should be barred to the previous patients and all articles that may have been in contact with them. Only thus can the effectiveness of the disinfection be assessed.

If the organisms are of different types, it is futile to engage in exhaustive searches for carriers. If the infection occurred in the theatre, it is far better to investigate the ventilation system and to check details of general hygiene as regards the patients' bedclothes and the movements of spectators. In ward infections of this type the various hospital routines should be critically examined.

GENERAL READING

WILLIAMS, R. E. O., BLOWERS, R., GARROD, L. P. & SHOOTER, R. A. (1966) *Hospital Infection*, 2nd edn, 386 pp. London: Lloyde-Luke.
LOWBURY, E. J. L., AYLIFFE, G. A. J., GEDDES, A. M. & WILLIAMS, J. D. (1975) *Control of Hospital Infection*. London: Chapman and Hall.

REFERENCES

1. INGLIS, B. (1965) *A History of Medicine*, p. 152 *et seq.* London: Weidenfeld and Nicolson.
2. Leading Article (1970) Herpesvirus infection in burned patients. *British Medical Journal*, 2, 618.
3. DREWETT, S. E. *et al.* (1972) Eradication of *Pseudomonas aeruginosa* infection from a special-care nursery. *Lancet*, 1, 946.
4. Leading Article (1970) The surgical scrub. *British Medical Journal*, 3, 418.
5. Leading Article (1976) Preventing infection at the operation site. *British Medical Journal* 2, 773.
6. Leading Article (1972) Surgical ritual. *British Medical Journal* 3, 543.
7. PRICE, D. J. E. & SLEIGH, J. D. (1970) Control of infection due to *Klebsiella aerogenes* in a neuro-surgical unit by withdrawal of all antibiotics. *Lancet*, 2, 1213.
8. LOWBURY, E. J. L., BABB, J. R. & ROE, E. (1972) Clearance from a hospital of Gram-negative bacilli that transfer carbenicillin-resistance to *Pseudomonas aeruginosa*. *Lancet*, 2, 941.
9. WILLIS, A. T. *et al.* (1976) Metronidazole in prevention and treatment of bacteroides infections after appendicectomy, *British Medical Journal*, 1, 318.
10. RUBBO, S. D., STRATFORD, B. C. & DIXSON, S. (1962) Spread of a marker organism in a hospital ward. *British Medical Journal*, 2, 282.
11. Leading Article (1963) Prevention of catheter infections in women. *British Medical Journal*, 2, 332.

Chapter 20.   Tuberculosis, Syphilis, and Actinomycosis

Whereas the acute pyogenic infections produce an inflammatory reaction which may or may not terminate in resolution, there are many other infections which commonly proceed to chronicity. In these there is usually such great tissue destruction that resolution is impossible and a chronic course invariable. During the progress of these infections acute exacerbations of an exudative type may occur, and these are usually due to allergy. Tuberculosis, syphilis, actinomycosis, and the fungal, protozoal, and helminthic infections all come into this category.

There are no histological features common to all these infections: in tuberculosis, leprosy, histoplasmosis, and leishmaniasis the macrophage is the prominent cell type and the infiltrate may be either diffuse or tuberculoid (p. 125); in actinomycosis and sporotrichosis there is a polymorph infiltration; in syphilis there is an infiltration of lymphocytes and plasma cells. The helminthic diseases are often associated with heavy eosinophil accumulations.

In the acute bacterial infections the causal organisms appear to produce damage by some direct action often by producing powerful toxins. From many of the micro-organisms responsible for chronic infection no definite toxin has been isolated. Their pathogenic action is probably the result of allergy of the cell-mediated type. Skin tests of a type similar to the Mantoux test are used in their diagnosis (see Ch. 14). Erythema nodosum, which sometimes accompanies these conditions, is an allergic vasculitis of the skin and subcutaneous tissues due, at least in leprosy, to a deposition of immune complexes on the vessel walls.[1] In other instances it is probably due to delayed-type hypersensitivity.

In many acute bacterial infections a long-lasting immunity is produced, and this is due to circulating immunoglobulins. In chronic infections there may also be antibodies in the circulation, but though these can be of value in diagnosis, e.g. in the serological diagnosis of syphilis, they do not necessarily produce immunity against the disease. In some of these infections, notably tuberculosis, a degree of immunity is acquired after an infection; it is not due to immunoglobulins, but is mediated by lymphocytes.

If these infections are generalised there is pyrexia; severe constitutional disturbances are invariable in miliary tuberculosis, leishmaniasis, and trypanosomiasis. The ESR is considerably raised, and there is usually hypergammaglobulinaemia. The white-cell count often indicates the course of the local infection. In active tuberculosis and protozoal diseases there is often a monocytosis, in actinomycosis a neutrophil leucocytosis, and in the helminthic infections an eosinophilia. Secondary syphilis may be accompanied by an absolute lymphocytosis, a change also noted on occasions in healing tuberculosis (see Ch. 53).

TUBERCULOSIS

There are at least five distinct strains of Mycobacterium tuberculosis as well as a sixth group of unclassified mycobacteria. The *human* and *bovine* strains are potential human pathogens, and the *murine* strain ('vole bacillus'), which is endemic in wild voles, has been used as an alternative to BCG in active immunisation against tuberculosis. *Myco. avium* is pathogenic to birds and may occasionally cause human infection. The fifth strain of mycobacteria affects the *cold-blooded vertebrates*, and is of little human importance. The bovine organism is excreted in the milk of infected cows, and was once an important cause of intestinal and tonsillar infection in childhood. Nowadays bovine tuberculosis in the human subject has almost completely disappeared in civilised countries following the eradication of tuberculous herds and the pasteurisation of milk. It therefore follows that nearly all tuberculosis is caused by the human strain. The mode of infection is by the inhalation of organisms present in fresh droplets or the dust of dried sputum expectorated from an open case of pulmonary tuberculosis. There are three possible methods of acquiring infection: inhalation, ingestion, and inoculation. Inhalation is all-important, since ingestion is now rare and inoculation of the skin from *post-mortem* material is little more than a curiosity. Congenital tuberculosis has been described in a few cases as a result of transplacental spread.

Bacteriology. *Myco. tuberculosis* is a slender bacillus about 3 μm long, non-motile and non-sporing. Its most conspicuous feature is its waxy content which makes it impermeable to the usual stains. It slowly takes up heated stains, e.g. carbol fuchsin in the Ziehl-Neelsen method (see Appendix 2), and then resists decolorisation even by strong acids and alcohols, i.e. it is acid-fast and alcohol-fast. It is Gram-positive, but Gram-staining is not performed because the methyl violet penetrates only with great difficulty.

It grows very slowly, and then only on very complex artificial media which should contain, amongst other things, egg-yolk and glycerol. The Löwenstein-Jensen medium is one that is commonly used, and it takes several weeks at 37°C in an aerobic atmosphere for any growth to appear. It is necessary to wait 6 weeks before discarding the culture as negative. Colonies can be recognised much earlier than this if micro-methods are used. Growth is faster in fluid media, such as the Dubos medium. This contains 'Tween 80' (polyoxyethylene sorbital mono-oleate, a wetting agent) and bovine serum albumin among its constituents.

The organism is pathogenic to the guinea-pig, and when injected subcutaneously, it leads to the animal's death within a few months. Necropsy reveals widespread miliary tuberculosis. A greatly enlarged spleen is characteristic; it contains many caseous foci crowded with acid-fast bacilli. Rabbits are highly susceptible only to the bovine strain.

The bovine strain grows less readily than the human strain, and glycerol does not favour its growth as in the human strain.

Myco. tuberculosis is very resistant to drying, and it can survive in dust for several months. It is, however, very sensitive to the effect of ultraviolet radiation, and is rapidly killed in sunlight.

Atypical or anonymous mycobacteria. Occasionally cases of human tuberculosis are encountered in which atypical bacilli are isolated. They differ from *Myco. tuberculosis* in being non-pathogenic to guinea-pigs and resistant to anti-tuberculous drugs, especially isoniazid. In the past such organisms have often been discarded as non-pathogens, but it is now accepted that they can cause disease, generally milder than classical tuberculosis. This is a good example of the futility of attempting to define pathogenicity in terms of one or two properties of an organism without considering its host. The atypical bacilli have been subdivided provisionally into four groups.

Group I, Photochromogens. These organisms produce a yellow pigment if the culture is grown continuously in light. *Myco. kansasii* is the best known.

Group II, Scotochromogens. Pigment is produced regardless of whether the growth is in the light or dark.

Group III, Nonchromogens. The Battey bacillus is in this group; it was named after the Battey Tuberculosis Sanatorium in Georgia where it was first isolated. Organisms in this group are closely related to the avian bacillus. No pigment is produced and, like groups I and II, growth in culture is slow and occurs at 37°C.

Group IV, Fast-growing Organisms. This group differs from the others in that there is rapid growth at 25°C as well as at 37°C. It includes *Myco. phlei* and *Myco. smegmatis*. Organisms in this group are the least pathogenic, but occasionally cause adenitis in children.

Some idea of the frequency of infection with these atypical organisms has been obtained by testing US Naval recruits with tuberculin derived from the various strains.[2] Whereas only 8·6 per cent reacted to tuberculin of *Myco. tuberculosis*, 35 per cent gave a positive reaction to that of the Battey bacillus. There is considerable cross-reaction to tuberculins derived from the various strains, and it has been suggested that subclinical infection with an anonymous mycobacterium may give a degree of immunity to tuberculosis.

Mycobacteria causing skin infection. In addition to the cutaneous infections with *Myco. tuberculosis*, such as lupus vulgaris, two other organisms have been implicated in chronic ulcerations of the skin. Both organisms are characterised by growing best at 31 to 33°C, a property which was responsible for them being overlooked until 1948.

Myco. ulcerans.[3] This organism causes chronic ulceration most commonly of the limbs. The lesion commences as a subcutaneous nodule in which there is necrotic fat but little inflammatory reaction. The necrosis spreads laterally and deeply, and the undermined skin breaks down into an ulcer with an overhanging edge.[4] After several weeks healing commences, but may take several months or even years for completion. The disease is remarkable for the lack of in-

flammation considering the extent of the necrosis. It bears little resemblance histologically to tuberculosis. The disease was first recognised in Australia but is known to occur elsewhere. It is common in Uganda, where in retrospect it was probably described as long ago as 1897; it is called Buruli ulcer.

Myco. marinum (balnei).[5] This organism causes infection of abrasions, and may be acquired in swimming pools (hence its name) or occasionally from tropical fish tanks.[6] The ulcers are usually solitary, and the elbow or knee is a common site. Microscopically a chronic inflammatory reaction, perhaps with a non-caseating tuberculoid reaction, is seen. The lesions tend to heal spontaneously.

Pathogenesis of the tuberculous lesion. The following sequence of events occurs when tubercle bacilli are introduced into the tissues:

1. A transient acute inflammatory reaction with an infiltration of polymorphs. These cells are rapidly destroyed by the organisms.

2. A progressive infiltration of macrophages derived mostly from the monocytes of the blood. The macrophages are responsible for the destruction of the organisms.

3. The macrophages phagocytose the bacilli. In a short time their character changes: their cytoplasm becomes pale and eosinophilic and their nuclei elongated and vesicular. Their appearance bears a resemblance to the epithelial cell, and they are called *epithelioid cells* (see p. 126).

4. Some macrophages, instead of becoming epithelioid cells, fuse to form Langhans giant cells (see p. 127).

5. Surrounding this mass of altered macrophages there is a wide zone of small round cells, mostly lymphocytes and fibroblasts.

6. Within 10 to 14 days necrosis begins in the centre of this mass, which consists of altered macrophages and cells peculiar to the tissue of the part. This is a firm, coagulative necrosis called *caseation*, and it is characterised by a high content of lipid and a tendency to resist autolysis and demolition. Histologically the necrosis is structureless and eosinophilic, but with silver stains reticulin fibres can sometimes be demonstrated.

The caseation is due primarily to hypersensitivity to products of the bacilli, notably tuberculoprotein. Ischaemia plays some part also, inasmuch as the blood supply becomes inadequate for the heavy infiltration of cells into the affected area.

There is now produced the *tubercle follicle* (Figs. 20.1 and 20.2), which consists of a central mass of caseation surrounded by epithelioid and giant cells, which in turn are enclosed in a wide zone of small round cells. The appearance is characteristic of tuberculosis, but a rather similar picture is seen in some of the deep-seated mycoses (see Ch. 21). For a diagnosis of tuberculosis organisms must be found in the lesion. This is difficult at this stage, and culture must be employed in parallel with Ziehl-Neelsen staining of smears or sections.

Variations in the reaction to the tubercle bacillus. The common type of lesion described above is called *productive* or *proliferative*, because its main components are cells rather than a fluid exudate.

Another type of lesion is the *exudative* form of tuberculosis. It is characterised by the out-pouring of an inflammatory

Figure 20.1
A tubercle follicle. There is a small area of caseation in the centre, and it is surrounded by an ill-defined zone of epithelioid cells, in the midst of which a Langhans giant cell is present. There is a diffuse infiltration of small round cells in the periphery. × 120.

Figure 20.2
A tubercle follicle. The large central area of structureless caseous necrosis is surrounded by a zone of epithelioid cells in which a Langhans giant cell is present. In the periphery there is a small round cell infiltration. × 230.

exudate rich in fibrin. There is a considerable infiltration of lymphocytes, and often polymorphs are present, but epithelioid and giant cells are rather scanty (Fig. 20.3). Exudative lesions are typical of tuberculosis of serous cavities. They are not necessarily more serious than productive ones. It was well recognised in the pre-antibiotic era that the so-called 'primary pleural effusion' of young adults was one of the most favourable types of pulmonary tuberculosis, and that recovery usually occurred. Tuberculosis involving epithelial surfaces also assumes an exudative character. This accounts for the 'sterile' pyuria that is such an important diagnostic feature of open renal tuberculosis.

In compact organs like the liver and kidney the lesions are almost always productive. In the lungs either type of reaction is possible, but here exudative phenomena are particularly serious, because they are attended by extensive caseation and a rapid spread of infection. Indeed, it is usual to classify pulmonary tuberculosis into the following categories, depending on the reaction of the tissue:

Acute caseous tuberculosis. There is confluent caseation of much of a lobe, producing caseous bronchopneumonia (Fig. 20.4). This is seen when large amounts of caseous debris are insufflated down a large bronchus, and a vigorous response is elicited as the result of intense hypersensitivity. A similar type of reaction may occur if the host's immunity is feeble, or if the organism is particularly virulent. The constitutional effects are very severe ('galloping consumption').

Chronic tuberculosis. Here the immunity of the host is adequate to cause some destruction of the bacilli, and healing by repair (fibrosis) occurs side by side with caseous destruction. Three types of chronic pulmonary tuberculosis are recognised: caseous, fibro-caseous, and fibroid, depending on the relative degrees of caseation and fibrosis. In longstanding fibroid tuberculosis the lung may be converted into a contracted mass of dense fibrous tissue in which there may be little recognisable evidence of active tuberculous infection. Bronchiectasis is a frequent complication of this type of disease.

The most serious type of lesion is *non-reactive tuberculosis.* This consists of extensive foci of caseation teeming with bacilli, but with virtually no cellular reaction around them. This type of disease is seen as a complication of leukaemia, and is also met with from time to time in elderly people. It may be associated with severe aplasia of the bone marrow (see Ch. 53), and the presenting symptoms may be those of an

Figure 20.3
Tuberculous meningitis. In this section of the meninges of the base of the brain a small central vessel is seen to be surrounded by small round cells (perivascular cuffing), and in the proximity there is a large area of dense cellular infiltration, much of which is the seat of early caseous necrosis. In the periphery there is an open space meshed with strands of fibrin, in which there are collections of small round cells. This is a typical example of the exudative type of tuberculous reaction seen in a serous cavity. The absence of giant cells is noteworthy. × 70.

Figure 20.4
Confluent tuberculous bronchopneumonia. The whole of the lower lobe and much of the upper lobe shows caseous consolidation. (R 36.2, *Reproduced by permission of the President and Council of the R.C.S. Eng.*)

obscure blood dyscrasia. The tuberculin reaction is sometimes negative; this may be due to an overwhelming infection impairing the immune response or alternatively there may be an initial immunological deficiency that predisposes to a non-reactive state. In either event the prognosis is very grave. Protein malnutrition also depresses the tuberculin reactivity of patients with pulmonary tuberculosis due to the generalised impairment of cell-mediated immunity it produces.[7]

The fate of the tuberculous lesion. The caseous focus may either cease to progress and heal by fibrosis, or it may soften and spread.

The hallmark of healing is fibrous tissue, and this is produced by the proliferating fibroblasts at the periphery of the lesion. In due course the area of caseation may be replaced by a solid fibrous nodule. Sometimes only a rind of fibrous tissue forms around the periphery, while the central mass of caseation undergoes slow dystrophic calcification. In this calcareous nodule organisms can still survive, and years later, when the resistance of the host breaks down, they may become active again. Sometimes the nodule ossifies.

The hallmark of activity is caseation and softening. If the lesion is spreading, bacilli are carried by macrophages into the surrounding lymphatics and tissue spaces. There they settle and set up satellite follicles, which by fusing with the primary

enlarging lesion, produce a conglomerate tubercle follicle. Caseous material does not soften rapidly, due possibly to phosphatides that inhibit autolytic enzymes. Sometimes, however, liquefaction does occur, and this is attended by serious consequences.

There is no really satisfactory explanation for this softening. There is no doubt that it is associated with spread, and that the liquefied debris contains many bacilli, but it is not known whether this multiplication of organisms is the cause or the result of the softening. It has been suggested that the liquefaction is due to secondary infection, but this is untrue. Pyogenic infection may certainly complicate a tuberculous lesion, but liquefaction often occurs in the absence of such infection. Hypersensitivity is probably of considerable importance.

Once liquefaction has occurred, the debris contains large numbers of tubercle bacilli, and the whole is called a *cold abscess*. Unlike a pyogenic abscess it contains few cells, and most of these are disintegrating. The term 'pus' is therefore inapplicable, as there are no pus cells. The term 'cold abscess' is equally inapplicable. In practice it is reserved exclusively for tuberculous lesions, even though other suppurative lesions such as actinomycosis may also be 'cold', inasmuch as neither the heat, pain, nor redness of acute pyogenic infection is marked in them. The liquefied debris ('pus') tracks towards a free surface and discharges there. In a lesion of the lung rupture soon occurs into a bronchus, and the disease spreads to other parts of the lung; much infectious material is also coughed up.

In areas such as the bones and joints, lymph nodes, and epididymis, where there are no immediately available passages, large cold abscesses often accumulate, e.g. the collar-stud abscess of the neck secondary to infection of a cervical lymph node. In due course these abscesses track through the tissues, the substance of which is destroyed in the path of the advancing tuberculous lesion. In this way sinuses are formed, which are lined by *tuberculous granulation tissue*. This consists of systems of tubercle follicles irregularly disposed in a mass of newly-formed fibrous tissue which is heavily infiltrated with lymphocytes and macrophages. Sometimes the 'pus' may track for long distances, e.g. it may enter the psoas sheath from an infected vertebra, spread down as a psoas abscess, and finally point below the inguinal ligament.

Whenever a tuberculous abscess opens to the exterior, the disease becomes more serious, firstly because of its *open*, infectious character, and secondly because the tubercle bacillus is an aerobic organism and proliferates much more profusely in an atmosphere of air. These features are well illustrated in the open, cavitating type of pulmonary tuberculosis. Much of the value of artificial pneumothorax therapy was due to its effect in preventing the aeration of the affected lung.

Spread of tuberculosis in the body. The principles differ in no significant way from those of other infections.

Local spread by macrophages has already been described.

Lymphatic spread is a continuation of local spread. The result is a regional tuberculous lymphadenitis which is typical of childhood infections. The primary focus with its attendant lymphangitis and lymphadenitis is called the *primary complex*. Nowadays nearly all primary complexes are pulmonary.

Blood spread occurs as an extension of lymphatic involvement. In an overwhelming infection the organisms escape from the lymph nodes and enter the blood stream to produce *miliary tuberculosis*, which in extreme cases is of the non-reactive type. The lungs, spleen, liver, kidney, and to a lesser extent other organs, are seeded with tubercle bacilli which produce numerous follicles of millet-seed size. Blood spread also occurs when caseous hilar nodes directly implicate an adjacent pulmonary vein. If there is a discharge of large numbers of organisms into the blood stream, miliary tuberculosis occurs, but the lungs are often spared.

Miliary tuberculosis is seen in young children as an extension of a primary complex. However, tuberculosis is now less frequent in children and it is not rare to encounter miliary tuberculosis in adults, especially the elderly and those on glucocorticoid therapy.[8] It produces fever, wasting, hepatosplenomegaly, leucopenia, and thrombocytopenia. The absence of classical miliary mottling in the chest radiograph and a negative tuberculin test render diagnosis difficult. Bone-marrow examination, liver biopsy, or a therapeutic trial with specific antituberculous drugs such as PAS and isoniazid, are the most successful diagnostic procedures. *Tuberculous meningitis* is a very frequent accompaniment of miliary tuberculosis, and is due either to direct involvement of the choroid plexus, or else to a small subcortical lesion (*Rich's focus*) rupturing into the subarachnoid space.

Figure 20.5
Tuberculous epididymitis. The enlarged, cowl-shaped epididymis shows diffuse caseous necrosis. (M 5.3, *Reproduced by permission of the President and Council of the R.C.S. Eng.*)

In older children and adults it sometimes happens that a tuberculous focus implicates a small pulmonary vein in the vicinity, and then only a few bacilli invade the systemic circulation. These may be destroyed by the RE system, or else become lodged in various sites to give rise to metastatic disease. Such a lesion may progress immediately to produce clinical effects, or else remain quiescent, only to undergo reactivation years later. This type of lesion is called *local metastatic tuberculosis*, and it accounts for most of the disease seen in surgical practice (Fig. 20.5). Organs sometimes involved in this way are the kidneys, adrenals, uterine tubes, epididymes, and the bones, joints, and tendon sheaths. Curiously enough, the thyroid, pancreas, heart, and voluntary muscles are seldom affected. The spleen is not commonly the seat of extensive caseous tuberculosis, though in miliary tuberculosis it is almost invariably affected.

Spread in serous cavities is seen in the pleurisy that may complicate lung lesions, the localised peritonitis found around tuberculous salpingitis, and in tuberculous meningitis.

Spread along epithelial-lined surfaces is typified by the intrabronchial spread of tuberculosis that occurs when sputum is inhaled into adjacent lung segments. If the sputum is coughed up it can produce tuberculous laryngitis, and when swallowed, the bacilli may infect the ileo-caecal area of the bowel and lead to tuberculous enteritis. Rectal involvement is manifested by ischiorectal abscesses.

Likewise tuberculosis of the kidney can spread down the

ureter to implicate the trigone of the bladder, and tuberculous salpingitis can lead to endometrial disease.

Factors determining the response of tissues to tuberculous infection. It is apparent that sometimes there is healing by fibrosis of a small caseous focus, and on other occasions a rapidly spreading fatal disease. The factors that determine the tissue response are:

(*a*) The dose and virulence of the organism. Virulent strains tend to produce rough colonies, and when cultivated on solid media aggregate to grow in long cords. Pathogenicity is not, however, closely correlated with growth characteristics. Pathogenicity to animals is discussed on page 239.

(*b*) The innate and acquired resistance of the body. This is a very important consideration.

Innate immunity is of great importance in tuberculosis and is discussed on page 162. Amongst the most susceptible groups are Black Africans, American Indians, and Australian Aborigines.

Age and sex. During the first 5 years of life the body's resistance is poor and the mortality rate is high. From 5 to 15 years resistance is at its peak, but it breaks down during the early adult period of 15 to 30 years, particularly in women. After the age of 30 years resistance is quite high, but it breaks down again in old age, particularly in men.[8]

General health of the individual is also of great importance. Malnutrition and overcrowding in prison camps and slums predispose to spreading tuberculosis. Psychological stress and chronic debilitating diseases also lower the resistance. Diabetes mellitus is particularly notorious in predisposing to a rapidly spreading type of infection. Likewise glucocorticoid therapy can activate previously quiescent tuberculous foci. Glucocorticoids should be used with great caution in tuberculosis.

Occupational factors influence the resistance: for instance, those whose work carries the hazard of silicosis, e.g. tunnellers, miners, and quarrymen, are liable to a spreading type of disease. Asbestosis is a less serious predisposing factor.

The effect of previous infection. A second infection shows a completely different pathogenesis to the primary one. This was demonstrated by Koch in guinea-pigs, and the *Koch phenomenon* is described in detail on page 183. It will be remembered that the secondary response is accelerated, a manifestation of bacterial allergy, and that it does not spread to the lymph nodes but remains localised and heals, an indication of acquired immunity. The animal becomes hypersensitive to a protein fraction of the organism called *tuberculoprotein* or *tuberculin*. Koch's *Old Tuberculin* (*OT*) is now superseded by *Purified Protein Derivative* (*PPD*). The administration of tuberculin to a hypersensitive person produces a local area of inflammation within 48 hours. Necrosis may ensue in very hypersensitive people, therefore a very small initial dose should be used. The *tuberculin unit* (*TU*) has been introduced to standardise the relative doses of OT and PPD. A standardised tuberculin consisting of a purified protein derivative of *Myco. tuberculosis* with 'Tween 80' as stabiliser is now available through the WHO. The intradermal injection of a measured amount, usually 1 to 3 tuberculin units, allows comparison of the results obtained at different times and in different countries to be made. This is the *Mantoux test*. An alternative method makes use of a multiple-puncture apparatus which pricks the skin through a film of stronger

tuberculin. This is the *Heaf test*, and it is read in grades from 1 to 4 according to the degree of reaction; grade 1 is probably a non-specific response. It is a speedier method than the conventional Mantoux test, but is less easily standardised.

It is evident that when a sensitised person is exposed to tuberculoprotein, whether in a skin test or through a second infection, a delayed hypersensitivity reaction occurs, which in extreme cases (when the dose of tuberculoprotein is great or if it is given intravenously) produces fever and a flare-up of other foci. Indeed, the reaction may be so severe that it kills the patient, an event sometimes noted when tuberculin was used therapeutically in the belief that the allergic inflammation helped to destroy the bacilli. Tuberculous allergy develops within a month to 6 weeks of infection, and is of cell-mediated type (see p. 183). It has been found that the hypersensitivity declines with age, especially from the fifth decade onwards.[9] This may be due to decreased contact with the organism.

It is the acquired immunity of the Koch phenomenon which is particularly interesting. It is not as effective as that which follows smallpox or diphtheria, and furthermore is not due to circulating immunoglobulins; though these are present and can be demonstrated serologically, they play no part in immunity. The immunity of tuberculosis is cell mediated: the altered lymphocytes enable the macrophages to destroy the bacilli more effectively than they do in a primary infection. The macrophages of rabbits previously immunised with BCG, when grown in tissue culture, withstand parasitisation by tubercle bacilli, whereas the macrophages from unimmunised animals have no such power. The precise nature of these cellular changes is unknown. In addition, the sensitised lymphocytes liberate lymphokines in the vicinity of the tubercle bacilli; these by inhibiting the random movement of the macrophages probably augment their local phagocytic activity. It is possible that the lymphokines have a directly lethal effect on the organisms as well.

Although allergy and acquired immunity are clearly closely related, they are also distinct; thus it has been found that the degree of immunity that follows BCG vaccination is not related to the degree of tuberculin sensitivity induced.[10] It has also been noted that guinea-pigs can be immunised with methyl-alcohol extracts of tubercle bacilli without the development of allergy,[11] whereas hypersensitivity without immunity can be induced by injecting a mixture of tuberculoprotein and a waxy extract from the bacilli. It would appear that allergy is harmful in that, by causing caseation, it leads to the destruction of fibrous tissue barriers which might limit the spread of infection. On the other hand, it has been argued that the inflammation it induces does bring macrophages into contact with the bacilli—and these are the cells that destroy them. It appears that following BCG immunisation the protective value of an accelerated macrophage response far exceeds any tendency to necrosis and spread of the infection engendered by the allergy.

It should finally be noted that the acquired immunity is only of partial degree, and has no effect in overcoming the primary infection. Despite Koch's phenomenon, the guinea-pig still dies of its first infection. This may indicate that an important mechanism of the immunity is the localisation of the organism at a very early stage of the infection.

Morphology of Tuberculous Infection

It is well recognised that the morbid anatomy of pulmonary tuberculosis in children differs from that of adults. At all ages the lung is the organ principally affected.

(*a*) *Childhood.* In childhood the primary focus (Ghon focus) is a small, wedge-shaped area situated at the periphery of the lung field usually in the mid-zone. This subpleural focus may heal, or else the infection spreads to the hilar nodes, which become greatly enlarged and caseous. A conspicuous primary complex is the result. It either heals and calcifies, or else it spreads, and the child dies of miliary tuberculosis with meningitis. The lung lesion is usually of little importance in causing death, but the enlarged hilar nodes may compress a bronchus sufficiently to lead to segmental collapse.

In days gone by the alimentary tract was frequently the site of childhood tuberculosis, and this was due, of course, to infection by bovine bacilli. In abdominal disease the primary focus in the bowel is so small that it is rarely identifiable, and the first manifestation of the infection is great enlargement of the mesenteric lymph nodes, giving rise to the clinical picture of *tabes mesenterica*. The nodes may occasionally rupture into the peritoneal cavity, and cause acute tuberculous peritonitis. Usually calcification ensues and recovery follows, but otherwise there is a progressive lymphatic spread to the thoracic duct culminating in miliary tuberculosis.

Rarely the primary focus is tonsillar. This usually passes unnoticed, until progressive enlargement of the cervical lymph nodes and their softening and discharge through the skin (*scrofula*) make the disease obvious.

In all childhood lesions the feature in common is the small size of the primary focus, and the tendency to extensive lymph-node involvement (as in the guinea-pig).

(*b*) *Adult life.* In adult life the focus is almost always apical or subapical (*Assmann focus*), particularly involving the right lung. The reason for this apical situation is unknown. The lesion either heals, or else it progresses, softens, and develops into a cavity. Depending on the resistance of the patient, there is a tendency either to fibrosis or extensive cavitation. In severe cases great destruction of lung tissue results. A large cavity may be produced, and a vessel in its wall may be eroded, leading to haemoptysis. If caseous debris is inhaled into other bronchi tuberculous bronchopneumonia develops. This may occur on a small scale and result in local extension of the disease, but if widespread it causes massive caseation of a great area of lung tissue. This is a fulminating allergic response, and the disease remains localised to the lungs. Lymph-node involvement is inconspicuous, and blood-spread dissemination is unusual. Death is due to destruction of lung tissue (Fig. 20.6).

A similar pathogenesis occurs in other organs in the adult. Tuberculous enteritis due to swallowing infected sputum is characterised by ulceration of the wall of the ileum (Fig. 20.7). There is a localised peritonitis and an insidious tendency for strictures and fistulae to develop, but local lymph-node involvement is only slight. The contrast between this and the childhood abdominal lesion is obvious.

Renal tuberculosis usually starts as a cortical focus, which spreads to destroy the surrounding renal parenchyma. Other lesions develop in the medulla due to the passage of bacilli down the renal tubules, and eventually cavitation into the

Figure 20.6

Caseous tuberculosis of lung. In this section the entire upper lobe is consolidated with extensive tuberculous bronchopneumonia, and at the apex there is a large, ragged-walled cavity. The adjacent upper part of the lower lobe is also affected. (R 37.1, *Reproduced by permission of the President and Council of the R.C.S. Eng.*)

pelvis ensues. The destructive lesion of tuberculous pyelonephritis ultimately converts the kidney into a ragged cavity lined by tuberculous granulation tissue, and spread down the ureter may follow (Fig. 20.8). If it is occluded, a large tuberculous pyonephrosis is produced.

Skeletal tuberculosis usually starts in the metaphyseal area of a bone, and it causes great local destruction (Fig. 20.9). Unlike pyogenic osteomyelitis, it destroys the epiphyseal cartilage with great ease, and soon the neighbouring joint is affected.

The feature that all these adult lesions have in common is the tendency to extensive local destruction with little lymphatic involvement.

It is traditionally believed that the adult lesion is always secondary to a primary lesion acquired during childhood, and that the difference in course of the two infections can be explained on the basis of allergy and immunity acquired during the primary infection. Just as in the Koch phenomenon, where the second dose of organisms remained localised and did not spread to the regional nodes, so it is that the

Figure 20.7
Tuberculous ulceration of ileum. In this specimen of ileum there are several extensive tuberculous ulcers. They have arisen from Peyer's patches, but unlike typhoid ulcers they have spread laterally and have encircled the lumen; this is due to lymphatic involvement. (A 51.1, *Reproduced by permission of the President and Council of the R.C.S. Eng.*)

Figure 20.8
Tuberculous pyelonephritis. Most of the kidney has been destroyed, and is replaced by large ragged cavities full of putty-like caseous debris. The pelvis is greatly dilated and filled with similar material. (U 16.1, *Reproduced by permission of the President and Council of the R.C.S. Eng.*)

secondary adult lesion remains localised to the lungs and does not spread further afield.

It has, however, become apparent that even when a previously Mantoux-negative young adult develops tuberculosis, the lesion approximates more to the adult type than the 'primary' Ghon type with prominent hilar lymphadenopathy. Thus there is usually an apical focus without much lymph-node enlargement. Furthermore, there are very definite differences between the adult lesion and the Koch phenomenon. There is lymph-node involvement in the adult, though it is of microscopic extent only; also the lesion shows no particular tendency to heal. The difference in behaviour between childhood and adult lesions appears to be due to tissue maturation; the older the patient the less is the tendency towards marked lymph-node involvement. The effect of a previous infection, perhaps with a relatively avirulent atypical bacillus, as an additional modifying factor cannot be excluded, but it is unjustifiable to label all adult lesions as secondary. The terms *childhood* and *adult* tuberculosis are much more accurate than primary and secondary tuberculosis.

The source of the organisms causing adult-type tuberculosis has been the centre of much discussion in the past. The

pulmonary lesions have been regarded as due either to *reactivation* of a quiescent primary lesion or to the development of a new lesion produced by a *reinfection* from some external source. In the past reinfection was probably of great importance, but nowadays it seems that many adult-type lesions are themselves primary infections. In other organs, e.g. kidney and bone, it is almost certain that tuberculosis is due to the reactivation of small lesions which were produced during a bacteraemic phase of an earlier primary infection.

Incidence of tuberculosis. Tuberculosis is still widespread despite the great advances that have been made both chemotherapeutically and immunologically. It is the poorer countries that show the highest incidence, and as most of these are in Africa, Latin America, and Asia, tuberculosis has now the predominant distribution of a tropical disease. Its incidence continues to be an accurate reflection of the social standards of a community.

In Britain it would appear that most of the population is infected during some period of life, but that the disease usually remains subclinical. This is induced from the high frequency of positive tuberculin reactions in adults who have not been immunised with BCG. However, it is now re-

Figure 20.9
Tuberculosis of the spinal column (Pott's disease of the spine). Two adjacent vertebral bodies have been partially destroyed by progressive caseous necrosis, and the intervening intervertebral disc has almost disappeared in the debris. Tuberculosis not only destroys bone, but also invades and destroys cartilage. The result has been collapse of the two vertebrae with acute angulation of the spine (gibbus). (S 49a.4, *Reproduced by permission of the President and Council of the R.C.S. Eng.*)

cognised that infection with other mycobacteria, especially the avian bacillus and *Myco marinum*, can also cause Mantoux conversion, though usually the reaction is weak.[12] A strongly positive reaction to the standard PPD is considered good evidence of past infection with the human bacillus; indeed, it calls for further investigation of overt infection, especially in children, young adults, and the elderly. The interpretation of a weakly positive reaction is difficult, and a differential skin test using tuberculin made from *Myco. avium* and other atypical bacilli might be of help. Other evidence of past infection is the presence of calcified hilar lymph nodes, but in North America these may be due to mycotic infection, often histoplasmosis. Likewise calcified mesenteric nodes in the elderly bear witness to infection from contaminated milk in their childhood.

Clinical tuberculosis is infrequent in Britain. Amongst the indigenous population the reservoir is predominantly in the elderly, particularly old men. It is, however, constantly being reinforced by younger immigrants who bring their infection in with them.[13]

The Registrar-General's Statistical Review for England and Wales for 1973 reveals that 964 men and 388 women died of the disease. In the first 35 years of life the mortality rate was very low in both sexes. After this age there was a much greater mortality. The peak death rate in both sexes occurred in the age-group 45 to 75 years, and it was three times greater in men than in women. Nearly all fatal tuberculosis nowadays is pulmonary, but amongst the less common extrapulmonary types of disease the sex incidence is almost equal. It is probable that some tuberculosis in the elderly is due to the reactivation of foci acquired at an earlier period of life, but the breakdown in immunity in old age as well as poor social conditions make reinfection an important alternative.

The Eradication of Tuberculosis

There are three main principles:

A general improvement in social conditions. The importance of overcrowding and malnutrition in the spread of tuberculosis has already been indicated.

The treatment of patients. There are no 'carriers' of tuberculosis comparable with the nasal carriers of staphylococci or the faecal carriers of typhoid bacilli. The source of infection is always an 'open' case, and the sputum, sometimes after drying into dust in the atmosphere, is inhaled by another person. It is therefore important to diagnose the disease as early as possible. Mass radiography is very useful especially in screening large populations. Patients must be isolated and treated as expeditiously as possible.

Streptomycin, para-aminosalicylic acid (PAS), and isonicotinic acid hydrazide (isoniazid) have been the main antituberculous drugs, but they are being supplemented or replaced by other agents, e.g. ethambutol (to replace PAS) and rifampicin. If possible the patient should not be allowed back into the community until the sputum is negative for tubercle bacilli on repeated examinations.

Prophylactic active immunisation. The strain commonly used is the BCG (*Bacille-Calmette-Guérin*), a bovine strain attenuated by prolonged culture on a bile-potato medium.* It is administered intradermally and it produces a mild localised infection. A successful result is indicated by a conversion in the tuberculin reaction. This is, of course, purely an indication of hypersensitivity, but it is assumed that there is also a concomitant acquisition of immunity.

There is now a general consensus of opinion that BCG vaccination is a valuable method of establishing immunity to tuberculosis and that it should be offered to all tuberculin-negative reactors. The reports of the Medical Research Council Clinical Trials Committee indicate that in Britain the incidence of tuberculosis in vaccinated children is a fifth that in tuberculin-negative controls.[14,15] Those whose profession brings them in contact with the disease and who are tuberculin negative should be immunised without delay. The value of BCG vaccination in other communities is still being assessed.[14,15] The question of weak tuberculin reactors is arousing interest; as already noted, many of these may have been infected with avian and other mycobacteria. These infections may conceivably add their quota to the patient's

*Vole bacillus is an effective alternative. Earlier batches occasionally produced severe local lesions, and the vaccine has never been as popular as BCG.[14]

immunity to tuberculosis, but it seems to be quite in order to offer them BCG in addition. Data are needed about the relative efficiency of BCG and other mycobacterial infections as immunisers against tuberculosis. In strongly tuberculin-positive reactors BCG is both unnecessary and potentially harmful.

The complications of BCG are a tuberculous abscess at the site of inoculation, sometimes with associated axillary lymphadenitis severe enough to require chemotherapy, and very rarely a generalised infection with progressive pulmonary lesions.[16]

SYPHILIS[17]

The causative organism *Treponema pallidum* is a delicate spiral filament, or spirochaete, about 10 μm long. It cannot be stained by the usual techniques, and is demonstrable in the exudate of chancres and secondary lesions by means of dark-ground illumination and fluorescent antibody techniques (Fig. 1.1, p. 2). In histological sections it is stained by special silver impregnation methods (Fig. 1.5, p. 5).

The organism has never been cultured artificially even in fertile eggs or tissue-culture systems, nor does animal inoculation play any part in the diagnosis of the disease. In fact, rabbits develop acute orchitis after the intratesticular inoculation of the organisms. This method is used to obtain a supply of spirochaetes for such procedures as the *Treponema pallidum immobilisation (TPI) test* and the *fluorescent treponemal antibody (FTA) test*.

During the course of infection the patient develops immunoglobulins of great importance. Two groups are recognised:

The Wassermann antibody. This antibody, formerly called reagin, was described by Wassermann as a complement-fixing antibody to an antigen present in extracts of human syphilitic liver. Subsequently an alcoholic extract of normal tissue was found to contain a similar antigen, and nowadays an extract of beef heart, to which cholesterol and lecithin have been added, is used. It is called *cardiolipin*, and the active component has been identified as *diphosphatidylglycerol*. This antigen is used in the *standard tests for syphilis*, namely the *Wassermann complement-fixation test* and the *flocculation tests*, of which the *Kahn* and the *Venereal Disease Research Laboratory (VDRL) tests* are the most widely used. They are more sensitive than the complement-fixation test but are no more specific.

Whether the Wassermann antibody is induced in the patient by an antigen of the treponeme or of damaged host tissue is not clear. The antigen is certainly not specific for *Tr. pallidum*, since not only are the serological tests positive in other treponemal diseases, such as yaws, pinta, and bejel, but false positive reactions may occur in non-treponemal diseases, notably malaria, leprosy, infectious mononucleosis, mycoplasmal pneumonia, trypanosomiasis, systemic lupus erythematosus, and autoimmune haemolytic anaemia, as well as occasionally in pregnant women, and in over 25 per cent of normal subjects after vaccination with vaccinia. In one epidemic of Coxsackie B infection there was a remarkably high incidence of positive reactions.[18] The occurrence of these false positive reactions suggests that tissue damage by a variety of agents can stimulate the formation of Wassermann antibodies. This correlates well with the observation in experimental syphilis in rabbits that the standard tests tend to be positive during active phases of the disease but negative during the latent periods, when presumably tissue damage is at a minimum. In human disease the flocculation tests are often positive even when the disease appears inactive.

Treponemal antibody. The second group of antibodies which is formed reacts with treponemal protein. Some antibody activity is directed against protein common to several treponemes (group protein), whereas others are more specific. The following tests are employed.

Reiter Protein Complement-Fixation (RPCF) Test. The Reiter strain, unlike the pathogenic *Tr. pallidum* strains, can be cultured artificially under strictly anaerobic conditions, and so the antigen can be obtained quite easily. The RPCF test is more specific than the standard tests for syphilis and therefore gives fewer false positive results.

Treponema Pallidum Immobilisation (TPI) Test. This employs the ability of antibody to immobilise *Tr. pallidum* in the presence of complement. A concentrated suspension of organisms is incubated for 18 hours with guinea-pig complement and serum, and motility is assessed under dark-ground illumination. Positive sera can be adsorbed with cardiolipin without diminution of the titre, thereby showing that the antibody detected is not the same as the Wassermann antibody. The TPI test becomes positive a little later in the disease than do the standard tests, but it remains positive for the remainder of the patient's life with the exception of some cases in which the disease has been successfully treated early in its course. Being more specific, it is useful when there is a suspected false serology. Unfortunately the test is technically difficult to perform and needs a supply of pathogenic organisms.

Fluorescent Treponemal Antibody (FTA) Test. Specific antibody adheres to *Tr. pallidum*, and can be detected by applying fluorescein-labelled anti-human γ-globulin. Two antibodies are involved; one is group specific, reacting with *Tr. pallidum* and other treponemes, but the other is specific for *Tr. pallidum*. Both are formed in syphilis. The group-specific antibody can be absorbed by Reiter treponemes, and the test (FTA-ABS) is as sensitive and specific as the TPI. These two specific tests are performed only when the standard tests are equivocal, or when the results do not correlate with the clinical features of the case. No test is absolutely reliable, and none can distinguish between syphilis and yaws, which is caused by *Tr. pertenue*, morphologically identical with *Tr. pallidum*.

Treponemal Passive Haemagglutination (TPHA) Test. Formolised, tanned sheep red cells sensitised with material from disrupted *Tr. pallidum* are used as the antigen. This is a simple, effective technique, and is an alternative to the FTA-ABS and TPI tests.

The disease. The infection is almost always acquired venereally, though on rare occasions the primary lesion may occur on the lips, tongue, or even on a finger. Unlike the tubercle bacillus, *Tr. pallidum* is very rapidly destroyed both in water and by drying. Intimate direct contact is therefore necessary for infection to occur. The spirochaete is one of the most invasive organisms known. Once it penetrates the surface integument, it spreads along the lymphatics to the regional lymph nodes, and finally reaches the blood stream within a matter of hours. There is therefore systemic dissemination long before any local manifestation appears.

Syphilis may also be transmitted by blood transfused from an infected donor. The organisms are destroyed after storage of the blood in a refrigerator for about 4 days, but, of course, in practice a syphilitic donor should not be accepted.

The disease is divisible into three stages with a latent period between each of them.

Primary syphilis. The typical lesion of primary syphilis is the *chancre*, which usually appears 2 to 4 weeks after exposure to infection. It is an indurated papule which breaks down to form an ulcer. It is characteristically painless, and is accompanied by a considerable regional lymphadenitis which is also painless.

The histological appearance is non-specific, consisting merely of a dense infiltration of lymphocytes, plasma cells, and a few macrophages in the dermis. There is a tendency towards a perivascular accumulation or 'cuffing' of these cells, but this is not peculiar to syphilis. Even without treatment the chancre gradually heals, and it leaves little scarring.

The painlessness of the chancre (and the later lesions of syphilis) is best explained in terms of its cellular, or proliferative, nature. There is little fluid exudate, which contains pain-producing substances in acute inflammation. The digital chancre is painful—it is called a syphilitic whitlow—due to raised tissue tension in a confined space.

The fact that the spirochaetes become disseminated in the blood stream long before there is any local lesion suggests that hypersensitivity plays an important part in the process. The chancre is not comparable with a boil, for it is not a local inflammatory reaction tending to limit the infection. A possible explanation is that sensitising antibodies are first formed in the cells at the site of entry and in the regional lymph nodes. During the incubation period the spirochaetes multiply in the RE system, and when liberated react with the sensitised tissue. This would explain the chancre and the lymphadenopathy quite well.

At a later stage the other tissues of the body become sensitised, and then the generalised lesions of secondary syphilis become manifest.

Diagnosis. The laboratory diagnosis depends on demonstrating spirochaetes in the exudate from the chancre by darkground illumination.

One to 3 weeks after the appearance of the chancre both Wassermann and antitreponemal antibodies first appear in the blood. Blood serology should never be neglected in practice.

Secondary syphilis. Within 2 to 3 months after exposure the disease becomes clinically generalised. When syphilis was first introduced into Europe, this stage was severe enough to warrant the name 'the great pox'. Nowadays it is much milder, and is characterised by the development of a skin eruption. This is widespread, symmetrical, usually not pruritic, and commonly present on the face, palms, and soles. The lesions are generally erythematous papules, but may be of any type except vesicular or bullous. Mucosal lesions in the form of condylomata lata, mucous patches, and snail-track ulcers are less frequent. The muco-cutaneous lesions may be accompanied by constitutional symptoms which include low-grade fever, myalgia, arthralgia, moderate anaemia, iridocyclitis, and a generalised painless lymphadenopathy. Histologically the secondary lesions show an infiltration by lymphocytes, plasma cells, and macrophages. They resolve spontaneously and do not form scars. This is the phase of maximal infectivity; spirochaetes ooze out of condylomata and mucous patches.

Diagnosis. The standard serological tests are always positive in overt secondary syphilis. If a negative result is reported in the face of strong clinical indications of syphilis, *the prozone phenomenon should be suspected* (p. 145) and the test repeated with suitable dilutions, so that the titre of antibody can be measured. The TPI test may be negative during the early stages of secondary syphilis, but in practice it is rarely necessary to perform it at this stage.

Organisms can be demonstrated with ease in the exudates from mucosal lesions and condylomata. They can also be shown in histological sections of primary and secondary lesions using silver impregnation methods. But in practice it is unnecessary to demonstrate the spirochaete in secondary syphilis.

The occurrence of the *Jarisch-Herxheimer reaction*[19] is confirmatory evidence of a correct diagnosis of syphilis. It consists of a transient episode of fever and malaise, with an accentuation of the skin eruption within 12 hours of the commencement of treatment—generally an injection of penicillin. The reaction is presumed to be due to the massive release of bacterial antigens as the organisms are killed.

Tertiary syphilis. Local destructive lesions of a truly chronic inflammatory nature may begin to appear 2 to 3 years after exposure, and may continue to erupt sporadically for at least 20 years. The lesions are presumably due to marked hypersensitivity, since spirochaetes are few and the reaction is excessive. Two forms of lesions occur: localised gummata and diffuse inflammatory lesions characterised by parenchymatous destruction.

Localised gummata. The *gumma* is the classical lesion of tertiary syphilis (Fig. 20.10). It is usually solitary, and consists of a large area of coagulative necrosis very similar in appearance to caseation, except that the tissue destruction is usually not quite so complete. Details of architecture can therefore still be faintly distinguished amid the debris. It is surrounded by an extensive zone of lymphocytes, plasma cells, and macrophages. Giant cells, sometimes in follicles with epithelioid cells, may be present, but they are much less frequent than in tuberculosis. Proliferating fibroblasts are plentiful, and much reparative fibrous tissue is laid down. The arteries in the vicinity show marked endarteritis obliterans.

Gummata are particularly liable to occur in the liver, testes (Fig. 20.11), subcutaneous tissues, and in bones, notably the tibia, ulna, clavicle, calvaria of skull, and the nasal and palatal bones. The destruction produced by gummata is exemplified by the perforated palate and the saddle-shaped nasal deformity so characteristic of tertiary syphilis. In the liver gummata are often multiple, and as they heal by fibrosis, a scarred, deformed *hepar lobatum* is left.

The necrosis in a gumma is probably due primarily to hypersensitivity to products of the spirochaete. The ischaemia engendered by the endarteritis obliterans no doubt augments the necrosis.

Spirochaetes are demonstrated only with great difficulty in the wall of a gumma. Tertiary syphilis is much less infectious than are the two preceding stages of the disease.

Figure 20.10
Gumma of brain. The top part of the figure consists of a large area of coagulative necrosis lightly infiltrated by small round cells. In the lower part there is a much heavier infiltration of lymphocytes, plasma cells, and a few macrophages in fibrous tissue. A foreign-body giant cell is present in the middle of the figure at the junction of the necrotic area and the fibrous tissue. × 100.

Figure 20.11
Gumma of testis. The testis is enlarged, and its substance is replaced by a diffuse area of gummatous necrosis, the edges of which are irregular. (EM 6.1, *Reproduced by permission of the President and Council of the R.C.S. Eng.*)

Diffuse lesions of tertiary syphilis. The really baneful effects of tertiary syphilis fall on the cardiovascular and nervous systems. In the former it is the ascending part of the thoracic aorta which usually suffers first. An infiltration of lymphocytes and plasma cells accumulates around the vasa vasorum of the tunica adventitia, and soon spreads inwards into the tunica media, where it destroys much of the elastic tissue on which the integrity of the aorta depends. Occasionally there is frank gummatous necrosis in the area of cellular infiltration, but usually the tissue of the aorta appears to disintegrate in front of the advancing cells.

The *syphilitic aortitis* that results weakens the media sufficiently to produce aneurysmal dilatation. Sometimes the disease extends to the aortic ring, which dilates and leads to aortic regurgitation. If the ostia of the coronary arteries are occluded at the same time there is also severe myocardial ischaemia. It is hardly surprising that cardiovascular complications are responsible for most of the deaths directly attributable to syphilis. The abdominal aorta is rarely attacked in syphilis.

Cerebral syphilis may be *meningovascular* or *parenchymatous*. In the former type there is focal meningitis and vascular occlusion due to endarteritis obliterans of the small vessels. Isolated cranial nerve palsies are quite common.

Parenchymatous neurosyphilis comprises *general paralysis of the insane* and *tabes dorsalis*. General paralysis of the insane is a chronic syphilitic meningo-encephalitis, and spirochaetes can be demonstrated in the frontal lobes, which are particularly severely affected. Tabes dorsalis is a degenerative condition of the posterior columns of the spinal cord and the posterior roots of the spinal nerves. There is severe demyelination of the posterior columns which is followed by gliosis.

The bones are also frequently affected by a diffuse type of syphilitic inflammation. There may be widespread periostitis involving especially the tibia and the calvaria of the skull. The irregular thickening that is very apparent clinically is due to the laying down of new bone. This gives rise to the classical *sabre tibia*. Unlike the tibial deformity of rickets or Paget's disease, where there is true bowing due to softening of the bone, the lesion of syphilis is a mere 'pseudo-bowing' due entirely to the irregular deposition of new periosteal bone. In the skull a worm-eaten appearance is produced by the concurrent effects of gummatous destruction and new-bone formation.

Diagnosis. The diagnosis of tertiary syphilis is primarily clinical, but it may often be substantiated by serological examination of the blood and cerebrospinal fluid. In most cases of overt syphilis this examination is strongly positive, and in neurosyphilis the cerebrospinal fluid is generally more helpful than the blood. In at least 20 per cent of cases of tabes dorsalis serological examination both of blood and cerebrospinal fluid is negative. An additional aid is the presence of spirochaetes in histological sections of gummata, but as already mentioned these are very scanty.

Congenital syphilis. An untreated syphilitic mother is very liable to transmit the disease to her fetus during the first 2 years of infection, particularly after the fourth month of pregnancy, when the Langhans layer of the placenta disappears. Abortion may result, or else a severely affected infant may die soon after birth. There is marked syphilitic inflammation of most of the organs, notably the liver, pancreas, lungs, and bony epiphyses. A characteristic lesion is *pericellular fibrosis of the liver*, in which innumerable groups of liver cells are isolated and surrounded by syphilitic granulation tissue.

More frequently the child survives, and it may then show early stigmata of infection like skin eruptions, snuffles, epiphysitis of the elbows, and marasmus. Sometimes stigmata appear only in later childhood. The notched, peg-shaped Hutchinson's incisor teeth due to syphilitic infection of the tooth germs during fetal life are well-known examples of this type of lesion, as are also interstitial keratitis, tibial periostitis (sabre tibia), and eighth-nerve deafness.

The histological appearances of these various lesions are all very similar, being combinations of the heavy cellular infiltration of secondary syphilis together with the gummatous destruction typical of the tertiary phase. In fact, congenital syphilis may be regarded as a combined secondary and tertiary syphilis occurring in a child whose primary lesion was placental.

Diagnosis. This depends on serological examination of the blood of the child and its parents. In the more florid lesions spirochaetes abound, and are demonstrated with ease.

Immunity to syphilis.[20] There appears to be a resistance to further infection while treponemes are present in the tissues. Two chancres may develop if the second infection precedes the appearance of the primary lesion, but once this has appeared, further exposure to infection fails to produce another chancre. There is no doubt that asymptomatic infection may coexist with the presence of treponemes in the tissues; these can produce syphilis when transferred to other individuals. There is no spontaneous cure of the disease, and therapeutic cure occurs only in the early stages.

In some patients with good immunity the infection remains latent for long periods, its existence being indicated by the specific serological tests. In the tertiary stage there is good

evidence that treponemes are sequestered in the tissues,[21] often remaining latent, but always liable to flare up in new lesions. In a case of tabes it has been possible to demonstrate treponemes in the anterior chamber of the eye, the cerebrospinal fluid, and the liver despite completely negative serology.[22] The immunity is presumably cell mediated, but macrophages are not as prominent as they are in tuberculosis. There is little evidence that immunoglobulins are important. The maximum immunity develops in the later stages—after 2 years in the human being—and it is never absolute.

Incidence of syphilis. After a prolonged period of decline, the incidence of syphilis has recently risen in many parts of the world. Due to the great therapeutic value of penicillin, syphilis accounted for the death of only 131 people in 1973 in England and Wales, the Registrar-General's Statistical Review revealing that 74 men and 57 women died of the disease. Of these 65 per cent succumbed to cardiovascular syphilis and 29 per cent to neurosyphilis.

ACTINOMYCOSIS[23, 24]

Actinomycosis is characterised by chronic, loculated foci of suppuration occurring particularly in the region of the lower jaw. It is seen in cattle, dogs and cats, and human beings. The causal organisms are *Actinomyces bovis* (in cattle), *Actinomyces baudeti* (in dogs and cats), and *Actinomyces israeli* (in human beings).

The disease in cattle is called *lumpy jaw*. It is often confused with another chronic suppurative condition of cattle called *woody tongue*. This is caused by a completely different organism, *Actinobacillus lignieresi*, a small Gram-negative bacillus. Actinobacillosis has many points of similarity to actinomycosis, but it does not usually invade bones, and it has a tendency to spread along the lymphatics.

Bacteriology. Actinomyces organisms are Gram-positive, branching filaments which show a tendency to break up into bacillary and twig-like forms. The filaments are much thinner than those of the fungi, and the organism is now classified as a bacterium of the family *Actinomycetaceae*, which also includes the genus *Nocardia* (Table 20.1). In animal tissues the organisms grow in colonies consisting of a densely felted mass of filaments* matted together in an amorphous matrix. Such a colony appears in the pus of actinomycotic lesions in the form of a small granule which is greyish-yellow in colour. This is

*Often called a *mycelium*, although this term is usually restricted to fungal growth.

TABLE 20.1 Members of the order Actinomycetales

Order	Family	Genus
Actinomycetales	*Mycobacteriaceae*—no mycelium, acid fast	*Mycobacterium.*
	Actinomycetaceae—branching filaments which break up into bacillary elements	*Actinomyces*—not acid-fast *Nocardia*—somewhat acid-fast
	Streptomycetaceae—mycelium with filaments which do not break up readily. Not acid-fast	*Streptomyces*—spores formed in chains

called a *sulphur granule*. In artificial culture this colonial tendency is less pronounced, and the individual filaments remain more separate.

A colony formed in the tissues tends to be surrounded by a radially projecting fringe of club-shaped excrescences (*clubs*). These 'clubs' are Gram-negative, and are not formed in artificial culture. It is believed that they are produced as the result of deposition on to the colony of lipid material derived from the host's tissues. This radiating fringe around the colony gave rise to the alternative name *ray fungus* which has been loosely applied to *Actinomyces* organisms.

The pathogenic actinomyces organisms are anaerobic or, at the most, micro-aerophilic. They grow best at 37°C on ordinary media like blood agar or glucose agar, but a few days may elapse before colonies appear. Aerobic actinomyces organisms, e.g. *Actinomyces graminis*, may sometimes also be found in actinomycotic lesions, but they are apparently secondary contaminants.

Diagnosis. The diagnosis of actinomycosis depends on finding sulphur granules in the copious pus that exudes from the abscess sinuses. These are then crushed between two slides and stained, and also cultured anaerobically on blood agar (see Appendix 3). The demonstration of antibodies plays no part in the diagnosis.

Pathogenesis. *Actinomyces israeli* is a normal commensal of the mouth, and it is found especially in the tonsils and carious teeth. Actinomycosis is an endogenous infection, and is not transmitted by contaminated pieces of straw and grass that have been sucked by cattle. It can follow a dental extraction, though considering the widespread distribution of the organism, the disease is surprisingly infrequent. It is not understood what local conditions must be fulfilled before the organism can invade the tissues of the gingiva and set up a progressive inflammatory reaction. It has been known to produce infection in a hand wound caused by hitting an assailant in the teeth ('punch actinomycosis').

The actinomycotic lesion starts as an acute suppurative inflammation, which then persists and progresses to intractable chronicity. As the organisms spread by direct continuity, large numbers of abscesses are produced. Some of these fuse together, but there is a tendency for individual foci of suppuration to remain discrete owing to the persistence of fibrous septa. This produces a characteristically loculated appearance, which is seen most typically in actinomycotic lesions of the liver (*honeycomb liver*).

Histologically the abscess cavities are crowded with pus cells which surround actinomycotic colonies (sulphur granules— Fig. 20.12). The narrow septa between the abscesses are composed of fibrous tissue which is heavily infiltrated by polymorphs with small numbers of lymphocytes, macrophages, and plasma cells. These fibrous septa are not merely the remains of destroyed parenchyma; they represent attempts at repair, and the entire lesion is surrounded by a dense zone of fibrous tissue.

Spread of infection. About 65 per cent of clinical actinomycosis starts in the cervico-facial area, 20 per cent is primarily ileo-caecal, and the remainder commences in the lungs.

The main mode of spread of the disease is by direct contact. Whereas other organisms move in the tissue spaces along

Figure 20.12
Actinomycotic pus. The section shows a dense infiltration of pus cells, in the centre of which there is a colony of actinomyces (sulphur granule). The peripheral clubs are evident as areas of darker staining. × 100.

preformed planes, the actinomyces extend slowly and inexorably ever onwards. In cervico-facial actinomycosis there is direct spread to the adjacent muscles and bones, so that eventually the spinal column and skull are invaded. There is also progressive cutaneous involvement, and the abscesses discharge through multiple sinuses. In the pus that exudes numerous pin's-head sized, yellowish or greyish sulphur granules are discharged. The appearance of a diffuse, indurated, painless area of suppuration in the region of the neck, discharging to the exterior through multiple sinuses, is characteristic of actinomycosis.

Similarly ileo-caecal actinomycosis spreads through the anterior abdominal wall with the development of discharging sinuses, and pulmonary actinomycosis erupts through the wall of the chest. When tuberculosis implicates a serous sac, there is usually a widespread involvement; actinomycosis, on the other hand, spreads directly from visceral to parietal layers and then invades the body wall and discharges externally. In abdominal actinomycosis fistulae develop between loops of bowel as in Crohn's disease.

Lymphatic spread does not occur in actinomycosis; perhaps the filaments are too large to be accommodated in the lymphatic channels. Any regional lymphadenitis that may occur is attributable to secondary bacterial infection.

Blood-borne spread, on the other hand, is important, and is typified by the spread of ileo-caecal disease by the portal vein to the liver, where the loculated actinomycotic abscesses of *honeycomb liver* are produced. Likewise pulmonary actinomycosis may disseminate *via* the systemic circulation and produce lesions in the kidneys, brain, bones, and other parts. Occasionally a honeycomb liver implicates the lung above it by direct spread of infection through the diaphragm.

Treatment. Actinomyces organisms are very sensitive to the commonly-used antibiotics, especially penicillin and lincomycin. The prognosis of cervico-facial disease is very good, but the abdominal and pulmonary infections are sometimes fatal.

Incidence. This is a rare disease in Britain. The Registrar-General's Review for 1973 has recorded no deaths.

Mycetoma[25,26]

The term mycetoma is used to denote a localised infection of the subcutaneous tissues, usually of the hands or feet, that follows the introduction of the specific causal organisms from the exterior. The organisms responsible fall into two groups, one bacterial and the other fungal.

Bacterial mycetoma. Nocardia and streptomyces of the order *Actinomycetales* are involved. Nocardia are aerobic, Gram-positive, and often acid-fast. They grow as branching filaments which tend to break up into bacillary forms. *N. asteroides* and *N. brasiliensis* are the best known. The streptomyces, e.g. *S. madurae*, grow as stable filaments, and are on the borderline of the bacteria and fungi.

Fungal mycetoma (maduromycosis). At least 13 species of fungi have been identified as causes of mycetoma. These include *Madurella mycetomi*, *Allescheria boydii*, and *Aspergillus nidulans*.

The habitat of all these organisms is the soil, and they may be introduced into the skin and subcutaneous tissues as the result of trivial injury. The condition occurs mainly in tropical countries, and is endemic in India. The foot is most commonly involved (*Madura foot*).

The pathogenesis and spread of the disease is similar to that described in actinomycosis except that blood-spread does not occur. There is widespread destruction of tissue and the appearance of multiple sinuses through which coloured granules are discharged. These are large and often black in colour. If the disease is left unchecked, the patient eventually dies of cachexia.

Sulphonamides are useful in *Nocardia* infections but are of no value against fungi. The affected part may have to be amputated (Fig. 20.13).

Figure 20.13
Mycetoma of hand. The hand has been sectioned to show the widespread ramifications of the infection in the deeper tissues, which have been destroyed by masses of black material. (S 52.2, *Reproduced by permission of the President and Council of the R.C.S. Eng.*)

GENERAL REFERNCES

See Chapter 17, page 228.

REFERENCES

1. Leading Article (1972) Mechanisms of reaction in leprosy. *Lancet*, **2**, 580.
2. EDWARDS, L. B. (1963) Current status of the tuberculin test. *Annals of the New York Academy of Sciences*, **106**, 32.
3. CONNOR, D. H. & LUNN, H. F. (1966) Buruli ulceration. *Archives of Pathology*, **81**, 183.
4. BARKER, D. J. P. (1974) Mycobacterial skin ulcers. *British Journal of Dermatology*, **91**, 473.
5. PHILPOTT, J. A. *et al.* (1963) Swimming pool granuloma. *Archives of Dermatology and Syphilology*, **88**, 158.
6. Leading Article (1970) Hazard from the home aquarium. *British Medical Journal*, **2**, 438.
7. HARRISON, B. D. W., TUGWELL, P. & FAWCETT, I. W. (1975) Tuberculin reaction in adult Nigerians with sputum-positive pulmonary tuberculosis. *Lancet*, **1**, 421.

8. Leading Article (1969) Miliary tuberculosis in the elderly. *British Medical Journal*, **2**, 265.
9. JOHNSTON, R. N., RITCHIE, R. T. & MURRAY, I. H. F. (1963) Declining tuberculin sensitivity with advancing age. *British Medical Journal*, **2**, 720.
10. Leading Article (1969) B.C.G. and the tuberculin test. *Lancet*, **1**, 192.
11. WEISS, D. W. & WELLS, A. Q. (1960) Vaccination against tuberculosis with nonliving vaccines 3. Vaccination of guinea-pigs with fractions of phenol-killed tubercle bacilli. *American Review of Respiratory Diseases*, **82**, 339.
12. GALBRAITH, N. S. *et al.* (1972) Interpretation of positive reactions to Heaf tuberculin test in London schoolchildren. *British Medical Journal*, **1**, 647.
13. SPRINGETT, V. H. (1972) Tuberculosis—epidemiology in England and Wales. *British Medical Journal*, **1**, 422.
14. Leading Article (1972) BCG vaccination. *Lancet*, **2**, 168.
15. Leading Article (1975) BCG vaccination. *British Medical Journal*, **4**, 603.
16. MARKS, J. *et al.* (1971) Pulmonary tuberculosis due to B.C.G. *British Medical Journal*, **3**, 229.
17. Sparling, P. F. (1971) Diagnosis and treatment of syphilis. *New England Journal of Medicine*, **284**, 642.
18. Leading Article (1971) An epidemic of false positives. *Lancet*, **1**, 1170.
19. Leading Article (1977) The Jarisch-Herxheimer reaction. *Lancet*, **1**, 340.
20. Leading Article (1974) Vaccines for syphilis. *British Medical Journal*, **2**, 346.
21. Leading Article (1968) Persistence of treponemes after treatment of syphilis. *Lancet*, **2**, 718.
22. SMITH, J. L. & ISRAEL, C. W. (1967) The presence of spirochetes in late seronegative syphilis. *Journal of the American Medical Association*, **199**, 980.
23. COPE, V. Z. (1938) *Actinomycosis.* London: Oxford University Press.
24. BRONNER, M. & BRONNER, M. (1971) *Actinomycosis*, 2nd edn, pp. 355. Bristol: John Wright.
25. OCHOA, A. G. (1962) Mycetoma caused by *Nocardia braziliensis*; with a note on the isolation of the causative organism from soil. *Laboratory Investigation*, **11**, 1118.
26. MACKINNON, I. E. (1962) Mycetomas as opportunistic wound infections. *Laboratory Investigation*, **11**, 1124.

Chapter 21. Some Interesting Chronic Inflammatory Conditions

In the previous chapter the inflammatory reactions associated with tuberculosis, syphilis, and actinomycosis were studied, and three responses were described:

The tuberculoid reaction, which consists of an epithelioid cell–giant cell follicle sometimes with central caseation and surrounded by lymphocytes. It is seen in tuberculosis.

The small round cell reaction, which consists of a diffuse lymphocyte–plasma cell infiltration. It is seen in syphilis.

The pyogenic reaction, which consists of a loculated abscess crowded with polymorphs. It is seen in actinomycosis.

It was noted that none of these reactions was strictly specific. Indeed, they can all be produced by different types of foreign bodies introduced into the tissues, though admittedly caseation is peculiar to tuberculosis and a few uncommon fungal diseases. In the conditions about to be described these reactions are often reproduced and sometimes combined, while on other occasions there may be very little tissue reaction at all. The theme of this discussion is the versatile response of the body to noxious agents of various types.

SOME DEEP-SEATED FUNGAL INFECTIONS

Fungi.[1] In the past fungi were regarded as plants without roots, stems, and leaves, and being incapable of photosynthesis because they lack chlorophyll. They are now regarded as neither plants nor animals, but are placed in a separate group. For practical purposes four varieties can be recognised:

Moulds, which grow as long filaments (*hyphae*), and which branch and interlace to form a meshwork, or *mycelium*.

Yeasts, which grow by budding only.

Yeast-like fungi, which grow partly as yeasts and partly as long filamentous forms called pseudohyphae.

Dimorphic fungi, which can grow either as hyphae or as yeasts depending on the cultural conditions.

Infection of the skin by fungi is very common, and is called ringworm. This will not be described. The first part of this chapter will deal with some fungi that can invade widely and produce a wide range of tissue responses.

The first three infections considered are cryptococcosis, histoplasmosis, and coccidioidomycosis. They are all caused by organisms present in the soil, which when inhaled may produce a pulmonary lesion. It usually heals, but occasionally there is systemic spread to the viscera and the outcome is often fatal. The parallel between these diseases and tuberculosis is very close; many of the histological features of tuberculosis are encountered in the deep-seated mycoses. Candidiasis is also described because the systemic variety is becoming increasingly common.

CRYPTOCOCCOSIS[2–4]

Cryptococcus neoformans (formerly called *Torula histolytica*) is a yeast. It is a spherical cell, 5 to 20 μm in diameter, Gram-positive, and surrounded by a thick gelatinous capsule which stains for mucus using the PAS or mucicarmine methods. This characteristic makes it easily demonstrable in histological sections.

The organism has been found in soil, in the droppings of birds, particularly pigeons, and also on fruit and in milk. It causes sporadic disease in horses, cattle, and pigs, and is characteristically pathogenic to mice. In animals and human beings it is rarely isolated except from overt lesions. The human disease has a world-wide distribution and occurs at all ages. The sporadic cases that occur are probably due to inhalation of organisms from the soil. The condition is not infectious.

The primary lesion is pulmonary, usually a single subpleural mass called a 'toruloma'. It is very chronic and is usually symptomless; it occasionally undergoes cavitation. Spread to the hilar nodes is very uncommon. Healing by fibrosis without much calcification may occur, but sometimes the disease is disseminated by the blood stream. The central nervous system is then usually invaded, and more rarely lesions may be encountered in the skin, bones, and lymph nodes.

The leptomeninges of the base of the brain are usually first affected. There is widening of the infiltrated subarachnoid space, and the colonies of cryptococci may proliferate so rapidly as to rupture through the pia arachnoid into the brain substance. The exudate is gelatinous in consistency, and there may be cystic spaces in the underlying brain, filled with aggregations of the organisms and their mucoid capsules. Clinically the disease resembles tuberculous meningitis, and the effects are due to a raised intracranial pressure. Untreated cases always die.

The tissue reactions to the cryptococcus.[4] Most commonly there is no reaction at all. Masses of organisms resembling a pure culture are found in the subarachnoid spaces, and there is no inflammatory or glial reaction (Fig. 21.1).

Occasionally there is an accumulation of giant cells both of foreign body and Langhans type, containing many phagocytosed organisms.

Sometimes a collection of organisms is surrounded by a diffuse small round cell infiltration composed of lymphocytes and plasma cells. This is common in pulmonary torulomata.

An epithelioid-cell infiltration with Langhans giant cells and a surrounding zone of small round cells is occasionally seen in cryptococcosis. This tuberculoid reaction is diffuse, and lacks the circumscribed follicular pattern typical of tuberculosis. Caseation is uncommon except in conglomerate torulomata. The cryptococci are present in the inflammatory tissue.

Figure 21.1
Cryptococcosis. In the meninges overlying the brain there is a gelatinous inflammatory exudate in which the conspicuous yeast *Cryptococcus neoformans* abounds. As there are virtually no inflammatory cells in this exudate, the nucleate structures are nearly all cryptococci. × 170.

Figure 21.2
Histoplasmosis. This is a section of spleen from a patient who died of generalised histoplasmosis. There is a profuse infiltration of macrophages which are crammed with *Histoplasma capsulatum* organisms. × 400.

In addition to producing primary disease, cryptococci are important causes of opportunistic infection in cases of T-lymphocyte deficiency (see p. 170). There may be a generalised infection or else the disease may remain localised to a few lymph nodes.

The diagnosis of cryptococcosis depends on isolating and culturing the organisms from the sputum or cerebrospinal fluid. Serological methods are not helpful diagnostically, but may be of some value in epidemiological surveys. Skin testing is of no value.

HISTOPLASMOSIS[5]

The causative organism *Histoplasma capsulatum* is a dimorphic fungus which exists in yeast form when cultured at 37°C and in animal tissues and in mycelial form in saprophytic life. It is a small, oval yeast cell, 1 to 4 μm in diameter, surrounded by a thin capsule which consists of mucoid material. Like the cryptococcus it is found in the soil, and it produces disease in various animals, e.g. dogs, rodents, cattle, and horses.

The disease has a world-wide distribution, and is endemic in the Mississippi Valley area of the USA. A special African type of histoplasmosis due to *Histoplasma duboisi* has been described.[6] This organism is distinctly larger than *Histoplasma capsulatum*.

Infection may occur at any age, but children are particularly susceptible. The inhalation of contaminated soil dust appears to be the mode of infection. The disease is not infectious.

The primary lesion is pulmonary. There is a transient infection with hilar-node involvement, usually followed by rapid healing with residual calcification; only occasionally does a chronic lesion with cavitation persist. Rarely the disease becomes disseminated by the blood stream, and the organisms are carried to various viscera. Systemic histoplasmosis is a fatal disease, and it resembles leishmaniasis, a protozoal disease that is also spread throughout the body by macrophages. The organs most heavily involved are the spleen, liver, lymph nodes, and bone marrow, and therefore severe anaemia and leucopenia are prominent features. Mucosal ulceration of the mouth and gut is a common manifestation. Adrenal destruction may lead to Addison's disease.

The tissue reaction typical of histoplasmosis[4] is intracellular parasitisation within macrophages (Fig. 21.2). In the African variety giant cells may also be formed. In the liver and spleen there are usually large areas of necrosis surrounded by the parasitised macrophages.

A tuberculoid reaction is rather uncommon, but occasionally affected lymph nodes may contain follicles reminiscent of sarcoidosis. Caseation is most uncommon except in solitary lung lesions. Like cryptococcosis, histoplasmosis may occur as an opportunistic infection where there is T-lymphocyte deficiency.

The diagnosis is made by finding the yeast-form of the organism as an intracellular parasite. Smears made from the blood, bone marrow, sputum, and scrapings from mucosal lesions may also show parasitised macrophages. The organism is easily cultured.

Serological methods help to confirm the diagnosis. Within a few weeks complement-fixing antibodies appear in the serum, and their titre is an indication of the activity of infection. At the same time hypersensitivity to the antigens of the organism develops, and this forms the basis of the *histoplasmin* skin test. A positive result indicates past or present infection.

COCCIDIOIDOMYCOSIS[7, 8]

The causative organism *Coccidioides immitis* is a dimorphic fungus. It grows as a fungus both at room temperature and at 37°C, producing a white cotton-like colony. The hyphae are septate, and lateral branches break up into arthrospores which are highly infectious when they become air-borne. Coccidioidomycosis is notorious for the ease with which laboratory workers may become infected.

In the tissues the organism appears typically as a large, spherical, non-budding structure about 60 μm in diameter. It has a thick wall and is called a sporangium. In it there are many small, spherical endospores from 2 to 5 μm in diameter. When the sporangium ruptures, these spores are released and then develop into new sporangia. This mode of reproduction contrasts sharply with the simple budding encountered in the *Cryptococcus* and *Histoplasma* species.

It too is a soil saprophyte, and it causes disease in rodents, dogs, and cattle. The distribution is fairly widespread, but the great bulk of the disease occurs in the South-West of the USA, especially Arizona and California where it is endemic. It is estimated that over three-quarters of the population of the San Joaquin Valley of California have had the disease as indicated by skin tests. It is also seen in South America and Italy.

As in the other two mycotic diseases infection is due to the inhalation of soil dust. All age-groups are afflicted, and patients are not infectious.

The primary lesion is a pulmonary complex very similar in morphology to tuberculosis. There is considerable mediastinal lymphadenopathy. The condition is generally benign and heals with calcification. It is often subclinical, but sometimes it is attended by a mild febrile illness called 'valley fever' or 'desert fever'. About 3 weeks after this there is often a sharp attack of erythema nodosum. This is much less common in cryptococcosis and histoplasmosis. The patient usually recovers completely, but in a few instances progressive coccidioidomycosis follows with destructive lesions in the viscera, skin, and bones. This is usually fatal, there often being a terminal meningitis. Generalisation is said to occur most frequently in darkskinned races. Opportunistic infections may occur, but are less common than with cryptococcosis and histoplasmosis.

The tissue reaction of coccidioidomycosis.[4] Of all the fungal diseases coccidioidomycosis resembles tuberculosis most closely in histological appearance. Complete tuberculoid systems with variable amounts of caseation are present, especially in lung lesions.

Often, however, there is a suppurative element: microab-scesses filled with pus cells lie centrally, and are surrounded by epithelioid cells and scanty giant cells. Such lesions are encompassed by extensive infiltrations of small round cells, and may fuse to form large conglomerate masses. Organisms may be found in the central abscesses.

Diagnosis. This depends on the isolation and culture of the organism.

Complement-fixing antibodies appear in the serum after a few weeks, and a skin test using an extract of organism (*coccidioidin*) gives a positive result. Patients with the progressive disease may not react, a state of affairs that is reminiscent of fulminating tuberculosis.

CANDIDIASIS[9, 10]

Infection with the *Candida* species is becoming one of the most frequent human fungal diseases. The organism most frequently involved is the yeast-like fungus *Candida albicans*. The common yeast form is found in superficial lesions, and it is 2·5 to 4·0 μm in diameter and intensely Gram positive. It reproduces by budding, but sometimes the bud elongates to form a pseudohypha. This form can occur in cultures, and is also seen in invasive candidal infections, especially in systemic candidiasis.

The organism is a common commensal of the mouth, alimentary tract, and vagina. The superficial infections of the mucous membranes appear as white patches called *thrush*. In the *mouth* this is very common in infants, especially premature ones, and it may be accompanied by perianal lesions. Oral candidiasis can occur at any age in the course of a debilitating illness. *Vaginal thrush* is common during pregnancy, in women who take the contraceptive pill, and in those with diabetes mellitus. In all these conditions there is excess glycogen in the vaginal cells; this the fungus ferments, and the acidity of the vagina increases. The organism grows well in an acid pH, and is in fact best cultured on an acid medium (Sabouraud's medium, see p. 665). The glycosuria in diabetics also favours the growth of *Candida albicans* in the vagina. Vaginal thrush is also sometimes a troublesome side-effect of tetracycline therapy for acne vulgaris. *Cutaneous candidiasis* occurs around the mouth (perlèche), in other moist intertriginous areas, and in the nail folds (chronic paronychia).

The importance of candidiasis is that it is a serious opportunistic infection. In any condition of impaired cell-mediated immunity, e.g. lymphomata and after the administration of glucocorticoids or cytotoxic drugs, oral lesions can extend down the alimentary or respiratory tracts to produce fatal results. The most serious type is *generalised systemic candidiasis*, in which there is haematogenous spread to many organs; renal lesions are prominent, but almost any organ may be affected and endocarditis is sometimes seen. Generalised candidiasis is sometimes a salient feature of those immunological deficiency syndromes in which there is a T-lymphocyte defect, e.g. Nezelof's syndrome (see p. 171). Less extensive candidal infections are seen in particular circumstances. *Endocarditis* can occur as an isolated event, particularly in addicts who inject themselves intravenously with narcotics. Oral lesions can spread to produce extensive *gastrointestinal infection* following the prolonged use of oral broad-spectrum antibiotics.

Finally there are some types of primary immunological deficiency disease affecting T lymphocytes in which widespread *chronic mucocutaneous candidiasis* is seen.[10,11] The type of defect varies from case to case. In some patients there is a lymphocyte defect such that the cells are unresponsive to phytohaemagglutinin. In others, such stimulation produces a normal transformation but the cells are unresponsive to *Candida* antigen. The treatment of this latter group with transfer factor may be successful. In some patients endocrine abnormalities, particularly hypoparathyroidism, may coexist. Chronic mucocutaneous candidiasis is therefore a manifestation of several distinct disease processes. It lasts for many years and does not terminate in generalised spread, nor is there usually a tendency for other infections to occur.

The tissue reaction to *Candida* varies. In minor and superficial infections there is some tissue necrosis accompanied by a pyogenic response; intra-epithelial pustules are seen in the cutaneous lesions. When the infection is overwhelming, as in generalised candidiasis, there is much necrosis and very little inflammatory reaction. Indeed, the lesions show massive accumulations of fungus and few host cells.

Treatment of Fungal Infections

The pulmonary lesions of the deep-seated mycoses usually heal spontaneously, but a toruloma, if diagnosed clinically, should be resected in view of the danger of systemic spread. For generalised infections the antibiotic *amphotericin B* can be given systemically with good effect. A less toxic drug is *5-fluorocytosine*; it is potent but unfortunately liable to induce drug-resistant strains.

For candidal infection these drugs can also be used.[12] The imidazole derivatives *clotrimazole* and *miconazole* are also useful, and can be used both topically and systemically. The antibiotic *nystatin* is very effective for local treatment, but is not absorbed when taken by mouth, and cannot be given parenterally.

SOME PROTOZOAL INFECTIONS

The most important human protozoal diseases are malaria, leishmaniasis, trypanosomiasis, and amoebiasis. These are not discussed here because detailed accounts of their pathology are available in standard text-books of tropical medicine. Instead, two rather uncommon diseases are touched on, toxoplasmosis and pneumocystis pneumonia, both of which are encountered in Britain from time to time.

TOXOPLASMOSIS[13–17]

The causative organism *Toxoplasma gondii* belongs to the subphylum *Sporozoa* and probably to the genus *Isospora*. It is crescentic in shape and about 7 μm long. It is stained by the usual Romanowsky methods used for malarial and leishmanial parasites; the nucleus is red and the cytoplasm blue. When introduced into an animal host, it penetrates and then multiplies in the cytoplasm of a nucleated cell, most often a reticuloendothelial cell. By repeated fission it soon proliferates and kills the cell, whereupon the liberated organisms infect other cells both locally and by carriage in the blood and lymph.

This stage of parasitaemia is accompanied by focal cell necrosis. The animal either dies, or else becomes immune to the organism. In this case the intracellular parasites encyst themselves in the tissues. Such a cyst may at first be less than 10 μm in diameter, but soon the parasites inside it start dividing, and the cyst may eventually attain a size of 100 μm. Cysts are found especially in the brain, but may also be encountered in the heart muscle, liver, lungs, spleen, and lymph nodes. As immunity increases, so the number of cysts decreases. A breakdown of immunity may be followed by a recrudescence of overt disease.

A sexual phase of development has been described in cats:[18,19] if they are fed on toxoplasma-infected mice, the organisms parasitise the cells of the bowel mucosa where both schizogony and gametogony occur. Oöcysts are produced which are excreted in the cat's faeces. These can then divide into two sporocysts each containing four sporozoites when the cyst is ingested by another animal. It would seem that cats (and other Felidae) are the definitive hosts of this parasite and that other mammalian species, including the human, are the intermediate hosts. People become infected through ingesting oöcysts from the excreta of cats, and the released sporozoites penetrate the bowel wall and are carried by the blood and lymph to different organs. Here they end their existence as cysts. Well over half the populations of many communities have been exposed to infection, usually during later childhood and at adolescence, by the evidence of serological tests.

The vast majority of human infections are subclinical, a state of affairs reminiscent of tuberculosis. Occasionally an adult may suffer from overt toxoplasmosis. Very rarely this may take the form of a fulminating typhus-like disease, and such features as interstitial pneumonia and encephalitis may be superadded. A much more usual event, however, is a mild, though prolonged, febrile illness in which lymphadenopathy is a prominent manifestation. The disease is easily mistaken for infectious mononucleosis, but the Paul-Bunnell reaction is negative.

The histological changes seen in an affected lymph node are those of pronounced reactive hyperplasia (see Ch. 30). In addition there are often small collections of epithelioid cells scattered throughout the lymph node. The appearance may resemble sarcoidosis, except that the aggregations are smaller, and there are no giant cells. Very occasionally a toxoplasma cyst may be included in the section. Both clinically and histologically toxoplasmosis may be confused with Hodgkin's disease.

The tragedy of toxoplasmosis lies in its tendency to be transmitted transplacentally to the fetus. The mother is usually healthy though infected, and there is often no transmission in succeeding pregnancies.

The effects on the fetus vary. A very severe infection may precipitate abortion, but this is not common. More often the child survives, and develops a severe generalised disease a few weeks after birth. The lungs, liver, spleen, and lymph nodes are severely affected. Acute peritonitis and pleurisy are common features, and there may also be skin eruptions of various types.

In other cases the disease appears later, when central nervous system and ocular lesions predominate. A severe choroidoretinitis is characteristic, and this may proceed to microphthalmos and blindness. On the other hand, a focal scotoma may be the only residual feature. Toxoplasmosis is a very important cause of posterior uveitis, and recrudescences are common. It is possible that some toxoplasmal uveitis is secondary to disease acquired in adult life.

The cerebral infection produces necrotic nodules in the meninges and brain substance, particularly around the walls of the lateral ventricles. Necrotic material may be shed into the ventricles and lead to obstructive hydrocephalus, which may also be produced as a result of fibrinous meningitis around the base of the brain. Sometimes necrosis is so extensive that microcephaly ensues. In patients who survive calcification in the area of the necrotic tissue is prominent. It is seen radiologically as sharply-outlined, curved ridges situated in the paraventricular areas of the cerebral hemispheres. Severe cases die in a few months, while others may be left with various residua, including paralysis and idiocy.

Pyrimethamine (Daraprim) and *sulphonamides*, especially sulphadiazine, are of some value in treatment.

The histological features of these severe congenital lesions are not pathognomonic. Focal necrosis may be found in the liver, spleen, and lungs, and this is surrounded by non-specific small round cell infiltrations that include polymorphs. Haemorrhagic extravasations are common, and the fibrinous pleurisy that often occurs may also be haemorrhagic. The brain likewise contains necrotic foci surrounded by small round cells and proliferating glial tissue. Dystrophic calcification is a prominent sequel.

The lymph nodes show no necrosis, but only a reactive change similar to that of the adult lesion.

Diagnosis. *Demonstration of the organism in lesions.* It is uncommon to find the toxoplasms in histological section, and they are furthermore very difficult to identify. Occasionally cysts may be found in areas that are quiescent.

Isolation of the organism. The mouse is very susceptible to infection. It is inoculated with a test suspension, and a rapidly fatal disease usually ensues. Smears of the spleen, lung, liver, and brain should reveal large numbers of organisms within the cells of the organ.

A rising titre of antibodies is the most important diagnostic test. These can be demonstrated by means of complement-fixation tests using a toxoplasmal antigen. The *dye-test* is also very useful. Normally extracellular toxoplasms stain easily with a methylene-blue buffer solution, but in the presence of the specific antibody and free complement, staining is impaired, due apparently to a modification induced in the cytoplasm of the organisms. The organisms for this test are obtained from the peritoneal exudates of infected mice.

A skin test can also be done, and is said to be especially useful in epidemiological surveys.

PNEUMOCYSTIS PNEUMONIA[20–24]

Pneumocystis carinii, like the plasmodia of malaria and the toxoplasma organism, belongs to the subphylum *Sporozoa*. The organisms are widely distributed in nature and are normal inhabitants of the respiratory tracts of rodents.

When they invade the lung they form cysts measuring about 4·5 μm in diameter in the alveolar septal cells. Within these cysts there is a proliferation and maturation of trophozoites,

and when the septal cells disintegrate within the alveolar spaces, the break in the cyst wall enables the trophozoites to escape into the alveoli. The trophozoites are initially about 1·5 μm in diameter, and they enlarge to about 2·5 μm. It is possible that the more developed trophozoites undergo budding or conjugation, but this stage of the life cycle of the parasite is still uncertain. In due course the large trophozoite acquires a thickened pellicle as it undergoes a precyst stage preliminary to encystment.

The lungs in pneumocystis pneumonia are firm and dry, and have a homogeneous consistency. On section the alveoli are seen to be filled with a foamy, reticulated, eosinophilic exudate. If examined carefully this apparently acellular, honeycomb exudate is found to contain many punctate bodies. Special stains, e.g. Gomori's methenamine silver method, the PAS method, and the Romanowsky stains (e.g. Giemsa's stain), reveal that the exudate is crowded with parasites. There is also hypertrophy of the alveolar cells and, provided there is no immunological abnormality, a considerable interstitial infiltration of plasma cells and lymphocytes. Where there is immunodeficiency, plasma cells may be absent and lymphocytes very sparse indeed.

Pneumocystis pneumonia first made its presence felt in Europe after the Second World War, when it was endemic in marasmic infants confined to orphanages where there was overcrowding and malnutrition. By 1960 the European endemics had subsided as social conditions improved, but at this time sporadic cases began to occur in the more affluent populations of North America who were being treated for malignant disease with various cytotoxic agents. Nowadays the disease is found almost exclusively as an opportunistic infection in patients with an immunological defect involving the T lymphocytes. It is much less common in cases of Bruton's congenital sex-linked agammaglobulinaemia. A valuable therapeutic agent in pneumocystosis is *pentamidine isethionate*. More recently combined therapy with *trimethoprim* and *sulphamethoxazole* has been used with success.

SOME CHRONIC INFLAMMATIONS OF DOUBTFUL AETIOLOGY

CAT-SCRATCH DISEASE[25]

This is an unusual inflammatory condition of lymph nodes, and it has been suggested that it is caused by a virus, but the aetiology remains obscure.

The disease is found almost invariably in people who come into contact with cats, and there is often a history of a cat-scratch. About a week later a sore develops locally, and there may be variable constitutional symptoms. About 3 weeks later there is painful regional lymphadenitis with considerable reddening of the skin over the nodes, and suppuration may occur if these are not excised.

The histological picture approximates closely to that described in coccidioidomycosis, namely a suppurative tuberculoid reaction. It starts with collections of epithelioid cells in the substance of the node, and these soon undergo central necrosis while a polymorph infiltration develops in their midst. After a few weeks these foci increase greatly in size and number. The larger ones collapse due to the extensive central

Figure 21.3
Cat-scratch disease. In this lymph node there are follicles typical of cat-scratch disease. In the centre there is a large area of necrosis in which the nuclei of disintegrating polymorphs are barely recognisable, and surrounding this there is an exuberant zone of epithelioid cells. There are few giant cells in this area. The evenly palisaded arrangement of the epithelioid cells perpendicular to the surrounding lymphoid tissue is very characteristic of the condition, and is in marked contrast to the irregular disposition of the cells in tuberculosis. × 40. (*Photograph by courtesy of Dr A. D. Thomson*)

Figure 21.4
Sarcoidosis. In this section of lymph node there are semi-confluent follicles consisting of epithelioid cells. A large giant cell is present in one follicle; it resembles a foreign-body cell rather than a Langhans one. There is no central caseation. × 230.

necrosis, and so tend to assume a flattened shape. The surrounding layers of epithelioid cells arrange themselves in a palisade around the collapsed centre. A few Langhans giant cells may appear among them, but they are never numerous (Fig. 21.3). Associated with this destruction of the node there is severe periadenitis with an infiltration of lymphocytes, plasma cells, and macrophages into the surrounding connective tissue. There is eventual healing by fibrosis, but suppurative foci persist for many months.

This picture is seen also in lymphogranuloma venereum, and in the acute mesenteric adenitis caused by *Yersinia enterocolitica* that resembles acute appendicitis clinically. An extract of pus from a lymph node removed from a case of cat-scratch disease produces a positive reaction when injected intradermally into a fresh case. This closely resembles the Frei test of lymphogranuloma venereum.

SARCOIDOSIS[26, 27]

This is a systemic disease of unknown aetiology in which characteristic epithelioid-cell follicles are scattered throughout many organs. It is quite common in Northern European communities.

The unit of sarcoidosis is a discrete follicle composed of plump epithelioid cells, in the midst of which a few Langhans giant cells may be found. Sometimes these giant cells contain star-shaped acidophilic bodies, or *asteroids*, and spherical basophilic masses, or *Schaumann bodies*. These inclusions are in no way pathognomonic of sarcoidosis, being found in the Langhans giant cells of other conditions from time to time. They are believed to be non-specific end-products of the active metabolism and secretion that takes place in these cells. The follicle is surrounded by a narrow rim of lymphocytes. It is very like the tubercle follicle, but differs in that there is never any true central caseation (Fig. 21.4). In very florid cases of sarcoidosis some of the follicles may contain small central areas of necrosis. The extensive small round cell infiltration of tuberculosis is lacking in sarcoidosis. Individual follicles often undergo partial coalescence to form conglomerate masses, a feature seen particularly in pulmonary sarcoidosis. The course of the lesions is towards healing. In them there are many reticulin fibres, and the follicles are gradually replaced by dense fibrous tissue. Ultimately a hyalinised scar remains, or else there is complete resolution.

Though the lesions are generalised,[28] the lungs bear the brunt of the disease. Chest radiography reveals miliary (and sometimes conglomerate) mottling of both lung fields with considerable hilar lymphadenopathy. The pulmonary symptoms are often initially very mild in comparison with the extent of the disease. In appearance the sarcoid tissue is pearly-grey in colour, and forms discrete or confluent masses in the lungs, especially in the mid-zones and bases. Other organs frequently involved are the lymph nodes, spleen, and liver, all of which may be clinically palpable. In the bones small cysts may be produced (*osteitis cystica multiplex*). The phalanges are most commonly affected. A considerable range of cutaneous lesions is due to sarcoidosis; a well-known one is *lupus pernio*, in which soft, infiltrated, violaceous plaques with superficial telangiectasia are present, especially on the nose, ears, or fingers ('chilblain lupus'[29]). Furthermore, *erythema nodosum* is a common accompaniment: indeed, in Northern European countries sarcoidosis and tuberculosis are the most frequent precipitating factors of erythema nodosum. Patients who develop erythema nodosum have a good prognosis, and their lung lesions tend to heal without the severe fibrosis which is a common sequel to sarcoidosis.[30] Other important manifestations of sarcoidosis are uveitis and salivary-gland and lacrimal-gland enlargement (when the three occur together it is called *Heerfordt's syndrome*).[31] The central nervous system is occasionally implicated, and diabetes insipidus due to involvement of the posterior pituitary may occur. Despite the benign course of the lesions, sarcoidosis can be a serious condition attended by an appreciable mortality rate.

An occasional feature is hypercalcaemia. This is due to an increased sensitivity to the action of vitamin D, which is absorbed in normal amounts from the bowel. The nature of this sensitivity is unknown. A more constant biochemical finding is hypergammaglobulinaemia.

A noteworthy feature of sarcoidosis is a tendency to depression of delayed-type hypersensitivity tests; the tuberculin reaction is frequently negative. On the other hand, there does not appear to be any significant impairment of cell-mediated immunity to infection. The sarcoid lesion is an immunological granuloma (see p. 130), such as is found in tuberculoid leprosy, where there is, however, an increased delayed-type hypersensitivity. The similarity between the two disease processes is emphasised by the delayed Mitsuda reaction (see p. 183) and the Kveim test described below. The paradox of good cell-mediated immunity and impaired delayed-type hypersensitivity tests in sarcoidosis cannot at present be explained. Two possible suggestions are (a) a pre-emptive diversion of T-cells to the agent causing the disease (if indeed there is such an agent), so that not enough T-cells are available to respond to the cutaneous tests of hypersensitivity, and (b) that the anergy of sarcoidosis is only skin deep.

An important diagnostic adjunct is the *Kveim test*, in which an extract of sarcoid tissue (usually obtained from a patient's spleen) produces a very delayed inflammatory reaction composed of sarcoid lesions when injected intradermally into a patient with sarcoidosis. The test is virtually pathognomonic when positive (it is occasionally negative in longstanding disease), but it is important to use a reliable source of sarcoid tissue. Confusion has been produced by numerous falsely positive results obtained from faulty batches of sarcoid splenic tissue, but the classical Chase-Siltzbach suspension remains completely reliable, as do other batches of Kveim material prepared correctly according to the method laid down by Siltzbach.[32–34] The test is read by sectioning a biopsy of the lesion 4 to 6 weeks after injection.

It has been found that if immunologically deficient mice (thymectomised a few weeks after birth and then subjected to whole body radiation) are injected with extracts of sarcoid material in their footpads, they develop disseminated granulomatous lesions resembling sarcoidosis, and the Kveim test becomes positive. Material from one mouse may be transmitted to another immunologically deficient one in this way, and the lesions are reproduced.[35, 36] This technique is very valuable for infecting mice with organisms that they would not tolerate in a healthy state, and has been used for the cultivation of *Myco. leprae*. It remains to be seen whether a specific infective agent is responsible.

Many different agents can produce local sarcoid tissue reactions. The lymph nodes draining cancerous foci occasionally contain follicles indistinguishable from those of sarcoidosis, and a similar appearance is sometimes encountered in the outlying lymph nodes in Hodgkin's disease. Various organs occasionally contain sarcoid follicles in the course of chronic inflammatory conditions. Sometimes tuberculosis, leprosy, leishmaniasis, histoplasmosis, and berylliosis give rise to focal lesions indistinguishable from sarcoidosis.[37] So also may zirconium compounds used in deodorant preparations,[38] and silica implanted in the skin.

It follows that the diagnosis of idiopathic sarcoidosis is a combined histological and clinical one, in which chest radiography plays an important part. It is particularly important to exclude tuberculosis and berylliosis before making a final diagnosis of sarcoidosis. The lesions of sarcoidosis are reversed by glucocorticoids. This forms a useful diagnostic test in distinguishing the hypercalcaemia of sarcoidosis from that of hyperparathyroidism, which is quite unresponsive to these drugs.

CROHN'S DISEASE[39]

This chronic granulomatous disease of unknown aetiology usually affects the terminal ileum, but it may also occur elsewhere in the small bowel and in the colon. It has even been described in the mouth, oesophagus, and stomach, and when it involves the colon, anal fistulae are quite common. These may cause extensive skin involvement.[40]

The affected bowel is swollen, its wall thickened, and its lumen considerably stenosed. A characteristic feature is a cobblestone mucosa between which linear ulcers extend into the bowel wall. These form the basis of fistulae between loops of bowel and to the abdominal skin. The mesentery is thickened and the local lymph nodes are enlarged. A feature of the disease is the tendency to affect several areas of the bowel—with normal intervening *skip areas*. There is often a sharp line of demarcation between diseased and healthy segments (Fig. 21.5).

Histologically there is a chronic inflammatory reaction involving the whole wall, but it is the submucosa that is especially involved. It is widened by oedema and later fibrosis, and there are many plasma cells and lymphocytes infiltrating it. Polymorphs, macrophages, and eosinophils are more scanty. A conspicuous feature in many cases is the development of lymphoid follicles in the submucosa and deeper in the wall. These may assume a tuberculoid character with epithelioid cells and Langhans giant cells, as in sarcoidosis, but the circumscribed arrangement of follicles seen in this disease is

Figure 21.5

Resected specimen of the terminal ileum, ileo-caecal junction, caecum, and a small portion of the ascending colon from a man aged 22 years. The terminal ileum shows great thickening and rigidity of its wall and the lumen is reduced in size. The mucosa has a characteristic cobblestone appearance, and the disease stops sharply at the ileo-caecal valve. Microscopically, the affected bowel showed transmural oedema, fibrosis, and the presence of non-caseating tuberculoid granulomata. (*Photograph by courtesy of Dr J. B. Cullen*).

not found in Crohn's disease. The lymph nodes may also contain tuberculoid granulomata. The mucosa is often fairly normal apart from the intersecting fissures that may be lined by epithelioid cells or polymorphs. Crohn's disease closely resembles intestinal tuberculosis, and it is important to rule out this infection by repeated faecal cultures. Ileo-caecal disease in the dark-skinned races is more often due to tuberculosis than to Crohn's disease.

When it affects the colon alone it may be difficult to distinguish from ulcerative colitis, but the mucosal lesions of this disease, particularly the crypt abscesses, contrast with the generalised involvement of the wall in Crohn's disease. In addition, there are no fistulae or giant-cell systems in ulcerative colitis. Thus in ulcerative colitis the inflammatory changes are mainly confined to the mucosa. In Crohn's disease, on the other hand, the changes are *transmural*. Hence in Crohn's disease there is peritoneal involvement, and this is responsible for adhesion and eventual fistula formation.

The nature of Crohn's disease is obscure.[41-44] It is generally believed that cell-mediated immunity is impaired and that anergy is common, but this is not always true. Using the footpad technique in immunologically deficient mice as described in sarcoidosis, a transmissible agent, possibly a slow virus, has been demonstrated by some workers, but others have not found any such agent. On the other hand, claims have also been made that a rather similar type of transmissible agent can be demonstrated from homogenates of material from patients with ulcerative colitis. If this is substantiated, it may link ulcerative colitis with Crohn's disease, which share a number of features, closer together. But the transmissible agent may be merely a non-specific component derived from the inflamed bowel. Even if a slow virus is implicated in these diseases, there are probably other factors involved also. A dietary one is a distinct possibility.

Both ulcerative colitis and Crohn's disease, especially that variety that affects the colon severely ('granulomatous colitis'), may show a number of extra-intestinal complications.

(*a*) *Arthritis*, either an episodic *synovitis* affecting chiefly the large weight-bearing joints, or the more serious *ankylosing spondylitis* with sacro-iliitis. This second type is closely associated with transplantation antigen HLA-B27, and it is probable that those patients with ankylosing spondylitis bear a hereditary predisposition which is precipitated by the chronic bowel disease.

(*b*) *Anterior uveitis* (*iridocyclitis*). This too is closely associated with transplantation antigen HLA-B27.

(*c*) *Skin lesions*, notably erythema nodosum and pyoderma gangrenosum. *Erythema nodosum* is characterised by tender, erythematous, ill-defined nodules that do not ulcerate. They occur in the subcutaneous tissues of the anterior surfaces of both legs, and are due to a vasculitis involving the panniculus. *Pyoderma gangrenosum* is characterised by papules, nodules, or pustules which subsequently ulcerate. They occur commonly on the legs but are also seen elsewhere. The lesions may be single or multiple, and the edge of the ulcer is characteristically purplish red and undermined. The pathogenesis is not clear, but the lesion usually responds to glucocorticoid therapy.

(*d*) *Aphthous stomatitis*.

Among less common complications of both conditions are *pericholangitis* and *chronic active hepatitis*. A rare biliary complication is *sclerosing cholangitis* with a danger of *bile-duct carcinoma*. *Amyloidosis* occasionally complicates Crohn's disease, and more rarely ulcerative colitis.

On the other hand, *bowel cancer* is a greater hazard of ulcerative colitis than of Crohn's disease (see p. 374). Whether this will also prove to be true of the colonic type of Crohn's disease remains to be seen.

Complications more specific to classical Crohn's disease of the small bowel are the *malabsorption syndrome, gallstones* (see p. 596), *hydronephrosis and hydroureter* (especially of the right side) due to obstruction caused by a retroperitoneal inflammatory mass, and *renal stones*. These are usually of the oxalate type, and it is believed that they are the result of an increased absorption of dietary oxalate with consequent hyperoxaluria. There is also often a tendency to hyperuricaemia, possibly due to an increased breakdown of tissue.

These widely-ranging complications show how a disease that appears to be localised to one system of the body can produce disturbances of a generalised type and play an important role in many processes generally considered to be the special preserve of general pathology.

REFERENCES

1. CRUICKSHANK, R., DUGUID, J. P., MARMION, B. P. & SWAIN, R. H. A. (1973) *Medical Microbiology*. 12th edn, Vol. 1, Ch. 53. Edinburgh: Churchill Livingstone.
2. LITTMAN, M. L. & WALTER, J. E. (1968) Cryptococcosis: current status. *American Journal of Medicine*, **45**, 922.
3. POWELL, K. & CHRISTIANSON, C. (1973) Pulmonary cryptococcosis: clinical forms and treatment: a center for disease control cooperative mycosis study. *American Review of Respiratory Diseases*, **108**, 116.
4. SYMMERS, W. StC. (1960) In *Recent Advances in Clinical Pathology*, Series III, p. 304. ed. Dyke, S. C. London: Churchill.
5. SCHWARZ, J. & BAUM, G. L. (1963) Histoplasmosis, 1962. *Archives of Internal Medicine*, **111**, 710.
6. COCKSHOTT, W. P. & LUCAS, A. O. (1964) Histoplasmosis duboisii. *Quarterly Journal of Medicine*, **33**, 223.
7. FIESE, M. J. (1958) *Coccidioidomycosis*. Springfield, Illinois: Thomas.
8. AJELLO, L. (1967) *Coccidioidomycosis*. Tucson: University of Arizona Press.
9. STIEHM, E. R. *et al.* (1972) Diseases of cellular immunity. *Annals of Internal Medicine*, **77**, 101.
10. KIRKPATRICK, C. H. *et al.* (1971) Chronic mucocutaneous candidiasis: model-building in cellular immunity. *Annals of Internal Medicine*, **74**, 955.
11. HOLT, P. J. L. *et al.* (1972) Chronic mucocutaneous candidiasis: a model for the investigation of cell mediated immunity. *British Journal of Clinical Practice*, **26**, 331.
12. Trends in candidal vaginitis (1977) *Proceedings of the Royal Society of Medicine*, Vol. 70, Supplement Number 4.
13. REMINGTON, J. S. (1974) Toxoplasmosis in the adult. *Bulletin of the New York Academy of Medicine*, **50**, 211.
14. DESMONTS, G. & COUVREUR, J. (1974) Congenital toxoplasmosis: a prospective study of 378 pregnancies. *New England Journal of Medicine*, **290**, 1110.
15. FELDMAN, H. A. (1974) Toxoplasmosis: an overview. *Bulletin of the New York Academy of Medicine*, **50**, 110.
16. GLEASON, T. H. & HAMLIN, W. B. (1974) Disseminated toxoplasmosis in the compromised host. *Archives of Internal Medicine*, **134**, 1059.
17. BEVERLEY, J. K. A. (1973) Toxoplasmosis. *British Medical Journal*, **2**, 475.
18. HUTCHISON, W. M. *et al.* (1970) Coccidian-like nature of Toxoplasma gondii. *British Medical Journal*, **1**, 142.
19. Leading Article (1970) Transmission of toxoplasmosis. *British Medical Journal*, **1**, 126.
20. ROSEN, F. S. (1972) Immunity deficiency in children. *British Journal of Clinical Practice*, **26**, 315.
21. BURKE, B. A. & GOOD, R. A. (1973) Pneumocystis carinii infection. *Medicine (Baltimore)*, **52**, 23.
22. CROSS, A. S. & STEIGBIGEL, R. T. (1974) Pneumocystis carinii pneumonia presenting as localised nodular densities. *New England Journal of Medicine*, **291**, 831.
23. CAMPBELL, W. G. (1972) Ultrastructure of pneumocystis in human lung. *Archives of Pathology*, **93**, 312.
24. PRICE, R. A. & HUGHES, W. T. (1974) Histopathology of Pneumocystis carinii infestation and infection in malignant disease in childhood. *Human Pathology*, **5**, 737.
25. HARRISON, C. V. (1960) In *Recent Advances in Pathology*, ed. Harrison, C. V. 7th edn, p. 36. London: Churchill.
26. SCADDING, J. G. (1967) *Sarcoidosis*. London: Eyre and Spottiswoode.
27. MITCHELL, D. N. *et al.* (1977) Sarcoidosis: histopathological definition and clinical diagnosis. *Journal of Clinical Pathology*, **30**, 395.
28. MAYOCK, R. L. *et al.* (1963) Manifestations of sarcoidosis. *American Journal of Medicine*, **35**, 67.
29. Leading Article (1977) The chilblain wolf. *British Medical Journal*, **1**, 930.
30. Annotation (1967) Prognosis of sarcoidosis. *Lancet*, **1**, 373.
31. Leading Article (1967) Uveoparotitis. *British Medical Journal*, **2**, 459.
32. SILTZBACH, L. E. *et al.* (1971) Is there Kveim responsiveness in Crohn's disease? *Lancet*, **2**, 634.
33. Leading Article (1972) Kveim-Siltzbach test vindicated. *Lancet*, **1**, 188.
34. JAMES, D. G. (1975) Kveim revisited, reassessed. *New England Journal of Medicine*, **292**, 859.
35. MITCHELL, D. N. & REES, R. J. W. (1969) A transmissible agent from sarcoid tissue. *Lancet*, **2**, 81.
36. MITCHELL, D. N. & REES, R. J. W. (1971) Sarcoidosis and Crohn's disease. *Proceedings of the Royal Society of Medicine*, **64**, 944.
37. JONES WILLIAMS, W. (1971) The beryllium granuloma. *Proceedings of the Royal Society of Medicine*, **64**, 946.
38. EPSTEIN, W. L. & ALLEN, J. R. (1964) Granulomatous hypersensitivity after use of zirconium-containing poison oak lotions. *Journal of the American Medical Association*, **190**, 940.
39. Various Authors: Symposium on Crohn's disease. (1971) *Proceedings of the Royal Society of Medicine*, **64**, 157.
40. Leading Article (1972) Unusual symptoms of Crohn's disease. *British Medical Journal*, **3**, 658.
41. Leading Article (1977) Chasing the cause of Crohn's disease. *British Medical Journal*, **1**, 929.
42. HEATLEY, R. V. *et al.* (1975) A search for a transmissible agent in Crohn's disease. *Gut*, **16**, 528.
43. SACHAR, D. B., TAUB, R. N. & JANOWITZ, H. D. (1975) A transmissible agent in Crohn's disease? New pursuit of an old concept. *New England Journal of Medicine*, **293**, 354.
44. Leading Article (1976) Crohn's disease. *Lancet*, **2**, 1284.

Chapter 22. Some Smaller Pathogenic Organisms: Rickettsiae, Chlamydiae, Mycoplasmas, and Viruses

INTRODUCTION

It is useful at the outset, before considering the properties of viruses, first to define those of other small organisms which might be confused with them.

Bacteria

These are generally unicellular, but even the smallest is within the range of the light microscope (which resolves up to about 0·2 μm in diameter). They grow with variable ease on artificial cell-free media, exceptions being *Mycobacterium leprae* and *Treponema pallidum*, which have not been cultured artificially. The bacterial cell contains DNA in its nuclear body and RNA in its cytoplasm (see Appendix 2).

An extremely small bacterium is the genus *Bartonella*. *Bartonella bacilliformis* can be cultivated quite easily on cell-free media, but in nature prefers an intracellular environment. It causes *Oroya fever* in the Andean area of South America; this fever is accompanied by a severe haemolytic anaemia, and the organism parasitises red cells and tissue cells. There is also a benign cutaneous variant called *verruga peruana*.

Rickettsiae

These are very close to Gram-negative bacteria, but are small (300 to 700 nm in diameter and 0·8 to 2·0 μm in length) and are obligatory intracellular parasites. They are stained well with Macchiavello's stain.*

The genus *Rickettsia* causes the typhus fever group—epidemic louse-borne (*R. prowazeki*) and murine (*R. mooseri*), which is flea-borne; the spotted fever group—including Rocky Mountain spotted fever (*R. rickettsi*) and Queensland tick 'typhus', (*R. australis*), all of which are transmitted by ticks; and scrub 'typhus', which is mite-borne and caused by *R. tsutsugamushi*.

The *Rickettsiae* share a heterophile antigen with a strain of *Proteus*, and give a positive Weil-Felix reaction (see p. 169). They are obligatory intracellular parasites, and are cultured in various rodents, the yolk-sac of fertile eggs, and in tissue-culture systems.

Coxiella burneti is a rather smaller organism which causes Q (query) fever. It is antigenically distinct from the *Rickettsia* organisms, and gives a negative Weil-Felix reaction. It is very resistant to environmental adversity and disinfectants. It is nearly always transmitted by the inhalation of aerosols from the products of conception of infected cattle, sheep, or goats, or by the ingestion of their milk, in this respect resembling the transmission of brucellosis.

*In this method a smear is stained with basic fuchsin, decolorised by citric acid, and counterstained with methylene blue. Rickettsial organisms are stained red and the cells blue.

Rochalimaea quintana, which causes trench fever, has been reclassified because it differs in several respects from the rickettsiae. It proliferates in the lumen of the louse gut rather than in the epithelial cells, and it can be cultivated on blood agar.

The pathological features of the rickettsial diseases have much in common. In the *typhus* and *spotted fever* groups, as well as in *scrub typhus*, there is a rickettsiaemia with parasitisation of the endothelial cells of the capillaries. These swell and proliferate, and there is capillary occlusion with thrombosis. Around the vessels there is an infiltration of lymphocytes and macrophages producing the so-called typhus nodules. In fatal cases there are few noteworthy macroscopic features, apart from the typical petechial skin eruption which is sometimes grossly haemorrhagic.

In *scrub typhus* the capillary occlusion is less severe, and the skin eruption is morbilliform and seldom haemorrhagic. On the other hand, the lungs are frequently involved, and there may be a mild rickettsial peritonitis, pleurisy, and pericarditis. Another feature of scrub typhus is the frequent presence of a localised area of necrosis and ulceration of the skin at the area of attachment of the mite.

Q fever is a rather different condition. It usually presents itself as an acute febrile condition without localising signs, but with radiological features in the chest out of all proportion to the clinical symptoms. Most cases recover completely, but sometimes the infection becomes chronic. These cases are nearly always associated with a *Cox. burneti* subacute infective endocarditis, which may be very difficult to eradicate. There is no skin eruption. In Q fever there is a much milder capillary parasitisation than in the other rickettsial infections. The main feature is a 'primary atypical pneumonia' (see p. 226). There may also be focal necrosis of the liver.

Trench fever is characterised by the sudden onset of fever and severe pains in the muscles and bones—particularly of the shins. The condition abates temporarily, but recurs in cycles of 5 days (hence the name quintana). Trench fever was first encountered in the First World War, and reappeared on Germany's Eastern Front during the Second World War.

These diseases respond well to tetracycline. It should be combined with lincomycin in the treatment of Q fever endocarditis. There is no reliable information concerning the effect of antibiotics on trench fever.

Chlamydiae

These organisms have much in common with the rickettsiae, but are smaller and more rudimentary. They exist in two forms, a small nucleoid structure called an 'elementary body', about 300 nm in diameter, which is extracellular and highly infectious, and an intracellular, non-infectious, reticulate 'initial body', 800 to 1200 nm in diameter, which does not have a dense nucleoid and is the dividing form (division is by binary fission as with rickettsiae and bacteria). All these organisms are obligatory intracellular parasites, and they are stained by Macchiavello's method. They are cultivated in mice, yolk-sacs of fertile eggs, and in tissue-culture systems. Parasitised cells contain characteristic inclusion bodies, which are microcolonies of the organisms. The *Chlamydiae* are classified into subgroups A and B. In subgroup A the inclusion bodies contain glycogen, and the organisms are sensitive to sulphadiazine and D-cycloserine (as well as tetracycline, to which all chlamydiae are sensitive). The inclusions of subgroup B do not contain glycogen, and the organisms are insensitive to sulphadiazine and only mildly sensitive to D-cycloserine.

Subgroup A chlamydiae, called *Chlamydia trachomatis*,[1] cause 5 eye diseases—hyperendemic trachoma, inclusion conjunctivitis, TRIC ophthalmia neonatorum (neonatal inclusion blennorrhoea), TRIC punctate keratoconjunctivitis, and endemic trachoma—and 2 infections of the genitourinary tract—lymphogranuloma venereum (LVG) and chlamydial urethritis and cervicitis in the male and female respectively. The word TRIC is derived from the first letters of *TR*achoma and *I*nclusion *C*onjunctivitis.

Chlamydia trachomatis includes the following serotypes:
Lymphogranuloma venereum agents 1, 2, and 3.
TRIC agents A, B, and C, generally responsible for hyperendemic trachoma.
TRIC agents D, E, F, G, H, I, J, and K, responsible for the other ocular infections, called collectively *paratrachoma*, and for chlamydial urethritis and cervicitis.

Whereas hyperendemic trachoma is transmitted from eye to eye, paratrachoma is usually associated with chlamydial urethritis and cervicitis,[2] which are the commonest venereal diseases in the developed countries. The infection is transmitted sexually from genital tract to genital tract, and occasionally from genital tract to eye.

TRIC ophthalmia neonatorum is an acute muco-purulent conjunctivitis that is acquired during the infant's passage through the infected birth canal. It may become chronic and lead to corneal pannus and scars. There may be an associated chlamydial pneumonia.[3,4]

The most severe ocular disease of chlamydial origin is *hyperendemic trachoma*, which is responsible for blinding several million people, especially in Africa and Asia. It starts as a chronic conjunctivitis with proliferation of the epithelium and a heavy infiltration of the subepithelial tissue with lymphocytes, macrophages, and ultimately discrete lymphoid follicles so that granular elevations (follicles) are visible on the conjunctiva. The epithelium later undergoes necrosis, and there is scarring of the underlying tissue, so that the lids become distorted by contracture. Ectropion or entropion often follows. Furthermore, the inflammatory process invades the cornea, which becomes ulcerated. The deeper layers are infiltrated by inflammatory cells, and they are progressively vascularised (pannus) and replaced by scar tissue which renders the cornea opaque.

Inclusion conjunctivitis, TRIC punctate keratoconjunctivitis, and *endemic trachoma of sexual transmission*—the adult forms of paratrachoma—are chronic follicular conjunctival infections, usually of acute onset and commonest in young adults.

Eventually follicles develop as in hyperendemic trachoma. In TRIC punctate keratoconjunctivitis there is a subepithelial punctate keratitis consisting of discrete, large infiltrations of lymphocytes and macrophages in the superficial stromal area of the cornea. The epithelium desquamates to leave small ulcers that heal rapidly. In sexually transmitted endemic trachoma corneal pannus and scars develop.

It is apparent that these three conditions are all manifestations of a single disease. Inclusion conjunctivitis has been seen to change to TRIC punctate keratoconjunctivitis and then to a typical picture of trachoma. Furthermore, different conditions may be present in each eye, and trachoma may be associated with subepithelial punctate keratitis.

The treatment of chlamydial ocular infections consists of topical tetracycline or rifampicin eye ointment 3 times a day for 5 to 6 weeks. In paratrachoma, because of the probable associated genital infection, systemic tetracycline or sulphonamide must also be given for 3 weeks.

Lymphogranuloma venereum starts as a small papule or ulcer in the area of the external genitalia which is followed in about a week by regional lymphadenitis, usually of a suppurative nature. There may be systemic effects, such as fever, skin eruptions, arthritis, and generalised lymphadenitis, but the major effect is local destruction of tissue. The female suffers worse than the male, because the female genitalia drain to the perirectal lymph nodes, whereas the male genitalia drain to the inguinal nodes. In the male the destruction of lymph nodes is comparatively superficial and does not usually implicate the large lymphatics draining the lower extremities and genitalia. In the female there is extensive lymphatic destruction with residual lymphoedema of the external genitalia. The end-result may be elephantiasis with ulceration and fibrosis, leading to vaginal stenosis. There is also often rectal stenosis following suppurative destruction and fibrosis of the perirectal lymph nodes. Another complication is squamous-cell carcinoma in the affected area of the external genitalia.

The pathology of the initial lesion is non-specific, but the lymph nodes show a tuberculoid suppurative reaction similar to that of cat-scratch disease.

Subgroup B chlamydiae, called *Chlamydia psittaci*, cause *psittacosis* and *ornithosis* in the human subject, and similar diseases in other animals. These are febrile infections with a predominantly respiratory emphasis. They are acquired by inhaling the infected aerosol or dust from birds which may have been handled as pets or killed and prepared for eating. The incubation period is about 10 days, and the disease may resemble influenza with rapid recovery or else proceed to a severe pneumonia with a typhoid state and death.

The pathological features are those of a severe pneumonia of 'primary atypical' morphology, similar to that found in Q fever. There may be focal necrosis of the liver and spleen.

Mycoplasmas

These organisms are amongst the smallest of the bacteria. They are remarkable in lacking a rigid cell wall and being enclosed by a thin cytoplasmic membrane only. This membrane is rich in lipid, and unlike the membranes of other bacteria, contains cholesterol or carotenol. These organisms are vulnerable to fat solvents. Their morphology varies according to the species: some are small and roughly spherical,

200 to 250 nm in diameter; others are somewhat larger, and there may also be short or long branching filaments. They are Gram-negative, but are stained best with Giemsa's stain. They can be grown on cell-free media; on solid media the colonies are very small and have a 'fried-egg' appearance. The mode of reproduction is by binary fission, but in filamentous species nuclear division may not be synchronous with that of the bacterial cell, so that an appearance of several organisms is found in one cell. These bodies are liberated when the cell disintegrates. Many species of mycoplasmas grow in tissue-culture systems and also in the lung and yolk-sac of chick embryos.

The important human pathogen is *Mycoplasma pneumoniae*, which causes *mycoplasmal pneumonia*, a febrile disease with no localising signs, and in which the radiological features in the chest are out of all proportion to the pulmonary symptoms. Patients have a high titre of autohaemagglutinins (directed against the I antigen widely present in adult red cells) in from 30 to 60 per cent of cases, and agglutinins against *Streptococcus MG* (a non-haemolytic, non-pathogenic variety) in about 15 per cent of cases. These two reactions are due to shared haptens (glycolipids) between the mycoplasma, the streptococcus, and the I antigen of the red cells. The Coombs test and the serological reactions for syphilis may also be positive. All these are autoimmune phenomena following tissue damage by the mycoplasma. The infection responds well to tetracycline.

Other mycoplasmas, e.g. *Mycoplasma hominis* and T-mycoplasmas (T indicates the tiny colonies formed), have been isolated in some cases of genito-urinary infection, but they can be found in the genito-urinary tract of both sexes, and it is doubtful whether they are pathogenic. There is likewise no evidence that these organisms play a role in cancer or rheumatoid arthritis, although they are sometimes cultured from lesions.

Viruses. These are smaller than rickettsiae, but some of them are about the same size as the mycoplasmal organisms; size, therefore, is not an absolute criterion in defining a virus. Like rickettsiae they are obligatory intracellular parasites. The one feature common to all viruses is a conversion to a non-infective form during the process of multiplication; this non-infective 'eclipse phase' is the essential difference between viruses and rickettsiae. Viruses do not possess all the enzyme systems necessary for the synthesis of new viral material; they are therefore dependent on the parasitised cell for survival and multiplication. Indeed, the essential difference between viruses and other organisms is that the synthetic processes that attend multiplication take place within the protoplasm of the infected cell in viruses, but in the body of the organism itself in all other infective agents.

THE PRINCIPLES OF VIROLOGY

PROPERTIES OF TRUE VIRUSES

Size and Shape

Amongst the largest of the true viruses are the pox group responsible for smallpox, vaccinia, and similar diseases in other species of animals. These are between 250 and 300 nm in size, and a single virus particle, or elementary body (called a *Paschen body* in vaccinia), is just visible under the light microscope using special staining techniques, e.g. Gutstein's method.*

The remainder cannot be seen by light microscopy, and therefore other methods of measurement are used.

(*a*) Their size can be assessed by their capacity to pass through specially graded filters. This is rather inaccurate.

(*b*) A more precise method is ultracentrifugation using high-speed centrifuges. The larger the particle, the faster it falls.

(*c*) The most accurate method at present available however, is direct observation under the electron microscope, which is capable of demonstrating objects as small as 0·5 nm in diameter. Electron microscopy has imparted fundamental information about virus size, shape, and chemical configuration. Most viruses are less than 200 nm in size: the herpesvirus group and the viruses of measles and rabies are 120 to 150 nm, the orthomyxovirus group 80 to 120 nm, the adenoviruses 70 to 90 nm, the reoviruses 70 to 80 nm, the togaviruses 30 to 50 nm, the enteroviruses 25 to 35 nm, and the foot-and-mouth disease virus is only 20 to 25 nm.

Many viruses are spherical in shape, e.g. enteroviruses, herpesviruses, and adenoviruses. Some are filamentous, e.g. tobacco-mosaic virus and myxoviruses. Bacteriophage has a characteristic tadpole shape (Fig. 22.1) and poxviruses are brick-shaped.

Chemical Constitution

A single virus particle, alternatively called a *virion* or an *elementary body*, consists basically of a core of a single nucleic acid and a surrounding protein shell called a *capsid*. Plant viruses all contain RNA, whereas nearly all bacteriophages contain DNA. Of the animal viruses affecting human beings, some, e.g. the adenoviruses, poxviruses, herpesviruses, and papovaviruses, contain DNA, whereas others, e.g. the picornaviruses, orthomyxoviruses, paramyxoviruses, togaviruses, and reoviruses, contain RNA.

Most RNA viruses contain a single strand of nucleic acid (reoviruses are an exception), whereas the great majority of DNA viruses contain a double strand of nucleic acid (the parvoviruses, which cause a number of animal diseases but no known human infection, are an exception). It is this nucleic acid that controls the synthesis of new viral material in an infected cell.

The capsid is composed of a specific number of identical subunits called *capsomeres*, which are built up regularly to form a compact mass. Spherical viruses have their capsomeres arranged in the form of a regular solid with 20 equilateral triangular faces. This is called an *icosahedron*, and the symmetry is described as being *cubical* (Figs. 22.2 and 22.3). Rod-shaped, filamentous viruses have their core of nucleic acid in the form of a spiral, and this is invested by a capsid composed of wedge-shaped capsomeres; the nucleocapsid is said to have *helical* symmetry. The tadpole-shaped bacteriophage has a *binal*

---

*This method is admirable for staining Paschen bodies in skin scrapings. The smear is fixed in methyl alcohol and stained with a mixture of methyl violet and sodium carbonate. The Paschen bodies are stained purple.

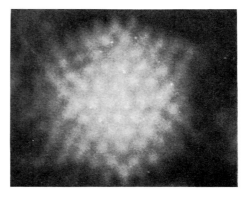

Figure 22.2
A single particle (elementary body) of adenovirus embedded in electron-opaque phosphotungstate. The negatively-stained particle viewed under the electron microscope is seen to be composed of morphological units (capsomeres) of spherical shape packed in a symmetrical arrangement. It has been calculated that the total number of capsomeres around the central core of an adenovirus is 252. × 480 000. (*From Horne, R. W., Brenner, S., Waterson, A. P. and Wildy, P.* (1959), Journal of Molecular Biology, **1**, 84)

Figure 22.1
The bacteriophage particle viewed under the electron microscope after negative staining. The following structures are visible:
  The head, a bipyramidal hexagonal prism. This contains the viral DNA.
  A central rigid core.
  The tail sheath which surrounds the central core. In this picture the sheath is contracted to the upper part of the core. The sheath has a helical symmetry. It is attached to a hexagonal plate structure at the extreme end of the tail—in this picture it is diffuse and unrecognisiable.
  Tail fibres (6 altogether) associated with the plate structure.
  × 300 000. (*From Brenner, S.,* et al. (1959), Journal of Molecular Biology, **1**, 281)

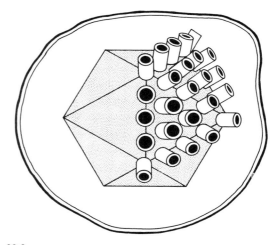

Figure 22.3
Diagrammatic representation of a typical virus showing cubical symmetry. The core of the virus has the form of an icosahedron having 20 facets. It is covered by symmetrically arranged capsomeres, each consisting of a short tube. The covering of capsomeres constitutes the viral capsid. The virion (consisting of the genetic material and the capsid) has an outer membrane that is derived from the altered host plasma membrane or nuclear membrane. Not all such viruses possess an outer membrane. (*Drawing by Frederick Lammerich, Department of Art as Applied to Medicine, University of Toronto.*)

symmetry in its capsid, meaning that it is arranged differently around the head as compared with the tail (see Fig. 22.1).

Some viruses are also ensheathed in one or more outer membranes, or envelopes, composed predominantly of lipid, derived in part from the host cell or nuclear membrane prior to the release of the virus. Enveloped viruses, e.g. herpesviruses, myxoviruses, and togaviruses, are vulnerable to fat solvents such as ether and bile salts. The larger viruses, especially poxviruses, also contain carbohydrates, co-enzymes, and even some enzymes, e.g. lipase, catalase, and phosphatase, but none contains all the enzymes necessary for the metabolism of its own substance. It is for this reason that viruses are obligatory intracellular parasites.

The Life-Cycle and Reproduction

The life-cycle of a virus is intracellular, and the details vary according to the virus, but the basic steps are similar for all viruses.

Attachment. The first step is the attachment of the virus to a specific *cell receptor*, or *receptor site*, on the cell membrane. This appears to be a necessary precursor of penetration and is related to the adsorption of complementary areas of the virus coat on to the cell receptors. Influenza virus attaches to the cell membrane by the action of neuraminidase which combines with mucopolysaccharide on the cell surface. Bacteriophage (Fig. 22.4) attaches by its tail fibres to specific receptor sites on the bacterial wall, which are weakened by a hydrolytic enzyme present in the phage tail.

Figure 22.4
Diagrammatic representation of the entry of bacteriophage into a bacterial cell. The bacteriophage consists of a head containing DNA, a rigid core surrounded by a sheath to which is attached a tail piece, and tail fibres. *A*. The first event in the entry of the phage is the attachment of the tail fibres to the receptors of the bacterial cell wall. *B*. Contraction of the sheath results in the injection of viral DNA into the bacterial cell substance. *C*. The protein component of the phage shown attached to the cell wall is subsequently lost, leaving the viral DNA within the substance of the bacterium. Here it can replicate and lead to lysis of the bacterial cell, or it can remain latent as prophage. (*Drawn by Sue Reynolds.*)

Penetration. With bacteriophage the naked DNA is injected into the interior of the bacterium, while the protein coat, which acts as a microsyringe, remains exterior attached to the bacterial wall. The mode of penetration of animal viruses is different, and both pinocytosis and phagocytosis are involved. With vaccinia virus in tissue cultures, the next step is removal of the protein coat and release of the nucleic acid.

Eclipse phase. Once the nucleic acid has been released it becomes unidentifiable for a few hours. This is the all-important *eclipse phase* characteristic of viruses, and the nucleic acid is not infectious during this period.

It appears that the free nucleic acid is engaged in redirecting the cell's metabolism so that more viral nucleic acid and protein are produced. The eclipse phase takes from 1 to 30 hours. In DNA-containing viruses the DNA directs the formation of mRNA as well as virus-specific enzymes which take part in the formation of new virus material. With RNA-containing viruses the single-stranded RNA appears to act as mRNA. In some instances it directs the formation of DNA (p. 378). It is remarkable that a minute quantity of foreign nucleic acid can so dominate the cellular metabolism that, instead of forming normal cell substance, the cell is perverted into forming large amounts of the virus. This mode of reproduction (or replication) contrasts strongly with the binary fission of higher organisms.

Maturation and replication of the virus. In some viruses, e.g. the adenoviruses, the components are formed in the nucleus, in others e.g. the poxviruses, in the cytoplasm, and in yet others in both cytoplasm and nucleus. When the components are assembled into mature infective virus, they are soon recognisable as elementary bodies and escape from the cell either in a dramatic burst—as with poliovirus—or in a steady release from the cell surface—as with herpesviruses and orthomyxoviruses—or else very tardily after accumulating in the cell, as with adenoviruses.

Enveloped viruses receive an additional coat from a cell membrane (Fig. 22.5). With herpesviruses the envelope is derived from the nuclear membrane; this membrane is not completely normal nuclear membrane, but one that has been modified by the presence of the virus and containing viral type antigens. The orthomyxoviruses incorporate modified cell membrane during the period of release, which takes about an hour. After release the virus enters other cells either by direct contact or after carriage by body fluids.

Some viruses produce globular intracellular masses which are easily visible under the light microscope. These are called *inclusion bodies*. Some, like the intranuclear inclusions of herpesviruses, are formed as a result of cell degeneration. A few, like the inclusions of adenoviruses and reoviruses, are crystalline aggregates of virions. Most are composed of aggregations of developing virus particles bound together in a gelatinous matrix (Fig. 22.6). Unlike *elementary bodies*, which are single mature virus particles, inclusion bodies are large (up to 20 μm in size). Some are acidophilic and others basophilic; some intracytoplasmic and others intranuclear. At one time they were of great moment in the diagnosis of viral disease; nowadays they are mostly of historical interest. Nevertheless, a few are worth noting:

(*a*) *Negri body*, an acidophilic body found in the cytoplasm of neurons in cases of rabies. The hippocampus is particularly involved.

(*b*) *Guarnieri body*, an acidophilic body seen in the cytoplasm of epidermal cells in vaccinia and smallpox.

(*c*) The enormous intranuclear body seen in various parenchymatous cells in *cytomegalic inclusion disease* (Fig. 22.7).

(*d*) The intranuclear bodies found in the epidermal cells in *zoster* and *herpes simplex*, the respiratory mucosal cells in *adenovirus infections*, and the anterior-horn-cell neurons in the later stages of *poliomyelitis*.

The nucleic-acid composition of the virus does not determine whether the inclusion body is intranuclear or intracytoplasmic, or whether the virus is formed predominantly in the cytoplasm or the nucleus.

Reaction to Environment

Unlike bacteria, most viruses are easily inactivated even at room temperature, and care must be taken to keep specimens frozen, if possible at −70°C. A few viruses are much more stable than this, however, and the viruses of poliomyelitis and vaccinia can survive at ordinary atmospheric temperatures for some weeks. The viruses of hepatitis are very resistant to heat (see p. 656), but the most resistant virus is that of scrapie, which withstands boiling for 3 hours.

Reaction of Chemicals

Viruses are rapidly destroyed by disinfectants used against bacteria; the scrapie virus is an exception, surviving in strong formalin solutions. It is noteworthy that viruses are resistant to a 50 per cent solution of glycerol—vaccinia virus is preserved in it—while non-sporing bacteria are killed quite rapidly. Antibiotics and sulphonamides are powerless against viruses, but some chemotherapeutic agents are now known (p. 275).

Inactivation of Viruses

The question of virus destruction is, in fact, less simple

Figure 22.5
Small areas of cytoplasm from HeLa cells infected with herpesvirus. Immature particles can be seen in various stages of budding out through cell membranes, from which they acquire in the process an outer covering, and thus the morphology of the free virus. ×120 000. (*From Epstein, M. A. (1962), Journal of Cell Biology, 12, 589)

than would appear at first sight. If activity is defined as the ability of a single virus particle to multiply in and produce lesions in a cell, there is no doubt that inactivation is quite easily achieved. But inactivated virus can undergo reactivation under certain circumstances. A bacteriophage inactivated by ultraviolet light and then introduced into a bacterium can sometimes be reactivated if the bacterium is exposed to visible light. Again, ultraviolet-light inactivated bacteriophage, ortho-myxoviruses, and poxviruses can sometimes achieve activation if a large dose is introduced into a cell system. This is called *multiplicity reactivation*. The explanation is that the nucleic acid which carries the genetic information of the virus is damaged by ultraviolet light, so that the *genome* (complete set of hereditary factors) is disrupted. If a large number of ultraviolet-light inactivated viruses are in close contact, a common pool of nucleic acids is produced. As these are likely to show different disturbances of their genomes, it is possible for two nucleic acids to mate and constitute an uninjured genome by complementing each other's deficiencies. Another genetic type of reactivation is *cross-reactivation*, in which an

Figure 22.6
Nuclear inclusion induced by adenovirus 12. The virus crystals in the centre are surrounded by very dense material with irregular contours. Many virus particles are dispersed in the nucleoplasm. ×24 000. (*From Bernhard, W. (1964), In 'Cellular Injury', a Ciba Foundation Symposium, p. 215. Edrs de Reuck, A. V. S. and Knight, J. London: Churchill*)

inactivated particle is rendered active by a closely related active virus. The explanation is as described above. It is an example of *recombination* (a phenomenon also described in bacteria and important in the transference of drug resistance).

A non-genetic type of reactivation is seen in the case of heat-inactivated myxoma virus injected into a rabbit with active fibroma virus (both are poxviruses). The animal dies of myxomatosis, and does not develop a fibroma (*Berry-Dedrick phenomenon*). The essential transfer factor is a protein.

Cultivation of Viruses

As viruses multiply only in susceptible living cells, the provision of suitable systems is of great importance. At first the only living systems that could be used were experimental animals and chick embryos. The discovery by Enders and his colleagues in 1949 that the virus of poliomyelitis could proliferate in tissue cultures of non-neuronal origin, e.g. human prepuce, made modern virus research possible. Nowadays the vast majority of viruses are cultivated in tissue culture, a method which is cheap, simple, and efficacious.

(*a*) At present *animal inoculation* is reserved for those viruses which do not grow satisfactorily in tissue culture. Most Coxsackie A viruses do not grow in any cell systems, but when injected into suckling mice produce a characteristic fatal myositis. There is still a place for the use of suckling mice in isolating togaviruses. An intracerebral injection of material from a rabid animal into adult mice produces a characteristic encephalitis. Animal isolation is slow, expensive, and useful for only a limited number of viruses.

(*b*) The *chick embryo* has been a very useful medium for virus cultivation. Orthomyxoviruses can be cultured in the amniotic cells, while the poxviruses and herpes-simplex virus produce characteristic lesions on the chorioallantoic membrane. The fertile egg is used comparatively infrequently in virology nowadays.

(*c*) The method of choice is *tissue culture*. In this technique

Figure 22.7
Cytomegalic inclusion disease. This is a section of the pancreas of an infant who died of this condition. The acinar cells are enormously swollen, and their enlarged nuclei are distended with darkly-staining inclusion bodies, while the remainder of the nuclear chromatin is pushed out to the nuclear membrane. Surrounding these cells there is an inflammatory reaction. ×260.

Figure 22.8
Normal HeLa cells. The confluent sheet is composed of plump, polygonal cells derived from a malignant epithelial cell line. A giant form is conspicuous in the field. (McCarthy phase contrast ×200)

living cells are grown on the sides of test-tubes (see p. 9). Many viruses are able to multiply in the cells, in which they produce destructive changes (*cytopathic effects*). These are sometimes characteristic of a certain virus, but in any case the virus must be accurately identified by complement fixation and neutralisation tests using specific rabbit antisera. If, for instance, a specific antiserum prevents a cytopathic effect in a cell system (or for that matter, if it prevents a lesion in an egg or a test animal), the virus is typed accordingly. The fluid in the tissue culture system provides the virus material, which is also used as the source of antigen for complement fixation tests. The cell systems commonly employed in this way are derived from monkey kidney, human amnion, and strains of cancer cells, e.g. the 'HeLa cell' derived from a carcinoma of the cervix of a woman named *He*len *La*ne. Among the many viruses that can grow in such systems are the enteroviruses, adenoviruses, herpesviruses, and poxviruses (Figs. 22.8–22.10).

Organ culture can be used to cultivate some viruses that do not flourish in cell systems. Thus some rhinoviruses have been isolated in organ cultures of adult and fetal trachea. Some viruses produce damage to the epithelium which can be determined histologically after the culture is fixed. The respiratory syncytial virus and some para-influenza viruses grow in the tracheal cells and cause the cilia to cease moving.

Infectivity

Viruses produce disease even in minute quantities, and their degree of infectivity is so high that epidemics are very common, e.g. smallpox, influenza, and the common viral diseases of childhood.

Viral disease is by no means confined to vertebrates; there are insect infections like silkworm jaundice and sacbrood of bees, plant diseases like tobacco-mosaic disease, and also the

Figure 22.9
HeLa cells infected with adenovirus. The sheet is broken up, and the swollen, refractile cells have fused to form irregular masses. (McCarthy phase contrast ×200)

Figure 22.10
HeLa cells infected with poliovirus. The cells have undergone profound disintegration, so that only a few shrunken survivors are still present. The polioviruses have a much more destructive effect on cell cultures than the adenoviruses. (McCarthy phase contrast ×200)

very important group of bacterial infections due to bacteriophage. Sometimes a viral disease of an animal may be transmitted to a person. A harmful transmission is rabies from a dog, whereas a beneficial one is cow-pox as in the classical Jennerian vaccination technique.

Of the viruses pathogenic to humans many seem to attack one organ specifically, but the once fashionable concept of *tropism* is no longer acceptable. A 'neutrotropic' virus like poliovirus multiplies in the cells of the small intestine, and the 'dermatotropic' virus of herpes simplex can produce encephalitis. It is helpful to enumerate the main viruses pathogenic to human beings in terms of the organ principally attacked:

Viruses attacking the skin: vaccinia, herpes-simplex, varicella-zoster, and the viruses of verruca vulgaris and molluscum contagiosum.

Viruses attacking the central nervous system: enteroviruses, varicella-zoster, rabies, lymphocytic choriomeningitis, arthropod-borne viruses causing encephalitis, mumps, and occasionally herpes simplex, measles, influenza, and vaccinia. A special group are the slow viruses responsible for kuru and related diseases.

Viruses attacking the liver: hepatitis and yellow fever.

Viruses attacking the respiratory tract: orthomyxoviruses, paramyxoviruses, adenoviruses, coronaviruses, and rhinoviruses.

Viruses attacking the conjunctiva: herpesviruses and adenoviruses.

Viruses attacking the salivary glands and other secreting organs: mumps virus and cytomegalovirus.

Generalised viral diseases often producing character- istic skin eruptions: smallpox, measles, rubella, chickenpox, dengue, and some enterovirus infections.

TISSUE REACTIONS TO VIRUSES

The effects of viruses on the tissues of the body all start at a cellular level; viruses are intracellular parasites, and the damage they produce is directed primarily at the cell. This is followed secondarily by a local inflammatory reaction.

Cellular reaction. A cell infected with a virus may die at once, or it may undergo proliferation which may or may not be followed by later necrosis, or it may show no change whatsoever.

This last effect is typical of *latent virus* infection. It is well known, for example, that herpes-simplex virus may remain latent and show no clinical evidence of its presence until an infective episode, e.g. a common cold or an attack of pneumonia, precipitates an attack of herpes febrilis (p. 289). It clears up, and recurs when the precipitating factor operates again. Similarly, many children are infected with certain types of adenoviruses early in life. These remain in their tonsils and adenoids without producing conspicuous lesions, but if such organs are grown in tissue culture, the emerging cells rapidly disintregrate because the virus released is now active and destructive.

Whether a cell undergoes necrosis or proliferation depends on the type of cell involved and on the nature of the infecting virus. Labile cells like those of the epidermis undergo continuous division throughout life, and if infected with virus may exhibit a proliferative tendency, e.g. verruca vulgaris. On the other hand, the foot-and-mouth disease virus causes rapid necrosis of the epidermal cells. Other cells described as permanent, e.g. neurons, cannot divide after birth, and viral infection of these is necessarily always destructive in tendency.

The skin is an organ in which the whole range of changes from rapid necrosis to neoplastic proliferation is seen. In *foot-and-mouth disease* the epidermal cells swell up and undergo rapid necrosis. In *vaccinia, smallpox, zoster, chickenpox*, and *herpes simplex* there is an initial phase of cellular proliferation lasting from 1 to 4 days according to the infection before necrosis occurs. In *fowl-pox* the proliferation is more marked and lasts several weeks before necrosis occurs, whereas in *molluscum contagiosum* and especially *verruca vulgaris* there is a degree of proliferation sufficient to suggest a benign tumour, and the lesion may persist for many months before it involutes spontaneously. The *Shope papilloma of wild cottontail rabbits* exhibits this neoplastic tendency even more clearly, and squamous-cell carcinoma may develop.

It is noteworthy that viral diseases of human beings tend to cause necrosis rather than cell proliferation, apart from the skin lesions mentioned above. There is still no certain causal relationship between a virus and a human neoplasm, comparable with the viral tumours of animals. The primarily necrotising tendency of human viral disease is seen in the way the respiratory viruses, especially those of influenza, destroy the surface epithelium, the viruses of hepatitis and yellow fever produce liver-cell necrosis, mumps virus and the cytomegalovirus lead to cellular destruction of the salivary and other exocrine glands, and the polioviruses and some togaviruses cause permanent neuronal loss as a result of poliomyelitis and encephalitis respectively.

Once the infection is overcome there is rapid regeneration due to proliferation of neighbouring cells. The focal necrosis of virus A hepatitis heals so rapidly that needle biopsy of the liver performed after a few months may reveal no abnormality whatsoever. Neuronal destruction can be healed only by gliosis, and hence permanent paralysis, or sensory loss in zoster, must sometimes be expected. However, not every neuron infected with poliovirus is doomed. Many recover completely after undergoing the degenerative change of chromatolysis (disappearance of Nissl granules from the cytoplasm).

Inflammatory reaction. Secondary to the cellular damage (and sometimes to allergy) there is an acute inflammatory reaction in the vicinity. This consists of vascular dilatation and an exudate containing moderate numbers of lymphocytes and macrophages. Polymorphs are scanty except in superficial skin lesions like smallpox and herpes simplex, where they are present even before secondary bacterial infection complicates the picture.

Viral disease of the central nervous system, typified by poliomyelitis, is accompanied by an active phagocytosis of neuronal debris by macrophages, some of which are mobilised microglial cells. This is called 'neuronophagia'. In the vicinity the blood vessels are dilated, and there is a heavy small round cell infiltration. This also accumulates around small blood vessels, especially those under the meninges, and is called 'perivascular cuffing'; it is by no means diagnostic of viral infection, occurring also in cerebral syphillis and tuberculous meningitis. Most of these cells are lymphocytes and macrophages, but sometimes a few polymorphs are also present.

Similarly the focal necrosis of viral hepatitis is accompanied by a moderate small round cell infiltration, not so much in the area of damage as in the portal tracts.

One of the few viral diseases that produces a diagnostic lesion is measles. There is generalised lymphoid hyperplasia, most marked in the tonsils and appendix. In the midst of the active germinal centres there are characteristic giant cells with bunched-up, hyperchromatic nuclei. These are called *Warthin-Finkeldey giant cells*, and are pathognomonic of measles (Fig. 22.11).

Viral infection of epithelial surfaces is usually complicated by secondary bacterial infection, and this is accompanied by a pyogenic reaction.

Many of the common viral infections run an acute course, either terminating in rapid death or else being followed by complete recovery. However, there are a number of chronic viral diseases. One example is the group of oncogenic viral infections in animals (to which the much milder human molluscum contagiosum and verruca vulgaris can be added). Another example is the progressive neurological disease associated with slow viruses and recrudescent measles and varicella-zoster viruses. A third is virus B hepatitis proceeding to chronic hepatitis and cirrhosis.

It is noteworthy that viral infections, even the chronic ones, do not bring forth a predominantly macrophage response. Epithelioid-cell formation is never seen, nor indeed is any viral infection characterised by a granulomatous reaction.

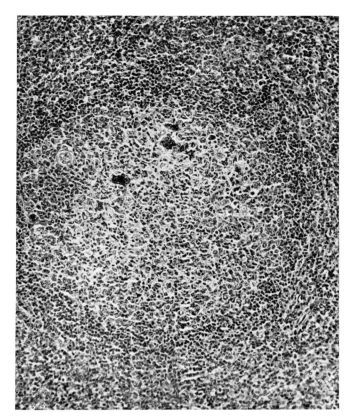

Figure 22.11
Lymphoid hyperplasia in measles. The germinal centre is enlarged, and amid the palely-staining lymphoblasts there are several giant cells with crowded, darkly-staining nuclei. These hyperchromatic Warthin-Finkeldey giant cells are typical of measles. × 150.

THE GENERAL BODY REACTION TO VIRAL INFECTION

Localisation. Like all foreign organisms viruses first contaminate and infect a surface integument, either by inoculation (e.g. vaccinia), or by ingestion (e.g. poliomyelitis), or by inhalation (e.g. influenza), or by the bite of an arthropod vector (e.g. yellow fever). Some viruses remain localised to their tissues of entry, e.g. that of verruca vulgaris and rhinoviruses, whereas others become disseminated throughout the blood stream and produce lesions in an organ remote from the sites of primary infection, e.g. poliomyelitis and yellow fever, or else lead to a generalised infection involving many organs, e.g. smallpox and measles. The systemic type of infection is associated with much more pronounced constitutional symptoms than is the localised one, and a characteristic feature is the presence of high fever during the early viraemic phase followed by a remission, which is then succeeded by another spurt of pyrexia when the virus becomes clinically fixed at its organ of destination. Localised diseases like upper respiratory tract and eye infections cause little constitutional upset. Systemic viral infection is associated with leucopenia during the prodromal period. Once the typical lesion appears (e.g. the eruption in smallpox or jaundice in hepatitis) the white-cell count returns to normal, and there may be a moderate neutrophil leucocytosis.

Dissemination. The mode of dissemination of a virus in the body has been investigated in mouse-pox. This virus enters the mouse's body through an abrasion on its skin, and multiplies there. Within 8 hours the virus reaches the local lymph nodes, from where after further multiplication it invades the blood stream* and is taken up by the RE cells of the liver and spleen. There it multiplies once more, invades the blood stream in large amounts, and settles selectively in the epidermal cells of the skin. This process takes about 6 days; still another 4 days elapse before the skin eruption appears. Before this, however, inclusion bodies can be demonstrated in these cells.

The 6 days prior to final skin localisation constitute the *incubation period*, and the 4 days of severe illness, which may prove fatal in overwhelming infections, are the *prodromal period*. During this time the virus may still be cultured from the blood, but once the eruption appears there is a rapidly rising level of neutralising antibody in the circulation. Human diseases like smallpox and measles probably have a somewhat similar pattern of dissemination, but the route of infection is apparently through the respiratory tract.

Transplacental infection of the fetus is important in rubella infections and in addition may lead to congenital abnormalities (p. 290). The other generalised viral diseases in the mother do not appear to be teratogenic, but it may be that they kill the fetus, and the subsequent abortion is dismissed as 'inevitable'. Other viral diseases that may be transmitted across the placenta are cytomegalic inclusion disease, Coxsackie myocarditis of the newborn, herpes infection, and vaccinia. In mice the lymphocytic choriomeningitis virus is likewise transmitted transplacentally.

Antibody response. Viral infections are accompanied by a high titre of immunoglobulins during the period of convalescence. The highest antibody response is encountered in those viruses which are widely disseminated in the circulation, and a life-long *immunity* may be expected after poliomyelitis, smallpox, measles, and mumps. Localised infections, like the common cold, herpes simplex, and verruca vulgaris, also induce antibodies, but probably because the virus does not enter the blood stream in large amounts, the degree of immunity is small and recurrence is common. Some viruses, e.g. adenoviruses and rhinoviruses, have many serotypes, and these add to the tendency to recurrent upper respiratory-tract infections.

Allergy is also noteworthy in viral infections. The accelerated reaction following a second vaccination is a good example. The lesion appears within a day or two and resolves after about a week, whereas a primary vaccination reaction appears only on the fourth or fifth day and reaches its zenith on about the tenth day. It takes about 3 weeks to heal, and is occasionally complicated by systemic lesions. The close resemblance of this to the Koch phenomenon is obvious, except that here the immunity is much greater than in tuberculosis. There is a strong allergic element in the exanthem that occurs in the course of generalised infections like smallpox and measles. In these there is an incubation period of about a fortnight, and it seems likely that the skin is sensitised to viral

---

*This stage corresponds to the primary bacteraemia of typhoid fever. The next stage of blood-borne spread corresponds to septicaemia.

products before the virus reaches it in full force. The analogy to the later intestinal ulceration of typhoid fever is very close.

There are certain occasions when antiviral antibody appears to augment the damage inflicted by a virus. Thus lymphocytic choriomeningitis virus produces a very severe disease in normal adult mice: many die, but the survivors have a permanent immunity to the virus. On the other hand, neonatal or fetal mice, or adults who have been given X-irradiation or glucocorticoids, or have been subjected to neonatal thymectomy, when similarly infected get a symptomless condition and may indeed develop tolerance. Thus delayed hypersensitivity has been invoked as the major cause of the effects of this virus. In postvaccinal encephalomyelitis the immune response also appears to be involved, since the condition occurs late in the course of the vaccination reaction. Another important example concerns respiratory syncytial virus infection; the presence of IgG antibody augments the damage caused by the virus to the lower respiratory tract. Specific immunoglobulins may be detrimental in another way: viral antigen acting in excess with antibody can be the cause of some immune-complex reactions (p. 181).

The pathogenic effects of viruses. Viruses produce their harmful effects by virtue of the cell destruction they cause; no factors comparable with bacterial toxins have been demonstrated. The cytotoxic effect of viruses is due in part to complex biochemical disturbances that accompany virus replication. The cause of death in acute virus disease is obvious enough when vital organs are damaged, e.g. the liver in hepatitis, and the central nervous system in poliomyelitis and encephalitis. In the pox diseases the mode of death is less easily explained. Clinically there is 'shock' reminiscent of the toxaemia of invasive bacterial infections, and it is suggested that this is due to viral invasion and damage of vascular endothelial cells.

In addition, viruses can also cause tissue damage by immunological means, as described above. Chronic virus infection has its own pathological spectrum (see p. 273).

IMMUNITY TO VIRAL INFECTIONS

The mechanism of immunity to viral infection is complex and has several components.

(*a*) **Immunoglobulins** play an important part. Viruses have a number of antigens, some associated with the nucleoprotein and others with the capsid and outer envelope. It is against these last two antigens that immunoglobulins act; by neutralising them they prevent the virus attaching itself to a cell receptor. The extracellular complex is phagocytosed and destroyed. Intracellular virus is invulnerable to antibody.

The classes of antibody that act against viruses are IgG and IgA; in the circulation the virus-neutralising antibodies are IgG, whereas the antibodies in the secretions that prevent infection of the mucous membranes belong to class IgA (see p. 144). In this respect it is noteworthy that an attack of poliomyelitis or the administration of the oral vaccine confers a local intestinal immunity as well as a circulating one, whereas the parenteral vaccine has no effect on the local proliferation of the virus, but merely intercepts it when it has become systematised. This is because the live oral virus, whether virulent or attenuated, stimulates IgA as well as IgG, whereas the dead parenteral vaccine stimulates only IgG. A similar state of affairs holds for viral infections of the respiratory tract, except that in this situation IgA is more immediately important than IgG, because the effects of these viruses are more localised than are those of the enteroviruses.

(*b*) **Cell-mediated immunity** plays an even more important role in viral infections than do the immunoglobulins. Thus in states of pure immunoglobulin deficiency (hypogammaglobulinaemia) there is usually an effective host response to systemic viral infections, whereas in states of T lymphocyte deficiency chronic, progressive, fatal viral infections, e.g. vaccinia, chickenpox, herpes simplex, and cytomegalic inclusion disease, are extremely common. The part the lymphocyte plays in viral infection is still obscure. It is known that a sensitised lymphocyte secretes interferon among the lymphokines; in addition, it is possible that the lymphocyte destroys the virus-infected cell directly, thereby killing intracellular virus.

(*c*) **Interferon.** The interferons are a family of antiviral proteins varying in molecular weight from 20 000 to 160 000 daltons which are produced by cells infected with a virus. This protein is non-toxic and non-antigenic to the host (and only feebly antigenic to other species), and has a remarkable effect in making the cells resistant to further viral infection. It 'interferes' with the proliferation of a second virus in the affected cell, and this effect has a very broad spectrum of activity. Inactivated virus is as effective in stimulating interferon production as is living virus. Interferon can be produced in many tissue culture systems, but its action is specific for the animal from which it was derived. There can be little doubt that it is important in checking the course of many viral infections. Whether it plays any part in the acquired cellular immunity of viral disease is uncertain. The administration of glucocorticoids inhibits the production and action of interferon; pyrexia, on the other hand, stimulates it. Interferon is thought to act by inhibiting the translation of viral mRNA. This it does not directly, but by inducing the formation of a second cellular protein called translation-inhibitory protein. Translation of host-cell mRNA is not interrupted; this explains why interferon is non-toxic.

Interferon is potentially an important therapeutic agent, and there have recently been a few encouraging reports of its use in human disease. Unfortunately the active interferon for such investigations must come from a primate source, preferably human. It has also been found that many substances other than live virus induce the formation of interferon. Among these are some bacteria, rickettsiae, mycoplasmas, malarial parasites, and *Toxoplasma gondii*. A few chemicals are also active, notably bacterial endotoxin and phytohaemagglutinin. None of these could be used therapeutically because of their toxicity. Two products of fungal fermentation called *helenine* and *statolon* (derived from *Penicillium funiculosum* and *Penicillium stoloniferum* respectively) are powerful interferon inducers, and in both the active principle is a double-stranded RNA molecule, which is a fungal virus. Synthetic double-stranded RNA molecules are also important interferon inducers; the most effective is a complex of polyinosinic acid and polycytidylic acid called *poly I:C*. These agents have given promising results in animal viral infections, but their effect in the human subject is still under trial. It should be noted that interferon is not only actively formed by cells, but can also be released preformed from lymphocytes and possibly RE cells. This method of promoting interferon formation seems better than the administration of extraneous interferon, but it must be instituted about a day before the infection starts.

Chemotherapy of Viral Diseases

Virus multiplication is so intimately bound up with normal cell metabolism that the possibility of finding effective chemotherapeutic agents seemed remote a few years ago. This gloomy forecast has proved to be ill founded and a number of effective agents have been discovered. Unfortunately many of them are unsuitable for systemic use in human beings, but there is every indication that new, less toxic agents will be found.

Chemotherapeutic agents may act at any stage in the lifecycle of the virus from its initial attachment to the cell to the final stage of assembly of mature virus particles and their subsequent release. Some agents appear to act at different or several stages according to the particular viral infection. The following account must therefore be regarded as provisional.

Interference with virus entry into cells. *Amantadine* (*α-adamantanamine*) inhibits the penetration of influenza virus in tissue culture and in mice. Preliminary trials in human subjects indicate that it can prevent contacts from developing clinical influenza. The main side-effect is somnolence.

Inhibition of replication of viral nucleic acids. Some agents may block the formation of viral nucleic acid for viral replication, the formation of mRNA, or in the RNA oncogenic viruses, the production of viral DNA.

5-Iodo-2'-deoxyuridine (*IUDR*, *5-IDU*, or *Idoxuridine*) has two actions. It inhibits the enzyme thymidic acid synthetase which converts deoxyuridilic acid to thymidilic acid, which is necessary for DNA synthesis. In addition, 5-IDU is incorporated into DNA instead of thymidine to produce a non-functional DNA. This is an example of Peters's lethal synthesis (p. 47). The drug inhibits the growth of vaccinia and herpes-simplex viruses *in vitro*. It has been used in herpetic encephalitis, but its toxicity is a grave disadvantage. Locally 5-IDU finds its greatest use in the treatment, and prevention of spread, of herpes-simplex infection of the cornea (dendritic ulcers).

Cytosine arabinoside (*cytarabine*) is another nucleoside analogue which acts on DNA-core viruses. It has been tried with some success in severe, progressive, herpes-simplex and varicella-zoster infections and in congenital cytomegalovirus infections. Like 5-IDU it is too toxic to be a useful systemic agent except in desperate situations.

2-(α-hydroxybenzyl) benzimidazole (*HBB*) is active against picornaviruses and inhibits viral RNA synthesis. It is less active in the intact animal and has not been used clinically.

Inhibition of synthesis of viral proteins. *N-methylisatin β-thiosemicarbazone* (*methisazone* or *marboran*) inhibits the formation of viral protein necessary for completing the assembly of viral particles. It is active against smallpox, and its administration prevents the development of clinical disease in contacts; when once the disease has developed, methisazone is much less effective. It has also been tried in vaccinia gangrenosa and eczema vaccinatum. Toxic effects include vomiting, skin eruptions, and jaundice.

Rifampicin is a derivative of rifamycin. Both drugs are used in the treatment of tuberculosis and leprosy, and are relatively non-toxic. Rifampicin is effective against a number of viruses and appears to act at various points; with vaccinia virus it interferes with the final assembly of viral particles. It also inhibits DNA-dependent RNA polymerase. Another derivative, N-demethylrifampicin, inhibits RNA-dependent DNA polymerase in RNA oncogenic viruses, and is therefore being studied as a possible agent in cancer chemotherapy.

Interferon and the *interferon inducing agents* have been described on page 275.

THE DIAGNOSIS OF VIRAL DISEASE[5,6]

In only a few viral infections can the agent be demonstrated in the lesions by the presence of typical inclusion bodies, e.g. rabies and cytomegalic inclusion disease, or by characteristic histological features, as for example the measles giant cell.

Electron microscopy is playing an increasing role in the rapid identification of viral particles from infected material. With negative contrast techniques virus may be detected within a few minutes of collecting the specimen, provided it is present at concentrations greater than about 10^6 per ml. For practical purposes this limits its use to examining specimens obtained from readily accessible sites which contain high concentrations of virus, e.g. poxviruses and herpesviruses from skin lesions (Fig. 23.1, p. 279) and rotaviruses, adenoviruses, and hepatitis A virus from the faeces. The technique of immune-electron microscopy can distinguish between antigenically distinct but morphologically identical viruses; it consists of the detection of immune complexes after the specimen has been pre-incubated with a virus-specific antiserum.

Immunofluorescence techniques are also valuable in the rapid diagnosis of viral disease, and they are more sensitive than electron microscopy especially now that the quality of the reagents is satisfactory enough to minimise the amount of non-specific fluorescence. They are particularly useful in examining brain material for herpes-simplex virus and rabies virus and nasopharyngeal secretions for respiratory viruses. Measles antigen may be detected in the ciliated epithelial cells as well as the multinucleate giant cells present in the nasopharyngeal secretions. This technique is far more sensitive and reliable than isolating measles virus in cell culture.

An important diagnostic procedure is the isolation of the virus from the patient's secretions using the living cell systems already described. The virus may then be typed by means of complement fixation and neutralisation tests using specific rabbit antisera.

In convalescent patients there is invariably a rise in titre of antibodies against the agent, and these too may be demonstrated by complement fixation, haemagglutination inhibition, and neutralisation tests against the specific viruses. It is important to collect a specimen of the patient's serum during the acute phase so that a rise in antibody titre can be recognised. The greatest rise is encountered in systemic infections like smallpox, mumps, measles, and poliomyelitis. In clinical practice it may be difficult to isolate the causal virus from the patient or his secretions during the acute phase, because it is often so evanescent that no virus is demonstrable by the time the clinician's attention is drawn to the necessity of searching for it.

It follows that retrospective diagnosis made on serological grounds is still the most important clinical method of diagnosing viral disease.

GENERAL READING

CRUICKSHANK, R., DUGUID, J. P., MARMION, B. P. & SWAIN, R. H. A. (1973) *General Microbiology*, 12th edn. Edinburgh: Churchill Livingstone. Chapters 50 to 52 give an account of rickettsiae, chlamydiae, and mycoplasmas. Chapters 12 to 14 give an account of the general properties of viruses. All of Part III is devoted to a detailed account of viral diseases.

FENNER, F. J. & WHITE, D. O. (1976) *Medical Virology*, 2nd edn, 487 pp. London: Academic Press. This is a good working account of viral disease from a clinical as well as a microbiological point of view.

WILSON, G. S. & MILES, A. A. (1975) In *Topley and Wilson's Principles of Bacteriology, Virology and Immunity*, 6th edn, Vol. 1, pp. 1195 to 1247; Vol. 2, pp. 2343 to 2603. London: Arnold. Volume 1 is devoted to the microbiological aspects and volume 2 to the clinical implications.

REFERENCES

1. Leading Article (1977). Chlamydial infections of the eye. *Lancet*, **2**, 857.
2. McCORMACK, W. M. (1975) Aetiology of nongonococcal urethritis. *New England Journal of Medicine*, **292**, 1239.
3. Leading Article (1977) Chlamydia trachomatis and the respiratory tract. *Lancet*, **1**, 787.
4. HAMMERSCHLAG, M. R. (1978) Chlamydial pneumonia in infants. *New England Journal of Mediciene*, **298**, 1083.
5. Leading Article (1975) Rapid diagnosis in virus diseases. *Lancet*, **1**, 1411.
6. Leading Article (1976) Rapid identification of virus infections. *British Medical Journal*, **2**, 601.

Chapter 23.   Viral Infections of Human Beings

It is useful to consider some pathogenic viruses briefly with special reference to their mode of infectivity, their spread in the body, and methods that may be employed in producing active immunity against them.

ENTEROVIRUS INFECTIONS

The enteroviruses are a group of small, spherical, single-stranded, RNA-containing viruses found particularly in the cells of the intestine. They are members of a larger group called the *picornaviruses* (pico = small + RNA), to which the foot-and-mouth disease virus of cattle and the rhinoviruses that cause the common cold also belong. The enteroviruses are especially associated with neurological diseases. There are three subgroups:

The polioviruses, of which there are three types. These cause poliomyelitis.

The Coxsackie viruses were first isolated in the town of Coxsackie in New York State in 1948. Some can be grown in tissue-culture systems. All are pathogenic to suckling mice and two groups are recognised by the lesions they produce. Group A (24 types) produce a fulminating myositis, while group B (6 types) attack the brown fatty tissue, the nervous system, and to a lesser extent muscle. Coxsackie A viruses are frequently found in the faeces of healthy children, but there are no normal carriers of Coxsackie B viruses.

Diseases caused by Coxsackie A viruses

(*a*) *Herpangina*, a febrile disease of childhood in which the mouth and fauces are the seat of shallow, greyish ulcers.

(*b*) *An upper respiratory, cold-like condition.* The virus responsible is the Coe virus (Coxsackie A21), so named after the first patient from whom it was isolated.

(*c*) *Hand-foot-and-mouth disease*, caused by Coxsackie A16, usually occurring in children in whom bullae develop on the parts mentioned in the name, and a maculopapular eruption appears on the buttocks. Usually there is no fever. It is not to be confused with foot-and-mouth disease, which rarely affects the human being; the bullae are larger and the constitutional disturbance is more severe.

Other macular or maculopapular exanthemata are seen in outbreaks of both A and B strain viruses.

Diseases caused by Coxsackie B viruses.

(*a*) *Epidemic myalgia*, also called *epidemic pleurodynia* and *Bornholm disease*, because it was first described in the Danish island of Bornholm. It is characterised by fever and agonising pains in the chest and abdomen.

(*b*) *Neonatal myocarditis* and *pericarditis*, a fatal condition, transmitted to the fetus by the mother. In adults *acute pericarditis* may occur.

(*c*) Cases of *lymphocytic meningitis* (aseptic meningitis) and *paralysis mimicking poliomyelitis* are caused by Coxsackie B and

some A strains. They may occur in epidemics. Severe *necrotising encephalitis* is a rare event.

The ECHO (Enteric, Cytopathogenic, Human, Orphan) viruses, of which there are at least 34 types. They are found quite commonly in children's faeces, and for a long time they could not be associated with any disease, hence the name 'orphan' (a virus in search of a disease). Many have now found their parents, and it is known that they can produce:

(*a*) *Aseptic meningitis* and *paralysis* similar to the Coxsackie viruses.

(*b*) *An epidemic febrile disease*, sometimes accompanied by meningoencephalitis. It is often associated with a diffuse maculopapular rash. Viruses incriminated are ECHO types 9, 16, and 18.

(*c*) *Acute haemorrhagic conjunctivitis.*[1] This has occurred in epidemics in many African and Asian countries, with a small outbreak in England. The agent is an enterovirus of a distinctive character, best included among the ECHO group until it is further classified. Neurological complications may occur after infections with this agent, which is tentatively called the AHC virus.

(*d*) *Acute respiratory disease* of a cold-like nature.

(*e*) *Diarrhoea.* The association is unproven, since ECHO viruses are often found in healthy children's faeces.

This group grows in monkey kidney cell culture, but is not pathogenic to mice.

Poliomyelitis is caused by the three types of polioviruses, of which type 1 produces the most severe disease. It is also the commonest of the three types of infection in unimmunised populations. The disease follows the ingestion of material that has been contaminated by virus-containing faeces, e.g. water from swimming-baths or for drinking, and also food exposed to house flies. Indirect contact with excretors, whose dirty hands contaminate fomites, is another source of infection. The mode of transmission is similar to that of typhoid fever.

Spread in the body. The virus proliferates first in the cells of the pharynx and the lower part of the small bowel.

If it is not arrested at this stage, it enters the general circulation *via* the lymphatics, and it then multiplies in various extraneural sites like the spleen and kidneys. This marks the end of the incubation period, which usually lasts 7 to 14 days, but may extend up to 30 days. The viraemic phase is accompanied by a febrile reaction, and even at this stage the infection may be overcome.

If the condition proceeds, the virus settles finally in the central nervous system which it reaches by the blood stream. It localises itself specifically in the anterior horn cells and their medullary counterparts, and paralysis ensues.

A second mode of spread is directly up the peripheral nerve endings of the bowel and especially the pharynx. Opinions vary about the importance of this method of spread; it probably accounts for the bulbar type of disease that sometimes follows tonsillectomy.

It is evident that many people can be infected with poliovirus, and either show no illness at all or else have a mild febrile reaction. Only a small unlucky minority develop paralysis. Poliomyelitis is an excellent example of an infection that tends to be subclinical.

Factors aggravating the disease. The incubation period is shortened, and the liability to nervous-system involvement increased by the following factors: heavy exercise and fatigue, pregnancy, operative procedures, and active immunisation. When the disease follows immunisation it is called *provocation poliomyelitis*; it is believed that alum and other adjuvants in the vaccines and toxoids are the important factors. The pathogenesis is unknown, but it has been suggested that the focus of inflammation acts as a nidus for proliferation of the virus during the period of viraemia. It might then travel up the local nerve to the spinal cord. The incidence of provocation poliomyelitis is about 1 per 37 000 inoculations. Active immunisation procedures should be postponed during a poliomyelitis epidemic.

Excretion of virus. Faecal excretion of virus usually precedes the advent of symptoms by a few days, and it is usually present during the first two weeks of paralytic manifestations. After about 6 weeks only a quarter of patients still excrete the virus, and by 12 weeks excretion has usually ceased. Permanent carriage is unknown. The virus can be isolated from the throat just before and after the onset of symptoms. It cannot usually be isolated from the cerebrospinal fluid.

Infectivity. Poliovirus is remarkable for its narrow range of host infectivity; only primates are readily susceptible. Fortunately the virus flourishes with consummate ease in the usual tissue-culture systems, and it is from these that effective vaccines have been developed. A consideration of poliomyelitis immunisation is valuable as a general exercise in comparing the relative merits of dead suspensions to those of live, attenuated viruses.

Active immunisation. The first effective vaccine was devised by Salk, who used polioviruses grown in monkey-kidney cells and subsequently inactivated by formolisation. It was issued in trivalent form, and required at least three intramuscular inoculations, the second a month after the first and the third about 6 months after the second. A high titre of circulating immunoglobulin was produced, though often there was a disappointing response to type-1 virus, the most dangerous of the three. Immunity depended on the presence of IgG antibody. The resistance of the small bowel to subsequent infection by polioviruses was not altered.

Later Sabin produced a vaccine consisting of living, attenuated strains of poliovirus which had undergone mutation after passage through monkey-kidney cell cultures. These attenuated viruses are given orally, and the infection closely simulates the natural disease except that spread does not occur to the nervous system. The immunity produced depends not only on IgG but also on IgA present in the intestinal secretions, as has already been discussed. Two important drawbacks are (a) that the viruses might not enter the bowel cells. This might be due to one virus (notably type 2) interfering with the entry of the others, or to other enteroviruses or adenoviruses preventing the entry of all the attenuated viruses, or even more important to repeated attacks of infantile gastroenteritis preventing the virus settling in the small bowel. This last snag is of great moment in the tropics; (b) that these viruses, which show a great tendency to undergo mutation in the alimentary tract, might revert to a virulent type, and after excretion infect other people in the vicinity with poliomyelitis. It has been proved that these excreted viruses may be more virulent to monkeys than the original vaccine.

In practice it has been found that any interfering tendency is obviated by giving several doses of trivalent vaccine. There is no doubt that any attenuated viruses and their variants, which are excreted in the faeces, will readily infect other people.

Large populations have been adventitiously immunised in this way, and there are no reports of subsequent epidemics of poliomyelitis among these groups. Nevertheless, it seems that a certain amount of poliomyelitis at present in Britain is due to vaccine strains that have reverted to a degree of virulence.[2] This is induced from three findings: (a) type 1 virus is giving place to types 2 and 3; (b) there are fewer cases of paralysis in those patients with neurological disease; and (c) the recently isolated strains lack the ability to grow at temperatures above 37°C. This tendency for live virus vaccine to spread to other people in the vicinity of the person who has been immunised is peculiar to poliovirus. Other live vaccines, e.g. those of measles and rubella do not behave in this way, and vaccinia virus spreads only in people with widespread skin disease.

Despite this warning, there can be no doubt that the amount of poliomyelitis is very much less now than it was before the days of active immunisation. Furthermore, virulent wild strains of poliovirus have been replaced by much less dangerous organisms derived from vaccine strains.

The oral vaccine has supplanted the inactivated one because it gives a better, long-lasting immunity and it acts more rapidly in a threatened epidemic. Despite its general safety it should not be given within three weeks of tonsillectomy or any immunisation procedure. It is a trivalent vaccine and is given in three doses at monthly intervals.

A last consideration concerns the monkey kidney tissue on which the polioviruses are cultured. It has been known to harbour commensal simian viruses, and some of these are resistant even to formalin treatment. In the past, batches of vaccine have been contaminated with these simian viruses. Though no human disease has so far been attributed to these particular viruses, they must be regarded with concern when live vaccine is given; one at least is oncogenic to baby hamsters (see p. 377). The use of human cells would obviate this danger, but unfortunately these are more difficult to assemble in a large quantity, and they soon die out in repeated cultures. Exceptions are the strains of cancer cells, e.g. HeLa cells, but it would be unwise to use them for human vaccine production. At present diploid lines of human cells derived from fetal tissues are being investigated; some can undergo up to 50 subcultures before dying.

POXVIRUS INFECTIONS

The poxviruses are a group of large, brick-shaped, double-stranded, DNA-containing viruses. The capsid has a complex

Figure 23.1
A poxvirus particle. This is vaccinia virus from a case of eczema vaccinatum. Note the complex symmetry of the capsid. Variola virus has a similar appearance. (Negatively stained with phosphotungstate ×400 000). (*Photograph by courtesy of Dr T. H. Flewett*)

symmetry (Fig. 23.1). This group produces vesicular skin lesions, and the affected cells contain large intracytoplasmic inclusion bodies. Many animals have their own variety of pox disease, e.g. *cow-pox*, *mouse-pox*, and *fowl-pox*. The important human disease is *smallpox*. *Molluscum contagiosum*, a skin condition consisting of pearly, elevated papules containing a curd-like material, is also included in the pox group.

Smallpox and vaccinia. There are two closely related viruses that cause smallpox, the classical *variola major* virus, and the virus causing the milder disease *alastrim*, or *variola minor*.

Smallpox is acquired by the inhalation of infected particles from a patient directly or from fomites indirectly. The bedding is particularly dangerous, and numerous instances are on record where laundry workers have contracted the disease from contaminated bedclothes.

Spread in the body. It is believed that a primary lesion may actually occur in the nasal mucosa, and that this is followed by systemic spread to the RE system. This is followed in turn by a phase of secondary viraemia, in the course of which the virus finally settles in the skin and produces the typical intra-epidermal vesicle. At an early stage Guarnieri bodies are present in the epidermal cells, and the characteristic elementary bodies (Paschen bodies) can be demonstrated in large numbers in the vesicles, pustules, and their crusts (Fig. 23.1). The incubation period is from 10 to 14 days, and virus can

usually be demonstrated in the blood during the first 2 days of the prodromal period (which lasts 4 days). The patient is infectious only when the characteristic eruption appears, and remains so until desquamation is complete.

The viruses of variola major and alastrim are so similar that only painstaking tests can differentiate them, yet alastrim is a much milder disease with a mortality rate of under 1 per cent.

Variola virus produces characteristic pocks on the chorioallantoic membranes of fertile eggs. Its host range is very narrow; only primates develop typical smallpox lesions.

Active immunisation. The first really effective attempt at smallpox immunisation was performed by Edward Jenner, who discovered that the natural pox infection of bovine animals, *cow-pox*, could produce a similar lesion in human beings, and protect them against smallpox infection.

Since then a third virus has emerged, *vaccinia virus*. Its origin is obscure. It is believed to be a mutant of either variola or cow-pox viruses; probably most strains used nowadays were originally derived from cow-pox. It resembles cow-pox virus closely, not only morphologically and antigenically (the differences between the two in these respects are infinitesimal), but also in the disease it produces and the immunity it affords against smallpox. Cow-pox vesicles are more bloodstained than those of vaccinia. In fact, the viruses of smallpox, vaccinia, and cow-pox are separate though closely related. The lesions they produce on the chorio-allantoic membrane of the fertile egg are quite distinct.

Vaccinia virus produces lesions in many animals, and the strains used prophylactically are passed through calves and rabbits. A sequence recommended is calf-rabbit-calf-child-calf-rabbit, etc.

The dangers of vaccination, apart from local bacterial infection and later keloid formation, are:

(*a*) *Eczema vaccinatum*. This may vary from the presence of a few discrete lesions on the skin to a widely disseminated confluent eruption with a 30 to 40 per cent mortality rate. It occurs in subjects with a pre-existing skin disease, particularly atopic dermatitis, and is one variety of *Kaposi's varicelliform eruption*, the other being *eczema herpeticum*, in which a herpes-simplex virus infection is superimposed on a pre-existing skin disease.

(*b*) *Generalised vaccinia*. In this condition multiple skin lesions occur as a result of blood-borne spread. It is self limiting and responds well to immune-globulin therapy.

(*c*) *Progressive vaccinia* (*vaccinia gangrenosa*). In this condition the lesion does not heal, but continues to spread until large areas of skin are involved (Fig. 23.2). It is particularly liable to occur in patients with T-lymphocyte deficiency. It is usually fatal after several months.

(*d*) *Postvaccinal encephalomyelitis*. This usually occurs 12 to 14 days after vaccination and has a 50 per cent death rate. There is marked demyelination around blood vessels. Opinions vary as to whether it is due to the virus (which cannot be isolated from the brain), or a second latent virus, or to allergy.

(*e*) *Vaccinial osteitis*, a rare complication, mimicking pyogenic osteomyelitis.

(*f*) *Congenital vaccinia*. A fatal, generalised infection has occurred in fetuses whose mothers were vaccinated early in pregnancy. The first trimester is the dangerous period.

Figure 23.2
Vaccinia gangrenosa. This picture was taken $4\frac{1}{2}$ months after the lesion first appeared. The extensive tissue destruction is apparent. (*From Hansson, O. and Vahlquist, B. (1963), Lancet, ii, 687*)

Though these complications are rare, it has become apparent that in many Western European countries the mortality due to them is greater than the indigenous smallpox mortality. It has therefore become the policy in Britain to dispense with the routine vaccination of infants and children, and reserve vaccination for those in immediate contact with a case of smallpox. Such vaccination of contacts within 3 days of exposure is usually effective. Of course, those whose occupation brings them into possible contact with the disease, e.g. doctors, nurses, and members of the armed forces, should be vaccinated regularly as long as they are at risk. Likewise, there are many countries, entry into which necessitates prior vaccination.

The most important contra-indication to vaccination is the presence of any widespread skin disease, especially atopic dermatitis. Vaccination should also be avoided in patients with any immunological deficiency syndrome especially of cell-mediated immunity, and also in those who are pregnant or who are being treated with glucocorticoids (unless there is an emergency).

There had been recent reports that no case of smallpox had occurred in the world for many months. Since no known carrier exists, smallpox may well be on the way to becoming extinct. In this event vaccination against the disease will be a thing of the past, and Jenner's true claim to fame will be the eradication of a disease rather than the development of a vaccine.*

*According to a WHO press release of 25 May 1978, the last confirmed case of smallpox was in Merka town, Somalia, with the onset of the skin eruption on 26 October 1977. If no new cases had occurred during the 2 years following that date, smallpox would have been regarded as extinct. Unfortunately there remains the hazard of

VIRUSES AFFECTING THE RESPIRATORY TRACT

The number of viruses incriminated in respiratory infections is legion. Many of the agents produce acute infections of the upper respiratory tract. The most important of these are the orthomyxoviruses and paramyxoviruses (which include the influenza and para-influenza viruses), the adenoviruses, and some recently isolated viruses associated with the common cold.

Orthomyxoviruses

These are a group of medium-sized, filamentous, single-stranded, RNA-containing viruses (Fig. 23.3). The name myxovirus stresses their affinity for mucins. They grow well

Figure 23.3
An orthomyxovirus. An electron micrograph of influenza A/2, England 4272, which is demonstrated by negative staining. The irregular shape of the virus is clearly seen, and the well-marked covering membrane from which numerous prickles project is also observable. These projections are called peplomeres; they contain haemagglutinin, and it is to them that red cells become adherent. The RNA within the virion is not apparent in this photograph. × 120 000. (*Photograph by courtesy of Micheline Fauvel, Department of Medical Microbiology, Faculty of Medicine, University of Toronto.*)

reference laboratories that keep stocks of smallpox virus for research purposes. In September 1978 a woman died of the disease in Birmingham, England; it seems certain that she acquired the virus from the research laboratory which was located in the same building where she herself worked.

in the amniotic cells of chick embryos. They have a conspicuous tendency to agglutinate the red cells of many species, e.g. fowls and guinea-pigs. They do this by their strong attachment to mucoprotein surface receptors on the red-cell envelopes, from which they act as bridges to other cells. Specific antisera inhibit this *haemagglutination*, thus aiding in typing the viruses.

Orthomyxoviruses grow in tissue cultures of monkey kidney cells. If suspensions of guinea-pig red cells are introduced into the infected culture tubes, the cells are adsorbed on to the surface of the monkey kidney cells. This is called *haemadsorption*, and is also useful in typing procedures.

The important human orthomyxovirus is that of influenza.

Influenza. The causal agents are three quite distinct types of influenza virus, A, B, and C, of which type A and its variants are by far the most important from an epidemiological point of view (Fig. 23.3). Influenza is a disease predominantly of children and young adults. It is transmitted by inhalation just before and during the acute stage, but the possibility of transmission by healthy carriers has not been excluded. The incubation period is only 1 to 2 days. The disease is a systemic one, but the effects are predominantly respiratory, and there is much necrosis of the epithelium of the trachea and bronchi. The severe, underlying, acute, inflammatory response accounts for the deep-red, congested appearance of the tracheal mucosa at necropsy. It is probable that even in severe pandemics the horrifying death rate is due to secondary pneumonias of bacterial origin rather than to the influenza.

Immunology. The most interesting feature of influenza A virus is its tendency to undergo frequent antigenic variation. The 1918 pandemic was probably caused by a mutant of the A virus, and since then new strains have frequently emerged. There were localised epidemics in 1932, 1934, 1946, and in 1957, the year of the Asian influenza pandemic.

The nomenclature of these viruses is as follows:[3] The geographical name refers to the place of origin of the first-identified isolate of the new strain, the number that follows is the sequential laboratory number allocated to the virus, and the last number is the year of its isolation. The Asian epidemic was caused by the A/Singapore/57 virus, and in 1968–69 another epidemic was caused by the A/Hong Kong/68 virus. In Britain strains that have caused localised epidemics are A/England/42/72 in the 1972–73 winter, A/Port Chalmers/1/73 in 1973–74, and so forth.

Further subdivision of the influenza viruses is based on antigenic differences in their haemagglutinins (H) and neuraminidase (N). All the recently described epidemic A strains are designated H3 N2, which indicates that their haemagglutinins are related antigenically to that of the A/Hong Kong (H3N2) virus, and their neuraminidase antigens to those of the A/Hong Kong and the A/Singapore (Asian) (H2 N2) virus of 1957. This means that the different strains are characterised by definite but incomplete changes, or 'drifts', in their surface antigens.

Immunity to influenza is directed against these antigens, particularly the haemagglutinin, and it is antigenic drift that helps a virus cause outbreaks in populations that have become immune to its precursors. Such outbreaks are unlikely to be severe because population immunity to the preceding related viruses is good enough to damp down the effects of every new

strain. Nevertheless, these variants of the Hong Kong virus have caused influenza throughout most of the world. A fresh pandemic would probably require the appearance of a virulent strain that has a new haemagglutinin, one unrelated to the H3 antigen or to the previous H2 or H1 antigens. If the neuraminidase antigen should also undergo a complete antigenic 'shift', with the emergence of an H4 N3 virus, the pandemic could be particularly severe.

The swine influenza virus is believed to be derived from, or even identical with, that responsible for the 1918–19 pandemic, which is the most serious on record. The virus stopped circulating in human beings in the early 1930s, but has remained endemic in the pig population of the USA ever since. It has been identified in a few cases of human influenza in the intervening years, usually where there has been close contact with pigs. In 1976 an outbreak of influenza among armed-forces recruits in New Jersey was ascribed to a virus with surface antigens resembling those of the swine influenza virus.[4] The danger of this to the young who have no immunity to the 1918–19 strain is obvious.

Influenza B virus is endemic and causes more circumscribed outbreaks, and has a much slower, less pronounced tendency to antigenic variation. Type C infection is rather uncommon, and the virus appears to exist as a single, stable, antigenic type.

It is obvious that effective immunisation against influenza is beset with difficulties. No one can forecast the nature of the next mutant that may cause a pandemic, and as the incubation period is so short, it is very difficult to immunise whole populations in time. International co-operation is essential in providing information about the origin and geography of spread of such a pandemic, so that distant communities can be immunised in time. At present killed and attenuated living vaccines are being offered to the elderly and those with chronic respiratory infections in the winter, and some protection against influenza has been demonstrated. Unfortunately a number of cases of the Guillain-Barré syndrome have followed the use of influenza vaccine.[5]

Paramyxoviruses

These resemble the orthomyxoviruses in morphology and symmetry but are larger and more pleomorphic (Fig. 23.4). Furthermore their replication cycle cannot be interrupted by actinomycin D. They do not grow so easily in the chick embryo, but they produce haemagglutination and haemadsorption.

The main respiratory pathogens of this group are the parainfluenza viruses and the respiratory syncytial virus.

Parainfluenza viruses. There are four groups; group 1 is also called the Sendai virus (Japanese haemagglutinating virus), and it is distinctive in growing well in the allantoic membrane of the chick embryo. Group 2 is also called the croup associated, or CA virus. Both of these groups have been found in cases of respiratory infection, especially in children with croup, bronchitis, and bronchopneumonia. Group 3 virus has a similar range of pathogenicity, and also affects cattle with a respiratory disease called 'shipping fever'. Group 4 occasionally causes a mild respiratory infection.

Respiratory syncytial virus. This virus is distinctive in the cytopathic effect it produces on cell cultures: giant-cell forms develop and coalesce into syncytial masses. It is a cause

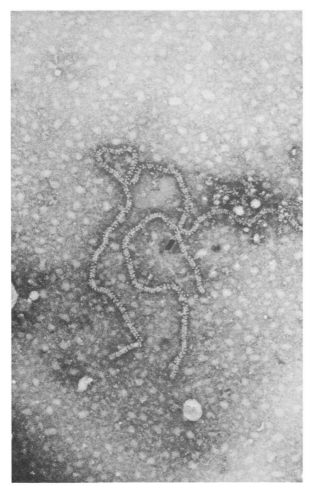

Figure 23.4
A paramyxovirus. The covering membrane of the paramyxovirus has been ruptured; its RNA content has been released. The long thread of nuclear protein is surrounded by the capsomeres arranged in a helical fashion. × 78 000. (*Photograph by courtesy of Micheline Fauvel, Department of Medical Microbiology, Faculty of Medicine, University of Toronto.*)

of colds and minor upper-respiratory-tract infections in adults, but in children, especially in young infants, the lower respiratory tract is also involved so that bronchiolitis and bronchopneumonia may occur.

Two other viruses of this group are those of measles (see p. 290) and mumps. **Mumps** is typically a bilateral parotitis, but the infection may involve the other salivary glands also (probably by direct spread from the mouth), and such distant organs as the testes or ovaries, pancreas, thyroid, breasts, and central nervous system (*via* the blood stream). Central nervous involvement is probably invariable, with an increase in lymphocytes in the cerebrospinal fluid, but occasionally there is a frank meningo-encephalitis. This may also occur in the absence of salivary-gland involvement, and is diagnosed serologically.

Adenovirus Infections

The adenoviruses are rather small, spherical, double-

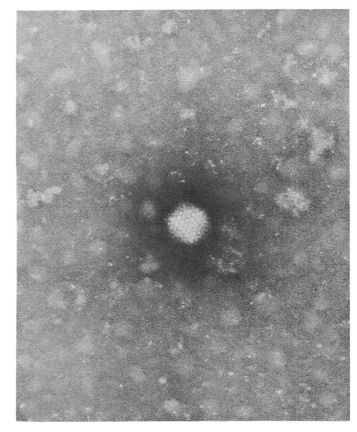

Figure 23.5
An adenovirus. This virus, which is demonstrated by negative staining, has the typical icosahedral form and no outer envelope. × 167 760. (*Photograph by courtesy of Micheline Fauvel, Department of Medical Microbiology, Faculty of Medicine, University of Toronto.*)

stranded, DNA-containing viruses (Fig. 23.5) which produce intranuclear inclusion bodies, and have a proclivity for the mucosa of the upper respiratory tract and the conjunctiva (Fig. 23.5). There are 33 human serotypes, and also many that are specific for other animals, e.g. monkeys, dogs, cattle, and mice. A few human strains cause tumours in newborn hamsters. Adenoviruses are cultured on the usual tissue-culture systems consisting preferably of the cells of the animal species affected.

(*a*) Types 1, 2, and 5 infect the tonsils and adenoids in early childhood. They seldom produce ill-effects, and tend to lie *latent*. It is unknown whether they play any part in the common hyperplasia of tonsils and adenoids.

(*b*) Types 3, 4, 7, 7a, and 14 produce explosive epidemics of *febrile pharyngitis* and other *acute respiratory diseases*. A primary atypical pneumonia syndrome may also occur. These infections occur most commonly in closed communities, and many epidemics have been described in military camps.

(*c*) These adenoviruses also have a strong proclivity for the conjunctiva and may cause *acute follicular conjunctivitis* in the course of the upper respiratory disease.

(*d*) *Epidemic keratoconjunctivitis* is caused by the type-8 adenovirus, and is seen in factory workers whose corneas are liable to be abraded by particles of dust and metal.

(*e*) Adenoviruses are swallowed and can be isolated in the faeces. They have been incriminated in some cases of *gastroenteritis* in children, and are probably of importance in *mesenteric adenitis* occurring in children. The lymphoid hyperplasia of the bowel may be an important factor in some cases of *intussusception*.

(*f*) Adenoviruses have been isolated from the urine, and type 11 has been associated with *acute haemorrhagic cystitis* in children.

Coronaviruses

These are a group of medium-sized, pleomorphic, single-stranded, RNA-containing viruses with a prominent envelope arranged into spikes, or *peplomeres*, which form a fringe of projections resembling petals. Their resemblance to a crown is the basis of the name coronavirus.

Many coronaviruses cause disease in animals, e.g. mouse hepatitis and avian infectious bronchitis. In the human being they are an important cause of upper-respiratory-tract infections of a cold-like type.

The Common Cold

The viruses that cause the common cold are called **rhinoviruses**. They are very small RNA-containing viruses, and are grouped among the picornaviruses.

The rhinoviruses are of interest in requiring a temperature of 33°C instead of 37°C for successful culture. Their habitat in the nose is probably related to this temperature requirement. They are cultured in human and monkey-embryo kidney tissue at a more acid pH than is usual.

Cold-like diseases are also caused by some coronaviruses, parainfluenza viruses, ECHO viruses, the Coe virus, and the respiratory syncytial virus. Possibly some reoviruses are also implicated (see p. 286).

ARTHROPOD-BORNE VIRAL INFECTIONS

There is a group of viruses that are distinctive in passing some part of their life-cycle in the tissues of an arthropod vector, where they actively multiply before being transmitted to a fresh host by the bite of the vector. The vector in turn acquires the viruses from the blood of an animal host.

Sometimes the life-cycle is very complicated, and implicates several vertebrate and invertebrate hosts. All these arthropod-borne viruses have been collectively called 'arboviruses', but although this comprises a logical epidemiological group, it is in fact made up of very different viruses that belong to several different families. The majority of the group are togaviruses and bunyaviruses, but a few are orbiviruses, and possibly other viruses are also involved.

Togaviruses. These are small, spherical, single-stranded, RNA-containing viruses. Their name derives from their cloak-like envelope (toga means a cloak). They infect a wide range of animals; the suckling mouse is very susceptible, and is used diagnostically. They also grow on fertile eggs and in tissue-culture systems, especially in chicken and mouse embryo cells.

The togaviruses are classified into two groups, largely on immunological grounds:

Group A (*alphaviruses*) are responsible for the equine types of encephalitis, chikungunya, and o'nyong-nyong.

Group B (*flaviviruses*) are responsible for most of the togavirus group of encephalitis, yellow fever (flavus means yellow), dengue, and some haemorrhagic fevers.

Bunyaviruses. These differ from the togaviruses in that their nucleocapsid has a helical, and not a cubical symmetry. The name derives from Bunyamwera, a locality in Africa. They are responsible for sandfly fever (Mediterranean), oropouche (South American), Rift Valley fever (African), Crimean haemorrhagic fever, and Californian encephalitis.

Orbiviruses. These are members of the reovirus family (see p. 286). They are responsible for Colorado tick fever.

The arthropod vectors are usually mosquitoes, but ticks and phlebotomus flies may also be implicated. It is not surprising that most of the diseases caused by these viruses have a distinctly tropical distribution. In human beings the chief arthropod-borne virus diseases are various types of *encephalitis, yellow fever, dengue fever, sandfly fever*, and a group of *virus haemorrhagic fevers*.

Arthropod-borne virus encephalitis varies in severity. Some types are mild, whereas others are severe and have a high mortality rate. The virus is widely disseminated throughout the central nervous system and affects the cerebral cortex particularly. There are different types of disease, which vary in geographical distribution. Eastern and Western Equine encephalitis occur especially in North America, whereas Japanese B, Murray Valley, and Russian spring-summer encephalitis are diseases endemic in Japan, Australia, and Russia respectively. St. Louis and West Nile encephalitis are other diseases of the same type occurring in the USA and the Middle East respectively. Most of these are mosquito-borne, but the Russian disease is transmitted by ticks.

Yellow fever is a disease primarily of monkeys, and is transmitted to them and to human victims by culicine *Aedes aegypti* mosquitoes. The disease is endemic in West Africa and Central America. Amongst the indigenous population subclinical infection is very common, though sometimes, especially in Europeans, virulent yellow fever develops. It appears that after the virus has been injected into the skin by the mosquito's bite, it spreads to the local lymph nodes where it multiplies. It then invades the blood stream, and settles in the viscera producing necrotic lesions. The incubation period is only about 4 days.

The typical lesion of yellow fever is midzonal hepatic necrosis. Shrunken necrotic cells with a hyaline, eosinophilic cytoplasm and pyknotic nucleus are seen amid the debris; these are called *Councilman bodies*, and are an example of apoptosis (see p. 299). Severe renal damage and a haemorrhagic tendency are also characteristic.

Nowadays yellow fever is rare in human beings, except in remote communities living in the tropics. Antimosquito measures and immunisation procedures have been responsible for this momentous eradication.

Active Immunisation. Active immunisation is mandatory for those travelling through endemic areas. It is performed by the subcutaneous or intramuscular injection of a suspension of living attenuated virus. This is the 17D strain, which was attenuated by passage through mice, and is now grown in chick embryos. These embryos are ground up and their juice is freeze-dried and placed in ampoules. The vaccine is reconstituted with normal saline immediately before use. The immunity is of a high degree, and lasts at least 6 years.

Diagnosis. The virus can be recovered from the blood during the first 5 days of illness, and when inoculated into suckling mice it leads to encephalitis. The mouse's brain is a good source of the virus, on which neutralisation tests can then be performed. The sera of convalescent patients contain high titres of complement-fixing and neutralising antibodies. These antibodies protect mice against the encephalitis caused by the virus. This is the basis of the *mouse protection test*, which has been employed in epidemiological surveys to ascertain the extent of subclinical yellow fever infection in a community.

Dengue fever occurs over a wide expanse of territory extending from the Levant to the Pacific Islands. The virus is transmitted by the *Aedes aegypti* mosquito, and is antigenically closely related to the yellow fever virus. The area of the mosquito bite is converted into a large red papule, which is the site of virus multiplication. The mode of dissemination is similar to that described in yellow fever, but the disease is quite different, consisting of a biphasic fever, severe headache and joint pains, and a variable maculopapular skin eruption. Pain in the acute phase is very severe, but death seldom occurs. There is, however, a severe variant with an often fatal haemorrhagic fever.[6] This may be due to infection by dengue serotype 1 (there are 4 serotypes) in persons partially immune as a result of infection with another serotype.

The virus produces encephalitis in suckling mice, and can be neutralised by specific antibodies. Active artificial immunisation is possible but seldom performed.

Two other togavirus diseases resemble dengue clinically, chikungunya and o'nyong-nyong. Both these words mean 'that which bends up' in the native African dialect, and they refer to the contorted position of the sufferer.

Chikungunya occurs in East Africa and South-East Asia, and is transmitted mostly by *Aedes aegypti* mosquitoes. It sometimes gives rise to a dangerous haemorrhagic fever.

O'nyong-nyong differs in that there is also lymphadenitis. It occurs in East Africa, and is transmitted by *Anopheles* mosquitoes. It is not associated with a haemorrhagic fever.

Sandfly fever is an example of a short-term pyrexial illness accompanied by agonising muscular pains and headache, which is encountered quite frequently in countries around the Mediterranean and in Iran and Pakistan. It is caused by a virus transmitted by the sandfly *Phlebotomus papatasi*. A lesion appears locally, and after an incubation period of about 4 days the virus becomes systematised. It too is pathogenic for suckling mice.

VIRAL HAEMORRHAGIC FEVERS[7]

Viral haemorrhagic fevers are a group of geographically widely-dispersed severe viral fevers in which a haemorrhagic tendency is prominent and the death rate considerable. Among the togavirus haemorrhagic fevers is the alphavirus *chikungunya* and the flavivirus *yellow fever*, dengue, *Omsk haemorrhagic fever* of Central Russia, and *Kyasanur forest disease* of India. These last two are transmitted by ticks, as is also the bunyavirus *Crimean haemorrhagic fever*. This virus was first associated with febrile conditions in the Congo.

Not all viral haemorrhagic fevers are transmitted by arthropod vectors. Two viruses are of considerable importance. Neither is associated with an arthropod.

Arenaviruses. These are medium-sized, pleomorphic, single-stranded, RNA-containing viruses. The name arena means sand, and it alludes to the presence of cellular ribosomes incorporated within the virion, which resemble grains of sand.

They cause *lymphocytic choriomeningitis* in mice and two serious diseases in human beings: *American haemorrhagic fever* in Argentina and Bolivia (the Junin and Machupo viruses are the important agents in human disease, and they are related to the Tacaribe viruses isolated from bats in Trinidad) and *Lassa fever*,[8] which was first described in Lassa, North-East Nigeria. This is a very serious haemorrhagic fever notorious for the high rate of transmission to contacts of the patient. Excreta, aerosols, and contaminated wounds are all means by which the infection can spread. The animal reservoir is the multimammate rat *Mastomys natalensis*, and the disease is probably spread by the contamination of foodstuffs by rodent urine.

The Marburg virus.[9] This agent was first imported into Germany in 1967 with a consignment of green Vervet monkeys, but it is now known that this animal is not the natural reservoir of the virus. It is distinct from all known groups of viruses, and consists of very long filaments with terminal blebs and regular surface projections on its envelope. It causes a very dangerous haemorrhagic fever with a high mortality rate. Outbreaks occurred in Germany in 1967 and in South Africa in 1975. More recently a similar virus has been isolated in the equatorial provinces of Sudan and Zaire, and is tentatively called the *Ebola virus*.[10]

VIRAL HEPATITIS

The two important diseases that come into this category are virus A hepatitis (previously called infective hepatitis) and virus B hepatitis (previously called serum hepatitis).

Virus A hepatitis occurs endemically in institutions like schools and military camps, and its main incidence is among children and young adults. The agent is excreted in the faeces, and infects other individuals after the ingestion of contaminated food. During the preicteric and early icteric phases of the illness it is present also in the blood. The disease is transmitted mainly by ingestion. No carrier state is known to exist.

Hepatitis A virus (HAV)[11] is small, 25 to 28 nm in size, and with cubical symmetry. Its nucleic acid is as yet unknown. It can be demonstrated in the faeces of patients for a few days after the onset of jaundice using electronmicroscopic techniques. It has not been grown in cell culture, but it produces virus particles in the cytoplasm of the liver cells of marmosets after experimental infection.

Virus B hepatitis is not usually acquired by the oral route, although it can be transmitted by ingesting contaminated blood. The virus is not usually present in the faeces, but it may be found in the blood for periods of over 5 years. It is transmitted not only by bood transfusion but also by the prick of a contaminated needle; the amount of blood or serum

Figure 23.6
Dane core antigen. A concentrated sample of Dane particles was treated with a detergent (polysorbate 80) in order to disrupt the outer coat and to release the internal component. This Dane core measures 27 nm in diameter. The suspension of particles was incubated with the serum of a patient who had recovered from an attack of virus B hepatitis. An anticore antibody causes the core particles to adhere to each other, and to form immune complexes. This method (immune electron microscopy) can be used to detect anti HBcAg. × 119 700. (*From Fauvel, M., Babiuk, L., Sheaff, E. T., and Spence, L. (1975), Preparation of a Dane core (hepatitis B) antigen from human plasma.* Canadian Journal of Microbiology, 21, 905.)

Figure 23.7
Hepatitis B virus. This is a negative-stained preparation of hepatitis-B positive serum. Three types of particles can be seen: spherical particles 20 nm in diameter; elongated, tubular filaments up to 230 nm in length; and Dane particles, 42 nm in diameter, and having a double shell. × 90 000. (*Photograph by courtesy of Micheline Fauvel, Department of Medical Microbiology, Faculty of Medicine, University of Toronto.*)

necessary to convey the infection need be as little as 0·01 ml. In the past the disease was common in venereal disease clinics after arsenical injections, and during the Second World War outbreaks followed yellow fever immunisation, because the vaccine was suspended in human serum at that time. Nowadays it is a major hazard among young drug-addicts, especially those who inject themselves intravenously ('mainliners'). People who handle blood, such as laboratory technicians, or work in haemodialysis units are also at risk.

Hepatitis B virus (HBV)[11,12] is double shelled and 42 nm in size. It used to be called the *Dane particle*. It contains double-stranded DNA. It clearly belongs to a new family of viruses. It is found in the serum of patients and carriers, but it has not been grown in cell culture (Fig. 23.6).

It possesses at least three separate antigens:

Hepatitis B surface antigen (HBsAg, which was first called *Australia antigen* because it was originally found in an Australian aborigine), which is found on the surface of the virus. It is also found on the 22 nm spherical particles and the long tubular forms, about 20 nm in diameter and of variable length, seen in the serum (Fig. 23.7). It displays antigenic heterogeneity: in addition to a common determinant 'a', all HBsAg particles possess two type-specific subdeterminants, either 'd' or 'y', and either 'w' or 'r'. Thus the four major serotypes are HBsAg/adr, ayr, adw, and ayw. Infection with one subtype may fail to confer immunity against a second infection with another subtype.

Hepatitis B core antigen (HBcAg), which is demonstrable only after disruption of the outer membrane of the virus. It is not found in the serum, but it may be found in the nuclei of the liver cells of monkeys that have been infected with HBV.

The e antigen (HBeAg), which has two subtypes HBeAg/1 and HBeAg/2. There appears to be a close association between the presence of HBeAg in HBsAg-positive serum and the presence of complete HBV particles, so that HBeAg is a good marker of the potential infectivity of HBsAg-positive serum.

The diseases these two viruses produce are pathologically very similar: a widespread focal necrosis which usually recovers by complete regeneration. Nevertheless, there are distinct clinical differences. Virus A hepatitis has a much shorter incubation period than virus B hepatitis (15 to 40 days as compared with 60 to 160 days). Although the clinical features of the two conditions are very similar, the mortality rate is 0·1 per cent with virus A hepatitis and up to 10 per cent, or even higher, with virus B hepatitis. Both can kill with a fulminating infection that leads to massive necrosis, but as yet there is no evidence that HAV infection leads to chronic liver disease.[11] On the other hand, about 10 per cent of cases of HBV infection progress to a chronic type of hepatitis, e.g. subacute or chronic active hepatitis, which may proceed to macronodular cirrhosis.[13,14] Adults are more vulnerable than are children, and pregnant and older women are especially endangered. The most dangerous type of virus B infection is post-transfusion hepatitis, which has a mortality rate of from 10 to 20 per cent. This is attributable to the large dose of virus received and the poor state of health of the patient which necessitated transfusion. The over-all mortality rate is much less than this (about 1 per cent).

Prophylactic passive immunisation with γ-globulin is useful against HAV, but is of much less value in HBV infection because of the low antibody against HBV. Special high-titre HBV immunoglobulin is now available, and promises to be of value.

After infection with HBV, HBsAg and HBeAg may be present in the blood for a month before the onset of symptoms.[14] Once symptoms have developed, HBs antigenaemia lasts about 6 weeks; normally antibody to HBsAg (anti-HBs) does not appear until convalescence. HBeAg is cleared more rapidly; once again clearance is associated with the appearance of anti-HBe. An antibody response to HBcAg (anti-HBc) occurs even earlier, about the time of the rise in the serum aminotransferase concentrations, but it seldom persists for over one year. Hence its detection in high titre is evidence of a recent infection with HBV.

When the course is atypical, there may be variations in these immune responses to the antigens. Progression to chronic hepatitis is normally associated with a failure to clear HBsAg and HBeAg from the serum, possibly because the patient fails to produce antibodies of high enough affinity to eliminate the virus. Fulminating hepatitis, on the other hand, is associated with an unusually rapid clearance of HBsAg from the serum, suggesting that the antibody response is enhanced.

Indeed, virus B hepatitis is a good example of a condition in which antibodies can play a dangerous role in the progress of the disease. Immune-complex hypersensitivity effects, e.g. serum-sickness phenomena (urticaria and arthralgia) occur in 10 to 20 per cent of cases some days or weeks before the symptoms of liver disease occur. Occasionally there may be glomerulonephritis or polyarteritis nodosa.

Furthermore, immunologically deficient people, e.g. lepromatous lepers, those on immuosuppressants, and especially those with chronic renal failure, carry the antigen for long periods. Such people do not appear to suffer from liver damage, but they are potent transmitters of the agent. Many cases of hepatitis have occurred in doctors and nurses working in renal dialysis units, and a disturbingly high mortality rate has occurred in some centres. This latency of infection in immunologically deficient hosts is clearly an exceptional state of

affairs in viral disease, but it has its analogy in lymphocytic choriomeningitis in mice (see p. 274).

It has been found experimentally in the infected monkey, that in the pre-icteric phase large numbers of liver cells contain HBV cores, surface antigen, and virions. It is possible that severe liver damage results from the immune cytolysis of cells that are not lethally infected with virus by the action of complement-fixing antibodies or sensitised T lymphocytes.

In chronic human carriers of HBsAg, some of the liver cells show a 'ground-glass' appearance of well-demarcated cytoplasmic zones of pale, eosinophilic granular material (Figs. 23.8 and 23.9). These areas can be shown to contain abundant HBsAg by immunological methods. On the whole, 'ground-glass cells' tend to be more abundant when the pathological lesions are slight, but there are exceptions.

In the general population the carrier rate varies from about 0·1 per cent in the USA to over 10 per cent in some of the Pacific Islands. Perhaps primitive conditions, including tattooing, play a part in carrying infection around the community. Transmission by mosquito bite is another possibility, as these insects have been shown to harbour HBsAg, but it is not known whether they can transmit it to another victim.

It has been shown that virus B hepatitis can spread naturally from person to person and that serum containing antigen is infectious when given by mouth. Thus the traditional teaching that virus B hepatitis be transmitted only by injection is not absolutely true; nevertheless, the great majority of infections are acquired parenterally. We know little about the excretion of the virus in the faeces and urine. The virus may also be present in the saliva, and be transmitted by kissing.

The detection of HBV antigens in the serum of blood donors has been a most important advance in blood-transfusion technique, and at last a means is available to protect recipients against this very unpleasant hazard. This is discussed in detail on page 653.

It should be noted finally that some episodes of acute viral hepatitis are not due to either HAV or HBV, nor even to such viruses as the Epstein-Barr virus or the cytomegalovirus, which occasionally produce a predominantly hepatic illness.

In the USA another as yet unidentified virus is the most common cause of hepatitis occurring after blood transfusion.[11,15] Indeed, it is probable that there are a number of such viruses, but as yet there is no laboratory test to identify them. Provisionally this has been called non-A non-B hepatitis, and there are indications that the infection can be acquired by routes other than by transfusion and that non-A non-B viruses are responsible for some cases of chronic hepatitis.[16]

REOVIRUS INFECTIONS[17,18]

Reoviruses are small, spherical, double-stranded RNA-containing viruses. The virus has a double icosahedral shell (it is not enveloped). There are three serotypes. Reoviruses grow slowly in cell culture, and produce characteristic eosinophilic, intracytoplasmic inclusion bodies. The name is derived from 'respiratory enteric orphan', for although the virus is often found in the respiratory and intestinal tracts of children, no disease has been associated with them.

The **orbivirus** (orbis means a ring) is another member of

Figure 23.8
Ground-glass liver cells. Many of the cells contain granular areas (arrows) rich in B HBsAg. ×465. (*From Scheuer, P. J.* (1977), *Chronic hepatitis: A problem for the pathologist.* Histopathology, **1,** 5.)

Figure 23.9
Ground-glass liver cells. In this example the ground-glass areas have been stained with orcein to show HBsAg. ×425. (*From Scheuer, P. J.* (1977), *Chronic hepatitis: A problem for the pathologist.* Histopathology, **1,** 5.)

the family. It is somewhat smaller than the reovirus, because there is only an indistinct outer layer covering the inner icosahedral capsid. There are at least 38 serotypes; most of these are arthropod-borne viruses of animals. Only one serotype is a human pathogen, causing *Colorado tick fever*, which occurs in North-West USA and resembles sandfly fever clinically. Orbiviruses grow in suckling mice and cell culture.

The **rotavirus** is another important member of the reovirus family. It is about the same size as the reovirus, but the circular outline of the outer shell of the capsid suggests the appearance of a wheel (rota means a wheel). The rotaviruses are responsible for diarrhoea in calves, mice, and piglets. The human pathogen causes *acute infantile gastroenteritis*, the main feature of which is severe diarrhoea. There may also be fever and vomiting, and although the condition is self-limiting, it can lead to serious dehydration. The condition is diagnosed by electron microscopy of the infected stools, which may contain vast numbers of virus particles (Fig. 23.10). Rotaviruses can be grown with difficulty in organ cultures of human fetal intestine, and then must be identified by electron microscopy or immunofluorescence.

It should be noted that at least two viral agents are firmly incriminated in the aetiology of acute gastroenteritis. The most important is the rotavirus. A second, that causes gastroenteritis in adults and children, is called the **Norwalk agent**. It is 27 nm in size and is an icosahedral virus, but its nucleic acid is still unknown, and it remains unclassified. It was first isolated after causing a winter vomiting disease in Norwalk, Connecticut. Coronaviruses, adenoviruses, ECHO viruses, and Coxsackie viruses have all been identified in stools by electron microscopy, but their significance is as yet unknown.

HERPESVIRUS INFECTIONS

The herpesviruses are medium-sized, spherical, double-stranded, DNA-containing viruses (Fig. 23.11). They produce large acidophilic, intranuclear inclusion bodies, and give rise to characteristic cytopathic effects in cells grown in tissue culture. The cells fuse into multinucleate giant forms.

A characteristic feature of herpesvirus infections is the tendency for the virus to lie latent in the tissues of its host after the primary infection. In this way the majority of human beings have, by adult life, come to terms with most, if not all the five, human herpesviruses—herpes-simplex and genital-herpes viruses, cytomegalovirus, Epstein–Barr virus, and varicella/zoster virus.[19]

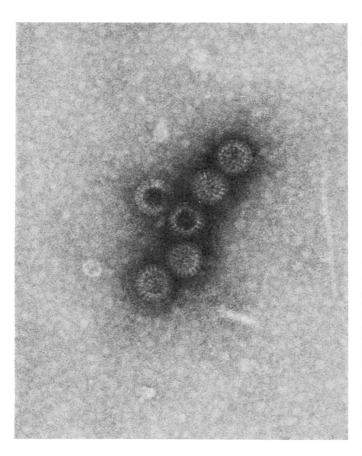

Figure 23.10
A rotavirus. The circular outline of the outer shell of the capsid suggests the appearance of a wheel. × 136 300. (*Photograph by courtesy of Micheline Fauvel, Department of Medical Microbiology, Faculty of Medicine, University of Toronto.*)

Figure 23.11
Herpes simplex virus. The envelope, which is clearly delineated, is derived from the modified nuclear membrane of an infected cell. The hollow capsomeres of the virion are clearly visible. × 139 800. (*Photograph by courtesy of Micheline Fauvel, Department of Microbiology, Faculty of Medicine, University of Toronto.*)

Varicella and zoster. Though the clinical features of these two infections are poles apart, there is good evidence that they are both caused by the same virus.

It has been recognized for a long time that children in contact with patients suffering from zoster tend to contract chickenpox, and this observation has been reproduced experimentally in susceptible children. The chickenpox so produced differs in no respect, either clinically or serologically, from chickenpox acquired from another child in the usual way, and the patient is subsequently rendered immune to chickenpox. A patient who already has had chickenpox will not acquire it after exposure to zoster.

Virus material derived from the vesicle fluids or crusts of chickenpox and zoster lesions produces identical cytopathic effects in tissue cultures of human amnion cells, and there is no antigenic difference between the two. The histology of zoster and chickenpox vesicles is also similar: the formation of multinucleate, giant, epithelial cells containing intranuclear inclusion bodies. There is no growth on the chorioallantoic membrane of fertile eggs.

After an attack of chickenpox the virus lies latent in the sensory ganglia of the nervous system, and is subsequently reactivated by some intercurrent episode, e.g. physical disease or psychological trauma. It produces lesions specifically in the posterior root ganglia of the spinal, trigeminal, or facial nerves, and from there infection spreads down the nerve fibres to the skin of the dermatome, and also sometimes upwards to the posterior columns of the spinal cord. Occasionally infection may spread to the anterior horn cells and produce permanent paralysis. A rare complication is encephalitis.

Herpes simplex. The virus of herpes simplex is one of the most widely distributed viruses in human beings. It is estimated that from 60 to 80 per cent of the population are affected. Of these only 10 per cent exhibit primary childhood lesions, such as *gingivostomatitis*, *keratoconjunctivitis*, and *vulvovaginitis*. *Eczema herpeticum* is described on page 279. In some cases the virus may invade the internal organs and produce *meningo-encephalitis*. Worst of all is *generalised visceral herpes simplex*, a fatal infection of the newborn, in which white, necrotic lesions are present in many organs.

Abrasions of the skin predispose to primary herpetic infection (*traumatic* or *inoculation herpes simplex*). A good example of this is the very painful *herpetic whitlow*, which is seen in people who come into contact with naso-bronchial secretions. About 30 per cent of young adults lack antibodies to herpes simplex, and are susceptible to infection. The herpetic whitlow is therefore usually seen in anaesthetists and young doctors and nurses who care for patients with a tracheostomy. It also occurs in dentists.

Usually, however, the primary infection remains subclinical, and the virus remains latent in the cells of the host. This symbiosis tends to be disturbed by intercurrent infections, e.g. the common cold, pneumonia, and malaria, and even, in very susceptible victims, by menstruation, emotional strain, and exposure to sunlight. There then develop typical *herpetic vesicles*, especially around the mucocutaneous junction of the lips and face. The skin of the genitalia is sometimes affected (*herpes genitalis*), and also occasionally the conjunctiva and cornea. Ocular involvement is serious because the keratitis leads to *dendritic ulceration*; scarring and impairment of vision

may follow. Uveitis is an occasional complication. Herpes infections are common in T-lymphocyte deficiency, where they tend to assume a generalised, visceral character and are often fatal.

The precise localisation of the virus during the latent periods has been a matter for speculation. It cannot be identified in the skin between attacks, but it has been isolated from sensory nerve-root ganglia—trigeminal or sacral[20]—examined at necropsy. It appears that the virus remains latent in nerve cells, but when conditions are favourable it is able to infect the skin or mucous membrane and produce typical herpetic vesicles. The mechanism is therefore analagous to that encountered in zoster.

The virus is easily grown on the usual tissue culture systems, and is pathogenic to suckling mice, in which a fatal encephalitis is produced. On the chorio-allantoic membrane of fertile eggs characteristic pocks are produced. The virus is present in large amounts in the fluid of herpetic vesicles, the epithelial cells of which contain large intranuclear inclusion bodies similar to those of zoster and varicella.

It has been discovered that there are two antigenically distinct types of herpes simplex, called 1 and 2. *Herpesvirus hominis type 1* causes typical herpes febrilis of the face, mouth, pharynx, and cornea, and is also responsible for eczema herpeticum and herpes meningo-encephalitis. *Herpesvirus hominis type 2* causes herpes genitalis and vulvovaginitis, and also neonatal herpes.

Cytomegalic inclusion disease. This is another herpesvirus infection, and it is caused by the *cytomegalovirus*. It occurs most often in newborn infants to whom it is transmitted transplacentally.

Cytomegalic inclusion disease may develop as a fulminating lethal infection in the newborn, and at necropsy the parenchymatous cells of many organs, e.g salivary glands, pancreas, liver, kidneys, and bronchial epithelium, are found to be distended by large intranuclear inclusion bodies (see Fig. 22.7, p. 271). The neonatal infection is not always fatal, but survivors are usually mentally retarded and microcephalic. Nevertheless, some infants infected with the virus are asymptomatic and appear normal.

Sometimes a congenital infection may pass unnoticed for some time and ultimately give rise to a moderate degree of auditory and mental dysfunction. These children may excrete the virus for long periods in their throat and urine, as may also young children below the age of five years who acquire a primary infection. Such children are often symptomless, but there may be evidence of hepatic damage from which they eventually recover, or else a protracted respiratory illness.

In older children and adults infection is usually subclinical, but a few develop a condition resembling infectious mononucleosis with a negative Paul-Bunnell reaction.[21] Finally cytomegalic inclusion disease is an important opportunistic infection in patients on immunosuppressive therapy. It is evident that the clinical presentation of the disease closely mimics that of toxoplasmosis. The condition is widespread, though clinical manifestations are rather uncommon; many adults have complement-fixing antibodies in their serum.

The virus, strains of which infect many different animals, grows on tissue-culture growths of fibroblasts derived from the same animal species.

Epstein-Barr virus (EBV). This herpesvirus was first isolated from cultures of lymphoblasts from *Burkitt's tumour* (p. 397). It is cell-associated, and cannot be transferred in series (in supernatant fluid) in the ordinary way. But if virus-infected cells are irradiated and then cultivated with normal lymphocytes, these lymphocytes undergo a lymphoblast transformation and can be shown to contain EBV by electron microscopy and EB viral antigens by immunofluorescence. Furthermore, these cells, unlike normal lymphocytes, will grow indefinitely in culture.

Cultures of the peripheral atypical lymphocytes of patients with *infectious mononucleosis* regularly develop into cell lines which can be shown to contain EBV, and antibodies to the viral capsid and membrane antigens can be detected in the sera of patients in the acute stage of the illness using immunofluorescence techniques against cell lines harbouring the virus (p. 621).

EBV has also been detected in cell cultures of *nasopharyngeal carcinoma* (p. 380).

MEASLES

Measles is probably the most infectious of all diseases, and it is transmitted by patients during the prodromal period, which is characterised by catarrhal inflammation of many mucous surfaces. The infected secretion is inspired by the next victim, and the virus appears to multiply in the lymphoid tissue of the respiratory tract for some time before it breaks out to produce a viraemia, which marks the beginning of the prodromal period lasting 3 to 4 days. Once the eruption appears, the patient rapidly becomes less infective. A characteristic feature of measles is the appearance of typical giant cells in the hyperplastic lymphoid follicles (Fig. 22.11). *Giant-cell pneumonia of infants*, in which a different type of giant cell is found in the interstitial tissue of the lungs, is a manifestation of measles, and the virus can be cultured from the lungs.[22]

The virus is a paramyxovirus, and is related antigenically to the viruses of canine distemper and rinderpest. It grows in cell cultures of human kidney and embryonic lung, and from these it can be adapted on to the more usual cell systems. It produces a typical cytopathic effect in which large giant cells are formed, similar to the Warthin-Finkeldey cells seen in the lymphoid follicles.

A rare, but fatal complication of measles is *subacute sclerosing panencephalitis*, in which intranuclear inclusion bodies are found in the cortical neurons. It is interesting that the patient usually has a high level of immunoglobulins to the measles virus both in the serum and the cerebrospinal fluid. It seems as if there is a continuous or repeated antigenic stimulus over a period of time and that there is a synthesis of immunoglobulins in the central nervous system. The disease may be the result of a persistent measles infection associated with an abnormal immunological response by the patient.

In view of the unpleasant pulmonary and neurological complications of measles, active immunisation is recommended, preferably near the beginning of the second year of life, since the efficacy of the live, attenuated vaccine used is less certain at a younger age.[23] The vaccine occasionally fails to prevent the disease, but even then the illness is less severe than usual. A common complication is a mild febrile reaction 5 to 12 days after immunisation.

An injection of measles immune globulin will prevent an attack of measles in an exposed individual if given within 5 days. Globulin given later following exposure will result in a mild attack, and this may be preferable since active immunity will then follow.

RUBELLA

German measles is a comparatively trivial acute infectious fever in children associated with an evanescent macular eruption. The virus has all the features of a togavirus, but it is not transmitted by arthropods. It produces rather feeble cytopathic effects in cell systems, and is usually detected by its interference with the cytopathic effect of an enterovirus. Amongst other animals only monkeys are susceptible to a mild degree.

The importance of rubella is that women who contract it in the first trimester of pregnancy sometimes bear congenitally deformed infants. The incidence of deformed children is about 25 per cent, and the first month of pregnancy is the most dangerous period. The usual abnormalities are heart lesions, cataract, and deafness; mental deficiency is not common.

Some of these infants are born with the *congenital rubella syndrome* consisting of thrombocytopenic purpura, hepatosplenomegaly, jaundice, and osteochondritis, and sometimes the typical eruption. Virus may be excreted from the nasopharynx and urine for over four months after birth, and doctors and nurses may be infected. Even this may not be the end of the tragedy, for a *progressive rubella encephalitis*[24] has been reported in children who had apparently become stabilised with the congenital rubella syndrome, only to develop deterioration of mental and motor function in the second decade of life.

Pregnant women exposed to rubella during the first trimester should be examined to assess their immune status. If rubella antibodies are present, infection of the fetus is unlikely. If antibodies are absent, the test should be repeated in 1 month's time. If there has been a rise in antibody titre, recent infection can be inferred and termination of pregnancy should be considered, the decision made depending upon the patient's moral and religious convictions. Human immune serum is available, but its value in prophylaxis is debatable.

Live, attenuated rubella vaccine is available, and it is recommended for children aged 5 to 10 years. It should not be given to pregnant women, nor to girls if there is any risk of them becoming pregnant.[23]

INFECTIOUS WARTS AND PAPOVAVIRUS INFECTIONS

The common wart *verruca vulgaris* appears as a sessile, discrete papillary mass on the skin, commonly that of the hands. Other variants are the flattened *plantar wart* on the soles of the feet, the fungating *condyloma acuminatum* on the labia and the penile sulcus, and also the *laryngeal papilloma* of children. The epidermis is thickened (acanthosis) and thrown into papillary folds. Vacuolation of the superficial cells in the stratum granulosum is characteristic.

These lesions may persist for many months, and then

disappear as rapidly as they arose. Genital warts (condylomata acuminata) may rarely become malignant.

In some warts there are eosinophilic intranuclear and intracytoplasmic inclusion bodies, whereas others do not contain any. Virus can be demonstrated by electron microscopy of thin sections of excised warts and of purified extracts. It is claimed that the virus can be cultivated with difficulty in organ cultures of human skin epithelium. Warts can be transmitted experimentally to human volunteers with an incubation period of 2 to 8 months.

The **papovavirus** is the family group responsible for viral papillomata in human beings and other animals, e.g. the Shope papilloma. Papovaviruses are small, spherical, double-stranded, DNA-containing viruses (Fig. 23.12). They are responsible for other important animal tumours, notably the *polyoma* lesions mentioned on page 377. Another papovavirus is the SV 40 virus, alluded to on page 278, which has been isolated from batches of monkey kidney used in tissue cultures; it belongs to the polyoma group, and is oncogenic. As it produces a typical vacuolation of the cells in culture, it has also been called *vacuolating agent*. It is the first two letters of these three viruses that have been put together to form the name papovavirus (*PA*pilloma, *PO*lyoma, and *VA*cuolating agent).

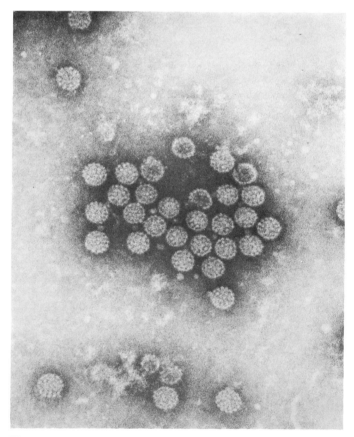

Figure 23.12

A papovavirus (SV 40). This organism was found as a contaminant in a culture of African Green Monkey kidney cells. × 136 000. (*Photograph by courtesy of Micheline Fauvel, Department of Medical Microbiology, Faculty of Medicine, University of Toronto.*)

Recently it has been discovered that a rare demyelinating disease of the central nervous system, *progressive multifocal leucoencephalopathy*, which is seen most often as a complication of lymphomata, is due to opportunistic infection by polyomaviruses of undetermined type. Some resemble the SV 40 virus. It is possible that these viruses lie latent in the tissues and are activated by states of immunosuppression, especially involving T lymphocytes. Progressive multifocal leucoencephalopathy is a rapidly fatal disease in which the white matter softens and disintegrates into a pulpy mass.

SLOW VIRUSES[25]

Sheep and goats are prone to a degenerative neurological disease called *scrapie*, the main features of which are severe pruritus, incoordination, paralysis, and death in a few weeks. The incubation period is several years, hence the name 'slow' virus. The disease can be transmitted to other animals (and also mice) from infected material, but the agent is so resistant to sterilising and other destructive procedures that it appears not to be a virus at all, for a nucleic acid or nucleoprotein could not withstand these procedures. At present the nature of the scrapie agent is under investigation. An interesting speculation is that it is a substance which complements an incompetent or incomplete virus which is present in, or part of, the normal cell.

There is a neurological disorder that affects certain remote tribes living in the highlands of New Guinea. It is called *kuru*, and its pathology resembles that of scrapie. The disease has been reproduced in chimpanzees inoculated with human brain material, and the incubation period is several years. It is suspected that cannibalism is responsible for transmitting the disease to each succeeding generation.

A rare encephalopathy of man, *Creutzfeldt-Jakob disease*, the main features of which are ataxia, dementia, abnormal movements, stupor, and death in a few months (as in kuru), can also be transmitted to species of laboratory primates, and it would appear that both conditions are slow virus infections.

The cardinal histological features of scrapie, kuru, and Creutzfeldt–Jakob disease are similar:—loss of nerve cells, marked astrocytic proliferation, and some microglial reaction without a conventional inflammatory response in the brain. The grey matter is predominantly affected, and it often has a finely-meshed spongy appearance (status spongiosus), due to the formation of innumerable closely-packed microcysts. These are apparently vacuoles that develop in the astrocytes and, less often, in the axons and dendrites of neurons.[26]

At present a slow virus is being investigated in the aetiology of multiple sclerosis, but the results are so far negative. The possibility of slow viruses being implicated in sarcoidosis and Crohn's disease is mentioned in Chapter 21.

Animal Viruses Transmissable Directly to Human Beings

Amongst viral diseases in this category are *cow-pox* and *contagious pustular dermatitis of sheep* (*orf*) (Fig. 23.13), poxvirus diseases, which produce characteristic lesions on the skin of farmworkers; *Newcastle disease of fowls*, a paramyxovirus infection, which produces severe conjunctivitis in laboratory workers and fowl-keepers; *Virus B infection of monkeys*, a

Figure 23.13
Orf. This warty lesion developed on the hypothenar eminence of the right hand of a shepherd, aged 25 years, at the site of a scar resulting from a cut sustained while paring sheep's hooves 5 weeks previously. The following day a similar lesion appeared on the inner aspect of the same forearm. The nodules bled easily but were painless and showed no induration or regional lymphadenitis. Since there was no evidence of regression in 3 weeks, the lesions were excised, and rapid healing resulted. (*I 13.2, Reproduced by permission of the President and Council of the R.C.S.Eng. The photograph was presented by Dr. T. V. Cooper, who also donated the specimen.*)

herpesvirus disease which produces a fatal encephalitis in animal-house keepers who are bitten by monkeys; *lymphocytic choriomeningitis*, an arenavirus disease endemic in mice and which causes a lymphocytic meningitis when the secretions of these animals are inhaled; *arthropod-borne virus disease; rabies*.

Rabies[27,28] virus is transmitted to human beings by the bite of a rabid animal, usually a dog or cat. Sometimes wolves, jackals, badgers, opossums, and vampire bats may be responsible, and of these only the bat harbours the virus in a latent form. Foxes and skunks are the main wildlife reservoirs in North America. The virus multiplies locally, and then travels up the damaged nerve fibres to reach the brain and spinal cord. The incubation period is prolonged, sometimes lasting several months, but an almost invariably fatal encephalitis follows (a few recovered cases have recently been reported[27]).

The **rhabdovirus** (rhabdos means a rod) is the family group responsible for rabies. It is a large, bullet-shaped, single-stranded, RNA-containing virus; one end is rounded and the other end truncated.

The virus spreads from the brain along the nerves to the secreting glands and the cornea, and the condition can be diagnosed during life by making corneal impressions and performing fluorescent antibody staining on them. A similar technique can be used on post-mortem brain smears. In addition, Negri bodies are present in the neurons, especially of the hippocampus. The diagnosis is confirmed by mouse transmission.

People bitten by a potentially rabid animal should be immunised.[27] Hyperimmune antirabies serum (horse) should be given, and a quantity of it may be infiltrated around the wound. Active immunisation must then be started if there is the slightest suspicion that the animal was rabid. At least 14 daily injections of vaccine are given subcutaneously into the abdomen at different sites to prevent local reactions. Semple's nervous-tissue vaccine prepared from rabbit brain and inactivated by phenol is still used in some countries, but is occasionally responsible for the development of allergic peripheral neuritis or the more serious encephalomyelitis (pp. 170

and 205). The duck-embryo vaccine is the one now recommended in Britain and the USA.[28] It gives far fewer neuroparalytic complications than the older vaccines prepared from nervous tissues. Another vaccine derived from virus grown on a strain of human diploid fibroblasts and then inactivated has recently been produced, and it promises to supplant the duck embryo since it does not produce neurological complications.[28]

Dogs, cats, and cattle in endemic areas should be immunised by the Flury strain of living, attenuated, egg-adapted virus. It is not licensed for human use.

CLASSIFICATION OF VIRUSES

Viruses are classified according to their nucleic acid, capsid symmetry, and the presence or absence of an outer envelope. The number of new groups of virus is steadily rising as more are isolated. The following list is limited to viruses causing human disease.

RNA-containing Viruses

Picornaviruses. These are small (20 to 35 nm in size), the capsid has a cubical symmetry, and there is no outer envelope. Important members are the enteroviruses and rhinoviruses.

Reoviruses. These are about 70 nm in size, the capsid has a cubical symmetry, and there is no outer envelope. Important members are the orbiviruses and rotaviruses.

Orthomyxoviruses. These vary in size from 80 nm to 120 nm, the capsid has a helical symmetry, and there is an outer envelope. These are the viruses of influenza.

Paramyxoviruses. These differ from the orthomyxoviruses in being larger (150 to 220 nm) and having a capsid with a wider diameter, but they are closely related.

Togaviruses. These vary in size from 40 nm to 80 nm, the capsid has a cubical symmetry, and there is an outer envelope.

Bunyaviruses. These are larger than the togaviruses (90 to 100 in size). The capsid has a helical symmetry, and there is an outer envelope.

Rhabdoviruses. These are large, varying in length from 130 nm to 220 nm and in diameter from 60 nm to 80 nm. The capsid has a helical symmetry, and there is an outer envelope.

Coronaviruses. These vary in size from 80 nm to 160 nm, the symmetry of the capsid is still undetermined, and there is a conspicuous outer envelope.

Arenaviruses. These vary in size from 50 nm to 200 nm, the capsid symmetry is still undetermined, and there is an outer envelope. A conspicuous feature is one or more electron-dense granules in the interior; these resemble ribosomes.

DNA-containing Viruses

Adenoviruses. These vary in size from 60 to 90 nm, the capsid has a cubical symmetry, and there is no outer membrane.

Papovaviruses. These are about 50 nm in size, the capsid has a cubical symmetry, and there is no outer envelope.

Herpesviruses. These are about 150 nm in diameter, the capsid has a cubical symmetry, and there is an outer envelope.

Poxviruses. These are large, varying in size from 200 nm to 300 nm, the capsid has a complex symmetry, and there are outer envelopes.

Unclassified Viruses

There are a number of viruses which defy classification at present. Hepatitis A and hepatitis B viruses are one example, so is the Norwalk agent that causes viral gastroenteritis, and so also is the Marburg agent that causes a dangerous haemorrhagic fever.

Two recent viruses have been described in the faeces of healthy children—the **astroviruses**, which are spherical, about 28 nm in diameter, and show upon their surface a 5- or 6-pointed star structure when they are negatively stained, and the **caliciviruses**, which have a characteristic structure, with small depressions ('calices'), upon their surface. Their systematic position awaits elucidation.[29]

It will be some time before we have a definitive classification of viruses, since new ones are being constantly discovered, and new features of well-established viruses sometimes make it necessary to reclassify them.

GENERAL READING
See Chapter 22.

REFERENCES
1. Leading Article (1973) Acute haemorrhagic conjuctivitis. *Lancet*, **1**, 86.
2. Leading Article (1977) Polio vaccines and polioviruses. *British Medical Journal*, **1**, 1617.
3. World Health Organization (1971) A revised system of nomenclature for influenza virus. *Bulletin of the World Health Organization*, **45**, 119.
4. Leading Article (1976) Pandemic and interpandemic influenza. *British Medical Journal*, **1**, 730.
5. Leading Article (1977) Guillain–Barré syndrome and influenza virus. *British Medical Journal*, **1**, 1373.
6. Leading Article (1976) Dengue. *Lancet*, **2**, 239.
7. Leading Article (1975) Viral haemorrhagic fevers. *British Medical Journal*, **4**, 67.
8. Leading Article (1975) Lassa fever. *British Medical Journal*, **1**, 173.
9. GEAR, J. S. S. *et al.* (1975) Outbreak of Marburg virus disease in Johannesburg. *British Medical Journal*, **4**, 489.
10. Leading Article (1977) After Marburg, Ebola . . . . *Lancet*, **1**, 581.
11. Leading Article (1977) Hepatitis viruses—old and new. *British Medical Journal*, **1**, 985.
12. ROBINSON, W. S. & LUTWICK, L. I. (1976) The virus of hepatitis, type B. *New England Journal of Medicine*, **295**, 1168 and 1232.
13. Leading Article (1975) After type B hepatitis. *British Medical Journal*, **4**, 311.
14. WOOLF, I. L. & WILLIAMS, R. (1976) Significance of persistent HBs antigenaemia. *British Medical Journal*, **2**, 807.
15. Leading Article (1975) The several viruses of post-transfusion hepatitis. *British Medical Journal*, **3**, 663.
16. Leading Article (1978) Non-A non-B hepatitis. *British Medical Journal*, **2**, 942.
17. Leading Article (1975) Rotaviruses in men and animals. *Lancet*, **1**, 257.
18. Leading Article (1975) Classifying gastrointestinal viruses. *Lancet*, **2**, 806.
19. Leading Article (1975) Simian viruses again. *Lancet*, **1**, 667.
20. BARINGER, J. R. (1974) Recovery of herpes simplex virus from human sacral ganglions. *New England Journal of Medicine*, **291**, 828.
21. Leading Article (1974) Unsuspected cytomegalic mononucleosis. *British Medical Journal*, **1**, 340.
22. Leading Article (1976) Pulmonary complications of measles. *British Medical Journal*, **2**, 777.
23. DOWNHAM, M. A. P. S. (1976) Immunisations. *British Medical Journal*, **1**, 1063.
24. JOHNSON, R. T. (1975) Progressive rubella encephalitis. *New England Journal of Medicine*, **292**, 1023.
25. Leading Article (1974) Slow virus infections. *British Medical Journal*, **2**, 343.
26. BLACKWOOD, W. & CORSELLIS, J. A. N. (Eds.) (1976) *Greenfield's Neuropathology*, 3rd edn, pp. 317–321 and 827–832. London: Arnold.
27. Leading Article (1976) Pre-exposure prophylaxis of rabies. *British Medical Journal*, **2**, 197.
28. Leading Article (1975) Diagnosis and management of human rabies. *British Medical Journal*, **3**, 721.
29. FLEWETT, T. H. (1978) In *New Perspectives in Clinical Microbiology*, ed. Brumfitt, W., **1**, p. 106–107. London: Kluwer Medical.

Chapter 24. Disorders of Growth

Most organs of the body possess a considerable reserve of tissue which can be brought into play whenever additional work is demanded of them. At rest the inactive cells are maintained by an intermittent blood flow through their supplying capillaries. This mechanism results in an economical use of the circulation, and explains why noxious substances spread by the blood stream may nevertheless produce patchy effects. When more work has to be performed, the shut-down vessels dilate and the organ shows active hyperaemia. This is well illustrated by the tremendous increase in blood flow through the salivary glands which occurs during periods of active secretion.

Growth Potentiality of Cells

In addition to this reserve mechanism, organs or tissues subjected to prolonged excessive strain respond by increasing their bulk. This may be done by either increasing the size of each constituent cell, or increasing the total cell number; which of these occurs depends upon the growth potentiality of the cells involved. Usually both occur together. Three classes of cells are described.[1]

Labile cells. These cells, also called continuous replicators, undergo frequent division throughout life to replace those lost through differentiation and subsequent desquamation.

The cells of lymph nodes, bone marrow, and most of the covering or protective epithelia (skin, endometrium, alimentary, respiratory, and urinary mucosa) come into this category.

Stable cells. These cells, also called discontinuous replicators, likewise show a definite pattern of replication with cells lost by wear and tear being replaced by the mitotic activity of others. Since the life span of each cell is long, the term stable is appropriate. DNA synthesis, when it takes place, occurs at a rate similar to that of other cells. It is the interval between mitoses which is long, and therefore very few mitotic figures are seen in a section of tissue from a normal adult. However, the cells never lose the ability to divide and can do so with ease if suitably stimulated. This group includes most of the secretory epithelial structures (liver, kidney, pancreas, and endocrine glands).

Permanent cells (non-replicators). These non-replicating cells lose the ability to divide either at birth or shortly thereafter. Neurons and cardiac muscle provide the important examples. Although mitoses are not seen in these cells, DNA synthesis and renewal can occur (see p. 54). Striated, and especially smooth, muscle has a decided power of regeneration (see p. 119), but this cannot be compared with that of stable cells.

The factors which control the growth and differentiation of cells are largely unknown. Nevertheless, abnormalities of these two functions are frequent, forming an important part of many disease processes. They may be considered under three headings:

1. *Abnormalities of cellular growth*, which are either *excesses* (hypertrophy and hyperplasia) or *decreases*, either developmental (agenesis and hypoplasia) or acquired after full development (atrophy and aplasia).

2. *Abnormalities of cellular differentiation*, which comprise metaplasia and certain other dysplasias.

3. *Neoplasia*, a completely abnormal cellular growth considered in the chapters that follow.

Quantitative Abnormalities of Cellular Growth

Excessive growth. Tissues composed of labile or stable cells respond to an increased demand for work primarily by multiplication, but may also show some increase in size. Permanent cells either show no morphological change (neurons), or else only an increase in size (cardiac and skeletal muscle). An increase in the cell number is called *hyperplasia*, and an increase in individual cell size is *hypertrophy*. It therefore follows that both conditions can occur in the presence of a stimulus; which process occurs depends on whether the individual cells are capable of enlargement, multiplication, or both combined.

Both hyperplasia and hypertrophy are usually related to a recognisable stimulus, which is often a basically physiological one acting to excess. The most important stimulus is an *increased demand for function*. As will be seen, this may take the form of increased muscular work in response to an abnormal load, an increased production of blood cells in response to hypoxia or infection, a thickening of protective epithelium in response to external trauma, or an increased secretion of a gland in response to some external need.

Some hyperplasias are related to an increased secretion of hormones, either physiologically during puberty or pregnancy, or else pathologically as when the hormone is secreted by a tumour.

Finally, hyperplasia may be idiopathic. Many of the commonest glandular hyperplasias come into this category, e.g. senile prostatic hyperplasia, cystic hyperplasia of the breast, and primary hyperthyroidism (which is often associated with an autoantibody in the serum, p. 455).

HYPERPLASIA

Definition. Hyperplasia is the increase in size of an organ or tissue due to an increase in the number of its specialised constituent cells. Enlargements due to congestion, oedema, inflammation, amyloid infiltration, or tumour formation must be distinguished from hyperplasia.

It is important to note that those hyperplasias due to a specific stimulus persist only for so long as that stimulus is applied. When it is removed, the tissue tends to revert to its normal size. In this respect hyperplasia differs from neoplasia, for neoplastic tissue continues to grow even when the stimulus is withdrawn.

While the concept of hyperplasia is traditionally a morphological one, it must never be forgotten that the increase in size of the organ is accompanied by a corresponding increase in function. Nowhere is this more apparent than in hyperplasia of the endocrine glands.

Hyperplasia in the Endocrine Glands

In the endocrine glands hyperplasia may be either diffuse or focal. Often it starts by causing diffuse enlargement of the gland (or glands, as the case may be), but later one or more focal, circumscribed, discrete nodules appear. These are often called adenomata, but it is unlikely that they are neoplastic; nodular hyperplasia is a better term. Malignancy seldom supervenes.

Good examples of hyperplasia affecting the endocrine glands are: parathyroid hyperplasia occurring in chronic renal failure, thyroid hyperplasia in Graves's disease, and the enlargement of the islets of Langerhans sometimes encountered in the child of a diabetic mother (p. 428). Endocrine hyperplasia is described in Chapter 35.

Hyperplasia in the Target Organs of the Endocrine Glands

Breasts. Hyperplasia of the epithelial tissue and surrounding specialised connective tissue is a normal feature of the female breast at puberty, during pregnancy and lactation, and to a lesser extent towards the end of each menstrual cycle. These changes are brought about by oestrogens and progesterone. Gross enlargement ('hypertrophy') of the female breast, which occasionally occurs at puberty, is generally due to an excessive accumulation of fat rather than hyperplasia of specialised breast tissue.

An important idiopathic hyperplasia of the breast is *mammary dysplasia*. In the early stages there is overgrowth of connective tissue and some dilatation of the ducts. In the next stage there is epithelial overgrowth so that the ducts become filled with cells (*epitheliosis*), or contain papillary ingrowths. New formation of glandular tissue produces the picture described as *adenosis*. In the most advanced stage the ducts form large cysts, and they are often lined by thin atrophic epithelium. This is the classical cystic disease of the breast; the blue-domed cyst is an extreme example. The condition is believed to be due to imbalance of ovarian hormones, probably excess oestrogen and too little progesterone. It is not precancerous (but see p. 386).

The administration of oestrogen to the male (e.g. stilboestrol therapy in prostatic cancer or as part of a sex change procedure) leads to a marked enlargement of the breasts. This is called *gynaecomastia*. It is also seen in advanced liver disease (p. 568). Gonadotrophins can also lead to gynaecomastia, as in some cases of giant-cell lung cancer and germ-cell tumours with trophoblastic differentiation.

Prostate. Senile enlargement of the prostate is due to epithelial hyperplasia as well as an increase in the fibromuscular element. The condition is common over the age of 60 years, and is confusingly called 'benign prostatic hypertrophy'

Figure 24.1

Benign prostatic enlargement. This specimen of bladder and prostatic urethra has been opened from the front. The prostate is enlarged, and its nodular median lobe projects into the trigone of the bladder, thereby acting as a ball valve and obstructing the passage of urine. The bladder wall is greatly thickened. Hypertrophy of the muscle bundles is responsible for the ribbed, or trabeculated, appearance of its lining. (*Specimen from the Boyd Museum, Toronto.*)

or 'adenomatosis of the prostate'. The enlargement is confined to the lateral lobes and the middle lobe; the latter often projects over the urethral orifice and acts like a ball-valve (Fig. 24.1). The atypical proliferation that occurs in the posterior lobes of old men is described in Chapter 25 under 'latent cancer'.

Endometrium. The endometrium is capable of marked hyperplasia as a response to the stimulation of prolonged oestrogen secretion. It may reach a thickness of over 1 cm and be difficult to distinguish histologically from carcinoma. Such hyperplasia is seen in connexion with granulosa-cell tumour of the ovary, and more commonly in women given large doses of oestrogen therapeutically for menopausal symptoms.

An idiopathic endometrial hyperplasia is seen in metropathia haemorrhagica. There is an increased secretion of oestrogen, and the cause is probably ovarian dysfunction.

Changes of Puberty. The increase in size of the gonads and the secondary sexual organs may all be regarded as examples of physiological hyperplasia.

Covering Epithelia

The covering epithelia of the skin, mouth, alimentary tract, and respiratory passages are apt to undergo hyperplasia when confronted with any persistent traumatising agent ('chronic irritant'). The skin shows epidermal hyperplasia under the mechanical trauma of an ill-fitting shoe when a corn develops.

Figure 24.2

'Tumourlet' of lung composed of regular, evenly-staining cells. The appearances resemble those of an oat-cell carcinoma, but the lesion was small and localised and enclosed in scar tissue. There were no mitotic figures. × 120.

Likewise an ill-fitting denture leads to hyperplasia of the underlying mucosal epithelium.

Chronic inflammatory lesions lead to considerable hyperplasia of the involved epithelium. In the skin hyperplasia is a feature of many intrinsic diseases such as psoriasis, chronic dermatitis, and lichen planus. It is a feature of some viral infections, being evanescent in chickenpox and prolonged in verruca vulgaris. The most extreme example of such epithelial hyperplasia is called pseudoepitheliomatous hyperplasia and is described further on. The 'tumourlets' found in fibrotic lung bear some resemblance to bronchial carcinoid or carcinoma, but they are of small size, the cells are regular, and mitoses absent (Fig. 24.2). Likewise in cholecystitis glandularis proliferans seen in chronic cholecystitis, the excellent differentiation together with an awareness of the existence of the condition should prevent a mistaken diagnosis of carcinoma (see Fig. 11.6, p. 130).

Kidney

Removal of one kidney results in a compensatory enlargement of the other; although sometimes called hypertrophy, this is best considered as regeneration (see p. 124).

Bone Marrow

Pronounced hyperplasia is seen in the haematopoietic tissue when there is a demand for more blood cells. The erythroid series of cells proliferate in all types of anaemia except that due to primary bone-marrow aplasia. The cellular marrow extends into the long bones of the adult (normally filled with fatty marrow), and in childhood extramedullary foci of erythropoiesis may occur in the liver, spleen, and other organs. An extreme example of this is seen in haemolytic disease of the newborn.

Erythroid hyperplasia producing secondary polycythaemia occurs in hypoxic states, e.g. living at a high altitude, in pulmonary disease, and in congenital cyanotic heart disease.

In infection it is the white-cell precursors which are affected.

RE System and Lymphoid Tissue

Both undergo hyperplasia in chronic infection and following antigenic stimulation. This is well-illustrated by the splenomegaly of malaria, kala-azar, and subacute infective endocarditis (see Ch. 30).

Liver

Following liver necrosis mitotic activity results in rapid replacement of the lost tissue. This is regeneration. It is doubtful whether true hyperplasia of the liver cells ever occurs. In cirrhosis of the liver there is, however, frequently considerable bile-duct hyperplasia (see p. 122).

PSEUDONEOPLASTIC HYPERPLASIA

Reference has been made to the difficulties in distinguishing nodular hyperplasia from benign neoplasia, particularly in the endocrine glands, the prostate, and the breast. From a practical point of view the distinction is unimportant since both processes are benign. There are, however, many examples of hyperplasia in which the mass of cells produced closely resembles a malignant tumour. Experience has taught that they are benign, since they either resolve spontaneously or respond to simple treatment. Their importance lies in their recognition, for a mistaken diagnosis can result in grave therapeutic errors. Almost any tissue can show such lesions and for their detailed descriptions special texts should be consulted.

Pseudomalignant Connective Tissue Hyperplasia

Pseudolymphoma. Pseudolymphoma of the skin[2] (Spiegler-Fendt sarcoid) appears as nodules of lymphoid tissue containing prominent follicles of large cells giving a histological picture which closely resembles that of the nodular type of lymphocytic lymphoma as seen in lymph nodes (see p. 396). Unlike the latter, however, the cutaneous lesions never become systematised nor develop into an overtly malignant disease. A somewhat similar lesion is the pseudolymphoma of the orbit, which closely resembles lymphocytic lymphoma (diffuse or nodular) histologically,[3] but again the behaviour is not one of malignancy. A similar benign lymphomatous lesion occurs in the rectum and in the mediastinum.[4]

Pseudosarcoma in fibrous tissue. Examples of this are described on page 318.

Pseudomalignant Epithelial Hyperplasia

Skin. Epidermal downgrowth and an appearance of dermal invasion by squamous cells is seen from time to time in a great variety of chronic ulcerating skin lesions ranging from blastomycosis and insect bites to basal-cell carcinoma. At times differentiation of these lesions from squamous-cell carcinoma is not possible, especially when small biopsy specimens alone are available for study.

A particularly good example of pseudoepitheliomatous hyperplasia is seen in *keratoacanthoma (molluscum sebaceum)*. This lesion usually appears on the exposed parts, generally the face, grows for several months, and then involves spontaneously with scarring (Fig. 24.3). It consists of a central crater containing keratin surrounded by dysplastic squamous epithelium which closely resembles a squamous-cell carcinoma. The downgrowing epithelium extends to the level of

Figure 24.3
Keratoacanthoma. This lesion had been developing for a period of 6 weeks. Note the rolled edges covered by apparently normal epidermis. The central area of this volcano-like lesion is filled with a mass of keratin. The lesion continued to grow rapidly for a further month, and was then excised for cosmetic reasons.

the sebaceous glands and excites a surrounding inflammatory reaction. The nature of the process is debatable. It may be an exuberant epithelial hyperplasia in response to some external agent, or else an example of a self-healing carcinoma. In support of the latter view is the fact that both keratoacanthoma and carcinoma occur most frequently on the sun-exposed skin. Certainly the histopathological changes in the two lesions are so similar that if curettings alone are available for study, it is often impossible to distinguish the one lesion from the other (Figs. 24.4(a) and 24.4(b). The biological behaviour of the two lesions is, however, quite distinct.

Pseudoepitheliomatous hyperplasia is also seen over a *myoblastoma*, a somewhat controversial lesion found most often in the tongue and occasionally in the skin. It is composed of very large polygonal and strap-shaped cells, the cytoplasm of which contains coarse eosinophilic granules (Fig. 24.5). Some of these lesions are probably merely foci of degenerate muscle

cells damaged during the wear and tear of mastication. But others are true tumours and may occasionally metastasise. The cell of origin of the lesion is disputed; by some it is thought to be the Schwann cell rather than muscle. The cause of the overlying epithelial hyperplasia is unknown.

There is little doubt that in the past pseudoepitheliomatous

Figure 24.4(a)
Keratoacanthoma. During the early growth phase the proliferating epidermal cells have the pleomorphism and atypical mitotic activity (arrow) that is typically associated with carcinoma. The over-all configuration of the lesion and the short history help in arriving at a correct diagnosis. × 250.

Figure 24.4(b)
This area of a well-developed keratoacanthoma shows proliferating squamous epithelium with good differentiation. Only the cells at the periphery of the masses show atypicality. The more central cells are large, and have abundant ground-glass appearing cytoplasm. × 120.

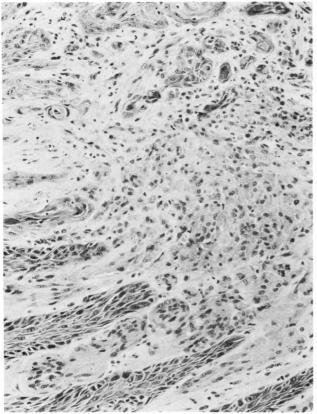

Figure 24.5
Granular-cell myoblastoma of skin. There is an extensive focus of large polygonal cells with a coarsely granular cytoplasm in the dermis. Dipping down towards them, and in part surrounding them, there are tongues of down-growing, hyperplastic epidermis. × 100.

hyperplasia has often been confused with squamous-cell carcinoma, and that the good prognosis encountered in some series of carcinomata of the skin and lip was due to the inclusion of many non-neoplastic lesions.

Pseudoepitheliomatous hyperplasia is also described in other epithelial-covered surfaces, e.g. the mouth and the stomach adjacent to chronic ulcers.

HYPERTROPHY

Definition. Hypertrophy is the increase in size of an organ or tissue due to increase in size of its constituent specialised cells. Pure hypertrophy without accompanying hyperplasia occurs only in muscle, and the stimulus is almost always a mechanical one.

Smooth Muscle

Any obstruction to the outflow of the contents of a hollow muscular viscus results in hypertrophy of its muscle coat. The following may be listed as examples.

Bladder.   Prostatic enlargement (Fig. 24,1).
Urethral stricture.

The bladder wall is greatly thickened, and shows trabeculation due to the arrangement of its muscle fibres.

Alimentary tract.

Oesophagus	Achalasia of the cardia.
	Carcinoma.
	Simple stricture.
Stomach	Pyloric stenosis due to peptic ulcer or carcinoma.
Intestine	Stricture following tuberculous enteritis or Crohn's disease.
Colon	Carcinoma

Hypertrophy is also seen in hollow organs when the wall is rigid and resists muscular contraction. This occurs in chronic inflammation, e.g. Crohn's disease, and in neoplastic infiltration. The hypertrophy in ulcerative colitis is not easily explained (p. 133).

Uterus. The myometrium shows the greatest hypertrophy known, and at a remarkably rapid rate. In pregnancy the muscle fibres eventually become ten times as long and five times as broad as those in the resting organ. The stimulus is partly mechanical and partly the effect of oestrogen.

Arteries. Muscular arteries show hypertrophy in hypertension.

A segment of vein, used to replace an artery, comes to resemble an artery.

Cardiac Muscle

Although the heart of a newborn child weighs only 30 g, it is believed that no further muscle cells are ever produced. The fibres increase in size seven-fold by the time adult life is reached. Any demand for increased work leads to hypertrophy of the fibres of the chambers affected. The stimulus is probably the stretching which results from the additional strain, and the ability of the heart to respond in this way constitutes part of the cardiac reserve (see Ch. 44).

Hypertrophy is best seen in the left ventricle (Fig. 24.6). Systemic hypertension, aortic valvular disease, and mitral regurgitation are common causes of enlargement. The biggest heart of all is the *cor bovinum*. This occurs when a heart with good coronary blood supply is subjected to overwork over a long period. Combined aortic and mitral regurgitation is the commonest cause.

Right ventricular hypertrophy occurs in left-to-right shunts (due to congenital heart disease), pulmonary and mitral valve lesions, pulmonary hypertension, and in chronic lung disease like emphysema and silicosis.

Hypertrophy of individual fibres is also seen in areas of myocardial fibrosis.

Microscopically the muscle fibres are increased in width from the normal 14 μm up to 25 μm. The nuclei are characteristically square-shaped. It is claimed that one capillary supplies approximately one fibre. In hypertrophy no new vessels are formed, with the result that the contractile tissue tends to be separated from its blood supply. The ischaemia may cause anginal pain, and on a morphological level muscle necrosis with replacement fibrosis.

Figure 24.6
Hypertrophy of the heart. The wall of the left ventricle is greatly thickened due to hypertrophy of its muscle. (C 20a.3, *Reproduced by permission of the President and Council of the R.C.S. Eng.*)

Skeletal Muscle

The village blacksmith's brawny arms provide a simple illustration of hypertrophy due to a mechanical stimulus. When he retires from work, his muscles return to a normal size.

Muscular dystrophy. A number of clinical syndromes exist in which specific groups of muscles undergo enlargement. Although in the early stages the muscle fibres become swollen, this is probably a degenerative change, because later on the fibres degenerate and are replaced by fibrous tissue. Much of the enlargement of the muscles is due to an increased deposition of fat, and is therefore not true hypertrophy. The syndromes are indeed characterised by muscular weakness. The common varieties are pseudohypertrophic muscular dystrophy (Duchenne type) and the facio-scapulo-humeral dystrophy of Landouzy and Dejerine.

Hypertrophy and hyperplasia compared. Both are cellular responses to an increased demand for work. The cells either enlarge or divide depending upon their growth potentialities. The stimulus for this is usually mechanical in hypertrophy, and chemical or hormonal in hyperplasia. When the stimulus is withdrawn, the condition regresses and the tissue reverts to normal. However, secondary structural alterations in the general architecture due to an accompanying degeneration may render a complete return to normal impossible.

DIMINISHED GROWTH

Nomenclature. A diminution in size may be of *developmental* origin due to a deficiency of growth, or it may be *acquired* after a period of normal growth.

Developmental diminutions of growth. These are usually present at birth, and the most extreme malformation of this type is *agenesis*, the complete failure of development of a part, which is therefore absent. A less severe condition is *hypoplasia*, in which there is a failure of development to a full, mature size. Such an organ (e.g. kidney) or tissue (e.g. enamel) is small in size or amount. Some hypoplastic kidneys are represented by only a fibrous nodule. Hypoplasia may become evident during childhood. Thus a testis that fails to mature at puberty is termed hypoplastic. These conditions are also noted on page 342.

Acquired diminutions in growth. *Atrophy* is an acquired diminution in size of a part due to a diminution in the number or size of its constituent elements. It is the antithesis of hyperplasia and hypertrophy combined. Only in muscle is a decrease in size the all-important feature; in all other instances there is also a decrease in the number of cells.

Another term sometimes used is *aplasia*. It has been used to describe extreme hypoplasia, but it is redundant in such a context. It is commonly used by haematologists to describe a condition of the bone marrow caused by the damaging effects of ionising radiation and certain drugs, in which the blood-cell precursors stop dividing and undergo destruction, and there is little or no regeneration. As no mature cells enter the blood, pancytopenia ensues (see p. 627). Clearly the destructive process is related to necrosis (especially if it is rapid) and to atrophy (if it is slow and sporadic). The term aplasia is preferably reserved for this usage in haematology.

ATROPHY

The Cellular Basis of Atrophy

In tissues composed of labile cells, and to a less obtrusive degree stable cells also, there is a constant loss of mature elements and their replacement by the mitotic activity of their fellows. The mechanism of this destruction of old cells is usually not obvious, since coagulative necrosis is not a feature of normal tissues.

Recently the concept of *apoptosis* (derived from the Greek and meaning 'dropping off' or 'falling off') has been introduced to describe the process by which cell numbers are reduced physiologically and also in some pathological conditions.[5-7] The cell condenses, apparently due to the loss of water, to form a pyknotic nuclear mass surrounded by a variable amount of cytoplasm in which the organelles are still easily recognisable. This is called an 'apoptotic body', and it undergoes nuclear fragmentation and the separation of protuberances that appear on the cell surface. These apoptotic bodies are then phagocytosed by histiocytes and also often by neighbouring epithelial cells, in which they are incorporated in lysosomes where they are digested, finally to form small, optically dense residual bodies (see p. 24). Apoptotic bodies derived from the epithelial cells lining free mucosal surfaces are also shed directly to the exterior.

Apoptosis, unlike coagulative necrosis, is not attended by an inflammatory reaction. The lysosomal residual bodies soon disappear, possibly as a result of 'cell defaecation'. The processs seems to be involved in the cell turnover in many healthy adult tissues, and has been shown to be very important in the later secretory and menstrual phases of the endometrial menstrual cycle when there is a considerable loss of cells from the glands. It is probably also responsible for the focal elimination of cells during normal embryonic development. Pathologically it is prominent in untreated malignant tumours, and it participates in some types of therapeutically induced tumour regression.

In cells undergoing atrophy there are abundant secondary lysosomes (autophagocytic vacuoles) and some residual bodies, and there is often evidence of apoptotic bodies also. This explains the progressive cell depletion in atrophy without evidence of frank coagulative necrosis.

The physiological death of cells described above has also been called 'necrobiosis', but apoptosis would seem to be a preferable term.

PHYSIOLOGICAL CAUSES

There are numerous examples of structures which are well developed at a certain period of life, but which subsequently undergo atrophy. The term *involution* is sometimes used synonymously with physiological atrophy. They may conveniently be considered under three age groups.

In the fetus, many structures form during embryonic development, and subsequently undergo regression. The branchial clefts, notochord, and thyroglossal duct are good examples.

In infancy, the ductus arteriosus and umbilical vessels either disappear or remain as fibrous cords. Soon after birth the fetal layer of the adrenal cortex undergoes involution.

Later life. From adolescence onwards the lymphoid tissue undergoes a reduction in size. As a rule it is replaced by fibrous tissue: on occasions, however, fat is also laid down. This is particularly well-marked in atrophic lymph nodes, and is also seen in the thymus and appendix. Lymph nodes in the adult are frequently found to be composed of a nodule of fat with a thin surrounding demilune of lymphoid tissue. Atrophy is also seen in the uterus after parturition and the breasts after lactation.

After the menopause and in old age there is atrophy of the gonads themselves. Indeed, as age advances most tissues take part in the process, but this may be due in some measure to ischaemia.

PATHOLOGICAL ATROPHY

This may be generalised or local.

Generalised Atrophy

Starvation atrophy. During starvation the carbohydrate and fat stores are first used up. Later the proteins are metabolised, those of the brain and heart being the last to be removed (Ch. 34). Generalised atrophy, seen in the cachexia of malignant disease, is probably largely dependent upon an inadequate food intake.

In extreme starvation the heart may be reduced from its normal 250 to 350 g to 100 g, the epicardial fat is replaced by pale, translucent material ('serous atrophy'), and the vessels are tortuous. Lipofuscins present in the small muscle fibres impart a brown colour, from which the name *brown atrophy of the heart* is coined. Starvation atrophy is a condition rarely seen in civilised countries. Occasional examples are encountered in neglected patients, and those dying of carcinoma of the oesophagus or stomach. It was also seen amongst the emaciated inmates of Belsen Concentration Camp in Germany.

Senile atrophy. This is a marked accentuation of the process of physiological atrophy that has already been described as occurring in old age. Brown atrophy of the heart is especially prominent in senility, and other organs, e.g. the liver and brain, may also show a lipofuscin accumulation in their cells. It is not known how much ischaemia (due to cerebral arterial atheroma) contributes to the brain atrophy of old people.

Endocrine atrophy. Hypopituitarism leads to an atrophy of the thyroid, adrenal cortex, and gonads. In the most severe cases the whole body may become stunted and the patient cachectic (see Simmonds's disease, Ch. 35).

Osteoporosis[8]

Osteoporosis is a condition of bone atrophy. It has been aptly defined as a lesion in which the volume of bone tissue per unit volume of anatomical bone is reduced.[9] The generalised disorder is considered here; localised bone atrophy is mentioned in connexion with the effects of pressure and disuse. The essential feature of osteoporosis is a reduction in amount of the osteoid matrix, which, however, remains normally mineralised. It must be distinguished from osteomalacia, in which osteoid is present in abundance but is poorly calcified. In osteoporosis the bony trabeculae are greatly thinned, and the bone as a whole is weakened and liable to fracture (Fig. 24.7). The radiological appearance is a reduction of bone density. But it must be remembered that this can be detected in routine films with certainty only when the content of calcium is reduced by at least half. Refined techniques may be more sensitive.[10]

Although bone is a rigid structure, it is constantly being remodelled; bone resorption and bone formation are continuously in progress even in the adult. Osteoporosis is brought about in one of two ways. There is either excessive bone destruction by osteoclastic activity, or else there is a failure in bone formation by the osteoblasts. Frequently the imbalance which results in the development of osteoporosis is of minor degree, and the period of calcium loss from the body extends over many months. By the time the patient is seen, a steady balanced state has been reached and there is no evidence of excessive calcium loss. The plasma levels of calcium and phosphate are usually within the normal limits, as is also the alkaline phosphatase level.

Causes of generalised osteoporosis. No satisfactory aetiological classification of osteoporosis is available. In the great majority of cases it is probable that many factors contribute to the final outcome: these include hormones, nutrition (including calcium), physical stress and its lack, and the blood supply. For descriptive purposes osteoporosis will be considered under the following headings:

Figure 24.7
Normal and osteoporotic vertebral bodies. *A*. Normal vertebral bodies. *B*. Moderate osteoporosis. *C*. Severe osteoporosis. The vertebral bodies have been sectioned to show their internal structure. Note the well-formed cancellous bone of the normal vertebral bodies in *A* as well as the structure of the intervertebral discs. One small focus of degeneration can be seen (white arrow). In *B* the specimen shows well-developed osteoporosis, but the over-all shape of the vertebrae is preserved. The discs show severe degenerative changes (black arrows). In *C* the specimen shows severe osteoporosis. The vertebrae have been compressed by the bulging discs.

Prolonged Recumbency.

Failure in Collagen Formation:
  Protein deficiency.
  Glucocorticoid excess.
  Scurvy.

Other Endocrine Disorders.

Senile and post-menopausal osteoporosis, including the idiopathic variety.

Prolonged recumbency. The effects of immobilisation have been studied in healthy volunteers placed in plaster casts from the waist to the toes.[11] There was a slow, steady loss of calcium, tending to increase up to about 0·3 g per day. During the 6 to 7 weeks of the experiment 9 to 24 g of calcium were lost, but as this represents only 1 to 2 per cent of the total body calcium (about 1 kg), no effects were detectable on X-ray examination.

Hypercalciuria occurs during immobilisation, and this may be a factor in stone formation. It is more marked in children and in patients with active Paget's disease.

Albright and Reifenstein attribute the osteoporosis of disuse to a failure of formation of new bone, for they believe that osteoblastic activity requires the stimulus of stress and strain produced by movement. However, more recent work suggests that immobilised limbs have a normal or even increased rate of bone formation, and that the osteoporosis is due to increased osteoclastic resorption.[12,13]

Failure in collagen formation. Osteoporosis may occur in *starvation* and the *malabsorption syndrome*, and the bone lesions are sometimes complicated by osteomalacia due to vitamin-D deficiency. Osteoporosis sometimes complicates *chronic liver disease* and may be combined with osteomalacia. Malabsorption due to steatorrhoea, vitamin-D deficiency, impaired hydroxylation of the vitamin in the liver, and glucocorticoid therapy are all factors that play a part in its causation.[14]

Scurvy. In adults generalised osteoporosis occurs, while in infantile scurvy (Barlow's disease) osteogenesis at the epiphyses is affected.

Glucocorticoid excess. Severe osteoporosis is typical of Cushing's syndrome; an unusual feature is that the skull is involved. Prolonged administration of glucocorticoids, e.g. for asthma or rheumatoid arthritis, may likewise produce a disabling osteoporosis.

In these three conditions the inability to form collagen fibres results in a cessation of osteoid formation. Abnormalities in the ground substance (osseomucin) may also play a part. There is no evidence of excessive osteoclastic activity.

Other endocrine disorders. Osteoporosis is not uncommon in severe *thyrotoxicosis*, and, as in the osteoporosis of immobilisation, it is due to increased resorption rather than inadequate formation. Hypercalciuria is a manifestation of this. There may rarely be fractures.[15] The osteoporosis of *acromegaly* may have a similar pathogenesis.

Senile and post-menopausal osteoporosis. Senile osteoporosis is common in the elderly, and is to be regarded as an exaggeration of the atrophy which is part and parcel of the ageing process. A similar condition is not uncommon among women of a younger age-group, and is then called *post-menopausal osteoporosis*. When the condition afflicts individuals of either sex at an earlier age, it is called *idiopathic osteoporosis*.

The mechanism involved is obscure; neither bone formation nor resorption seems to be impaired, but, as already noted, the trouble may have occurred at some time in the past and a state of balance achieved at the time of diagnosis. Anabolic steroids, both oestrogens and androgens, cause symptomatic amelioration, but their mode of action is unknown. Deficiency of either male or female sex hormones has been incriminated as the cause of senile and post-menopausal osteoporosis, but proof is lacking. Long-term dietary deficiency of calcium can produce osteoporosis in rats, and it may play a subsidiary part in human senile osteoporosis.[16] It would seem that the best protection against excessive senile osteoporosis is the presence of a large skeletal mass in early adult life.

Effects of osteoporosis. Symptoms are generally referable to the spine and pelvis which are the parts of the skeleton most severely affected in generalised osteoporosis. Chronic backache and kyphosis are common, and collapse of the vertebrae may produce episodes of acute pain. Diminution in height is characteristic, and as much as 4 to 8 inches may be lost before being noticed by the patient. Fractures may complicate osteoporosis; the most important are those of the lower forearm in middle-aged and elderly women, the proximal femur in both sexes over 70 years old, and crush fracture of the vertebrae, especially in old women.[16]

Radiographs show diminution in bone density; enlargement of the intervertebral disc-spaces produces the 'codfish-spine' appearance. The ribs and to a lesser extent the long bones show rarefaction.

Conditions Simulating Osteoporosis

Osteogenesis imperfecta (Fragilitas ossium).[17] This is characterised by a defect in osteoid formation which causes the bones to be very thin and extremely fragile. In some cases multiple fractures are present at birth, but in others the disease first appears during infancy or rarely during adolescence. The sclera may be abnormally transparent, thereby allowing the underlying choroid to give it a blue colour. Otosclerosis is also common. The condition is inherited as an autosomal dominant character.

Hyperparathyroidism. The lesion here is an excessive osteoclastic activity which may be so great as to produce tumour-like masses ('brown tumours') and large cysts. There is also much fibrous repair and the laying down of new bone. The condition, called osteitis fibrosa cystica, is described on page 461.

These conditions have been mentioned as they may produce radiological appearances indistinguishable from osteoporosis. But the underlying pathology is different. In osteogenesis imperfecta there is a hypoplasia of osteoid, and in osteitis fibrosa cystica there is a gross destruction of bone by hyperactive osteoclasts with evidence of reparative osteogenesis. This leads to a characteristic rise in the level of alkaline phosphatase in the plasma, which, as already noted, does not occur in osteoporosis.

Local Atrophy

Ischaemic atrophy. This is simply a local form of tissue malnutrition in which hypoxia is predominant. With gradual vascular obstruction the parenchyma of many tissues undergoes atrophy, which is followed by fibrous (or glial) replacement. This is a feature of cerebral arterial atheroma. In the case of coronary arterial disease, atrophy of the heart is not a usual feature; there is overt necrosis, and the process merges into one of infarction.

Pressure atrophy. This is a variant of ischaemic atrophy. It is caused by pressure on a solid organ, the vessels of which are progressively occluded by compression. It is the capillaries that suffer most, and damage is caused both by malnutrition and hypoxia. In this way the capsule around a benign tumour or a cyst is formed (see Ch. 26).

Some of the best examples are provided by bone; cartilage, being avascular, is much less severely affected. This is well illustrated by the way epiphyseal cartilage is spared by an expanding simple bone cyst, and by the scalloped appearance produced by the protruding intervertebral discs following the atrophy of the spinal column caused by an aneurysm of the thoracic aorta. A meningioma growing from the dura mater and hollowing the underlying brain is another good example of pressure atrophy. So also is the atrophic kidney that forms a cap on an expanding hydronephrosis which develops as a result of partial or intermittent obstruction of a ureter.

Disuse atrophy. The best examples are seen in the locomotor system and in the exocrine glands. The atrophy of bone (local osteoporosis), ligaments, and muscles that follows joint immobilisation must always be borne in mind when limbs are encased in plaster. Atrophy may occur in bone adjacent to an inflammatory process. It also occurs when joints are ankylosed, or if movement is prevented by pain; the atrophy around rheumatoid and tuberculous arthritis is particularly marked.

Sudeck's acute bone atrophy is perhaps due to this. It follows quite trivial trauma to the hands, and more rarely the feet, and is associated with marked pain and swelling. Examples of this condition have also been noted in the mandible.[18] There is radiological evidence of patchy osteoporosis. The pain is usually out of all proportion to the extent of the injury, and in one series of cases abnormalities were found in the median nerve as it passed under the carpal tunnel.[19] The most likely explanation of both the osteoporosis and the oedema is disuse consequent on the pain; an alternative suggestion of 'neuropathic' bone atrophy is less convincing (see below).

When the duct of a secreting gland is suddenly and completely blocked, the parenchyma undergoes atrophy, e.g. after total obstruction of a ureter, a salivary duct, and the pancreatic duct. It is interesting to recall that it was this method of producing pancreatic atrophy which was employed by Banting and Best in the isolation of insulin.

Neuropathic atrophy. This term is sometimes applied to the pronounced wasting of paralysed limbs—particularly after lower motor neuron lesions, e.g. poliomyelitis, motor neuron disease, and syringomyelia, or following nerve section. It is certain that in the event of paralysis disuse atrophy ensues, affecting the muscles and the other tissues. Whether sensory denervation also plays a part is not known. Direct damage due to unnoticed trauma may sometimes be an additional factor as,

Figure 24.8
Neuropathic atrophy of fingers. This is a photograph of the hand of a victim of lepromatous leprosy. Note the severe trophic changes involving the skin of the fingers as well as the destruction of the phalanges and soft tissues of the fingers, which are thereby shortened by a concertina effect. Nails are still present at the tips of the fingers. This type of leprosy is associated with involvement of nerves causing a symmetrical peripheral neuropathy. In addition, there is infiltration and destruction of the tissues by bacteria-laden macrophages.

for example, in syringomyelia, leprosy (Fig. 24.8) and tabes dorsalis.

Whether there is a specific 'neuropathic atrophy' of tissues that is unrelated to either disuse atrophy or direct trauma is disputed. The 'succulent hand' of syringomyelia and the changes seen in Sudeck's acute bone atrophy have been cited as examples, but changes in blood supply may be the explanation rather than a direct nervous influence. In amphibia, the usual regeneration after an amputation does not occur if the limb is first denervated. Indeed, the stump may be absorbed, so that amputation of even a finger may result in complete resorption of the limb.[20] This nervous influence, whether for regeneration or for maintenance of structural integrity, is called *trophic*, or more specifically, *neurotrophic*.

Idiopathic atrophy. There are examples of atrophy where no cause is evident. The myopathies, progressive muscular atrophy (motor neuron disease), sterility due to testicular atrophy, thyroid atrophy in myxoedema, and Addison's disease due to adrenal atrophy are good examples. In some, an autoimmune basis has been suggested but as yet unconfirmed; in others, an inherited defect is indicated (Huntington's chorea and dystrophia myotonica), while in others the atrophy appears to be a presenile one, as in Alzheimer's disease.

This group of diseases is likely to be eroded by future research. Thus Alzheimer's disease has been linked with aluminium toxicity; a slow virus has also been incriminated.

ABNORMALITIES OF CELLULAR DIFFERENTIATION

As described in Chapter 4, cells which are subjected to abnormal influences can change their structure and function. The best defined of these changes, which can be recognised on light microscopy, is metaplasia.

Metaplasia

Metaplasia is a condition in which there is a change of one type of differentiated tissue to another type of similarly differentiated tissue. The importance of the word differentiated should be noted, because its use excludes tumour formation as a form of metaplasia. The persistence of a similar differentiated tissue implies that tissues do not radically change their character: thus one type of epithelium changes to another type of epithelium, and similarly connective tissue changes to connective tissue. However, as we shall see, epithelium and connective tissue are more interchangeable than was at one time thought, even in humans. This should occasion no great surprise, for in the lower animals some cells have a remarkable ability to alter their pattern of differentiation. Thus in the newt, following the removal of the lens of the eye, the cells of the adjacent iris can form a new lens.

TYPES

Epithelial Metaplasia

Squamous metaplasia. Many types of epithelium are capable of changing to a stratified squamous variety which may undergo keratinisation. It often appears to be the result of persistent trauma ('chronic irritation'). The following examples may be cited:

(*a*) Gallbladder (simple columnar epithelium) in chronic cholecystitis, especially if accompanied by stones.

(*b*) Renal pelvis and bladder (transitional epithelium) in chronic infection. It is more common if stones are present.

(*c*) Uterus (simple columnar epithelium). Squamous metaplasia of the endometrium is an occasional senile change, and occurs in the rare condition of chronic inversion of the uterus. The glands of the cervix frequently undergo squamous metaplasia in chronic cervicitis, and the change may mimic early squamous-cell carcinoma. This metaplasia is especially common during pregnancy.

(*d*) Bronchi (pseudostratified columnar ciliated epithelium) (Fig. 24.9). Squamous metaplasia is common, and there is no evidence that it is precancerous. It is seen in chronic bronchitis, bronchiectasis, in epithelialised abscess cavities, and in bronchi draining tuberculous cavities. The almost constant

Figure 24.9
Squamous metaplasia of bronchial epithelium. The normal pseudos-tratified columnar ciliated respiratory epithelium of the bronchus has been replaced by a stratified squamous type of epithelium. × 200.

occurrence of squamous metaplasia overlying a bronchial 'adenoma' is of some practical importance. A superficial biopsy may lead to the mistaken diagnosis of squamous-cell carcinoma, and the true nature of the tumour be missed.

(*e*) Prostate (simple columnar epithelium). Squamous metaplasia is seen in the ducts in patients treated with oestrogen.

Although in many of these examples 'chronic irritation' appears to be the cause of the metaplasia, there is one condition in which squamous metaplasia is common, but in which irritation plays no part. This is hypovitaminosis A (see Ch. 34).

Columnar metaplasia. Squamous epithelium rarely changes to a columnar type. Cervical erosion is often cited as an example. In this condition the vaginal portion of the cervix is covered by columnar epithelium instead of the normal squamous type. This may arise in one of two ways. The cervix is covered by columnar epithelium during development and normally this changes to a squamous type, probably under the influence of oestrogenic stimulation. If columnar epithelium persists during childhood, the condition is termed a *congenital erosion*. The second type of erosion occurs in adults, and usually follows childbirth. There is a pouting of the endocervical mucosa so that this becomes visible on the vaginal aspect. Subsequent squamous metaplasia may occur, and blockage of the mucous glands results in the production of retention cysts. These are the familiar nabothian follicles.* It

*Named after Martin Naboth, a Leipzic anatomist of the early eighteenth century.

is unlikely that columnar epithelium ever replaces a previously squamous-covered surface either by metaplasia or by growth over an ulcerated area.

Specialised columnar epithelia may change to a more simple type. The conversion of the pseudostratified columnar ciliated respiratory epithelium to a simple mucus-secreting columnar type is common in chronic bronchitis and bronchiectasis, and plays a part in predisposing patients with these conditions to bronchopneumonia (see p. 90).

The occurrence of patches of an intestinal type of epithelium complete with villi in the stomach is not infrequent, and some authorities regard these areas as being particularly liable to malignant change. Intestinal metaplasia also often occurs in a healed chronic gastric ulcer (see p. 121). The epithelium also functions like intestinal epithelium, and its absorptive capacity might provide an explanation of how carcinogens gain entrance to the gastric wall.[21]

The eosinophilic columnar epithelium, called 'pale' or 'pink' epithelium, often found lining some of the cysts in mammary dysplasia is another fine example of columnar metaplasia. It closely resembles the epithelium of the normal apocrine glands found most abundantly in the axilla, and serves as a reminder that the mammary glands are developmentally closely related to sweat glands.

Connective Tissue Metaplasia

Osseous metaplasia. The question as to whether fibroblasts can produce osteoid tissue or not is largely a matter of definition of fibroblasts and osteoblasts. They certainly exhibit morphological identity, and before the appearance of the intercellular substance, whether fibrous tissue or osteoid, they cannot be distinguished. 'Fibroblasts' do not normally produce osteoid, but under some conditions they may be regarded as undergoing metaplasia to 'osteoblasts'. Bone then makes its appearance. An alternative explanation is that the osteoblasts are derived from primitive stem cells (see p. 391). Marrow is often found in the metaplastic bone. It could either be the result of metaplasia of the local mesenchymal cells or else follow the deposition of primitive haematopoietic cells from the blood stream. The relationship between fibroblasts, chondroblasts, and osteoblasts is discussed on pages 117 to 119 in relation to fracture healing.

Osseous metaplasia occurs as an ageing process in cartilage, e.g. the costal and thyroid cartilages. A rare, interesting lesion is *tracheopathia osteoplastica*,[22] where cartilaginous and bony masses develop in the submucosa of the trachea and larger bronchi. Some of these foci apparently develop directly from the cartilage rings and bars, but others arise from the connective tissue by metaplasia.

Osseous metaplasia is also seen in soft tissue, e.g. in scars and areas of dystrophic calcification such as long-standing goitres, caseous foci, tonsils, and Mönckeberg's sclerosis. The ossification of such calcareous foci depends on the osteogenic potentiality of the adjacent fibroblasts.

Foci of ossification are sometimes found in muscle. It is probable that local trauma is a predisposing factor. The muscles most often involved are the gluteus maximus and the adductors of the thigh. Ossification in muscle and tendon has been reported after tetanus, and it is also a complication of paralytic poliomyelitis in which bone may develop in the wasted muscles. The most important example of metaplastic ossification in muscle, or *localised myositis ossificans* as it is often called, is seen in the bend of the elbow after a supracondylar fracture of the humerus. The bony mass forms in the insertion of the brachialis muscle. It would appear that traumatic myositis ossificans is due to the organisation and subsequent ossification of a haematoma. When this occurs in proximity to bone it may be that osteoblasts are derived from the periosteum.

There are two rare but interesting conditions, both inherited as dominant characteristics, in which widespread osseous metaplasia occurs. In *fibrodysplasia ossificans progressiva*[23,24] there is progressive laying-down of bone in aponeuroses, tendons, and fascia, so that the body eventually may become completely rigid. The disease is also called 'myositis ossificans progressiva', but in fact the muscles are only secondarily involved in this ossification, the nature of which is obscure. In the early stages painful swellings develop in the tissues, and these subsequently ossify. An associated feature is microdactyly (with monophalangy of the big toe as a usual concomitant). In *pseudohypoparathyroidism*, which is mentioned on page 559, the body is unresponsive to parathyroid hormone. In addition, there are skeletal deformities, mental retardation, and a tendency to widespread subcutaneous calcification and ossification. Osteoma cutis is quite common, and is not localised as after trauma or acne vulgaris. In *pseudo-pseudohypoparathyroidism* similar skeletal deformities and subcutaneous ossification may occur, but there is normal responsiveness to parathyroid hormone and therefore no disturbance in calcium and phosphate metabolism. It is probable that this condition is merely an incompletely expressed form of a genetically determined abnormality of which pseudohypoparathyroidism represents the complete clinical syndrome. It is suggested that the syndrome be called *Albright's hereditary osteodystrophy.*[25]

Changes in mesothelium. Squamous metaplasia may occur both in the pleura and peritoneum. We have encountered a patch of keratinising stratified squamous epithelium overlying a pulmonary infarct. Some rare cases of squamous-cell carcinoma appear to arise from the pleura; it might be that they are derived from such an area of squamous metaplasia, although the possibility of such a tumour arising from an underlying bronchiole is very difficult to exclude.

Under other circumstances pleural mesothelium may become columnar, and even form tubules (Fig. 24.10). It is not surprising therefore that malignant mesotheliomata of the pleura and peritoneum often have an epithelial component in which clefts and tubular spaces may be found. The pathogenesis of *endometriosis* is disputed, but it may be that this too represents a type of metaplasia of the mesothelial lining of the peritoneum—and occasionally the pleura. The potentialities of the mesothelial cells covering the ovary should also be remembered; they can form germinal follicles and epithelial-lined cysts, as well as give rise to frankly epithelial tumours. Synovial cells may also closely resemble columnar epithelium, and a synovioma may occasionally present the appearance of an adenocarcinoma.

It is apparent that mesothelium can form various cell types: herein lies one of the pitfalls in examining pleural or peritoneal exudates for malignant cells. Groups of cells arranged

Figure 24.10
Metaplasia in mesothelium. Section of thickened pleura shows groups of altered mesothelial cells. It is understandable that such groups of cells might become detached and appear in a pleural effusion. × 700.

in the form of an acinus are not necessarily malignant. Other cytological characteristics must be taken into account before a diagnosis of adenocarcinoma is made.

Finally, it should be noted that the metaplasia which can occur in mesothelium indicates that the division between connective tissue and epithelium is not as definite as is sometimes assumed. A striking example of this occurs in the lens of the eye. In some examples of cataract the epithelial cells of the anterior aspect of the lens undergo metaplasia and form fibrous tissue.

Tumour Metaplasia

The occurrence of mixed adenocarcinoma and squamous-cell carcinoma (adenoacanthoma) is not an uncommon event, and may be explained on the basis of tumour metaplasia (Fig. 24.11). The assumption is that the tumour commences as an adenocarcinoma, but that a change occurs in some of its cells leading to squamous differentiation. It should be noted that this change is not 'metaplasia' in the strict sense, because a tumour cannot be regarded as a completely differentiated tissue. It is therefore preferably called 'tumour metaplasia', and is believed to be quite common in cancer of the lung. About a fifth of lung adenocarcinomata show squamous elements. Indeed, tumour metaplasia may explain the origin of all squamous-cell carcinomata of lung if it is assumed that the squamous cells can outgrow and completely obliterate the adenocarcinomatous element. Another explanation may be that

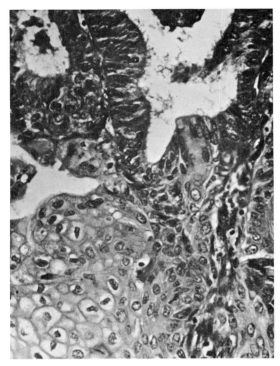

Figure 24.11
Squamous tumour metaplasia. This is a section of well-differentiated adenocarcinoma of the body of the uterus. Part of the columnar-cell lining of the malignant acinus is replaced by stratified squamous epithelium. ×250.

the tumours arise in areas of squamous metaplasia. These possibilities are shown diagrammatically in Figure 24.12.

Tumour metaplasia of squamous type is also seen in carcinoma of the gall-bladder, in endometrial adenocarcinoma, and transitional-cell carcinoma of urinary tract. It is occasionally seen in pleomorphic salivary gland tumours, carcinoma of the breast, and more rarely in adenocarcinomata of other sites.

Mucoid metaplasia is occasionally seen in adenocarcinomata of the breast.

The stroma of a tumour can also undergo metaplasia, e.g. osseous metaplasia is common in fibro-adenomata of the canine breast.

The question arises whether, in general, epithelial metaplasia, particularly the squamous type, is a precancerous condition. It is impossible to give a dogmatic answer. There is no doubt that squamous-cell carcinomata can arise from the bronchus, the urinary passages, and the gallbladder, but it is

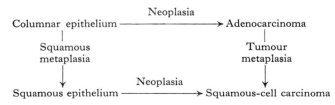

Figure 24.12

less certain whether they start on an area of metaplastic epithelium, or whether the tumour epithelium subsequently undergoes squamous change. The consensus of opinion is that the change succeeds neoplasia much more often than preceding it.

OTHER CELLULAR DYSTROPHIES

Dystrophy* may be defined as a disorder, usually congenital, of the structure or function of an organ or tissue due to its perverted nutrition. In its widest sense it includes agenesis, atrophy, hypertrophy, hyperplasia, and metaplasia, but in practice the term is usually applied to those disorders which do not readily fit into any of these other categories. The alternative term *dysplasia** may also be used for such an abnormal development of tissue, although strictly it should be applied to developmental disorders only. *Dyscrasia** literally means a bad mixture (of the four humours), and is now used only by haematologists to describe any blood disorder of uncertain aetiology.

One of the best examples of a dystrophy is the lesion found in pernicious anaemia. Although the abnormal nuclear maturation found in the red-cell precursors in this disease led Ehrlich to describe them as megaloblasts, it was not realised at that time that other cells showed similar changes. Examination of the cells of the gastric, buccal, nasal, vaginal, and other mucosae has revealed nuclear abnormalities presumably caused by vitamin-B_{12} deficiency. The changes include pleomorphism, giant nuclei, and large nucleoli. These observations have an important application: the exfoliative cytologist must avoid mistaking these cells for malignant cells in sputum, gastric washings, urine, etc. The premature greying of the hair and the degeneration of the spinal cord indicate that pernicious anaemia is more than merely a haematological disorder.

Another interesting dystrophy is seen in the skin, sometimes following a burn, or superimposed on some existing lesion, such as a solar keratosis or a seborrhoeic keratosis. The abnormal squamous epithelium produces excessive keratin which adheres to produce a cutaneous horn (Fig. 24.13).

Many special dystrophies involving muscle, bone, cornea, retina, etc., have been described, but these are outside the scope of general pathology.

It must be reiterated that the term dystrophy has no specific intrinsic meaning, but like dysplasia is used to describe a lesion whose nature is not understood and for which the author can find no other more appropriate name. In recent years dysplasia has acquired a specific meaning when applied to epithelium—most commonly that of the cervix uteri and epidermis of the skin. It is used to describe a type of hyperplasia that is accompanied by atypicality of the cells and their maturation. The condition progresses to *carcinoma-in-situ* in some cases and later to invasive squamous-cell carcinoma

*The Greek derivation of these words is as follows:
Dys—bad or difficult.
Krasis—a mingling.
Plasis—a forming.
Trophe—nourishment.

Figure 24.13
Cutaneous horn. This amazing horny excrescence was removed from the skin of the arm of a man who had been
severely burnt 20 years before. A skin graft had been
applied, and healing was excellent. Twenty years later this
truncated keratin horn developed at the site of the burn
after a minor injury to the part. On excision it was found
that the mass was not attached to the deeper structures, and
recovery was complete after another skin graft had been
applied.

Before the horn was excised, the patient's wife was wont
to saw off pieces with a hacksaw. The specimen comprises
the complete horn including the sawn-off portions. (I 18a.4,
*Reproduced by permission of the President and Council of the
R.C.S. Eng.*)

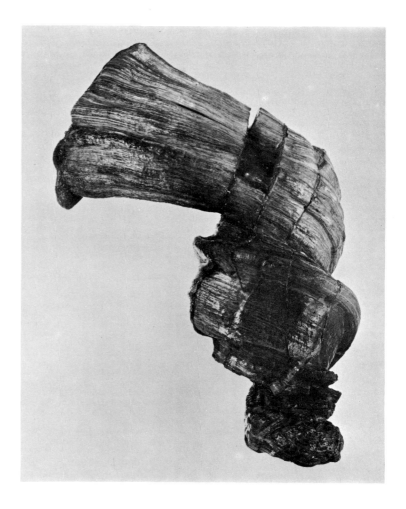

(p. 381). But dysplasia is also used in other contexts, e.g.
fibrous dysplasia of bone and mammary dysplasia, in which
there is no suggestion of incipient neoplastic change.

In this chapter many different perversions of cell growth
have been described. With few exceptions, the one thing they
all have in common is that they are self-limiting and reversible
if the stimulus is removed. In the following chapters neoplasia
is considered. Here the perversion of cell growth persists even
when the stimulus is eradicated.

REFERENCES

1. POST, J. & HOFFMAN, J. (1968) Cell renewal patterns. *New England Journal of Medicine*, **279**, 248.
2. LEVER, W. F. & SCHAUMBURG-LEVER, G. (1975) *Histopathology of the Skin*, 5th edn, p. 708. Philadelphia: Lippincott.
3. HOGAN, M. J. & ZIMMERMAN, L. E. (1962) *Ophthalmic Pathology*, 2nd edn, p. 765. Philadelphia: Saunders.
4. ANAGNOSTOU, D. & HARRISON, C. V. (1972) Angiofollicular lymph node hyperplasia (Castleman). *Journal of Clinical Pathology*, **25**, 306.
5. KERR, J. F. R., WYLLIE, A. H. & CURRIE, A. R. (1972) Apoptosis: a basic biological phenomenon with wideranging implications in tissue kinetics. *British Journal of Cancer*, **26**, 239.
6. Leading Article (1972) Apoptosis. *Lancet*, **2**, 1011.
7. HOPWOOD, D. & LEVISON, D. A. (1976) Atrophy and apoptosis in the cyclical human endometrium. *Journal of Pathology*, **119**, 159.
8. BARZEL, U. S. (1970) *Osteoporosis*, 290 pp. New York: Grune and Stratton.
9. Leading Article (1971) Osteoporosis. *British Medical Journal*, **1**, 566.
10. MEEMA, H. E., HARRIS, C. K. & PORRETT, R. E. (1964) A method for determination of bone-salt content of cortical bone. *Radiology*, **82**, 986.
11. DEITRICK, J. E., WHEDON, G. D. & SHORR, E. (1948) Effects of immobilization upon various metabolic and physiologic functions of normal men. *American Journal of Medicine*, **4**, 3.
12. HEANEY, R. P. (1962) Radiocalcium metabolism in disuse osteoporosis in man. *American Journal of Medicine*, **33**, 188.
13. Annotation (1963) Disuse osteoporosis. *Lancet*, **1**, 150.
14. SHERLOCK, S. (1975) *Diseases of the Liver*, 5th edn, p. 268. Oxford: Blackwell.
15. FRASER, S. A. *et al.* (1971) Osteoporosis and fractures following thyrotoxicosis. *Lancet*, **1**, 981.

16. NORDIN, B. E. C. (1971) Clinical significance and pathogenesis of osteoporosis. *British Medical Journal*, **1**, 571.

17. McKUSICK, V. A. (1972) *Heritable Disorders of Connective Tissue*, 4th edn, p. 390 *et seq.* Saint Louis: Mosby.

18. PHILLIPS, R. M., BUSH, O. B. & HALL, H. D. (1972) Massive osteolysis (phantom bone, disappearing bone). *Oral Surgery, Oral Medicine and Oral Pathology*, **34**, 886.

19. STEIN, A. H. (1962) The relation of median nerve compression to Sudeck's syndrome. *Surgery, Gynecology and Obstetrics*, **115**, 713.

20. THORNTON, C. S. (1968) Amphibian limb regeneration. *Advances in Morphogenesis*, Eds Abercrombie, M., Brachet, J. & King, T. J., Vol. 7, p. 2-5-249. New York: Academic Press.

21. RUBIN, W. *et al.* (1967) Some physiologic properties of heterotopic intestinal epithelium. *Laboratory Investigation*, **16**, 813.

22. Leading Article (1968) Rigid trachea. *British Medical Journal*, **2**, 4.

23. LUTWAK, L. (1964) Myositis ossificans progressiva. *American Journal of Medicine*, **37**, 269.

24. McKUSICK, V. A. (1972) *Heritable Disorders of Connective Tissue*, 4th edn, p. 687 *et seq.* Saint Louis: Mosby.

25. BROOK, C. G. D. & VALMAN, H. B. (1971) Osteoma cutis and Albright's hereditary osteodystrophy. *British Journal of Dermatology*, **85**, 471.

Chapter 25. Tumours: Introduction and Classification

It must be acknowledged that no completely satisfactory definition of a tumour exists. Since the exact nature and cause of tumour growth are unknown, the only existing definitions are in fact descriptions, and like most descriptions some are better than others.

To Powell White we owe the concept that 'a tumour proper is a mass of cells, tissues or organs resembling those normally present, but arranged atypically. It grows at the expense of the organism without at the same time subserving any useful function'. The cells of the tumour are sometimes arranged so atypically that their resemblance to the normal is difficult to recognise. Indeed, they may resemble those found during development rather than those present in post-uterine life. On the other hand, some tumour cells may so closely resemble the normal that a morphological distinction is scarcely possible. Thus the appearance of the cells is not of overriding importance.

Abnormal behaviour, on the other hand, is of greater significance than abnormal appearance. The continued growth at the expense of the host has been emphasised by such a trite definition of tumours as 'autonomous parasites'. Autonomy means self-government, and it is obvious that no tumour is entirely independent of the surrounding tissues; without a blood supply it would soon undergo necrosis. Benign tumours may show only limited autonomy, because growth often ceases when the tumour has attained a certain size. Some malignant tumours also, far from being completely autonomous, are under some controlling influence, for they may remain quiescent for many years: sometimes the control appears to be hormonal. The fetus is quite as autonomous as any tumour. It is a true parasite, but its natural history entails only a limited stay within its parent.

Nevertheless, it is probably true to say that a characteristic of all tumours is that the cells are behaving in an abnormal way, which indicates that they are escaping from some, if not all, the normal mechanisms that control cell growth and anatomical arrangement. Unfortunately we are ignorant even about these normal mechanisms.

This process of escape is often manifested by the production of a space-occupying mass or tumour, but this is not always the case. Sometimes the migration of cells outside the normal confining limits outweighs the abnormal proliferation; in this case no 'tumour' as such exists. An excellent example of this is the diffuse infiltrating carcinoma of the stomach ('linitis plastica').

A term which is therefore more suitable is *neoplasia*; it indicates an abnormal type of new growth which not only may be evident in the intact antimal, but which can also be seen and studied in tissue culture. Neoplasia differs from hyperplasia in several important respects:

(*a*) Neoplasia usually appears to arise spontaneously, but in those cases where the stimulus is known, it is not physiological, e.g. ionising radiation, chemical carcinogen, or viral infection. Hyperplasia, on the other hand, is usually produced by the excessive action of a normal stimulus, e.g. a hormone. Nevertheless, this is not an absolute distinction because hyperplasia can also be induced by agents similar to those which produce tumours. Epidermal hyperplasia is a marked feature in molluscum contagiosum and the common wart, both of which are caused by viruses. Epidermal hyperplasia is also seen in the skin's response to chemical irritants.

(*b*) The growth in hyperplasia is directly related to the degree of stimulation, while neoplasia, once it starts, proceeds irrespective of the stimulus.

(*c*) Once the stimulus is removed, hyperplasia regresses. Neoplasia, on the other hand, proceeds unabated.

The definition given by Willis embodies this concept: '*a tumour is an abnormal mass of tissue, the growth of which exceeds and is uncoordinated with that of the normal tissues, and persists in the same excessive manner after cessation of the stimuli which evoked the change*'. To this extent the tumour cells may be said to be autonomous and beyond normal growth control. It certainly seems that their continued growth is quite useless, and the neoplastic response to a stimulus appears to have no survival value in the evolutionary process. When it is remembered that most tumours occur during the post-reproductive years, this is not altogether surprising.

CLASSIFICATION

The difficulties encountered in the classification of neoplasias are those that are inherent in the classification of any condition of unknown aetiology. No single classification is wholly satisfactory; by examining tumours from different aspects various subdivisions are possible. While some classifications are more useful than others, none is more 'correct' than another. Some classifications are dependent on a microscopical examination of the tumour, while others are related to the naked-eye appearance or behaviour. The following bases for classification may be recognised:

1. Naked-eye appearance including the organ of origin.
2. Histogenetic classification (including embryological considerations).
3. Histological.
4. Behavioural.
5. Aetiological.
6. Functional.

Naked-eye Appearances and Regional Classification

When the patient is first seen clinically the organ of origin is the most striking feature of many tumours. There is a complaint of a lump or the effect of a lump in an organ.

Although tumours of widely differing behaviour and origin can arise in one particular organ, this classification is nevertheless of some importance. A tumour of the brain or its meninges is invariably more serious than a tumour of a finger: it produces a characteristic clinical picture, and whatever its nature, demands early treatment if life is to be saved.

A naked-eye examination of tumours frequently reveals characteristics which by experience are known to coincide with other properties. For example, the terms 'annular' and 'fungating' (cauliflower) growth are often applied to gut tumours, and are self-explanatory. The former produces constriction, while the latter ulcerates and bleeds. 'Scirrhous' tumours are hard, a feature due to the large amount of fibrous tissue present in the stroma. 'Encephaloid' or 'medullary' tumours are soft and brain-like due to the sparse stromal reaction. Mucoid tumours form another characteristic group.

Histogenetic Classification

The cell-type of origin forms an important feature of our present classification. The body has by convention been divided into epithelium and connective tissue, although the distinction between the two is by no means as clear-cut as is sometimes imagined. Two groups of tumours are therefore recognised:

Tumours of epithelial origin

Tumours of connective-tissue origin

Six main difficulties are apparent in this classification:

1. *The Nature of Endothelium, Mesothelium, and Synovium.* The flattened lining cells of the serous spaces present a problem. The endothelial or mesothelial cells, although ge- nerally classified as connective tissue, may on occasions give rise to tumours which resemble those of frankly epithelial origin. Thus, a mesothelioma of the pleura may closely resemble an adenocarcinoma, and indeed some tumours so labelled are in fact secondary lung cancers and not mesotheliomata. It is now accepted, however, that genuine mesotheliomata do occur, for some are composed of spindle-shaped cells of connective tissue type, while in others both types of cells are present.

In the peritoneum the same types of difficulty arise. Many suspected mesotheliomata are in fact secondary carcinomata. Nevertheless, it is generally accepted that the cells covering the ovary can give rise to frankly epithelial tumours. Perhaps the same is true of other sites. In joints the synovium may give rise to tumours which closely resemble adenocarcinomata. It is apparent that, although convention dictates that epithelial and connective tissue cells are quite distinct, the conversion of one type to another is not outside the realm of possibility. The subject has been further discussed in relation to metaplasia (see p. 305).

2. *Undifferentiated Tumours.* A second difficulty in a histogenetic classification is the occurrence of tumours so poorly differentiated that their cell of origin defies recognition, i.e. the parent tissue is very poorly reproduced.

Electron microscopy is sometimes of help in determining the origin of a tumour: the finding of melanosomes would indicate that an anaplastic tumour was a malignant melanoma. On the other hand, the presence of neurosecretory granules would point to an origin from cells of the APUD series (Figs. 25.1 to 25.4)

Figure 25.1

Malignant melanoma. A 16-year-old boy developed enlargement of the inguinal lymph nodes, and biopsy revealed an anaplastic tumour consistent with anaplastic carcinoma, lymphoma, or malignant melanoma. No melanin could be demonstrated by silver staining. Electron microscopy revealed cytoplasmic structures (mel), which on high magnification (inset) show the characteristic banding of melanosomes that is visible before the extensive deposition of melanin obscures this detail. On reviewing the patient's history it was found that a 'mole' had been removed from the leg two years previously. This had been reported as a benign naevus, but in fact was a malignant melanoma. × 8000. Insert ×107 000. (*Photograph by courtesy of Dr Y. C. Bedard*)

Figure 25.2
Oat-cell carcinoma of the lung. A 45-year-old woman developed features of Cushing's syndrome, and a scalene lymph-node biopsy revealed an anaplastic tumour consistent with the diagnosis of oat-cell carcinoma of the lung. The electron micrograph of the tumour shows typical neurosecretory granules. Note also the presence of free lipid and lysosomes, some of which contain myelin figures. × 8000. (*Photograph by courtesy of Dr Y. C. Bedard*)

Figure 25.3

Carcinoma of the breast. A 65-year-old woman developed enlarged axillary lymph nodes, and biopsy revealed an anaplastic tumour. Lymphoma was considered to be the most likely diagnosis, but electron microscopy revealed intracellular lumina with microvilli. This is a feature of poorly-differentiated glandular carcinoma. A blind biopsy of the ipsilateral breast of this patient showed infiltrating lobular carcinoma. Note the presence of numerous glycogen granules. × 8000. (*Photograph by courtesy of Dr Y. C. Bedard*)

Figure 25.4

Squamous-cell carcinoma of nose. A 50-year-old man developed a polypoid lesion of the nose. This was excised, and the specimen reported as consisting of inflammatory tissue. However, the lesion recurred, and a biopsy revealed a vascular lesion with many spindle cells consistent with a diagnosis of spindle-cell sarcoma. Electron microscopy showed typical features of an epithelial tumour. The figure shows several tight junctions with desmosome formation. In the cytoplasm tonofilaments are present as well as numerous free ribosomes, which are grouped as polysomes. The tumour was therefore regarded as a spindle-cell squamous-cell carcinoma. × 16 000. (*Photograph by courtesy of Dr Y. C. Bedard*)

3. *Tumour Metaplasia.* The occurrence of tumour metaplasia may further confuse the issue. For instance, a tumour of the lung may be undifferentiated, and yet have areas of squamous differentiation as evidenced by prickle-cell formation and keratinisation. The supposition is that the tumour is a poorly-differentiated growth of columnar bronchial epithelium, and should therefore be called a polygonal-cell carcinoma with squamous metaplasia. Regardless of the true origin of a tumour it must be admitted that the label given to a particular growth is frequently a matter of personal prejudice on the part of the pathologist. An anaplastic squamous-cell carcinoma to one authority may be called a transitional-cell carcinoma, an anaplastic carcinoma, a reticulum-cell sarcoma (histiocytic lymphoma), or merely an undifferentiated malignant tumour by other pathologists.

4. *Debatable Origin of a Tissue.* Another difficulty is the histogenetic classification of tumours arising from cells whose precise origin has been disputed. The best example of this is the melanocyte of the skin. Those who favour a neural origin (see p. 350) might call malignant tumours of melanocytes melanotic sarcomata. Those who favour an epithelial origin (now an outdated hypothesis) would support the name naevocarcinoma.

5. *Origin from highly specialised tissues.* A fifth difficulty arises with certain very specialised tissues which produce tumours that are distinctive and unlike those found elsewhere. For example, the nervous system, excluding the ependyma, and the haematopoietic tissues, although included in the broad group of connective tissue, are so different from other connective tissues that some authorities prefer to separate them from the others when classifying the tissues from which tumours may take origin. This serves to point out the distinctive features of malignant lymphoma, leukaemia, phaeochromocytoma, the gliomata, etc. It must, however, be appreciated that the number of 'basic' tissues recognised is an arbitrary affair. Bichat in fact recognised over 30, and indeed if each type of epithelium and connective tissue is regarded as separate the number could greatly exceed this.

6. *Origin from placental and embryonic tissues.* Finally, certain tumours arise from cells which are not normally present in the adult body. Two groups of tumours can be recognised:

(*a*) Those of placental origin like the hydatidiform mole and choriocarcinoma. Both are derived from chorionic tissue, and are of fetal origin.

(*b*) Tumours of germ-cell and embryonic origin. These include the teratomata and such tumours of infancy as the nephroblastoma, neuroblastoma, and medulloblastoma.

Teratomata arise from *totipotential cells*, i.e. cells capable of differentiating into any of the tissues of the body. This has given rise to the concept that representatives of each of the three germ-layers must be present before a teratoma can be diagnosed. In fact, in most of the benign teratomata one particular tissue, the skin with its appendages, outgrows all the others, so that it is difficult to find representatives of all three germinal layers. As will be shown, the concept of germ-layers is unhelpful in the classification of most tumours, and can be discarded without great loss. But even here there are exceptions; the concept of the APUD series of cells appears to provide an explanation of the hormonal secretion exhibited by some tumours (see p. 340).

The embryonic tumours of infancy arise from specific organs or areas of tissue during their development to a mature size, e.g. the pole of a kidney, the retina, or the area around the fourth ventricle. Some of the tumours consist only of the primitive cells pertaining to the part (e.g. retinoblastoma, medulloblastoma, and neuroblastoma), but others contain muscle fibres in addition (e.g. the Wilms tumour). Such tumours that consist of more than one element are called 'mixed tumours'. The teratoma is an extreme example of a mixed tumour. A cell capable of giving rise to several tissues is called *pluripotential*. It is obvious that these embryonic tumours of infancy and the teratomata are best explained on a developmental or embryological basis.

A further extension of an embryological classification was attempted, and finally abandoned as unsatisfactory.[1] Each tumour was described as *lepidic* if of epithelial origin or *hyalic* if from pulp or connective tissue. To this was prefixed either *epi-*, *meso-*, or *hypo-*, according to the germ-layer involved. Innocent tumours were designated *typical* while malignant tumours were regarded as *atypical*. Thus a squamous-cell carcinoma of the labium majus was called an atypical epilepidoma, while a similar tumour of the vagina was an atypical hypolepidoma. Such a cumbersome classification has little to recommend it. It is evident that the germ-layer of origin of tumour cells is of little importance in respect of tumour structure or behaviour. It should incidentally be noted that mesoderm can form epithelium as well as connective tissue, a fact which is not always appreciated. Renal tubules, ovary, (excluding the ova themselves), adrenal cortex, and endometrium are all mesodermal. Furthermore, ectoderm can form connective tissue: the muscle of the iris is ectodermal as is also the neuroglia.

Histological Classification

It sometimes happens that a malignant tumour consists merely of a diffuse mass of irregular cells which do not resemble any normal tissue. Such complete undifferentiation is called *anaplasia*. In this case the actual appearance of the neoplastic cells may be used as a basis for classification. A histological classification is used under the following circumstances:

When the tumour is so undifferentiated as to defy recognition of its site of origin. A tumour of glandular tissue which shows no evidence of glandular formation can be described only as polygonal-cell, spheroidal-cell, or anaplastic. The term actually used is frequently a matter of convention. A spheroidal-cell carcinoma at one hospital may be a polygonal-cell carcinoma at another. 'Carcinoma simplex' is another term frequently used to describe this type of tumour. Sometimes the anaplasia is so great that it is uncertain whether the tumour has arisen from connective tissue or epithelium. One of the best examples of this difficulty is seen in the lung tumour now known as oat-cell (or small-cell in North America) carcinoma. Before 1926 it was labelled oat-cell sarcoma of the mediastinum.

Small-cell, large-cell, pleomorphic-cell, giant-cell, spindle-cell, etc., are all self-explanatory terms when applied to tumours.

The occurrence of tumour metaplasia. Again pure description has to be used. The term 'squamous-cell carcinoma' is used to describe a tumour of lung with a squamous differentiation, rather than to indicate a tumour arising from a stratified squamous epithelium (see p. 305).

The histological grading of tumours is based upon the degree of differentiation, and sometimes also the degree of irregularity, number of mitoses, etc. (see Ch. 26).

Classification According to Behaviour

Although the classical division of tumours into the two main groups, benign and malignant, is of great practical importance, it must be appreciated that intermediate types of behaviour exist which do not fall properly into either of these categories. The characteristics of the two groups must first be considered.

Benign or innocent tumours. The cells which constitute this type of growth show no tendency to invade the surrounding tissues. The excessive accumulation of cells produces an expanding lesion which causes pressure atrophy of the surrounding tissues. The stroma that remains forms the capsule that is a characteristic feature of benign tumours situated in a solid organ or tissue.

Benign tumours proliferate slowly, and usually show few mitoses. The arrangement of the cells closely resembles that of the parent tissue—they are *well-differentiated*. It must be realised that a benign tumour is one which behaves in a characteristic way, rather than one which has a particular microscopical appearance. Other characteristics of benign tumours are considered in Chapter 26.

Malignant tumours. A malignant tumour always invades the surrounding tissues. It eventually enters channels like the lymphatics and blood vessels, and groups of cells are carried to other parts, where they set up secondary growths, or metastases. *Local invasion* and *embolic spread* are the two characteristics of malignant tumours. Both are probably related to the reduced cell adhesion which is a fundamental characteristic of cancer grown in tissue culture; the cells growing out of the explant do not resist mechanical separation as well as those of normal tissue. The power to invade and spread combined with the capacity for progressive growth make the term 'malignant' particularly suitable for this type of tumour. Death is inevitable in untreated cases although the rate of progression varies markedly from one case to the next (but see below).

Microscopically, malignant tumours tend to show less accurate reproduction of the parent tissue than do their benign counterparts. Other features of malignant tumours like irregularity, pleomorphism, etc., are described elsewhere (see Ch. 26).

In addition to the classical benign and malignant tumours there are other types which show noteworthy patterns of behaviour and fit into neither group.

Intermediate tumours. This category, named by Morehead,[2] includes tumours which are locally invasive, and therefore not benign, but which either show little or no tendency to metastasise (*locally malignant tumours* such as basal-cell carcinoma and ameloblastoma) or else sometimes give rise to metastases which progress slowly and usually cause little constitutional disturbance to the patient. These are the *tumours of erratic behaviour* which include pleomorphic tumour of the salivary glands, 'adenoma' of the bronchus, and

carcinoid tumours of the intestine. These are described in the next chapter.

Latent cancer. This is the name given to a proliferation of cells that has all the histological characteristics of carcinoma, including sometimes lymphatic and blood vessel invasion, and yet which remains clinically silent and does not metastasise. The most convincing examples of this condition have been described in the prostates of elderly men.[3] It is the outer zone that contains these lesions, and not the middle zone that is affected in benign hyperplasia and removed during partial prostatectomy. The nature of the condition is obscure. In some instances it may indeed be a carcinoma which is not progressing because the environment (e.g. hormonal) is not suitable, but most of the lesions are probably atypical epithelial hyperplasias associated with old age. The tendency for excessive epithelial hyperplasia to form pseudocarcinomatous downgrowths into the connective tissue has been noted on page 296.

Carcinoma-in-situ. This is a pre-invasive proliferation of the epithelium which has the cytological features of malignancy. It is considered on page 381.

Spontaneous Regressions.[4,5] These are amongst the most fascinating phenomena of malignancy. There is now a considerable literature of cases of cancer which have suddenly regressed spontaneously and permanently. This rare occurrence is most often seen in cases of malignant melanoma, hypernephroma, neuroblastoma, and choriocarcinoma. The Burkitt tumour may sometimes regress, apparently permanently, after a single dose of cytotoxic agent too small in amount to account for the result in terms of its known action.[6] The mechanism of these regressions is not known. It may be hormonal, thus relating it to the hormone-dependent tumours, or it may be immunological. The serum of cases of malignant melanoma that have regressed spontaneously has been noted to affect the course of malignant melanomata when administered to patients with this disease.[7] Sometimes the removal of a primary tumour leads to the regression of its metastases, a phenomenon most often seen in choriocarcinoma and malignant melanoma. Incomplete resection of an inoperable tumour, even one as malignant as an oat-cell carcinoma invading the left atrium, has been known to end in a complete cure of the condition.[8]

Another mechanism involved in the remission of a tumour is a maturation of its cells to a benign or non-neoplastic form. This event is best documented in some cases of neuroblastoma and teratoma of the testis.[9]

Dormant cancer. This is the late appearance of metastases after the primary tumour has been successfully removed. Its implications are considered on page 365.

Aetiological Classification

Since the cause of most human tumours is unknown, this is at present an impractical basis for classification. Furthermore, there is no indication at the present time that such a classification is likely to be very useful. Tumours induced by radiations, chemical carcinogens, etc., can all look alike, and behave in the same way. Likewise a single agent, e.g. ionising radiations, can induce carcinoma of the skin, osteosarcoma, and leukaemia. It seems that the type of tumour growth is independent of the initiating cause.

Functional Classification

The discovery that some tumours secrete hormones in sufficient quantity to produce characteristic clinical and pathological changes has led some authorities to name the tumour after the hormone, e.g. glucagonoma, insulinoma, etc. This cannot be regarded as a satisfactory basis for classification, since neither the site nor the behaviour of the tumour is included.

Classification Currently Used

The tissue of origin and the behaviour pattern form the basis of the present classification (see tables on pp. 314–315). This is supplemented by a histological description. The suffix -oma, is used to denote a neoplasm. Unfortunately it is also used in connexion with some non-neoplastic swellings, e.g. haematoma, granuloma, and hamartoma.

It will be seen that benign tumours of surface epithelia are called papillomata. Benign tumours of solid epithelia are adenomata. These may be cystic (cystadenoma), and into these cysts papillary ingrowths may occur (papillary cystadenoma).

The malignant epithelial tumours are all carcinomata, and a histological description is appended.

In the connective tissues the benign tumours are named after the tissue of origin, e.g. fibroma and osteoma, while the malignant tumours are sarcomata, e.g. fibrosarcoma and osteosarcoma. The term spindle-cell sarcoma is used to describe a sarcoma in which the tissue of origin cannot be recognised. Certain tumours of specialised cells have characteristics which have led to them being given names which do not conform to these rules. Thus the clear-cell carcinoma of the kidney is commonly called a hypernephroma, and a tumour derived from the argentaffin cells a carcinoid. Finally, it should be noted that the term neoplasia is applied in any type of tumour growth whether benign or malignant, while cancer is a colloquial term used to describe any type of malignant tumour whether carcinoma or sarcoma. However, in medical literature it is commonly used synonymously with carcinoma.

In conclusion it must be admitted that our present classification of tumours is far from satisfactory. The accepted division into benign and malignant is confounded by the existence of the group of intermediate tumours. When one adds the occasional instance of spontaneous regression of cancer and latent cancer, and the phenomenon of dormancy to the known unpredictable behaviour of cancer in any individual, it is obvious that there is still much to be learned about the behaviour and classification of tumours.

Classification of tumours

Tissue of origin	Behaviour		
	Benign	Intermediate	Malignant
Epithelium.			
1. *Covering and Protective Epithelium.*			
(*a*) Squamous.	Squamous-cell papilloma.		Squamous-cell carcinoma.
(*b*) Transitional.	Transitional-cell papilloma.		Transitional-cell carcinoma.
(*c*) Columnar.	Columnar-cell papilloma.		Adenocarcinoma.
2. *Compact Secreting Epithelium.*	Adenoma. If cystic, cystadenoma or papillary cystadenoma.		Adenocarcinoma. If cystic, cystadenocarcinoma.
3. *Other Epithelial Tumours include.*		Basal-cell carcinoma. Salivary and mucous gland tumours. Carcinoid tumours (argentaffinoma).	
Connective tissue.			
Fibrous tissue.	Fibroma.		Fibrosarcoma.
Nerve sheath.	Neurofibroma.		Neurofibrosarcoma.
Fat.	Lipoma.		Liposarcoma.
Smooth muscle.	Leiomyoma.		Leiomyosarcoma.
Striated muscle.	Rhabdomyoma.		Rhabdomyosarcoma.
Synovium.	Synovioma.		Malignant synovioma.
Cartilage.	Chondroma.		Chondrosarcoma.
Bone.			
Osteoblast.	Osteoma.	Giant-cell tumour.	Osteosarcoma.
Mesothelium.	Benign mesothelioma.		Malignant mesothelioma.
Blood vessels and lymphatics.	? Benign haemangioma and lymphangioma.		Angiosarcoma.
Meninges.	Meningioma.		Malignant meningioma.

Classification of tumours—*continued*

Tissue of origin	Behaviour		
	Benign	Intermediate	Malignant
Specialised connective tissue.			
Neuroglia and Ependyma	Astrocytoma; Oligodendroglioma; Ependymoma.*		
Chromaffin tissue.	Carotid body tumour.		Malignant carotid body tumour.
Lymphoid and	Benign lymphoma e.g. of		Lymphocytic lymphoma.
Haematopoietic tissue.	rectum and skin.		Histiocytic lymphoma
			Hodgkin's disease.
			Multiple myeloma.
		Myeloproliferative disorders†	Leukaemias.
Melanocytes.			Malignant melanoma.
Fetal trophoblast.	Hydatidiform mole.		Choriocarcinoma.
Germ cell.			Seminoma.
(*Totipotential cell*).	Benign teratoma.		Malignant teratoma.
Embryonic tissue.			
(*Pluripotential cell*).			
Kidney.			Nephroblastoma.
Liver.			Hepatoblastoma.
Unipotential cell.			
Retina.			Retinoblastoma.
Hind-brain.			Medulloblastoma.
Sympathetic ganglia and	Ganglioneuroma.		Neuroblastoma.
adrenal medulla.			
Pelvic organs.			Rhabdomyosarcoma (sarcoma botryoides).
Embryonic vestiges.			
Notochord.			Chordoma.
Enamel organ.		Ameloblastoma.	
Parapituitary residues.		Craniopharyngioma.	
Branchial cyst.			Branchiogenic carcinoma.
Hamartoma.			
Melanotic.	? Benign melanoma.		Malignant melanoma.
Angiomatous.	? Benign angioma.		Angiosarcoma.
'Exostoses' and			
'Ecchondroses'.			Chondrosarcoma.
Neurofibromatosis.	Neurofibroma.		Neurofibrosarcoma.
Tuberous sclerosis.	Glioma.		Malignant glioma.

*These tumours are difficult to classify. The common types are locally malignant, but some also metastasise within the central nervous system. Rarely, and most often in children, they appear to be benign.

†These include polycythaemia vera, haemorrhagic thrombocythaemia, and myelosclerosis (see p. 631).

REFERENCES

1. ADAMI, J. G. (1909) *Principles of Pathology*. London: Oxford University Press.
2. MOREHEAD, R. P. (1965) In *Human Pathology*, p. 181. New York: McGraw-Hill.
3. FRANKS, L. M. (1954) Latent carcinoma. *Annals of the Royal College of Surgeons of England*, 15, 236.
4. BOYD, W. (1966) *The Spontaneous Regression of Cancer*, Springfield, Illinois: Thomas.
5. EVERSON, T. C. & COLE, W. H. (1966) *Spontaneous Regression of Cancer*. Philadelphia: Saunders.
6. DAVID, J. & BURKITT, D. (1968) Burkitt's lymphoma: remissions following seemingly non-specific therapy. *British Medical Journal*, 4, 288.
7. NATHANSON, L., HALL, T. C. & FARBER, S. (1967) Biological aspects of human malignant melanoma. *Cancer (Philadelphia)*, 20, 650.
8. SMITH, R. A. (1971) Cure of lung cancer from incomplete surgical resection. *British Medical Journal*, 2, 563.
9. SMITHERS, D. W. (1969) Maturation in human tumours. *Lancet*, 2, 949.

Chapter 26. Structure and Effects of Some Common Tumours

BENIGN EPITHELIAL TUMOURS

Epithelial tumours may grow in one of two ways: either as sheets of neoplastic cells covering a surface (*papilloma*), or as solid masses of cells separated into groups by stromal connective tissue (*adenoma*). A tumour may show both types of growth. As in normal tissue the epithelial cells tend to adhere firmly to each other and be distinctly separate from the connective tissue. Epithelial cells are soft, therefore the consistency of their tumours depends upon the quantity and type of the supporting stroma; when this is abundant and collagenous the tumour is hard, but when it is scanty or cellular the tumour is soft.

Papillomata

Benign tumours of surface epithelia appear as warty or papillary overgrowths. Some papillomata are sessile, but most are pedunculated, and these are loosely called *polyps*, a morphological term applied to any pedunculated mass attached to a surface, and not necessarily neoplastic. Sometimes the papilloma is composed of many delicate finger-like processes, or fronds, and it is then called a *villous papilloma*.* These tumours are supplied by a core of connective-tissue stroma containing blood vessels, lymphatics, and nerves. The stroma is an integral part of the tumour and its growth is subservient to that of the epithelium. The stroma is therefore not considered to be primarily involved in the neoplastic process, and these tumours are not regarded as mixed. There is seldom any evidence of an inflammatory reaction in the stroma of a benign tumour, unless there is infection, ulceration, or necrosis.

The tumour is covered by a profuse neoplastic epithelium, which is regularly arranged and shows little evidence of mitotic activity. The basement membrane is always intact, but frequently in histological preparations the complex frond-like structure gives a false impression of invasion; the presence of inflammation due to trauma or infection may disrupt the basement membrane, and further add to the illusion of malignancy. Three main types of papilloma are described according to the nature of the epithelium involved:

Stratified squamous-cell papilloma. This tumour is found on the skin and other stratified squamous epithelial surfaces, e.g. tongue, larynx, and anus. There is invariably an increase in thickness of the prickle cell layer (acanthosis), an increase in the amount of adherent keratin (hyperkeratosis), and retention of the nuclei of the desquamating keratinised cells in some areas (parakeratosis).

*For reasons that are obscure the villous papilloma of the large intestine is known as a villous adenoma in North America. This term has now been recommended by the WHO (International Histological Classification of Tumours). Tubular adenoma is the recommended term for the solid tumour previously called an adenoma. Mixed forms are also recognised—tubulovillous adenoma.

Papillary lesions of the skin in fact form a heterogeneous group and it is often difficult to state which of them are truly neoplastic. Some are of developmental origin (*epithelial naevus* or *naevus verrucosus*), whereas others are caused by a virus—the common wart *verruca vulgaris* being the usual lesion. Papillary lesions on the exposed parts are not uncommon in elderly people (*actinic* or *solar keratoses*), and are important because the epithelium shows dysplasia and the lesions can progress to *in-situ* and ultimately invasive carcinoma. Similar lesions are found in those people who have ingested inorganic arsenic. These *arsenical keratoses* occur on the palms, soles, and trunk, and are premalignant and often multiple. A very common papillary lesion of the skin in elderly people is the basal-cell papilloma, or *seborrhoeic keratosis*. The proliferating cells tend to retain their basal-cell morphology. The lesion appears to be growing on the skin surface, there is no invasion of the dermis, and malignancy is almost unknown.

Transitional-cell papilloma. This occurs throughout the urinary passages, most frequently in the bladder. Multiple growths are characteristic. The villous character of the tumour is often so pronounced that it resembles a sea-anemone. The delicate fronds are easily torn, and haematuria is a common symptom. After these tumours are removed recurrence commonly takes place, and from a practical point of view they are best regarded as malignant. Since there is a poor correlation between the histological appearance of the biopsied material and the clinical behaviour of the lesion, some pathologists report all transitional-cell papillomatous lesions as carcinoma regardless of whether or not there is any cellular anaplasia or tissue invasion in the tissues available for study.

Columnar-cell papilloma. This occurs on any surface covered by columnar epithelium; in the colon the surface mucus-secreting epithelium may occasionally produce a villous papilloma, but this is an uncommon tumour and should not be confused with the pedunculated tubular adenoma.*

Papillomata are also found in cystic adenomata (papillary cystadenoma), in the breast ducts, and occasionally in the gallbladder and bronchi (Fig. 26.1).

Adenomata

A simple tumour of a solid glandular tissue is called an *adenoma*. It consists of dense masses of acini lined by exuberant epithelium which may be columnar or cuboidal in shape (Fig. 26.2). Adenomata of endocrine glands often show no acini, but are merely composed of uniform polygonal or spheroidal cells arranged in solid groups.

Adenomata arising in glands opening directly on a surface often become pedunculated and form polyps. This is particularly common in the large intestine, and the tumours are frequently multiple. In the hereditary condition of *polyposis coli* thousands of tumours are present, and they may involve

Figure 26.1
Intraductal papilloma of breast. This is a portion of a complex columnar-cell papilloma in a breast duct. The central stromal core is prolonged into an extensive framework which is surmounted by neoplastic epithelium. × 30.

Figure 26.2
Tubular adenoma of stomach. There are numerous acini lined by an exuberant columnar epithelium, the cells of which show only mild pleomorphism and little mitotic activity. The tumour was pedunculated, and there was no evidence of invasive activity. × 75.

the rectum also. The exuberant epithelium of the tumours closely resembles that of the normal, except that the cells are usually larger and the nuclei more hyperchromatic. Any marked degree of irregularity (dysplasia) should be viewed with suspicion, as malignant change is quite common.

If an adenoma arises at a distance from a surface it assumes the form of a spherical nodule with a capsule. This is produced as the result of pressure atrophy on the surrounding parenchyma: the more resistant connective tissue remains and condenses to produce a capsule. Adenomata may be found in any glandular organ; the breast, prostate, and endocrine glands are the most common sites, but they are also found in the secreting glands of the skin and bronchi. In the thyroid, adrenal cortex, and prostate the tumours are frequently multiple, and it is difficult to decide whether the condition is neoplastic or merely a nodular hyperplasia (see p. 295).

Two variants of adenoma should be noted:

Cystadenoma. Sometimes adenomata form elaborate cystic spaces into which papillary ingrowths of neoplastic epithelium protrude. These papillary cystadenomata are most common in the ovary. Two types are found—one in which the epithelium secretes a serous fluid (serous cystadenoma) and the other in which mucin is produced (mucinous cystadenoma).

Cystadenomata are also found in the pancreas, salivary glands, and kidney (Fig. 26.3).

Fibro-adenoma. In the breast the specialised connective tissue surrounding the glandular epithelium is almost invariably involved when an adenoma develops. This overgrowth is more than an excessive stromal reaction, and is probably a true connective tissue neoplasia, because under rare conditions in which malignancy supervenes, a sarcoma, and not a carcinoma, is usually produced. The tumour is probably a truly 'mixed' one.

Two types are described although mixed examples occur, and in practice the distinction is seldom made. In the *hard pericanalicular type* the ducts are small and are surrounded by dense connective tissue, whereas in the *soft intracanalicular type* the ducts are elongated and slit-like, because they are impinged on by looser connective tissue (Fig. 26.4). In this variety the connective tissue sometimes shows such rapid growth that the overlying stretched skin may ulcerate. This is called *Brodie's tumour* (giant fibro-adenoma), and may be mistaken clinically for carcinoma, and histologically for a sarcoma. It is interesting that during pregnancy and lactation, not only does the normal breast epithelium undergo hyperplasia, but similar changes also occur in the epithelial element

Figure 26.3
Cystadenoma of kidney. The tumour consists of intricate papillary ingrowths of cuboidal epithelium into a cystic space on the surface of a kidney. At the bottom of the section some renal tubules are present. The tumour has arisen from this tubular epithelium. It is the benign counterpart of the clear-cell carcinoma shown in Fig. 26.21. × 100.

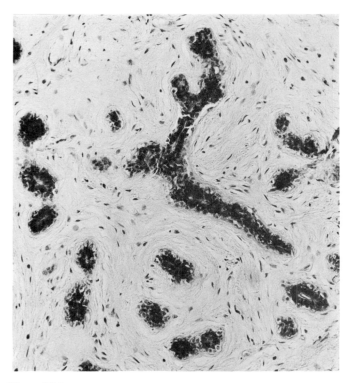

Figure 26.4
Intracanalicular fibro-adenoma of breast. There are a number of proliferating ducts surrounded by a loose connective-tissue stroma. Most of the ducts are small and round, but there is also a more elaborate, elongated, slit-like duct into which the stroma impinges, giving the tumour an intracanalicular pattern. × 100.

of a fibroadenoma. The tumour is thus subject to hormonal influence. It undergoes atrophy and fibrosis after the menopause.

BENIGN CONNECTIVE TISSUE TUMOURS

On the whole this group is rather less important clinically than the epithelial one. Nevertheless the commonest of all tumours belongs to this category, the uterine myoma.

The structure of these tumours is easily predictable in terms of the constituent tissue. There is merely a neoplastic overgrowth of the tissue (bone, muscle, etc.), and the individual cells are separated from each other by intercellular substance which they themselves have produced. The consistency of the tumour depends upon the nature and quantity of this substance rather than that of the stroma (cf. epithelial tumours). Thus a chondroma is harder than a fibroma. The stroma consists of blood vessels and perhaps some surrounding connective tissue. It tends to merge with the neoplastic tissue, particularly so in fibromata. A poorly delineated stroma is, however, a characteristic of all connective-tissue tumours.

Fibroma. Fibromata are not common tumours. They consist of circumscribed collections of fibroblasts between which

there is a variable amount of collagen. 'Hard' fibromata have much collagen, whereas the 'soft' variety are predominantly cellular. They are found in many sites, e.g skin, stomach, ovary, etc.

An unusual type is the *desmoid tumour*,* also known as the *recurring fibroma of Paget*. This is a tumour of musculo-aponeurotic origin, arising most commonly from the rectus sheath of parous women. It is not encapsulated and invades the surrounding muscles, recurring if not completely excised, but it is well differentiated and does not metastasise. It is best regarded as an intermediate tumour of fibrous tissue. Similar tumours are known to occur in other sites and have been given unnecessarily complicated names, e.g. recurring dermatofibroma of Darier and dermatofibrosarcoma protuberans of the skin.

There are, in fact, a number of curious proliferative conditions of fibrous tissue, sometimes grouped as the *fibromatoses*, in which histological assessment of malignancy is difficult.[1] In *nodular fasciitis*, which affects the subcutaneous tissues and deep fascia, there is the rapid growth of a highly vascular mass which diffusely infiltrates the surrounding tissues; in spite of the malignant microscopic appearance the lesion is quite benign. Similar benign lesions are *juvenile fibromatosis* and *pseudosarcomatous dermatofibroma* of the skin.

*The word is derived from the Greek *desmos*, a band or tendon, and alludes to the tendon-like consistency of the tumour.

Palmar(Dupuytren's contracture) and plantar fibromatosis are in a similar category, for they are ill-defined fibromatous overgrowths which may appear malignant microscopically, but which never behave so clinically. *Idiopathic mediastinal fibrosis*, which causes superior-vena-caval obstruction, and *retroperitoneal fibrosis*, which frequently obstructs the ureters, may both fall into this same group. It is of interest that the latter appears to be caused by the ingestion of the drug methysergide used in the prophylaxis of migraine.[2] The association of Dupuytren's contracture with chronic alcoholism may be a further indication that a chemical agent can cause a localised fibromatous overgrowth.

Myxoma.[3] This is an uncommon tumour of connective tissue consisting of scattered stellate cells disposed in an expanse of connective-tissue mucin in which there is a network of reticulin fibres. Its histological and biochemical features resemble those of Wharton's jelly, which is found in the umbilical cord of the mature fetus.

The myxoma may be found in the jaw (where it is probably of odontogenic origin) and arising from the interatrial wall of the heart and from soft tissues, usually in association with striated muscle and neighbouring tissues. In appearance it is well circumscribed, oval or spherical, and of translucent grey colour. Its cut surface is glistening and slimy, and it may exude a mucoid material. It probably arises from a fibroblastic cell that has not differentiated enough to produce collagen but is capable of forming acid mucopolysaccharides. Alternatively it may be of primitive mesenchymal origin.

It should be noted that areas of myxomatous change are common in a variety of connective-tissue tumours, e.g. fibromata, neurofibromata and schwannomata, lipomata, and chondromata. When a tumour of myxomatous type shows malignant characteristics, it is placed in the category of *myxoid liposarcoma* rather than myxosarcoma, for nearly all such tumours show liposarcomatous features in addition.

Myoma. Tumours of muscle are of two types:

Leiomyoma (Fig. 26.5). This is the commonest of all tumours, being found in the uteri of about 20 per cent of women over 30 years of age. Leiomyomata of the skin, stomach, and intestine are also not uncommon. These tumours are often multiple. A leiomyoma is composed of whorls of smooth muscle cells, interspersed among which there is a variable amount of fibrous tissue. In due course the muscle element may be replaced by the fibrous tissue, and a fibroleiomyoma (or 'fibroid') is produced. Such a tumour may undergo cystic change or else become densely calcified. On section the whorled interlacing pattern of glistening, white bundles resembling watered-silk is characteristic.

Rhabdomyoma. A tumour of striated muscle is very uncommon. Most examples are malignant rhabdomyosarcomata occurring in young children (see Ch. 27). Rhabdomyomata of the heart are described, but most of these are malformations occurring in tuberous sclerosis.

Tumours of Nerve Sheath Origin[4]

The literature on this subject is confusing because of the uncertainty regarding the parent cell of origin. Two types of lesion can be recognised, but it is not known whether they are distinct entities or merely variations of a single process.

Neurofibroma. This tumour is now thought to arise from

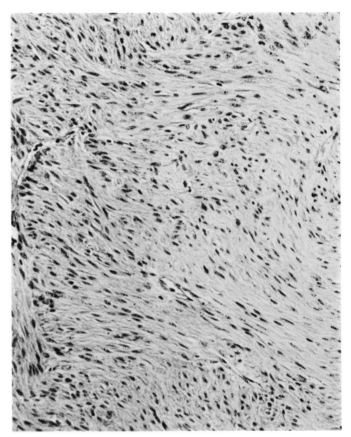

Figure 26.5
Leiomyoma of stomach. The tumour consists of sheaves of elongated, spindle-shaped smooth-muscle cells arranged in interlacing whorls. ×80.

Schwann cells rather than fibroblasts. It causes a diffuse fusiform enlargement of a nerve, and is composed of spindle cells arranged in flowing streams with a varying amount of intervening reticulin and collagen. Nerve fibres pass through the tumour, and myxomatous change is not infrequently present. The tumours may be solitary, and can occur on a spinal nerve root or a peripheral nerve. Often they are multiple, and their presence constitutes a major feature of von Recklinghausen's disease. Whether all the nodules in this disease are true neoplasms is debatable—it might be more reasonable to regard them as hamartomatous or areas of dysplasia. Nevertheless, meningiomata, schwannomata, and even gliomata can also be found in this disease, and these are classified as tumours. Malignant change is not uncommon especially in patients with multiple lesions. Another lesion on the borderline of neoplasia is the *plexiform neuroma*, a diffuse overgrowth of the connective tissue of a nerve which produces great thickening, coiling, and distortion of the nerve. When occurring in a limb there may be other developmental anomalies, e.g. local gigantism. This too may occur as part of von Recklinghausen's disease.

Schwannoma. This tumour is usually solitary and may arise from any cranial or peripheral nerve. It is encapsulated and appears to arise focally on a nerve trunk, so that the nerve itself is stretched over the tumour rather than running through it as in the neurofibroma. A common site for schwannomata is the auditory nerve, and they may be bilateral. The tumour may occur on spinal nerve roots and indeed on any large nerve trunk. A mediastinal location is not uncommon. Apart from arising on large nerve trunks, these tumours may appear in relation to a small peripheral nerve of the skin or an internal viscus, e.g. stomach.

Macroscopically and microscopically the tumour is very similar to a leiomyoma, the whorled arrangement of spindle cells being common to both. Sometimes these spindle cells

thereby resembling adult Schwann cells.[5] The same cell type is seen in neurofibromata, and this argues against them being fibroblasts, which have no surrounding basement membrane. Both neurofibromata and schwannomata therefore arise from this cell type, and it is not surprising that both types of lesion may occur in the same patient or even in the same tumour mass.

Meningioma. This is a tumour of the arachnoid cells that lie on the deep surface of the dura and on the arachnoid granulations. Meningiomata are usually situated in relation to the superior sagittal sinus, the transverse sinus, and the falx

Figure 26.6
Schwannoma. Note the palisaded, or regimented, appearance of the long, spindle-shaped cells; their nuclei form a continuous sinuous column, and on each side there is a similar column composed of clear cytoplasm. × 200.

Figure 26.7
Meningioma. It is composed of circumscribed, whorled aggregations of plump, epithelial-like cells surrounded by a vascular stroma. A few darkly-staining, calcareous spherules (psammoma bodies) are present amid the cellular clumps. × 150.

have a palisaded, or regimented, appearance, all the nuclei being aligned in one strip, and the clear cytoplasm of the cells in an adjacent strip (Fig. 26.6). This appearance may be seen in leiomyomata, but it can be distinguished by phosphotungstic-acid haematoxylin staining, which is taken up by muscle cells.

As the name suggests, the schwannoma is thought to arise from the Schwann cells of the nerve sheath. Neurilemoma is an alternative name, but is falling into disuse on the objection that the neurilemma signifies the sheath or basement membrane of the Schwann cells rather than the cells themselves. The schwannoma can produce collagen, and on electron microscopy the neoplastic cells have a basement membrane,

cerebri, and by pressure on the underlying brain a hollow is formed. Sometimes the calvaria is implicated by the tumour, and excessive bone formation results. In structure these tumours consist of plump epithelial-like clumps of arachnoid cells, usually arranged in a whorled pattern. There is a variable fibrous stroma, and sometimes a vascular element is prominent. Spherules of calcification are common in the arachnoid cell clumps (psammoma bodies), and this brain 'sand' is alluded to in the alternative name 'psammoma' which is applied to these tumours (Fig. 26.7).

Lipoma. This common tumour is composed of adult adipose tissue. It is usually subcutaneous, but may be retroperitoneal or subserosal. In appearance it is yellow in colour, lobulated, and well encapsulated, so that enucleation is usually easily performed.

Giant-cell tumour of bone. This is composed of fusiform fibroblastic cells and numerous giant cells, some of which have enormous numbers of nuclei (Fig. 26.8). These giant cells are believed to be neoplastic osteoclasts, but as some authorities dispute this, the alternative name 'osteoclastoma' is best avoided. It is usually found at the metaphysis of the long bone. It produces pressure atrophy of the bone. It occurs in young adults up to about the age of 30 years. It frequently undergoes central cystic change, and appears radiologically as

Figure 26.8
Giant-cell tumour of bone. It is composed of many large giant cells, interspersed among which there are smaller, spindle-shaped fibroblastic cells. × 200.

an osteolytic tumour in which a few bony trabeculae are still recognisable. Macroscopically it is an expansive haemorrhagic cyst with an egg-shell covering of bone. Although this tumour is generally classified as benign, some examples are locally malignant and a small percentage metastasise.

In hyperparathyroidism tumour-like lesions may develop in the bones, and they closely resemble giant-cell tumours. These *brown tumours*, as they are termed, are usually multiple but can occasionally occur as a solitary lesion. Hence recurrence after treatment should always lead to an investigation of calcium metabolism.

Chondroma. A benign chondroma is comparatively uncommon, for most examples are really skeletal malformations involving the epiphyseal cartilage. One type involves the hands, and by its expanding nature leads to great deformity. It consists of mature cartilage with regular chondrocytes.

Osteoma. Many osteomata, e.g. the common exostoses, are malformations, but now and again solitary tumours of this type are encountered, especially in the skull. They may consist of compact bone (hard or ivory osteomata) or of spongy bone (cancellous osteomata).

Characteristics of Benign Tumours

Shape. Benign tumours are usually circumscribed, and apart from surface growths like papillomata, they usually possess a capsule. Their shape is usually round, but they tend to be moulded by surrounding structures. Thus a particular arrangement of fascia may make them oval. On the other hand, a neurofibroma of a posterior nerve root tends to expand into the spinal canal in one direction, and into the thoracic cavity in the other: the result is a dumb-bell shaped tumour.

Size. Although *benign tumours are usually smaller* than malignant ones, they may at times attain enormous proportions. Some of the largest tumours reported are ovarian cystadenomata and uterine fibroids, and the largest tumour in the museum of the Royal College of Surgeons of England is a fibroma of the kidney weighing 82 pounds (37 kg). A malignant tumour would have killed the patient long before reaching this size.

Ulceration and haemorrhage. These complications are rare except in surface tumours, e.g. papillomata and submucous fibroids, and even in these they are infinitely less severe than in their malignant counterparts.

The rate of growth. The rate of growth of benign tumours is generally slow. It is often erratic, and usually tends to cease after a period.

Degree of differentiation. *Both structurally and functionally the tumour cells tend to copy the parent tissue.* The cells themselves are regular, and mitotic figures are few. Tumours of the endocrine glands, in addition, may secrete an excess of hormone which can have serious and sometimes even fatal results. Although both benign and malignant tumours can produce hormones, the most marked effects are usually seen in adenomata.

Secretory Activity by Tumours of Endocrine Origin

(i) *Pancreatic islet-cell tumours* are associated with several characteristic syndromes due to their secretion of hormones. These are considered in Chapter 35 together with the effects of other APUD-cell tumours.

(ii) Tumours of the adrenal medulla (*phaeochromocytomata*) secrete noradrenaline and adrenaline (see p. 450).

(iii) Tumours of the *adrenal cortex* produce a wide range of steroid hormones. The following syndromes may be produced by such tumours: (*a*) the adrenogenital syndrome, (*b*) Cushing's syndrome, (*c*) Conn's syndrome (see p. 449).

(iv) *Pituitary tumours* produce several different syndromes: (*a*) *Gigantism* in children and *acromegaly* in adults due to acidophil adenomata, (*b*) *Cushing's syndrome* due to basophil adenomata (see p. 448).

(**v**) *Parathyroid tumours* are associated with osteitis fibrosa cystica (von Recklinghausen's disease of bone).

(vi) *Thyroid adenomata* and carcinomata rarely produce hyperthyroidism.

(vii) In the ovary *granulosa-cell tumours* are oestrogen producers and lead to endometrial hyperplasia with uterine bleeding, while the *arrhenoblastoma* is androgenic and causes virilisation. The *choriocarcinoma* and *hydatidiform mole* produce large quantities of placental gonadotrophic hormone.

(viii) The *interstitial-cell adenoma* of the testis may secrete either androgens or oestrogens. When it occurs in boys there may be premature puberty; others develop gynaecomastia.

(ix) *Carcinoid tumours* produce a specific syndrome, see page 452.

Other Effects of Benign Tumours

Benign tumours may produce serious mechanical effects by virtue of their position. In this way intracranial and spinal tumours like meningiomata and neurofibromata are dangerous. Natural passages may be blocked, and extensive damage results. Thus obstruction to a bronchus leads to bronchiectasis, while an occluded ureter produces a hydronephrosis with secondary infection. Tumours of the gut, e.g. polypoid adenomata and lipomata, may produce intestinal obstruction by precipitating an intussusception. Occasionally the heart's action is impaired by a benign growth. These effects are, of course, also produced by malignant tumours.

Distant spread. Benign tumours do not metastasise.

MALIGNANT EPITHELIAL TUMOURS— CARCINOMATA

The carcinomata are the commonest of all malignant tumours, probably because epithelium is a continuously dividing tissue. Some carcinomata involve covering non-secreting epithelium, and are called squamous-cell or transitional-cell carcinoma. Carcinoma of secretory epithelium is called adenocarcinoma provided it is sufficiently well differentiated to show glandular structure.

Three main types are recognised as with the papillomata:

Squamous-cell Carcinomata

These tumours arise at any site normally covered by stratified squamous epithelium—skin, mouth, oesophagus, anus, ectocervix, etc. At other sites they may occur as a result of tumour metaplasia, or possibly neoplasia in an area of squamous metaplasia (see p. 305), e.g. lung, urinary tract, gallbladder, etc.

Macroscopic types. Two are usually described:

The papillary carcinoma appears as a warty outgrowth with an infiltrating base; this type may arise in a papilloma.

The nodular type produces a hard, nodular mass beneath the surface, and shows more rapid infiltration and dissemination. Both types usually ulcerate to form a typical *carcinomatous ulcer*. This has a raised, craggy, rolled edge which is fixed to surrounding skin and deeper structures. The base is composed of white, necrotic tumour, which is usually friable and bleeds easily.

Histological type. In considering the histological structure of a squamous-cell carcinoma it is necessary first to understand its formation (Fig. 26.9).

A

B

C

Figure 26.9

Three types of neoplasia of a keratinising squamous stratified epithelium, e.g. epidermis.

(A) Benign neoplasia results in an excessive production of regular epithelium, which is thrown into a complicated, folded structure in order to be accommodated. This formation is called a *papilloma*. The epidermal cells mature in an orderly way from the basal cells to the superficial squames.

(B) In *carcinoma-in-situ* there is excessive growth of epithelium, which thereby becomes thickened (acanthosis). Maturation of the cells is disorderly; foci of keratinisation are found within the epidermis instead of being present only on the surface (dyskeratosis).

(C) In *carcinoma* the atypical epithelial cells break through the basement membrane and invade the underlying tissues.

(*Drawings by Margot Mackay, Department of Art as Applied to Medicine, University of Toronto.*)

Formation. When epithelium shows malignant propensities, there is a progressive, irregular proliferation of the prickle-cell layer. Cellular pleomorphism, atypical mitotic activity, and other features of *dysplasia* may become so marked that the epithelium gives the impression of malignancy even though the cells have not broken through the basement membrane and invaded the connective tissues. To this condition the name *carcinoma-in-situ*, or *intraepithelial carcinoma*, is applied. Whether all such 'carcinomata' do in fact proceed to frank invasive malignancy is questionable, and the subject is considered in detail in Chapter 29.

The criterion of truly invasive carcinoma is the penetration of the basement membrane by masses of malignant cells, which then spread into the connective tissues and muscle. As they proceed, they tend to break up into separate groups or columns. These clumps may comprise hundreds of cancer cells, or else only a few. In the most anaplastic tumours there may be no attempt at any splitting up, and the tumour cells proceed in one diffuse mass.

As the tumour infiltrates, so it destroys the tissue with which it comes in contact, and this is replaced by a fibrous stroma which may be dense and acellular as in scirrhous cancers, or else loose and vascular, and infiltrated with lymphocytes, plasma cells, and even polymorphs and eosinophils. Nearly all malignant tumours excite an inflammatory reaction around them; the lymphocytic component of this is very important, because cell-mediated immunity is especially involved in checking the spread of malignant tumours. Lymphocytes are present around tumours of low-grade malignancy and during the early stages of malignant change (see p. 353). Once ulceration of the surface occurs, there is a more acute type of response due to secondary bacterial infection.

In those carcinomata that break up into discrete columns, each individual clump may then differentiate partly or completely to resemble the normal epithelium from which it has arisen.

Differentiation. Squamous-cell carcinomata vary considerably in the degree of differentiation which they show. When differentiation is good, *epithelial pearls* (also called *keratin pearls*, *horn pearls*, or *cell nests*) are formed. These are groups of cells, which by differentiating produce a central whorl of keratin (Fig. 26.10). Surrounding this there are prickle cells, and occasionally a stratum granulosum is recognisable. A basal-cell layer is not well formed. In this way there is a fairly accurate reproduction of the upper layers of normal stratified squamous keratinising epithelium. The cells are usually fairly uniform in size and shape, their nuclei are evenly staining, and mitoses are scanty. On the whole spread is slow. The skin is the commonest site, but sometimes well-differentiated cancers occur in the oral cavity and bronchus.

The more undifferentiated tumours contain no keratin, but groups of prickle cells may still be recognisable (Fig. 26.11).

Highly undifferentiated, anaplastic tumours show no attempt at prickle-cell formation. There is a diffuse sheet of neoplastic cells supported by a scanty, vascular stroma with no separation into groups. The cells themselves show great variation in size and shape, their nuclei are darkly-staining and irregular in morphology, and mitotic figures abound (some of these are bizarre). Tumour giant cells may be present (Fig. 26.12). It may be impossible to distinguish the tumour from a

Figure 26.10
A cell nest or epithelial pearl. This is a group of cells from a well-differentiated squamous-cell carcinoma. In the centre of the group the cells have differentiated so well that they resemble stratum corneum with keratin in the midst. ×100.

Figure 26.11
Poorly-differentiated squamous-cell carcinoma. In this section there are well-formed clumps of squamous cells which show considerable pleomorphism. There is no attempt at keratin formation. ×150.

Figure 26.12
Anaplasia. This is part of an anaplastic squamous-cell carcinoma from the maxillary antrum. The cells are arranged in irregular sheets surrounded by a vascular stroma. Cellular pleomorphism is very marked. In the centre of the field there are two tumour giant cells. Elsewhere there is much variation in cell size and shape and in nuclear size and staining intensity. × 200.

connective tissue neoplasm. This type of tumour is found usually in the mouth, bronchus, and cervix.

Variations of Squamous-cell Carcinoma

'Transitional-cell' papillary carcinoma. Some squamous-cell carcinomata of the nasopharynx and lung have a papillary structure, and are composed of a transitional type of epithelium similar to that of the urinary passages. It is better not to call this type of tumour transitional-celled, as it simply causes confusion.

Verrucous Carcinoma.[6] This papillomatous, well-differentiated tumour occurs in the mouth, larynx, and genital region. Histological evidence of invasion is sometimes difficult to find, particularly in biopsy material. The tumour is noteworthy for its very good prognosis.

A rare variety of verrucous carcinoma occurs on the sole of the foot. It masquerades as a plantar wart, but burrows deeply into the underlying tissues. It is called *epithelioma* (or *carcinoma*) *cuniculatum* (from the Latin cuniculus, meaning an underground passage).[7]

Spindle-cell squamous-cell carcinoma. Occasionally the cells of a squamous-cell carcinoma are fusiform or spindle-shaped. This is a very undifferentiated type of tumour, and it may be impossible to distinguish from a sarcoma or an amelanotic

melanoma. Electron microscopy is of value in this connexion (pp. 310 to 311).

Grading. Histological grading as described by Broders is of some help in assessing prognosis. Four grades are recognised, according to the degree of differentiation.

Grade I	More than 75 per cent cell-differentiation.
Grade II	50 to 75 per cent cell-differentiation.
Grade III	25 to 50 per cent cell-differentiation.
Grade IV	Less than 25 per cent cell-differentiation.

Accurate grading on a numerical basis is seldom used, because (*a*) it is time-consuming and difficult, and there is bound to be a difference of opinion among pathologists as to what constitutes a differentiated cell; most pathologists would agree about grades I and IV, but not about grades II and III, and (*b*) to be done accurately, the whole tumour should be serially sectioned. This is impossible in practice. It not infrequently happens that one area of a tumour is better differentiated than another. The same often applies to metastases of the tumour. It is obvious that the painstaking grading of a few sections is quite inadequate. (*c*) Prognosis is not infallibly related to the grade. The relationship is only approximate.

It is therefore more reasonable to define three grades—well-differentiated, poorly-differentiated, and undifferentiated. On the whole, the higher the grade, the worse is the prognosis, but the greater is the degree of radiosensitivity.

Unfortunately many exceptions to these rules are found, and some authorities are not convinced that grading is of any great help in the individual case. Certainly the site of the tumour is of great importance. A grade-I squamous-cell carcinoma of the skin usually has an excellent prognosis, while in the lung the outlook is poor. Similarly, a grade-IV tumour of the cervix has a much better prognosis than a similar tumour of the lung or pharynx. The prognosis can also be related to the cause of a tumour; for instance the prognosis of squamous-cell carcinomata of the skin arising in actinic keratoses is much better than that of similar tumours arising *de novo* or in Bowen's disease.

Carcinomata of Glandular Epithelium

These tumours arise from surface, secreting epithelia as well as from underlying glands. They may on occasions arise from columnar-cell papillomata and adenomata.

The pattern of invasion of neoplastic epithelium beneath the basement membrane into the deeper tissue is similar to that already described; in this case the groups of cancer cells, instead of producing keratin, tend to arrange themselves into acinar structures containing a central lumen into which secretion pours. The cells surrounding this lumen may be columnar, cuboidal, polygonal, or spheroidal (Fig. 26.13). The best differentiated cancers show excellent acinus formation, which may mimic normal glandular structure. These tumours are called adenocarcinomata (Fig. 26.14).

In less well differentiated tumours there are merely clumps of cells surrounded by a stroma. There is no attempt at central cavitation to produce acini. To this type of cancer the name *carcinoma simplex* is applied. It is seen most commonly in the breast, where the cancer clumps are often surrounded by a dense fibrous stroma. There may be acinus formation else-

Figure 26.13

Tumours derived from glandular epithelium. The normal gland (1) is contained within a sheath of connective tissue. Benign neoplasia results in the formation of an adenoma (2) with well-differentiated structure and encapsulation. Cystic dilatation of acini and complicated infolding of the epithelium produce a cystadenoma (3). The remainder of the tumours are malignant. The adenocarcinomata show some tubular differentiation which may be good (4) or poor (5). Lack of differentiation results in a carcinoma simplex (6). The most anaplastic tumours form a sheet of loosely attached cells (7). Giant-cell forms may predominate (8). These anaplastic tumours may be difficult to distinguish from sarcomata, melanomata, and tumours of squamous epithelial origin. Abnormal differentiation results in squamous metaplasia (9) or the formation of signet-ring cell carcinoma (10).

Figure 26.14

Columnar-cell adenocarcinoma. This is a well-differentiated adenocarcinoma of the stomach. It consists of large, well-formed acini containing secretion, and is lined by exuberant columnar cells. It is infiltrating the muscle diffusely. × 100.

where in the tumour (Fig. 26.15). Electron microscopy may reveal evidence of differentiation that cannot be detected in the routine paraffin section (Figs. 25.1 to 25.4).

The most undifferentiated examples cannot be distinguished from other anaplastic tumours.

Mucoid cancer. Sometimes the cells of a carcinoma simplex contain demonstrable mucus. This is evidence of glandular function, and it is not unreasonable to call such a tumour an adenocarcinoma even if there is no evidence of acinus formation. However, most pathologists restrict the term

adenocarcinoma to tumours showing structural glandular differentiation. Sometimes there is so large an accumulation of mucus in the cytoplasm that the nucleus is compressed on to the cell wall. This type of cell is called a *signet-ring cell*, and it bears a morphological resemblance to an adult fat cell. If mucus secretion is marked, the tumour is called a *mucoid cancer*.

In some adenocarcinomata so much mucus is formed that it infiltrates into the stroma, which appears as a basophilic lake, in the midst of which lies disintegrating tumour tissue (Fig. 26.16). This forms another type of mucus-secreting, or mucoid, carcinoma, and both types may be found in the stomach, large bowel, lung, and rarely in the breast. Mucoid breast cancer is an example of mucus-secreting tumour metaplasia of neoplastic breast epithelium; mucous glands are not normally found in the breast.

Mucoid cancers are commonly miscalled 'colloid' cancers; this is a bad term because it carries the false association of thyroid tissue.

Mucoid cancer presents a characteristic naked-eye appearance of a bulky, gelatinous, mucoid mass. The mucus tends to stimulate a considerable fibrous-tissue reaction in its vicinity.

Figure 26.15
Poorly-differentiated tumour of lung. This is in fact a section of an adenocarcinoma of the lung; in some parts it contained tubules and in others mucus-secreting cells. In this field there is complete undifferentiation—the cells are pleomorphic and there are three abnormal mitotic figures. If the whole tumour were of this type of cell, it would be termed a polygonal-cell carcinoma. ×910. (*From Walter, J. B. and Pryce, D.M.* (1955), Thorax, **10**, 107)

Figure 26.16
Mucoid cancer. This is a mucus-secreting carcinoma infiltrating the muscular coat of the stomach. Most of the space between the muscle fibres consists of lakes of mucus, in the midst of which the disintegrating cancer cells are still recognisable. ×250.

Grading of glandular carcinomata on a system similar to that of Broders has been used to assess malignancy. In cancer of the breast a system based upon that first described by Greenough in the USA has proved of some value. Three features were taken into account when grading a tumour:

(*a*) Tubule formation.
(*b*) Regularity in size, shape, and staining of nuclei.
(*c*) Number of mitoses.

The prognosis in relation to stage (see p. 364) and grade of tumour is shown in Figure 26.17.

Stromal reaction. The reaction of the invaded tissue to the carcinoma cells varies; it may be so stimulated to grow that a fibrotic, hard (*scirrhous*) type of tumour is produced. Most breast cancers are of this type (Fig. 26.18). The dense fibrosis appears to be associated with a contracting tendency, which is ill understood. In the breast there is an accompanying retraction of the nipple and dimpling of the skin. Eventually a stony fixation to the chest wall ensues.

Scirrhous tumours are also commonly found in the alimentary tract. In the stomach a pyloric cancer may cause thickening of the wall and obstruction. In the diffuse infiltrating form of gastric cancer (linitis plastica) the fibrous tissue response is so marked that a careless histopathologist may miss the scanty carcinoma cells scattered throughout. The annular, or pursestring, type of cancer of the colon is another example of a scirrhous cancer, and it too causes obstruction (Fig. 26.39). It

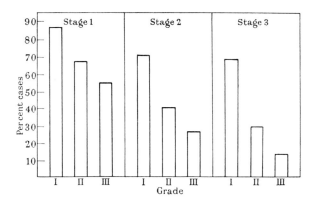

Figure 26.17
Stage, grade, and prognosis in cancer of the breast. Percentage of cases alive at 5 years (all treatments). (*From Bloom, H. J. G.* (1950), *Prognosis in carcinoma of the breast*, Brit. J. Cancer, **4**, 259)

should be noted that, although the fibrosis seen in scirrhous tumours gives the impression of an attempt by the host to strangle the tumour cells, this does not appear to be the case in practice. The prognosis of scirrhous cancer is quite as poor as that of the encephaloid type. The metastases of scirrhous cancer also tend to have the same dense fibrous stroma.

Figure 26.18
Carcinoma of the breast. The section through the breast shows a typical scirrhous carcinoma. Its outline is irregular and ill-defined for it spreads sinuously into the surrounding fibro-fatty tissue. (EB 10.1, *Reproduced by permission of the President and Council of the R.C.S. Eng.*)

When the tumour has little stroma in relation to the cell bulk, the growth is soft and is described as medullary, or *encephaloid*. Some breast cancers, e.g during lactation, and the 'cauliflower' cancer of large bowel, e.g. caecum, are of this type.

Transitional-cell Carcinoma

These tumours occur in the renal pelvis, ureter, and bladder. They are often papillomatous in appearance. Microscopically the structure varies from well-differentiated columns of transitional epithelial cells (Fig. 26.19) to highly anaplastic cell sheets differing in no way from other undifferentiated neoplasms. Squamous metaplasia is common.

Special Types of Carcinoma

It is useful at this stage to consider the structure of a few special carcinomata in greater detail.

Carcinoma of kidney. This common tumour has a characteristic naked-eye appearance: situated usually at one pole of a kidney (more commonly the upper) it has a variegated appearance due to areas of orange colour interspersed amid white stroma with contrasting red areas of haemorrhage (Fig. 26.20).

Figure 26.19
Transitional-cell carcinoma. This tumour consists of fronds of well-differentiated transitional epithelial cells showing considerable proliferative change, but minimal invasive activity. The tumour arose from the ureter, and appeared macroscopically as a large papilloma with associated hydronephrosis. × 80.

Microscopically it is composed of large, polygonal, clear cells arranged in groups, and sometimes disposed in tubules (Fig. 26.21). The resemblance of these cells to those of the adrenal cortex led to the belief that these tumours arose from the ectopic adrenal rests which are found quite frequently on the surface of the kidney. The traditional name 'hypernephroma' is a relic of this erroneous hypothesis. The tumour is certainly renal in origin. Small adenomata of the kidney are not uncommon, and in many of these similar clear cells are found. Furthermore, 'hypernephromata' are not found outside the kidney in the other sites where adrenal rests are known to occur.

The clear appearance of the cells is due to their high content of glycogen and lipid, which tend to be removed during histological preparation. The orange colour of the tumour is due to the lipochrome content of these cells. The correct name is *clear-cell carcinoma of the kidney*.*

Lung carcinoma. Tumours may arise from the large bronchi (central) or small bronchioles (peripheral). Peripheral cancer is thought by some (including the authors)[8] to be the commoner type, but the classical view is that central growths are the more frequent. Four main histological types are usually recognised.[9]

*Clear-cell tumours are typical of the adrenal cortex and parathyroid also. Occasionally adenocarcinomata of other organs, and even squamous-cell carcinomata, consist of clear cells. It is apparently related to glycogen content in these cases.

Figure 26.20
Clear-cell carcinoma of the kidney. The lower pole of the kidney has been replaced by an encephaloid tumour, which is infiltrating into the upper pole and is occluding the ureter. The substance of the mass has a typical variegated appearance. (EU 30.1, *Reproduced by permission of the President and Council of the R.C.S. Eng.*)

Figure 26.21
Clear-cell carcinoma of the kidney. The tumour consists of sheets of large round and polygonal cells with a copious clear cytoplasm and darkly-staining nuclei. × 100.

(1) The *adenocarcinoma*, which tends to occur peripherally, is more frequent in women, and apart from a tendency towards squamous metaplasia does not differ from similar tumours elsewhere. A mucoid variant occasionally occurs.

'*Alveolar-cell carcinoma.*' This uncommon type of lung cancer presents a characteristic radiological and naked-eye appearance. Both lungs show numerous small discrete foci of growth, which radiologically give a 'snow-storm' effect. The tumour appears to arise multifocally, but inhalation metastasis from a small localised primary tumour cannot be absolutely excluded.

Microscopically the tumour is a well-differentiated adenocarcinoma; tumour cells may be seen lining the alveoli, but there is no evidence to suggest that it arises from the alveolar cells themselves. In fact, it does not differ microscopically from many localised, well-differentiated, lung adenocarcinomata, and it therefore presumably arises from bronchiolar epithelium.

It is important to note that many apparent examples of 'alveolar-cell carcinoma' are in fact secondary deposits from adenocarcinomata arising elsewhere, e.g. thyroid, ovary, or pancreas. Indeed, it is important to exclude secondary tumours before diagnosing primary lung cancer, even when there is a solitary mass.

(2) The *squamous-cell carcinoma* affects the larger bronchi more frequently (Fig. 26.22), but even in this type peripheral growths are common.

(3) *Oat-cell carcinoma.* This type is variously called the small-cell (USA) or oat-cell carcinoma (Britain). The naked-eye appearance is often characteristic in advanced cases: masses of fleshy, white tumour are seen invading the lung and the lymphatics around the blood vessels and bronchi (Fig. 26.23). The lymph nodes of the mediastinum are massively involved, which accounts for the misconception that the tumour was a mediastinal sarcoma. Microscopically the growth is composed of sheets of small, basophilic cells with hyperchromatic nuclei, which are either round, oval, or 'oat-shaped' (Fig. 26.24). The cytoplasm is scanty, and superficially the cells resemble lymphocytes. Rosettes or tubular structures are not infrequently present amid the diffuse sheets, and these are evidence of the epithelial origin of the tumour.

Oat-cell carcinoma appears to be a distinct tumour, and is probably derived from neurosecretory cells of the bronchial mucosa akin to the argentaffin cells of the intestine and of the APUD series. In this respect it shares a common origin with the carcinoid tumour of the bronchus (see Ch. 35). It is found predominantly in men, and is highly malignant and equally highly radiosensitive.

Figure 26.22
Carcinoma of the lung. Thus tumour has arisen from the left lower lobe main bronchus. Not only has it infiltrated into the lower lobe extensively, but it has also led to distal bronchiectasis. The hilar lymph nodes are also involved in the tumour. The tumour proved to be a squamous-cell carcinoma. (R. 45.1, *Reproduced by permission of the President and Council of the R.C.S. Eng.*)

Figure 26.23
Carcinoma of the lung. The tumour has arisen from the right main bronchus, and has infiltrated extensively into all the lobes. The hilar lymph nodes are enlarged and invaded by the tumour. The tumour was proved to be an oat-cell carcinoma. (R 45.3, *Reproduced by permission of the President and Council of the R.C.S. Eng.*)

(4) *Polygonal-cell carcinoma (large-cell carcinoma).* This type of tumour is undifferentiated, and consists of sheets and groups of large, eosinophilic polygonal cells (Fig. 26.15).

Carcinoma of the testis. The commonest testicular cancer is derived from the seminiferous epithelium, and is called a *seminoma*. As with most malignant testicular tumours, the seminoma occurs between the ages of 20 and 50 years—somewhat earlier than is the case with many carcinomata. It has a very typical microscopical appearance: columns of large spheroidal cells with prominent, round, darkly-staining nuclei and scanty cytoplasm. These cells are clearly neoplastic spermatocytes (germ cells). The columns are separated by thin fibrous trabeculae in which there are often many lymphocytes (Fig. 26.25). Macroscopically it is a white, encephaloid tumour which tends to spread up the spermatic cord to the regional lymph nodes.

The *teratoma* occurs usually in a somewhat younger age-group, and is considered in Chapter 27.

Carcinoma of the skin. The common skin cancer is a *squamous-cell carcinoma*, which is usually well differentiated. It usually ulcerates early and becomes secondarily infected. Spread is slow, and as the tumour is very radiosensitive, cure

may be achieved with comparatively little cosmetic disturbance (see also p. 324).

The other important invasive skin tumour is the *basal-cell carcinoma* described below.

Adenocarcinomata of the accessory skin appendages (sweat and sebaceous glands) are occasionally encountered. Some sweat-gland tumours resemble pleomorphic salivary adenomata microscopically, but are usually benign.

The *malignant melanoma* is usually found in the skin. It is considered in Chapter 27.

Intermediate Epithelial Tumours

Some tumours, although locally invasive, very seldom show distant metastases; these are the locally malignant tumours, of which the basal-cell carcinoma is the typical example. Another group of tumours is characterised by a more erratic type of behaviour, some being benign, some locally malignant, and others frankly malignant.

Locally malignant tumours. *Basal-cell carcinoma*, or *rodent ulcer*, occurs most frequently on the skin of the face of fair-skinned people exposed excessively to the sun. It is much commoner than squamous-cell carcinoma.

Microscopically the dermis is infiltrated by groups of small, basophilic, round or fusiform cells with prominent, darkly-staining nuclei (Figs. 26.26 and 26.27). These cells resemble 'oat cells', and there is often considerable mitotic activity in their midst, yet the prognosis of the lesion is excellent. The

Figure 26.24
Oat-cell carcinoma of lung. The tumour is composed of sheets of uniform, small, darkly-staining cells, nearly all the substance of which is nuclear. Many have a fusiform shape which gives rise to the descriptive term 'oat cell'. × 320.

Figure 26.25
Seminoma. The tumour is composed of columns of large, round cells which are neoplastic spermatocytes. These columns are separated by thin fibrous trabeculae containing lymphocytes. × 150.

layer of cells at the edge of each clump is sometimes arranged in the form of a 'palisade', perpendicular to the surrounding connective tissue. It resembles the germinative layer of the epidermis very closely, and is not found in squamous-cell carcinoma. Degenerative changes within the clump may produce central cystic spaces (Fig. 26.27).

The origin of the tumour is debatable. The appearance of tongues of growth protruding downwards from the surface epithelium has given rise to the concept that it is a 'basal-cell carcinoma'. The continuity of the basal germinal cells with the outer, palisaded, tumour cells confirms this. Nevertheless, squamous-cell carcinoma must also ultimately arise from the basal cells. It seems that basal-cell carcinoma is derived from basal cells tending towards differentiation into hair follicles, sweat glands, and sebaceous glands. When it is remembered that the adnexae are formed as buds of epithelial cells into the dermis, a close similarity between their genesis and that of basal-cell carcinoma is apparent. It is not surprising therefore that areas of squamous differentiation, sometimes with keratinisation, are commonly found in basal-cell carcinoma. These represent attempts at hair-follicle formation. Less commonly glandular spaces are present, and occasionally there is recognisable sebaceous differentiation. Whatever the histogenesis of this tumour, there is no doubt that it is distinct from the squamous-cell carcinoma in its biological behaviour. It invades locally, but growth is generally very slow and can extend over many years. Metastasis almost never occurs. Occasionally the tumour can be more aggressive locally and invade adjacent

Figure 26.26
Basal-cell carcinoma. Separated from the epidermis there is a well-defined group of basal-cell carcinoma cells. In this section the peripheral palisading of the cells perpendicular to the dermal stroma is well shown. × 135.

Figure 26.27
Basal-cell carcinoma. A collection of basal-cell carcinoma cells underneath the thinned epidermis is present in this section. The cells are small and fusiform, and have a scanty cytoplasm and relatively large, darkly-staining nuclei. In this section peripheral palisading is not well marked. A central cystic area due to degeneration is present. × 120.

structures. In neglected cases there can be destruction of the nose and eyes, and eventually the tumour can erode through the skull and lead to meningitis.

Cylindroma. This tumour has a structure which resembles that of a basal-cell carcinoma but in spite of this it is almost invariably benign. It is composed of small, darkly-staining cells arranged in clumps. Outer palisading around each clump is a well marked feature, and external to this there is a conspicuous hyaline sheath. This consists of the basement membrane proper and an associated layer of collagen fibres. Occasional tubule formation is present and thought to indicate apocrine differentiation. Cylindromata usually occur on the face or scalp. They are sometimes multiple and inherited as an autosomal dominant characteristic (turban tumours). The name cylindroma is unsatisfactory because it refers merely to the microscopic appearance of the groups or cylinders of cells. Cylindroma has also been applied to the adenoid cystic carcinoma of the salivary glands and a type of bronchial tumour (p. 332), both of which are malignant, and a similar appearance can be seen in basal-cell carcinoma and even oat-cell carcinoma of lung.

Trichoepithelioma. Like the cylindroma of the skin, this tumour is usually benign and also occurs on the face or scalp. If multiple it is inherited as a dominant trait. Both types of tumour may co-exist. Trichoepithelioma consists of groups of cells not unlike basal-cell carcinoma, but the centre of each

clump is occupied by a well-marked whorl of keratin. This gives the tumour a cystic appearance and an alternative name is *epithelioma adenoides cysticum.*

It should be noted that the term epithelioma is often used as a synonym of squamous-cell carcinoma in Britain. However, in the North American continent it has no such malignant connotation, and is used to include other epithelial tumours of the skin, benign as well as malignant, e.g. benign calcifying epithelioma. The term should therefore never be used without qualification.

Ameloblastoma. This is a tumour derived from the enamel organ, and is considered in Chapter 27. It too has considerable powers of local destructive spread, but seldom metastasises. A peculiar tumour of the tibia, also called an ameloblastoma, is described. Like the dental tumour it bears some histological resemblance to a basal-cell carcinoma, but unlike it there is a tendency to lung metastasis. Whether it is an atypical synovioma or an aberrant epithelial tumour is not known.

Tumours of erratic behaviour. *Pleomorphic salivary gland tumours.* These tumours, found most commonly in the parotid, tend to behave for the most part like adenomata. They consist of acini, cords, and thin strands of epithelial cells suspended in a stroma which often has a myxomatous appearance (Fig. 26.28). This was once regarded as true cartilage, and the tumour was called a 'mixed salivary tumour'. It

Figure 26.28
Pleomorphic salivary gland tumour ('adenoma'). The structure consists of masses of epithelial cells, some of which are disposed in well-formed ductules. The stroma is copious and dense, and much of it has a cartilaginous appearance. × 80.

is now realised that the mucoid appearance is due to a sero-mucous secretion from the tumour acini into the stroma. True cartilage is very rarely found, and when present, it is due to chondral metaplasia of the altered stroma. The epithelium itself often shows squamous metaplasia.

The tumour may appear encapsulated, but the capsule is often infiltrated by lateral extensions of growth. Simple en-ucleation is likely to be followed by recurrence. Furthermore, local invasion may sometimes occur. Rarely distant, blood-borne metastases are encountered, even in tumours which in one area 'look benign'. There are all degrees of transition from adenoma to frank carcinoma in this type of neoplasm.

Other pleomorphic adenomata. Tumours of similar type are found in the palate, nasopharynx, and bronchi, and are derived from mucous glands. Pleomorphic lacrimal gland tumours are recognised, and finally some sweat-gland tumours of the skin have a similar appearance. In them the mucoid stromal change is less in evidence. Their behaviour is very similar to that of the salivary variety. In the skin they are invariably benign.

Mucoepidermoid carcinoma. This tumour commonly arises in the parotid gland. It consists of cells that show both mucus formation and areas of squamous differentiation. An abundance of mucous cells is found in tumours of low-grade malignancy; these grow slowly and rarely metastasise. Extensive squamous differentiation and anaplasia are found in tumours of high-grade malignancy; in these widespread metastasis is likely to occur. As with the pleomorphic salivary gland tumours, clinical behaviour cannot reliably be predicted from the microscopic appearances.

*Adenoid cystic carcinoma.** This tumour also occurs in the parotid gland, but more frequently arises in the other major salivary glands or from the mucosal glands of the nose, mouth, pharynx, or respiratory tract. The tumour consists of columns or clumps of cells which often contain a central cavity containing PAS-positive material. A cribriform pattern is common. The tumour is locally invasive and tends to recur unless widely excised. In some locations this is technically difficult, e.g. in the trachea: hence in this location the prognosis is poor. Lymph-node metastases and blood-borne spread ultimately occur in some cases.

Bronchial 'adenoma'. This term, which now serves no useful purpose and should be dropped, has been applied to a group of bronchial tumours which forms about 1 per cent of all pulmonary neoplasms.[10] Four distinct entities are included. The rarest is a mucous-gland adenoma of the bronchus. The other three are best classified as tumours of intermediate type since they tend to grow slowly, invade locally, sometimes spread to the regional lymph nodes, and rarely disseminate by the blood stream. The carcinoid tumour is the most common and arises from neurosecretory cells. Occasionally it gives rise to hormonal effects like its highly malignant counterpart, the oat-cell carcinoma. The two other types are the adenoid cystic carcinoma and the mucoepidermoid carcinoma, which his-tologically resemble similar tumours occurring in the salivary glands. These tumours may occur peripherally, but more commonly they are central and involve one of the major bronchi. They bulge into the lumen and produce obstruction,

and invade the bronchial wall between the cartilage rings, leading to an 'iceberg' effect. Endoscopic removal is therefore unlikely to be curative.

Carcinoid tumour (argentaffinoma). This is found most com-monly in the bowel, especially in the appendix, and rather less frequently in the terminal ileum and the large intestine. But it has also been described in the stomach, and it forms one type of bronchial 'adenoma'. Rarer sites are the thymus, ovary, and testis—in the last two it may be of teratomatous origin. It arises from the argentaffin cells of Kultschitzky. It has a characteristic yellow colour, and tends to stimulate a scirrhous reaction so that a stricture forms around the bowel.

The small, round, darkly-staining cells are arranged in solid clumps or cylinders; acinar differentiation is unusual (Fig. 26.29). If the cells are fixed freshly in formalin, special granules can be demonstrated with silver stains. The tumour is locally invasive, and may metastasise to the regional lymph nodes and the liver, especially in lesions of the small and large bowel. Despite multiple metastases the patient may survive for many years in comparatively good health.

In about 1 per cent of all cases and in 20 per cent of those with metastases an endocrine syndrome, the *carcinoid syn-drome*, develops. It consists of paroxysmal facial flushing, diarrhoea, bronchospasm with dyspnoea, and sometimes or-ganic heart disease—usually pulmonary stenosis or tricuspid regurgitation.[11] The tumour produces large amounts of 5-hydroxytryptamine (5-HT), which is excreted in the urine

Figure 26.29
Carcinoid tumour of colon. There is an infiltration of the submucosa and muscular coat of the colon by groups of tumour cells. These are small, spherical, and of uniform appearance, and are arranged in cylinders and elongated trabeculae. At one edge a few mucous glands are present. × 80.

---

*The tumour has also been called a cylindroma, but this term is best avoided since other tumours, e.g. of the skin, have also been given this name.

mostly as 5-hydroxyindoleacetic acid (5-HIAA). The 5-HT is not the main cause of symptoms, for an intravenous injection of it does not produce them. Adrenaline, on the other hand, does induce an attack in these patients, and it appears that catecholamines act as a trigger while the actual mediator is a kinin, probably bradykinin.[12] It is known that some carcinoids secrete kallikrein. Alcohol can also induce an attack, perhaps by leading to the release of catecholamines.[12] The most recent evidence suggests that 5-HT plays a subsidiary part, especially in the diarrhoea, and 5-HT antagonists are very useful in relieving it. Some gastric carcinoids produce 5-hydroxytryptophan, and these also show a relief of gastrointestinal symptoms when treated with antagonistic drugs. Carcinoids of the stomach and bronchus sometimes also secrete histamine, in which case there is a tendency to peptic ulceration. The valvular lesions in the heart probably develop from subendothelial fibrosis produced by kinins and possibly 5-HT.

Medullary carcinoma of the thyroid. This uncommon tumour consists of solid sheets and cords of uniform cells in a hyaline stroma rich in amyloid material. Despite its anaplastic appearance the tumour behaves very similarly to the carcinoid tumour, often causing death many years after metastases have developed. It arises from the parafollicular (C) cells of the thyroid, and is quite distinct from other thyroid carcinomata. These cells secrete calcitonin (see p. 459), but so far no case of hypocalcaemia has been reported in association with the tumour. On the other hand, a carcinoid syndrome has been noted, and the tumour may elaborate 5-HT, a kinin-forming enzyme, and prostaglandins. The explanation of the stromal amyloid is not understood. A familial tendency is noteworthy in this tumour.[13]

Figure 26.30
Hydatidiform mole. There is an oedematous placental villus surmounted by regularly proliferating chorion epithelium. ×80.

TUMOURS OF CHORION-EPITHELIUM

Choriocarcinoma (chorion-epithelioma) is a distinctive tumour of fetal origin, being derived from the trophoblast. It may be considered together with the carcinomata, for it has much in common with highly malignant tumours of other epithelia.

The well-known *hydatidiform mole* is the benign counterpart of this tumour: the characteristic grape-like clusters that are expelled from the uterus consist of oedematous placental villi surmounted by proliferating chorion-epithelium (Fig. 26.30).

Sometimes there are foci in which the cells are extremely pleomorphic, and these may invade the wall extensively. This is called an *invasive mole (chorio-adenoma destruens)*, but in spite of its appearance it rarely metastasises. It is important in this respect to realise that even normal chorionic tissue invades the uterine veins, and fragments are found in the lungs in pregnancy and especially during parturition.

In the rare *choriocarcinoma* there is an anaplastic proliferation of chorionic cells which are large and irregular. Many fuse to form syncytial masses, which are in fact a type of tumour giant cell. (Fig. 26.31). The tumour actively invades blood vessels and therefore bleeds easily; massive haemorrhage is a notable feature of the condition. Metastases occur early, and the lung is usually the first site of secondary deposits. These tumours are interesting in that they secrete a large amount of gonadotrophic hormone (of placental type). This produces bilateral theca-lutein ovarian cysts. The pregnancy tests are strongly positive. Very rarely a choriocarcinoma is found as a germ-cell tumour occurring in either sex. It should be noted that other anaplastic neoplasms may produce a histological appearance of pleomorphic giant cells which is very similar in appearance to that of a choriocarcinoma.

MALIGNANT TUMOURS OF CONNECTIVE TISSUE—SARCOMATA

Sarcomata are much less common than carcinomata, and unlike them, they occur at all ages. Whereas the cells in a carcinoma tend to be arranged in discrete cellular clumps surrounded by a variable stroma (this does not apply to the most anaplastic of them), those in a sarcoma are disposed in diffuse sheets, in which the neoplastic cells merge inseparably into the stroma.

On the whole, sarcomata spread more rapidly than carcinomata, and the prognosis is correspondingly more grave. Early blood-borne metastases are typical, and the lungs are often riddled with secondary deposits. Radical resection affords the best hope of cure, for these tumours are very radioresistant. Even when complete removal of a sarcoma is possible, e.g. osteosarcoma and malignant synovioma of an extremity, later pulmonary metastases are the rule.

Fibrosarcoma. This is the malignant counterpart of the fibroma. It differs from the benign tumour in that it infiltrates the surrounding tissues and metastasises. Although it is not

Figure 26.31
Choriocarcinoma. This section shows a large, central vascular space lined by extensive syncytial masses of tumour cells. These are large and pleomorphic, and many have prominent, darkly-staining nuclei. ×80.

encapsulated, in practice it is very difficult to assess infiltration until the tumour is quite large. An important diagnostic feature that distinguishes a fibrosarcoma from a cellular fibroma is the irregular, pleomorphic appearance of the individual cells. There is always evidence of mitotic activity, but it is often difficult to arrive at a decision which is of the utmost importance from the patient's point of view.

The more malignant varieties of fibrosarcoma show greater cellular pleomorphism, nuclear hyperchromatism, and mitotic activity; giant cells are quite common. Collagen formation is scanty (Fig. 26.32).

The most anaplastic tumours show no collagen, and the cells are either spindle-shaped (*spindle-cell sarcoma*) or plumper, and are then scarcely distinguishable from anaplastic carcinomata. Haemorrhage and necrosis are common features of most sarcomata, because the stroma is delicate and the vascular supply inadequate to meet the demands of the tumour.

Liposarcoma. This is one of the commoner types of sarcoma. It arises usually from the deeper connective-tissue planes of the limbs, especially the thighs, and has considerable invasive potentialities. It metastasises rather late. Histologically it consists of malignant lipoblasts which may assume giant proportions. A conspicuous tendency is the production of myxomatous tissue, which may overshadow the lipomatous element of the tumour.

Osteosarcoma. This is another common form of sarcoma. It tends to occur in later childhood, and is notoriously malignant. It may also occur as a complication of Paget's disease in older patients. The cell of its origin is the osteoblast. As in other sarcomata the tumour cells are very pleomorphic, and giant cells are often numerous. If the tumour is well differentiated there is osteoid formation which may or may not calcify to produce bone (Fig. 26.33). Sometimes islets of

TABLE 26.1   A comparison of malignant epithelial tumours (carcinomata) and connective tissue tumours (sarcomata, excluding the lymphomata)

Carcinoma	Sarcoma
Age incidence Commonest in middle and old age. A very common tumour.	Occurs at all times of life; common in young people. A much less common tumour.
Structure (a) Typically arranged in groups and columns, except in the most anaplastic tumours. (b) Stroma often well-formed.	(a) Arranged in diffuse sheets intimately related to the stroma. (b) Stroma nearly always poorly-formed and inadequate for the growth of the tumour.
Haemorrhage and necrosis less extensive, except in anaplastic tumours.	Haemorrhage and necrosis extensive.
Growth pattern Often somewhat slowly-growing.	Growth usually very rapid.
Metastases (a) Early lymphatic metastases. (b) Blood-borne metastases usually evident a little later. (c) Commonest seat of blood-borne metastasis is the liver. Other organs often involved are the lungs, brain, bones, kidneys, and adrenals.	(a) Lymphatic spread uncommon. (b) Blood-borne metastases appear very early. (c) Commonest seat of metastasis is the lung. Other organs may also be involved. Skeletal deposits are rare.
Radiosensitivity Many are highly radiosensitive.	Much more radioresistant.

Figure 26.32
Fibrosarcoma. The tumour is composed of sheets of large spindle-shaped cells with a minimal amount of intervening stroma. There is some pleomorphism and nuclear irregularity. × 300.

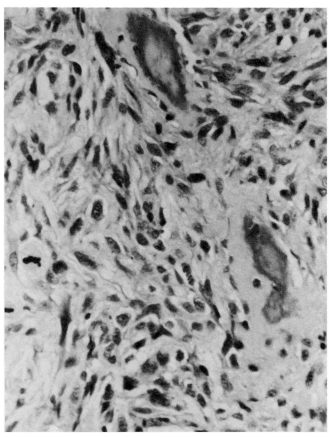

Figure 26.33
Osteosarcoma. The section consists of sheets of spindle-shaped cells intimately connected with the intervening stroma. In their midst there are two spicules of osteoid. There is a conspicuous mitotic figure at the left side of the section. × 300. (*Photograph by courtesy of Dr. A. D. Thomson*)

cartilage are formed, but the osteosarcoma should be distinguished from the chondrosarcoma, in which neoplastic cartilage is laid down in large amounts. It is a less malignant tumour.

As an osteosarcoma grows (it usually starts at the metaphysis of a long bone), it tends to elevate the periosteum. A fusiform swelling is produced, and bone forms under the periosteum and around the stretched-out periosteal vessels. In this way the characteristic sun-ray appearance of bony spicules is produced. It is interesting that the epiphyseal cartilage forms a barrier to the spread of the tumour, and that most osteosarcomata do not invade joints (Fig. 26.34).

THE LYMPHOMATA

These tumours, together with the leukaemias, constitute the commonest type of malignancy after the carcinomata. It is the 'labile' lymphoid and haematopoietic tissues which are respectively involved. It is better not to class them with the sarcomata, as their behaviour and radiosensitivity are quite distinctive (see Ch. 30).

THE GLIOMATA

Three main types are recognised:

1. *Astrocytoma.*
2. *Oligodendroglioma.*
3. *Ependymoma.*

The astrocytoma is the commonest glioma (Fig. 26.35). The differentiated tumours are composed of cells which closely resemble astrocytes with abundant glial processes. Although only locally invasive, their situation renders them very lethal tumours. In the more anaplastic tumours the cells have fewer glial processes and show the pleomorphism and mitotic activity characteristic of malignant tumours. The old name glioblastoma multiforme emphasises this feature. At one time it was thought that the tumour cells resembled the spongioblasts present during embryonic development, and it has also been called a spongioblastoma. It is now believed that this is a purely fortuitous feature of anaplasia, and in reality the tumour is derived from adult astrocytes. There is, however, a school of thought that still classes the glioblastoma multiforme as a distinct tumour.

Figure 26.35
Malignant glioma. The left cerebral hemisphere contains a large haemorrhagic tumour. It is poorly demarcated, and the swelling it has occasioned has partly occluded the lateral ventricle which is pushed over to the opposite side. (N 33.5, *Reproduced by permission of the President and Council of the R.C.S. Eng.*)

Figure 26.34
Osteosarcoma. The lower end of the femur has been destroyed by an osteosarcoma which has spread almost as far as the knee joint. The tendency for the tumour to lift up the periosteum and assume a fusiform shape is well shown in this specimen. (S 72a.5, *Reproduced by permission of the President and Council of the R.C.S. Eng.*)

Astrocytomata are generally classified according to their degree of differentiation and described as being well-differentiated, poorly-differentiated, or undifferentiated (Figs 26.36 and 26.37).

The oligodendroglioma consists of uniform sheets of rectangular, box-like cells with a clear cytoplasm and darkly-staining nuclei. Malignancy is, as usual, indicated by pleomorphism and mitotic activity.

The ependymoma consists of irregular spaces lined by exuberant ependymal cells similar to those seen in the walls of the ventricles and the central canal of the spinal cord.

Both oligodendrogliomata and ependymomata are rare tumours, and their growth potentiality resembles that of the astrocytoma.

Dystrophic calcification is prominent in these brain tumours (especially the oligodendroglioma), and is useful in radiological diagnosis.

Figure 26.36
Astrocytoma. This is a well-differentiated example. The astrocytic element is uniform, mitotic figures are not present, and there is abundant glial formation. × 100.

Figure 26.37
Astrocytoma. This is an undifferentiated example. There are sheets of anaplastic cells without any glial elements. A thin-walled sinusoidal vessel is present at one edge. × 80.

CHARACTERISTICS OF MALIGNANT TUMOURS

The criterion of malignancy is *invasiveness*. The tumour edge is therefore ill-defined, contrasting with the encapsulation of benign tumours. It is this infiltrative capacity which gives the name 'cancer' (the crab). Some rapidly-growing tumours may indeed show evidence of expansive growth, and a false appearance of encapsulation may be produced. Clear-cell kidney carcinomata, for instance, may appear to be well circumscribed: microscopy, however, reveals invasion.

Excluding the locally malignant group, all malignant tumours *metastasise*. The spread of tumours is considered in detail in Chapter 28.

Malignant tumours usually undergo a *rapid increase in size*. Therefore, unless death occurs very early in the course of the condition, a greater size is attained than with benign tumours. Enormous size is, however, uncommon.

Microscopical Features

Microscopically several important features should be noted. The tumour tissue may resemble the parent tissue to a considerable extent, but the similarity is not as great as in benign tumours. Differentiation is not so well developed, and recognition of the tissue of origin is sometimes difficult or impossible. It is the estimation of the degree of differentiation which forms the basis of tumour grading. At one time it was thought that normal differentiated cells could undergo neoplasia and revert to a more primitive state and appearance. This process of 'dedifferentiation' is nowadays discredited. Primitive cell-forms are now ascribed to a basically primitive cell-origin with a subsequent failure of normal differentiation. Neoplastic cells do differentiate, but frequently the differentiation is abnormal and does not conform to that found normally in the tissue. To describe a tumour as poorly differentiated is probably inaccurate, but it is a common practice and means that to the observer the neoplastic cells are making little attempt to resemble the structure of those found normally in the tissue.

Malignant tumours usually show much mitotic activity. The synthesis of DNA prior to division results in nuclear enlargement and hyperchromatism. This factor together with the formation of aneuploid and polyploid cells accounts for the irregularity in size, shape, and staining which is so characteristic of malignant tumours. Mitoses are not only numerous, but also sometimes abnormal. The number of chromosomes formed during division often diverges from the normal 46. Such aneuploid cells usually contain an excess of chromosomes, some perhaps with abnormal forms. A histogram of the DNA content of malignant cells therefore shows a wider scatter than normal. No single, constant change in chromosome form or number is characteristic of malignancy. However, in a few tumour types an abnormality of a particular chromosome has been reported. The best known example is the Philadelphia chromosome that is found in chronic myeloid leukaemia (see p. 44). Triradiate mitoses with the formation of three daughter cells is particularly characteristic of malignancy, but the authors have also noted it in *carcinoma-in-situ* such as may occur in actinic keratoses.

Anaplasia. This term was introduced by Hansemann to describe new cells which deviated from the normal and resembled those of embryonic tissue. The term is generally restricted to the abnormalities seen in tumours and can be applied widely to all the variations that occur. One may therefore have architectural anaplasia when the cells produce an abnormal structure, such as when smooth muscle cells produce an irregular interwoven myoma rather than an orderly sheet of smooth muscle. Likewise when applied to individual cells the term may be used to indicate the structural and functional aberrations ranging from the degree of differentiation and the cellular pleomorphism to the production of an abnormal hormone. Nevertheless, in practice the term anaplasia is used in respect of the microscopic cellular changes of neoplasia. An anaplastic tumour is one which has little or no normal differentiation and which exhibits the cellular changes depicted in Figure 26.38.

Giant cells. Giant cells may occur in malignant tumours under a variety of circumstances:

1. They are seen in some tumours as a regular occurrence due to the nature of the growth, e.g. giant-cell tumour of bone, osteosarcoma, Hodgkin's disease, and choriocarcinoma.

2. They occur as a feature of anaplasia in any malignant tumour. Giant-cell variants of many neoplasms are known, e.g. carcinoma of the lung and thyroid.

3. Giant cells may form in a tumour which is growing under adverse conditions, e.g. a tongue of lung cancer growing into the lumen of a bronchus.

4. Finally, foreign-body giant cells may form in relationship to necrotic tissue, cholesterol, keratin, etc.

Malignant tumours are thus characterised by a failure of the cells to differentiate normally, by their irregular disposition, by the number of mitoses, by prominent nucleoli, and finally by abnormalities in cell shape, size, and staining. These features are frequently relied upon in the clinical diagnosis of cancer. When small biopsies are taken, the arrangement of a few groups of cells may be sufficient to establish a diagnosis; in exfoliative cytology a few abnormal cells may suffice.

Figure 26.38
Anaplastic tumour of lung. This section shows the main features of malignant cells—pleomorphism, nuclear irregularity in size and staining capacity, giant cells, and a bizarre mitotic figure. × 450.

Although in practised hands diagnoses based upon these cellular changes may be reliable, it must never be forgotten that the only absolute criterion is tumour behaviour. *It is only by the detection of spread that cancer can be diagnosed with absolute certainty.* In clinical practice the tumour is often inoperable by the time this stage is reached. Morphological changes may be extremely useful in early diagnosis, but they are never an absolute indication of malignancy. For example, mitoses may be seen in hyperplastic lesions and some benign tumours, and abnormal cell-forms can occur in irradiated tissue.

The clinician and the patient are anxious to know the behavioural characteristics of a particular tumour. The pathologist has to rely on the morphological appearance of the tumour and the accumulated wisdom of past experience. A pathological diagnosis of malignancy is generally substantiated clinically unless effective treatment is available. Exceptions occur, but it is remarkable that these are so infrequent considering our ignorance about the basic nature of malignancy. There is indeed no reason for complacency, because the prognosis for an individual patient with a tumour, especially a 'malignant' one, is always in doubt.

Effects of Malignant Tumours

Malignant tumours produce their ill-effects in a large number of ways:

Figure 26.39
Carcinoma of colon. This resection specimen from a man aged 66 years shows an adenocarcinoma at the recto-sigmoid junction. The tumour involves the whole circumference of the gut, and has produced stenosis. The pericolic fat has been invaded, and several regional lymph nodes contained metastatic carcinoma. (*Photograph by courtesy of Dr. J. B. Cullen*).

Like benign tumours by causing mechanical pressure and obstruction. The obstruction produced by a malignant tumour is more pronounced and complete than that of a benign tumour, e.g. a carcinoma of the colon soon leads to intestinal obstruction (Fig. 26.39), and a bronchial carcinoma may rapidly cause collapse of a lobe. Pressure is also greater, and vessels may be occluded at an early stage.

Destruction of tissue. In addition, malignant tumours infiltrate and destroy vital structures. Their metastases similarly destroy vital organs. This is the usual mode of death in cancer. A carcinoma of the cervix eventually implicates the ureters and leads to uraemia; a breast cancer metastasises to the spinal column and damages the cord; a prostatic cancer metastasises to the bones and causes marrow destruction leading to anaemia, etc. It is this destructive character of cancer that is the root of the havoc wreaked by the disease. In addition, there are other subsidiary factors.

Haemorrhage. Carcinomata of surface epithelia eventually ulcerate and bleed. Usually the haemorrhage is occult, e.g. in gastrointestinal tumours, but large arteries may be eroded. This leads to a final fatal bleed.

Secondary infection. All ulcerative cancers undergo secondary bacterial infection, and this aggravates the clinical condition. The element of obstruction already mentioned is also complicated by infection, e.g. bronchopneumonia and bronchiectasis distal to a bronchial cancer, pyelonephritis and cystitis in prostatic cancer, etc. Cancer of the mouth interferes so much with deglutition that in due course food and saliva are inspired into the respiratory passages. It is not surprising that suppurative bronchopneumonia is the commonest cause of death in this condition.

Starvation. In cancers of the mouth, oesophagus, and stomach there may be a directly nutritional effect due to a failure of intake. In cancer of the colon there may be diarrhoea, and if there are intestinal fistulae, there will be a severe malabsorption syndrome.

Pain. In advanced malignancy pain may be severe. It occasions anxiety, and leads to insomnia.

Haematological changes. *Anaemia* is common in cancer. Apart from such obvious causes as haemorrhage, malabsorption, and bone-marrow replacement, it is not infrequently due to increased red-cell destruction. This haemolytic anaemia may be accompanied by autoantibodies in the serum, especially in the lymphomata, but sometimes these are not present. Pure red-cell aplasia is an occasional complication of thymoma.

There is commonly a *neutrophil leucocytosis* in progressive cancer, and occasionally an *eosinophilia* also.

Cachexia. Most patients with advanced cancer are emaciated and have an earthy skin pigmentation, but a few remain obese to the end. The generalised body atrophy of malignant disease is attributable to secondary factors, such as infection, starvation, malabsorption, liver involvement, and serous effusions, as well as anxiety, pain, and insomnia. Another possibility is that the neoplastic tissue secretes an ectopic product that leads to cachexia. This may also be the explanation of the *raised basal metabolic rate* and *pyrexia* that are frequently found in advanced cancer, but care must always be taken first to exclude the possibility of hidden infection.[14]

Immunological effects. On the whole there is little impairment in the immune response in cancer except perhaps terminally. Lymphomata, however, do depress the immune response—Hodgkin's disease the cell-mediated part, multiple myeloma the immunoglobulins, and chronic lymphatic leukaemia sometimes both. An occasional occurrence is *amyloidosis*, especially in Hodgkin's disease and renal carcinoma; more frequently it complicates multiple myeloma.

Cases of the *nephrotic syndrome* have been found in association with cancer.[15,16] Effective treatment of the tumour has led to a reversal of the renal condition, and in some cases deposits of IgG and IgM have been demonstrated on the glomerular basement membrane. The lumpy appearance of these deposits is that of non-specific antigen-antibody complexes, and on one occasion the antigen eluted from the glomeruli was found to be similar to that extracted from the lung tumour.[16]

CARCINOMATOUS SYNDROMES[17]

A variety of syndromes have been reported in association with neoplasms which are not explicable in terms of infiltration either by the primary tumour or its metastases.

Neuropathic effects. Some cancers, especially those of the lung, stomach, breast, and ovary, may be accompanied by progressive destruction of neurons throughout the central nervous system. This occurs in the absence of metastases in the brain and cord, and the nature of the degenerative process is unknown. Sometimes the clinical picture is one of cortical cerebellar degeneration and at other times it resembles peripheral neuritis. Encephalomyelitic forms are also described.

Myopathic effects. Some tumours, especially oat-cell lung cancer and cancer of the breast and colon, may produce a *myopathy* involving the limb girdles and proximal limb muscles. Sometimes, especially in lung cancer, there are also features of *myasthenia gravis*. Another occasional complication of visceral cancer is *dermatomyositis*, which is considered in Chapter 16. The possibility of these intriguing neurological and myopathic manifestations being due to an immunological mechanism is suggested by some authorities.

Dermatological effects. Sometimes an internal neoplasm first makes its existence known by the production of a widespread skin lesion. A good example is the condition of *acanthosis nigricans*, in which profuse, black, warty lesions develop in the axillae and groins in the course of an adenocarcinoma of the stomach, pancreas, lung, or other internal organ. Sometimes a figurate erythematous eruption with elaborate gyrate lesions may herald the clinical onset of malignancy, as may also urticaria, erythema multiforme, and bullous pemphigoid. Recurrent attacks of *zoster* are not uncommon in patients with a lymphoma, and are no doubt an expression of impaired cell-mediated immunity. Heavy *pigmentation* of the skin has been ascribed to the secretion of melanocyte stimulating hormone by the tumour—particularly carcinoma of the pancreas.

Thrombotic complications. *Thrombophlebitis migrans* (see p. 493) in an occasional concomitant of deep-seated cancer, usually of the pancreas, lung, and stomach. It may affect superficial or deep veins in any part of the body, and though the tumour is usually inoperable, cases have been reported in which removal of the cancer has been followed by relief of the phlebitis. Another occasional thrombotic complication of visceral cancer is *non-bacterial thrombotic endocarditis*. This type of endocarditis is also found at necropsy in patients dying of many other diseases,[18] but it does seem to be unusually common in cases of cancer, especially the mucoid variety.[19]

The onset of Raynaud's syndrome and ischaemic necrosis of fingers may be the first sign of occult carcinoma.[20]

Afibrinogenaemia. This is a rare occurrence in visceral cancer, usually of the prostate. This organ normally secretes a fibrinolysin, and occasionally in metastatic prostatic carcinoma there occurs a bleeding syndrome due to fibrinolysis (see p. 643).

Hormonal effects.[21] These come into two categories: (*a*) tumours of endocrine tissue secreting their own hormones, a topic considered in Ch. 35, and (*b*) tumours of non-endocrine origin producing a hormonal effect. The most important of these are *Cushing's syndrome* often with pronounced hypokalaemic alkalosis (usually with oat-cell lung cancer, islet-cell tumours of the pancreas, carcinoid tumours, and medullary carcinoma of the thyroid), *hypoglycaemia* (usually with mesothelioma and liver cancer), *hypercalcaemia*[22] (usually with squamous-cell lung cancer and carcinoma of the kidney), and water retention with *hyponatraemia* (with oat-cell lung cancer).

TABLE 26.2   A comparison of the main features of benign and malignant tumours

Benign	Malignant
1. Growth.	
(a) Slowly-growing.	(a) Rapidly-growing.
(b) Expansive type of growth.	(b) Invasive type of growth.
(c) The progress of growth is erratic with a tendency to cease.	(c) The progress is usually relentless until death occurs.
2. Metastases never occur.	Metastases frequent.
3. Size.	
Usually of small size, but occasionally enormous.	Usually of large size.
4. Histological structure.	(a) Less well-differentiated and sometimes completely anaplastic.
(a) Well-differentiated.	(b) Stroma often poorly formed. Haemorrhage and necrosis common.
(b) Well-formed stroma with little tendency to haemorrhage and necrosis.	(c) Cells are often pleomorphic. Mitosis often numerous.
(c) Cells regular. Few mitoses.	
5. Cause of death.	
Usually not fatal. If death occurs, it is due to mechanical pressure and obstructive effects. Endocrine adenomata may have hormonal effects.	Almost invariably fatal if untreated. Cause of death a combination of mechanical and destructive effects, together with blood loss, secondary infection, starvation, ectopic secretions, etc.

Two other hormonal effects worth noting are *polycythaemia* associated with renal carcinoma and a few other lesions mentioned on page 616 and *hyperthyroidism* associated with hydatidiform mole and choriocarcinoma. This is produced by a specific thyrotrophic hormone secreted by molar tissue; it differs from pituitary TSH, chorionic TSH secreted normally during pregnancy, and the LATS of Graves's disease.[23, 24]

The mechanism of these curious syndromes is the production by the tumours of a hormone or hormone-like substance. The hyponatraemia is due to the production of antidiuretic hormone, and the hypercalcaemia sometimes to parathyroid hormone (prostaglandins and other osteoclast-activating factors are also involved).[23] The Cushing syndrome is probably caused by the secretion of ACTH, since adrenocortical hyperplasia is usually present, and the hypoglycaemia may be due to the inappropriate secretion of insulin. An increasing number of syndromes are being described, and it seems that almost any tumour can produce any hormone. Cancer of the lung seems to be particularly adept at this perverted behaviour; in addition to the syndromes already noted, the occurrence of *gynaecomastia* has been described due to the production of a gonadotrophin. The tumour is usually anaplastic with many giant cells.[25] It has been noted that ACTH-secreting lung tumours have a particularly bad prognosis, due apparently to the immunosuppressive action of the cortisol the ACTH releases.[26] By contrast, ADH-secreting lung tumours do not have a worse prognosis than that of tumours not secreting hormones.[26]

Apart from the amines produced by the carcinoid type of tumour (p. 333), all these hormones are of polypeptide nature. A number of the above-mentioned tumours are composed of APUD cells,[27] and it is to be expected that they might produce other polypeptide hormones in addition to their own when their cells became malignant, e.g. the medullary carcinoma of the thyroid can be associated with a carcinoid syndrome and even Cushing's syndrome in addition to its secretion of calcitonin, and pancreatic islet-cell tumours have been known to produce corticotrophins and 5-hydroxytryptamine as well as insulin and gastrin. The same explanation might apply to some of the secretions of the oat-cell lung cancer.

It is probable, however, that the production of ectopic secretions by a wide variety of tumours is fundamentally a functional aspect of anaplasia. It is, for instance, now known that ectopic ACTH secretion is much more widespread than was previously thought, but that it is frequently not sufficient to produce the changes of Cushing's syndrome. Likewise high plasma calcitonin levels have been found in patients with a variety of tumours, including a number of cases of lung and breast cancer. The ectopic production of polypeptides by tumours is probably due to the activation or derepression of genetic information contained in the nuclear DNA, which should normally be inactive. Such purposeless, undirected activity would be more likely to lead to the production of simple-coded polypeptides than of steroid hormones, the formation of which is complex and due to the sequential action of a number of enzymes.[27] It is interesting, nevertheless, that specific tumours of an organ often produce a specific hormone, e.g. squamous-cell lung cancer produces a parathyroid hormone but seldom ACTH, melanocyte stimulating hormone, or antidiutetic hormone, all of which are often produced by the oat-cell cancer.[21]

The production of polypeptides with biological activity is possibly an explanation for the death of some patients with cancer in whom the extent of the tumour seems too limited to be lethal.[26] Such a polypeptide might interfere with a vital biological process by inhibiting other active peptides or by altering the protein binding of biologically active substances. Thus cases of lung cancer have been known which have had all the clinical features of Addison's disease and yet the plasma cortisol level has been very high. It would seem that the cortisol has been largely bound to peptides secreted by the tumour, and free, biologically-active cortisol almost absent. There is thus physiological adrenal insufficiency despite an excess of cortisol. The administration of a glucocorticoid with low protein binding, e.g. prednisolone, relieves the adrenal symptoms without, of course, altering the ultimate prognosis of the tumour.[26]

Pulmonary osteoarthropathy. This is seen in lung cancer and also fibrous mesothelioma of the pleura and chronic suppurative lung disease (bronchiectasis and empyema). There is marked finger clubbing with pain and swelling of the wrists and ankles, sometimes sufficient to simulate rheumatoid arthritis. There is subperiosteal new-bone formation and often mild synovitis. In cases due to lung cancer the tumour is often small and peripheral, and its resection causes rapid amelioration of the arthropathy. In inoperable cases cervical vagotomy similarly relieves the condition, suggesting that it is mediated through the afferent fibres of the vagus. The condition has not been found in association with oat-cell cancer.

The osteoarthropathy has been associated with the ectopic secretion of growth hormone by the tumour, but the causal relationship is not established, because some cases of the condition do not have raised levels of the hormone. Conversely, a raised level of growth hormone has been found in cases of lung cancer without osteoarthropathy.

The ectopic secretion of various substances by tumours, once a clinical curiosity, is now becoming one of the most rewarding studies in cancer. Not all these secretions are hormones, and therefore do not necessarily produce a clinical effect. But their presence in the blood can be a useful marker, not so much in the diagnosis of cancer, as in its follow-up after therapy. For instance, α-fetoprotein is secreted by some hepatomata and teratomata, whereas carcinoembryonic antigen (CEA) is secreted by a number of carcinomata, especially of gastrointestinal origin. A rise in the level of these proteins may be the first herald of a recurrence many months before a clinical relapse becomes apparent. This interval might afford an opportunity for the clinician to try cytotoxic or other therapies while the recurrence was still small.

GENERAL READING

ACKERMAN, L. V. & ROSAI, J. (1974) *Surgical Pathology*, 5th edn. Saint Louis: Mosby.
U.S. Armed Forces Institute of Pathology: *Atlas of Tumor Pathology*. Many fascicles have been published, and each covers the tumours of a particular organ or system. Series 1 and 2, Washington, D.C., 1949–1976.
International Histological Classification of Tumours. (1967–1978). WHO Series. 19 sections have now been issued, each dealing with the classification of a group of tumours. Each is accompanied by a set of 35 mm colour projection slides.

REFERENCES

1. MACKENZIE, D. H. (1972) The fibromatoses: a clinicopathological concept. *British Medical Journal*, **4**, 277.
2. GRAHAM, J. R. *et al.* (1966) Fibrotic disorders associated with methysergide therapy for headache. *New England Journal of Medicine*, **274**, 359.
3. Leading Article (1974) Myxoma of soft tissues. *British Medical Journal*, **1**, 170.
4. RUSSELL, D. S. & RUBINSTEIN, L. J. (1977) *Pathology of Tumours of the Nervous System*, 4th edn, p. 372. London: Arnold.
5. FISHER, E. R. & VUZEVSKI, V. D. (1968) Cytogenesis of schwannoma (neurilemoma), neurofibroma, dermatofibroma, and dermatofibrosarcoma as revealed by electron microscopy. *American Journal of Clinical Pathology*, **49**, 141.
6. LUCAS, R. B. (1976) In *Pathology of Tumours of the Oral Tissues*, 3rd edn, p. 145. Edinburgh: Churchill Livingstone.
7. LEVER, W. F. & SCHAUMBURG-LEVER, G. (1975) In *Histopathology of the Skin*, 5th edn, p. 476. Philadelphia: Lippincott.
8. WALTER, J. B. & PRYCE, D. M. (1955) The histology of lung cancer. *Thorax*, **10**, 107.
9. KREYBERG, L., LIEBOW, A. A. & UEHLINGER, E. A. (1967) *Histological Typing of Lung Tumours*, International Histological Classification of Tumours, No. 1. Geneva: World Health Organisation.
10. Leading Article (1973) Malignancy of bronchial adenoma. *British Medical Journal*, **2**, 378.
11. Leading Article (1975) Diagnosis of malignant carcinoid syndrome. *British Medical Journal*, **3**, 122.
12. ADAMSON, A. R. *et al.* (1969) Pharmacological blockade of carcinoid flushing provoked by catecholamines and alcohol. *Lancet*, **2**, 293.
13. Leading Article (1974) Familial medullary carcinoma of thyroid. *British Medical Journal*, **2**, 461.
14. Leading Article (1974) Fever in malignant disease. *British Medical Journal*, **1**, 591.
15. LOUGHRIDGE, L. W. & LEWIS, M. G. (1971) Nephrotic syndrome in malignant disease of non-renal origin. *Lancet*, **1**, 256.
16. LEWIS, M. G., LOUGHRIDGE, L. W. & PHILLIPS, T. M. (1972) Immunological studies in nephrotic syndrome associated with extrarenal malignant disease. *Lancet*, **2**, 134.
17. AZZOPARDI, J. G. (1966) Systemic effects of neoplasia. In *Recent Advances in Pathology*, 8th edn, pp. 98–184, ed. Harrison, C. V. London: Churchill.
18. Leading Article (1967) Nonbacterial vegetations on the heart valves. *British Medical Journal*, **3**, 812.
19. Leading Article (1978) Non-bacterial thrombotic endocarditis. *British Medical Journal*, **1**, 197.
20. HAWLEY, P. R., JOHNSTON, A. W. & RANKIN, J. T. (1967) Association between digital ischaemia and malignant disease. *British Medical Journal*, **3**, 208.
21. Leading Article (1976) Ectopic secretion by tumours. *British Medical Journal*, **1**, 1300.
22. TASHJIAN, A. H. (1974) Tumor humors and the hypercalcemias of cancer. *New England Journal of Medicine*, **290**, 905.
23. Leading Article (1971) Hydatidiform mole and hyperthyroidism. *British Medical Journal*, **2**, 606.
24. Leading Article (1976) Hyperthyroidism of hydatidiform mole. *British Medical Journal*, **1**, 179.
25. NEVILLE, A. M. (1972) Pathological aspects of the para-endocrine syndrome. *Proceedings of the Royal Society of Medicine*, **65**, 55.
26. ROSS, E. J. (1972) Some clinical aspects of the para-endocrine syndromes. *Proceedings of the Royal Society of Medicine*, **65**, 59.
27. ELLISON, M. L. & NEVILLE, A. M. (1973) Neoplasia and ectopic hormone production. In *Modern Trends in Oncology*, ed. Raven, R. W.—1: Part I, p. 163. London: Butterworth.

Chapter 27. Developmental Tumours and Tumour-like Conditions

INTRODUCTION

It is remarkable that in the course of a few months a single cell, the fertilised ovum, can proliferate and differentiate into the complex system of organs and tissues that characterises the mature organism. The science of embryology has revealed in great detail how these tissues originate, and has thrown suggestive sidelights on the mode of production of the various malformations that may blight the development of the growing embryo. A *malformation* is essentially an anatomical error arising during the development of an organism to its final adult proportions. Most malformations are manifest when the fetus is born, but quite a number first make their presence obvious during the actively growing period of childhood and adolescence. In such cases it must be assumed that the fundamental defect was already present at birth, but that it was of such a nature that it first became apparent during post-natal life. Sometimes the malformation is concealed in the depths of the tissues, and comes to light only in later life as the result of some secondary change in it, e.g. a chordoma developing from the notochordal remnants, or a branchial cyst appearing as the result of excessive secretion of the cells of the residual branchial vestige.

Malformations may take many forms. There may be complete failure of development of a part (*agenesis*), or the part may never attain a full, mature size and remain rudimentary (*hypoplasia*). Sometimes there may be a *failure of fusion* of parts (e.g. cleft palate and spina bifida), and sometimes there may be a *failure of separation* (e.g. webbed digits, Fig. 27.1) *or of canalisation* (e.g. imperforate anus and vaginal atresia).

Some malformations may consist of a simple overgrowth (e.g. an enlarged digit or limb in neurofibromatosis), and this is often rather dubiously called 'hypertrophy' or 'hyperplasia'. It should be called *local gigantism* because the organ has never been normal in relation to the remainder of the body. In true hyperplasia the part is initially normal in size, and subsequently undergoes enlargement (see Ch. 24). Sometimes there is a superfluity of parts resulting in the production of *supernumerary organs* (e.g. double ureter, polydactyly, and accessory spleens or spleniculi).

Sometimes organs and tissues are found in abnormal sites. This is called *ectopia*, *heterotopia*, or *aberrance*. It may come about in one of three ways: (*a*) *Persistence* or growth of a tissue which normally atrophies or remains vestigial. In this way thyroid tissue may be found at the upper end of the thyroglossal duct. Patent ductus arteriosus, Meckel's diverticulum, and branchial cysts are further examples. (*b*) *Dislocation* of part or all of a developing organ. Thus an ectopic testis may be found in the perineum or the pelvis. (*c*) *Heteroplasia*. This is the anomalous differentiation of tissue. A well-known example is the presence of gastric mucosa in a Meckel's diverticulum or in part of the oesophagus.

Figure 27.1
Syndactyly. The third and fourth fingers of the hand are completely fused. (*Photograph by courtesy of Mr. V. S. Brookes.*)

Heteroplasia must be distinguished from metaplasia, in which the alteration of tissue occurs after it has already differentiated normally. In heteroplasia the abnormal differentiation is a primary affair. It is of interest in illustrating the varied growth potentialities of a particular tissue. Thus there are many examples of cysts or masses in the region of the bladder, alimentary tract, or bronchi in which a wide variety of tissues is present. A cystic facial mass has been described which contained intestinal, gastric, and respiratory epithelium together with differentiated liver and pancreatic tissue.[1] Such a mass could be derived by heteroplasia in a portion of displaced endoderm. The term *choristoma* is applied to these non-neoplastic, tumour-like masses of developmental origin in which there are found tissues foreign to the part.

A more common lesion is the *hamartoma*; it consists of a tumour-like mass composed of a haphazard mixture of the tissues normally found in the part. Finally, the malformed tissues may assume the independent proliferative activity of a true tumour. It is these last two varieties of malformation, the *developmental tumours* and the hamartomata, that this chapter discusses in greatest detail.

Before leaving the subject of malformation it is worth completing the list by including those many malformations which manifest themselves primarily at a *cellular* or even a *biochemical level*. An inherited defect in an amino-acid sequence of the globin moiety of the haemoglobin molecule may lead to a sickle-cell or target-cell malformation of the erythrocytes (see p. 603), and a failure in the tubular reabsorption of phosphate may lead to a variety of osteomalacia (see p. 558).

All malformations are either congenital or else arise in the early years of life. Some are also hereditary, e.g. cleidocranial dysostosis and hereditary haemorrhagic telangiectasia, but the majority show no particularly familial tendency.

TUMOURS DERIVED FROM GERM CELLS[2, 3]

The germ cells first appear in the embryo in the wall of the yolk sac, from where they migrate around the posterior end of the primitive gut to the genital ridge on the posterior abdominal wall. Here they congregate and are incorporated into the developing gonad which later descends into the pelvis or the scrotum. It is now believed that some germ cells may either remain behind or stray from their final path and come to rest at various sites along the posterior wall of the embryo near the mid-line. If these cells do not die but remain viable, they could later give rise to tumours in just these situations: *the retroperitoneal area, the sacral region, the mediastinum,* and *the pineal region.* The greatest number of germ-cell tumours would, of course, be expected in the *gonads.*

The following are considered to be the tumours derived from germ cells:

(*a*) Seminoma
(*b*) Teratoma
(*c*) Extra-uterine choriocarcinoma
(*d*) Yolk-sac tumour.

Seminoma

This has been described on page 329. In the ovary a similar tumour is called a *dysgerminoma,* and when found in extragonadal sites it is called a *seminoma* or a *germinoma.*

Teratoma

A *teratoma* is a tumour consisting of multiple tissues foreign to the part from which it arises. This definition, derived from Willis, is subject to the rider that it is most aptly applicable to well-differentiated benign teratomata. Some, e.g. the testicular variety, may be so undifferentiated that their bulk is composed of bizarre anaplastic cells, which cannot be said to be forming any recognisable tissues at all. A careful inspection may be necessary to find elements that are recognisably foreign to the testis.

The vast majority of teratomata occur in the gonads, the ovary being much more often affected than the testis.

Ovarian teratomata are usually well-differentiated and benign. They are encountered chiefly in young and middle-aged women, and they constitute a variety of 'ovarian cyst'. In structure they usually comprise a thin-walled cystic mass which is filled with sebaceous, keratinous debris and matted hair. In one portion of the wall there is an eminence, or *umbo*, which may bear teeth and a tongue-like structure, and contain bone and cartilage (Figs. 27.2 and 27.3). Histologically the cyst is lined in most cases by stratified squamous epithelium, and skin appendages are prominent in the wall. This appearance has given rise to the erroneous name of 'dermoid

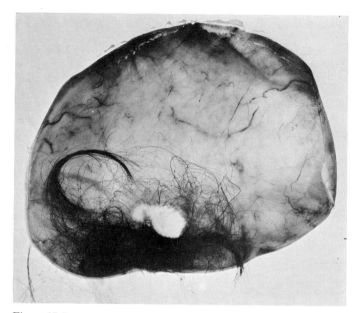

Figure 27.2
Ovarian teratoma. This cystic mass has a thin wall. At the base of the tumour there is a prominent umbo from which a mass of dark hair sprouts. (EF 13.1, *Reproduced by permission of the President and Council of the R.C.S. Eng.*)

Figure 27.3
Ovarian teratoma. The patient was a woman aged 32 years who was admitted to hospital with pain in the right iliac fossa. X-rays showed an ovarian cyst containing teeth.
The cyst was X-rayed after excision; it shows an irregular plate of bone bearing three teeth embedded in the projecting ridge. (F 13.1, *Reproduced by permission of the President and Council of the R.C.S. Eng.*)

cyst', but unlike a true dermoid cyst other tissues are also present, especially in the area of the umbo. Here various types of epithelium may be identified (e.g. intestinal and respiratory), bone and cartilage abound, and foci of nervous tissue can often be distinguished. Rarely the entire teratoma may be composed of one such tissue, e.g. the *struma ovarii*, which consists of mature thyroid tissue, and the *ovarian carcinoid tumour*. These teratomata are true tumours: they grow and gradually destroy the surrounding ovary. Malignant change is uncommon, and when it occurs it usually takes the form of a squamous-cell carcinoma. A much less common solid teratoma is also described, and is similar in malignancy to its testicular counterpart.

Testicular teratomata afflict young and middle-aged men chiefly, and the majority are highly malignant tumours. However, some are *well differentiated* and behave in a benign manner; these occur most often in children. The malignant varieties may show some organoid differentiation in association with undifferentiated tissue (*malignant intermediate type*), but the most malignant show only undifferentiated tissue (*malignant undifferentiated type*).

The less malignant types are solid but often with cystic spaces (Fig. 27.4). Histologically they consist of irregularly dilated gland-like spaces lined by atypical cells which may resemble squamous, respiratory, and intestinal epithelium in different places. There are also masses of bone, cartilage, and muscle interspersed among the epithelial elements, and the whole is supported by a primitive connective-tissue stroma.

The highly malignant type may be composed of sheets of large anaplastic cells. Such a tumour has in the past been called an 'embryonal carcinoma' of the testis, but the term has also been used for the yolk-sac tumour, and is best discarded.

The fourth testicular teratoma is the *malignant trophoblastic type*, in which there is trophoblastic tissue in addition to the other elements. It too is highly malignant, and merges into the testicular choriocarcinoma.

Malignant teratomata metastasise rapidly, both by the lymphatics and the blood stream, and their deposits may be as complex in structure as the primary lesion.

Much less frequently teratomata are found in the *anterior mediastinum, the retroperitoneal tissues*, and *intracranially*. These are usually benign, but carcinomatous change may supervene. *Sacrococcygeal teratomata* appear as enormous masses in the newborn, and they often contain at least one malignant component. Another rare neonatal teratoma is the large *epignathus* which arises from the base of the skull and protrudes from the mouth. It is usually well differentiated, but it soon kills because of mechanical interference with the functions of this part of the body.

The *histogenesis* of the teratoma has caused much debate in the past. At one time it was thought to represent the frustrated development of a conjoined twin, but this is unlikely because in even the best differentiated teratomata the tissues are not arranged in composite organs, e.g. there may be teeth and even a tongue, but there is no mouth. Furthermore, there is no vertebral axis in a teratoma such as is essential for the diagnosis of a fetus.

Another theory was that the teratoma developed from totipotential cells of somatic origin that became separated from the primitive streak and head process during very early

Figure 27.4
Teratoma of testis. The substance of the testis is replaced by a large, fleshy mass consisting of areas of bone, cartilage, fibrous tissue, and many cysts. Some of these contain blood and others a mucous fluid. (M 12.2, *Reproduced by permission of the President and Council of the R.C.S. Eng.*)

embryogenesis, and were scattered into surrounding areas during embryonic life. This suggestion does not account for the great predominance of gonadal teratomata.

The germ-cell theory, though still lacking definitive proof, is the most widely held, for the germ cell is the only truly totipotential cell in the body. Apart from explaining the frequency of gonadal teratomata, it also explains the not infrequent association of testicular (and ovarian) teratomata and seminomata, and the also well-recognised association of the four tumours in certain specific anatomical sites either alone or in combination.

Other Germ-Cell Tumours

If the seminoma can be regarded as the primary germ-cell tumour and the teratoma as a germ-cell tumour that has differentiated towards the formation of embryonic structures, there are two rare germ-cell tumours that appear to have differentiated towards the formation of extra-embryonic structures.

Choriocarcinoma. This has been described on page 333 as a uterine tumour associated with pregnancy. It occurs rarely in the gonads and other sites mentioned on page 344 as a germ-cell tumour of trophoblastic nature.

Yolk-sac tumour. This is a highly malignant tumour occurring in children and young adults. It has the structure of a complex adenocarcinoma with characteristic cystic areas and much mucin formation. Prominent mantles of cells are often found around blood vessels producing the appearance of glomeruli. In the testis the tumour has also been called the 'orchioblastoma' and 'embryonal carcinoma of juvenile type', and in the ovary it is known as the 'endodermal sinus tumour'; the name 'yolk-sac tumour' is preferable.

THE EMBRYONIC TUMOURS OF INFANCY

Unlike the teratomata, which contain a wide assortment of the body's tissues, this group of tumours consists only of those elements present in a particular part of the body, e.g. the kidney, retina, liver, and brain. It would appear that during the development of these particular areas a perversion of organogenesis occurs. A part of the developing organ undergoes neoplastic transformation, and a tumour, usually highly malignant, may result. Some of these lesions are present at birth, but most develop within the first 5 years of life at a time when the tissues are continuing their development. Very rarely authentic cases have been reported in adults, and it must be assumed that the lesion has remained latent until later life in such instances, or that it has developed from a 'cell rest'.

Nephroblastoma (Wilms's Tumour)

This tumour manifests itself as an abdominal mass in infancy and early childhood. It is very malignant, metastasising both by the lymphatics and the blood stream. Macroscopically it is a large, pinkish-white, soft tumour that replaces most of the kidney.

The neoplastic tissue is composed of both epithelial and connective tissue elements. The epithelium may form tubules, and also be arranged in the form of primitive glomeruli (proglomeruli). In fact, the tumour usually contains easily recognisable renal elements, such as would be expected in the kidney of a normal 4 to 5 months old fetus (Fig. 27.5). The tumour may contain bone, cartilage, or adipose tissue, and of greater interest, striated muscle fibres. Sometimes striated muscle cannot be demonstrated, and at other times it forms the bulk of the tumour. Some tumours are undifferentiated, and are composed of small darkly-staining cells with little or no attempt at tubular differentiation.

There is no doubt that this is a tumour of the renal blastema, but the origin of the striated muscle has aroused some controversy. It is generally believed to be due to a simple heteroplasia of the tissue of the blastema (comparable with the bone and cartilage which may also be present). Such a blastema would then be truly *pluripotential*, and responsible for the development of the 'mixed tumour'. It is not impossible, of course, that the muscle is derived from an adjacent myotome.

Figure 27.5
Nephroblastoma. Most of the tumour consists of undifferentiated embryonic tissue, but there is a primitive tubule in one part of the section, and evidence of very early glomerulus formation nearby. ×80.

An interesting feature of the nephroblastoma is that it is sometimes associated with other malformations.[4] There is a strong positive association with *sporadic aniridia* (a failure of development of the iris), and a weaker one with microcephaly, genito-urinary malformations, malformed ears, and lumbosacral spina bifida. Another interesting condition associated with nephroblastoma is *hemihypertrophy* (there is no correlation between the side of the tumour and that of the hemihypertrophy). Adrenocortical carcinoma and hepatoblastoma have also been associated with hemihypertrophy. The *Beckwith-Wiedemann syndrome* (macroglossia, omphalocele, adrenal cytomegaly, and visceromegaly) is closely related to the hemihypertrophy-visceral neoplasia syndrome, and has been associated with nephroblastoma also.

Neuroblastoma

This tumour arises almost invariably from the adrenal medulla or one of the sympathetic ganglia. It is doubtful whether it ever develops from the central nervous system. It often appears as an abdominal swelling in infancy, but its most characteristic feature is its capacity to metastasise to predictable sites. If the liver is extensively involved (and this may occur as the result of direct extension from a tumour of the right adrenal), hepatomegaly accounts for much of the abdominal swelling (*Pepper's syndrome*). Sometimes osseous metastases predominate, and a characteristic feature is the presence of enormous deposits in the skull especially around the orbits. Exophthalmos and bruising around the eyelids are early signs of this tendency (*Hutchison's syndrome*). Lymphatic metastases are also frequent.

Histologically the neoplasm consists of tightly-packed masses of darkly-staining round cells easily mistaken for lymphocytes. Sometimes these cells are disposed in rosette-like clusters, and if differentiation is particularly good, it may be possible to recognise tiny fibrils in the centres of the rosettes. These represent primitive nerve fibres, and the rosettes themselves resemble those seen in the normally developing sympathetic ganglia of a 4 to 5 months old fetus. Sometimes the round cells become pear-shaped and may actually develop into young nerve cells, in which case the fibres extrude from them like axons. If all the tumour cells differentiate into neurons, the tumour regresses; cure has been known to occur spontaneously.

True *ganglioneuromata* are often silent, or else they may manifest themselves in later childhood and during adult life. They consist entirely of mature nerve fibres and cells which closely resemble normal ganglion cells, even to the extent of containing brown pigment in their cytoplasm. The fibres may form interlacing bundles which may be provided with plentiful Schwann cells (Fig. 27.6). These tumours are benign, and once again demonstrate that as differentiation proceeds, so malignancy recedes. Many neuroblastomata contain well-formed ganglioneuromatous tissue in their midst. It is generally believed that all ganglioneuromata arise from primitive neuroblasts, because it does not seem likely that mature nerve cells would start proliferating to form a tumour. It is sometimes possible to diagnose these tumours biochemically, for there may be an increased secretion of catecholamines, e.g. dopamine, noradrenaline, and vanilmandelic acid, in the urine.

Medulloblastoma

This highly malignant brain tumour is found in the region of the fourth ventricle near the cerebellum. It occurs predominantly in young children, but it has been reported occasionally in adults. Like other malignant cerebral neoplasms it does not metastasise outside the central nervous

Figure 27.6
Ganglioneuroma. The tumour consists of aggregations of mature ganglion cells interspersed among which there are well-formed nerve fibres. × 240.

system, but intrathecal seedlings right down the spinal cord are quite common. The histological appearance is very similar to that of a poorly-differentiated neuroblastoma: sheets of small dark cells, round or elongated in shape, and arranged in clumps or rosettes.

These primitive cells are probably mostly neuroblastic in origin, but some may be spongioblastic (the spongioblast is the primitive glial cell which differentiates into the astrocyte, the oligodendroglia, and the ependymal cell) or even bipotential (capable of forming either neuroblasts or neuroglia). The medulloblastoma is therefore classified most satisfactorily as a *primitive bipotential tumour*.[5] Some authorities believe that the tumour arises from the granular layer of the fetal cerebellum. Another possible site is the neuro-epithelial roof of the fourth ventricle.

Retinoblastoma

This developmental tumour has the distinction of exhibiting a definite hereditary incidence. It is usually sporadic, but when familial it is transmitted as a dominant characteristic with variable penetrance, as the condition may be transmitted through apparently unaffected people. About a third of cases are bilateral, and this tragedy is most likely to occur in the hereditary group. There is a relationship between retinoblastoma and a deletion of the long arm of a D chromosome, and some of these cases also show mental deficiency and a tendency to develop other tumours, especially osteosarcoma.[6]

It is a disease of infancy and early childhood. Unless enucleation is performed expeditiously, widespread lymphatic and blood-borne metastases ensue. Histologically the rosette pattern of the neuroblastoma and medulloblastoma group is reproduced (Fig. 27.7). The centre of the rosette may be demarcated by a distinct membrane. Rod-shaped processes from the inner margins of the cells may project into the central cavity in a manner exactly reminiscent of the rod and cone cells and the external limiting membrane of the normal retina.

Hepatoblastoma

This is a very rare developmental tumour which like the nephroblastoma (and unlike the other three described) is truly 'mixed'. It consists of primitive liver-cell parenchyma, and often there is an admixture of connective tissue elements including bone, cartilage, and striated muscle. Whether the last is derived from the septum transversum (which eventually forms the diaphragm), or whether it develops as a result of heteroplasia from the hepatic blastema, is not certain.

A mixed tumour similar to the hepatoblastoma occurs in the lung. This pulmonary blastoma is very rare.[7]

Embryonic Sarcomata

A rare group of rhabdomyosarcomata usually involving the vagina, urethra, bladder, prostate, or orbit is well recognised. These highly malignant tumours occur in young children, and are due to a neoplastic proliferation of mesenchymal connective tissue. There is often a non-neoplastic proliferation of the surface epithelium, with the result that these tumours have a polypoid or grape-like appearance (hence the name *sarcoma botryoides*). Histologically the picture is one of spindle-cell or

Figure 27.7
Retinoblastoma. The tumour consists of small, darkly-staining fusiform cells which tend to be arranged in rosettes. Some of the rosettes enclose a well-formed central cavity. ×140.

pleomorphic-cell sarcoma in a myxomatous type of stroma. Striated rhabdomyoblasts are usually easily demonstrable, especially if an iron-haematoxylin stain is used to demonstrate their stripes. Very undifferentiated tumours may show no evidence of muscle fibres at all. It is probable that this rhabdomyosarcomatous differentiation is due to heteroplasia, but once again the alternative possibility of derivation of primitive rhabdomyoblasts from a neighbouring myotome cannot be discounted.

THE HAMARTOMATA

A *hamartoma* is a tumour-like malformation in which the tissues of a particular part of the body are arranged haphazardly, usually with an excess of one or more of its components. The term was coined by Albrecht in 1904,* and the concept it embodies is of great importance, since a large number of common lesions fall into the general category of hamartomata.

A typical example of a hamartoma is the isolated cartilaginous mass not infrequently found in the substance of a lung. This is usually 2 to 3 cm in diameter and has a white, pearly appearance and a hard consistency. On section it is found to be composed of mature hyaline cartilage, similar to that present in the bronchi. In the substance of the cartilage there are clefts lined by respiratory epithelium, and surrounding the

*It is derived from the Greek *hamartion*, a bodily defect.

cartilaginous masses there is connective tissue and smooth muscle. There is no true capsule between the lesion and the surrounding lung parenchyma. It is evident that this lesion contains several different elements (i.e. it is 'mixed'), but that all of these are normally found in the lung. It seems likely that it is a malformation derived from a developing bronchus, for all the tissues of a bronchus are present in it, though they are grossly misaligned, and there is an excess of cartilage (Figs. 27.8 and 27.9).

It is very important to distinguish this type of lesion from a teratoma.

(*a*) The tissues present are those specific to the part from which it arises.

(*b*) The lesion has no tendency towards excessive growth. Its growth is co-ordinated with that of the surrounding tissues, and it stops after adolescence. There is no capsule around a hamartoma; as its growth proceeds *pari passu* with that of its surroundings, there is no pressure atrophy and therefore no connective tissue condensation. Hamartomata are not tumours, but it is possible for a tumour to develop in a hamartoma. In the pulmonary lesion just described this does not happen.

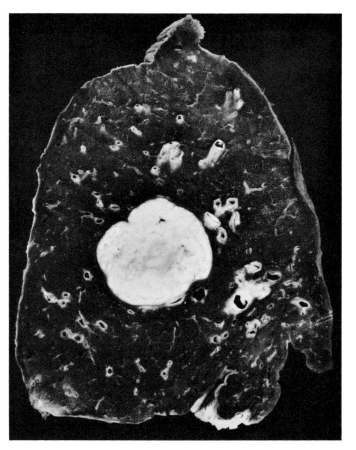

Figure 27.8
Hamartoma of lung. In the centre of the upper lobe there is a circumscribed, pearly-white, round mass. It consists predominantly of mature hyaline cartilage, and there is no obvious capsule around it. (ER 22.1, *Reproduced by permission of the President and Council of the R.C.S. Eng.*)

Figure 27.9
Hamartoma of lung. This specimen consists mostly of masses of compact connective tissue containing deep clefts lined by respiratory epithelium. Foci of adipose tissue are also conspicuous, and at the top there is a mass of hyaline cartilage. ×55.

It should be noted that many hamartomata are given 'tumour-sounding' names. These are so much part and parcel of pathological nomenclature that they are bound to persist, e.g. angioma and chondroma of the lung.

Most hamartomata are present at birth or in the early years of childhood, but only those on exposed areas like the skin and mouth will be recognised as early as this. The cartilaginous hamartoma of the lung is always described in adults, though no doubt the original nidus was present at birth, and thereafter underwent steady growth to its final mature size. It is usually discovered during a routine radiological examination of the chest, and if misdiagnosed as carcinoma may be the cause of a completely unnecessary pneumonectomy.

Vascular Hamartomata

The very common **haemangioma** is a hamartomatous malformation and not a true tumour. It is usually present at birth or else appears soon afterwards, and though its growth is sometimes quite active in early childhood, it soon becomes quiescent, and may even undergo regression as the result of interference with its vascular supply. This is particularly true of the strawberry naevus, which starts as an inconspicuous lesion on an infant's face, grows rapidly to giant proportions, and then after a few years regresses and finally disappears leaving an area of scarring.

Figure 27.10
Haemangioma of tongue. This specimen of the sagittal section of skull comes from a child who survived 4 days. The tongue is enormously enlarged, and protrudes from the mouth as a dark mass. It is almost completely replaced by cavernous vascular tissue. (A 7.2, *Reproduced by permission of the President and Council of the R.C.S. Eng.*)

The commonest type of haemangioma is seen on the skin where it forms a variety of *naevus*. This word is used to describe any type of developmental blemish of the skin (birthmark), e.g. hairy, melanotic, or sebaceous. Sometimes vascular naevi are small and spider-like, sometimes raised (strawberry naevi), and sometimes flattened and extensive, covering a considerable expanse of skin (*naevus flammeus*). Characteristically they blanch on pressure due to an emptying of their contained blood. Haemangiomata are also often found in the mouth and on the lips, and their frequency in solid organs like the liver, brain, bones (especially the vertebrae), and muscles is well recognised (Fig. 27.10).

Microscopically they consist of poorly-demarcated, non-encapsulated masses and leashes of vascular channels, most of which contain blood. Sometimes the channels are capacious and confluent—like the erectile tissue of the penis (*cavernous haemangiomata*), sometimes they are narrow and well-formed (*capillary haemangiomata*), and sometimes they are provided with large tortuous arterioles and venules (*plexiform haemangiomata*). All three types may occur together. Sometimes there are extensive areas of endothelial cells arranged in uncanalised clumps. It is the subsequent canalisation of these areas that often gives the clinical impression of rapid growth of an angioma. Large haemangiomata occurring in infancy may rarely selectively trap circulating platelets, and lead to thrombocytopenic purpura (see also Ch. 54). There are all degrees of angiomatous malformations from single, small, flat naevi up to extensive cirsoid aneurysms (Fig. 27.11).

Some haemangiomata enlarge and undergo progressive fibrosis, probably as a result of repeated haemorrhage into their substance. These *sclerosing haemangiomata* contain much free haemosiderin pigment and also foci of foamy macrophages and

Figure 27.11
Haemangioma. This is a typical cavernous haemangioma. It consists of loose strands of connective tissue lined by endothelium enclosing extensive vascular spaces. It resembles normal erectile tissue. ×120.

giant cells reminiscent of a xanthoma. The final picture is indistinguishable from a dermatofibroma, a common lesion variously regarded as a benign neoplasm or a reaction to injury, such as an insect bite. In heavily pigmented lesions it is necessary to stain for haemosiderin, otherwise the pigment may be mistaken for melanin and an incorrect diagnosis of blue naevus or even malignant melanoma made.

Angiomatous syndromes.[8] A very important feature of the haemangiomata is their tendency towards multiplicity. Some very characteristic syndromes are produced in this way, e.g. (*a*) *Hereditary haemorrhagic telangiectasia* (Rendu-Osler-Weber disease—see Ch. 54). (*b*) *Sturge-Weber syndrome*, in which there is a combined naevus flammeus over one half of the face and a haemangioma of the ipsilateral cerebral hemisphere. (*c*) Haemangiomatosis of the retina and central nervous system (*von Hippel-Lindau disease*).

There are sometimes other malformations present as well, e.g. *Kast's* or *Maffucci's syndrome*, in which there is enchondromatosis of the bones as well as multiple cutaneous haemangiomatosis.[8]

Angioblastic tumours. Although the great majority of tumour-like lesions of blood vessels are merely angiomatous malformations, true angiomatous neoplasms also occur but are uncommon, except for the peculiar Kaposi tumour, which is usually included in the category of haemangiosarcoma.

(*a*) *Haemangiosarcoma* also called *haemangio-endothelioma* may arise either spontaneously,[9] or very rarely in a congenital angioma. When an angioma undergoes malignant change, the endothelial cells show variations in size and shape, and there are numerous mitotic figures. To diagnose a haemangiosarcoma it is necessary to establish the vasoformative nature of the tumour, for many undifferentiated tumours with an abundant sinusoidal vasculature can mimic it. In haemangiosarcoma (and lymphangiosarcoma) a reticulin stain demonstrates that the proliferating tumour cells lie within the reticulin sheaths. This also distinguishes the tumour from a haemangiopericytoma, in which the neoplastic cells lie external to the silver-impregnated, endothelial basement membrane zone.

There are two interesting tumours that come into the category of haemangiosarcoma: (1) *Post-mastectomy angiosarcoma*, which is a remote complication of breast cancer. These cases first develop severe lymphoedema of the arm due to the occlusion of the axillary lymphatics following their permeation by cancer cells and their further obliteration by radiotherapy. Several years later multiple angiosarcomata develop in the skin of the arm, and these may metastasise to the lungs. The condition is called the *Stewart-Treves syndrome*, and it has a combined haemangiomatous and lymphangiomatous element (Fig. 27.12).

Some authorities doubt the existence of the postmastectomy angiosarcoma, and attribute the tumour to a metastasis of the original breast cancer. However, authentic angiosarcoma has also been reported arising in chronic congenital and idiopathic lymphoedema where there has been no question of coincidental carcinoma.[10] The current view is that the Stewart-Treves syndrome is a definite entity.

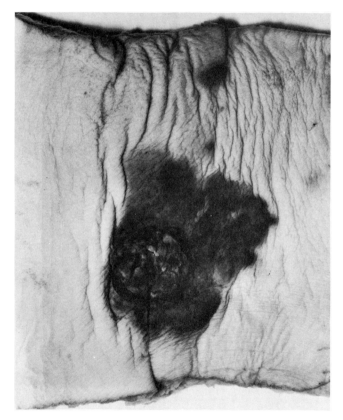

Figure 27.12
Post-mastectomy angiosarcoma of skin of arm. The patient had had a radical mastectomy 5 years before. Immediately after operation her arm became oedematous, and there was also a severe reaction over the neck and shoulder following radiotherapy. The swelling of the arm persisted, and about 2 years later a red spot was noticed on the inner aspect of the arm. It continued to enlarge and became pedunculated at one point. Biopsy revealed an angiomatous tumour resembling Kaposi's sarcoma, and a forequarter amputation was performed. The specimen consists of a portion of the skin of the inner aspect of the arm. The main lesion is an irregular dusky area 7.5 cm in diameter, projecting from the surface of which there is an ulcerated, pedunculated mass about 2.5 cm in diameter. (127.2, *Reproduced by permission of the President and Council of the R.S.C. Eng.*)

(2) *Kaposi's sarcoma.* This consists histologically of proliferating plump spindle cells and angiomatous tissue. It has been described as an 'idiopathic haemorrhagic sarcoma' and is often classified with the angiosarcomata, but the histogenesis of the neoplastic spindle cells is not known. The tumour is seen in Eastern Europeans, but its maximum prevalence is in the Black population of Eastern and Southern Africa, where it is one of the commonest types of cancer.

The disease appears to be of multicentric origin, and generally affects both legs and later the arms also. It can run a protracted, indolent course for many years, but ultimately tumour nodules appear. Sometimes the disease is fulminating and associated with visceral lesions. In European cases there is not infrequently an association with neoplasms of the lymphoreticular system, but in Black people this is exceptional.

Glomangioma (glomus tumour). This is a completely different tumour of blood vessels, and is always benign. It is found most often in the skin of the extremities where it gives rise to paroxysms of severe pain. It arises from the arterio-venous anastomosis, or glomus, which contains a thick layer of cuboidal cells in its wall. These cells are of myoneural origin, and their ultrastructure resembles that of the smooth muscle cell.[11] Glomangiomata consist of irregular vascular spaces which are surrounded by many layers of characteristic cuboidal glomus cells.

Another type of vascular hamartoma is the **lymphangioma**. It differs in no important respect from the commoner haemangioma, except that it contains no blood. A well-known extensive lymphangioma of infancy is the *cystic hygroma of the neck.* It infiltrates the vital surrounding structures so intimately that complete removal is seldom possible.

Melanotic Hamartomata (Naevocellular Naevus*)[12]

The common *naevocellular naevus* of the skin is another important example of a hamartomatous malformation, which, unlike the angioma, shows a more definite tendency towards malignant change. The parent cell, the melanocyte (the melanin-producing cell of the body, see Ch. 50), is believed to originate in the region of the neural crest and to migrate to the epidermis with the peripheral nerves.

By the time of birth there are moderate numbers of melanocytes in the basal layer of the epidermis, though in fair-skinned individuals the DOPA reaction may be necessary to

*Many terms are used to describe this lesion: benign melanoma, pigmented mole, pigmented naevus, naevocellular naevus, etc. The last is perhaps the most precise. The word melanoma should never be used unqualified, because to many people it has a malignant connotation. The term naevus may be used alone provided it is the naevocellular variety which is being described (e.g. compound naevus).

Figure 27.13

Sketches to show the various types of melanotic naevi: the only cells drawn are melanocytes and naevus cells. In the normal skin melanocytes are present only in the basal layer of the epidermis. A focal proliferation of these cells produces a junctional naevus (b) which may be regarded as a stage in the development of a compound and intradermal naevus. Such junctional activity is of little importance in a young person, but in an adult is to be regarded as dangerous; (c) shows the formation of a compound naevus by the invasion of the dermis by melanocytes. When the junctional activity regresses, the naevus cells remain in the dermis as an intradermal naevus (d); (e) shows a malignant melanoma which in addition to junctional activity, shows invasion of the epidermis as well as the dermis and deeper structures. Atypicality of the cells serves as a further distinguishing feature from the compound naevus, which an early malignant melanoma may resemble. (f) The strap-like naevus cells situated deep in the dermis impart the colour to the blue naevus.

(a) Normal skin.

(d) Quiescent intradermal naevus.

(b) Junctional naevus with activity.

(e) Malignant melanoma.

(c) Developing compound naevus.

(f) Blue naevus.

reveal them. There is surely not a single individual who does not have a number of pigmented 'moles', or melanotic naevi, on his skin. These are simply excessive accumulations of melanocytes which have developed during infancy and childhood. They may be associated with malformations of the epidermis, hair follicles, and sebaceous glands, so that large, papillomatous, hairy naevi are sometimes present as well as the flatter, darker lesions that are composed only of *naevus cells*, as the altered melanocytes of a pigmented mole are usually called (see Fig. 27.13).

The focal proliferation and accumulation of melanocytes, usually containing much melanin, at the junction of the epidermis and dermis is invariable in infancy, and the lesion so formed is called a *junctional naevus*. It is flat and deeply pigmented. As the child grows older, there is a tendency for the naevus cells to be shed from the basal layer of the epidermis into the dense connective tissue of the dermis, where they lie characteristically in inert clumps which are completely unencapsulated. The cells are cuboidal in shape, and have a somewhat basophilic cytoplasm which usually contains little or no melanin pigment. The appearance of these cells 'invading' the dermis is disconcerting, but must be regarded as a normal event in the evolution of the naevus.

By the time adult life is reached, all the naevus cells in many naevi have left the epidermis and are sequestered in the underlying dermis. The flesh-coloured papule so produced is described as an *intradermal naevus*, and is believed to be perfectly harmless (Fig. 27.14). The naevus cells often become

spindle shaped, especially in the deeper part of the lesion, and this is interpreted as differentiation into Schwann cells. Indeed, old naevi may contain areas resembling a neurofibroma. In some naevi, some or even all the naevus cells retain their attachment to the epidermis, so that the naevus is either partly in the dermis and partly junctional (*compound naevus*), or else it remains completely junctional.

Junctional activity. It is the junctional component of a naevus which is potentially dangerous, because it is these cells which are liable to undergo proliferation from time to time. During childhood a naevus often manifests signs of active growth of a degree rather greater than would be expected of a truly hamartomatous lesion, and histologically such a naevus may show quite an alarming degree of active proliferation of its junctional component, even with mitotic figures and general pleomorphism. This is called *junctional activity*. Experience has taught us that such junctional activity is quite common and should not arouse undue alarm. When, however, similar activity occurs in a naevus of a person over the age of 30 years, the matter is much more serious, for it may indeed be the first indication of malignancy (Fig. 27.15). Even in adult life, however, junctional activity is sometimes a phasic affair, and does not necessarily terminate in malignancy.

Figure 27.14
Intradermal naevus. There is a focal accumulation of naevus cells in the deeper layer of the dermis, but they are well separated from the overlying epidermis. ×120.

Figure 27.15
Junctional naevus. There are considerable aggregations of naevus cells in contact with the basal layer of the epidermis, but there is no evidence of invasion of the epidermis. × 80.

Juvenile melanoma. This is a type of compound naevus which generally occurs in young people and because of its rapid growth mimics a malignant melanoma. Histologically the predominant cell type is usually spindle shaped, and the presence of mitoses can easily lead to a diagnosis of malignancy. Nevertheless, the lesion is entirely benign.

Regression of naevi.[13,14] Occasionally one or more naevi undergo spontaneous regression and are surrounded by a zone of depigmentation. Such a lesion is called a *halo*, or *Sutton's, naevus*. Histologically there is a lymphocytic infiltrate, and this must not be misinterpreted as evidence of malignancy in a naevus (see p. 353). The halo phenomenon can also be seen in malignant melanoma and is generally interpreted as evidence of an autoimmune reaction.

MALIGNANT MELANOMA OF THE SKIN AND MUCOUS MEMBRANES

This is a malignant tumour derived from melanocytes and may arise *de novo* or else in some pre-existing lesion, such as a naevus or an *in-situ* melanoma (Fig. 27.16). Estimates of the number that arise from naevi vary considerably, due in part to the fact that most patients are poor historians and in part to the varying criteria used by pathologists in recognising malignant change in a naevocellular naevus.

Some put the figure at about 40 per cent,[15] while others regard it as occurring in less than 10 per cent.[16] Nevertheless, malignant change in a naevus should be suspected if any of the following changes occur: increase in size; change in colour whether darker, lighter, or mottled; bleeding; ulceration; crusting. When any of these changes occur, excisional biopsy is recommended before radical treatment is considered, since clinical misdiagnosis is common.

Aetiology. It is doubtful whether trauma or hormonal changes, such as occur in pregnancy, are important. *Ultraviolet light* is however important.[17] Malignant melanoma is common in fair-skinned people living in the northern parts of Australia and in the southern states of the USA.[18] It seems, like other actinic skin cancers, to be particularly common in the Celtic group of people, and its frequency among those of Irish stock in Australia is noteworthy. *Areas of ectopic pigmentation*, e.g. of the soles, mouth, and nose, are particularly vulnerable to melanomatous change in Blacks.[19] Indeed, melanoma of the plantar region is common in the Black population of Africa. The subungual melanoma is usually malignant by the time it is diagnosed. There is also a *hereditary element* in some cases of malignant melanoma; these tend to be multiple, and they occur at an earlier age than that at which sporadic melanomata develop (which is about 50 years).[20] There is one type of naevus which is definitely premalignant: the *giant*, or *bathing-trunk, naevus*, which is truly congenital and of massive proportions. It may be associated with meningeal melanosis, and malignant melanoma develops in up to 25 per cent of cases.[14]

Two other rare but definitely premalignant conditions should be noted; both may be regarded as examples of *in-situ* melanoma.

Conjunctival melanosis.[21] This consists of the appearance of a diffuse brown patch on the conjunctiva, usually in middle-aged people whose conjunctivae were previously normal. This patch spreads and may implicate the surrounding skin. Histologically it is a proliferation of atypical melanocytes in the epithelium, and invasive melanoma tends to supervene, though this often takes many years to occur.

Lentigo maligna, or *Hutchinson's freckle*,[22] is a similar condition and is generally seen on the face of elderly individuals. There is marked junctional activity with proliferation of bizarre atypical melanocytes and disorganisation of the deeper layers of the epidermis but no dermal invasion. Invasion and metastasis can occur, often after 10 years or even longer.

Types of melanoma. The unpredictable behaviour of malignant melanoma has led to many attempts at classification. These have been designed to relate macroscopic and histological features to prognosis. The classification of Clark and his colleagues is currently favoured.[16,23] Three types are recognised:

(*a*) *Lentigo-maligna melanoma.* This tumour develops slowly

Figure 27.16
Malignant melanoma. The dermis is diffusely infiltrated by pleomorphic tumour cells, some of which are pigmented. The epidermis is considerably thinned, its deeper layers having been destroyed. Adjacent to this area there was extensive ulceration. × 80.

at the site of a previous Hutchinson's freckle. It has a relatively good prognosis (Fig. 27.17).

(*b*) *Superficial spreading melanoma.* This is a flat lesion which can occur on any area of the skin and histologically shows a wide area of proliferation of atypical melanocytes at the dermo-epidermal junction. Dermal invasion occurs later, and nodular lesions can then develop (Fig. 27.18).

(*c*) *Nodular melanoma.* Early dermal invasion produces a nodular lesion, and there is no flanking junctional component as is seen in the superficial spreading variety. The prognosis is worst in this type (Fig. 27.19).

Any of these three types of melanoma may show different types of cells. These may be of epithelial appearance (sometimes exhibiting considerable pleomorphism with giant forms), spindle shaped, or small. It is the occurrence of the small cells together with the presence of junctional proliferation in the superficial spreading melanoma that makes it difficult to recognise the pre-existence of a benign naevus in an established malignant melanoma.

The detection of malignancy in a pre-existing naevus is often a matter of great difficulty. The presence of atypical, pleomorphic cells, mitoses, and epidermal invasion leading to ulceration are points in favour of diagnosing such a change (Fig. 27.15). So also is a dermal inflammatory reaction, but it must be remembered that inflammation is not uncommon in response to trauma, an infected hair follicle, or the regressive changes seen in a halo naevus.

Regardless of the type of tumour, the prognosis of malignant melanoma of the skin is related to the level of tumour invasion; five levels are described:[23]

Level I Tumour confined to the epidermis, i.e. *in-situ* melanoma.

Level II Tumour has penetrated the basement membrane zone of the epidermis and extended into the papillary dermis.

Level III Tumour has filled the papillary dermis and accumulated at the junction of the papillary and reticular dermis.

Level IV Invasion of the reticular dermis.

Level V Invasion of the subcutaneous fat.

More recently the prognosis of cutaneous melanoma has been related to tumour thickness.[24]

When a malignant melanoma enters into an aggressive phase, there is a rapid invasion of local lymphatics which may sometimes show black streaking due to melanomatous permation. Early lymph-node and blood-borne metastases are the

Figure 27.18
Superficial spreading type of malignant melanoma. Two black nodules of tumour are surrounded by superficial, barely palpable, growth. Some areas are pigmented, whereas others show erythema. The pale areas of depigmentation are due to foci of tumour regression. (*Photograph by courtesy of Dr. Wallace H. Clark, Jr.*)

Figure 27.17
Lentigo-maligna type of malignant melanoma. It has the best prognosis of the three. (*Photograph by courtesy of Dr. Wallace H. Clark, Jr.*)

Figure 27.19
Nodular malignant melanoma. This black lesion had recently appeared, and it showed superficial ulceration. It has the worst prognosis of the three. (*Photograph by courtesy of Dr. Wallace H. Clark, Jr.*)

rule, and the condition is a fearful one. Metastases may occur in unusual sites, e.g. bowel, heart, and spleen. Often both the primary tumour and its metastases are well-pigmented, but sometimes they contain very little pigment. Such an amelanotic melanoma is difficult to distinguish from an anaplastic carcinoma or sarcoma; the DOPA reaction may help in the diagnosis, but to be of value the tissue must be processed after a short period of fixation. In practice, some melanin can be found in routine sections provided an adequate amount of tumour is available for examination. Electron microscopy may reveal typical melanosomes in cases in which melanin cannot be demonstrated (Fig. 25.1, p. 310).

It is important to be aware that not all skin tumours pigmented with melanin are malignant melanomata. Apart from naevocellular and blue naevi, basal-cell carcinomata and seborrhoeic keratoses often show heavy melanin pigmentation due either to hyperactivity or to hyperplasia of the melanocytes. This is much less common in squamous-cell tumours and Bowen's disease.

The blue naevus.[14] This is a special type of melanotic naevus which is intradermal from the start, and blue in colour because its melanocytes are deeply situated in the skin. They are elongated dendritic cells scattered in the deep layers of the dermis. The epidermis itself is normal. This is the one type of naevus which may undergo malignant change in its intradermal portion. Nevertheless malignant change is very rare. The cells of the blue naevus are derived from a dermal pigmentary system in addition to the epidermal system of melanocytes, that is normally present in other mammals and especially the higher apes, but usually vestigial in humans. Collections of such cells are to be found normally only in the sacral area at birth, especially in the Mongolian and Black races, and are called the *mongolian spot*. This usually involutes completely at puberty, but sometimes there are heterotopic collections of dermal melanocytes, and these may give rise to blue naevi, which are not truly congenital. The commonest sites for a blue naevus are the face, dorsum of the hand and foot, and the buttock. The histogenesis of the dermal melanocyte is uncertain; it may either be neural in origin or else develop locally.

Mucosal melanomata. Malignant melanomata may rarely occur in the nasal cavity, mouth, oesophagus, rectum, vagina, and vulva. These lesions are extremely malignant. It is not certain whether they arise in pre-existing naevi or whether they develop on normal epithelium.

Uveal melanoma. Malignant melanoma is one of the most common intraocular tumours. It usually arises in the choroid, but it may affect any part of the uveal tract. It is much commoner in White races than Black, in whom it is a rare tumour.[19] The melanoma may arise from pre-existing melanotic hamartomata in the choroid and iris, but it often develops spontaneously. Some tumours are composed of large spindle-shaped cells which are usually heavily pigmented, and this type has a better prognosis than the tumours which are composed of plump epithelial-type cells ('epithelioid'). A characteristic feature is late metastasis, especially to the liver; this is a classical example of dormant cancer (see p. 365). It is generally accepted that the choroidal melanocytes are neural in origin. It is of interest that malignant melanoma of the iris has a particularly good prognosis, and often responds well to local excision in spite of its malignant histological appearance.

Other melanomata. Melanocytes are present in the *pia arachnoid* especially around the base of the brain, and from these a diffuse melanomatous infiltration may envelop the brain. Similarly the *adrenal medulla* contains melanocytes which may give rise to a malignant melanoma.

Skeletal Hamartomata

The common *solitary exostosis* which grows out from the epiphyseal cartilage of a long bone is a good example of a cartilaginous hamartoma. It stops growing after puberty, when it becomes completely ossified. The rarer condition of multiple exostoses is a generalised hamartomatous disorder of the same nature, and it involves most of the bones derived from cartilage. In addition to the exostoses there is a general failure of bone remodelling, and the name *diaphysial aclasis* is aptly applied. These lesions may sometimes undergo chondrosarcomatous change (this applies to a solitary exostosis also). Diaphysial aclasis is inherited as an autosomal dominant characteristic.

Generalised Hamartomatous Dysplasias

Neurofibromatosis (von Recklinghausen's Disease). In this condition there is a widespread hamartomatous overgrowth of nerve-sheath tissue. It is characterised by neurofibromatous masses surrounding the peripheral nerves of the limbs and the skin. Histologically the masses of nerve-sheath tissue are much more diffuse in extent and arrangement than those found in solitary neurofibromata. Palisading is usually very poorly developed (see p. 320). Other interesting features are *regional gigantism* due to a congenital overgrowth of tissues, and the rather frequent *café-au-lait spots* on the skin. The disease is inherited as an autosomal dominant characteristic.

Typical schwannomata of the auditory nerves commonly complicate neurofibromatosis. Of even greater importance is the tendency for neurogenic sarcomata to arise in the hamartomatous lesions involving the larger peripheral nerves of the limbs. Histologically these tumours resemble fibrosarcomata, and pulmonary metastases may occur.

Tuberous sclerosis (epiloia). This is another familial hamartomatous condition inherited as a dominant trait. There are focal overgrowths of the glial tissues in the central nervous system and the retina. On the face multiple papules due to focal fibroangiomatous overgrowth are characteristic.* Subungual 'fibromata' also occur. A similar focal overgrowth of fibrous tissue occurs in the kidneys (forming large tumour-like masses) and the lungs (leading to fibrosis and cystic change with a danger of spontaneous pneumothorax). Areas of malformed myocardium (so-called 'rhabdomyomata'), the fibres of which are rich in a type of glycogen, are also characteristic of this disease. Occasionally the renal lesions become sarcomatous, and gliomata may develop in the central nervous system on the basis of a pre-existing glial hamartoma.

---

*These lesions are often erroneously referred to as 'adenoma sebaceum'. In fact, there is atrophy of the sebaceous glands, and the lesions are not related to the true sebaceous adenoma, which is a benign tumour of sebaceous glands.

Cysts Developing on the Basis of Pre-existing Malformations

A **cyst** (derived from the Greek *kustis*, a bladder) is a pathological fluid-filled sac bounded by a wall. The fluid may be secreted by cells lining the wall or it may be derived from the tissue fluid of the area. It is often clear and colourless, but it may be thick and turbid, or contain shimmering crystals of cholesterol. If it contains pus or blood, the lesion is preferably called an abscess or a haematoma as the case may be, but, of course, a cyst may be the seat of secondary infection or haemorrhage.

Where the cyst wall is lined by an epithelium, this may be derived from developmental residues such as the epithelial rests of Malassez in the periodontal ligament or epithelial residues lying in planes of embryonic fusion. On the other hand, it may arise from a normal anatomical structure, such as the cells lining the ducts and acini of an exocrine gland. Usually the stimulus that evokes the epithelial proliferation is not known, but sometimes chronic inflammation is a factor, as in the development of the dental cyst (also called an apical, radicular, or periodontal cyst). Here the chronic inflammation in the periapical tissues around a dead tooth stimulates the epithelial rests of Malassez to proliferate and line the liquefied apical granuloma, thus forming part of the wall of the cyst, the contents of which are turbid and characteristically contain cholesterol crystals, which are a product of tissue breakdown.

A classification of cysts is difficult, but the most practical one is based on the pathogenesis of the lesion.

(*a*) *Developmental.* These are described below.

(*b*) *Inflammatory*, e.g. the dental (or radicular) cyst, encysted pleural effusions, and pancreatic 'pseudocysts' following acute pancreatitis.

(*c*) *Degenerative*, e.g. cystic change in goitres, in solid tumours like the uterine leiomyoma, and in other pathological lesions like fibrous dysplasia of bone. The precipitating factor is necrosis, nearly always ischaemic in origin, with liquefaction of the necrotic debris. The ischaemia may be due to general vascular disease, as in brain cysts following infarction, or to a locally inadequate blood supply in a tumour or other lesion.

(*d*) *Retention*, e.g. mucous cysts of the mouth. The ranula, a cystic dilatation in the submandibular or sublingual gland, is believed to form as a result of obstruction of the duct (the Latin *ranula*, a little frog, alludes to the shape of the swelling produced).

(*e*) *Implantation.* This is the epidermoid cyst mentioned below and on page 113.

(*f*) *Parasitic*, e.g. the hydatid cyst, found especially in the liver and lungs, is due to the proliferation and growth of the larval form of the canine tapeworm *Echinococcus granulosus*. The germinative layer secretes the 'hydatid fluid'.

(*g*) *Hyperplastic*, e.g. mammary dysplasia (blue-domed cyst of the breast).

(*h*) *Neoplastic*, e.g. the cystadenoma and the cystic teratoma.

Developmental cysts arise in several different ways.

(*a*) *The persistence of normally vestigial remnants.* Examples of this type of cyst are the branchial and thyroglossal cysts. A branchial cyst is due to the persistence of a portion of the cervical sinus, and it is lined by stratified squamous epithelium which is heavily invested in lymphoid tissue. It contains turbid material which is rich in cholesterol crystals.

Some cysts of dental origin (e.g. primordial and dentigerous cysts) are due to changes in the enamel organ during the development of a tooth. The juxta-testicular vestiges, e.g. the appendix testis and paradidymis, sometimes undergo cystic dilatation in old men.

(*b*) *Ectopia of various tissues.* Ectopia is frequently due to the dislocation of a tissue into a neighbouring area where it tends to form a cyst. A good example of this is the *dermoid cyst*, which is due to the sequestration of a piece of skin beneath one of the lines of fusion of the various embryonic body processes. Such cysts occur most commonly in the subcutaneous tissue of the face, usually near one of the angles of the orbit. Sometimes they are intracranial, in which case it appears that the dislocation of the skin must have occurred before the bony skull was laid down. A dermoid cyst is lined by stratified squamous epithelium, and in its wall there are hair follicles, sebaceous glands, and sweat glands. It contains sebaceous debris and matted hairs. Unlike a teratoma it does not include any other tissues in its wall.

An *epidermoid cyst* is also lined by a layer of stratified squamous epithelium, but external to this there is only connective tissue. Skin appendages are not present, and its cavity contains only keratin. Some epidermoid cysts are due to the implantation of a piece of epidermis into the deeper layers of the skin and subcutaneous tissue as the result of trauma or acne vulgaris, and a few are true congenital ectopias of epidermis e.g. the intracranial epidermoid cyst. Most epidermoid cysts are, however, derived from plugged pilosebaceous follicles, and form the common variety of 'sebaceous cyst'.

Enterogenous cysts are the result of an ectopia of the intestinal mucosa. They occur not only in the bowel wall, but also in the mesentery and the retroperitoneal tissues.

(*c*) *A failure of connexion of tubular elements.* Polycystic kidney is probably due to a failure of fusion of the metanephric tubules with the collecting tubules. Another widely-held view is that it is due to the persistence of earlier generations of nephric tubules (pronephros and mesonephros). Polycystic disease, which in the common adult variety is often inherited as an autosomal dominant characteristic, sometimes affects the liver and pancreas as well as the kidneys, and it is probably due to a malformation of the biliary and pancreatic ducts in an early stage of development. The same explanation is probably true of congenital cystic lung, in which there appears to be severe bronchiolar maldevelopment.

(*d*) *As a hamartomatous process.* Cystic dilatations may occur in haemangiomata and lymphangiomata. The cystic hygroma of the neck and the lymphatic cysts occasionally found in the greater omentum are good examples.

TUMOURS DEVELOPING IN PRE-EXISTING MALFORMATIONS

I. Tumours Developing in Hamartomata

This topic has already been mentioned (see table on p. 315).

II. Tumours Arising from Vestigial Remnants

Chordoma. Vestiges of the embryonic notochord may be found throughout the vertebral axis, and are commonest in the spheno-occipital area of the skull and the sacrococcygeal

Figure 27.20
Chordoma. The tumour is composed of polygonal cells arranged in a dense stroma which is heavily infiltrated by a mucopolysaccharide secreted by the cells themselves. The empty, vacuolated cytoplasm of many of the cells is quite conspicuous; these are the physaliferous cells. The over-all appearance resembles that of a tumour of cartilage, both because of the mucoid nature of the stroma and the vacuolated tumour cells. ×110.

Figure 27.21
Ameloblastoma. The tumour consists of aggregations of small epithelial cells, the outer layers of which form a palisade as is found in the basal-cell carcinoma. In the midst of the central clump there is an open meshwork reminiscent of the stellate reticulum of the developing tooth germ ('enamel organ'). ×80.

region. Occasionally a recognisable button-like remnant, or 'ecchordosis', may be found under the dura mater of the dorsum sellae in the course of a necropsy. The chordoma is a rare tumour derived from these remnants, and is found most frequently in the two sites already mentioned. It is a pale pink, soft, gelatinous tumour which infiltrates the bone and surrounding soft tissues. Histologically it consists of groups of polyhedral cells, the larger ones of which contain large vacuoles in their cytoplasm. These are called *physaliferous cells* (i.e. bubble-bearing cells), and they may coalesce to produce a blurred vacuolated syncytium. The gelatinous consistency of the tumour is due to its mucoid nature (Fig. 27.20).

A chordoma is a slowly-growing malignant tumour which only occasionally metastasises by the blood stream. It is commonest in middle-aged and elderly people. By virtue of its situation it can seldom be eradicated surgically, and it is not very sensitive to X-rays.

Ameloblastoma (adamantinoma). This is a yellowish, cystic tumour of the jaws, which is slowly-growing and only locally malignant. Both in behaviour and in structure it resembles the common basal-cell carcinoma quite closely. It usually occurs in the mandible, and is commonest in young adults. It consists of angular clumps of small epithelial cells, and in the centres of these aggregations there is often an open meshwork resembling the 'stellate reticulum' of the enamel organ (Fig. 27.21). In between the cells there may be accumulations of fluid, which give rise to the cystic appearance so typical of this tumour. Despite its name the tumour does not form enamel. It probably arises from remnants of the dental lamina and the enamel organ.

Craniopharyngioma. Foci of epithelium (usually squamous) derived from Rathke's pouch are often found in the body of the sphenoid bone and around the pituitary itself.

These epithelial residues may occasionally give rise to cysts and also to slowly-growing, locally malignant tumours called craniopharyngiomata. These usually have the structure of ameloblastomata, but sometimes they resemble squamous-cell carcinomata. Extensive foci of ossification are characteristic of these tumours, and cystic change is also conspicuous.

Branchiogenic carcinoma. This is a highly malignant squamous-cell carcinoma developing in the tissues of the front of the neck. The majority of reported tumours are probably secondary lymph-node metastases from undetected primary pulmonary or oropharyngeal carcinomata, but it is possible that very occasionally a carcinoma may develop on the basis of a branchial cyst.

Urachal tumours. The urachus is the intra-abdominal part of the allantois, and it extends from the vertex of the bladder to the umbilicus. Occasionally vestiges persist, and these may give rise to cysts and also to papillary and mucus-secreting adenocarcinomata.

III. Tumours Arising from Ectopic Organs and Tissues

Squamous-cell carcinomata very occasionally arise in dermoid cysts, and enterogenous cysts occasionally form the sites of origin of adenocarcinomata, usually of a mucus-secreting type.

Cryptorchidism is due either to the imperfect descent of a testis or to its malposition in neighbouring areas (ectopia). In either event these testes are notoriously liable to undergo malignant change, both of a seminomatous and a teratomatous nature. It appears that there is some fundamental abnormality in such testes which predisposes them to neoplasia.

CONCLUSION

A study of perverted embryogenesis is one of the most fascinating facets of pathology, and an enthusiast may well be tempted to attribute many morbid processes to a fundamental developmental defect. As it is often impossible to deny the possibility of such a pathogenesis in respect of many lesions appearing in adults, a type of reasoning may easily be fostered in which all morbid processes are believed to be basically developmental in origin. This approach gave rise to Cohnheim's 'cell rest' theory of the origin of tumours, which is mentioned in Chapter 29.

It is nevertheless a challenging thought that some diseases of adult life may have their basis in a defect that first arose during the course of embryogenesis. Such a defect may come about in a variety of ways.

Malformations may be due to *genetic factors*. These may vary from gross *chromosomal abnormalities*, e.g. the syndromes of Down, Turner, and Klinefelter, to *single point mutations* involving biochemical mechanisms. For example, galactosaemia leads to abnormalities of liver, kidney, brain, and eye. In many hereditary diseases the actual defect is unknown, e.g. in achondroplasia. Sometimes the malformation becomes evident only in adult life, e.g. hereditary haemorrhagic telangiectasia.

Most malformations, however, are not genetic in origin, but are due apparently to external factors. Many of these are unknown, but among the important *teratogenic agents* are the following:

Drugs.[25] The most notorious is the sedative *thalidomide* which leads to the absence of limbs (amelus) or parts of limbs, haemangiomatosis of the upper lip and nose, and severe malformations of the alimentary tract, heart, and genito-urinary system.[26-28] *Cytotoxic agents* also produce malformations, and the use of large doses of *progesterone* can produce genital deformities in female infants. *Cortisol* given to pregnant mice leads to cleft palate in the offspring in certain strains but not in others. This is yet another example of how genetic and environmental factors can interact. The anticonvulsant drug *phenytoin* may also be added to the list of teratogenic drugs.[29]

The effects of these agents depend upon two factors:

(*a*) The specific action of the agent itself.

(*b*) The susceptibility of the organ or tissue of the fetus. Organs are particularly vulnerable during the period of rapid growth and differentiation. Thus the human fetus is most sensitive to thalidomide 20 to 40 days after conception, while the heart is liable to be affected during the short period 40 to 45 days after conception.

Ionising radiations.

An even more serious hazard to fetal development is *maternal alcoholism*.[30-32] Expectant mothers who consume large amounts of alcohol tend to give birth to infants that are short and below average weight. There is often hypoplasia of the maxilla with prominence of the forehead and lower jaw, short palpebral fissures, microcephaly, and mental retardation. The failure of growth and mental development persists even if the child is later cared for by foster parents. Other typical malformations are ventricular septal defect and various joint abnormalities. It is evident that excessive amounts of *alcohol* in the fetal blood constitute a very real teratogenic hazard, and it is important to be aware of the condition as soon as possible in order to protect subsequent newborn infants.

Infections of the fetus in utero, e.g. toxoplasmosis, syphilis and certain viral diseases, notably rubella.[33]

Rhesus incompatibility, i.e. haemolytic disease of the newborn.

It is in this group of acquired defects that success is most likely to attend measures designed to reduce the incidence of congenital malformations.

REFERENCES

1. WILLIS, R. A. (1968) Some unusual developmental heterotoplas. *British Medical Journal*, **3**, 267.
2. BROWN, N. J. (1976) Teratomas and yolk-sac tumours. *Journal of Clinical Pathology*, **29**, 1021.
3. FOX, H. & LANGLEY, F. A. (1976) In *Tumours of the Ovary*, p. 172 *et seq.* London: Heinemann Medical.
4. BENNINGTON, J. L. & BECKWITH, J. B. (1975) In *Tumors of the Kidney, Renal Pelvis, and Ureter*, Second Series, Fascicle 13, p. 50. Washington: Armed Forces Institute of Pathology.
5. BARNARD, R. O., LOGUE, V. & REAVES, P. S. (1976) In *An Atlas of Tumours Involving the Central Nervous System*, p. 60. London: Baillière Tindall.
6. JENSEN, R. D. & MILLER, R. W. (1971) Retinoblastoma: epidemiologic characteristics. *New England Journal of Medicine*, **285**, 307.
7. MINKEN, S. L., CRAVER, W. L. & ADAMS, J. T. (1968) Pulmonary blastoma. *Archives of Pathology*, **86**, 442.
8. BEAN, W. B. (1958) *Vascular Spiders and Related Lesions of the Skin*. Oxford: Blackwell.
9. KESSLER, E. & KOSENITZKY, I. L. (1971) Haemangiosarcoma of breast. *Journal of Clinical Pathology*, **24**, 530.
10. MACKENZIE, D. H. (1971) Lymphangiosarcoma arising in chronic congenital and idiopathic lymphoedema. *Journal of Clinical Pathology*, **24**, 524.
11. HARRIS, M. (1971) Ultrastructure of a glomus tumour. *Journal of Clinical Pathology*, **24**, 520.
12. McGOVERN, V. J. (1976) *Malignant Melanoma*. New York: Wiley.
13. WAYTE, D. M. & HELWIG, E. B. (1968) Halo nevi. *Cancer (Philadelphia)*, **22**, 69.
14. LEVENE, A. (1972) Moles and melanoma: the pathological basis of clinical management. *Proceedings of the Royal Society of Medicine*, **65**, 137.
15. Leading Article (1967) Malignant melanoma. *British Medical Journal*, **2**, 129.
16. CLARK, W. H. *et al.* (1969) The histogenesis and biological behavior of primary human malignant melanomas of the skin. *Cancer Research*, **29**, 705.
17. Leading Article (1971) Sunlight and melanomas. *Lancet*, **1**, 172.

18. Leading Article (1972) Epidemiological approach to malignant melanoma. *British Medical Journal*, **1**, 130.
19. Leading Article (1968) Malignant melanomas. *Lancet*, **1**, 76.
20. Leading Article (1967) Hereditary malignant melanoma. *British Medical Journal*, **3**, 191.
21. JAY, B. (1964) A follow-up study of limbal melanomata. *Proceedings of the Royal Society of Medicine*, **57**, 497.
22. LEVER, W. F. & SCHAUMBURG-LEVER, G. (1975) *Histopathology of Skin*. 5th edn, p. 665. Philadelphia: Lippincott.
23. MIHM, M. C., CLARK, W. H. & FROM, L. (1971) The clinical diagnosis, classification and histogenetic concepts of the early stages of cutaneous malignant melanomas. *New England Journal of Medicine*, **284**, 1078.
24. BRESLOW, A. (1977) Problems in the measurement of tumor thickness and level of invasion in cutaneous melanoma. *Human Pathology*, **8**, 1.
25. SMITHELLS, R. W. (1966) Drugs and human malformations. *Advances in Teratology*, ed. Woollam, D. H. M., **1**, 251. London: Logos Press.
26. Leading Article (1962) Thalidomide and congenital malformations. *Lancet*, **1**, 307.
27. Leading Article (1962) Thalidomide: part 2. *Lancet*, **2**, 336.
28. LAWRENCE, D. R. (1973) *Clinical Pharmacology*, 4th edn, pp. 667–670. Edinburgh: Churchill Livingstone. This provides a fascinating account of the thalidomide disaster.
29. LOUGHNAN, P. M., GOLD, H. & VANCE, J. C. (1973) Phenytoin teratogenicity in man. *Lancet*, **1**, 70.
30. Leading Article (1976) The fetal alcohol syndrome. *British Medical Journal*, **2**, 1404.
31. Leading Article (1976) Fetal alcohol syndrome. *Lancet*, **1**, 1335.
32. CLARREN, S. K. & SMITH, D. W. (1978) The fetal alcohol syndrome. *New England Journal of Medicine*, **298**, 1063.
33. BROWN, G. C. (1966) Recent advances in the vital aetiology of congenital anomalies. *Advances in Teratology*, **1**, 55, *loc cit*.

Chapter 28.   Spread of Malignant Tumours

The mode of spread of cancer cells has given rise to much speculation, but there is still little understanding of the process. The reduction in cell adhesiveness (see p. 313) may play a part, and furthermore some tumour cells are feebly motile in tissue culture. It has been suggested that tumours may secrete toxins or enzymes that facilitate spread in the tissues; hyaluronidase is favoured by some workers, but the evidence is far from convincing. Others stress the importance of fibrin in providing a network on which the tumour cells grow, and they claim that fibrinolysins may inhibit the spread of the tumour.[1] Be this as it may, infiltration into the surrounding tissues is the salient feature of all malignant tumours. The invading cells penetrate various natural passages which afford an easy route for further spread. The most important of these are the lymphatics and blood vessels, and in both the malignant cells may become detached as emboli which are carried to distant sites. If the cells survive and multiply a secondary isolated mass of tumour is produced. This is a *metastasis*. *Direct invasion* and *embolisation* are thus the two main methods of spread.

DIRECT SPREAD

Local spread. The direct infiltration of the surrounding tissues common to all malignant tumours means that the microscopic extent of a tumour exceeds what is macroscopically apparent. For this reason any excision which aims at removing all the neoplastic cells must incorporate a wide extent of the surrounding tissue. The invading cells tend to follow natural clefts or tissue planes, and to move in the line of least resistance. Dense fascial sheaths may confine malignant cells for some time. This is well shown in osteosarcoma of a long bone: the tumour reaches the periosteum, but is there held up; it invades in the subperiosteal plane to produce a fusiform swelling. Cartilage is resistant to tumour infiltration; osteosarcoma seldom destroys the epiphyseal cartilage until late in its course. Likewise, secondary cancer and myeloma in a vertebra do not invade the intervertebral disc.

The tendency of carcinoma cells to invade along tissue septa is demonstrated in the breast; particularly characteristic is the appearance of a column of cells in single file invading between collagen bundles. Infiltration often occurs in the ligaments of Astley Cooper, causing the tumour to become attached both to the dermis and the deep fascia. The fibrous reaction caused by the scirrhous tumour leads to the contraction which is responsible for the skin dimpling seen clinically. Why this contraction should occur is not easily explained. In cancers of the stomach and colon the invasion of the septa between the muscle fibres produces the characteristic appearance of *segmentation* of the muscle layer (Fig. 28.1).

Infiltration can also occur into individual cells. Thus

Figure 28.1
Infiltrating carcinoma of the stomach. The pyloric portion is greatly thickened, and the wall is diffusely infiltrated by pale tumour tissue. There is extensive invasion of the septa between muscle fibres by the tumour. This is most pronounced in the wall of the distal part of the lesser curvature where segmentation is evident. (EA. 42.1, *Reproduced by permission of the President and Council of the R.C.S. Eng.*)

squamous-cell cancers of the cervical lymph nodes may infiltrate into the fibres of the adjacent striated muscles.

Infiltration can also proceed into the epidermis from a nearby duct which is the seat of neoplasia. Paget's disease of the nipple has been explained in this way, but it is probably a primary intra-epithelial lesion (p. 382). Epidermal invasion is a prominent feature of malignant melanoma, particularly the superficial spreading variety, and is also seen in malignant lymphoma of skin. Its detection is a useful diagnostic feature of mycosis fungoides (p. 399), and the collections of lymphoma cells within the epidermis are known as Pautrier micro-abscesses.*

Evidence of local invasion is an important sign, for its detection is tantamount to a diagnosis of malignancy. The basal-cell carcinoma is the prototype of a group of tumours the spread of which is entirely local. Nevertheless, some benign hyperplastic lesions may show a local invasive tendency. Several cases of mammary dysplasia have been reported in which there was perineural or neural invasion. Rarely there may be infiltration of the walls of veins or even arteries. In these cases the invading elements are obviously not malignant in appearance, but are simply part of the hyperplastic process.[2]

Invasion of lymphatics. Carcinoma shows a particular tendency to invade the local lymphatics at an early stage. Sarcomata only occasionally spread *via* the lymphatics.

*This is an unfortunate misuse of the term abscess, but being time honoured, is likely to persist.

Sampson Handley drew attention to the spread which may occur along these vessels in breast cancer. The tumour cells grow progressively within the lumen of the lymphatics as a solid cord which extends in all directions to involve an ever-widening area of tissue. This process is called *permeation* (Fig. 28.2). The central area of the malignant cord may undergo necrosis and even disappear while the advancing end proliferates. Eventually the cord of cells reaches the draining lymph nodes. By blocking the main ducts, the lymph is diverted to adjacent channels, and in this way there may be retrograde deviation of tumour cells. It is not surprising that numerous outlying nodules of tumour may be found in the skin of such a breast. In extreme cases the entire skin of the chest wall may be the seat of confluent carcinoma, producing *cancer en cuirasse*. Lymphatic permeation also causes the local dermal oedema which produces the *peau d'orange* appearance seen in breast cancer.

In the lung the major lymphatics run with the bronchi and the main pulmonary vessels. If they are infiltrated with cancer, these other structures may be cuffed with the tumour; oat-cell cancer is the usual cause of this. Extensive invasion of the pulmonary lymphatics produces the condition sometimes

Figure 28.2
Lymphatic permeation of cancer. This is a section of skin showing dilated lymphatic vessels filled with spheroidal carcinoma cells arranged in solid cords. There was an advanced carcinoma of the breast. ×150.

known as 'lymphangitis carcinomatosa'. The tumour-filled vessels give the lung a reticulated appearance both macroscopically and radiologically. This almost always denotes a secondary carcinoma arising from the breast, and is curiously uncommon in primary lung cancer. Malignant melanoma is also liable to invade lymph vessels, which may appear clinically as black streaks emerging from the primary tumour. In some cases of cancer of the lung and colon permeation of the subpleural and subperitoneal lymphatics is so marked that these distended vessels are easily visible to the naked eye.

Perineural invasion and spread. This is seen in many types of carcinoma, and is a useful diagnostic feature when the possibly malignant nature of a lesion is being assessed, e.g. in a section of prostate or pancreas. It is usually attributed to lymphatic spread, but it is doubtful whether there are any perineural lymphatics. The appearance of malignant cells lying in a space is often taken to indicate lymphatic invasion, but unless a clear endothelial lining is present, one cannot be sure that the cells are not lying in a tissue space.

Venous invasion. The invasion of large veins is seen most frequently in lung cancer because of the large number of vessels available. The tumour becomes covered by thrombus, and this venous extension is easily missed.

Clear-cell carcinoma of the kidney is another tumour in which venous invasion is common. A solid mass of growth may be found growing in the renal vein, and cases have been described in which this has extended into the vena cava and up to the right atrium. Occasionally a left-sided varicocele is the first indication of a tumour of the left kidney which has spread into the renal vein. As the left spermatic vein drains into the renal vein (the right drains directly into the inferior vena cava), it is to be expected that there would be a back-pressure effect.

Arterial invasion. It is generally stated that the thick elastic wall of large arteries effectively prevents tumour ingrowth. In the lung, however, careful examination not infrequently reveals invasion of the pulmonary arteries. Arterial obstruction may be responsible for tumour necrosis as well as infarction of the adjacent lung.

Small vessels. It is probably true to say that small vessels are invaded in every case of malignant disease. This is particularly noticeable in sarcomata, since the tumour cells may actually line the vascular spaces. An extreme example of this is found in angiosarcomata. Choriocarcinoma is another tumour notorious for the ease with which it invades blood vessels; the tumours are typically haemorrhagic and necrotic.

Serous spaces. Tumours reaching a serous surface like the visceral pleura tend to erode the mesothelium. Fibrinous adhesions may then form to the parietal surface. Tumour cells can thus traverse the space; in this way some peripheral lung cancers invade the chest wall directly.

SPREAD BY METASTASIS

Lymphatic Spread

The detachment of groups of tumour cells in an invaded lymphatic leads to the production of emboli, which become lodged in the subcapsular sinus of the regional lymph node. If the cells survive and grow, the node soon becomes replaced by the tumour, and further spread occurs to the next group of nodes by way of the efferent channel. This is a familiar event in carcinoma and melanoma, but is rare in sarcoma. The extent of the lymphatic involvement is important in assessing the prognosis, and is one of the factors taken into consideration in the staging of tumours.

Retrograde embolism is a term used to denote spread in a reverse direction to the usual flow. If a lymphatic is blocked (nearly always due to permeation), the flow of lymph may be reversed, and subsequent embolism produces metastases in unusual sites. The importance of the phenomenon has been greatly exaggerated. A well-known example is the involvement of the left cervical lymph nodes (Virchow's node) in gastric cancer (Troisier's sign). This is probably due to blockage of the thoracic duct near its entry into the left subclavian vein.

Some carcinomata, e.g. of the breast and lung, appear to spread very rapidly to the regional nodes, whereas those of the skin and lip do so at a late stage. Tongue carcinoma, on the other hand, is usually attended by early cervical-node involvement. This has been attributed to the mobility of the tongue, and the massaging of cancer cells into the lymphatics during speech and mastication. In fact, the spreading tendency of malignant tumours is probably an inherent property of the cancer itself, and for some reason at present unknown cancers of the mouth are generally more malignant in their course than are those of the skin and lip.

Blood Spread

The occurrence of blood-spread metastasis is the feature of malignant disease which is responsible for death in most cases. It is also the factor which limits the surgical and radio-therapeutic treatment of cancer.

At first sight the mode of production of secondary tumours is easy to understand. Malignant cells invade small vessels or veins, become detached, and are then carried by the blood stream to some distant site where they reach a capillary network. There the emboli become impacted, proliferate, and develop into secondary tumours. A second method of blood-borne metastasis is by way of the lymphatics. Eventually all the lymph drains into the venous circulation, and the first capillary network the tumour cells meet is in the lung. It is difficult to assess how much blood spread is due to primary venous invasion, and how much is secondary to lymphatic involvement. In the sarcomata, which spread into the blood stream at a very early stage, there is no doubt that invasion is primarily venous, as lymphatic spread is most uncommon. In the carcinomata blood spread usually manifests itself some time after lymphatic involvement, and it is quite possible that much of the blood stream invasion is secondary to regional lymphatic spread. It is often said that sarcomata spread by the blood stream and carcinomata by the lymphatics; this is a half-truth, because carcinomata also spread by the blood stream, although the first metastases usually appear in the lymph nodes.

As would be expected, one of the commonest sites for secondaries from most tumours is the lung. Likewise, primary tumours arising from the area of tissue drained by the portal vein regularly metastasise to the liver. Purely anatomical factors would appear to account for this distribution, but closer examination makes such an explanation inadequate.

Many tumours, e.g. of the breast and kidney, give rise to secondaries not only in the lungs, but also in the liver, bones, and other organs. Systemic metastases sometimes occur in the absence of apparent lung deposits. It is possible that these are really present, but have been missed because of an inadequate *post-mortem* examination by the pathologist. Alternatively the cells may be able to pass through the lung capillaries, and become arrested elsewhere. Another explanation is the possibility of a direct venous communication between the primary and secondary sites.*

The distribution of secondary tumours might be expected to be related to the blood supply, but this is not the case. Cardiac and skeletal muscle have an abundant blood supply, and yet are rarely the site of metastasis. The spleen likewise is not usually involved. The liver, on the other hand, is frequently the site of secondary tumours regardless of the site of the primary.

It has been found that tumour cells are present in the blood stream in cases of malignant disease, but the frequency of this event is undecided. The cells are not plentiful, and many techniques for concentrating them have been devised. Considerable difficulty is experienced in distinguishing imma-ture blood cells from malignant cells, and different investi-gators report widely divergent results. Thus, the reported incidence in known cases of cancer has varied from 100 per cent to 0 per cent. Perhaps 10 per cent is a realistic figure.[3] There is no general agreement as to the significance of finding cells in the blood, for it does not seem to be related to prognosis. It is probable that many of the cells die. Only the selected few are able to take root to grow into secondary deposits. What factors govern this are not known, but it appears likely that certain sites are particularly favoured. The 'seed' may be widespread, but only where the 'soil' is suitable does growth occur. Some examples of this *selective metastasis* must now be examined.

(*a*) The commonest organ in which blood-borne metastases occur is the *liver* (Fig. 28.3). Not only do gastrointestinal cancers regularly metastasise there, but also carcinomata of the genitourinary system, lungs, and breast, melanomata, and sarcomata. Apparently the liver affords an excellent nutritional medium for tumour cells. It may even be the seat of transpla-cental metastases, as shown in Figure 28.4. Placental metastases are very rare.[4]

(*b*) The next most common site for metastases is the *lung*; it is especially frequently involved in sarcomata, and carcinomata of the thyroid, breast, and kidney. Testicular tumours and choriocarcinomata also favour the lungs (Fig. 28.5).

(*c*) *Bone Metastases*. After the liver and lungs, the bones are the most frequent sites of secondary deposits. The primary tumour is usually a carcinoma of lung, breast, prostate, kidney (clear-cell tumour), or thyroid. The neuroblastoma also spreads in this way (see Hutchison's syndrome, p. 345). Of the lung cancers it is the oat-cell carcinoma that is particularly liable to metastasise to the skeleton;[5] by contrast the squamous-cell carcinoma, adenocarcinoma, and undifferen-tiated carcinoma only occasionally produce skeletal deposits. It

---

*In cases where there is extensive venous invasion, e.g. in clear-cell kidney cancer, there may be retrograde venous embolism comparable with that described in regard to the lymphatics. This accounts for the occasional metastases in the left spermatic cord, vulva, and vagina in the course of a carcinoma of the left kidney.

Figure 28.3
Metastatic carcinoid tumour in liver. The top part of the figure contains large trabeculae of carcinoid tumour surrounded by a fibrous stroma. Below there are atrophic cords of liver cells separated from the tumour deposit by a thin layer of fibrous tissue only. × 100.

Figure 28.4
Transplacental metastasis of malignant melanoma. In this remarkable case a woman suffering from extensive malignant melanomatosis gave birth to a child shortly before her death. The placenta was massively involved in the tumour. The infant progressed well at first, but at about 9 months developed marasmus, hepatomegaly, and secondary infection. It soon died, and at necropsy the liver was found to contain metastases of malignant melanoma. (A 110.1, *Reproduced by permission of the President and Council of the R.C.S. Eng.*)

Figure 28.5
Metastatic carcinoma in lung. Note the circumscribed white deposits, apparently encapsulated from the parenchyma. Primary lung cancer infiltrates into the surrounding tissue much more obviously. The primary site in this case was the breast. (R 47.3, *Reproduced by permission of the President and Council of the R.C.S. Eng.*)

is the follicular carcinoma of the thyroid that produces metastases in bone most commonly;[6] the papillary carcinoma rarely spreads this way, and the anaplastic carcinoma only occasionally. These distinctive patterns of metastasis indicate the biological individuality of different cancers arising from a single organ.

Secondaries from prostatic cancer are particularly liable to occur in the pelvic bones and vertebrae. The communications between the prostatic venous plexus and the various vertebral plexuses are believed by some to account for this, since often there is no evidence of pulmonary involvement, but selective metastasis would seem a more likely explanation.

Bone metastases almost always develop from within the sinusoids of the red marrow, from which they spread into marrow spaces and the canal system of compact bone and subsequently invade the cortex.[7] Osseous metastases may be osteoplastic (osteosclerotic) or osteolytic. In the former there is much new bone laid down, and as a result the secondaries are hard and radio-opaque. The osteogenesis is reflected in a raised level of plasma alkaline phosphatase, while the plasma calcium and phosphate levels remain normal (occasionally the plasma calcium falls). Most osteoplastic secondaries are due to prostatic cancer, when there is usually a raised level of plasma acid phosphatase as well. Both the primary lesion and the widespread skeletal metastases produce this enzyme, which may possibly be responsible for the characteristic osteosclerosis of prostatic cancer.

Occasionally other secondary tumours, e.g. neuroblastoma

and carcinoma of the breast or colon, cause new bone to be produced, but much more frequently they, and the other tumours mentioned, cause osteolysis. This is seen radiologically as an area of translucency in the bone, and it may lead to spontaneous fracture. The plasma alkaline phosphatase level is normal, but sometimes there may be sufficient demineralisation to lead to severe hypercalcaemia and renal failure (see Ch. 36).

Early on in this invasive process there appears to be a considerable activation of osteoclasts, which resorb the bone in advance of the developing tumour. Later the tumour cells seem able to produce bone destruction even without osteoclastic mediation.[7]

It has been found that many tumours secrete substances that induce osteolysis. The most important are prostaglandins, especially prostaglandin E_2; aspirin and indomethacin inhibit the action of prostaglandins, and may delay or even prevent the development of osteolytic metastases from breast cancer.[7] Other secretions from tumours that may also promote osteolysis are ectopic parathyroid hormone, osteolytic activating factor, and active vitamin-D metabolites or related compounds. In addition, the leucocytes that infiltrate malignant tumours can also secrete prostaglandins and other osteolytic factors.

If much of the bone marrow is replaced by tumour tissue leuco-erythroblastic anaemia may result.

(*d*) The *brain* is sometimes a site for secondary tumours, and here the usual primary source is the lung. Whenever a middle-aged or elderly man suddenly develops neurological or psychiatric symptoms, it is most important to X-ray his chest before proceeding with other investigations. Carcinomata of the breast and melanomata sometimes also spread to the brain. It has been postulated that there is a direct communication between the bronchial veins and the vertebral plexus, but the importance of this has not been proven.

(*e*) Of the *endocrine glands* the adrenal is the one which most frequently contains metastases; usually the medulla is involved, but discrete cortical deposits are not uncommon. Lung cancer, especially the oat-cell variety, frequently metastasises to this site, and some authorities believe that the route of spread may be lymphatic rather than haematogenous in some instances. It is estimated that about a third of all fatal lung cancers show adrenal deposits. Cancer of the breast also often spreads to the adrenals, as is noted in adrenalectomy specimens (see p. 376). The ovaries also often harbour metastases in this condition.

The other endocrine glands are less often involved in metastases. The thyroid may harbour secondary tumours of various types, and it is interesting that a goitrous gland is more vulnerable than a healthy one. It may be that the vascular arrangement in a goitre is more prone to entrap emboli than that of a normal gland.

(*f*) The *skin* is occasionally the site of metastases, which tend to erupt as discrete nodules. The primary source is usually the lung or the breast. Multiple cutaneous deposits are also characteristic of malignant melanoma.

(*g*) Occasionally metastases occur within *benign tumours*. Widespread cancer of the breast may rarely metastasise to uterine fibroids, and occasionally a deposit of oat-cell lung cancer is found in association with a colonic adenoma.

The metastasising powers of tumours vary widely. Amongst those with the greatest tendency are carcinomata of the breast and lungs. The lethal effects of breast cancer are attributable almost entirely to its widespread blood-borne metastases which are found especially in the lungs, liver, and vertebral column. Cancer of the lung, especially the oat-cell variety, is also notorious for the speed with which it metastasises. In addition to the common sites, e.g. liver, adrenals, and bones, it may spread in a more bizarre way. Sometimes whole organs, e.g. pancreas, gonads, and thyroid, are replaced by the tumour, while the usually affected organs remain free. The spleen and bowel are also occasionally implicated. When a lung tumour metastasises to the brain there is often little evidence of other blood-borne deposits; perhaps the cerebral lesion kills too rapidly for these to develop.

Sarcomata metastasise early, and the lung is by far the most heavily implicated organ. The liver and brain are also frequently affected, but bone deposits are uncommon.

Malignant brain tumours rarely metastasise outside the cranial cavity. The absence of lymphatic metastases is attributable to the lack of a lymphatic drainage in the brain. The absence of blood-borne deposits may be related to the raised intracranial pressure occluding the adjacent cerebral veins; the larger venous sinuses are so well separated from the brain that the tumour kills the patient before it can spread to invade them. Extracerebral metastases may occasionally follow surgical procedures, especially decompression operations leaving large gaps in the dura and skull so that the tumour comes into direct contact with the surrounding soft tissues. Shunting operations for obstructive hydrocephalus, in which the cerebrospinal fluid is drained into the right atrium, may also lead to such metastases.[8,9] The very rare glioma arising in an ovarian teratoma may also metastasise.

Although tumour emboli are very common, most of them, after impaction in a small vessel, become covered by thrombus and die. The vascular occlusion may itself produce damage; thus right-sided heart failure may follow the obliteration of many lung vessels.

Occasionally a large vein is invaded by growth; this may break off to produce a large embolus. In cancer of the lung a large piece of tumour growing in a pulmonary vein has been known to break off and produce a massive systemic embolus. Similarly massive tumour pulmonary embolism may occur in limb sarcoma, testicular teratoma, and clear-cell kidney cancer, tumours which tend to invade the large systemic veins.

Secondary tumours are usually multiple; the solitary, cannon-ball lung metastases sometimes seen in clear-cell kidney cancer and seminoma are obvious exceptions. Metastases in liver and lung frequently grow so rapidly that expansion exceeds local infiltration. The growths then give the impression of being sharply demarcated.

Transcoelomic Spread

When a tumour invades the serosal layer of a viscus, it excites a local inflammatory response with a small effusion into the serous cavity. Malignant cells become incorporated into the local fibrinous exudate, and are then detached. They are swept into the effusion, and carried by it into the cavity. They settle widely on its wall, proliferate, and set up innumerable 'seedlings'. These excite the formation of more inflammatory exudate, and in due course the space may contain a great deal of fluid. Sometimes the exudate is more fibrinous, and the viscera are bound together by dense adhesions.

The commonest example of transcoelomic spread is seen in the peritoneal cavity in cases of primary gastric, colonic, and ovarian carcinomata. The greater omentum may be so massively infiltrated that it is converted into a thick, spongy, gelatinous mass of tumour (omental cake). Metastases are common in the pouch of Douglas, doubtless due to a gravitational effect.

In gastric and colonic cancer there may also be transperitoneal spread to the ovaries. The best-known example of this is the *Krukenberg tumour*. This is usually bilateral: both ovaries are enlarged, their surfaces are smooth and thickened, and their substance is completely replaced by a mass of mucoid carcinoma. There is usually a primary mucoid cancer elsewhere, most often in the stomach or colon, but occasionally in the breast. The mode of metastasis has caused much speculation. Some authorities attribute it to retrograde lymphatic spread, because the surfaces of the ovaries are smooth and free of seedling deposits. However, some cases may be true examples of transcoelomic spread. It is known that mucoid cancer penetrates very easily, and it is therefore possible that the cells deposited on the surface invade the ovary without destroying the tunica albuginea. Mucoid cancer tends to stimulate a dense stromal reaction, and this may account for the thickened surface. In those cases secondary to breast cancer a haematogenous metastasis is the most likely explanation, but in the gastric and colonic cases there is often little evidence of extensive blood-borne or lymphatic deposits elsewhere. Occasionally a carcinoma similar to a Krukenberg tumour appears to be of primary ovarian origin.

Transpleural spread occurs in some cases of lung and breast cancer, and in both these examples there may also be pericardial involvement. Secondary tumours in the lung can spread likewise.

A related type of spread is the metastasis of primary cerebral tumours down the subarachnoid space to the spinal theca. Seedlings of this type are characteristic of medulloblastoma, oligodendroglioma, and ependymoma.[9] They may be seen in anaplastic astrocytomata and also in secondary tumours involving the brain.

It is important to note that peritoneal effusions are not confined to malignant tumours. A benign tumour in close proximity to a serous surface can also excite an inflammatory reaction. A good example of this is the ovarian fibroma, which sometimes gives rise to a considerable ascites. If there is also a pleural effusion, the condition is called *Meigs's syndrome*. The mechanism of this pleural effusion is still not understood.

An even more spectacular condition is *pseudomyxoma peritonei*, in which a mucus-secreting lesion, usually of the appendix or the ovary, ruptures and discharges its contents into the peritoneal cavity. The secreting cells take root, and secrete large amounts of mucinous material which produces a chronic peritonitis. In most cases the initial lesion is a low-grade adenocarcinoma, but the cells in the peritoneal cavity show no tendency to invade the deeper tissues. If the material is removed and the primary lesion extirpated, life may be preserved for many years.[10]

Another example of implantation of cells on to a serous surface is the very rare condition called *peritoneal gliomatosis*, or *benign glial implants*,[11] that may occur when mature brain tissue is extruded through a defect in the capsule of an ovarian teratoma. There are small implants, consisting of mature neuroglial tissue, in which neurons or cerebellar tissue may be recognised, which may be scattered throughout the peritoneal cavity. The condition is benign, since there is no progress in growth; all that needs to be done is to remove the ovarian tumour.

Spread Along Epithelial-lined Spaces

It is common in papillary tumours of the renal pelvis to find other similar tumours scattered along the ureter and even in the bladder. Likewise it is sometimes noted that a cancer on the lower lip may be associated with a cancer on the apposing upper lip. At one time this was attributed to the transfer of malignant cells from one surface to another. It seems very unlikely that tumour cells can penetrate intact epithelia in this way. Although the possibility of epithelial implantation cannot entirely be excluded, these tumours are best explained as examples of multicentric neoplasia on a preconditioned field of growth (see Ch. 29).

A different type of spread by implantation can occur during an operation on a tumour-bearing area, for example a carcinoma of the bladder. Clumsy surgical technique may allow the implantation of cancer cells on to the adjacent incised tissues, from which a new tumour may subsequently develop. Likewise tumour cells may be implanted in the needle track following the aspiration of a malignant ascites.

STAGING OF MALIGNANT TUMOURS

Staging is an important method of documenting the spread of a tumour, which can then be related to the prognosis. A well-known scheme is that used in breast cancer:

STAGE I   Tumour confined to the breast including the skin immediately over it.

STAGE II   The tumour involves the axillary lymph nodes on the same side, but both breast and nodes are mobile.

STAGE III Spread to the chest wall or the supraclavicular nodes of the same side.

STAGE IV   Further spread than Stage III including blood-borne metastases.

A very important staging of rectal cancer is that devised by Dukes:

STAGE A   Tumour confined to the muscular coat of the wall of the rectum.

STAGE B   Tumour invading the pararectal tissues, but without lymph-node metastases.

STAGE C   Involvement of lymph nodes.

The prognosis after abdomino-perineal resection has been related to the three stages.[12]

STAGE A   80–90 per cent survive for 5 years.

STAGE B   60–70 per cent survive for 5 years.

STAGE C   Less than 25 per cent survive for 5 years.

This example shows how the prognosis of a tumour can be predicted by assessing its degree of spread. But it does not necessarily follow that a Stage I tumour is always an 'early' one. It might be of long standing, but of such low-grade malignancy that it progresses very slowly and does not metastasise. Likewise a Stage IV tumour is not necessarily a 'late' one. It might be one of high-grade malignancy which metastasises widely before it produces a conspicuous local lesion. Though nobody would advocate delay in treating cancer, it must be remembered that the most important factor in the prognosis is the intrinsic malignancy of the tumour. The degree of spread is an external manifestation of this. The good prognosis that follows the resection of a Stage I cancer is probably due more to its low-grade character than to the speed of detection. If left alone it might remain at this stage for a considerable time, causing the patient little trouble. But, of course, it might also advance to Stages II, III, and IV, and it is this possibility which makes immediate treatment necessary. This consideration is relevant when the results of operative treatment are assessed in relation to the stage of the tumour, especially when radical resections are advocated for Stage I lesions.

In order to standardise the staging of tumours, the *TNM system* is internationally recommended:

T_1, T_2, T_3, T_4 indicate the size of the tumour and its extent of local spread.

N_0, N_1, N_2, N_3 indicate the absence or presence of involvement of the regional lymph nodes and the extent of that involvement.

M_0, M_1 indicate the absence or presence of distant metastases.

The actual measurements of tumour size and spread and lymph-node involvement are standardised for each particular tumour. The value of the TNM system is that the extent of a patient's cancer can be accurately imparted to medical workers in all parts of the world, and the results of a particular treatment can be correlated internationally with the stage of the tumour.

Dormant cancer. This is the appearance of metastases many years after the primary tumour has been successfully removed. The phenomenon of dormancy is seen most often in carcinoma of the breast and kidney and malignant melanoma (especially of the uveal tract), when some 10 to 35 years after the resection of the organ affected the patient may suddenly develop metastases (usually in the bones following breast and kidney carcinoma, and in the liver following uveal melanoma). In these cases there is no local recurrence, and the patient is quite well during the dormant period. The eruption of metastases is usually unheralded, but it sometimes follows a severe intercurrent illness, an operation, or an accident. Psychological trauma is another precipitating factor.

Once the metastases appear they develop rapidly, and if not treated will lead to the patient's death. It is evident that for reasons not yet understood the tumour cells have lain dormant in distant sites. Perhaps the hormonal environment was not suitable or else the patient's immunological state prevented the growth of metastases. At any rate it must be assumed that at a certain time the environment becomes propitious for the growth of tumour cells, and then metastases develop.

The phenomenon of dormancy is obviously of importance when the prognosis of a tumour is being considered. A 5-year survival rate, a fair measure of cure in many types of malignancy treated by radical surgery, is of much less use in the cancers mentioned above. Indeed, no woman who has had a mastectomy for breast cancer can ever be certified as cured; metastases have been known to develop more than 30 years after resection. The natural history of cancer is still poorly understood, and until it is studied with care and dispassion, many erroneous assumptions will be made about the efficacy of various forms of treatment.

SURGICAL TREATMENT IN RELATION TO SPREAD OF TUMOUR

The surgical treatment of cancer is based on the following time-honoured assumptions:

1. That cancer commences as a local disease and remains so in many cases, even though the tumour has progressed sufficiently to produce clinical signs or symptoms.
2. That the common carcinomata spread first *via* the lymphatics and later by the blood stream.
3. That cure is attained by removing all malignant cells, and that with suitably designed operations this is possible in many cases.

As lymphatic routes of spread were mapped out, so the magnitude of the operations increased. This is well illustrated by the super-radical mastectomy which has been practised by some surgeons for cancer of the breast. Another approach to improving the results of treatment was to attempt to detect cancer at an early stage; the earlier the disease is diagnosed and treated the greater should be the chance of cure.

There is now considerable evidence that these views are an oversimplification of the situation.[13] Thus, in cancer of the stomach, some series show that the relationship between the prognosis and the duration of symptoms is the reverse of what would be expected: the longer the history, the greater the survival-rate. In cancer of the breast it has been found that early diagnosis has not appreciably altered the death-rate. Nor are the results of various forms of treatment greatly different. Furthermore, in view of the fact that blood-borne metastases may lie dormant for long periods, it can no longer be accepted as proven that blood spread occurs after lymphatic involvement. All that is known is that lymphatic metastases are usually apparent before those derived from blood-borne emboli. It is evident that in cancer of the breast, occult haematogenous spread presents a hazard which can neither be totally assessed nor guarded against. Bony metastases can now be looked for by scanning procedures before major surgery is performed in cases of lung and breast cancer.

The factors determining whether a particular tumour will progress or not are its intrinsic malignancy and the host's immunity. Unfortunately, neither can be measured with precision. Histological grading gives some indication of the malignancy of a particular tumour, but is in general unreliable. A lymphocytic infiltration around the tumour is associated with a better prognosis in some instances, e.g. breast and stomach,[14,15] but in other tumours an admixture of lymphocytes does not appear to be particularly favourable prognostically, e.g. in carcinoma of the pharynx and seminoma. The presence of anti-tumour immunoglobulins has been claimed to indicate immunity in malignant melanoma, but this principle has not been extended to other tumours. Hormonal environment is important in certain tumours. The phenomena of dormancy and spontaneous regression emphasise this defence mechanism.

In cancer of the breast the phenomenon of dormancy indicates that the seeds of the secondary deposits were already sown at the time of operation, and that, in this event, radical surgery can offer no more in terms of survival than less mutilating procedures designed to remove the local tumour, including its field of growth. It is not known how frequent 'occult metastases' are when the patient is first seen, nor is it known what forces hold them in check. Until this information is available, therapy can be based only on information obtained by observing the results of different forms of treatment. Unfortunately there are so many variables to consider in assessing these results that no satisfactory conclusion can yet be reached.[16,17] Commonly a course of treatment which appears to be superior to another in one centre is found by others to offer no advantage.

The treatment of many cancers is based largely on the concepts derived from the study of breast cancer. It is apparent that the subject of surgery in relation to the treatment of malignant disease needs a fresh appraisal.

GENERAL READING

WILLIS, R. A. (1973) *The Spread of Tumours in the Human Body*, 3rd edn, 417 pp. London: Butterworth.

REFERENCES

1. Leading Article (1971) Fibrin and cancer. *British Medical Journal*, **4**, 641.
2. Leading Article (1976) Benign proliferative lesions of the breast. *British Medical Journal*, **1**, 1106.
3. Leading Article (1967) Circulating cancer cells. *Lancet*, **2**, 84.
4. JONES, E. M. (1969) Placental metastases from bronchial carcinoma. *British Medical Journal*, **2**, 491.
5. HANSEN, H. H., MUGGIA, F. M. & SELAWRY, O. S. (1971) Bone-marrow examination in 100 consecutive patients with bronchogenic carcinoma. *Lancet*, **2**, 443.
6. FRANSSILA, K. (1971) Value of histologic classification of thyroid cancer. *Acta Pathologica et Microbiologica Scandinavica*, A, Supplement No. 225.
7. Leading Article (1976) Osteolytic metastases. *Lancet*, **2**, 1063.
8. RUSSELL, D. S. & RUBINSTEIN, L. J. (1977) In *Pathology of Tumours of the Nervous System*, 4th edn, pp. 341–345. London: Arnold.
9. EADE, O. E. & URICH, H. (1971) Metastasising glioma in young subjects. *Journal of Pathology*, **103**, 245.
10. LITTLE, J. M., HALLIDAY, J. P. & GLENN, D. C. (1969) Pseudomyxoma peritonei. *Lancet*, **2**, 659.
11. FOX, H. & LANGLEY, F. A. (1976) In *Tumours of the Ovary*, p. 226. London: Heinemann Medical.
12. DUKES, C. E. (1958) In *Cancer*, ed. Raven, R. W., Vol. 2, p. 136. London: Butterworth.
13. BROOKE, B. N. (1968) Early detection of cancer. *Lancet*, **2**, 1289.
14. PAILE, A. (1971) Morphology and prognosis of carcinoma of the stomach. *Annales Chirurgiae et Gynaecologiae Fenniae*, **60**, Supplement No. 175, 1.
15. Leading Article (1971) Prognosis of gastric cancer. *British Medical Journal*, **4**, 67.
16. Leading Article (1972) Treatment of early carcinoma of breast. *British Medical Journal*, **2**, 417.
17. BAUM, M. (1976) The curability of breast cancer. *British Medical Journal*, **1**, 439.

Chapter 29. *The Aetiology and Incidence of Tumours*

Research into the aetiology of cancer has both a clinical and an experimental approach. It has been recognised for a long time that some types of malignancy are particularly common in certain occupations, while on a more individual level, certain families have been known to bear the trait of rare neoplastic diseases. More recently it has been noted that local environmental factors predispose large groups of people to the risk of cancer. Now that medicine is moving from the field of treatment to that of prevention, social and industrial medicine are assuming ever-increasing importance in cancer prophylaxis. The result has been the recognition of many exogenous carcinogenic agents. Furthermore, precancerous lesions are being detected with greater frequency.

The experimental side of cancer research concerns the artificial production of tumours in animals. At first only substances carcinogenic to human beings were used, but now their range is much greater than this. They include innumerable chemical agents, radiations of various types, hormones, and viruses. The object of this work is to elucidate the nature of the change that heralds malignancy in a cell. Furthermore, it is hoped that the results may eventually be applied to human beings, in respect of the prevention not only of occupational and environmental tumours but also those which seem to bear no relationship to these factors.

THE ORIGIN OF TUMOURS

The mode of origin of a tumour is still not completely understood. An early theory introduced by Cohnheim in 1875 was that tumours arose from 'cell rests' sequestered during embryonic life, that underwent neoplastic change many years later. This theory may explain the development of the germ-cell tumours and the embryonic tumours of infancy, but there is no evidence that the common adult tumours arise from cell rests, the very existence of which has not been proved.

The current evidence suggests that most tumours arise from a **single clone of cells**, or perhaps only a few such clones, that have undergone malignant transformation. This evidence is derived from the following sources:[1-3]

(a) In the monoclonal gammopathies, described in Chapter 49, of which multiple myeloma is the typical example, there is good evidence that a single clone of B lymphocytes (which have developed into plasma cells in the case of multiple myeloma) have become malignant, and by metastatic spread as well as local proliferation have crowded out the many normal clones of immunoglobulin-forming B lymphocytes. These neoplastic cells produce only one type of immunoglobulin molecule, and so can be easily identified.

The same argument applies to those tumours of B lymphocyte origin which, although not producing a circulating immunoglobulin, nevertheless have a specific cell-surface immunoglobulin. Chronic lymphatic leukaemia is a good example.

(b) According to the Lyon hypothesis (p. 40), one of the X chromosomes in each cell of a female becomes inactivated early in fetal life. This random inactivation may affect either the maternal or paternal X chromosome, and the progeny of the cell inherits this change. If the two X chromosomes differ at a particular locus, the clone derived from a single cell will show only the allele present on the X chromosome which was active in the parent cell. The enzyme glucose-6-phosphate dehydrogenase (G6PD) is coded for by a gene on the X chromosome, and in Black populations two allelic forms, called A and B, are commonly found. Some 40 per cent of Black females are heterozygous, so that extracts of blood, skin, and other tissues contain a mixture of enzyme types A and B. It is apparent that if only one type of enzyme, whether A or B, is found in an extract of a tumour from a person whose normal tissues contains both types, the inference is that the tumour arose from a single clone of cells.

On the basis of G6PD typing a clonal origin has been demonstrated for uterine fibroids, common warts, and thyroid adenomata among other benign tumours. Among malignant tumours those with a single enzyme phenotype have included melanoma, reticulum-cell sarcoma (histiocytic lymphoma), and carcinoma of the cervix and thyroid. The findings in the haematological neoplasias chronic myeloid leukaemia and polycythaemia vera[4] have also tended to substantiate this clonal derivation, and G6PD typing has confirmed it in multiple myeloma and Burkitt's tumour.

This emphasis on a clonal derivation does not mean that many tumours develop from a transforming event affecting only a single cell. It is probable that successive waves of neoplastic clones emerge during the course of malignancy, but that one particular clone dominates and forms the overwhelming mass of tumour by the time the condition is clinically evident. In some tumours there is a strong suggestion of two separate clones of cells that have independently undergone malignant transformation. The evidence does, however, indicate that most tumours grow by the proliferation of one or a few 'committed' cells rather than by continuous recruitment of normal cells through the horizontal transmission of some oncogenic factor. At present the search continues for a usable X-linked polymorphism in White populations.

If it appears that most tumours arise from one or a few clones of cells, there is also compelling clinical evidence that many tumours tend to arise on a restricted area of tissue which is called a **field of growth**. The field of growth theory is based on the frequency of origin of multiple tumours on a restricted site and for apparently recurrent tumours to develop near the site of removal of a primary tumour. It is exceptional for a whole field of growth to become malignant; much more usually there are circumscribed foci of neoplasia on it, developing no doubt from individual clones of cells that have undergone transformation.

There are numerous examples of *multiple primary tumours* arising in a particular field:

(*a*) Transitional-cell tumours of the urinary tract, from the pelvis and ureter to the bladder (Fig. 29.1).

(*b*) Polyposis coli (see p. 373). In ulcerative colitis multiple malignancy is also the rule.

(*c*) Squamous-cell and basal-cell carcinomata of the skin in those exposed to sunlight and in xeroderma pigmentosum.

(*d*) Uterine leiomyomata.

(*e*) Breast cancer is bilateral in about 9 per cent of cases. It is particularly frequent with the lobular type of carcinoma. Sometimes there are multiple fibro-adenomata of the breast.

(*f*) Hepatoma developing on cirrhosis of the liver is often multicentric.

(*g*) Sometimes there is a widespread malignancy in an expanse of epithelium with a common embryological derivation, e.g. carcinoma involving the gall-bladder, bile ducts (intrahepatic as well as extrahepatic), and pancreatic ducts in a continuous wave. Another example is cloacogenic cancer,[5] in which multiple tumours arise in epithelium that derived from the primitive cloaca, e.g. vagina, vulva, and anus.

The origin of some types of *recurrence* can also be explained in terms of a preconditioned field of growth. Thus it is not uncommon to find an area of early basal-cell or squamous-cell carcinomatous change close to an excised basal-cell or squamous-cell cancer of the skin or mouth, as the case may be, but separated from it by a variable extent of healthy epidermis (Fig. 29.2). It is such unnoticed areas of early neoplasia that provide the basis for a later recurrence, but, of course, some recurrences are due to an inadequate resection of the primary tumour. Whatever the origin of local recurrences, there is no doubt that whenever possible the whole field should be removed at the time of resection of the tumour. This is often impossible, as in the case of cancer of the exposed areas of skin, but in such a localised area as a burn or varicose ulcer from which a carcinoma has arisen, that whole site must be excised if recurrence of the tumour is to be prevented. This may necessitate an amputation. The pleomorphic salivary tumour also tends to recur after enucleation, but whether this is due to local infiltration or to seedling tumours in the capsule is undecided. The right treatment is subtotal parotidectomy.

Figure 29.1
Multiple papillary tumours of the ureter. The ureter shows extensive areas of sessile tumours. This is a good example of neoplasia occurring on a field of growth. (U 49.2, *Reproduced by permission of the President and Council of R.C.S. Eng.*)

Figure 29.2
Multifocal origin of basal-cell carcinoma. The mode of origin of the tumour as a downgrowth from the basal-cell layer is apparent, and its resemblance to an embryonic hair follicle is quite marked. The surrounding epidermis is normal, but at the edge of the section there is part of a much larger basal-cell carcinoma. × 50.

Factors Producing a Field of Growth

The probability of neoplasia developing in a previously conditioned area of tissue leads to a consideration of the factors that may be responsible for this malevolent predisposition. This is in fact the *precancerous state*. A field of growth may bear a recognisable lesion, but often it appears completely healthy until at some stage of the individual's life a succession of tumours arise on it.

Most cancers in adults arise spontaneously in response to an unknown stimulus, but a few can be attributed with certainty to some tangible preceding cause. The three factors generally recognised as causes of human neoplasia are:

Extrinsic physical and chemical agents.
Hereditary predisposition.
Chronic disease, usually of an inflammatory nature.

Two additional factors have to be considered: *hormones* and *viruses*.

EXTRINSIC CARCINOGENIC AGENTS[6]

These can be divided into chemical and physical carcinogens.

Chemical

The first chemical agents to be incriminated in human cancer were derived from soot, coal tar, and mineral oils. The first occupational cancer to be carefully documented was *chimney-sweep's cancer* of the scrotum which was described by Percivall Pott in 1775. Later on the high temperature destructive distillation of coal yielded coal tar, which produced cancer of the skin of the head, neck, and arms of exposed workers. The crude distillation products of mineral oils, particularly shale-oil mined in Scotland, led to *shale-oil cancer* of the hands and arms. When this oil was used as a lubricant in the Lancashire cotton-spinning industry, *mule-spinner's cancer** of the abdominal wall and scrotum occurred due to seepage of the splashed oil through the workers' clothing. Scrotal cancer[7] also occurs in road workers and coal-gas and coke makers, who are exposed to coal tar, and in automatic lathe operators and chain makers, whose clothes may be penetrated by the low-viscosity cutting oils used in these trades. Manufacturers of coal-tar dyes may be similarly endangered. All these types of cancer are due to specific polycyclic aromatic hydrocarbons which have been the source of much experimental work.

In 1895 bladder cancer was first described amongst manufacturers of synthetic dyestuffs, and it was subsequently discovered that specific *aromatic amines* were responsible.

It was also found that workers using *arsenic* were prone to develop cancers of the skin of the limbs and face. This followed the ingestion of the arsenic, and people who took the inorganic form of the metal medicinally as Fowler's solution (usually for recalcitrant psoriasis) have been similarly endangered. Furthermore there is evidence that it may cause lung cancer.

Cancer of the lung is also seen in those whose occupation brings them into contact with *hot tar fumes, chrome ores, nickel*

*A 'mule' is a spinning machine used in the Lancashire cotton industry.

ore, and *asbestos*, all of which presumably produce a local reaction following inhalation.

A recently discovered occupational hazard is adenocarcinoma of the nasal sinuses occurring in *hardwood furniture makers*. This association has been noted in the High Wycombe area of Buckinghamshire. Apparently it is the inhaled dust that contains the carcinogenic factor, but its nature is still not known.[8] Other occupational groups also liable to cancer of the nasal sinuses are *leather workers* (once more the factor is not known), isopropylene manufacturers (the factor is believed to be *isopropyl oil*), and those who work with *nickel ore*.[9]

Another chemical agent that has recently proved to be carcinogenic is *vinyl chloride* (CH_2CH_2Cl).[10–12] This, as the monomer, is a gas at normal temperatures and pressures, but in its liquefied form under pressure readily polymerises into polyvinyl chloride, a white, solid plastic which is widely used. In addition to the triad of Raynaud's phenomenon, sclerodermatous skin changes, and osteolysis of the distal phalanges, there is also a greatly increased incidence of angiosarcoma of the liver in those working with vinyl chloride monomer.

There is also an increased incidence of cancer of the lung, larynx, nasal sinuses, and oropharynx amongst those who manufacture *alkylating agents*, e.g. mustard gas, chloromethyl ether, and bis(chloromethyl)ether. This is not surprising, since the alkylation of DNA is thought to be an important mechanism of carcinogenic action.

Physical

The important physical agents associated with neoplasia are ionising and ultraviolet radiations.

The relationship between *ionising radiations* and cancer is considered in detail in Chapter 31. It will suffice at this stage to note that pioneer X-ray workers, radiotherapists, patients who have been treated with radioactive materials or X-rays, and the victims of nuclear fall-out have all developed malignant conditions.

Ultraviolet radiations exert their harmful effects in the strong sunlight continually acting on the exposed skin of fair-complexioned people. Farmers in Australia and South Africa, sailors, and others habitually exposed to the elements tend in later life to develop actinic (solar) keratoses on their faces and hands. These may develop into multiple squamous-cell carcinomata. Basal-cell cancers are also frequently encountered in this group of people. Cancer of the lip, typically seen in elderly agricultural workers, is probably also related to prolonged exposure of the face to sunlight. Exposure to sunlight also predisposes to malignant melanoma.

It is questionable whether *thermal radiation* acting alone is ever adequate to produce neoplasia. It probably acts as a 'promoter' of cancer in an area that has already been 'initiated' by carcinogenic agents like ultraviolet light or the tar products from burning coals or tobacco. This would account for the increased incidence of lip cancer in pipe-smokers, and also for the cancers of the abdominal skin seen in the Kangri basket-carriers.

The latent period. An important factor notable in all the occupational and environmental cancers mentioned above is the long latent period that elapses from the time of application of the agent to the time of first appearance of the neoplasm. It varied from about 20 years in chimney-sweeps and 10 years in pioneer X-ray workers to about 5 years in those developing leukaemia as the result of whole-body irradiation. There is ample time for the initiating stimulus to be completely forgotten by the patient. This is of great importance both in research work and in the question of the workman's compensation.

Experimental Carcinogenesis

This is best considered in the light of occupational cancer. Carcinogenic substances are given to animals in order to produce tumours, but two basic pitfalls must be remembered.

Firstly, there is a tendency for many animals to develop spontaneous tumours. Of the laboratory animals mice tend to develop tumours of the breast, lungs, and lymphoid tissue, whereas rats are prone to mammary fibro-adenomata, bone and skin sarcoma, lymphocytic lymphoma, and thymic tumours. The tumour incidence in mice may vary according to the strain: C_3H mice have a high incidence of breast cancer but a low one of leukaemia, whereas Ak mice have a high leukaemia incidence but seldom get breast cancer.

Secondly, animals react specifically to carcinogenic stimuli. Many fruitless years were spent trying to induce coal-tar cancers in rats and dogs, animals which are almost completely resistant. Likewise β-naphthylamine induces bladder tumours in dogs and human beings, but is without effect in rats and rabbits. The necessity for the most scrupulous controls in animal experiments is obvious. It is interesting in this respect that arsenic is carcinogenic only to the human subject.

The most important chemicals employed in experimental work are the *polycyclic hydrocarbons* responsible for soot, tar, and oil-induced tumours, the *aromatic amines* used in the aniline-dye industry, and the *azo-compounds*, which are used to colour foods.

The aromatic polycyclic hydrocarbons. Credit is due to the Japanese workers Yamagiwa and Ichikawa who, in the second decade of this century, first produced skin cancers in rabbits by painting their ears with tar. It was then found that mice were also susceptible to such treatment.

The next step was the isolation of the actual substances in the tar which were responsible for carcinogenesis. It was found that these were present in the higher-boiling fractions obtained during distillation, and that the fluorescent spectra of these fractions resembled that of the polycyclic hydrocarbon 1:2 benzanthracene.

This substance itself is only feebly carcinogenic, but Kennaway experimented with allied hydrocarbons, and found that *1 : 2 : 5 : 6-dibenzanthracene* was powerfully carcinogenic. This discovery in 1930 is of historical importance, as it was the first of a long list of chemical carcinogens to be isolated in a pure form. In fact it is not an actual constituent of tar.

Since then many more potent hydrocarbon carcinogens have been isolated, the most important of which are *9 : 10-dimethyl-1 : 2-benzanthracene*, the most powerful of them all; *methylcholanthrene*, which is related chemically to the bile acids; and **3 : 4 benzpyrene**, which is certainly the most important carcinogenic constituent of coal tar and the most significant hydrocarbon carcinogen to the human being. The structural formulae below indicate how the carcinogenic potency of these polycyclic hydrocarbons is increased by substitution groups at the positions 10, 9, 6, and 5 of the benzanthracene complex. The structural formulae of some of these chemicals are given below.

The tumours these hydrocarbons produce generally appear at the site of application of the agent. Squamous-cell carcinoma follows application to the skin, while subcutaneous injections induce sarcoma formation. It has been found, however, that the agents may also be absorbed, and produce neoplasms in sites remote from the area of application. Tumours of the lung have followed surface applications of these agents in mice. It is also noteworthy that pure polycyclic hydrocarbons have a much more extensive species range than crude coal tar; dogs, rats, and even guinea-pigs may develop tumours after exposure.

The aromatic amines. The important carcinogens of this category are *α-naphthylamine*, *β-naphthylamine*, *benzidine*, and *4-aminobiphenyl*, and those most likely to come in contact with these substances are workers in the aniline-dye industry. More recently bladder tumours have been noted unusually frequently in those working in the rubber and cable industries. This has been attributed to the addition of an antioxidant to the rubber to prevent it perishing. Before 1949 this antioxidant contained a trace of β-naphthylamine (which is much

1:2-BENZANTHRACENE

1:2:5:6-DIBENZANTHRACENE

9:10-DIMETHYL-1:2-BENZANTHRACENE

3:4-BENZPYRENE

METHYLCHOLANTHRENE

more powerfully carcinogenic than α-naphthylamine), so that workers with rubber and cables (which contain rubber) exposed before that date are endangered. Other occupational groups that are endangered, though to a much lesser degree, are pigment and paint manufactures, textile dyers and printers, gas workers, patent fuel, tar, and pitch workers, laboratory workers, and rodent controllers.[9]

Bladder tumours can also be produced in dogs fed on β-naphthylamine, yet the local application of this substance to a dog's bladder mucosa produces no effect. An intermediary metabolic product, *2-amino-1-naphthol*, is the carcinogenic agent. It is produced in the liver, where it is at once detoxified by conjugation with glucuronic acid. The resulting 2-amino-1-naphthyl glucuronide is harmless when excreted in the urine, but unfortunately the bladder mucosa of human beings and dogs secretes the enzyme β-glucuronidase which splits the compound and releases free carcinogen. Saccharolactone inhibits this enzyme, and can protect dogs against bladder cancer. It has also been used in exposed workers. Induction of bladder tumours by the aromatic amines is a good example of *remote carcinogenesis*, for the agent is taken by mouth yet produces its effects on the bladder. It may be that intermediary aminophenol substances produced during the metabolism of tryptophan are of importance in the aetiology of spontaneously occurring bladder tumours.

Another important aromatic amine that has been used extensively in experimental work is *2-acetylaminofluorene*, which was nearly marketed as an insecticide. Fortunately its powerful carcinogenic activity was discovered in time. It too is a remote carcinogen, but unlike the naphthylamines it produces a wide range of cancers in different animals. Tumours of the liver, breast, lung, bladder, and intestines are produced in mice, rats, dogs, and rabbits, and a rather surprising addition is carcinoma of the external auditory meatus. Once again some unidentified intermediary product apparently produces tumours at its sites of excretion. The structural formulae of some of these chemicals are given below.

The azo-compounds. Azo-dyes like *scarlet red* (which contains in its molecule 2′ : 3-dimethyl-4-aminoazobenzene) and *butter yellow* (4-dimethylaminoazobenzene), when fed to

rats, produce different varieties of liver tumours, e.g. hepatomata and cholangiomata, usually without the supervention of previous necrosis or cirrhosis. Mice are much less susceptible. This is yet another example of remote carcinogenesis. Azo-dye carcinogenesis is greatly facilitated by a diet deficient in riboflavin. Some of these azo-compounds have been used commercially as dyes for leather and in foodstuffs, but there is no definite evidence that human cancer has been caused by these compounds.

CARCINOGENS OF NATURAL ORIGIN[13]

Certain natural foodstuffs also carry a carcinogenic hazard, indicating that a return to a 'natural' way of living advocated by enthusiasts need not necessarily eliminate cancer. Two important carcinogens are:

Aflatoxin.[14] This is the toxic principle of the mould *Aspergillus flavus* which may contaminate foodstuffs such as ground-nut meal. Aflatoxin is a powerful liver carcinogen in a wide variety of animals, and it may well be that the human liver cancer so prevalent in Africa and elsewhere is due to it rather than to the effects of malnutrition.

Human liver cells contain the enzymes necessary to produce the epoxy-metabolites of aflatoxin, which are the active agents. It has been shown both in Africa and South-East Asia that the incidence of liver cancer increases in proportion to the amount of aflatoxin in the diet.[9]

Cycasin. This is a glycoside isolated from a palm-like tree *Cycas circinalis*, which grows in certain areas of the Far East. Cycasin is a general carcinogen producing neoplasms at various sites in different animals; liver cancer is frequently produced.

Both aflatoxin and cycasin act by interference with DNA synthesis, an effect they share in common with the **nitrosamines,**[15] a chemical carcinogen of great potency and closely related in intermediate metabolism to cycasin. The nitrosamines are little used in industry, but occur in food, drink, and tobacco smoke. They are found in only minute amounts, and there is no present evidence of their carcinogenicity in the human. Nevertheless, they produce a wide range of tumours in many animal species, including primates. Some act as transplacental carcinogens, and they can also act synergistically with other known carcinogenic agents.

IMMUNOLOGICAL ASPECTS OF CARCINOGENESIS[16]

Tumours can differ antigenically from their host and therefore may excite an immune response.

Loss of antigen. Some tumours lose tissue-specific antigens because of their poor differentiation, but the transplantation antigens are retained.

Development of new antigen. The development of new transplantation antigens on the surface of tumour cells is an important feature of neoplasia. In virus-induced tumours the new antigen is a tumour-specific transplantation antigen, and is the same in all tumours produced by the particular virus. It is quite distinct from the antigens of the mature virions. In carcinogen-induced tumours the new transplantation antigen is weak and is individual for the particular tumour; it is different

2 – NAPHTHYLAMINE

BENZIDINE

2 – AMINO – 1 – NAPHTHOL

2 – AMINO – 1 – NAPHTHYL GLUCURONIDE

2 – ACETYLAMINOFLUORENE

from antigens present in other tumours produced by the particular carcinogen.[17-19] Radiation-induced tumours likewise are individual.

Tumours may also produce antigens which are not transplantation antigens. Thus distinctive antigens have been found with some human tumours, e.g. the Burkitt tumour antigen and the carcino-embryonic antigen (see below). Specific antiviral antibodies are found in animal virus-induced tumours.

The effects of antigenic difference between host and its tumour may be immunological or non-immunological.

IMMUNOLOGICAL EFFECTS

Immunoglobulin formation may be associated with enhancement of tumour growth or tumour rejection. Immune cells can cause tumour destruction. Finally there may be no antibody production due to the induction of tolerance.

In animal tumours transplanted to genetically non-identical recipients there is a homograft reaction and the tumour is promptly rejected, unless a privileged site is used.

It is noteworthy that immunologically tolerant animals, for example newborn mice, and especially those that are thymectomised, develop most virus-induced tumours much more rapidly than do adult animals. An exception is the group of oncogenic viruses that proliferate in the lymphocyte before causing tumour formation, e.g. the Bittner factor and the mouse leukaemia virus, in which neonatal thymectomy decreases the incidence of tumours by causing severe lymphocytic depletion.

The part played by the immune response in the restraint and rejection of human tumours is much less certain, although the graft rejection phenomenon is explained teleologically as a homeostatic mechanism devised to recognise and destroy aberrant mutant cells that develop transplantation antigens unnatural to the individual. This function is called *immunological surveillance*. The findings supporting an immunological restraint on tumours are:

(a) The increased incidence of tumours in the immunological deficiency syndromes (see p. 170) and after immunosuppression for homografts. Most of these tumours are lymphomata.

(b) The heavy lymphocytic infiltration around tumours of low-grade malignancy. Indeed, the evidence points to the great importance of cell-mediated immunity in solid tumours, and lymphocytes from such patients are destructive to tumour cells grown in tissue culture.

(c) Circulating immunoglobulins have been demonstrated against some tumours. The difficulty here lies in the assessment of the specificity of the tumour antigen; as yet none has been proved to be specific for the tumour. One antigen that has aroused much attention is found in some colonic carcinoma cells. Both antigen and corresponding antibody have been found in patients' serum. The antigen is found in fetal tissues, and has therefore been called *carcino-embryonic antigen* (*CEA*).[20] It is present in small quantities in other tissues, e.g. liver, bowel mucosa, and lung, and in the sera of pregnant women as well as in many patients with primary gastrointestinal tumours. Smaller amounts of CEA are found in sera of patients with other tumours and occasionally in non-neoplastic diseases, such as cirrhosis of the liver, ulcerative colitis, Crohn's disease, pancreatitis, and chronic bronchitis. The finding of carcino-embryonic antigen in the blood is therefore not diagnostic of cancer of the large bowel; however, following surgery the level of CEA drops, and a return to preoperative levels is an indication of the tumour's recurrence.[21] Some other fetal antigens have been reported in human tumours, but these too are non-specific. It would seem that the numerous antibodies to tumours that patients may have in their sera are autoantibodies to normal adult or fetal components that are exposed or are in greater concentration than in normal tissue.

The antibodies probably play no part in the control of tumour growth. Nevertheless, since both antibody and antigen (e.g. CEA) can be present in the blood, it is possible that antigen-antibody complexes can lead to a type of immune-complex disease.[22] This may be the explanation of weight loss, fever, raised ESR, nephrotic syndrome, arthralgia, skin eruptions, and other obscure features of human malignant disease.

There are, however, a few tumours in which immunological mechanisms do appear to be very important.[23,24] In Burkitt's tumour autoantibodies to the tumour cells are invariable, and they appear to react against antigens associated with the EB virus (see p. 380). In this tumour many apparently permanent cures have followed the administration of totally inadequate doses (even one) of cyclophosphamide. It would seem that when the main bulk of the tumour is killed, the immunoglobulins can destroy the remainder. A similar situation may occur in choriocarcinoma treated with methotrexate. Specific anti-tumour immunoglobulins are found in the early stages of malignant melanoma, but these tend to disappear as the tumour metastasises.[25]

It should be noted that some immunoglobulins formed against tumours actually enhance the growth of the neoplasm, presumably by inhibiting the immune response in its afferent limb or preventing cytotoxic antibody (whether immunoglobulin or lymphocyte) acting in the efferent limb (see p. 152). Thus at least two types of immunoglobulin are produced: a deleterious enhancing one and a beneficial cytotoxic one that activates complement. Perhaps there is also an unblocking antibody to reverse the enhancement of the first immunoglobulin mentioned. Serum from patients who have recovered from malignant melanoma and clear-cell renal carcinoma has occasionally helped other victims of these tumours.

There is evidence in both animal and human tumour victims that cell-mediated immunity develops against specific tumour antigens. The lymphocytotoxic effect can be blocked by serum factors—probably complexes of tumour antigen and immunoglobulin.[26] Unblocking antibodies have also been identified.[27]

The status of immunotherapy is slight at present. It is agreed that the bulk of the tumour must first be destroyed by conventional methods, so that only a small residuum of tumour cells is left. Non-specific stimulation of the RE system with BCG or *Corynebacterium parvum* is worth trying.[28-30] Mathé has combined this with immunisation using irradiated leukaemic cells, and has achieved noteworthy remissions in acute lymphatic leukaemia (he already used conventional treatment on these patients). However, subsequent trials have failed to substantiate this claim. In acute myeloid leukaemia various trials suggest that survival may be prolonged.[28]

Specifically stimulated lymphoid cells are not very satisfactory, and the casual use of antisera may well enhance the growth rather than destroy it.

NON-IMMUNOLOGICAL MECHANISM IN TUMOUR CONTROL[31, 32]

If allogeneic cells are made to grow in close proximity to each other in tissue culture, each type of cell inhibits the growth of the other. This is called *allogeneic inhibition*, and appears not to be immunological because the phenomenon can be demonstrated using immunologically incompetent cells. Tumour cells which lack antigens can be shown to be at a disadvantage when in company with normal cells. This can be demonstrated by injecting tumour cells into a histocompatible host and *in vitro*. The inhibitory effect can be swamped if a large inoculum is used. The reaction seems to be well adapted to the destruction of small groups of tumour cells.

HEREDITARY PREDISPOSITION[33, 34]

There is little significant hereditary predisposition to most of the common types of cancer, and statistical surveys amongst relations of cancer patients have not yielded convincing evidence of an increased incidence of tumours in them. Cancer of the breast, however, is somewhat commoner in the relatives of affected women than in the population at large.

There are nevertheless a number of uncommon neoplastic diseases which are inherited, and the affected tissue could be considered a field of growth predisposed to cancer from the time of its conception, though the lethal tendency may manifest itself only in adult life.

The three important examples of such a tendency are polyposis coli, xeroderma pigmentosum, and retinoblastoma (see p. 346).

The trait of *polyposis coli* is transmitted as an autosomal dominant. The condition is not present at birth, but usually first manifests itself at puberty with the passage of blood and mucus in the faeces. The colon and rectum are studded with innumerable adenomata (Fig. 29.3), and by the age of 30 years multiple carcinoma develop. Total resection of the colon and rectum will alone ensure cure. In a related condition, *Gardner's syndrome*, colonic polyposis is found in association with sebaceous cysts, osteomata of the face and skull, desmoid tumours, and multiple fibromata. This too is inherited as a dominant trait and terminates in colonic cancer.

There is some evidence that a few cases of polyposis coli also have benign duodenal and gastric polyps, and occasionally there may be a periampullary carcinoma. This tendency is more marked in Gardner's syndrome.[35]

Xeroderma pigmentosum is inherited as an autosomal recessive trait. In this condition the skin is abnormally susceptible to the effects of sunlight. Within the first few years of life exposed areas show blotchy pigmentation which is followed by atrophy of the skin and telangiectasia. Multiple basal-cell and squamous-cell carcinomata (and more rarely malignant melanomata) then develop, and unless the patient is protected from sunlight by covering up all the exposed parts, death occurs within the first decade.

The mechanism of xeroderma pigmentosum has now been elucidated.[36] Ultraviolet light gives rise to dimer formation between neighbouring thymidine radicles in DNA, and when

Figure 29.3
Polyposis coli. These are portions of the descending colon and rectum resected from a patient with polyposis coli. The mucosa is studded with innumerable polyps, some of which are pedunculated and others sessile. There is no evidence of carcinomatous change in any of the polyps. (A 74.4, *Reproduced by permission of the President and Council of the R.C.S. Eng.*)

such DNA replicates, the dimer causes a mutation. In normal cells there are enzymes that can excise the dimer and replace it by the correct nitrogen bases. In xeroderma pigmentosum one such enzyme is lacking, and the disease is an inborn error of metabolism. This mechanism also explains actinic skin cancer; without DNA-repairing enzymes the frequency of skin cancer among fair-skinned people would be extremely high even in youth.

Rarely xeroderma pigmentosum is associated with mesodermal and angiomatous tumours, and there may also be malformations of the nervous system with microcephaly, athetoid movements, and mental subnormality.[37]

Some varieties of basal-cell carcinoma also show a hereditary pattern. In the *naevoid basal-cell carcinoma syndrome*[38] multiple carcinomata occur on the exposed parts at a very early age, and there is often an association with cysts of the jaws, malformations of the skull, spine, ribs, and extremities, and calcification of the falx cerebri. The condition is inherited as an autosomal dominant trait, as are also two adnexal skin tumours (in some patients). These are the *trichoepithelioma* and the *cylindroma*. Multiple tumours are present, on the face with trichoepithelioma and on the scalp with cylindroma (turban tumour). Both tumours may occur in the same patient. Hereditary aspects of *malignant melanoma* and *multiple endocrine adenopathy* are mentioned on pages 352 and 452.

A somewhat different relationship between genetics and cancer is seen in a number of conditions in which there is a chromosomal abnormality.[39]

In *trisomy 21 (Down's syndrome)* there is an increased

frequency of acute leukaemia, but probably not of any other type of malignancy.

In the three conditions mentioned on page 31, in which there is a tendency to spontaneous chromosomal breakage in both lymphoid and fibroblastic cells, there is also an increased tendency to cancer. In *Fanconi's anaemia* this is confined to leukaemia and lymphoma only, but in *ataxia telengiectasia* and *Bloom's syndrome* the tendency includes other types of neoplasms also. All three conditions are probably inherited as autosomal recessive characteristics. The cause of this malignant propensity is much more likely to be related to the chromosomal anomaly than to any possible failure of immunosurveillance.

CANCER FOLLOWING CHRONIC DISEASE

Virchow believed that cancer was the result of prolonged stimulation of the tissues through 'chronic irritation'. The concept of chronic irritation is too imprecise now that a large number of specific carcinogenic agents have been isolated. It is doubtful whether physical irritation acting alone can ever produce cancer, though it may certainly 'promote' a tumour in a field already 'initiated' by a carcinogenic substance. Corns on the toes of those who wear ill-fitting shoes and callosities on the fingers of string instrumentalists do not become malignant, nor does cancer tend to supervene on a hyperplasia of a gum subjected to the friction of a jagged tooth or an ill-fitting denture. These are true examples of hyperplasia of protective epithelium in response to trauma, and once the stimulus is removed, regression may be expected. Nevertheless, there are a number of chronic diseases which may from time to time be complicated by malignancy, and these must be included in the list of precancerous lesions.

Chronic Inflammatory Conditions of Surface Epithelia

Chronic varicose ulcers, the sinuses of chronic osteomyelitis particularly of the tibia (Fig. 29.4), and *old burn scars* occasionally give rise to squamous-cell cancers. These are nowadays collectively called *Marjolin's ulcer*, though the name should properly be reserved for cancer developing in a chronic leg ulcer. *Tropical ulcers* (non-specific chronic skin ulcers found in Black Africans, the cause of which is obscure) may also become malignant. Marjolin's ulcer is more malignant than actinic skin cancer.

Tertiary syphilis of the mouth was said to have been frequently complicated by dysplastic leucoplakia and carcinoma, but there may have been other factors acting also.

Gastric ulcers may occasionally be the site of origin of cancer of the stomach. Probably less than 4 per cent of ulcers are complicated by cancer, and only 6 per cent of cancers arise in pre-existing ulcers, and the opinion generally held is that there is no significant causal relationship between the two. Duodenal ulcers are never complicated by cancer, which is in keeping with the mysterious resistance of the duodenum to carcinoma, except when involved in neoplasia of the ampulla of Vater.

Ulcerative colitis is an important precancerous condition. About 4 per cent of all cases develop carcinoma, but it is those with repeated relapses that are most at risk; at least a third of

Figure 29.4

Carcinoma of chronic osteomyelitis sinus. There is chronic osteomyelitis of the upper part of the tibia; the bone is sclerotic, and there is an abscess cavity in its neck. At the site of a sinus there is an extensive squamous-cell carcinoma, which has infiltrated completely through the shaft of the bone. (I 19.10, *Reproduction by permission of the President and Council of the R.C.S. Eng.*)

all cases lasting 12 years develop cancer, usually multifocally. The incidence is greatest when the disease starts before the age of 25 years and when the entire large bowel is affected.

Crohn's disease is also a precancerous condition, but probably less so than the closely related ulcerative colitis. A number of cases have developed small-bowel carcinoma after a mean duration of 15 years and at a considerably earlier age than is usual for this uncommon tumour.[40]

Gallstones are found in about three-quarters of cases of cancer of the gallbladder. Nevertheless, carcinoma is a rare complication of this very common condition.[41]

Cancer of the renal pelvis is occasionally associated with calculi, but these may have arisen secondarily to the tumour.

Schistosomiasis may be a predisposing factor to bladder cancer in areas of heavy infestation, e.g. Egypt, for the age incidence is lower than usual and the lesion is nearly always squamous-celled and not transitional-celled. Nevertheless the association is not proven, for there is still no evidence of a higher incidence of bladder cancer in Egypt than elsewhere.[42]

Metabolic and Deficiency Disease

About 90 *per cent of primary liver-cell cancer (hepatoma) in humans* (Fig. 29.5) is superimposed on a previous cirrhosis; in

Figure 29.5
Hepatoma. This is a primary liver-cell carcinoma. It is well differentiated, since the cancer cells are of uniform appearance and are arranged in solid cords, not altogether dissimilar to those of normal liver cells. There was also a micronodular type of cirrhosis. × 100.

the bile-duct type of liver cancer the figure is only 25 per cent. Liver-cell cancer is prevalent in Black African races in whom there is usually a preceding cirrhosis considered nutritional in origin, but the possibility of aflatoxin being the cause is now preferred as an alternative explanation. The incidence of liver cancer is very much less in the Black population of the USA, proving that exogenous factors rather than racial constitution are important in causing the disease. White groups with cirrhosis (including that due to alcoholism) likewise have a high incidence of liver cancer; the fine, 'Morocco-leather' cirrhosis of haemochromatosis is complicated by cancer in at least 10 per cent of cases.

Thyroid cancer is traditionally associated with the goitre of iodine deficiency, and it was common in Switzerland, where goitre was very rife; a survey in the USA revealed a higher incidence in a goitre-belt than elsewhere. Nevertheless, the current view is that cancer arises independently of previous thyroid disease. Though found in goitrous glands, it occurs more frequently in glands that are otherwise normal. Indeed, considering the frequency of goitre, cancer is a rare complication. Furthermore, it is possible that in some cases the tumour lay latent and masqueraded as a nodular goitre.

Post-cricoid carcinoma may be associated with an iron-deficiency anaemia, characteristically in middle-aged women,

in whom there is also glossitis and dysphagia. This is the *Plummer-Vinson syndrome*.* The pathological basis is obscure: atrophic changes in the mucosa and underlying muscle of the mouth and pharynx are described, with later web formation and strictures. Malignancy commonly ensues.

In Paget's disease of bone osteosarcoma is an occasional complication, occurring in about 1 per cent of clinically apparent cases. More rarely a fibrosarcoma or chondrosarcoma develops.

Chronic lymphatic oedema is occasionally complicated by an angiosarcoma of the skin (see p. 349).

Hamartomatous Malformations

There are a number of localised and generalised hamartomatous lesions which occasionally become malignant (see Ch. 27). A congenitally abnormal organ, e.g. an imperfectly descended testis, is more liable to malignancy than a normal one.

Benign Tumours

There is no doubt that an apparently benign tumour, e.g. a uterine myoma or a bladder papilloma, which has been quiescent may suddenly assume malignant potentialities. The question arises whether the tumour was malignant from the start, but in a latent phase, or whether there is indeed true malignant transformation. At present there is no definite solution to this problem.

HORMONES AND NEOPLASIA

The relationship between hormones and neoplasia is complex.

Earlier workers had noted that ovariectomised mice seldom developed breast cancer, and in 1932 Lacassagne successfully produced mammary cancers in mice of both sexes by administering large doses of *oestrogen*. This was a noteworthy finding, being the first example of neoplasia related to an endogenous agent.

Since then it has been discovered that mice can be divided into low-cancer and high-cancer strains. The latter develop cancer of the breast at a comparatively early age due to the presence of a virus first described by Bittner in 1936, and called the *milk factor*. It is transmitted to the young in the mother's milk, and is not effective after the first few days of life. If the suckling mice are fed by foster-mothers of a low-cancer strain, they do not become infected with the tumour-inducing virus, and do not develop cancer. In high-cancer strain mice oestrogen induces mammary tumours, but in those of low cancer strain only cystic hyperplasia of the breast. Conversely, castration serves to decrease the liability of a high-cancer strain mouse to mammary neoplasia. The hormone merely 'promotes' a tumour in a breast already 'initiated' by a tumour virus. Certain polycyclic hydrocarbons can similarly initiate a mouse's breast to malignancy, which may then be promoted by oestrogen.

Large doses of oestrogen in mice also lead to hyperplasia of the endometrium, interstitial cells of the testis, and the pi-

*This syndrome was first described in 1906 by Paterson, and soon afterwards by Kelly; both were laryngologists. It should rightly be called the Paterson-Kelly syndrome.

tuitary acidophils, and if the stimulus is continued indefinitely, true adenomata may develop. Occasionally endometrial carcinoma may supervene.

The *pituitary hormones* have also been the subject of much experimental work. A classical method of subjecting a mouse to an excess of *gonadotrophic hormone* is to remove one ovary and transplant the other into its spleen. The ovarian hormones are inactivated by the liver, and can no longer inhibit the secretion of pituitary gonadotrophins, which are then free to act on the transplanted ovary. Ovarian cancer may sometimes be produced in this way.

Similarly rats and mice can be subjected to large doses of *thyrotrophic hormone* if they are given thiouracil derivatives and fed on a low-iodine diet. Thyroxine formation is curtailed, and once again the inhibitory effect on the pituitary is lost. The excess thyrotrophic hormone produces great thyroid hyperplasia which is often accompanied by discrete adenomata. Occasionally thyroid cancer supervenes.

Castrated animals develop marked hyperplasia of the pituitary basophil 'gonadotrophic cells', and thyroidectomised animals develop a comparable hyperplasia of the pituitary 'thyrotrophs'. Large adenomata composed of these cells are frequently produced if the animal lives long enough. The pituitary acidophil tumours induced by oestrogen are mammotrophic in effect. It is doubtful whether any of these pituitary tumours ever becomes malignant.

It would therefore appear that animal tumours are produced only after massive doses of hormones administered over a long period of time. The effect is one of hyperplasia merging imperceptibly into circumscribed adenomatous formations in the affected organs. Malignancy may occur, but its supervention is not common. In the human being hormones are not usually an important factor in causing cancer. There are a few exceptions:

(*a*) There is a positive association between granulosa-cell tumour of the ovary, which secretes large amounts of oestrogen and leads to great endometrial hyperplasia, and *endometrial carcinoma*. There is also a slightly increased risk of endometrial cancer developing in women treated with oestrogens during the menopause. It is, however, felt that this hazard is insufficient to preclude the use of oestrogen in patients with severe menopausal symptoms, but that synthetic oestrogens and oestrone sulphate should be avoided.[43]

(*b*) Men who have undergone artificial sex change and have taken large doses of oestrogen to produce enlargement of their breasts occasionally develop *breast cancer*.[44] There is also an increased incidence of breast cancer in cases of Klinefelter's syndrome.

(*c*) There is an association between *clear-cell adenocarcinoma of the vagina* in young women (which is a rare tumour at any age) and the administration of diethylstilboestrol to their mothers during the first trimester of pregnancy for threatened abortion.[45,46] Fetal tissue is apparently more sensitive to this carcinogen than is the adult, and the transplacental passage of drugs is a factor to be reckoned with in carcinogenesis. Nevertheless, this is an uncommon complication of oestrogen therapy during pregnancy. It has been calculated that the over-all incidence amongst the offspring of mothers who took the hormone was 4 per 1000, and when it was given in the first trimester 9 per 1000.

(*d*) The administration of androgens in rarely complicated by *hepatocellular carcinoma (hepatoma)*.[47] *Hepatic adenoma* has also been reported.

(*e*) The use of oral contraceptives containing oestrogen is occasionally complicated by two benign tumours of the liver,[48,49] *hepatic adenoma* and a lesion called *focal nodular hyperplasia*. This consists of nodules of liver cells separated by fibrous trabeculae in which there are aggregates of proliferated bile ducts; it resembles a hamartoma. Both of these lesions are often vascular, and haemoperitoneum is a serious, and sometimes fatal hazard. A few cases of *hepatoma* have also been reported.[50,51]

There is some doubt as to whether these instances constitute a positive association between the contraceptive pill and liver tumours. They are so infrequent that the occurrence may have been fortuitous. A non-neoplastic lesion of the liver that is known to follow both androgen and oestrogen administration is *peliosis hepatis*. This consists of blood-filled spaces without any endothelial lining scattered throughout the liver, and it too may lead to intraperitoneal bleeding.

Hormone Dependency

While hormones play only a small role in the aetiology of human cancer, they are of great importance in maintaining the growth of some tumours. These are called *hormone dependent tumours*. Such neoplasms depend on specific hormones for their continued growth, and if deprived of them undergo regression, only to recur when the hormone is restored. It seems that during a stage in the development of certain tumours a propitious hormonal *milieu* is essential for their continued growth. This is a transient phase, however, for these tumours eventually progress to complete hormone independence. Nevertheless, a patient suffering from such a cancer may enjoy some years of amelioration of symptoms if the responsible hormone is eradicated from the body. Both in this respect and from the further light that is shed on the nature of carcinogenesis, hormone dependence is worth careful study.

Prostate. Prostatic cancer was the first human neoplasm to be successfully repressed by hormonal therapy. It is often androgen dependent, and following castration there is dramatic relief with regression of the tumour and its metastases and a fall in the acid-phosphatase level of the plasma. Nowadays large doses of stilboestrol are given, either as an adjunct to orchidectomy or else alone. Unfortunately such large doses may lead to cardiovascular complications, so that although the tumour may regress for a considerable time, the patient's life is sometimes not substantially prolonged by the therapy.[52]

Breast. Breast cancer manifests hormone dependency in about 30 per cent of cases. The hormones on which it may depend are oestrogens, progestins, androgens, prolactin, growth hormone, and placental lactogen.

In pre-menopausal women oophorectomy often produces a remission usually lasting about 6 months, but occasionally up to several years. It removes the major source of oestrogens and progestins. Bilateral adrenalectomy is sometimes performed at the same time to eliminate the other source of these hormones. In this respect it is noteworthy that breast cancer is particularly lethal during pregnancy and lactation.

If a relapse follows oophorectomy, hypophysectomy may be

performed. This is the most radical endocrine operation for breast cancer, and a further remission lasting up to 18 months may follow.

In post-menopausal women hypophysectomy is sometimes recommended. There is an interesting variation of response to hormone therapy amongst these cases. Some respond well to large doses of oestrogens, some to progestins, and some to androgens. In some these hormones cause remissions of from 6 to 12 months, whereas in others they lead to sudden exacerbations and rapid death. Glucocorticoids also sometimes have an ameliorative effect, probably in part by inhibiting the adrenals.

Since most cases of breast cancer are hormone independent from the start, much research has been undertaken to determine which patients are most likely to respond to hormone therapy. At present most interest in centred on the hormone receptors that are often present in the cancer cell.[53] If there are many receptors in a particular tumour to a particular hormone, the tumour might, at least theoretically, be dependent on that hormone. In fact, the correlation is imperfect, and a number of breast cancers with oestrogen receptors are clinically not responsive to oestrogen deprival.

Thyroid. Some cancers of the thyroid, usually the well-differentiated ones, are under the control of pituitary thyrotrophic hormone. Treatment of the tumour by excision or with ^{131}I may cause excessive pituitary secretion and so stimulate any remaining growth to activity. The administration of thyroid hormone, on the other hand, can cause a remission due to its inhibitory effect on the pituitary.[54]

Other tumours.[55] Progestins sometimes produce remissions in metastatic endometrial carcinoma and renal carcinoma. Clear-cell carcinoma of the kidney seems sometimes to be under definite hormonal control, and may respond to oestrogen also.

A somewhat different type of dependence is seen with the amino acid L-asparagine. Normal cells do not require an external source, whereas some neoplastic cells cannot grow without it in tissue culture. The systemic administration of L-asparaginase (derived from *Esch. coli*) has been tried as a treatment for malignant disease, in particular leukaemia.[56]

Pregnancy and Tumours

Some tumours may increase in size in pregnancy, and may even show an increased tendency to become malignant. The melanotic hamartoma tends to darken during pregnancy, an effect probably related to the increased secretion of oestrogen (see p. 587). It is commonly held that malignancy is especially liable to occur at this period, though detailed studies have not substantiated this view. Nevertheless, metastases occurring during pregnancy have been known to regress after its termination.[57] Neurofibromatosis is another hamartomatous disorder in which the lesions tend to grow during pregnancy, and during which sarcomatous change may occasionally supervene. The bad effect of pregnancy on breast cancer has already been noted, and the same is true of cancer of the cervix.

VIRUSES AND NEOPLASIA[58, 59]

Tumour-producing (oncogenic) viruses are of great importance not only in the aetiology of some animal tumours but also because some human tumours are associated with, if not actually caused by viruses. Some are DNA viruses, and others RNA viruses (see Table 29.1). The first virus-induced animal tumour to be discovered was fowl leukaemia (Ellerman and Bang, 1908), and it was followed by fowl sarcoma (Rous, 1911),* rabbit papilloma (Shope, 1932), renal adenocarcinoma in frogs (Lucké, 1934), and mammary cancer in mice (Bittner, 1936).

Gross (1951) isolated the virus of mouse leukaemia by transmitting the disease from an animal of a high-incidence strain, Ak, to the newborn of a low-incidence strain, C_3H. In 1953 a second, unrelated virus was found in Gross's material—this produced tumours in mice, rats, hamsters, and many other animals. The salivary glands were especially vulnerable, but tumours of the connective tissues, breasts, and kidneys were also encountered. This agent is now called polyoma virus.

TABLE 29.1 Oncogenic viruses

DNA-CONTAINING VIRUSES	
Papovaviruses	Shope papilloma
	Warts and laryngeal papillomata in human beings
	SV 40
	Polyoma virus
Adenoviruses	Experimental (baby hamsters)
Herpesviruses	Lucké renal carcinoma of frogs
	Marek's disease of chickens
	Lymphoma of marmosets and Owl monkeys
	Epstein–Barr virus in human beings (?)
	Herpes simplex in human beings (?)
Poxviruses	Molluscum contagiosum

RNA-CONTAINING VIRUSES	
Oncoviruses	Lymphomata and leukaemia in birds, mice, cats, and human beings (?)
	Rous sarcoma
	Mammary carcinoma in mice (Bittner factor)…and in other species, including human beings (?)

One of the many viruses present in a latent form in monkey kidneys is oncogenic to newborn hamsters. This agent, simian virus (SV) 40, has been adventitiously inoculated into human beings who were given poliomyelitis vaccines (see p. 278). In addition, a number of human and animal adenoviruses are oncogenic to baby hamsters. Some more recently proven animal tumours of viral origin are feline leukaemia (which may present with lymphomata also),[60] Marek's disease of chickens (a lymphoma), and a lymphoma of New World subhuman primates. The main groups of viruses that are oncogenic to animals are classified in Table 29.1. It is noteworthy that successful vaccination has been achieved against Marek's disease, felin leukaemia, and the lymphoma of subhuman primates.[61]

The factors involved in the induction of tumours by these viruses are complex. The agents concerned in mammary

*It is an interesting but sad reflection of the remarkable resistance of contemporary medicine to new ideas, that had Rous not lived to be an octogenarian he would not have received the Nobel Prize for Medicine in 1966.

cancer and leukaemia in mice are infinitely more pathogenic to newborn animals than to adults. The strain of animal is also important; thus although the Bittner virus can cause mammary cancer in low incidence strains when introduced early in life, the virus becomes less potent in successive generations and ultimately dies out. The hormonal environment is also important: oestrogen accelerates tumour production, as already explained. Mouse leukaemia can be induced both by the virus and by ionising radiations (radiation-induced leukaemias in mice have been shown to yield a leukaemia-producing virus which was apparently latent). When both factors act together the incidence of leukaemia is much increased. The Shope papilloma virus assumes malignant propensities much more rapidly when the ears of the rabbits have been tarred beforehand. The polyoma virus is widely distributed in nature, apparently lying latent in many mice. When grown in tissue culture (as was done with Gross's material) it acquires greatly enhanced virulence.

In order to establish the viral aetiology of a tumour, it is necessary to transmit the lesion by means of bacteriologically sterile, cell-free filtrates to other animals. It has also been found that some of these viruses, notably polyoma and SV 40, induce changes in cells grown in tissue culture. This phenomenon, *cell transformation*, is indicated by a rapid, unruly proliferation of the cells with copious, irregular mitotic activity, and when they are transplanted into animals they exhibit malignant propensities.

It is important to realise that the mere presence of a virus in a cancer is no indication of its causal role. Cancers frequently harbour 'passenger viruses'; these lie latent there, because neoplastic cells produce less interferon than do normal ones. Some of these passengers may be quite dangerous pathogens, but in respect of the tumour they are irrelevant. Conversely, in some virus-induced tumours the agent itself cannot be demonstrated—this applies especially to transplanted tumours caused originally by the Shope papilloma, polyoma, and SV 40 viruses. The Rous virus, on the other hand, is usually recoverable from its sarcomata. Even when the virus which induced the tumour cannot be isolated from a transplanted tumour, it is often possible to demonstrate antibodies against the virus in question. Furthermore, if an animal is first inoculated with the virus, and then has the corresponding tumour transplanted into it, it tends to reject the tumour due to the immunity already acquired.

The DNA Oncogenic Viruses

In an infection with DNA oncogenic viruses, the cell undergoes transformation, and infective virus can no longer be detected. The viral DNA becomes incorporated into the cell's genome and replicates with it; mRNA of viral type is produced, and subsequently viral-type protein is synthesised by the cell. One early product is the *T-antigen*, which is found in the nucleus of infected cells. Another is the *tumour-specific transplantation antigen*, which is present on the cell's surface. The situation is not unlike that of lysogeny in bacteria, when bacteriophage may remain latent in the organismal DNA during a temperate phase; so far it has not been possible to induce the DNA tumour viruses to multiply excessively and kill the tumour cells as occurs with bacteriophage in a virulent phase. Perhaps this takes place when tumours regress spon-

taneously or as a result of X-ray therapy; there is, however, no evidence for it. The poxviruses, although containing DNA, behave somewhat differently; they remain in the cytoplasm and replicate there.

The RNA Oncogenic Viruses

The RNA oncogenic viruses, called *oncoviruses* (alternatively called *oncornaviruses*) are one of three genera within the family of *retroviruses*.[*][62,63] These are single-stranded, RNA-containing, enveloped viruses that are characterised by the occurrence of *RNA-dependent (or directed) DNA polymerase*, also called *reverse transcriptase* (the first syllables of these two words are the origin of the word retrovirus), within the virion. The enzyme transcribes the viral RNA into *DNA provirus*, which is then integrated with the DNA of the chromosomes of the host cell. This process is of great theoretical interest in being a reversal of the usual sequence of DNA control of RNA and protein formation in the cell (see pp. 20 and 268). The provirus encodes for further viral RNA, and free virus particles are released from the infected cells. These can then infect adjacent cells, and the tumour can grow by local recruitment. It follows that if a tumour is transplanted from one animal to another, the transplanted tumour soon becomes replaced by tumour cells of host origin.

Oncoviruses behave like temperate bacteriophage, and never cause a cytopathic effect as do some of the DNA oncogenic viruses. They can transform a normal cell into a genetically stable cancer cell because of the presence of their reverse transcriptase. The oncoviruses are associated with leukaemia and sarcoma in birds, mice, and cats, and with mammary tumours in mice. Historically these conditions have been associated with particles, subdivided into A, B, and C types on the basis of their location and electron-microscopic structure.[64,65] *A particles* are found in the cytoplasm of mammary tumours, and appear to have a double shell giving them a doughnut-shaped form with a diameter of about 70 nm. *B particles* are found only outside cells, from which they arise by budding (Fig. 29.6). They have an envelope derived from altered cell membrane, and negative staining reveals regularly-spaced projections from the surface (these are called peplomeres). In early forms the B particles contain a double-shelled structure (similar to that of A particles), but this soon alters to form an electron-dense, eccentrically-placed core, or nucleoid. It is uncertain whether B particles are derived from A particles or whether they are separate structures; both occur in mammary tumours. *C particles* are also extracellular, and are associated with avian, murine, and feline leukaemia and sarcomata.[66] They also develop by budding from the cell surface, and their envelope encloses a centrally-placed electron-dense core (Fig. 29.7). It seems certain that B and C particles are the causative agents of some animal tumours, and the finding of similar particles in human tissue has lent weight

---

*The two other genera of the retroviruses are the *lentiviruses* and the *spumaviruses*. The lentiviruses (lentus is Latin for slow) cause slowly progressive brain and lung diseases in sheep, called respectively visna and maedi. The lentiviruses are not to be confused with the slow viruses that cause kuru and related diseases (p. 291). The spumaviruses (spuma is Latin for foam) produce a foamy appearance in cells grown in culture. They lie latent in various animals.

Figure 29.6
Type B virus. This section is from a C_3H mouse mammary carcinoma. Virus particles are seen to be budding from the tumour cells. The mature virus particles have an eccentric core (arrows). × 35 000. (*Photograph by courtesy of Dr. A.F. Howatson, University of Toronto.*)

to the concept that viruses also cause some human malignancies.

Oncoviruses contain a *group-specific* (*gs*) *antigen* which is common to the viruses that infect a particular species of animal. Thus mammalian oncoviruses have a common gs antigen distinct from that of avian viruses. It has been found that the gs antigen can be a component of the normal cells in the appropriate species, and that its presence is determined by a dominant autosomal gene. This remarkable finding has led to a number of hypotheses. Perhaps infective virus could be generated by apparently uninfected cells. Possibly the DNA provirus exists in all normal cells as part of a normal gene pool—the so-called oncogene. Another possibility is that informational transfer from DNA to RNA, and back to DNA, is a normal process. Disruption of this transfer mechanism, e.g. by radiation or chemical damage, could result in an alteration of the genetic information encoded in a cell during its lifetime.

It is not certain whether oncogenic viruses merely initiate the cells, which then pursue an independent course of neoplasia (as with chemical agents), or whether the presence of the virus (perhaps in an unrecognised form) is necessary for the continued propagation of the tumour. It is certain that Koch's postulates (Appendix 2) have to be modified in respect to establishing the viral aetiology of tumours, inasmuch as it is common to find no virus at all in such a tumour, at least by currently available methods.

At present much research is being done in investigating a viral aetiology for certain human tumours. The essential criterion, the inoculation of suspected viruses into human beings, is clearly impracticable. Instead, a train of circumstantial evidence is necessary:

Figure 29.7
Type C virus. This preparation of type C virus has been stained with uranyl acetate. Both the envelope and the core are well shown. The bar indicates 100 nm. (*From Lo, R. and Howatson, A.F. (1975) Positive staining of type C viruses. Microscopical Society of Canada, 11, 56.*)

(a) The isolation and titration of virus or viral nucleic acid in human tumours.
(b) Its effects on cells grown in tissue culture with special reference to transformation. This applies to the DNA viruses; the RNA viruses do not cause transformation.
(c) Its oncogenic effect in animals.
(d) The presence of antibodies in the affected individual and in the population in general.
(e) The epidemiology of the lesion.
(f) The prophylactic effect of a vaccine against the virus in reducing the incidence of the tumour. There are, however, formidable problems in assessing safety and evaluating effectiveness in the preparation and use of any such vaccine.

Of human tumours, four seem to have an association with viruses. (a) *Burkitt's tumour*, which is described on p. 397, is associated with a herpesvirus called the EB virus, after the two workers Epstein and Barr who first isolated it in 1964. This virus has been cultured from the neoplastic lymphocytes of the tumour, and all patients have high-titre antibodies to the virus. The picture is, however, complicated by the fact that antibodies are present in lower titre in many normal controls, and that the virus is established as the cause of infectious mononucleosis with a positive Paul-Bunnell reaction. It is therefore impossible to incriminate EB virus as the cause of Burkitt's tumour without serious reservations. It might be merely a passenger. Another possibility is that it produces infectious mononucleosis in healthy people, but in children with chronic infections that have already caused RE and lymphocytic hyperplasia, the added assault of the EB virus leads to lymphocytic neoplasia. This suggestion would explain the geographical distribution of the tumour—it is found where there is a high incidence of endemic malaria. There is experimental evidence that mice given *Plasmodium berghei yoelii* malaria suffer immunological suppression, and are particularly susceptible to a lymphoma from Maloney leukaemogenic virus.[67] Immunosuppression has also been reported in children with malaria.[68]

In vitro, the EB virus confers the property of continuous growth on normal human B lymphocytes in culture in a way that is analogous to malignant transformation, and it has been shown to cause malignant lymphoma in South American cotton top marmosets.

(*b*) *Nasopharyngeal carcinoma.*[69] Some patients with this tumour have a high titre of antibodies to the EB virus, but as with the Burkitt tumour the precise relationship between the virus and the tumour is complex and poorly defined.

(*c*) Virus particles identical electron microscopically with the Bittner factor have been found in human *breast cancer* cells.[70-72] Of even greater significance, the milk of women with a close family history of cancer of the breast contains similar virus particles much more frequently (60 per cent) than does the milk of normal women (5 per cent). In the Parsi community of Bombay there is a very high incidence of breast cancer, much greater than in the Hindu and Moslem population, and once again virus particles have been frequently found in the milk of Parsi women (39 per cent).[71]

The murine (Bittner) RNA virus contains RNA-dependent DNA polymerase which catalyses the synthesis of DNA. This DNA has a base sequence which is complementery to that of the viral RNA and will hybridise with it. Thus the DNA may be used as a specific agent for detecting viral RNA. It has been found by Spiegelman that DNA synthesised under the influence of murine virus will hybridise *in vitro* with RNA extracted from human mammary cancers (67 per cent), but not with extracts from normal breasts or benign tumours.[72,73] This is very strong evidence that human tumours contain an oncogenic RNA virus very similar to the Bittner factor, but nevertheless its precise relationship to the tumour remains to be determined. The technique of detecting molecular hybridisation of RNA from human tumours with DNA formed by known animal oncogenic RNA viruses is being extended. Thus human sarcomata[74] and lymphomata[75] contain RNA related to mouse leukaemia virus.

(*d*) Women with *carcinoma of the cervix*[76] have a higher incidence of antibodies to herpes simplex virus type 2 than do normal women. There is a close relationship between cervical cancer and sexual intercourse. The tumour is almost unknown in nuns and is commonest in prostitutes and those who are promiscuous.

Summary

It is apparent from the above discussion that most tumours arising in adult life have no known cause. Some, however, can be related to occupational and environmental factors, some are associated with pre-existent disease of a particular area of tissue, and finally there is a group of rare conditions in which there is an hereditary predisposition to tumour formation at a particular site. Hormones do not appear to play a very significant role in causing cancer, but are of great importance in the life-history of some tumours that depend on them for their survival. The role of viruses in human cancer is still problematic.

THE PRECANCEROUS STATE: INITIATION AND PROMOTION

It was already noted in the early years of experimental coal-tar carcinogenesis that when the skin of a mouse had been painted with tar it was peculiarly prone to develop tumours at the site of any wound inflicted on the painted area. In the decade 1940 to 1950 there was enough evidence to indicate that carcinogenesis was a multiple stage phenomenon. When the skins of mice or rabbits were treated with carcinogenic hydrocarbons and later with croton oil, many tumours developed on that area. The concept arose that a subthreshold dose of carcinogen had *initiated* a group of cells, so that they became 'latent' tumour cells which were finally *promoted* to overt cancerous activity by a non-specific traumatising agent like croton oil. The interesting hypothesis of initiation and promotion has received much support from the work of Berenblum and his colleagues, who found that after painting an area of mouse skin with one application of a carcinogen and then subjecting it to numerous applications of croton oil, a latent period elapsed, after which a specific number of tumours appeared. If the croton oil treatment was delayed, the development of tumours was equally delayed, but the final number that developed was the same as when the croton oil had been applied at once. Initiating agents have a dose-dependent, irreversible, and additive effect which is transmissable to the cell's progeny. Cell proliferation is next needed, and after a number of divisions, the cancer cell emerges. Injury, such as that produced by the action of a promoting agent, speeds up this process. Promoting agents are therefore non-specific and act slowly. It is postulated that carcinogens, or their activated products, alter DNA either by binding to it directly or by modifying RNA-dependent DNA polymerase.[77] When the concept of initiation and promotion is applied to occupational cancer, the long latent period between leaving employment and developing the tumour becomes readily understandable.

In fact the processes of initiation and promotion are less clearly divisible than has been described above. No pure chemical promoter has yet been isolated, for even croton oil has a mildy carcinogenic action on mouse skin. Nearly all initiators are also promotors, but urethane is said to be a pure initiator for mouse skin. As most local carcinogens, even the polycyclic hydrocarbons, tend to be absorbed, they are capable of initiating a wider area of tissue than would be expected at first sight. Nowadays the concept of *cocarcinogenesis*, the collaboration of a number of different factors in the production of cancer, is often used instead of initiation and promotion.

Thus a whole field of tissue could be so altered by an initiating agent that, when subjected to non-specific promoting agents, like croton oil, heat, or physical trauma, it tends towards multicentric malignancy. During the phase of initiation the tissue shows no changes to indicate a cancerous transformation. It is normal microscopically. Only later promotion indicates its latent malignant potentiality.

There is a similar two-stage mode of carcinogenesis in respect of remotely-acting agents. Croton oil promotes cancer in skin initiated with oral 2-acetylaminofluorene. Likewise, oestrogen will promote cancer in mouse breasts initiated by hydrocarbons or the Bittner virus.

EARLY MALIGNANT LESIONS

In the early days of experimental tar carcinogenesis it was noted that areas of hyperplasia and even discrete papillomata appeared at the sites of treatment, but that they tended to disappear if the agent was discontinued in time. They recurred rapidly, however, if the agent was reapplied. The nature of these lesions is obscure.

In the human the question of early malignant change is of great importance, for it is at this stage that complete eradication is easiest. In recent years a number of interesting lesions involving epithelial surfaces have been recognised. In these areas the epithelium is undergoing atypical proliferation. The orderly maturation of cells as they reach the surface is lost. The cells vary in size and shape, have large, darkly-staining nuclei, and show an increased amount of mitotic activity. The term *dysplasia* is applied to this change. When it is severe, the cells appear anaplastic, tend to lose their polarity, and lie haphazardly in relationship to one another. They have the microscopic changes usually associated with malignancy, and since there is no invasion of the underlying connective tissue, the terms *carcinoma-in-situ* or *intraepithelial carcinoma* are used (Fig. 29.8). In stratified squamous epithelium there may be foci of abnormal keratinisation within the area of cell proliferation, and this is called *malignant dyskeratosis*.

The natural history of these premalignant changes is not known for certain. Dysplasia may progress to *carcinoma-in-situ* and ultimately invasive tumour. The progression from one stage to the next is often slow, and the possibility exists that some lesions regress.

Carcinoma-in-situ has been described in most epithelia, and it is encountered most typically in the stratified squamous covering epithelium of the skin, mouth, and cervix. Some clinical examples are worth noting:

Bowen's disease of the skin. This occurs in the middle-aged and elderly, and appears as discrete, red plaques which are sometimes mistaken for superficial basal-cell carcinoma, or resistant chronic dermatitis or psoriasis. Any area of the skin may be implicated. Invasive carcinoma may finally ensue, sometimes after many years.

Figure 29.8
Carcinoma-in-situ. This is a skin biopsy from a case of Bowen's disease. The cells are pleomorphic, and the orderly arrangement of the upper layers of the prickle-cell layer is disrupted. A number of cells have large, darkly-staining nuclei, and elsewhere in the section there were mitotic figures. There is a heavy lymphocytic infiltration in the dermis. Serial sections of the block failed to show any evidence of invasion. × 200.

Actinic, or solar, keratoses. All gradations of changes are seen varying from mild atypicality of the epithelial cells to *carcinoma-in-situ* and on occasions invasive squamous-cell carcinoma. This rarely metastasises, but it is advisable to treat all senile keratoses.

Erythroplasia of Queyrat. This is a rare condition almost always involving the penis, and it manifests itself as a red, velvety plaque of *in-situ* carcinoma.

Leukoplakia with Dysplasia.* This appears as dead-white shiny plaques on a mucous membrane. The mouth and tongue are commonly affected, and the vulva is another favourite site. Microscopically the epithelium shows all degrees of cellular atypicality ranging from mild dysplasia to *carcinoma-in-situ*. Invasive squamous-cell carcinoma may develop, especially in the vulva.

Cervical erosions. Most of these are quite benign, but occasionally *carcinoma-in-situ* and even an early invasive carcinoma is found to co-exist. For this reason all erosions should be examined cytologically.

Similar changes may be encountered in adenomatous polyps

---

*The term leukoplakia is often used clinically in its literal sense to describe any white plaque on a mucosal surface. This may include candidiasis, epithelial naevi, simple keratoses due to trauma, dysplasia, carcinoma, and lichen planus, as well as other less common conditions. To some pathologists the term implies a dysplastic condition that will in due course progress to invasive cancer. Hence the term should never be used without qualification.

of the uterus and colon that are undergoing early cancerous transformation. The gastric and bronchial epithelia may also be affected.

Paget's disease of the skin.[78] This has its greatest incidence on the nipple, but may also occur on extramammary sites such as the vulva, anal region, and axilla. Clinically there is an eczematous lesion which consists histologically of large, round Paget cells with pale, clear cytoplasm (often containing much mucoprotein in the extramammary lesions but not always in the breast lesions) and large, vesicular nuclei with prominent nucleoli infiltrating the lower part of the epidermis (Fig. 29.9). In many instances, especially in the mammary and anal lesions, there is an underlying adenocarcinoma which may be contiguous with the skin lesion, and it was originally suggested that this was the result of intra-epithelial invasion of the deeper cancer. However, in many cases elsewhere in the skin there is no underlying malignancy, and the breast tumour itself is sometimes too deep to be in contact with the skin lesion. It is now widely held that Paget's disease is an example

Figure 29.9
Paget's disease of the nipple. The epidermis is thickened; its prickle-cell layer contains numerous, large, palely-staining round cells with prominent vesicular nuclei. These are typical Paget cells. Clinically there had been an eczematous eruption of the skin of the left breast for over a year. Although no tumour could be palpated, mammography showed a suspicious mass, and carcinoma was confirmed after mastectomy. × 120.

of *carcinoma-in-situ*, and that, where there is an underlying tumour, it is to be regarded as a second primary neoplasm in a field of growth.

Whenever *carcinoma-in-situ* is encountered histologically, it is important to examine multiple sections of the tissue in order to exclude the possibility of invasive cancer in an adjacent area.

EXFOLIATIVE CYTOLOGY[79, 80]

When cancer involves a lining epithelium, some of the neoplastic cells are shed on to the surrounding surface. If the surface is internal, these cells are trapped in the secretion of the part, and ultimately discharged to the exterior. Bronchial carcinoma cells may be coughed up in the sputum, gastric carcinoma cells may be aspirated in the gastric juice, and cervical carcinoma cells may be shed into the vaginal secretions. In recent years much progress has been made in recognising clumps of cancer cells in such secretions, and sometimes this allows for an early diagnosis of malignant disease. The technique of exfoliative cytology has its greatest value in the diagnosis of cervical cancer, where an area of early carcinoma may be so small that it is missed in a routine examination of the part.

Cancer of the Cervix Uteri

Papanicolaou and his colleagues first described the use of vaginal and cervical smears in the diagnosis of uterine cancer, and they have shown that malignancy can be diagnosed by the recognition of abnormal exfoliated cells (Fig. 29.10). In addition to obvious cancer cells, other abnormal forms are sometimes found. These cellular abnormalities have been called *dyskaryosis* by Papanicolaou, because the principal changes are found in the nucleus. The nuclei are enlarged and show variation in size and shape. Hyperchromatism is present, and the nucleoli are enlarged. A careful comparison of the smears with subsequent biopsy specimens has confirmed that the morphology of the cells accurately reflects the changes in the cervical mucosa. The varying degrees of dysplasia, *carcinoma-in-situ*, and invasive carcinoma may therefore be diagnosed by the exfoliative cytologist.

The significance of these cervical lesions is at present under review, but there is convincing statistical evidence from the USA that many cases of epithelial dysplasia progress to *carcinoma-in-situ* and finally invasive cancer. In the cervix at least, cancer appears to develop over a period of many years, and the appearance of invasive tumour heralds the final act of a long drama which commences with mild atypia and progresses through dysplasia and *carcinoma-in-situ*. Extensive projects are now under way in which whole populations are being routinely screened for cervical disease, and the treatment of these early lesions already appears to be reducing the incidence of invasive cancer. Before such campaigns are started, there are two prerequisites: firstly, there must be an adequate number of trained diagnostic cytologists, and secondly, the surgeons must be aware of the nature of the lesions which they will be called upon to treat.

When a Papanicolaou ('PAP') smear is found to be positive for abnormal cells, it should be repeated to exclude errors of interpretation or labelling. The precise course of action varies

Figure 29.10
Cancer cells in a vaginal smear. There is a clump of large, darkly-staining cancer cells surrounded by numerous pus cells. Note the size and irregularity of the cells. This patient had an anaplastic carcinoma of the cervix. × 320.

from one centre to another. Patients with mild dysplasia can be followed for evidence indicating that their disease is progressing. Severe dysplasia and *carcinoma-in-situ* demand more active treatment. The experienced and equipped gynaecologist can detect abnormal areas of the cervix by using the colposcope: these areas can be biopsied (to exclude invasive carcinoma) and treated by cryotherapy. Another course of action is to biopsy a large cone of cervical tissue and search for abnormal areas. This form of treatment can lead to complications due to scarring. When invasive cancer is detected, the choice of treatment lies between hysterectomy and radiotherapy, or a combination of both. It is evident that the management of carcinoma of the cervix involves technical skills and good judgement. There are few other areas in medicine where the technician, the pathologist, and the clinician must collaborate if their patients are to receive the best treatment. Over-diagnosis and over-treatment can result in unnecessary surgery that may prevent young women from bearing children. Under-diagnosis and under-treatment, on the other hand, can lead to the patient's death.

Sputum, gastric contents, urine, and the fluid obtained by prostatic massage can all be examined for malignant cells. A similar technique can be used to investigate pleural and peritoneal effusions. Those secondary to cancer may contain numbers of neoplastic cells, and the method is useful both

diagnostically and prognostically. Care must be taken not to mistake metaplastic serosal cells for malignant cells.

THE INCIDENCE OF TUMOURS

Incidence of tumours in plants.[81] True tumours are described in plants, and form a fascinating subject. The best known is *crown gall* caused by the bacterium *Phytomonas tumefaciens*; the organism is present in the primary but not in the secondary growths. Mushrooms develop tumours when treated with tar, and in clover tumours can be induced by a virus acting after injury.

Incidence of tumours in animals.[81] Tumours have been described in most species which have been studied. Thus melanoma and lymphoma occur in *Drosophila*. So far as vertebrates are concerned, the best-known tumours occur in species valued as pets, or used for food or experimental purposes. The following may be cited:

DOGS: Mammary fibro-adenoma, interstitial-cell tumours of testis, carcinoma of skin, tonsil, and breast. Boston and Scottish terriers have a high incidence of mast-cell tumours.

PARAKEETS AND BUDGERIGARS: Pituitary tumours.

HORSES: Teratoma of testis, melanoma of skin, carcinoma of skin, mouth, and nasal sinuses.

BOVINE ANIMALS: Carcinoma of skin, adrenal cortical tumours.

PIGS: Nephroblastoma.

Incidence of Tumours in Human Beings

Age. In European children the incidence of malignancy is small, the commonest tumours being acute leukaemia and the rather uncommon embryonic tumours mentioned in Chapter 27. Nevertheless, cancer is the most important cause of childhood mortality in civilised countries now that infections have been so well combated. In adolescence and early adult life malignancy is also uncommon, the most frequent tumours being osteosarcoma, leukaemia, and Hodgkin's disease. At this age carcinoma occurs sporadically, but its incidence does not become significant until the fifth decade is reached, when it rapidly assumes its lethal role especially between the ages of 60 and 75 years. The Registrar-General's figures for England and Wales for the year 1973 reveal that 65 406 males and 55 891 females died as the result of tumours (including leukaemia), and that about 80 per cent of the victims were over the age of 55 years. The question repeatedly arises as to whether there is an actual increase in the incidence of tumours in the world's population as a whole, or in the population of any country in particular. It is extremely difficult to give a straight answer to this. In only the most civilised countries are the statistics of tumour incidence of any value, and even in such areas many fatal tumours are not confirmed by histological examination. It is amongst civilised communities that the medical services are the most adequate, and many tumours are revealed in them which would remain undiagnosed in primitive, under-privileged groups. On the other hand, as cancer incidence increases with age, it is the civilised groups who, by living longer, are more prone to develop neoplasms. Cancer is widespread in many primitive communities, in whom the age of onset is often earlier than in Europeans. As will be seen, the pattern of tumours is different. The age expectancy of such groups is also less due to the effects of poverty. It will be interesting to see whether this tumour pattern will approximate more closely to the European one when the fundamental causes of disease have been removed by education and economic progress.

Sex. Apart from the malignancy of those organs peculiar to each sex it seems that most neoplasms are commoner in men than in women. According to the Registrar-General's Statistics for 1973 fatal cancer of the oral cavity, tongue, and bladder was about twice as common in men as in women, while cancer of the respiratory tract four times more common in the male sex: in the kidney, pancreas, stomach, and rectum there was a slight male predominance. A few noteworthy exceptions to this rule were cancers of the breast, gallbladder, and thyroid. Breast cancer was 150 times commoner in women than in men, and it accounted for about a fifth of all fatal neoplasia in women. Cancer of the biliary passages and thyroid cancer were 1.5 to 3 times as common in women as in men. Hypopharyngeal carcinoma was the one malignancy in the oropharyngeal region which was slightly commoner in women than in men, and much of it is associated with a pre-existing Plummer-Vinson syndrome. Cancer of the colon, excluding the rectum, was distinctly more common in the female sex (6086 fatal cases in women as opposed to 4222 in men). The commonest fatal neoplasm in women was cancer of the breast (11 428 cases), and in men cancer of the lung (25 997 cases).

Over the age of 75 years there was a moderate decrease in the incidence of malignancy, a tendency more marked in men than in women. An exception was cancer of the prostate, which was most prevalent in old men (2243 of the total 4236 occurred over the age of 75 years). In extreme old age cancer was distinctly commoner in the female sex, a trend accentuated by the greater longevity of women as compared with men.

Social class. Apart from specific occupational factors already discussed there is statistical evidence that cancer of the skin, penis, mouth, oesophagus, and stomach is commoner in the 'lower' social groups, whereas cancer of the breast is decidedly more prevalent in women of the 'higher' social groups.

Heredity. This has already been discussed.

The Incidence of Specific Tumours

It is by investigating the incidence of specific tumours in a community that aetiological factors are most likely to be discovered. Detailed surveys have now established that lung cancer is much commoner in heavy smokers than in those who smoke moderately or not at all. Likewise the danger of leukaemia has been proved to be much greater in those who have been exposed to large doses of ionising radiation than in the population at large. The data of geographical pathology have thrown much light on the incidence of tumours in different countries.[82-84] For instance, the commonest malignancies in White Europeans affect the lung, breast, stomach, and colon, but in black Africans these types of cancer (other than the breast) are generally not at all common, whereas cancer of the skin, penis, cervix, and liver predominate. But even this statement is too vague—there are millions of Black

Africans, and in even one country the incidence of tumours may vary according to locality. A survey in Uganda[85] showed inexplicable concentrations of penile, gastric, oesophageal, and skin cancers in various localities; where one tumour was common another was hardly ever seen. It was particularly interesting that the incidence of penile cancer varied tremendously despite the fact that nearly all the men were uncircumcised. Similarly Kaposi's tumour, generally regarded as one of the commonest neoplasms in Black Africans, shows great regional variations, and is much commoner in East and Southern Africa than in West Africa. Nasopharyngeal cancer is very common in South-East Asians, especially those of Chinese origin, and is also frequent in some East Africans. It must be admitted that there is no explanation of these facts.

In order to rationalise the knowledge about the geographical incidence of tumours, the following factors may be cited:

External environment. This may be of some importance in stomach cancer, for in Britain there is an excess of cases in North Wales and the Fen District of East Anglia,[86] and the high peat content of the soil has been incriminated.[87] The actual effect of this is unknown. Actinic skin cancer is another example.

Nutrition. Liver cancer in Black Africans and Asians has been attributed to nutritional cirrhosis. Aflatoxin is a more likely factor.

Occupation. This has already been discussed.

Cultural and religious customs. The rarity of penile cancer in those groups who practice ritual circumcision, and the liability to oral cancer of those South-East Asians who chew betel quid are good examples of regional variations of tumours due to national habits.

Racial constitution. A good example is the virtual immunity of the dark-skinned races to the carcinogenic action of sunlight on the skin. Carcinoma of the testis is almost unknown in the Black African, and carcinoma of the prostate and chronic lymphatic leukaemia are very uncommon in the Japanese and Chinese.[88] By contrast chronic lymphatic leukaemia is common in Israeli Jews.[88] The explanation of these findings is not known. It seems probable that in all tumours genetic factors play some part even when there is overwhelming evidence of an exogenous cause.

It will be useful to conclude this discussion of the aetiology of tumours by briefly considering some factors that are of importance in the incidence of various neoplasms.

Cancer of the skin. *Geographical factors.* Actinic skin cancer is discussed on page 369. Regional examples of skin cancer are the *Kangri cancer* of Kashmir and the *Kang cancer* of North-West China (Fig. 29.11). The Kangri is a charcoal heater carried to the abdomen, and following its continual use carcinoma of the abdominal skin may develop.

The Kang is a hollow bed heated from below by burning coals. People who sleep on such a bed may develop cancer of the skin of the thigh and leg. It is probable that carcinogenic agents in the soot initiate the tumour, and the heat of the burner merely acts as a promoting agent. Melanoma of the feet is common in Black Africans as is also Kaposi's tumour.

Occupational factors. Ionising radiations and the application of hydrocarbons may produce squamous-cell cancers of the skin. Ingested inorganic arsenic is also carcinogenic, and may lead to cutaneous cancer many years after exposure has ceased.

Figure 29.11
Kang cancer. A portion of skin removed from the trochanteric region of the thigh. There is an extensive area of fungating squamous-cell carcinoma. (I 19.6, *Reproduced by permission of the President and Council of the R.C.S. Eng.*)

Keratoses on the palms are characteristic, and these may show malignant change. Bowen's disease and invasive squamous-cell carcinomata are also common.[89]

Genetic factors. Xeroderma pigmentosum has already been mentioned. Another condition inherited as a recessive character which is liable to be complicated by skin cancer is albinism (p. 588).

Chronic skin lesions, e.g. varicose ulcers and old osteomyelitis sinuses, have already been described as precursors of squamous-cell cancer.

Cancer of the penis. Penile cancer is almost unknown in Jews, who practise circumcision soon after birth, and uncommon in Moslems, who perform it later in childhood. However, it is an uncommon form of cancer in uncircumcised white Europeans, especially of the higher social groups, and even in uncircumcised black Africans its incidence varies greatly according to locality (see p. 384). It is probable that the semgma acts as a solvent for carcinogenic agents in the environment. The cancer is commonest in those whose standard of personal hygiene is low, and is probably always preceded by chronic balanitis.

Cancer of the lip. This is commonest in elderly, White, pipe-smoking, agricultural workers. The sunlight probably initiates the tumour, and the heat of the pipe promotes it to activity on the basis of a preceding actinic cheilitis.

Cancer of the mouth. *Geographical factors.* Oral cancer is very common amongst some communities in South-East Asia who indulge in the habit of betel chewing. The quid, which is kept in the mouth for long periods of time, consists of betel nut, spices, tobacco, lime, and buyo leaves. The carcinogenic principle probably resides in the betel nut.[90] The buccal aspect of the cheek and lower jaw is the usual site, but the tongue may also be involved. Another peculiar habit associated with oral cancer is reverse-cigar smoking, which is practised in parts of India, Sardinia, and Latin America. The lighted end of the cigar is held in the mouth which is burned in consequence. Cancer of the palate may ensue.

There is evidence that the consumption of alcohol interacts with tobacco smoke and other agents to cause cancer of the mouth, pharynx, larynx, and oesophagus. Pure alcohol is not carcinogenic to animals, and it seems probable that alcohol renders some other agent soluble, or that the agent is another component of alcoholic drinks.[9]

Chronic disease. There is little evidence that hot food or chronic dental disease predispose to oral cancer, but tobacco smoking is of importance. Women with the Plummer-Vinson syndrome show an increased incidence of oral cancer.

Cancer of the oesophagus.[91] *Geographical factors.* The interesting feature of the epidemiology of oesophageal cancer is its tendency to occur in almost epidemic proportions in circumscribed areas, while elsewhere it is quite uncommon.[9,88] Areas of high incidence include the Transkei in the Easter Cape Province of South Africa, the area of Bulawayo in Rhodesia, that part of the USSR around the Caspian sea, Northern Iran, south of the Taihang Mountains in Northern China, and around the Kenyan coast of Lake Victoria. The reason for these local areas of high incidence is not known.

The highest incidence of oesophageal cancer in Europe is found in France in Brittany and Normandy, where the population consumes large amounts of cider and cider-based liqueurs. Investigations have shown that the highest incidence of oesophageal cancer is found in men who drink a large amount of alcohol and smoke many cigarettes.[9]

Genetic factors. There is an interesting association between a type of congenital tylosis (thickening of the epidermis of the palms and soles) and oesophageal cancer.[92]

Chronic disease. Long-standing achalasia of the cardia is sometimes complicated by cancer. The relation of the Plummer-Vinson syndrome to postcricoid and upper oesophageal cancer has already been noted.

Cancer of the stomach. *Geographical factors.* Cancer of the stomach is most prevalent in the Japanese, and is also common in parts of Siberia. Its incidence falls through Eastern Europe to the West, and it is low in the White community of the USA, South Africa, and Australasia. Japanese and Black African groups conform to the White population's incidence of stomach cancer in Hawaii and the USA respectively.[9,88] There is no known dietary association with the condition. The possibility that soil conditions may be important has been noted, but at present the evidence is unimpressive.

Genetic factors. There is an increased incidence of blood group A in cases of gastric cancer.

Chronic disease. As already noted, there is no causal relationship between peptic ulceration and cancer. On the other hand, it is accepted that pernicious anaemia (Ch. 52) may predispose to malignancy, for the incidence of cancer is three times that found in normal stomachs. In one series it was found that 10 per cent of patients with pernicious anaemia eventually developed gastric cancer.[93] Gastric adenomata sometimes become malignant. There is no positive proof that alcohol, hot food, or imperfectly masticated material are important factors in the aetiology of gastric cancer.

Cancer of the colon. *Geographical factors.* These are not as definite as in gastric or oesophageal cancer, but the tumour is common throughout Western Europe, North America, and Australasia.[88] Its relative uncommonness in Africans may be due to the high-fibre diets they take. Colonic cancer is seven times commoner in people on a low-fibre diet, and this may be due to the effect of constipation in allowing carcinogens in the diet to remain for a longer period in contact with the colonic mucosa than would be the case in those with regular bowel actions.[94]

It has been found that the faeces of groups in whom colonic carcinoma is common contain large numbers of anaerobic bacteriodes organisms, unlike the faeces of vegetarians, which contain *Sarcina ventriculi.* Furthermore, anaerobic bacteroides degrade steroids by dehydrogenating the α-hydroxyl groups, and the amount of metabolic products in pooled faeces, especially the hydroxycholanic acids, correlate very closely with the incidence of cancer of the colon in the community.[9]

Genetic factors. The classical example of polyposis coli has already been discussed.

Chronic disease. The relationship between ulcerative colitis and cancer has already been mentioned. Solitary and multiple benign polyps (tubular adenomata and villous adenomata) also tend to become malignant. In some there is a familial tendency.[95]

Cancer of the lung. *Geographical factors.* Lung cancer has its maximum incidence in Britain, especially Scotland. It is common in Western Europe, especially Finland and Germany, but is not nearly so common in the USA, Canada, Australia, and South Africa despite the large number of cigarettes smoked in these countries. It is very common in the Maoris and Hawaiians.[88]

Occupational factors are of importance in the aetiology of the disease. The peculiar pulmonary malady that afflicted the miners of Schneeberg and Joachimstal for so long has now been diagnosed as lung cancer, and it is generally attributed to radioactive substances, like *radon*, rather than metallic ores present in the inhaled dust. *Nickel workers* are prone to cancer of the nasal sinuses and the lungs, and there is evidence that *chromium* may have a similar effect. *Arsenical sheep-dip workers* are also predisposed to lung cancer.

Some of the pneumoconioses predispose to cancer; *asbestosis* is by far the most important, the tumour being either a squamous-cell carcinoma or else a diffusely spreading pleural lesion described as a mesothelioma. Similar lesions of the peritoneum have also been found. Where there is cancer of the lung associated with the inhalation of asbestos, there is always a degree of preceding asbestosis, and the incidence is greatest in cigarette smokers. All commercial types of asbestos are liable to lead to lung cancer.[96] On the other hand, mesothelioma is strongly associated with the inhalation of blue asbestos (crocidolite), there need be no associated pulmonary fibrosis, and there is no relation to cigarette smoking. It is possible that people who have been unwittingly exposed to crocidolite fibre may later develop mesothelioma, but only about 200 mesotheliomata are diagnosed per year in Britain, and of these at most 60 occur in people with no known exposure to asbestos.[96]

There is some tendency for *haematite-worker's lung (siderosilicosis)* to undergo malignant change, but uncomplicated silicosis and coal-miner's pneumoconiosis are not precancerous.

There can be little doubt that *heavy tobacco smoking* predisposes to lung cancer, and that the danger is greater in cigarette users than in pipe smokers. The malignancy is usually of squamous-cell or oat-cell type, but not adenocarcinoma. At present no adequate cause has been found to explain the dangerous effects of tobacco smoking. Another factor of undetermined importance is atmospheric pollution with soot and smoke: it probably acts in concert with tobacco smoking in producing lung cancer. Since the incidence of lung cancer drops even if smoking is discontinued late in life, it may be that the tobacco acts more as a promoter than an initiator.

There is no evidence that chronic inflammatory disease, such as tuberculosis, bronchiectasis, or fungal disease, is precancerous. Bronchitis is, however, commoner in patients with cancer. This is no doubt attributable to smoking (see p. 544).

Cancer of the liver. The importance of preceding cirrhosis has already been mentioned. Other inflammatory diseases of the liver, such as schistosomiasis and syphilis, do not appear to be precancerous. However, cancer of the larger intrahepatic bile ducts (malignant cholangioma) is very common in the Far East, and is attributable to infestation of the bile ducts with liver flukes.

Cancer of the breast. The incidence of breast cancer is greatest in the USA and Canada and in Western Europe. It decreases in Eastern Europe and the USSR and is uncommon in Central Asia and Japan—indeed, its incidence is the reverse of that of gastric cancer. While not very common in the Black African, it is as common in the Black as in the White population of the USA. It is traditionally held that childlessness and inadequate lactation are important predisposing causes of breast cancer, but more recent investigations have not substantiated this theory. Perhaps a dietary factor is implicated on the same basis as postulated in regard to colonic cancer. It may be that in susceptible groups conditions in the colon are suitable for the productions of steroidal oestrogens.[9]

Mammary dysplasia is not regarded as a premalignant condition, since the lesions do not commonly progress to malignancy. Nevertheless, cancer is more liable to develop in a breast that is also affected by dysplasia, suggesting that the two diseases share a common contributory factor—probably a hormonal imbalance.

Cancer of the uterus. The relationship between cervical cancer and coitus has already been noted. The tumour is generally a common one, but is rare in Jewesses.[88] The circumcision of the Jewish husband may be an important factor. Cancer of the body of the uterus is much less common than cervical cancer; it has a fair incidence in Canada and the USA. The relationship between ovarian granulosa-cell tumour and endometrial cancer has been mentioned.

Cancer of the bladder. The relation to aromatic amines has been noted. Tobacco smoking predisposes to bladder cancer, particularly in the male.[97,98]

Cancer of the thyroid. Its relationship to goitre has already been noted. It has also followed the exposure of the area to ionising radiation (see p. 408).

Testicular tumours. A considerable increase in the incidence of testicular tumours has taken place recently in Denmark, and probably also elsewhere.[99] The reason for this is unknown.

Osteosarcoma. Radioactive elements that are stored in the bones are possible agents in producing osteosarcomata. The case of the girls who swallowed radium and mesothorium in the luminous paint used for painting watch-dials is mentioned on page 408. A more current hazard is the pollution of the atmosphere with radioactive strontium following nuclear explosions. Strontium, like radium and calcium, is stored in the bones. The relationship of Paget's disease to osteosarcoma has already been noted.

THE NATURE OF CANCER

Neoplasia is generally assumed to be related to the uncontrolled growth of cells.[100] Whether the change is in the cells themselves or in the local tissue environment is not known. Thus it is possible that carcinoma is due not to a change in the involved epithelial cells but to a disturbance of the epithelial-connective tissue arrangement. Such interaction is well known in embryogenesis,[101] and there is some evidence that the same is true in neoplasia. When skin is treated with methylcholanthrene, an early change is fragmentation and reduplication of the basement membrane and destruction of the superficial connective tissue. Such changes are not seen in skin treated with non-carcinogenic irritants.[102] Furthermore, polyoma virus will produce tumours in the submandibular gland tissue in embryo mice only if epithelial and connective tissue are both present.[103]

In spite of these interesting observations it is currently believed that the events responsible for the development of malignancy reside in the affected neoplastic cells, and it is convenient at this point to summarise the known properties of malignant cells. The variations from the normal which they exhibit have been extensively studied in the hope that this would explain the fundamental nature of the malignant process itself, and provide the basis for rational treatment.

Changes in Appearance

The pleomorphism and bizarre appearances of malignant cells have already been considered in detail, as have also the nuclear changes, chromosomal abnormalities, and variations in DNA content (see p. 337). There is, however, no constant variation characteristic of all tumour cells.

Changes in Chemical Content

Nucleic acid. Whether the change in DNA content noted above is a reflection of an abnormality in the molecular structure is not known, i.e. there is no definite evidence of a mutation. The incorporation of viral DNA or virus-produced DNA has been described previously. The RNA content of malignant cells tends to be as high as in any actively growing tissue. The endoplasmic reticulum is usually poorly formed and the mitochondria tend to be sparse.

Enzymatic activity[104] The early studies on tumour metabolism *in vitro* led Warburg to conclude that tumour cells obtained their energy by glycolysis, even in the presence of oxygen. Exceptions to the rule have since been found, and furthermore some normal tissues, e.g. retina, have a similar type of metabolism. Extensive investigations into the enzyme contents of cancer cells have shown that tumour cells tend to contain the same enzymes as the parent tissue, but that the quantity is usually reduced. Numerous quantitative biochemical abnormalities have been described in cancer cells and in patients also. So far no reliable tests have materialised, though many have been tried. Thus, an increase of β-glucuronidase activity has been found in the vaginal secretions of women with cervical carcinoma, but the test is unreliable.

Antigens. This has already been discussed (p. 371).

Changes in the Cell Membrane[105]

Many chemical differences in the cell membrane of normal cells as opposed to malignant cells have been catalogued, but little insight into the fundamental nature of neoplasia has been attained. Thus there is an increased protease activity in malignant cells, and normal cells treated with protease temporarily acquire many properties of transformed (malignant) cells. Malignant cells exhibit an increased mobility of their surface receptors, and this may be associated with changes in the membrane-associated cytoskeletal components (p. 15). Anti-tumour antibodies, by becoming attached to these receptors, could induce them to form clusters or patches (p. 16). Subsequent endocytosis would remove the antigenic receptors from the surface, thereby allowing the cell to escape from further damaging effects of the antibody. Proof that this mechanism is of any significance in the control of tumour growth is lacking.

Changes in Behaviour

In vivo. Progressive growth is the characteristic of neoplasia; malignant tumours invade and metastasise. Even so, the phenomena of dormancy and regression indicate that some tumours undergo phases of retrenchment.

Inappropriate secretion.[106] This is a common phenomenon. Epidermal cells can produce mucus, as in Paget's disease, and respiratory epithelial tumours can form keratin (see metaplasia p. 305). The inappropriate secretion of hormones is described on page 339. Tumour cells may revert to activities normally seen only in their parents during embryonic life. The formation of carcino-embryonic antigen has been noted on page 372. Another example of considerable practical importance is seen in cancer of the liver. *Alpha-fetoprotein* is a globulin which normally forms about 50 per cent of the total plasma proteins of the fetus. Its formation ceases in the third trimester, and it is therefore absent from the serum at birth. In 50 to 79 per cent of cases of hepatoma α-fetoprotein reappears in the plasma, and its presence has proved to be a useful diagnostic test. It is also found in cases of yolk-sac tumour.

In vitro. Malignant cells do not, on the whole, grow nearly so well as cells from normal tissues. However, a few lines of cancer cells have so adapted themselves to cell culture that they are now well established and grown in many laboratories; the HeLa cell is a good example. Such cells lack the alignment of normal cells grown in tissue culture, and tend to heap up into several layers. Normal cells (with the exception of lymphocytes and haematopoietic cells) form monolayers, and will grow only on a firm surface such as glass or solid agar: they are described as *anchorage dependent*. Growth ceases if the concentration of cells becomes too high, a phenomenon described as *contact inhibition of growth*. Normal cells also need an unidentified factor present in normal serum for their growth. Virus-transformed malignant cells are less anchorage dependent, and will grow in soft agar. They show less contact inhibition of growth and require little or no serum factor. Finally, normal cells have a finite life-span (p. 28), whereas some neoplastic cells have acquired the property of indefinite life provided suitable growth facilities are provided either in tissue culture or in a host animal.[107]

This brief survey of the properties of the cancer cell is sufficient to indicate that although there are often many points of difference from the normal, there is no single characteristic by which it can be recognised. Perhaps it is wrong to expect that this should be so. The well-documented morphological features of cancer cells are of great importance to the cytologist, but researches into cell metabolism have been essentially sterile both as regards a reliable cancer test and the elaboration of an effective chemotherapeutic agent. Studies of the antigenic composition and the *in-vitro* behaviour of tumour cells may perhaps yield more fruitful results.

CONCLUSION

It is humiliating to reflect that the vast majority of tumours arising in adults have no apparent cause, and appear to develop spontaneously. While some geographical factors are suggestive and a few occupational hazards have been successfully unmasked and controlled, there is still no indication as to the cause of cancer or the nature of its perverted growth. At present all that can be hoped for in the treatment of cancer is a radical removal using surgical resection or radiotherapy.

These measures are effective only when the tumour is localised, but there is much evidence that cancer is not a local disease. Even if removal of the entire field of growth is feasible, the presence of secondary deposits presents an unknown hazard. Since these may remain dormant for many years, it is evident that the assessment of the effects of local treatment is very difficult. When the disease is clinically generalised, the cytotoxic agents may be used as the means of attack. Hormone therapy may produce some alleviation of symptoms.

The most successful approach to the control of cancer at the present time lies in its prevention.[108] The many known physical and chemical carcinogenic agents have already been described, and their avoidance can appreciably reduce the incidence of cancer. Each tumour must be considered separately, e.g. a reduction in the amount of cigarette smoking and atmospheric pollution would undoubtedly reduce the incidence of lung cancer, while the elimination of aflatoxin and the control of malnutrition might diminish that of liver cancer. The careful screening of drugs for carcinogenic activity in animals is an important aspect of public health. It is impossible to foretell the carcinogenicity of a substance from its chemical formula alone.

A second method of cancer prophylaxis is the treatment of known precancerous lesions. In the previous chapters a point of view has been expressed that cancer must be defined and diagnosed in terms of its invasive behaviour. The observations on the development of uterine cancer indicate that invasive tumour is the final development of a sequence of precancerous lesions. These are sometimes reflected in the abnormal appearance of the cells, and in the cervix can be detected and treated with relative ease. Cancer of the cervix uteri is therefore a preventable disease. It is probable that all invasive cancers commence in a similar manner, but in the vital organs treatment is not so easy. Thus in the case of the lung, *carcinoma-in-situ* can be diagnosed and located with the aid of the exfoliative cytologist, but even if it is practicable to excise the lesion, it is impossible to remove the whole field of growth, i.e. both lungs. The avoidance of carcinogens is obviously a more practical method of controlling the tumour. So far, no effective methods have been devised to control the common gastric, colonic, and mammary cancers.

The failure of workers in basic cancer research to produce any results which can be translated into action in the treatment of human disease has encouraged clinicians to adopt a more experimental approach to cancer therapy. The ritual of applying standard treatment to cases where the outlook is hopeless is being augmented or replaced, in well-controlled series, by other methods—for instance those based on an immunological concept, but here too the results are not encouraging.

REFERENCES

1. FIALKOW, P. J. (1971) Single or multiple cell origin for tumors? *New England Journal of Medicine*, **285**, 1198.
2. FIALKOW, P. J. (1974) The origin and development of human tumors studied with cell markers. *New England Journal of Medicine*, **291**, 26.
3. Leading Article (1976) Cell tracers in disease. *Lancet*, **2**, 1181.
4. BECK, W. S. (1976) New outpost on the trail of polycythaemia vera. *New England Journal of Medicine*, **295**, 951.
5. STERN, B. D. & KAPLAN, L. (1969) Multicentric foci of carcinomas arising in structures of cloacal origin. *American Journal of Obstetrics and Gynecology*, **104**, 255.

6. GOLDBLATT, M. W. (1958) Occupational carcinogenesis. *British Medical Bulletin*, **14**, 136.
7. Leading Article (1972) Scrotal cancer continues. *British Medical Journal*, **4**, 3.
8. HADFIELD, E. H. (1970) A study of adenocarcinoma of the paranasal sinuses in woodworkers in the furniture industry. *Annals of the Royal College of Surgeons of England*, **46**, 301.
9. DOLL, R. (1977) The prevention of cancer. *Journal of the Royal College of Physicians of London*, **11**, 125.
10. Leading Article (1974) Vinyl chloride and cancer. *British Medical Journal*, **1**, 590.
11. Leading Article (1974) More facts on vinyl chloride and cancer. *British Medical Journal*, **4**, 486.
12. Leading Article (1976) Vinyl chloride: the carcinogenic risk. *British Medical Journal*, **2**, 134.
13. BONSER, G. M. (1967) Factors concerned in the location of human and experimental tumours. *British Medical Journal*, **2**, 655.
14. Leading Article (1975) More on the aflatoxin-hepatoma story. *British Medical Journal*, **2**, 647.
15. Leading Article (1968) Nitrites, nitrosamines, and cancer. *Lancet*, **1**, 1071.
16. FAIRLEY, G. H. (1971) Immunity to malignant disease in man. *British Journal of Hospital Medicine*, **6**, 633.
17. KLEIN, G. (1968) Tumor-specific transplantation antigens. *Cancer Research*, **28**, 625.
18. KLEIN, G. (1968) Summary: antigens of chemically induced tumors; and search for tumor-specific antigens in other human cancers. *Cancer Research*, **28**, 1354.
19. PREHN, R. T. (1968) Tumor-specific antigens of putatively nonviral tumors. *Cancer Research*, **28**, 1326.
20. ZAMCHECK, N. *et al.* (1972) Immunologic diagnosis and prognosis of human digestive-tract cancer: carcinoembryonic antigens. *New England Journal of Medicine*, **286**, 83.
21. MACH, J. -P. *et al.* (1974) Detection of recurrence of large-bowel carcinoma by radioimmunoassay of circulating carcinoembryonic antigen (C.E.A.). *Lancet*, **2**, 535.
22. SMITH, R. T. & ADLER, W. H. (1970) Human tumor immunity. *New England Journal of Medicine*, **282**, 1320.
23. Leading Article (1971) 'Unblocking' factors in antitumour immunity. *Lancet*, **2**, 753.
24. Leading Article (1971) Antibodies against tumours. *British Medical Journal*, **4**, 505.
25. LEWIS, M. G. *et al.* (1969) Tumour-specific antibodies in human malignant melanoma and their relationship to the extent of the disease. *British Medical Journal*, **3**, 547.
26. HELLSTRÖM, K. E. & HELLSTRÖM, I. (1972) Some aspects of the cellular and humoral immune response to tumour antigens. *Triangle*, **11**, 23.
27. BANSAL, S. C. & SJÖGREN, H. O. (1972) Counteraction of the blocking of cell-mediated tumor immunity by inoculation of unblocking sera and splenectomy: immunotherapeutic effects on primary polyoma tumors in rats. *International Journal of Cancer*, **9**, 490.
28. Leading Article (1976) BCG in cancer. *British Medical Journal*, **1**, 1487.
29. Leading Article (1975) Immunological control of cancer. *Lancet*, **1**, 502.
30. Leading Article (1976) Immunostimulation. *Lancet*, **2**, 349.
31. HELLSTRÖM, I. & HELLSTRÖM, K. E. (1966) Recent studies on the mechanisms of tha allogeneic inhibition phenomenon. *Annals of the New York Academy of Sciences*, **129**, 724.
32. MÖLLER, G. & MÖLLER, E. (1966) Interaction between allogeneic cells in tissue transplantation. *Annals of the New York Academy of Sciences*, **129**, 735.
33. LYNCH, H. T. (1969) Genetic factors in carcinoma. *Medical Clinics of North America*, **53**, 923.
34. KNUDSON, A. G. (1974) Heredity and human cancer. *American Journal of Pathology*, **77**, 77.
35. Leading Article (1976) Polyposis coli and the stomach. *British Medical Journal*, **2**, 900.
36. SWANBECK, G. (1971) Aetiological factors in squamous cell skin cancer. *British Journal of Dermatology*, **85**, 394.
37. Leading Article (1974) Xeroderma pigmentosum. *Lancet*, **1**, 792.
38. ANDERSON, D. E. *et al.* (1967) The nevoid basal cell carcinoma syndrome. *American Journal of Human Genetics*, **19**, 12.
39. HARNDEN, D. G. (1976) Chromosome abnormalities and predisposition towards cancer. *Proceedings of the Royal Society of Medicine*, **69**, 41.
40. Leading Article (1976) Crohn's disease. *Lancet*, **2**, 1284.
41. Leading Article (1975) Dangers of silent gallstones. *British Medical Journal*, **1**, 415.
42. WYNDER, E. L. ONDERDONK, J. & MANTEL, N. (1963) An epidemiological investigation of cancer of the bladder. *Cancer (Philadelphia)*, **16**, 1388.
43. Leading Article (1976) Oestrogen as a cause of endometrial carcinoma. *British Medical Journal*, **1**, 791.
44. SYMMERS, W. St. C. (1968) Carcinoma of breast in trans-sexual individuals after surgical and hormonal interference with the primary and secondary sex characteristics. *British Medical Journal*, **2**, 83.
45. HERBST, A. L. *et al.* (1972) Clear-cell adenocarcinoma of the genital tract in young females: registry report. *New England Journal of Medicine*, **287**, 1259.
46. Leading Article (1974) Vaginal adenocarcinomas and maternal oestrogen ingestion. *Lancet*, **1**, 250.
47. FARRELL, G. C. *et al.* (1975) Androgen-induced hepatoma. *Lancet*, **1**, 430.
48. Leading Article (1975) More on liver tumours and the pill. *British Medical Journal*, **4**, 484.
49. Leading Article (1976) Oral contraceptives and liver nodules. *Lancet*, **1**, 843.
50. DAVIS, M. *et al.* (1975) Histological evidence of carcinoma in a hepatic tumour associated with oral contraceptives. *British Medical Journal*, **4**, 496.
51. O'SULLIVAN, J. P. (1976) Oral contraceptives and liver tumours. *Proceedings of the Royal Society of Medicine*, **69**, 351.
52. Veterans Administration Co-operative Urological Research Group: Treatment and survival of patients with cancer of the prostate (1967). *Surgery, Gynecology and Obstetrics*, **124**, 1011.
53. Leading Article (1976) Hormone receptors and breast cancer. *British Medical Journal*, **2**, 67.
54. CRILE, G. (1960) Endocrine dependency of tumours of the thyroid. *American Journal of Surgery*, **99**, 533.
55. Leading Article (1971) Progestogens and cancer. *British Medical Journal*, **1**, 360.
56. Leading Article (1969) Asparaginase. *British Medical Journal*, **2**, 465.
57. ALLEN, E. P. (1955) Malignant melanoma; spontaneous regression after pregnancy. *British Medical Journal*, **2**, 1067.
58. EPSTEIN, M. A. (1971) The possible role of viruses in human cancer. *Lancet*, **1**, 1344.
59. ALLEN, D. W. & COLE, P. (1972) Viruses and human cancer. *New England Journal of Medicine*, **286**, 70.
60. Leading Article (1975) As in cats, so in man. *Lancet*, **1**, 503.
61. Leading Article (1975) Vaccination against an oncogenic herpesvirus. *Lancet*, **1**, 504.
62. FENNER, F. J. & WHITE, D. O. (1976) *Medical Virology*, 2nd edn, p. 170. New York: Academic Press.
63. FENNER, F. (1976) Classification and Nomenclature of Viruses: *Second Report of the International Committee on Taxonomy of Viruses*. Basel: S. Karger.

64. DALTON, A. & HAGUENAU, F. (1973) *Ultrastructure of Animal Viruses and Bacteriophages*, Chs 13, 15, and 16. New York: Academic Press.
65. DE HARVEN, E. (1968) In *Experimental Leukemia*, p. 97. (Morphology of murine leukemia viruses), ed. Rich, M. A. New York: Appleton-Century-Crofts Inc.
66. GROSS, L. (1976) The role of C-type and other oncogenic virus particles in cancer and leukemia. *New England Journal of Medicine*, **294**, 724.
67. WEDDERBURN, N. (1970) Effect of concurrent malarial infection on development of virus-induced lymphoma in Balb/c mice. *Lancet*, **2**, 1114.
68. GREENWOOD, B. M. *et al.* (1972) Immunosupression in children with malaria. *Lancet*, **1**, 169.
69. Leading Article (1976) Aetiology of nasopharyngeal carcinoma. *Lancet*, **2**, 1393.
70. MOORE, D. H. *et al.* (1971) Search for a human breast cancer virus. *Nature (London)*, **229**, 611.
71. Leading Article (1971) A virus in human breast cancer? *Lancet*, **1**, 741.
72. Leading Article (1972) Viruses and human breast cancer. *Lancet*, **1**, 359.
73. AXEL, R., SCHLOM, J. & SPIEGELMAN, S. (1972) Presence in human breast cancer of RNA homologous to mouse mammary tumour virus RNA. *Nature (London)*, **235**, 32.
74. KUFE, D., HEHLMANN, R. & SPIEGELMAN, S. (1972) Human sarcomas contain RNA related to the RNA of a mouse leukemia virus. *Science*, **175**, 182.
75. HEHLMANN, R., KUFE, D. & SPIEGELMAN, S. (1972) Viral-related RNA in Hodgkin's disease and other human lymphomas. *Proceeding of the National Academy of Sciences of the United States of America*, **69**, 1727.
76. Leading Article (1976) Herpesvirus and cancer of uterine cervix. *British Medical Journal*, **1**, 671.
77. RYSER, H. J-P. (1971) Chemical carcinogenesis. *New England Journal of Medicine*, **285**, 721.
78. Leading Article (1972) Paget's disease of the skin. *British Medical Journal*, **1**, 707.
79. WAY, S. (1963) *The Diagnosis of Early Carcinoma of the Cervix*. London: Churchill.
80. KOSS, L. G. (1968) *Diagnostic Cytology and its Histopathological Bases*, 2nd edn. Philadelphia: Lippincott.
81. McMANUS, J. F. A. (1966) *General Pathology*, p. 64 *et seq.* Chicago: Year Book Medical Publishers.
82. DAVIES, J. N. P. *et al.* (1964) Cancer in an African community, 1897–1956. *British Medical Journal*, **1**, 259 and 336.
83. BARUAH, B. D. (1964) Cancer in Assam: observations based on a study of 2,493 biopsy specimens of malignant tumours. *Cancer (Philadelphia)*, **17**, 413.
84. FARAGO, C. (1963) Report of 1,160 registered tumor cases in Papua and New Guinea. *Cancer (Philadelphia)*, **16**, 670.
85. HUTT, M. S. R. & BURKITT, D. (1965) Geographical distribution of cancer in East Africa: a new clinicopathological approach. *British Medical Journal*, **2**, 719.
86. LEGON, C. D. (1951) A note on geographical variations in cancer mortality, with special reference to gastric cancer in Wales. *British Journal of Cancer*, **5**, 175.
87. STOCKS, P. & DAVIES, R. I. (1960) Epidemiological evidence from chemical and spectrographic analyses that soil is concerned in the causation of cancer. *British Journal of Cancer*, **14**, 8.
88. DOLL, R. (1972) Cancer in five continents. *Proceedings of the Royal Society of Medicine*, **65**, 49.
89. LEVER, W. F. and SCHAUMBURG-LEVER, G. (1975) In *Histopathology of the Skin*, 5th edn, p. 246. Philadelphia: Lippincott.
90. SURI, K., GOLDMAN, H. M. & WELLS, H. (1971) Carcinogenic effect of a dimethyl sulphoxide extract of betel nut on the mucosa of the hamster buccal pouch. *Nature (London)*, **230**, 383.
91. Leading Article (1976) Cancer of the oesophagus. *British Medical Journal*, **2**, 135.
92. CLARKE, C. A., HOWEL-EVANS, A. W. & McCONNELL, R. B. (1957) Carcinoma of oesophagus associated with tylosis. *British Medical Journal*, **1**, 945.
93. ZAMCHECK, N. *et al.* (1955) Occurrence of gastric cancer among patients with pernicious anaemia at the Boston City Hospital. *New England Journal of Medicine*, **252**, 1103.
94. BURKITT, D. P. (1971) Epidemiology of cancer of the colon and rectum. *Cancer (Philadelphia)*, **28**, 3.
95. MORSON, B. C. (1971) Precancerous conditions of the large bowel. *Proceedings of the Royal Society of Medicine*, **64**, 959.
96. Leading Article (1976) Exposure to asbestos dust. *British Medical Journal*, **1**, 1361.
97. Leading Article (1971) Smoking and cancers of the bladder and kidney. *Lancet*, **1**, 635.
98. Leading Article (1972) Bladder cancer and smoking. *British Medical Journal*, **1**, 763.
99. Annotation (1968) An epidemic of testicular cancer? *Lancet*, **2**, 164.
100. ROSE, S. M. (1970) *Regeneration: Key to Understanding Normal and Abnormal Growth and Development*, Ch. 9, p. 229 (tumor formation—a case of never-completed regeneration). New York: Appleton-Century-Crofts.
101. FLEISCHMAJER, R. & BILLINGHAM, R. E. (Eds.) (1968) *Epithelial–Mesenchymal Interactions*, p. 326. Baltimore: Williams and Wilkins.
102. TARIN, D. (1968) Further electronmicroscopic studies on the mechanism of carcinogenesis: the specificity of the changes in carcinogen-treated mouse skin. *International Journal of Cancer*, **3**, 734.
103. DAWE, C. J., MORGAN, W. D. & SLATICK, M. S. (1966) Influence of epithelio-mesenchymal interactions on tumour induction by polyoma virus. *International Journal of Cancer*, **1**, 419.
104. GREENSTEIN, J. P. (1954) *Biochemistry of Cancer*, 2nd edn, pp. 327–506. New York: Academic Press.
105. NICOLSON, G. L. & POSTE, G. (1976) The cancer cell: dynamic aspects and modifications in cell-surface organization. *New England Journal of Medicine*, **295**, 197 and 253.
106. SMITH, J. B. (1970) Alpha-fetoprotein: occurrence in certain malignant diseases and review of clinical applications. *Medical Clinics of North America*, **54**, 797.
107. STOKER, M. (1970) New growth and viruses. *British Medical Journal*, **3**, 541.
108. RAVEN, R. W. & ROE, F. J. C. (1967) *The Prevention of Cancer*. London: Butterworth.

Chapter 30. *The Stem Cell and the Reticulo-Endothelial System: Their Pathological Associations*

The connective tissues of the body, apart from those of the central nervous system, differentiate from mesenchyme. This embryonic connective tissue consists of stellate cells embedded in a gelatinous ground substance in which there are reticulin fibres. While mesenchyme, as thus defined, is found only in the fetus, there are nevertheless primitive connective tissue elements that persist throughout life, and are capable of proliferation and differentiation as the necessity arises. These elements exist as large cells with a pale, basophilic cytoplasm and a round or indented nucleus containing prominent nucleoli. They are multipotential and are called *stem cells*. Though probably scattered throughout all the tissues, they are found in greatest number in the lymph nodes, spleen, and bone marrow, where they are closely associated with the reticulin framework of the organs.

The cellular content of the lymphatic organs includes stellate *reticular cells* responsible for laying down the reticulin framework, *histiocytes*, and *lymphocytes*. Among these cells there are large forms that used to be called 'reticulum cells', and were regarded as primitive mesenchymal cells. At present the view is that these 'reticulum cells' have no independent identity, and are probably of histiocytic origin. Indeed, many of them may be transformed lymphocytes rather than histiocytes (see p. 400).

It is now considered that morphologically a stem cell can be a small lymphocyte. The precise morphology of bone-marrow stem cells is less clear (see p. 600). Allogeneic small lymphocytes labelled with tritiated thymidine have been seen to enlarge and undergo mitosis when administered to an animal,[1] and in irradiated animals lymphocytes not only repopulate the lymph nodes but also provide fresh lymphoid tissue.[2] It should be noted that, although the immunologically competent cell is also a lymphocyte, it does not follow that every lymphocyte is immunologically competent. The body's content of lymphocytes probably includes a number of different types of cell, each with a similar appearance but of dissimilar function. The immunologically competent cell may be regarded as a lymphocyte that has differentiated towards an immunological function.

The stem cell is capable of giving rise to the following cells:

The reticulo-endothelial system, which is endowed with phagocytic powers.

The haematopoietic cells.[3]

Connective tissue cells, i.e. fibroblasts, chondroblasts, osteoblasts, and synovial cells. A stem cell which is differentiating in this direction first starts to lay down reticulin fibres, and is called a reticular cell. Stem cells may also give rise to fat cells and mast cells.

Vascular endothelial cells, at least during embryonic development. The newly formed blood vessels so prominent in granulation tissue are believed to be derived from the proliferation of adjacent endothelial cells.

Smooth muscle cells. It is possible that the muscle forming the wall of arterioles which develop in a healing wound is derived from the local fibroblasts or pericytes which have dedifferentiated during the repair process. This may be the basis of connective tissue metaplasia, when fibroblasts assume an osteoblastic or synovial potentiality.

The stem cells of the adult are found predominantly in the spleen, liver, bone marrow, and lymph nodes, where they give rise to the lymphoid, haematopoietic, and reticulo-endothelial cells of these organs. They also lay down the reticulin framework. The development of the blood cells is described in Chapters 52, 53, and 54, while the connective tissue elements are discussed in Chapter 5. At this stage it is therefore necessary to consider the reticulo-endothelial system.

THE RETICULO-ENDOTHELIAL SYSTEM

The term *reticulo-endothelial system* was coined by Aschoff in 1924 to delineate a large collection of cells that shared a common origin, morphology, and phagocytic function. The characteristic phagocytic functions he regarded as essential for grouping these cells into a single system were the uptake of a vital dye, e.g. trypan blue, and the scavenging of a particulate marker e.g. colloidal carbon. In fact neither of these two functions provides an acid test, for poorly phagocytic cells, like reticular cells, endothelial cells, and fibroblasts, can also become labelled by pinocytosis, and if the markers are released from strongly phagocytic cells, e.g. when these cells die, they can be taken up by other more feebly phagocytic cells. The cells that have been included in Aschoff's reticulo-endothelial system are the 'reticulum cells' of the spleen and lymph nodes, the cells lining the lymphatic and blood sinuses, e.g. of the lymph nodes, spleen, and liver (where they are called Kupffer cells—Fig. 30.1), the monocytes of the blood, and the tissue histiocytes. The name reticulo-endothelium was derived from the close relationship of some of these cells to the reticulin framework that intersects the lymph nodes and spleen, and their endothelium-like appearance when lining sinuses in these organs. But the cells of this system are very different both morphologically and functionally from both endothelial cells and reticular cells, and the name reticulo-endothelial (RE) system is inappropriate. It is retained in this book because it is in general use by pathologists.

At a conference held in Leiden in 1969 a group of workers proposed a new classification of this system of cells, which they call the *mononuclear phagocyte system*.[4] They propose that the following cells form part of this system:

Precursor cells from the bone marrow.

Promonocytes from the bone marrow.

Figure 30.1
Sinus-lining cells of liver (Kupffer cells). These are well delineated because they have taken up particles of black malarial pigment. × 320.

Monocytes from the bone marrow and the blood.

Macrophages, which include the connective-tissue histiocytes, the liver Kupffer cells, the alveolar macrophages of the lung, the sinus-lining cells and free macrophages of the spleen and lymph nodes, the pleural and peritoneal macrophages and those of the bone marrow, and probably also the osteoclast which is believed to arise by coalescence of monocytes. The microglial cell of the central nervous system is also regarded as a probable candidate for membership of this system.

The functional criteria for including the macrophages, monocytes, and promonocytes in a single system are avid phagocytosis and pinocytosis (especially phagocytosis), and the ability to attach firmly to a glass surface. Monocytes and macrophages have receptor sites for immunoglobulins and complement at the cell surface. They are to be regarded as 'professional' phagocytes as opposed to such 'facultative' phagocytes as the fibroblast, endothelial cell, and reticular cell, which can ingest particles at a low rate independent of immunoglobulins or complement, and probably have no receptors for these components.[4]

Morphologically these cells tend to vary considerably. Thus macrophages have many more lysosomes and mitochondria than do monocytes. But they are fairly large cells, 10 to 25 μm in diameter with kidney-shaped or oval nuclei which are single and contain nucleoli. Sometimes they are difficult to distinguish from lymphocytes, which, of course, differ in function, life span, and origin. A lymphocyte should not be called a phagocytic mononuclear cell.

The cells of the mononuclear phagocyte system originate from precursor cells in the bone marrow, are transported in the blood as monocytes, and eventually become tissue macrophages. This sequence is described on page 126 in respect of chronic inflammation. There is no evidence that mononuclear phagocytes are derived from lymphocytes. The most immature member of the system that can be recognised in the bone marrow is the promonocyte, but presumably there is an even more immature precursor cell. The monocytes are a pool of relatively immature cells in the blood, and when conditions are favourable for phagocytosis, these cells become macrophages and develop the necessary equipment for digesting phagocytosed material. Thus the monocyte is the origin of the macrophage populations in the various organs mentioned above. Whether the fixed macrophages of the spleen, lymph nodes, and bone marrow (the sinus-lining cells) are also derived from monocytes is not certain, but the probability is that they are. In the spleen and lymph nodes both free and fixed macrophages lie in close association with the reticulin fibres—the free ones lie in the interstices of the framework formed by reticular cells, while the fixed ones are attached to cytoplasmic extensions of the reticular cells, but unlike these cells, the fixed macrophages do not form reticulin fibres.[4]

While the RE (or mononuclear phagocyte) system is widely dispersed throughout the tissues of the body, most of its content is present in the liver, bone marrow, lymph nodes, and spleen. They are sometimes called the *reticulo-endothelial organs* on this account. They are also sometimes described as the *lymphoreticular tissues* because of their reticulin framework and the predominance of lymphocytes, though in the marrow the granulocytic and normoblastic elements far outnumber the lymphocytic ones.

FUNCTIONS OF THE RETICULO-ENDOTHELIAL SYSTEM

Phagocytosis

LOCAL. The appearance of large phagocytic cells is characteristic of the demolition phase that follows acute inflammation (Fig. 30.2). It is seen during the stage of resolution, and also in the early phases of repair by granulation tissue. These macrophages ingest cell debris, broken-down red cells, fibrin, and organisms, e.g. *S. typhi*, *Myco. tuberculosis*, *Myco. leprae*, and many of the fungal and protozoal pathogens. Macrophages are the predominant cells of foreign-body reactions.

GENERAL. Once an organism gains access to the lymphatics and blood stream, the sinus-lining cells of the lymph nodes, liver, spleen, and bone marrow provide an effective defence. In bacteraemia these last three organs are able to eliminate the offending organism quite rapidly, but in septicaemia they are inadequate (see Ch. 8).

On some occasions the organisms are engulfed by the RE cells, and enter into a state of virtual symbiosis. This occurs in histoplasmosis and leishmaniasis (Fig. 30.3). Inevitably some damage is produced by the organism, but the disease runs a very protracted course. Either the patient or the organism may finally win the battle.

The Immune Response

The relationship between the RE system, the lymphocyte, and the formation of antibodies is described in detail in Chapter 12.

Figure 30.2

Microglial reaction in an area of cerebral softening. There is almost complete disintegration of brain substance, and an infiltration of round, swollen macrophages. These are phagocytosing the debris, and the granular appearance of their cytoplasm is due to its content of fat and haemosiderin. These cells are called compound granular corpuscles. × 330.

Figure 30.3

Leishmania donovani in a macrophage. This is a bone-marrow smear taken from a sternal puncture. In the centre there is a large macrophage stuffed with parasites. Each organism has one large nucleus and a smaller, rod-shaped structure called a *kinetoplast*. The membrane surrounding each individual organism is not clearly seen. The patient was a Maltese man, aged 25 years, who had visceral leishmaniasis (kala-azar). × 700.

Red-Cell Destruction and Iron Metabolism

Effete red cells are broken down by the RE cells, especially in the spleen, after fragmentation in the circulation (see Ch. 52). The haem moiety of the haemoglobin is divested of its iron, which is stored in the RE cell. It is combined there with apoferritin to form *ferritin*, which consists of about 23 per cent ferric iron. Where there is massive blood breakdown, e.g. following a local extravasation, the iron-binding protein is supersaturated with ferric iron (over 35 per cent) to form *haemosiderin*. The tetrapyrrolic ring structure of the haem is broken up, and eventually bilirubin is formed.

Storage

The RE system stores excess amounts of lipids and mucoproteins, and the cells become swollen. In the event of cholesterol storage the cytoplasm assumes a foamy appearance in paraffin sections (Fig. 30.4).

PROLIFERATIVE LESIONS OF THE STEM CELL AND ITS DERIVATIVES

Proliferation of the stem cell and its derivatives is a very common condition, and, when generalised, it is manifested clinically by an enlargement of the liver, spleen, and lymph nodes. Such a proliferation may be an apparently purposeful response to some stimulus, e.g. infection, when it comes into the category of hyperplasia, or else it may entail the purposeless progressive multiplication of neoplasia. These proliferations have in the past been assembled under a single heading of *reticulosis*, but fortunately this term and the unwieldy classifications that were derived from it are no longer in vogue.

Hyperplasia

INFECTIVE ('REACTIVE') HYPERPLASIA. This very common condition is seen to its best advantage in the lymph nodes. Proliferation involves not only the reticulo-endothelial elements but also the cells involved in the immune response. When immunoglobulin production is evoked, the lymphoid follicles are enlarged and increased in number, and in their midst there are large pale germinal centres. Coincidentally many plasma cells are formed in the medulla. Hyperplasia occurs in the paracortical zone when cell-mediated immunity

Figure 30.4
Xanthoma. This tumour arose from the skin, and the section through the dermis shows an extensive accumulation of 'foam cells', which are macrophages filled with lipid material (mostly cholesterol). During the histological processing of the tissue, the fat is dissolved out of the cells by the clearing agent, e.g. xylene or chloroform; this accounts for the appearance of clear cytoplasm surrounding the central nuclei. A Touton giant cell is also present. (See Figs. 11.2a and 11.2b.) × 250.

is stimulated. The reticulo-endothelial hyperplasia is evidenced by proliferation of the sinus-lining cells, producing accumulations of macrophages in the dilated sinuses ('sinus catarrh').

Reactive hyperplasia may produce such marked distortion of lymph-node structure that lymphoma is sometimes closely simulated. This has been described in *toxoplasmosis*,[5] *infectious mononucleosis*,[5] in the lymph nodes draining a site of vaccination (*post-vaccinal lymphadenitis*),[6] and in epileptic patients who take *anticonvulsant drugs* such as dilantin[7] and methoin, and develop a morbilliform eruption, arthropathy, hepatosplenomegaly, and lymphadenopathy.

In chronic widespread pruritic skin diseases there is often a marked regional lymphadenopathy. The characteristic feature is a dense accumulation of RE cells especially in the periphery of the nodes. Some of these cells contain droplets of fat and granules of melanin. This condition of *dermatopathic lymphadenitis* (*lipomelanic reticulosis*) is merely a florid variation of reactive hyperplasia.

Sometimes the RE cells play a very active part in the response against the agent: in sarcoidosis, tuberculosis, cat-scratch disease, and the deep-seated mycoses there are dense focal accumulations of altered macrophages (epithelioid cells), which tend to be arranged in discrete follicles.

The most exuberant examples of infective hyperplasia of the RE system are met with in the systematised (disseminated) conditions of visceral leishmaniasis (Fig. 30.3) and histoplasmosis, where they are vast accumulations of parasitised macrophages in many organs.

In chronic infective hyperplasia of a lymph node there is an ever-increasing thickening of the reticulin framework, and in due course this is converted into dense collagen fibre. Once again the versatility of the proliferating stem cell is demonstrated. In this instance it is giving rise to reticular cells and fibroblasts.

HAEMATOPOIETIC HYERPLASIA. In conditions which demand an increased formation of one of the elements of the blood, there is a hyperplasia of its precursor cells in the bone marrow, e.g. *normoblastic hyperplasia* of the marrow after severe haemorrhage or in people who live at high altitudes, and *leucoblastic (myeloid) hyperplasia* in acute pyogenic infections. If all the marrow space is occupied (as in children in whom there is no reserve of fatty marrow), or if it is replaced by fibrous tissue (as in myelosclerosis), foci of haematopoiesis will be found in extramedullary sites like the spleen, liver, and lymph nodes. This myeloid differentiation is yet another example of the ease with which the multipotential stem cell diverts its development towards one particular line in response to a specific stimulus.

STORAGE HYPERPLASIA. This is of greatest importance in conditions of lipid excess; the RE cells proliferate to accommodate the load. Generalised disorders of lipid storage are called the *lipidoses*. The following are important:

Hyperlipoproteinaemia. Following prolonged hyperlipoproteinaemia there may be sufficient RE cell hyerplasia to cause moderate splenomegaly. Focal accumulations of fat-laden macrophages with occasional Touton giant cells may also be seen in the skin, and are called *xanthomata* (Fig. 30.4). These yellow-orange lesions are not tumours. They are found particularly on the extensor aspects of the limbs and on the eyelids. Plaques of xanthomata on the eyelids of elderly people are called *xanthelasma*; this common lesion may be encountered also in people who have normal plasma lipid levels.

Hypercholesterolaemia with splenomegaly is seen as a rare complication of diabetes mellitus (untreated) and prolonged obstructive jaundice. In addition, there are various types of *familial hyperlipoproteinaemia* which are described in Chapter 49. Xanthomata are common, and in some types there is splenomegaly and hepatomegaly due to the accumulation of lipid-laden macrophages.

In the other lipidoses, of which Gaucher's disease and Niemann-Pick disease are by far the most important examples, the RE cells are filled with abnormal lipids. Both of these conditions are usually inherited as autosomal recessive characteristics, and both are found most frequently in Jewish people.

Gaucher's disease.[8,9] In the common *adult form* of this disease, which runs a protracted course, there is a particularly massive accumulation of macrophages in the spleen which is enormously enlarged, and may be the site of marked overactivity (Fig. 30.5). The liver is also enlarged and the bone marrow is extensively involved, but the lymph nodes show much milder changes. Gaucher's disease is accompanied by a generalised haemosiderosis which gives rise to a brown pigmentation of the skin. A characteristic feature of the disease is

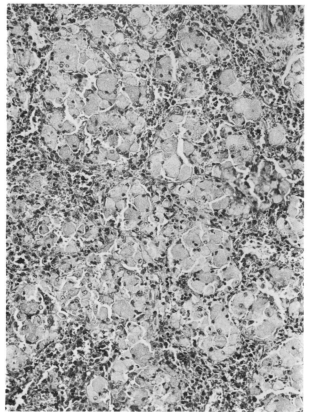

Figure 30.5
Gaucher's disease. In this section of spleen the red pulp contains large numbers of swollen macrophages. Their cytoplasm is full of abnormal lipid which produces a pale, reticulated appearance in histological section. × 100.

the presence of wedge-shaped pingueculae (pigmented scleral thickenings) on each side of the corneae, and these too contain the characteristic cells. The *Gaucher cell* is a grossly enlarged macrophage about 50 μm in diameter with a pale fibrillary cytoplasm somewhat reminiscent of a spider's web. It is not vacuolated, and the usual fat stains are negative, but it is PAS-positive. The lipid contained in the Gaucher cell is a glucocerebroside, and it accumulates because of a deficiency of glucocerebrosidase. Glucocerebroside is probably derived from effete white and red cells in the RE system, and it is not surprising that it is here that the main accumulation of lipid is found. In the brain glucocerebroside is derived from gangliosides, which have a rapid turnover in infancy. It follows that central nervous involvement with severe mental retardation and death is a feature of the *acute neuropathic (infantile)* and *subacute neuropathic (juvenile)* forms of Gaucher's disease. Each type is probably determined by a separate recessive gene.

Niemann-Pick disease.[8,9] This is a more severe condition, which is usually fatal in infancy. The spleen, liver, lymph nodes, and bone marrow are all extensively infiltrated with lipid-laden macrophages, and the parenchymatous cells of the endocrine glands, lungs, bowel, and brain are also affected. Mental retardation is usually present, and about a quarter of the cases present the features of *amaurotic familial idiocy* (including the pathognomonic cherry-red spot in the macula of the retina).*

The cells are somewhat smaller than those of Gaucher's disease, and their cytoplasm is not wrinkled, but instead contains foamy droplets which stain positively with Sudan III and other fat stains. The lipid consists of cholesterol, its esters, and a phosphatide called sphingomyelin. Haemosiderosis is not a feature of this disease.

Both Gaucher's disease and Niemann-Pick disease are examples of inherited disturbances of lipid metabolism associated with a specific enzyme defect. Variants of each probably exist, and there are many other rare lipid storage diseases known, some affecting only the central nervous system.*

Mucopolysaccharide storage. There are a number of rare diseases in which mucopolysaccharide accumulates in phagocytic cells as well as parenchymal tissue. The best known is Hurler's syndrome (gargoylism) (see p. 61).

It is probable that the fundamental defect in most storage diseases is a deficiency in the associated lysosomal hydrolase. The progressive accumulation of adventitious material in the cell leads to dysfunction.

HISTIOCYTOSIS-X. This non-committal title describes a triad of diseases, Letterer-Siwe disease, Hand-Schüller-Christian disease, and eosinophilic granuloma of bone, in which there are focal accumulations of large macrophages in various organs. These cells often contain cholesterol, especially in the more chronic forms of the condition, but this is apparently secondary and not a storage effect. The condition is normocholesterolaemic, and it is not an example of lipid-storage disease.

The most severe of the three disorders is *Letterer-Siwe disease*, which is usually a rapidly fatal malady of infancy. Destructive accumulations of RE cells are found in many organs, especially the spleen, bone marrow, liver, lymph nodes, intestinal mucosa, skin, and lungs. The cells are large and pale, and contain phagocytosed debris. There is usually a mild infiltration of neutrophil and eosinophil polymorphs among these active macrophages.

Hand-Schüller-Christian disease affects a somewhat older age group, and the histiocytic lesions are usually confined to the bones, especially those of the skull. A classical triad of manifestations is produced: defects in the membranous bones of the skull, exophthalmos, and diabetes insipidus. The mandible is often affected, and loosening of the teeth is a common symptom. Occasionally diffuse pulmonary involvement leads to the condition of cystic lung which may be complicated by a spontaneous pneumothorax. Involvement of the liver, spleen, and lymph nodes may also occur, but is much less conspicuous than in Letterer-Siwe disease.

Eosinophilic granuloma of bone is the most benign of the three diseases. It usually affects older children and young adults, and it is typically confined to one bone. It produces a

---

Amaurotic familial idiocy is itself a fatal disease characterised by blindness, paralysis, and dementia. Only the nervous system is affected, and the ganglion cells show ballooning with ganglioside. In the infantile form (*Tay-Sachs disease*), which is confined to Jewish families, there is a characteristic cherry-red spot in the macula. Late infantile, juvenile, and adult forms are also recognised, and these are genetically and biochemically distinct.

painful bony swelling, which is seen radiologically as an area of destruction.

Histologically, in these last two diseases there are focal accumulations of foamy macrophages and giant cells with a variable admixture of eosinophils and polymorphs. The eosinophilia is particularly marked in eosinophilic granuloma of bone. The histiocytic lesions of Hand-Schüller-Christian disease are more proliferative than those of eosinophilic granuloma of bone. As the lesions heal, there is much dense fibrosis replacing the fat-laden macrophages.

The nature of the process underlying these three diseases is obscure. Although Letterer-Siwe disease has many of the features of a highly malignant neoplasm, its histology is rather like that of a chronic inflammatory lesion, and it sometimes merges into the Hand-Schüller-Christian syndrome, which is not clinically reminiscent of a tumour.

Neoplasia of the Stem Cell and its Derivatives[5, 10]

The neoplastic lesions of these cells are the *lymphomata* and the *tumours of the haematopoietic tissues*.

LYMPHOMATA

These are all malignant, and since they vary considerably in their clinical course, many attempts have been made to classify them so that behaviour may be correlated with histological type. There is still no agreed classification, and the nomenclature is confusing. Hence it is often impossible to compare the results of treatment in one centre with those in another.

In the classification most widely used at present, Hodgkin's disease, clinically the most important lymphoma, is separated from the others because of its distinctive histological features. The remaining 'non-Hodgkin's lymphomata' are classified according to the predominant cell type involved, whether lymphocytic or histiocytic, and according to whether the neoplastic cells are disposed in distinct nodules or in a diffuse manner. A nodular disposition is associated with a better prognosis than is a diffuse one. But, as will be pointed out later, there is increasing doubt about the true nature of the neoplastic histiocytes found in the lymphomata (including Hodgkin's disease). The great majority may well be transformed lymphocytes. The nodular lymphomata may become diffuse as the disease progresses, but the diffuse ones never become nodular. The lesions therefore always tend to become more malignant.

The following lymphomata are described:[10]
Histiocytic lymphoma—nodular or diffuse.
Lymphocytic lymphoma—nodular or diffuse. Each may be poorly, moderately, or well differentiated.
Lymphoma, mixed cell type—nodular or diffuse.
Hodgkin's disease. The subdivisions are described later.

Histiocytic lymphoma, also called *reticulosarcoma* and *reticulum-cell sarcoma*, is a disease predominantly of later life. It usually commences in one particular group of lymph nodes, but sometimes the tonsils or the small bowel are the sites of the primary lesion. It soon becomes systematised with splenic, hepatic, and bone-marrow infiltration. Deposits in the lungs, heart, and kidneys are not infrequent. The spread of this group of tumours to the lymph nodes and viscera is probably due both to lymphatic and blood-borne metastasis and to the development of new tumours in a field of growth that includes all the lymphoid tissues. Histologically there is complete obliteration of the normal architecture of the affected lymph nodes, which are massively infiltrated by large, pale, histiocytic cells (Fig. 30.6). On the whole these are uniform in size and shape, but mitotic activity is usually pronounced. Foci of necrosis are usually present, and capsular invasion is a conspicuous feature. Sometimes the histiocytic cells are pleomorphic with many giant cells among them, so that there may be a resemblance to Hodgkin's disease. It is sometimes difficult to distinguish between a histiocytic lymphoma and an anaplastic carcinoma. In some tumours the cells appear primitive and resemble stem cells. Pleomorphism is not marked and the tumour is called a *stem-cell sarcoma*.

Lymphocytic lymphoma. This tumour is commonly called a *lymphosarcoma*, a term which is deprecated by many experts in the field, but which may yet retain its place by virtue of common usage. The neoplastic cells can vary in differentiation and resemble mature lymphocytes (lymphocytic lymphosarcoma) or immature lymphoblasts (lymphoblastic lymphosarcoma). An intermediate group can also be recognised. The nodular variants of these tumours form the common type of the tumour previously called the *giant follicular lymphoma*. See Figure 30.9, page 399.

Lymphocytic lymphoma is about twice as common as histiocytic lymphoma. It too affects an older age group predominantly, and its mode of presentation is similar to that of histiocytic lymphoma. Histologically the architecture of the

Figure 30.6
Histiocytic lymphoma. There is a diffuse infiltration of sheets of uniform, rather palely-staining polygonal cells in this lymph node. × 80.

lymph node is destroyed by sheets or nodules of fairly uniform lymphocytes, either well or poorly differentiated. Mitotic activity and capsular invasion are both important features. This condition is clearly very similar to histiocytic lymphoma, and differs only in so far as the stem cell has differentiated into a neoplastic lymphocytic cell.

The histological appearance of the lymph nodes in chronic lymphatic leukaemia is indistinguishable from that of well-differentiated lymphocytic lymphoma. It is sometimes stated that mitotic activity is uncommon in leukaemia, and that capsular invasion is infrequent, but both these features are unreliable. The distinction between the two conditions rests entirely on an examination of the peripheral blood. In lymphoma the white-cell count should be within the normal range, whereas in chronic lymphatic leukaemia there is a great excess of circulating mature lymphocytes (see Ch. 53). A case of lymphoma occasionally develops the blood picture of chronic lymphatic leukaemia.

The *Burkitt tumour*[11] is a type of lymphocytic lymphoma found almost exclusively in children aged from 2 to 14 years. It has two distinctive features: (*a*) the lesions affect the jaws, ovaries, retroperitoneal lymph nodes, kidneys, and thyroid gland particularly, while the superficial nodes, liver, and spleen are much less severely affected, and (*b*) there is a great preponderance in low-lying, moist, tropical areas. It was first described in Central Africa, and indeed its greatest incidence is in tropical Africa, but it is also found in New Guinea and Colombia, and is met with from time to time in Europe and North America in areas that are temperate or even cold. Histologically it resembles other diffuse lymphocytic lymphomata; there are numerous palely-staining histiocytes amongst the lymphocytic cells producing a 'starry-sky' appearance (Fig. 30.7), but this is seen in some cases of lymphomata that do not fall into the category of Burkitt's tumour, and so is not diagnostic. The aetiology of the condition is discussed on page 379. It is interesting that in endemic areas of Africa the incidence of acute childhood leukaemia is much less than in Europe. There seems to be a reciprocal relationship between Burkitt's tumour and acute leukaemia.

Lymphoma, mixed-cell type. The lymph-node architecture is destroyed by neoplastic lymphoblasts and histiocytes. The histiocytes are not markedly phagocytic, a point which helps to distinguish the lesion histologically from extreme degrees of reactive hyperplasia. Sternberg-Reed cells are absent, and the lesion does not have the pleomorphism so commonly seen in Hodgkin's disease.

Hodgkin's disease. This is the commonest of this group of neoplasms, occurring at all ages, especially amongst young and middle-aged adults. It usually starts in a single group of lymph nodes, often the cervical or mediastinal ones, and after a variable time it becomes generalised to implicate the lymphoreticular tissues of the body including the spleen, liver, and bone marrow. There may be little constitutional disturbance at first, but later cachexia occurs and there may be considerable pyrexia. A more acute variety affects the abdominal nodes and spleen primarily, and manifests itself as a 'pyrexia of unknown origin', which is characteristically intermittent, the *Pel-Ebstein fever*. Abdominal Hodgkin's disease runs a rapid course and is usually fatal within 6 months.

Figure 30.7
Burkitt's tumour. Note the uniform lymphocytes, interspersed among which there are large histiocytes. This is the 'starry-sky appearance' stressed in Burkitt's tumour, though seen in other lymphocytic lymphomata also. × 400.

Other noteworthy features of Hodgkin's disease are a distressing generalised pruritus, sometimes accompanied by skin infiltrations of a type resembling mycosis fungoides. In some cases the ingestion of alcohol causes severe pain in the lesions, especially in the bones. There is no satisfactory explanation for this effect, which is also encountered in other types of cancer but much less often.[12]

Histologically the normal structure of the lymph node is replaced by a pleomorphic mass of cells that comprise (*a*) histiocytes, both normal and neoplastic, (*b*) lymphocytes, (*c*) neutrophil and eosinophil polymorphs, and (*d*) plasma cells. The neoplastic histiocyte is the most important element in Hodgkin's disease. It is large and pleomorphic, and may show mitotic activity. Giant forms are also present, including the pathognomonic *Sternberg-Reed cell* with its double mirror-image nuclei containing vesicular chromatin and a prominent nucleolus (Fig. 30.8). There is often a considerable excess of mature lymphocytes, especially in the early stages and in those types which are least malignant. In progressive disease the lymphocytic element is crowded out by neoplastic histiocytes, and this may account for the impaired cell-mediated immunity seen in the condition. This impairs delayed-type hypersensitivity and homograft rejection. The lymphocytic depletion is important in causing death, since these patients are very susceptible to opportunistic infection. Thus lymphocytic depletion is associated with a poor prognosis.

There is usually a variable infiltration of plasma cells and

Figure 30.8
Hodgkin's disease. This is the mixed cellularity type. In addition to the neoplastic macrophages there are several Sternberg-Reed giant cells. There is also an infiltration of lymphocytes, plasma cells, and a few granulocytes. × 250.
At the top right-hand corner there is an insert of a field showing two Sternberg-Reed cells. × 320.

polymorphs, amongst which eosinophils are often prominent. Sometimes there is extensive necrosis, and often there is fibrosis. Capsular invasion may occur, and considerable infiltration is seen in the abdominal type of disease where the retroperitoneal tissues may be diffusely involved.

Classification of Hodgkin's disease.[13,14] The important current histopathological classification was devised by Lukes,[13] and later simplified into four categories at a conference held at Rye, New York in 1965:[15]

(a) *Lymphocytic and/or histiocytic predominance* (Lukes). In this group either lymphocytes or normal histiocytes may predominate or there may be an equal mixture. Of each type there are nodular and diffuse variants. There are few plasma cells or eosinophils and typical Sternberg-Reed cells are scanty. There is no fibrosis or necrosis. This whole group is classified by the Rye conference as 'Hodgkin's disease, lymphocytic predominance', but there seems to be some virtue in retaining Lukes's nomenclature, since the lesions contain both lymphocytes and histiocytes. In some instances either lymphocytes or histiocytes form the dominant component. There is also some virtue in retaining the subdivision of nodular and diffuse, since the nodular variants have an appreciably better prognosis than do the diffuse types. The remaining four headings are those of the Rye conference:

(b) *Nodular sclerosis.* Collagenous bands circumscribe nodules of lymphomatous tissue containing neoplastic histiocytes and Sternberg-Reed cells. There is either a lymphocytic or a mixed lymphocyte-histiocyte predominance. In advanced disease eosinophils and neutrophils are present, and fibrosis increases.

A variant of the Sternberg-Reed cell, called the *lacunar cell*, is typical of nodular sclerosis. It is the same size as or a little larger than the Sternberg-Reed cell, and the cytoplasm tends to shrink away from the surrounding cells, leaving only

spider-like strands still attached. It usually has more than two nuclei, and these are quite small.

(c) *Mixed cellularity type.* Histiocytes (both normal and neoplastic), neutrophils, eosinophils, plasma cells, and a variable number of lymphocytes are present. There are numerous Sternberg-Reed cells, a moderate degree of fibrosis, and sometimes a little necrosis.

(d) *Lymphocytic depletion type.* This group is divided into two types by Lukes. In the *diffuse fibrosis type* there is diffuse fibrosis with necrosis and very few cells, those remaining being nearly all Sternberg-Reed cells. It represents the final stage of the disease. In the second type, described as *reticular* by Lukes, there is a heavy infiltration of Sternberg-Reed cells, with or without other cells, but always with few lymphocytes.

The prognosis is best in the lymphocytic predominance type, in which Lukes found a 43.5 per cent 15-year survival rate in nodular disposition and 27.5 in diffuse disposition. The nodular sclerosis type had a 15·4 per cent 15-year survival rate, mixed cellularity 10·3 per cent, and lymphocytic depletion less than 5 per cent.

As the disease progresses lymphocytic depletion intensifies, and the later grades are the most malignant. The nodular sclerosing type seems to be particularly common in the mediastinal lymph nodes, while the lymphocytic predominance and mixed cellularity types do not usually affect the chest markedly.[16] The granulocytic, histiocytic, and plasma-cell reactions are apparently secondary phenomena.

Course

A clinical staging based on the Rye conference is used in Hodgkin's disease.[17–19]

Stage I. Disease limited to one anatomical region or to two contiguous regions on the same side of the diaphragm.

Stage II. Disease in more than two anatomical regions or in two non-contiguous regions both on the same side of the diaphragm.

Stage III. Disease on both sides of the diaphragm, but restricted to involvement of the lymph nodes, spleen, or Waldeyer's ring of lymphoid tissue.

Stage IV. Involvement of extranodal sites (bone marrow, skin, liver, etc.) in addition to involvement of the nodes, spleen, or Waldeyer's ring.

Occasional cases are encountered in which the disease appears to be confined to one particular organ, e.g. the bowel or skin. These cases cannot be placed into any of the above stages, and are best listed separately in clinical reports.

These stagings were originally established following the introduction of lymphangiography as a means of diagnosing nodal involvement. Laparotomies were also often performed, and the spleen removed and examined. Each stage may usefully be subdivided into two groups, either A or B depending upon the absence or presence respectively of systemic manifestations (fever, night sweats, or pruritus).

In stage I disease there is a 40 per cent 15-year remission rate following adequate radiotherapy. Lymphangiography is an important investigation in assessing the extent of the disease. Once the condition becomes generalised the prognosis is very bad; eventually the disease becomes unresponsive to radiotherapy and cytotoxic drugs, and death occurs.

The lymphocytic predominance and nodular sclerosing types of Hodgkin's disease have the best prognosis. Follicular lymphocytic lymphoma also has a fair prognosis, over half the cases surviving for 5 years.

Localised types of lymphoma can involve such single organs as the bowel, stomach, lungs, and bones.* These lesions may have the histological features of any one of the 4 neoplasms mentioned above. They are important conditions to be aware of, because the prognosis is surprisingly good if the affected parts are resected and the areas then treated with radiotherapy. The follicular 'lymphoma' of the rectum appears to be completely benign, and may be regarded as reactive rather than neoplastic.[22]

The uncommon dermatological condition *mycosis fungoides*[23] has also been alluded to. It usually starts as an extensive, intractable, pruritic dermatitis which is followed by the appearance of many soft, necrotic tumours on the affected skin. Sometimes the tumours appear without prior dermatitis. The condition responds well to radiotherapy, but in due course systematisation usually occurs. It is a lymphoma primarily affecting the skin. Some cases are clearly related to Hodgkin's disease.

The morbid anatomy of these four conditions is basically similar. In lymphocytic and histiocytic lymphoma the affected lymph nodes are replaced by white, soft tumour which infiltrates into the surrounding tissues. Similar deposits are found in the spleen, liver, and other organs. In Hodgkin's

disease the lymph nodes are firmer and have a pinkish-yellow coloration. Deposits of Hodgkin's disease are sometimes rather diffuse in distribution. The spleen may be uniformly seeded with yellowish-white deposits, a few millimetres in diameter, and the appearance of the cut surface may closely resemble that of 'hardbake' (almond toffee). Nevertheless, *hardbake spleen* is an exceptional appearance in Hodgkin's disease, and usually the deposits occur as large, discrete masses indistinguishable from the other diseases of this type.

In practice it is not possible to distinguish between these conditions without the aid of the microscope, and considerable specialised knowledge is often needed to arrive at a correct diagnosis. The most difficult problem is to distinguish between reactive hyperplasia and one of these neoplastic conditions. From the patient's point of view the decision is one of life and death. The most important deciding factors in such cases are an assessment of the general structure of the lymph node and a detailed study of the proliferating macrophages.

Destruction of the normal architecture, such as loss of sinus structure or loss of definition between cortex and medulla, is an important feature of lymphoma and may affect a focal area or be diffuse and affect the whole node. In the nodular lymphomata, the nodules tend to be uniform in size, poorly delineated, and to occupy all parts of the node. Normal lymphoid follicles, on the other hand, are situated in the cortex, usually contain germinal centres, and do not compress the

Figure 30.9
Nodular type of lymphocytic lymphoma. The lymph node has been stained by a silver impregnation method to demonstrate its pattern of reticulin fibres. The numerous abnormal follicles are surrounded by compressed reticulin fibres, but themselves contain hardly any. Normal lymphoid follicles are not surrounded by compressed reticulin. × 30.

---

*A peculiar round-cell tumour of bone is *Ewing's tumour*. It is not osteogenic. It causes a raising-up of the periosteum. Its nature is obscure; some examples may be histiocytic lymphoma of bone or else metastases of an adrenal neuroblastoma or anaplastic carcinoma. It tends to spread to many bones, and is accompanied by marked fever.[20,21]

surrounding reticulin framework (see Fig. 30.9). Invasion of the capsule and the pericapsular fat points to lymphoma, but some infiltration by normal small lymphocytes is often seen in reactive hyperplasia. It is evident that it can be extremely difficult to interpret the histological features of some lymph nodes, and close clinico-pathological correlation is necessary (see also p. 296). Sometimes it is best to admit one's inadequacy and await events. In practice such lymph nodes are sent to experts in the field, and it is by the detailed follow-up of these cases that our knowledge of the natural history of these diseases becomes broadened. The recently acquired information about the more benign types of Hodgkin's disease is a triumph of this type.

Furthermore, other new entities have been recognised. *Benign sinus histiocytosis*[24] is a condition with fever and lymphadenopathy in which massive proliferation of sinus histiocytes can mimic a lymphoma histologically. *Angiofollicular lymph-node hyperplasia*[25] is usually a symptomless type of lymphadenopathy discovered coincidentally during a routine examination. The enlargement of the lymph nodes is due to aggregations of lymphoid nodules throughout the node, and in the centres of the nodules there are thick-walled arterioles surrounded by a cluster of histiocytes which do not show phagocytosis. There are also increased numbers of arterioles between the nodules.

Other Lymphomata

There are a number of malignant processes that fall into the category of lymphoma that should be noted.

(*a*) *Sézary syndrome.*[26] This is a generalised erythroderma with intense pruritus in which there is a lymphocytosis, although the bone marrow is usually spared. Two characteristic cells are seen in the tissues and blood; they are called *Sézary cells*: one is large and has a typically convoluted nucleus, the other is small and resembles a normal lymphocyte. A malignant lymphoma develops in 25 per cent of cases, and the condition bears a similarity to mycosis fungoides. Cytogenetic studies suggest that the Sézary cells are derived from T lymphocytes.

(*b*) *Leukaemic reticulo-endotheliosis*,[27] also called *hairy-cell leukaemia*, is a condition predominantly of middle-aged men. There is great splenomegaly, but usually no enlargement of the lymph nodes. The liver may be enlarged, and there is often anaemia and thrombocytopenia. The characteristic feature is a diffuse infiltration of the organs with a characteristic histiocytic cell that does not phagocytose red cells. It is also present in the blood, and its main morphological feature is the irregular cytoplasmic villi that give the cell a flagellated, or hairy, appearance. The condition responds badly to chemotherapy but well to splenectomy. It is not certain whether the hairy cell is of histiocytic or lymphocytic origin.

(*c*) *Histiocytic medullary reticulosis*[27] is another rare condition in which there is a proliferation of atypical histiocytic cells. These are found especially in the medullary sinuses of the lymph nodes, and also in the spleen, liver, and bone marrow. A characteristic feature of many of these cells is their tendency to phagocytose red cells (erythrophagocytosis). Clinically there is an acute onset of lymphadenopathy, hepatosplenomegaly, and often jaundice. The course is relentless, the response to treatment slight, and death occurs within a few months. Pancytopenia is a common finding. An interesting finding is that most of the cases have occurred in Chinese and Ugandans.

A New Classification of the Lymphomata[28,29]

Lukes and his colleagues have recently investigated the predominant cell types of the non-Hodgkin's lymphomata, and have found that in the great majority of them the cell involved is the lymphocyte. Using the specific immunological techniques to distinguish between B and T lymphocytes (see p. 149) and demonstrating histiocytes through their content of a non-specific esterase, Lukes and Collins have indicated that most of the lymphomata arise from B cells. They trace the normal transformation of the B cell in the centre of the lymphoid follicle of the lymph node through a probable plasmacytoid stage to a stage where the lymphocyte has a characteristically cleaved (split) nucleus. This 'cleaved cell' then enlarges, and eventually its nucleus loses its cleft, becoming a 'non-cleaved cell' with much pyroninophilic cytoplasm and a number of nucleoli. These follicular centre cell (FCC) types are accordingly classified as small cleaved, large cleaved, small non-cleaved, and large non-cleaved. This last cell resembles a fully transformed lymphocyte, and it is called an 'immunoblast' when it leaves the follicle and enters the interfollicular tissue.

On the basis of this development of the B cell, seven types of lymphoma are recognised: *chronic lymphatic leukaemia* from the small lymphocyte; *Waldenström's macroglobulinaemia*, which is closely related to chronic lymphatic leukaemia, from the plasmacytoid variant; *lymphomata from each of the four types of FCC*, of which the cleaved cells show the greater tendency to nodular dispositions and the better prognosis; and the *immunoblastic sarcoma*, which closely resembles a lymphoma arising from a large non-cleaved cell. It may occur as a complication of chronic abnormal immune states, in Sjøgren's syndrome, in patients on immunosuppressive therapy, or in the aged.

Lukes and Collins find that true histiocytic lymphomata are uncommon, because nearly all the cells that were previously called histiocytes are in fact transformed lymphocytes. They are not able to establish any lymphoma firmly in the T-cell class, but the indications are that the *Sézary syndrome, mycosis fungoides, a type of acute lymphatic leukaemia presenting with a mediastinal mass*, and *Hodgkin's disease* arise from T lymphocytes. Indeed, Lukes believes that the Sternberg-Reed cell is a polyploid transformed T lymphocyte rather than a histiocyte. He has encountered Sternberg-Reed cells in the course of viral infections, such as infectious mononucleosis.

At present this new classification must await confirmation, but it has the great merit of combining functional studies with the purely cytological description of the established classifications of the lymphomata.

Neoplasms of the Haematopoietic System

The commonest neoplasms of this group involve the white-cell precursors and are called *leukaemias*. Sometimes the neoplastic process affects the most primitive white cells, e.g. the myeloblasts, lymphoblasts, or even the marrow stem cell itself, and the marrow is crowded out with these cells. This condition is called acute leukaemia. On the other hand, the proliferation may affect the intermediate myelocytic cells, when chronic myeloid leukaemia will ensue. The relationship between lymphocytic lymphoma and chronic lymphatic leukaemia has already been mentioned.

Sometimes the neoplastic process is focused primarily on the erythroblastic series, and *polycythaemia vera* results. Rarely, a type of leukaemia occurs (erythroblastic leukaemia, or Di Guglielmo's disease). A similar megakaryocytic neoplasia leads to the rare *haemorrhagic thrombocythaemia*. All these conditions are considered in detail in the chapters devoted to disorders of the blood. They are all manifested by haematological abnormalities, but in some of the acute ('aleukaemic') leukaemias abnormal cells may be very scanty in the peripheral blood.

Haematological abnormalities may certainly occur in Hodgkin's disease and allied disorders, but they are never primary. If they occur, they are due to secondary processes, e.g. splenic overactivity causing haemolytic anaemia, or bone-marrow involvement leading to leuco-erythroblastic anaemia.

Multiple myeloma is a neoplasm of the bone marrow affecting the plasma cells primarily. Only rarely do these neoplastic myeloma cells enter the general circulation.

Incidence

The Registrar-General's figures for England and Wales reveal that 3837 men and 3243 women died of neoplastic diseases of the lymphatic and haematopoietic tissues in 1973. Of this about a fifth was due to lymphocytic lymphoma and histiocytic lymphoma, and an eighth to Hodgkin's disease.

A quarter of the deaths were attributed to acute leukaemia, and a little over a fifth each to chronic leukaemia and multiple myeloma.

There was a slight female predominance, except in leukaemia, where there was a slight preponderance of men.

The brunt was borne by the older age groups (from 45 years onwards), except in the case of leukaemia, which was fairly evenly distributed over all age groups; it killed 288 children under the age of 15 years.

Apart from the carcinomata, these neoplasms cause most of the mortality from malignant disease. They are also the most responsive to ionising radiations and cytotoxic drugs.

REFERENCES

1. PORTER, K. A. & COOPER, E. H. (1962) Recognition of transformed small lymphocytes by combined chromosomal and isotopic labels. *Lancet*, **2**, 317.
2. FORD, C. E., MICKLEM, H. S. & OGDEN, D. A. (1968) Evidence for the existence of a lymphoid stem cell. *Lancet*, **1**, 621.
3. Leading Article (1971) The enigmatic bone-marrow cell. *Lancet*, **2**, 304.
4. VAN FURTH, R. *et al.* (1972) The mononuclear phagocyte system: a new classification of macrophages, monocytes, and their precursor cells. *Bulletin of the World Health Organisation*, **46**, 845.
5. HARRISON, C. V. (1966) In *Recent Advances in Pathology*—8, p. 207. London: Churchill.
6. HARTSOCK, R. J. (1968) Postvaccinial lymphadenitis. *Cancer (Philadelphia)*, **21**, 632.
7. LE VAN, P. & BIERMAN, S. M. (1962) Idiosyncratic drug eruption to dilantin and trimethadione. *Archives of Dermatology*, **86**, 254.
8. STANBURY, J. B., WYNGAARDEN, J. B. & FREDRICKSON, D. S. (Eds.) (1972) *The Metabolic Basis of Inherited Disease*, 3rd edn, p. 730 *et seq.* New York: McGraw-Hill.
9. BLACKWOOD, W. & CORSELLIS, J. A. N. (Eds.) (1976) *Greenfield's Neuropathology*, 3rd edn, p. 500 *et seq.* London: Arnold.
10. ANDERSON, W. A. D. (Ed.) (1977) *Pathology*, 7th edn, Vol. 2, p. 1526 *et seq.* St. Louis: Mosby.
11. BERARD, C. *et al.* (1969) Histopathological definition of Burkitt's tumour. *Bulletin of the World Health Organisation*, **40**, 601.
12. JAMES, A. H. (1960) Hodgkin's disease with and without alcohol-induced pain. A clinical and histological comparison. *Quarterly Journal of Medicine*, **29**, 47.
13. LUKES, R. J. & BUTLER, J. J. (1966) The pathology and nomenclature of Hodgkin's disease. *Cancer Research*, **26**, 1063.
14. LUKES, R. J., BUTLER, J. J. & HICKS, E. B. (1966) Natural history of Hodgkin's disease as related to its pathologic picture. *Cancer (Philadelphia)*, **19**, 317.
15. LUKES, R. J. (1966) Report of the nomenclature committee. *Cancer Research*, **26**, 1311.
16. KAPLAN, H. S. (1972) Hodgkin's disease: prognosis as related to pathology, staging and treatment. *Proceedings of the Royal Society of Medicine*, **65**, 62.
17. ROSENBERG, S. A. (1966) Report of the committee on the staging of Hodgkin's disease. *Cancer Research*, **26**, 1310.
18. PETERS, M. V., ALISON, R. E. & BUSH, R. S. (1966) Natural history of Hodgkin's disease as related to staging. *Cancer (Philadelphia)*, **19**, 308.
19. AISENBERG, A. C. (1973) Malignant lymphoma. *New England Journal of Medicine*, **288**, 883 and 935.
20. BAIRD, R. J. & KRAUSE, V. W. (1963) Ewing's tumour: a review of 33 cases. *Canadian Journal of Surgery*, **6**, 136.
21. MARSDEN, H. B. & STEWARD, J. K. (1964) Ewing's tumours and neuroblastomas. *Journal of Clinical Pathology*, **17**, 411.
22. HARRISON, C. V. (1966) In *Recent Advances in Pathology*—8, p. 216, *loc cit.*
23. EPSTEIN, E. H. *et al.* (1972) Mycosis fungoides: survival, prognostic features, response to therapy, and autopsy findings. *Medicine (Baltimore)*, **51**, 61.
24. HARRISON, C. V. (1975) In *Recent Advances in Pathology*—9, p. 92. Edinburgh: Churchill Livingstone.
25. HARRISON, C. V. (1975) In *Recent Advances in Pathology*—9, p. 87, *loc cit.*
26. Leading Article (1975) Sézary syndrome. *British Medical Journal*, **1**, 590.
27. Leading Article (1974) Proliferating and phagocytic histiocytes. *Lancet*, **2**, 937.
28. LUKES, R. J. & COLLINS, R. D. (1975) New approaches to the classification of the lymphomata. *British Journal of Cancer*, **31**, Supplement No. 11, 1.
29. Leading Article (1975) Classification of lymphomata. *British Medical Journal*, **3**, 4.

Chapter 31. *The Effect of Ionising Radiation*

The ever-increasing use of radioactive substances both in industry and medicine has made the study of radiation damage of great practical importance. On the human body its effects vary from local tissue necrosis to genetic damage, cancer, and death. With such a perplexing array of effects, it is little wonder that the ionising radiations are regarded with fear and amazement. As their physical nature is so well understood, it might be expected that the mechanisms involved in the damage which they produce would be equally explicable. It is important to understand why this is not so.

The ionising radiations produce changes in the structure of the atoms through which they pass. These subatomic lesions produce effects at a chemical level. If these chemicals are part of a living cell, a 'biochemical lesion' similar in nature to that described in Chapter 4 is produced. The morphological and biochemical sequelae will be recognised as *radiation damage*, while the sum-total of the damage to all the cells and tissues will amount to the effects of *total body irradiation*. It is therefore understandable that with so many steps there are many gaps in our knowledge of the mechanism of radiation damage.

It is, however, no more of a mystery than is the damage produced by other agents. Formaldehyde causes mutations, staphylococci produce tissue necrosis, and arsenic initiates cancer. These changes are as mysterious as those of radiation damage, and differ only in that the exciting agents are more tangible.

Radiation damage will therefore firstly be described at a physical level; the chemical changes which it induces will then be examined. The effects on the living cell should be analysed in the light of this knowledge: the result of total body radiation represents the summation of damage to each cell and tissue.

Physical Considerations

In order to understand the primary effect of ionising radiations, the nature of the rays and the atoms through which they pass must be understood: these are considered in Appendix 3.

The energy absorbed by the tissue appears partly as heat, but this is of negligible quantity. The *ions* and *free radicals* are of much greater importance, and are presumed to be responsible for much of the radiation damage. Another effect which has been less studied is the *excitation of molecules*: this change renders the molecule unstable.

Chemical Considerations

There are two ways in which a chemical change may be induced in a molecule by radiation. The absorbed energy in the molecule itself may produce either ionisation or excitation, which then results in a chemical change. This is *direct action*.

Alternatively a chemical change may occur due to the action of free radicals or ions produced in other adjacent molecules, e.g. OH· from water. This is *indirect action*. Which of these actions is the more important in biological systems is of some significance. With indirect action chemical protection against radiation damage is possible, because the free radicals or ions could be intercepted before they attack vital molecules. With direct action protection is much less likely; it is, however, still theoretically possible, because a molecule could transmit its energy to the protector and thereby avoid any change within itself.

Both direct and indirect actions have been shown to affect viruses and many enzymes, but, whereas viruses are more easily killed by direct action, the indirect effect is more important in the inactivation of enzymes.

Effect of Radiation on Chemicals of Biological Importance

Enzymes. Although there is no doubt that ionising radiations can inactivate enzymes *in vitro*, the dose necessary is generally in excess of that needed to damage a cell. Some enzymes which depend upon a sulphydryl group, —SH, are oxidised to the inactive disulphide form, (—S—S—):

$$-SH + HS- + 20H^{\cdot} = -S-S- + 2H_2O$$

However, there seems no reason why this should not be reduced back to an active form in the body, for the addition of cellular material protects a solution of an enzyme from radiation inactivation.

Many enzymatic changes have been observed in irradiated cells, but it appears that they are the effect of cell damage rather than its cause. Thus, although a biochemical lesion may be postulated, we are quite ignorant of its nature.

DNA. The viscous solution of DNA is liquefied by radiation, and a direct effect is thought to be the most important factor; the changes produced are complex, and do not seem to be related to the observed cell damage. Thus, densely ionising rays, like α-particles, are very effective in producing cell damage, but less so in degrading DNA. Ionising radiation can break one or both chains of the DNA double helix. This is considered together with the repair mechanism on page 54.

Effects Upon the Cell[1]

Although it would be desirable to explain the cellular damage in terms of the known physico-chemical changes, it must be admitted that this is not yet possible. The effect of ionising radiation on cell cultures has been studied extensively. Suitable cell-lines can be plated in a Petri dish so that each cell produces a clone which is visible to the naked eye. If the culture has been irradiated previously, the effect on the reproductive activity of the cells can be assessed. Cells actually in mitosis tend to be less adherent to glass and may be separated from the remainder. By this and other techniques it is possible to obtain cultures in which the majority of the cells are at the same stage in the mitotic cycle. Hence the effect of irradiation at different stages of the cycle can be studied.

The effects of irradiation on cells may be summarised:

1. Immediate death of the cell occurs with very heavy dosage, i.e. 10 000 r or more. This effect occurs regardless of the stage of mitosis and is called *interphase death*. It is also seen in very sensitive cells, e.g. small lymphocytes, with moderate dosage.

2. DNA synthesis is inhibited.

3. Mitosis is delayed, usually due to a prolongation of the G_2 phase.

4. DNA synthesis may occur unrelated to mitosis, so that giant-cell forms are produced.

5. When mitosis does occur in irradiated cells, abnormalities such as chromosome breaks may occur. At this stage the cell may die. Nevertheless, a cell may go through several mitotic cycles before death finally occurs.

6. The growth rate may be slowed down even in sublethally irradiated cells.

7. Fractionated doses of radiation do not produce a strictly cumulative effect. Hence there appear to exist intracellular mechanisms whereby radiation damage can be reversed or 'repaired'.

8. The sensitivity of cells to damage varies according to the stage in the mitotic cycle when the radiation is given. Maximum sensitivity occurs in most cell-types during mitosis itself. They are relatively resistant during most of the G_1 phase, but radiosensitivity returns during the late G_1 and early synthetic (S) phases. They are most resistant during the late S and early G_2 phases (see p. 29).

Two main theories have been put forward to explain cellular damage.

The target theory supposes that the injury is due to damage at some specific sensitive spot in the cell. This may be caused either by direct or indirect action. If the action is assumed to be direct, and if one ionisation is assumed to cause damage, the size of the target can be calculated. In respect of virus inactivation the calculated target size and observed size of the organisms tally remarkably well. In larger cells, however, the evidence for there being a sensitive target is much less convincing. Attractive as it may be to conceive a chromosome or centromere as a target, there is little to support the theory.

The poison theory proposes that the ionisation leads to the production of poisonous substances—usually powerful oxidising agents, which then cause the damage. Such substances are known to appear. For instance, with α-particles the closely adjacent $OH^\cdot$ radicals unite to form H_2O_2. Alpha-radiation has thus been likened to multiple jets of hydrogen peroxide.

Effect on intracellular barriers. It has been suggested that ionising radiation may upset the highly complex system of membrane barriers in the cytoplasm. In this way enzymes may be released (presumably from lysosomes), and cause cell damage.

Effect on mitosis. As noted above mitosis is delayed, and in tissue-culture systems even a dose as small as 35 r will produce this effect.

When mitosis does occur, there may be various abnormalities. The chromosomes may appear to be 'sticky', and abnormalities in spindle-formation occur. A very characteristic effect is the production of breaks in the chromosomes or chromatids. The small fragments unite to form a small nuclear body, which, not being attached to the spindle, persists as a separate unit. A micronucleus formed in this way is very characteristic of irradiated tissue. The larger fragments may unite and form a bridge which interferes with the separation of chromatids at anaphase.

Although the chromosome abnormalities are striking, their significance is not clear. In some of the cells the abnormality is severe enough to cause death. Although at first sight the breaks would seem to indicate a visible change which might coincide with a genetic mutation, this is in fact unlikely. Thus, for the same total dose the number of chromosomal abnormalities increases with the dose rate; on the other hand, dose rate does not influence the number of genetic mutations.

Relative sensitivity of cells. *The law of Bergonié and Tribondeau:** 'The sensitivity of cells to irradiation is in direct proportion to their reproductive activity, and inversely proportional to their degree of differentiation.' This 'law' states in general terms the observed sensitivity of the various cells of the body—it does not explain the difference in sensitivity. The germinal cells of the ovary are most sensitive. Then follow the spermatogonia, lymphocytes, the erythropoietic and myeloid marrow cells, and the intestinal epithelium. Least sensitive are the neurons and muscle cells.

The differences in the sensitivity of various species are not understood. Thus, the LD_{50} for paramoecium is about 300 000 r, for amoebae 100 000 r, *Esch. coli* 5000 r, frogs 700 r, mice 400 to 650 r, pigs 275 r, and the human being 450 to 500 r.

Effect of oxygen tension. In the absence of oxygen the effect of X-rays and γ-rays is diminished by a factor of 2 to 3. The hypoxia must be present during the period of irradiation. The effect is invariable, i.e. it protects against all radiation effects in all species. This is strong evidence in favour of the importance of the indirect effect on biological systems: the formation of $HO_2^\cdot$ is described in Appendix 3.

This oxygen effect is of great importance when considering radiotherapy for cancer. The centre of a nodule of tumour is almost certainly hypoxic and its cells are therefore protected.

One way of overcoming this is to allow the patient to breathe oxygen under pressure. The results of this type of treatment are encouraging with some tumours, e.g. carcinoma of the nose and mouth, but few well-controlled series have been reported and the possible benefit of hyperbaric oxygen and radiotherapy is still under review.[2] One of the main difficulties is the technical problem of giving oxygen under pressure. Thus the patient must be given a general anaesthetic, and the dose-fractionation scheme has to be modified. An alternative approach would be to render the whole body hypoxic (possibly under hypothermia) and then give a larger dose of radiation. The oxygen effect is not nearly so marked with the densely ionising α-particles and neutrons.

---

*Translated by Spear, F. G. (1953), 'Radiation and living Cells'. London: Chapman and Hall.

Effect Upon Cells and Tissues in the Intact Animal

This most important aspect of radiology is also the most difficult. A feature which is outstanding is the remarkable *delay* in the appearance of radiation damage. The initial damage caused by radiation must be almost instantaneous, and yet the effect may not be apparent for days, weeks, or even months. Thus, if a single dose of 5500 r is applied to a small circular area of guinea-pig skin, erythema does not appear until about the tenth day, and necrosis not until after the third week.[3]

Experiments with amphibians help to explain this phenomenon. Frogs can be given a dose of radiation which will kill them within 6 weeks. If the irradiated animals are kept at 5°C, they remain alive for several months, but on being warmed up, die within 6 weeks like the control animals kept at normal temperature.[4] These and similar experiments on hibernating animals indicate that radiation damage is manifest only when cells are active. This lends strong support to the concept that a biochemical lesion is produced. Such a lesion is not in itself harmful, but produces effects when cellular activity commences. Unfortunately, we are ignorant of the nature of this biochemical lesion even assuming that it exists. The fact that radiation damage is manifested only after cellular activity helps to explain the differing radio-sensitivities of various tissues.

It may also explain why several phases of damage sometimes occur, inasmuch as different tissues have different rates of division and metabolic activity.[3] Irradiated tissue therefore shows changes which persist for many weeks or even months and have the characteristics of chronic inflammation even after a single exposure.

Effect of irradiation on skin. Following a single exposure to X-rays, an erythema may appear after 24 hours but is fleeting and may be missed. It reappears after about 10 days, and there are all the features of acute inflammation. Pigmentation is increased, giving the skin a red, dusky hue. With heavy dosage, necrosis of tissue occurs, collagen becomes 'fibrinoid', vessels thrombose, ulceration results, and subsequent healing is slow. Before necrosis occurs the epidermis shows degenerative changes, including the formation of giant cells and micronuclei (Fig. 31.1). Even when healed, ulceration may recur after trivial injury.

With lower dosage a smouldering chronic inflammation occurs. There is a proliferation of fibroblasts often with the production of *bizarre giant forms*. These are presumably produced by the failure of cell division to keep pace with DNA synthesis. Both the newly-formed and the original collagen become hyalinised, and the blood vessels show endarteritis obliterans. Although the tissue becomes devascularised, thin-walled telangiectases may develop. The epithelium becomes atrophic and lacks the normal rete ridges. The hair follicles and accessory glands are much more sensitive to radiation than is the less active surface epithelium. With a dosage above 700 r these structures undergo necrosis, and do not regenerate. In chronic radiodermatitis the skin appendages are therefore absent (Fig. 31.2).

Thus ionising radiation produces a type of chronic inflammatory reaction with ensuing dense fibrosis. In healing wounds radiation *delays* the growth of granulation tissue. Even doses as low as 500 r retard the growth in a rabbit ear-

Figure 31.1
Abnormal changes in epithelium following X-irradiation. This section was taken from a guinea-pig 16 days after a heavy irradiation. A multinucleate mass of epithelial cells is shown. On the left there is a cell with two nuclei and a micronucleus in between them. × 480. (*From Mellett, P. G., Walter, J. B. and Houghton, L. E.* (1960), British Journal of Experimental Pathology, **41**, 160)

chamber. The delaying effect on wound contraction is described on page 105.

One remarkable effect is that the adjacent normal skin has a protective action. Thus in experimental irradiation the ulcer produced by 5500 r is not as large as the area treated. The explanation is not known, but advantage is taken of this in clinical radiotherapy. The use of a grid helps prevent skin damage, and enables a larger tumour-dose to be given than would otherwise be possible (see p. 409).

Effect of irradiation on other tissues. This has been less intensively studied.

In the *testis* the seminiferous tubules undergo atrophy following the destruction of their spermatogonia. Mature sperms are not affected, so that sterility does not develop immediately.

Irradiation of the *lungs* produces inflammatory changes which culminate in fibrosis: this is sometimes seen as a complication of radiotherapy for breast cancer. The condition is characterised clinically by marked dyspnoea.

The *kidney* shows a progressive glomerular fibrosis, and malignant hypertension may develop.

Irradiation of *bone* produces changes which may persist for years, and are punctuated by episodes of painful 'radionecrosis'. This often complicates the irradiation of oral tumours; the effect of radiation on the mandible is greatly accentuated by the presence of infection. The late effects of radiation of bone are probably due to ischaemia; another area where this is

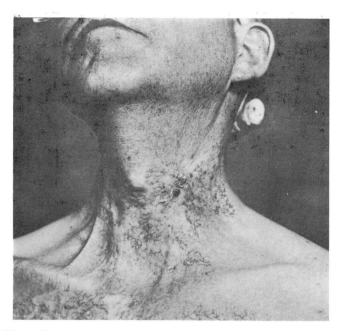

Figure 31.2
Chronic radiodermatitis. The skin of this patient's neck shows atrophy and a disturbance of pigmentation, areas of hypopigmentation alternating with areas of hyperpigmentation and telangiectasia. This triad is often called *poikiloderma*. In addition, there is scarring and early cicatrisation to complete the picture of chronic radiodermatitis. The persistent area of crusting on the left side of the neck indicates the development of a squamous-cell carcinoma.

important is the femur and pelvis. Since these bones are weight bearing, the radionecrosis is often complicated by the development of fractures. Doses of over 1000 r inhibit growth at the epiphysis, an effect which should be remembered when using radiotherapy in children. Thus scoliosis can follow the treatment of a Wilms's tumour or neuroblastoma.

The *intestine*, both large and small, is readily damaged by radiation, and ulceration, haemorrhage, perforation, and the late formation of fistulae, adhesions, and strictures are well-recognised complications of radiotherapy for cancer of the cervix uteri.

The *central nervous system* is generally regarded as being insensitive. Nevertheless, irradiation of the *brain* (2400 rad), as a prophylactic measure in the treatment of children with acute leukaemia in remission, has shown that this organ is not as insensitive as has been thought. Over a third of the patients develop anorexia, lethargy, and somnolence.[5] If the *spinal cord* is irradiated, damage, probably due to ischaemia, may develop 2 to 4 years later; it can lead to quadriplegia.

An unusual complication of radiotherapy is anuria due to the *blockage of the renal tubules* by uric-acid crystals. This follows the treatment of a large, highly sensitive tumour, and is due to the release of nucleoprotein following necrosis of the tumour cells.

When considering the action of radiation on any tissue, two main effects must be borne in mind. These have been called 'direct' and 'indirect', but the terms are best avoided, as they have already been used in another connexion (see p. 402). The *primary effect* is directly due to the irradiation of the tissue concerned; the *secondary effect* is due to damage to an adjacent tissue. For instance, epidermis irradiated on its own is more resistant than as part of the intact skin. Presumably therefore the epithelial damage is partly secondary to dermal injury. It seems likely that this damage is due to vascular occlusion; indeed, some authorities attribute much of the beneficial effect of radiotherapy in cancer to this mechanism.

TOTAL BODY IRRADIATION

During the last decade the applications of atomic science in both civilian and military fields have brought to the fore the hazards of total body irradiation in the human subject. A mass of data is available about the effects on animals, but since few human beings have been subjected to total body irradiation, our knowledge about its effects in the human is scanty. Many of the Japanese survivors of the Hiroshima and Nagasaki explosions were subjected to total body irradiation, but the exact dosage was unknown, and their exposure was probably uneven due to the shielding effects of buildings and other objects. Furthermore, the presence of burns and other injuries complicated the clinical picture.

In the H-bomb fall-out on the Marshall Islands the situation was complicated by β-radiation damage to the skin, and in the various civilian accidents the victims have usually been subjected to both γ-ray and neutron bombardment.

Our information is therefore seriously incomplete, and it is hardly surprising that even the LD_{50} dose is not known with any degree of certainty; 450 r is the figure generally quoted, but the actual level obviously depends upon many factors, the type of radiation being not the least important.

It is convenient to describe the effect of total body irradiation under two headings—those occurring during the first 2 months (immediate), and those occurring later.

Immediate Effects

These depend largely upon the dose received. Although no hard-and-fast rules can be given, three groups of cases may be recognised:

Very high dosage (over 5000 r single exposure). The first effects of high dosage are nausea and vomiting, which occur early and are subsequently followed by a state of shock and prostration. There is an initial rise in temperature which later drops, tremors and convulsions occur, and within a day or two death ensues. These symptoms are classified as the *cerebral syndrome*, because they occur not only with a very high single total body exposure, but also as a result of irradiation of the head alone. Only one human case has been recorded; animal experiments have proved that the cerebral syndrome is invariably fatal. Even if life is prolonged for a few days, gastrointestinal damage soon leads to death.

Moderate dosage (800 to 5000 r single exposure). Anorexia, nausea, and vomiting develop with 2 hours of irradiation for reasons which are not clear. The symptoms resemble motion sickness, and like it are easily influenced by psychological factors and individual susceptibility. These symptoms may persist, but are more likely to abate, only to recur after 2 or 3 days with intractable severity. This later episode of vomiting is accompanied by severe diarrhoea, and is due to necrosis of the gastrointestinal epithelium. This clinical picture is called the *gastrointestinal syndrome* and results in severe dehydration, haemoconcentration, and shock. Death may be averted by vigorous supportive measures, and the gastrointestinal epithelium regenerates in about 10 days. Nevertheless, 2 to 3 weeks later the effects of marrow aplasia appear, and death occurs.

Lower dosage (under 800 r single exposure). Initial nausea and vomiting are less severe, and the patient may then appear to make a complete recovery. 2 to 3 weeks later the results of bone-marrow aplasia become apparent. The serious effects of irradiation at this stage are due to damage to the haematopoietic tissues. White cells, platelets, and red cells are all affected, and their deficiency explains the clinical picture seen during this *haematological phase*. Epilation may also occur, but regrowth of hair is usual in those who survive.

Blood Changes Following Irradiation

Lymphocytes. Lymphopenia is the earliest blood change of total body irradiation, and is most marked after a day or two. In those who survive the count remains low, and does not return to normal for months or even years. The lymphocyte count is therefore no useful guide to prognosis.

Granulocytes. The granulocyte count may increase initially, but during the ensuing weeks it shows a marked decline. With heavy dosage neutropenia becomes severe by the end of the second week, but with smaller doses the lowest count occurs around the fifth or sixth week. The count may take a year or more to return to normal.

Platelets. There is an initial rise, but within a few days the number of platelets drops. In severe cases they are virtually completely absent after about 4 weeks.

The red cells. Because primitive erythroblastic cells are highly radiosensitive and the mature red cells resistant, the effect of marrow aplasia on the peripheral count is delayed, being manifested as an anaemia of gradual onset. The actual red-cell count may, however, be influenced by the effects of haemoconcentration during the gastrointestinal phase, and haemorrhage occurring later.

Although the changes in the white-cell and platelet counts commence shortly after irradiation, their effects on the patient do not become apparent for at least 2 to 3 weeks. The two most important manifestations are infection and haemorrhage.

Infection. Many factors play a part in this manifestation of marrow aplasia, the neutropenia and diminished phagocytic power of the polymorphs probably being the most important. The RE system is damaged, and although phagocytosis is not impaired, and may even be enhanced, the phagocytes are less capable of destroying bacteria. In addition, antibody production is impaired (p. 142). Organisms may gain access of the tissues through the denuded intestine, the mouth, and the respiratory tract. Treatment with antibiotics is worth trying, although experiments with germ-free animals given a lethal dose are reported to show that the avoidance of infection merely delays death.

Haemorrhage. The thrombocytopenia leads to a haemorrhagic tendency which may manifest itself either as trivial petechial haemorrhages into the skin and other organs or as severe intestinal and pulmonary bleeding. Death is not infrequently due to massive haemorrhage, and treatment with fresh blood or platelet transfusions may be of value.

Late Effects of Total Body Irradiation

Those exposed to a sublethal dose may show the following after-effects:

Premature ageing. Following one large sublethal dose, mice are found to die sooner than normal, but this effect does not seem to occur after slow, continuous exposure (e.g. 5 r per week). No data are available for the human being.

Cataract. In the human the development of cataract may occasionally follow a large dose especially after neutron irradiation.

Sterility. The sterility which occurs in those who survive total body irradiation is not permanent: in the male complete recovery is usual, but in the female the result is less predictable. Permanent sterility occurs only when the gonads have received a dose which would cause death if applied to the whole body.

Fetal abnormalities. Although the effects in the human are not known, mice irradiated *in utero* during early pregnancy have been shown to develop abnormalities.

Malignant disease (see p. 407)
Genetic effect (see p. 408).

PROTECTION FROM RADIATION DAMAGE

Marrow protection or replacement. One of the best ways of reducing the effects of radiation is to shield a part of the body which has a haematopoietic function, e.g. the bone marrow, or in some animals the spleen. This is because the destroyed marrow is repopulated by unaffected haematopoietic cells.

The use of high-energy X- and γ-radiation in radiotherapy reduces the bone dosage relative to that received by the soft tissues. Thus for a given soft tissue dose of 250 kV X-rays, the bones will receive about three times that received using a 2–4 MeV beam.

Animals exposed to moderate total body irradiation may be saved if injected with autologous, homologous, or even heterologous marrow cells. This method has been tried in human subjects for the treatment of leukaemia. Radiation chimeras are further described on page 194.

The oxygen effect has already been described.

Chemical protection. A large number of chemicals are known that protect against radiation; curiously enough, not only do they protect a wide range of living matter against the lethal effects of radiation, but some also preserve solutions of polymers, like polymethylmethacrylate, against degradation. The various test systems do not, however, always give the same quantitative results. Amongst known chemical agents, those which have been shown to afford protection are cyanides, nitrites, 5-hydroxytryptamine, and adrenaline. They probably act by producing tissue hypoxia, and are too toxic for animal use. So far the most effective compounds are derivatives of cysteine.

Cysteine itself, $HS—CH_2—CH\diagup^{NH_2}_{\diagdown COOH}$,

is an effective protector whether given by mouth or injection. Some of its derivatives are even more powerful and suitable for animal administration. Cysteamine, HS—CH$_2$CH$_2$NH$_2$,

and cystamine, $\begin{array}{l} S—CH_2CH_2NH_2 \\ | \\ S—CH_2CH_2NH_2 \end{array}$,

which is converted into cysteamine *in vivo*, have been used, and reduce the effect of X-rays by about 50 per cent. One of the most promising derivatives is AET.* Glutathione, a tripeptide containing one molecule of cysteine, is another related protector, but is only effective by injection.

The following features should be noted:

(1) All substances must be given before exposure to radiation; they are quite ineffective if administered afterwards, and therefore cannot be considered a curative form of treatment once radiation damage has been sustained.

(2) They are not very effective against high density ionising particles, e.g. α-particles.

(3) They are less effective under hypoxic conditions.

(4) Their action is almost universal. They protect a wide range of animals, infusoria, bacteria, and tissue cultures.

Although it is tempting to think that the —SH group is important, not all substances containing it are active. Reducing power may also be a factor, but not all protective substances are reducing agents. Ascorbic acid is a powerful reducing substance, but has little protective activity. Some compounds may act by producing hypoxia, but it seems unlikely that all chemicals protect in the same way. The following alternatives have been suggested:

(*a*) The protecting chemicals compete for the free radicals, e.g. OH· and HO$_2'$. As the powerfully oxidising HO$_2'$ is found only in the presence of oxygen, this theory would explain why the effects of hypoxia and chemicals overlap.

(*b*) The protector may convert the altered chemical, e.g. an enzyme, back to its normal state, e.g. by its —SH groupings.

(*c*) Protectors may combine with receptor groups of important molecules, and render them non-reactive to free radicals.

(*d*) Even if the effect of radiation is *direct*, the protector may prevent the transfer of energy from one part of a macromolecule to another part.

It is not yet possible to state which of these four is the most important. Topical applications of AET or DMSO (dimethylsulphoxide) have been shown to provide some degree of protection against local irradiation in animals.[6]

Most of the work done on chemical protection has been based on the lethal action of total body irradiation, and it is not known whether this applies to the other effects of ionising radiation, e.g. the carcinogenic and genetic hazards.

CARCINOGENIC EFFECT

It has been realised since the beginning of this century that tumours may develop after the application of ionising radiation. The first case, a carcinoma of the skin, was reported in 1902, and subsequently cancers of the skin of the hands have been seen frequently in X-ray workers.

In animals it has been found possible to produce tumours by the local irradiation of both normal and inflamed tissues.

*S-β-Aminoethyl*iso*thiouronium bromide hydrobromide.

In this way skin cancers, subcutaneous sarcomata, and osteosarcomata have been produced, frequently after a latent interval of many months.

Irradiation as a Cause of Human Malignant Disease

Skin. Irradiation of the skin, whether accidental as in the early radium workers, or therapeutic for some other condition, may be followed years later by the development of squamous-cell carcinoma (Fig. 31.3). Irradiated lupus vulgaris frequently underwent malignancy.

Bone. Osteosarcoma may develop following local irradiation. It usually appears several years after the treatment of either a benign tumour or an inflammatory lesion, like tuberculosis. Radiation-induced osteosarcoma more commonly follows the deposition of long-lived radioactive elements in the bone itself (internal irradiation). Certain metals, e.g. radium, mesothorium, and strontium, are treated like calcium, and

Figure 31.3
X-ray neoplasia of the skin. This specimen demonstrates many of the changes that the hands of pioneer radiologists underwent. The skin is scarred and the nail deformed. On the atrophic skin of the finger there are several large papillomata as well as many smaller ones. The neighbouring finger has already been amputated. (I 2.6, *Reproduced by permission of the President and Council of the R.C.S. Eng.*)

become deposited in bone, where the long-continued radiation causes neoplasia. A classical instance of this occurred in 1928 when some girls, who were employed in painting the dials of watches with a luminous paint containing radium and mesothorium, sucked the tips of the brushes, and swallowed quantities of the radioactive elements.[7] Tumours developed 1 to 5 years after exposure to the carcinogen. More recently anxiety has been expressed because the ^{90}Sr released from nuclear devices is taken up by the grass, and finally reaches human bones *via* ingested cows' milk. This may obviously lead to osteosarcoma and leukaemia, but it is probable that ^{90}Sr is eliminated more rapidly than was originally thought, and that the risk is not as great as was at one time feared.

Leukaemia. The steady increase in the incidence of leukaemia over the last 30 years has led to the investigation of ionising radiation of the bone marrow as a causative factor. An increased incidence has been noted in the survivors of the Nagasaki and Hiroshima atomic bomb attacks, and a statistically significant risk has been shown to attend treatment of ankylosing spondylitis with X-rays. Leukaemia was also more common in radiologists before strict protective standards were introduced. Statistical evidence suggests that irradiation of the abdomen for pelvimetry during pregnancy increases the incidence of leukaemia in the child. However, not all investigators have confirmed this finding. Diagnostic radiology in the adult also increases the incidence of leukaemia.

The latent period between irradiation and disease is seldom less than 2 years and usually 5 to 8. After 10 years the risk appears to diminish. The type of leukaemia induced is predominantly acute. Chronic myeloid leukaemia occurs much less commonly, and chronic lymphatic leukaemia is very rare. The increased incidence of the last disease is therefore unlikely to be due to the radiation hazard. Whether, in fact, the observed increase of acute leukaemia is due to the effects of irradiation is not known, but it is certain that the population is now exposed to more radiation than ever before. Diagnostic radiology constitutes the greatest hazard, but luminous watches, fluorescent shoe-fitting machines, radiotherapy, and bomb fall-out all contribute to the general increase. It would seem prudent to limit the exposure of all individuals to X-rays, especially if they are young or pregnant. It should, however, be borne in mind that the risk of leukaemia is very small. Common surgical operations, even under the best conditions, have a greater mortality risk than the complication of radiotherapy for spondylitis. The negligible risk of diagnostic radiography should therefore be seen in proper perspective.

Thyroid. Irradiation of the adult thyroid is not usually followed by malignancy, although a few cases have been reported. It was, however, the fashion at one time, in the USA especially, to treat children suffering from 'thymic asthma' with radiotherapy. The thyroid gland received considerable radiation, and some 3 to 18 years later cancer was found to develop in a number of these patients.

A 20-year review of medical findings in a Marshall Island population that was accidentally exposed to radioactive fallout has shown growth retardation in young children, myxoedema, and thyroid nodules (9 years after exposure). These nodules were usually benign, but carcinoma of the papillary type was also found.[8]

The rarity of thyroid carcinoma after radioiodine treatment for hyperthyroidism may be due to the high dose of radiation causing a great deal of local cellular destruction.

Liver. Thorotrast, a preparation of thorium dioxide, was at one time used as a contrast medium in angiography. It accumulates in the liver and spleen and there causes tumours, the most common of which is an angiosarcoma of the liver.[9] Other liver tumours may arise, as may also leukaemia.

Other organs. Cancer of the pharynx has been described following irradiation. Cancer of the lung in the Schneeberg miners is mentioned on page 386.

Irradiation of the scalp for ringworm may predispose to tumours of the head and neck. One series of approximately 11 000 children so treated was followed up for 12 to 23 years, and an excess of both benign and malignant tumours of the brain (including meningioma), parotid gland, and thyroid was noted. Interestingly, there was no increase in the incidence of leukaemia.[10]

GENETIC EFFECT OF IONISING RADIATION

The ability of ionising rays to increase the rate of mutation is well established in micro-organisms, plants, and animals. In somatic cells this effect is probably not important, but in the germ cells it is of potential significance, since the new factor may have a profound effect, and is handed down to subsequent generations. It is generally believed that the *type* of mutation is not influenced by radiation—it is only the *rate* which is changed. Within wide limits it is thought that the number of mutations is related to the total dose received by the gonads regardless of the rate at which it is given. However, with very low dosage it is probable that the genetic effect is much less than the calculations from the cumulative dose would lead one to postulate. In the human the genetic hazard is difficult to assess, since most of the abnormal genes produced are likely to be recessive, and may therefore remain hidden for generations. It is generally agreed that most mutations are harmful, although it should not be forgotten that in the heterozygous state 'harmful' genes may confer some advantage upon the individuals, e.g. sickle-cell trait in relation to malaria. Furthermore, if the improvement of species and the process of evolution itself are dependent upon the occurrence of mutations, then an increase in their frequency might in the long run be of benefit.

THE PERMISSIBLE DOSE[11]

It is probable that ionising radiation produces some effect on living matter, however small the dose. Whether the damage is of any consequence depends upon many factors, including dosage-rate and age. Evidence is accumulating to show that with slow dosage-rates damage is considerably lessened. The increased liability of children to ill-effects after irradiation is well known to radiotherapists, and was borne out by the experiences of those exposed to fall-out on the Marshall Islands in 1954. The problem of whether a threshold dose* exists is therefore complex: it depends not only upon factors like type of radiation, area of body exposed, dosage-rate, etc.,

---

*The term 'threshold' is used in the sense that a dose below it produces no detectable effect.

but also upon our ability to detect damage in exposed individuals or experimental animals. The permissible dose for X-ray workers is therefore chosen arbitrarily as a dose unlikely to cause appreciable damage to the worker, and at the same time which allows the work to be pursued.

The present trend has been to emphasise the importance of a cumulative dose. For radiation workers the maximum permissible dose to the gonads, the blood-forming organs, and the lens of the eye is 3 rem. in any period of 13 consecutive weeks. However, the maximum whole body radiation from the age of 18 to 65 is 235 rem. This corresponds to an over-all average of about 5 rem./year or 0·1 rem./week. Further details are available in the Medical Research Council's Second Report of 1960.

RADIOTHERAPY

The destructive effects of ionising radiations on living cells, particularly those in an active state, have led to the widespread use of these radiations in the treatment of malignant disease. Nowadays radiotherapy plays an important part in the curative treatment of some primary cancers as well as in the palliation of those which have already metastasised and are beyond the scope of surgical excision.

Tumours differ widely in their reaction to radiotherapy, and it is only after treatment has been commenced that the response can be assessed. However, some guide to the probable local results of treatment may be given by a consideration of the following factors:

Tissue of origin. The relative sensitivities of normal tissues are often reflected in the radiosensitivities of the tumours derived from them. Thus, seminoma of the testis and tumours of the lymphoreticular system are generally very radiosensitive; sarcomata are usually resistant. On the other hand, there are some exceptions to this rule: carcinomata of the gastriointestinal tract do not usually respond well, and the medulloblastoma, although of neural origin, is highly radiosensitive.

Degree of differentiation and mitotic activity. It is generally taught that within any tumour group, the most undifferentiated tumours are also the most radiosensitive. As a generalisation this is true, but nevertheless it is found that the histological appearances of an individual tumour are no sure guide to the results obtained in practice. It is found, for instance, that well-differentiated squamous-cell carcinoma of the skin and tongue frequently responds very well.

The tumour bed. The nature of the tumour bed is thought to play an important role in the response of a tumour to ionising radiation. Several factors are probably involved. An avascular bed rendering the growth hypoxic may make the tumour more resistant due to the oxygen effect (see p. 403). Irradiation damage to the stromal blood vessels may lead to the destruction of the tumour by a process of infarction.

There are some authorities who maintain that the connective tissues have an even more important role. It is possible that the tumour bed with its inflammatory response has a restraining effect upon the growth which can lead to its destruction. If the bed is itself damaged by excessive irradiation, the results of treatment are said to be poor. This concept has led to the development of sieve therapy, whereby a grid or sieve is placed in the X-ray beam and only parts of the tumour and its stroma are irradiated.[12] Whatever may be the merits of this approach, there seems little doubt that the effects of ionising radiation on a tumour are due only partly to a primary destructive effect on the malignant cells. Some viable cells remain, and in those cases where clinical success is apparent it is probable that the body defences either destroy the remaining tumour or else induce it to enter into a dormant phase.

Recurrent tumour following previous irradiation generally responds poorly. This may be a result of selection whereby resistant cells survive, but the ischaemia which accompanies the radiation fibrosis may also play a part.

Nature of the individual tumour. Certain tumours respond well, e.g. most basal-cell and squamous-cell carcinomata of the skin. Some squamous-cell carcinomata of the cervix respond well, but others are resistant. Squamous-cell tumours of the lung respond poorly. It is evident that tumours of identical histological appearances in different organs react very differently to irradiation. The reason for this is not apparent.

The cure rate to be expected from radiotherapy must, as with surgical treatment, be considered in relation to the general properties of the tumour. Many malignant conditions, e.g. those of the lymphoreticular system, cannot be considered as local diseases, and although a tumour mass may respond remarkably well to treatment, the disease usually progresses sooner or later. Some carcinomata, e.g. oat-cell carcinoma of the lung, appear to spread so early that treatment of any sort directed to the primary growth does not greatly influence the course of the disease.

TABLE 31.1 Prognosis in treated carcinoma of the cervix uteri

Stage	5-year survivals %
I	71.2
II	52.8
III	25.2
IV	11.7
Total	43.8

The figures are quoted from Raven, R. W. (1959), 'Cancer', vol. 5, p. 282. London: Butterworth. The classification of stages is the one recommended by W.H.O. (*see* Raven, R.W. (1958). 'Cancer', vol. 4, p. 4, London: Butterworth).

When the growth is localised, excellent results may be obtained, e.g. with basal-cell carcinoma of the skin. The results of treatment of cancer of the cervix illustrate the ability of ionising radiation to eradicate local disease (Table 31.1).

Radiotherapy is often useful as an effective palliative treatment. It can reduce the size of tumour masses and thereby produce great clinical relief; this is well seen in mediastinal tumours producing obstruction of the great vessels. It can control haemorrhage from a bleeding carcinoma of the bladder, and help to clear up fungating tumours, e.g. a carcinoma of the breast. Pain due to metastases in bone may be alleviated, and combined with surgery, radiotherapy can relieve compression of the spinal cord, thereby delaying the onset of paraplegia. Slowly-growing tumours, like carcinoma of the breast and Hodgkin's disease, can sometimes be held in check, and at times a tumour which appears hopelessly advanced may respond dramatically, thereby giving the patient several years of useful life. It may well be that radiotherapy and surgery are often both forms of palliation which allow the body to retard the growth of the tumour. Depending on whether the remaining malignant cells stay dormant for a short or a long period, one may speak of a '5-year cure', a '10-year cure', etc. There is increasing evidence, however, that on some occasions a thorough eradication of malignant cells is effected by the combined action of therapeutic measures, whether surgical excision, ionising radiation, or cytotoxic drugs, on the one hand, and the natural defences of the body on the other. In these cases the patient's life-span is no shorter than that of a healthy control, and we may speak with growing confidence of a complete cure.

GENERAL READING

ALEXANDER, P. (1957) *Atomic Radiation and Life*, 239 pp. Harmondsworth: Penguin Books Ltd. A simple account of ionising radiations and their effects.

BACQ, Z. M. & ALEXANDER, P. (1961) *Fundamentals of Radiobiology*, 2nd edn, 555 pp. Oxford: Pergamon Press. Both this and the first edition (1955, London: Butterworth) should be consulted for details on specific aspects of radiobiology.

CRONKITE, E. P. & BOND, V. P. (1960) *Radiation Injury in Man*, 200 pp. Springfield, Illinois: Thomas.

GLASSER, O., QUIMBY, E. H., TAYLOR, L. S., WEATHERWAX, J. L. & MORGAN, R. H. (1961) *Physical Foundations of Radiology*, 3rd edn, 503 pp. London: Pitman Medical.

MOLE, R. H. (1960) The toxicity of radiation. In *Recent Advances in Pathology*—7 ed. Harrison, C. V., pp. 339–383. London: Churchill.

RUBIN, P. & CASARETT, G. W. (1968) *Clinical Radiation Pathology*, Vol. 2, pp. 518–1057. Philadelphia: Saunders.

WARREN, S. (1970) Radiation carcinogenesis. *Bulletin of the New York Academy of Medicine*, **46**, 131.

REFERENCES

1. LITTLE, J. B. (1968) Cellular effects of ionising radiation. *New England Journal of Medicine*, **278**, 308 and 369.
2. Leading Article (1972) Hyperbaric oxygen and radiotherapy. *British Medical Journal*, **2**, 368.
3. MELLETT, P. G., WALTER, J. B. & HOUGHTON, L. E. (1960) Two-phase ulceration in guinea-pig skin following local irradiation with X-rays. *British Journal of Experimental Pathology*, **41**, 160.
4. PATT, H. M. & SWIFT, M. N. (1948) Influence of temperature on the response of frogs to X irradiation. *American Journal of Physiology*, **155**, 388.
5. FREEMAN, J. E., JOHNSTON, P. G. B. & VOKE, J. M. (1973) Somnolence after prophylactic cranial irradiation in children with acute lymphoblastic leukaemia. *British Medical Journal*, **4**, 523.
6. Annotation (1969) Local radiation protection. *Lancet*, **1**, 1039.
7. DAVIS, C., BROWN, R. G. & ALEXANDER, R. W. (1963) Osteogenic sarcoma in a luminous watch dial painter. *Archives of Surgery*, **86**, 190.
8. Leading Article (1976) Irradiation of the thyroid gland. *Lancet*, **1**, 1278.
9. DA SILVA HORTA, J. *et al.* (1965) Malignancy and other late effects following administration of thorotrast. *Lancet*, **2**, 201.
10. MODAN, B. *et al.* (1974) Radiation-induced head and neck tumours. *Lancet*, **1**, 277.
11. BARNES, D. E. & TAYLOR, D. (1963) *Radiation Hazards and Protection*, 2nd edn. London: Newnes.
12. JOLLES, B. (1953) *X-ray Sieve Therapy in Cancer*. London: Lewis.

Chapter 32. The General Reaction to Trauma: Haemorrhage and Shock

Following major trauma there ensues a complex series of changes from which scarcely any tissue of the body escapes. The nervous system responds promptly with an increased outflow of autonomic impulses. There is an immediate outpouring of catecholamines from the adrenal medulla, while the other endocrine glands respond more slowly: stimulation of the hypothalamus leads to an increase in the secretion of ACTH from the pituitary gland, which in turn results in adrenocortical overactivity. These changes assist the injured animal to withstand trauma; in fact, there is little doubt that the adrenalectomised animal is less equipped to withstand infection and trauma than is the normal. Continued stress in the intact animal leads to adrenal hyperplasia and an excessive secretion of its hormones.

One very obvious early effect of trauma involves the circulatory system. When the trauma is severe, a state develops from which recovery may or may not occur; this is called *shock*, and is characterised by inadequate perfusion of the tissues, hypotension, and depression of general metabolic activity.

If the patient survives, there ensue metabolic changes that terminate in complete recovery. This is called the period of *convalescence*.

For descriptive purposes therefore it is convenient to consider the response to injury under three headings:

The metabolic changes.
The circulatory changes.
Shock.

THE METABOLIC CHANGES[1]

These changes may be considered under the following headings:

The early, or ebb, phase.
Convalescence: (a) *Catabolic phase*
            (b) *Anabolic phase.*

THE EARLY OR EBB PHASE

The early response to injury is termed the low flow, or ebb phase. After severe injury it is an accompaniment of the state of shock. It is characterised by a reduction in the metabolic rate, a reduced body temperature, and an increased output of catecholamines from the adrenal medulla (see Table 32.1). The increased blood level of catecholamines has several effects:

(a) There is increased glycogenolysis in the liver.

(b) Lactic acid is released from the muscles and is converted into glucose in the liver (the Cori cycle). The result of all this is hyperglycaemia and possibly glycosuria.

(c) A reduction in insulin secretion promotes gluconeogenesis in the liver, and this contributes to the hyperglycaemia.

(d) Catecholamines have a lipolytic effect, and fatty acids are released from the adipose tissues. The plasma level of fatty acids is therefore raised. The metabolic acidosis that accompanies this ebb phase in shocked patients is considered on page 421.

TABLE 32.1 Metabolic changes following injury[a]

	Low-flow phase	High-flow phase
Metabolic rate	↓	↑
Body temperature	↓	↑
Catecholamine output	↑	Normal or slightly ↑
Blood insulin level	↓	↑
Blood glucose	↑	Normal or slightly ↑
Blood lactate	↑	Normal or slightly ↑
Blood fatty acid	↑	↓

[a]Modified from Ryan, N.T. (1976) Metabolic adaptations for energy production during trauma and sepsis. Surgical Clinics of North America, **56**, 1073.

CONVALESCENCE

Assuming that the patient survives the initial phase and does not die of shock, there ensues a period of metabolic upset that has been termed the *high-flow phase*, or simply the *flow phase*. This has two components: (a) a *catabolic phase*, which is characterised by excessive protein breakdown and a negative nitrogen balance, followed by (b) an *anabolic phase*, during which the body's stores are replenished. These important metabolic changes are highly complex and are incompletely understood. They have been studied extensively both in animals and the human subject.

The Catabolic Phase

During the catabolic phase there is increased glucose production in the liver (Table 32.1). This gluconeogenesis is fed by lactate, pyruvate, and alanine and other amino acids derived from muscle, which are used as substrates. The breakdown of muscle components, particularly the proteins, for use in energy generation leads to muscular atrophy and a consequent loss of weight. The nitrogen of the metabolised amino acids is excreted as urea, and the body enters a phase of negative nitrogen balance. The extent of this nitrogen loss varies according to the severity of the trauma; it may reach 20 g (expressed as urea) daily, but usually does not exceed 10 g. Its duration varies with the extent of the trauma: after a simple herniorrhaphy it may last only a day or two, but with severe burns it can continue for 10 days or more. Fractures cause more disturbance than might be supposed from the clinical condition; chronic suppuration may prolong the catabolic state for weeks. The following points should be noted:

1. The nitrogen loss cannot be abolished by increasing the protein intake; any extra protein in the diet is broken down and the extra nitrogen excreted. There is therefore no point in forcing patients to ingest protein during this phase.

2. The administration of carbohydrate does reduce the nitrogen loss very considerably.

3. Protein starvation prior to injury depletes the protein reserve of the body, and virtually abolishes the nitrogen loss.

4. Patients with Addison's disease and adrenalectomised animals do not show any post-traumatic nitrogen loss.

During the catabolic phase there is an increased production of insulin two or three times above normal. Nevertheless, the tissues appear to be resistant to the action of insulin, and gluconeogenesis is stimulated by the unopposed action of cortisol. The relative lack of insulin activity is the probable mechanism whereby amino acids are released from muscle. There is, however, sufficient insulin activity to inhibit lipolysis, hence fatty acids are not released from the adipose tissues, and while the muscles waste as a result of protein loss, the adipose tissues remain intact. This is in contrast to the situation encountered in simple starvation.

Mechanism of the protein loss. The following should be noted:

1. The metabolic effects of injury are closely simulated by the effects of glucocorticoids.

2. The adrenal glands are known to enlarge following injury.

3. There is an increased secretion of adrenal cortical hormones following trauma.

4. Adrenalectomised animals do not show this nitrogen loss.

It would therefore not be unreasonable to assume that excessive adrenal function explains the loss of nitrogen, but that this is not the case is shown by the finding that adrenalectomised animals (and human subjects) on a constant maintenance dose of cortisol still show the same negative nitrogen balance when subjected to trauma. It would therefore appear that adrenal hormones are necessary for this metabolic change but do not directly produce it. It may be that they play a permissive role, but the increase in cortisol production is not the direct mechanism involved in the metabolic changes.

Other metabolic changes. *Sodium and water metabolism.* During the early period after trauma the urine volume diminishes owing to an increased secretion of ADH, and sodium is retained by the kidneys as a result of increased aldosterone secretion. This phase of sodium retention is a little shorter than the catabolic phase; it has been held that this is obligatory, and that the body is defenceless against overdosage, because it cannot excrete sodium and water (see p. 422). However, this view has been disputed.

There is a later return of sodium to the urine; unless there was excessive administration during the oliguric phase, its excretion is little increased.

Potassium metabolism. A negative potassium balance occurs during the initial phase, and is most marked on the first day. Because potassium is intracellular, it is presumed to be liberated at the same time as protein is metabolised: the loss is

2·5 to 3·0 mmol per 1·0 g of nitrogen, and the total loss after a major operation, e.g. gastrectomy, is about 100 mmol.

The average daily intake is about 70 mmol, therefore there is little point in supplementing the diet during convalescence.

Other changes. There is an increased urinary excretion of *creatine* (derived from the muscles), *phosphate*, and *sulphur*. This occurs *pari passu* with the nitrogenous and potassium excretion, and is due to cellular breakdown.

Vitamin C is retained, its excretion in the urine being dramatically reduced. A scorbutic state may develop despite this careful guarding of the ascorbic-acid stores. *Riboflavin*, on the other hand, is excreted in excess.

During this catabolic phase there is a marked loss of weight. A moderate *pyrexia* is invariable, and is not due to concomitant infection.

The haematological changes are a moderate neutrophilia accompanied by a lymphopenia and eosinopenia. There is also a thrombocytosis (see p. 489). An interesting feature of severe trauma is the development of a progressive normocytic, normochromic anaemia. This is not due to iron deficiency; it may be that there is deficient haemoglobin synthesis during a period of general protein breakdown. Sludging may accentuate this anaemia (see p. 421).

The Anabolic Phase

The final stage of convalescence is characterised by a positive nitrogen balance and a resynthesis of muscle protein. The changes noted during the catabolic phase are reversed, and the body returns to normal.

THE CIRCULATORY CHANGES

The changes in the circulation are seen to their best advantage following acute haemorrhage; this will therefore be described first.

HAEMORRHAGE

Haemorrhage is the most dramatic of the circulatory disorders. The bleeding may occur externally or into the body tissues, usually a hollow viscus or one of the serous cavities. The blood loss may be large and sudden, or small bleeds may occur repeatedly. The changes which follow differ markedly in these two instances; chronic blood loss produces an iron-deficiency anaemia (see p. 607), whereas acute haemorrhage, which may be arterial or venous, leads to more serious immediate consequences.

Causes of Acute Haemorrhage

Trauma. Penetrating wounds involving the heart or large vessels may result in the very rapid loss of large quantities of blood. Bleeding from the large vascular spaces exposed during labour can be of frightening severity.

Abnormalities of the blood-vessel wall. *Inflammatory lesions* may cause weakening of a vessel wall, usually arterial, with subsequent rupture. Aneurysmal dilatation may occur before the final rupture. Bleeding from a chronic peptic ulcer, typhoid ulcers, Rasmussen's aneurysm traversing a tuberculous cavity in the lung, and syphilitic aortic aneurysm are well-known examples. The inflammation need not always be infective, e.g. polyarteritis nodosa.

Neoplastic invasion. Haemorrhage is a frequent terminal event in carcinoma of the tongue, and is due to rupture of the lingual artery; superimposed infection is a major factor in the weakening of the wall.

Other vascular diseases. Atheroma, either with or without aneurysmal dilatation, is the most common cause. Aneurysms due to trauma or persistent friction, e.g. subclavian aneurysm due to cervical rib, also fall into this category.

High pressure within the vessels. Systemic hypertension may precipitate haemorrhage at sites of arterial weakness. Raised venous pressure with varicose-vein formation, e.g. in the legs or oesophagus, is another important cause of severe haemorrhage.

Effects of Acute Haemorrhage

These depend mainly upon two factors:
1. The amount of blood lost.
2. The speed with which the loss occurs.

The general effects are slight when less than 20 per cent of the blood volume is lost. A sudden loss of 33 per cent may cause death, but if the bleeding extends over a period of 24 hours, a loss of over 50 per cent of blood volume is not necessarily fatal. However, with losses of over 50 per cent the effects are always serious. Individuals, both human and animal, show a considerable variation in their response to blood loss, even though the amount and rate are constant. It is therefore impossible to assess accurately the magnitude of any haemorrhage on purely clinical grounds.

The body response to acute haemorrhage may be divided into three phases:

PHASE I

The early changes. During the first few hours the manifestations are mostly due to nervous mechanisms. An immediate syncope may occur, and this is followed by important vascular changes which result in the redistribution of the remaining blood, the volume of which is considerably depleted.

Immediate syncope ('primary shock'). The vasovagal attack, or faint, is seen only in the human, and may perhaps represent an escape mechanism. It commences with yawning, sighing respiration, nausea, and vomiting. This is followed by loss of consciousness, but the attack rarely lasts for more than a few minutes. The condition is characterised by a fall in blood pressure, a slow pulse, and pallor and coldness of the extremities. The cardiac output remains unchanged, but there is a widespread dilatation of the arteries of the muscles which results in a dramatic fall in blood pressure and a reduction in the cerebral blood flow.[2] This leads to a loss of consciousness.

Emotional stress has been shown to lead to vasodilatation of muscular vessels in normal individuals, and an overaction of this mechanism in sensitive individuals can lead to fainting.[3] Thus, although syncope is more common after large haemorrhages than small ones, psychological factors such as fear and anxiety also play a large part. Healthy people may faint when only a few ml of blood are withdrawn, and even the sight of blood may be sufficient. Pain is also an important factor. It is possible that the fainting reflex helps to divert blood to the brain by causing the patient to fall to the ground. When the horizontal position is assumed recovery soon occurs.

The phase of redistribution of available blood to vital centres.[2] The changes are summarised in Figure 32.1. Following haemorrhage the venous return to the heart falls; cardiac catheterisation confirms that the right atrial pressure is low. In this way the cardiac output is reduced, and the blood pressure tends to fall. The tonic inhibitory impulses arising from the aortic and carotid sinuses are therefore reduced. Baroreceptors are also present in the atria. The increased activity of the vasomotor centre results in an increased peripheral resistance, and the *blood pressure is maintained*. The blood vessels of the brain are not affected by this generalised vasoconstriction, and the coronary vessels actually dilate. There is also *tachycardia*. Normally impulses from the carotid and aortic sinuses stimulate the cardiac centre, which is responsible for slowing the heart *via* the vagus. If the impulses drop, vagal activity is reduced.

Contraction of the spleen occurs in animals, and the reserve of blood injected into the circulation helps maintain the blood volume. This is of little importance in the human subject. The venous reservoir is of greater significance. In the human 60 to 70 per cent of the blood volume is contained in the veins and venules. Constriction of these vessels can readily increase the venous return to the heart; following a 10 per cent blood loss, contraction of the venous reservoir can prevent any change occurring in the cardiac output and blood pressure.

The arteriolar constriction is selective: the blood flow to the skin, salivary glands, intestines, liver, spleen, and kidneys is reduced. The skin becomes pale, clammy, and cold. Salivary secretion stops, the mouth becomes dry, and thirst results. The intestine manifests impaired digestion, and water is not well absorbed—a point to remember when treating patients.

The blood flow to essential organs is, however, maintained. These include the brain, heart, diaphragm, intercostal muscles and skeletal muscles generally. Although this selective vasoconstriction is mediated mainly by autonomic nerves, two additional mechanisms play some part:

(*a*) The *adrenal medulla* secretes excess adrenaline and noradrenaline.[4] Both are general vasoconstrictors, but adrenaline dilates skeletal muscular arteries while noradrenaline dilates the coronary vessels.

(*b*) There is also an increased secretion of *renin* by the kidneys, due to a decreased renal afferent arteriolar pressure (see Ch. 46).

These mechanisms tend to restore the blood pressure, and divert blood from the less essential organs to those of immediate importance, namely the heart and brain. With a blood loss of less than 30 per cent the blood pressure tends to remain almost unchanged. Blood-pressure measurements are therefore not an accurate guide to the severity of the bleeding. If the blood loss is of such a magnitude that these compensatory mechanisms are unable to maintain an effective blood pressure, *haemorrhagic shock* ensues.

Occasionally *hypertension* occurs soon after a haemorrhage, but this is usually a transient phase, and is presumably due to the overaction of the compensatory nervous adjustments already described. The pulse rate is either normal or slow, and the blood volume not reduced below 80 per cent.

Changes in respiration. The pulmonary blood flow is reduced

Figure 32.1
The cardiovascular effects of sudden haemor-
rhage. RC: Respiratory Centre. CC: Cardiac
Centre. VMC: Vasomotor Centre.

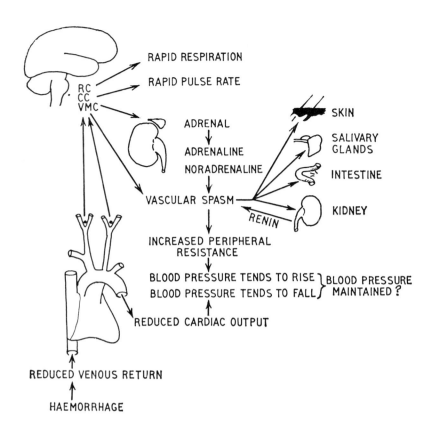

pari passu with the cardiac output. There is an increase in the physiological dead-space due to the under-perfusion of the upper parts of the lungs. The increase in dead-space ventilation in part explains the hyperpnoea which characteristically occurs after haemorrhage. The major factor causing this air hunger, however, is a fall in arterial blood pH due to metabolic acidosis.

Blood supply to the brain. The blood flow through the brain can be measured experimentally by the use of radioactive krypton. A quantity of the gas, dissolved in saline, is injected into the arterial supply, and on reaching the brain there is equilibration between blood and tissue. The ^{85}Kr which passes through into the venous blood is nearly all excreted in the lungs, and there is very little recirculation. The dissolved gas in the brain tissue is measured by an end-window Geiger-Muller tube, and its rate of disappearance is a measure of the cerebral blood flow in that area.

The blood flow to the brain is determined by the systemic blood pressure and the resistance of the cerebral vasculature. When the blood flow to the brain is reduced as a result of hypotension, the Po_2 of the brain tissue is reduced and the Pco_2 rises. These changes cause vasodilatation and a corresponding increase in blood flow. Thus, the cerebral blood flow is maintained at the expense of the other tissues. Any marked reduction of arterial Pco_2 due to hyperpnoea tends to impair the cerebral circulation, because the cerebral vessels are very sensitive to changes in CO_2 tension. The administration of morphine under these circumstances will so depress respiration that the arterial Pco_2 rises, the cerebral vessels dilate, and the blood flow to the brain is improved. When the

flow falls below a critical level for any length of time, the cortical neurons undergo necrosis. The neurons of the brain-stem appear to be less susceptible to hypoxia, and remain unaffected even in the presence of cortical damage. Blindness may occasionally follow acute haemorrhage, especially gastrointestinal. The mechanism involved is not well understood; spasm of the retinal arteries may be a factor.

Blood supply to the heart. The coronary blood flow is related to the systemic blood pressure and the duration of ventricular diastole. Tachycardia and hypotension both tend to produce myocardial ischaemia. Heart failure may therefore occur (see later).

Renal blood flow. There is intense renal vasoconstriction which leads to oliguria and even anuria (see Ch. 46). Prolonged ischaemia can cause severe damage to the kidneys. Antidiuretic hormone (ADH) secretion contributes to the oliguria. Moderate ischaemia can interfere with tubular function such that there is an inability to concentrate urine. Hence there may be an increased excretion of a dilute urine. This effect is ADH resistant.

Blood changes. A haemorrhage should be viewed in the same light as an amputation of any organ. Immediately after the trauma the remainder of the organ is unchanged. In other words, the haemoglobin level and the red-cell count are both normal immediately after haemorrhage. It is useless to use these estimations as immediate guides to the amount of blood lost.

The *platelet count* rapidly rises after haemorrhage, and may be 1000×10^9 per litre (1 000 000 per μl) within an hour. The *clotting time* decreases within a few minutes and the *fibrinolytic system* is activated. It is an old observation by William Hewson, a friend of the Hunters, that when animals are killed by bleeding, 'the blood which issued last coagulated first.[5] In one experiment with rabbits, a 15·4 per cent blood loss reduced the clotting time from 2·5 to 1·75 minutes, while a 30·9 per cent loss reduced it to 1 minute.[6] The accelerated clotting and increased fibrinolysis are transient phenomena which are soon succeeded by other important changes. Aggregation of red cells (sludging) is described as occurring within a few hours of injury, and this impedes the flow of blood in the small vessels.[7] Small clumps of platelets and fibrin further obstruct the circulation, and multiple micro-thrombi have been described in the lungs following haemorrhage, shock, and operations involving the use of an extracorporeal circulation. These changes last for 2 to 3 days. The blood fibrinogen level rises and with it the ESR; a peak is reached in 2 to 3 days, and this is followed by a slow return to normal.

The *white-cell count* rises within 2 to 5 hours, and may reach 35×10^9 per litre (35 000 per μl). The excess cells are neutrophil leucocytes released from the stores in the bone marrow. Many of the cells are young, and occasional myelocytes appear.

PHASE II

The restoration of blood volume. During this phase fluid is withdrawn from the tissue spaces into the blood stream. The mechanism is as follows: the arteriolar spasm results in a lowering of the capillary pressure. On Starling's hypothesis fluid therefore passes into the vessels, and this continues until the reduction in plasma osmotic pressure due to the dilution of the plasma proteins is sufficiently great to offset the forces tending to draw fluid into the blood. The lost plasma proteins are replaced within 2 to 3 days. As the blood volume is restored, so the vasospasm passes off, and the capillary pressure rises. Thus, extracellular fluid passes into the blood until the forces governing the interchange of fluid across the capillary wall are balanced. During this phase there is progressive haemodilution, rapid at first and complete by about 2 days (see Fig. 32.2).

Haemoglobin estimations are now of value, because they reflect the magnitude of the original blood loss. The importance of knowing the haemoglobin level immediately after the haemorrhage is apparent, for it provides a baseline from which subsequent changes can be assessed.

PHASE III

The replacement of lost red cells. *During the dilution phase anaemia becomes apparent, and is of a normocytic, normochromic type.* The dilute blood is an inefficient oxygenator of the tissues, and therefore more oxygen is extracted from it. The total amount of oxygen supplied to the tissues may be adequate, but the oxygen tension of tissue and venous blood is low. Sometimes the quantity of oxygen supplied to the tissues is insufficient; the anaemic hypoxia so engendered leads to anaerobic cell metabolism, resulting in the release of lactic acid. A metabolic acidosis follows, and is accompanied by hyperpnoea.

Within 4 to 7 days the *reticulocyte count* reaches 5 to 15 per cent, indicating active red-cell formation. The bone marrow shows normoblastic hyperplasia, the stimulus for which is probably erythropoietin (see p. 605). Generally the anaemia remains normocytic and normochromic; macrocytosis may develop due to the large number of reticulocytes. Microcytic, hypochromic anaemia does not generally occur, unless the patient is already suffering from iron deficiency due, for example, to previous haemorrhage. The reticulocytosis should abate after 10 to 14 days; failure to do so suggests recurrent haemorrhage. The white-cell count should return to normal after 3 to 4 days.

The rate of recovery of the red cells is dependent upon the severity of the anaemia. At first red cells are produced rapidly,

Figure 32.2
Haemoglobin levels after haemorrhage involving loss of 40 per cent of blood volume.

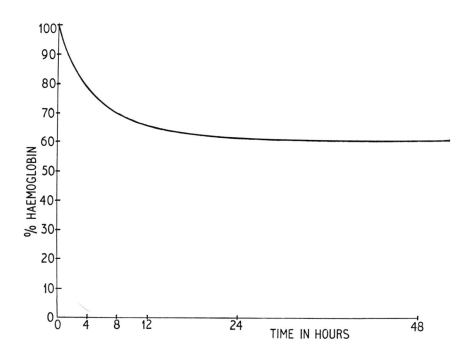

e.g. 2 per cent increase in haemoglobin each day, but as the count approaches normal, so the rate slows down. Complete recovery takes about 6 weeks regardless of the severity of the original haemorrhage. Of course, in practice the process is accelerated by blood transfusions.

SHOCK[8]

Shock is the name given to a clinical state in which the patient has a tachycardia, and is pale, ashen, and sweating. The transient *primary shock*, or vasovagal attack, which follows immediately after injury has already been described (see p. 413). Though the vasovagal attack is transient and benign, death has been attributed to it following certain surgical procedures, e.g. 'obstetric shock' following manual removal of the placenta, and 'pleural shock' after paracentesis. It has been reported that syncope occurring during the induction of anaesthesia may be fatal if the anaesthetic is administered with the patient in the upright position, e.g. in a dental chair. The remainder of this section will be devoted to the much more important *secondary shock*, which occurs as a complication of the ebb phase previously described.

The patient presents a characteristic appearance. He lies still and apathetic, his temperature is subnormal, his skin cold and clammy, and his face ashen-grey. Obvious cyanosis may be present. The blood pressure is low, and the pulse rapid and thready. Little or no urine is passed.

The clinical picture of shock may occur in many conditions, and these have been included in the general classification of 'shock':

Loss of blood (haemorrhagic shock).

Overwhelming infection, e.g. anthrax septicaemia and gas-gangrene.

Loss of plasma, e.g. burns.

Loss of fluid and electrolytes, e.g. diabetic coma, sodium and water depletion, etc.

Cardiogenic shock, e.g. after myocardial infarction.

Anaphylactic shock, see Chapter 14.

The inclusion of so many divergent syndromes under this one heading has tended to obscure our understanding of the condition. They all produce a similar clinical picture which is described as shock, but it is hardly to be expected that the mechanisms involved would be the same in each case. It should also be remembered that a state of shock frequently precedes death regardless of the cause, e.g. electrocution, overdose of drugs, drowning, or following massive total body irradiation (p. 405). To attempt to understand 'shock' it is necessary to consider each condition separately.

Methods of Investigating Haemorrhagic and Traumatic Shock

Attempts to produce a standard response to injury in animals have not been very successful. Many variable factors are involved, including the age and nutrition of the animal, temperature, etc. These often result in great variations in response even after a standard injury. The situation in fact is similar to that encountered in injured patients. The following standard injuries have been used:

1. Rats are placed in a drum, which on rotation throws the animals against fixed projections. The injury can be varied by altering the number of revolutions, but the use of this method on unanaesthetised animals is to be deprecated.

2. Bleeding.

3. Scalding.

4. Occluding the blood supply to a limb (tourniquet shock, see p. 419).

The simplest and most intensively studied is haemorrhagic shock.

Haemorrhagic Shock

The loss of blood volume and the reduction of cardiac output tend to lower the blood pressure. If the compensatory mechanisms described on page 413 are effective, the blood pressure is maintained and no 'shock' develops. This end-result of haemorrhage is familiar to any blood donor.

If the compensatory mechanisms fail to maintain the blood pressure, either as a result of their own inefficiency or the excessive load placed upon them by a large haemorrhage, the patient enters into a state of *shock*. Recovery may occur spontaneously or as a result of efficient treatment, e.g. transfusion; such shock is therefore said to be *reversible*. It sometimes happens that in spite of vigorous and efficient treatment the blood pressure continues to fall, the patient's clinical condition deteriorates, and death ensues. This is *irreversible shock* (Fig. 32.3).

The phenomenon can be demonstrated experimentally. If an animal is bled to the extent that its blood pressure is considerably reduced, immediate replacement of the blood restores the blood pressure to its previous level—the shock is reversible. If the experiment is repeated, but on this occasion the animal is allowed to remain in a hypotensive state ('shock') for some period before reinfusing the lost blood, it is found that the blood pressure is not restored to normal, but continues to fall. The animal is in a state of irreversible shock, and dies in spite of a full restoration of blood volume. Some other mechanism must be involved. This is one of the main problems that has to be solved before the cause of the irreversibility of shock can be explained.

Traumatic Shock

In spite of the considerable amount of research which has been done on the changes that follow trauma, no comprehensive account can yet be given.

The *circulatory changes* which occur resemble those already described following acute haemorrhage. In the human fainting may occur. This is related to many factors amongst which may be mentioned age, sex, extent of the injury, amount of blood loss, and pain.

Following this the various nervous mechanisms come into play to help maintain the blood pressure. If these are unsuccessful, a state of shock develops. The possible causes of this more dangerous secondary shock must now be considered.

Loss of blood. In the past it has not been fully recognised that there is considerable loss of blood from the circulation in all but the most trivial injuries. In closed injuries of the limbs an estimate of this blood loss may be made by measuring the extent of the swelling. Actual measurements of the blood volume following fractures have shown the magnitude of this

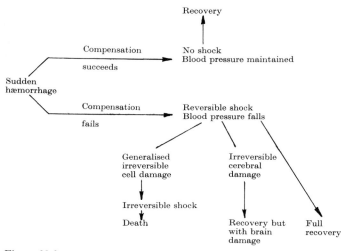

Figure 32.3
The possible end-results of a sudden haemorrhage.

blood loss. Thus, in simple closed fractures of the tibia and fibula 0·5 to 1 litre is usually lost, but it may exceed 3 litres in severe cases. An average closed fracture of the shaft of the femur loses about 2 litres into the surrounding tissues.

A practical rule which is a guide in traumatic surgery is to relate blood loss to wound size as measured in terms of a clenched fist.

		% Blood volume lost
Small wounds:	Less than 1 hand	20
Moderate wounds:	1–3 hands	20–40
Large wounds:	3–5 hands	40
Very large wounds:	Over 5 hands	50

Blood loss during operations is often quite considerable, and in all major surgery reliable methods must be employed to measure it. The amount on swabs can be estimated by weighing, or by extracting the haemoglobin and measuring it colorimetrically. Blood-volume measurements can now be made more easily (see p. 422).

It is evident therefore that the circulatory changes following physical trauma could be due largely to haemorrhage.

Toxins from the damaged area. Many toxic substances, including potassium and histamine, have been isolated from damaged tissue, but none has been proved to be of any great clinical importance in the pathogenesis of human shock.

Increase in vascular permeability to proteins. It has been postulated that loss of circulating plasma follows a generalised increase in vascular permeability. This has never been substantiated, although some loss must obviously occur into the wound itself due to the formation of an acute inflammatory exudate. Fluid loss into the injured area is thought to be a major factor in the production of tourniquet shock.

Infection of the wound. There is little doubt that the powerful exotoxins of the pathogenic clostridia exert a profound effect on the circulation. Gas-gangrene, even in the absence of substantial traumatic damage, causes a shock-like condition which may terminate in death. It is equally probable

that the toxins of other organisms contribute to shock: staphylococcal α-toxin may be cited as an example.

Experiments designed to show that damaged tissues liberate 'toxin' are often invalidated by the fact that normal tissues may be contaminated with bacteria. In the dog, for example, the muscles frequently contain *Clostridium welchii*. Furthermore, wounds in experimental animals frequently become infected from external sources.

Endotoxic factor in shock (Sanarelli phenomenon). It has been shown that bacterial endotoxins are capable of producing shock by some type of sensitisation. Experimentally it is known that an intravenous injection of a suspension of certain organisms, e.g. *Vibrio cholerae*, meningococci, and many members of the coli-typhoid group, will induce a state of 'sensitisation', such that if the injection is repeated intravenously *24 hours later*, a shock-like condition results. The reaction is most easily elicited in rabbits, and frequently results in death after a few hours. Many small vessels are blocked by fibrin, and bilateral cortical necrosis of the kidney is a characteristic *postmortem* finding in animals dying at about 24 hours (Fig. 32.4).

Some important features should be noted:

(*a*) Lipoprotein extracts ('endotoxins') can be used instead of whole organisms.

(*b*) The reaction is completely non-specific, i.e. the same organism need not be used for both injections.

(*c*) The state of sensitivity is of temporary duration; it remains for 1 to 2 days only, and is in no way connected with antibody production.

No certain explanation of this remarkable phenomenon is known. Probably a temporary blockade of the RE system is an important factor, and perhaps this defect, combined with the excessive formation of fibrin, is responsible for the production of intravascular fibrin plugs which are characteristic of the lesions seen in endotoxic shock. Such a pathogenesis would explain why the prior administration of heparin inhibits the reaction. Intravascular coagulation is probably initiated by the release of platelet factors which occurs when platelets interact with endotoxin.[9] Rendering animals thrombocytopenic protects them against the Sanarelli phenomenon, as does the administration of aspirin, which interferes with the platelet release reaction (p. 487). Complement is also involved, for the injection of venom from the cobra *Naja naja* is also protective, presumably by depleting the terminal components of complement *via* activation of the alternate pathway[10] (p. 160).

The original observations were made by Sanarelli at the end of the last century and a somewhat similar, non-specific, local sensitisation was later described by Shwartzman. For this reason the generalised response is sometimes known as the 'generalised Shwartzman phenomenon'.

It has been suggested that organisms of the coliform group normally pass from the gut into the portal blood stream and then to the liver. It is therefore possible that such continuous intravenous injections of organisms or their endotoxins could produce a Shwartzman-like state, if one postulates that the liver's normal function is to remove these, and that in shock this mechanism is impaired. It has been shown that the blood from a dog in shock contains a toxic substance which has the properties of bacterial endotoxin. Furthermore, oral antibiotics can markedly influence the severity of shock produced by bleeding. There is thus some evidence that toxic substances in

Figure 32.4
Cortical necrosis of kidney. This kidney came from a patient who died of bilateral symmetrical cortical necrosis following abruptio placentae. The outer two thirds of the cortex is pale and infarcted, while the inner part of the kidney is very congested. A similar appearance is seen in the rabbit kidney as a result of the Sanarelli phenomenon.

the intestine are concerned in the production of shock. However, some investigators have found that oral antibiotics are without protective effect on haemorrhagic shock. Furthermore, it has been shown that shock can be produced just as easily in germ-free rats as in normal ones. At first sight this argues against the importance of the bacterial factor. Nevertheless, bacterial products present in the food might be absorbed and produce a toxic effect. Whether bacterial endotoxin plays any part in the production of haemorrhagic or traumatic shock in the human has yet to be determined.[11]

The concentration of bacterial endotoxin in blood can be estimated by its ability to gel extracts of the blood amoebocytes of the horseshoe crab, *Limulus polyphemus*. This test is extremely sensitive, but Gram-negative endotoxin can also be detected in the blood in conditions other than shock. It seems therefore that the test is not of great value, since the levels of endotoxin do not closely parallel the clinical evidence of endotoxaemia.[12]

It should be noted that most of the experiments designed to illustrate the importance of the endotoxic factor in haemorrhagic or traumatic shock have been performed on the dog or

the rabbit. Both exhibit certain peculiarities: thus, the rabbit is particularly susceptible to the Sanarelli phenomenon, and the dog's intestine is very sensitive to ischaemia. Dogs dying of haemorrhagic shock show striking necrosis of the small intestine, and it is not surprising that toxic substances are absorbed.

Endotoxic shock in the human.[13] Sudden collapse may occur during a variety of infections, commonly those of the urinary tract. Usually the condition is precipitated by some manipulation or operation on the urethra or bladder. It is ascribed to the sudden entry into the blood of Gram-negative bacilli, and a positive blood culture may be obtained. An alternative name is therefore *bacteraemic shock*. The condition may also occur in cirrhosis of the liver, as a consequence of the portal-systemic venous shunts, and in patients on immunosuppressive therapy. Energetic steroid and antibiotic treatment may be life-saving.

Damage to the heart.[14] The heart extracts more oxygen from the blood than does any other organ, hence it is more vulnerable to the effects of hypoxia than other organs. Patchy myocardial necrosis is a common finding in the hearts of patients dying of shock, and may indeed be the cause of death.

Damage to the adrenal glands. Adrenal necrosis, sometimes accompanied by haemorrhage, may complicate shock, and acute adrenal insufficiency may contribute to death (p. 449).

Pancreatic damage. It is not uncommon to find patchy pancreatic necrosis with dystrophic calcification in necropsies on patients dying of shock. This is of little importance, but occasionally the necrosis is extensive enough to contribute to death.

Damage to the gastrointestinal tract. In the human ischaemia of the gastrointestinal tract after shock is less striking than in the dog. Acute *stress ulcers* of the stomach or duodenum may occur after any injury, but are best known in association with severe burns (*Curling's ulcer*).*[15] These acute ulcers may bleed profusely. Ischaemia of the intestine can lead to focal areas of mucosal infarction in both the small and large intestine (particularly the splenic flexure).[16] The ensuing ulceration causes loss of blood and fluid which adds to the patient's plight.

Liver damage. Quite apart from the effect on the RE cells causing undue susceptibility to bacterial endotoxin it has been suggested that the poor blood flow to the liver has other results. Impaired liver function may be detected by suitable clinical tests, and at necropsy focal necrosis, usually centrilobular, may be noted.

It has been claimed that the liver releases a vasodepressor material (VDM, which is reduced ferritin) which causes vasodilatation, and makes vessels unresponsive to adrenaline. The consensus of opinion is that this is not an important factor in shock. The release of lysosomal enzymes from the liver has also been postulated as a factor in the pathogenesis of

*The term *Cushing's ulcer* is usually reserved for the ulceration of the oesophagus, stomach, or duodenum that occurs in association with intracranial trauma or tumour, or after craniotomy. In contrast with the multiple superficial erosions of typical Curling's ulcers, the ulcers described by Cushing are deep and penetrating, with a tendency to perforation by a dissolution of the entire wall.

shock. The effect of glucocorticoids in stabilising the lysosomes could explain how this drug protects rabbits against endotoxic shock.

Lung damage. Pulmonary congestion and oedema are common in patients dying of shock and are also seen following cardio-pulmonary bypass procedures. The sequestration of polymorphs in the lung capillaries and the release of their lysosomal enzymes is one suggested mechanism in this 'shock-lung syndrome'.[17]

Fat embolism. An occasional feature of shock in the human is the occurrence of fat embolism. It has been shown experimentally in animals that the deliberate introduction of fat emboli into the circulation does not have any effect upon the degree of shock that is produced by trauma. This factor therefore can be discounted as an important cause of shock.

Conclusion. Although the causes of shock following mechanical trauma are poorly understood, the most important factor in the early stages is loss of blood. Local inflammation and the effects of infection may later aggravate this, but their relative importance probably varies from case to case.

Shock in Infections

In addition to Gram-negative endotoxic shock described above, a shock-like state followed by death has been described in many infections, including those produced by Gram-positive organisms, rickettsiae (Rocky mountain spotted fever and typhus), and viruses (dengue, Bolivian haemorrhagic fever, chickenpox, and measles). The pathogenesis is not necessarily the same in the two types.[18] It occurs in diphtheria and gas-gangrene, and can be produced experimentally by injecting animals with the respective exotoxins. In overwhelming infections with an invasive organism various factors play a part. In *Bacillus anthracis* septicaemia in guinea-pigs it has been shown that a toxin is produced, and that the rapid formation of oedema leads to hypovolaemic shock. In *Yersinia pestis* infections, on the other hand, oligaemia does not occur, and the shock appears to be due to a pooling of the blood in the splanchnic area. The mechanisms whereby shock is produced are complex, and probably vary in different infections. The possibility that bacterial toxins damage specific organs must also be considered: thus diphtheria toxin damages the heart and kidneys. Another example is acute adrenal haemorrhage. This occurs in the *Waterhouse-Friderichsen syndrome*, which is characterised by bilateral adrenal haemorrhages and confluent purpura occurring in patients with septicaemia (usually meningococcal) dying rapidly in a state of shock. Death has been ascribed to acute adrenal insufficiency, but this is most improbable. The normal levels of plasma electrolytes, the rapid course of the syndrome, and the inconstancy of the adrenal haemorrhages all point to the conclusion that the cause of death is the infection itself, while the haemorrhages are secondary. They are believed to be due to disseminated intravascular coagulation (p. 643).

It has been suggested that the Jarisch-Herxheimer reaction (p. 249) is a manifestation of endotoxic shock, and that the sudden release of bacterial toxins is the cause of the occasional fatality that is encountered in the treatment of syphilis and louse-borne relapsing fever.[19]

Shock due to Loss of Plasma

Rapid loss of plasma from the circulation occurs whenever an acute inflammatory reaction involves a large area of the body. This is seen experimentally in *tourniquet shock*. The blood supply to a limb is occluded by means of a rubber band for 5 hours, and when this is released the animal subsequently goes into a state of shock and dies. This is due to a leakage of plasma into the infarcted limb. A similar condition is seen in the human in the crush syndrome, following extensive burns, and when there is the rapid accumulation of an exudate, e.g. ascites. Generalised loss of plasma from the circulation is a factor in the shock of anaphylaxis and in the rare, but remarkable, case of cyclical oedema noted on page 525.

Burn Shock

The shock produced by extensive burning is very similar to that of haemorrhage. There are, however, certain differences. The early clinical picture is often misleading. A patient admitted with a 40 per cent burn may appear to be in excellent condition 1 to 2 hours after the accident; 10 hours later, however, there may be a state of irreversible shock. In general, the severity of the shock is proportional to the extent of the skin burned. Thus in children, if the area of burning exceeds 10 per cent of the surface area, or in adults 15 per cent, the patient is likely to need intravenous therapy. The area burned may be estimated by the simple *rule of nines*. This is shown diagrammatically in Figure 32.5.

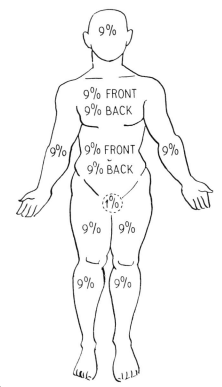

Figure 32.5
The rule of nines. The body surface of an adult may be divided into eleven areas each comprising 9 per cent approximately. (*After Wallace, A. B.* (1951), Lancet, **1**, 501)

The effect of heat on tissues has been studied experimentally. A temperature of 50°C leads to vasodilatation with an additional formation of protein-poor extravascular fluid. A temperature of 55°C causes, in addition, an increase in vascular permeability. This leads to the formation of a protein-rich exudate. Temperatures of 100°C or more simply coagulate the tissue, and cause complete cessation of blood flow. An important feature of burns therefore is the loss of fluid from the circulation, and much of that which exudes from the burned area has a composition similar to plasma. It has been shown in animals that the volume of fluid lost in a 50 per cent burn is equal to the entire circulating plasma volume. This fluid loss results in a low blood volume. In burns, unlike haemorrhage, the viscosity of the blood is increased; haemoconcentration occurs instead of dilution. Although the loss of plasma from the circulating blood is important in the causation of burn shock, other factors may also play a part and contribute to the over-all picture observed clinically:

Vomiting is not uncommon, and leads to dehydration.

Infection may occur in the wound.

Red cells may be damaged in the burned area. This results in a haemolytic anaemia, especially after extensive burning. Haemoglobinuria occasionally occurs.

Sludging of the blood is a prominent feature.

Anaesthetics may potentiate the shock.

Liver damage: this was usually seen following the application of tannic acid to the burns.

Gastrointestinal ulceration and bleeding: (see p. 418).

Cerebral damage:[20] burns may be followed, particularly in children, by psychiatric and neurological complications. These are often fatal, and those patients who survive may suffer permanent cerebral damage. The cause of these phenomena is not known, but cerebral oedema and hypoxia have been suggested.

Shock from Fluid Loss

Shock may be induced in animals by subjecting them to prolonged unnatural postures. If an anaesthetised dog is suspended with its feet hanging down it passes into a state of shock, especially if a small quantity of blood is removed at the same time. Haemoconcentration develops due to the loss of fluid through the vessels in the dependent parts.

Subcutaneous injections of hypertonic solutions, e.g. 40 per cent glucose, will also lead to the withdrawal of fluid from the circulating blood, thereby producing a shock-like state with haemoconcentration. In the human shock may result from dehydration due to inadequate fluid intake or excessive loss, such as may follow excessive sweating, vomiting, or diarrhoea. Infants are particularly vulnerable because they cannot secrete as concentrated a urine as can adults. Diarrhoea is therefore a serious condition in this age group. Dehydration is also a feature of diabetic coma.

It appears that the most important causative factor in the types of shock so far considered is the loss of circulating blood volume. A convenient term is therefore *hypovolaemic shock*. It is due to loss of blood, plasma, or fluid.

In other types of shock the blood volume is not primarily or greatly altered, and some other mechanisms must be invoked. These are not clearly defined at the present time; four aspects should be considered:

Cardiogenic shock.
Peripheral vascular failure.
The metabolic upset.
Poor capillary circulation due to sludging.

Cardiogenic Shock

Myocardial infarction may sometimes produce a clinical state which resembles that of hypovolaemic shock. The cardiac output is reduced, and the poor perfusion of tissues is responsible for a metabolic acidosis. This acidosis can lead to peripheral vasodilatation with pooling of blood and subsequent transudation; the loss of fluid tends to lower the blood volume and accentuate the shock. Cardiogenic shock is also seen in a number of other conditions: myocarditis, acute valvular dysfunction such as occurs following the rupture of a papillary muscle (itself often the result of infarction), serious cardiac dysrhythmias, cardiac tamponade, and tension pneumothorax with marked mediastinal shift.

Heart failure may be an important additional factor in the pathogenesis of hypovolaemic shock. In experiments with dogs, a state of haemorrhagic shock can be induced such that replacement of the lost blood does not save the animals. Further transfusion causes a rise in central venous pressure and a fall in cardiac output—a sure indication that the heart is failing. The administration of digitalis improves the state of the animals. Thus, heart failure may be an important factor in experimental irreversible shock.

In the human, focal microscopic or massive myocardial infarcts are sometimes found at necropsy in patients dying in shock, and in these cases heart failure appears to have been the immediate cause of death. Nevertheless, there is little evidence that heart failure contributes significantly to most cases of haemorrhagic, traumatic, or endotoxic shock, and digitalis is without beneficial effect.

Peripheral Vascular Failure

The concept of peripheral vascular failure embodies the idea that the circulation is impaired, not by a decrease in the blood volume, but by an increase in the capacity of the vascular system. This might occur in various ways. Blood could be *sequestered*, and in this way lost from a functional point of view. Thus, if rabbits are suspended erect they become unconscious in 20 to 120 minutes, and may die in a shock-like state within 24 hours. They show a low blood pressure, oliguria, and a metabolic acidosis. Haemoconcentration does not occur, and the condition is due to the pooling of the blood in the splanchnic area, with the result that the supply of oxygen to the vital organs is impaired. The fainting of guardsmen on parade is due to a similar mechanism—the blood becomes sequestered in the leg veins—but the condition is not serious, for the automatic assumption of the horizontal position effects a cure!

The contraction of arterioles and veins is an important compensatory reaction in hypotension, and a failure in this mechanism could be an additional factor in shock due initially to other causes. Furthermore, if the venous constriction is maintained while the arterioles relax, blood becomes sequestered or pooled in the capillary bed. This has been described in the shock of myocardial infarction, in some types of bacterial shock, e.g. in septicaemic plague, and as a complication of metabolic acidosis.

Metabolic Changes in Shock

In shock, although there is abundant evidence of an upset in carbohydrate metabolism and diminished energy production, the exact nature of the changes remains a mystery. The secretions of the adrenal medulla and cortex are probably important, and these have been considered previously.

Another important metabolic upset that develops during shock is *metabolic acidosis*. The cause is tissue hypoxia with resulting anaerobic glycolysis and the release of pyruvate and lactate into the circulation. Metabolic acidosis is very well marked in haemorrhagic shock, but is also seen in any condition in which there is *underperfusion of the tissues* with blood. Thus, it occurs in many types of shock, and is a well-recognised complication of inadequate blood flow in the extracorporeal cardio-pulmonary bypass.

Sludging

'Shock is not merely a problem of blood volume, blood pressure, and anaemia, but essentially a problem of flow'.[7] The concept has arisen since techniques have been devised to study the flow of blood in vessels of microscopic size. In shock it has been observed that the flow is poor and that the red cells are clumped together. That such clumping can occur *in vivo* is no new observation, but it is largely due to the work of Knisely and his associates that the phenomenon is now being more widely recognised. Working with malaria-infected monkeys they described thick, glassy precipitates between and around the blood cells, binding the red cells together in wads and masses, thus converting the 'circulating blood into a thick muck-like sludge'. The red cells are adherent to each other to form aggregates, more irregular than the 'pile of plates' appearance of rouleaux, but differing from true agglutination in that the masses can be broken up again. Some degree of aggregation occurs normally in the post-capillary venules when the flow is slow, and indeed some observers have regarded sludging as a result of stasis rather than its cause. However, there seems little doubt that under certain conditions a solid aggregation of red cells occurs, not only in the venules but also in the arterioles. In this way the blood-flow through the tissues is impaired and the tissue suffers accordingly. Micro-infarcts have been described.

Sludging occurs after trauma, especially burns, haemorrhage, and in shock. It is seen in many infections and also to a minor extent in pregnancy. It is a feature of the generalised Shwartzman phenomenon, and is a complicating factor in the use of extracorporeal circulation techniques.

The suspension stability of the red cells is determined by the composition of the plasma. An increase in the proportion of high-molecular-weight substances results in sludging; in practice a rise in fibrinogen is the most important factor. The administration of high-molecular-weight dextrans has a similar effect.

Low-molecular-weight substances, e.g. albumin and dextran, inhibit or reverse sludging. A low-molecular-weight dextran preparation* is now available for intravenous administration and its value has been proven. In shock it appears to diminish the amount of sludging and improve the circulation of blood through the small vessels.

Quite apart from impeding the circulation, sludging has been suggested as a cause of the anaemia of injury. The clumps of red cells may be trapped in the vessels and thereby become sequestered from the general circulation.

IRREVERSIBLE SHOCK

The reasons why shock becomes irreversible are poorly understood. Irreversibility means that the blood pressure continues to fall despite the compensatory mechanisms and also treatment. The patient's condition steadily deteriorates, and death ensues.

The present concept of shock is that the major abnormalitiy is the underperfusion of certain vital organs. If this ischaemia persists, irreparable damage is done and death becomes inevitable.

Cellular Changes during Shock[21]

The cellular changes are due to ischaemia; lack of oxygen and the accumulation of waste products cause a change in function of the cell membrane. Thus in muscle the resting transmembrane potential can change from -90 mV to -60 mV. Sodium and water enter the cell, and potassium leaves it. Similar changes occur in the liver. Initially the ATPase shows increased activity in response to the entry of sodium into the cell. ATP production by mitochondria is at first increased, but it later declines. The concentration of cyclic AMP decreases, a circumstance which may influence the effects of hormones on the cell. As cell injury proceeds, so the cell swells as do its mitochondria and endoplasmic reticulum (see p. 52). There is a shift from oxidative metabolism to anaerobic glycolysis; the result is the production of lactic acid. Fewer two-carbon fragments (acetyl-coenzyme A) enter the Krebs cycle to be burned and broken down to CO_2 and water. Finally the lysosomal membranes are damaged, and lysosomal enzymes join the scene as the cell dies and undergoes autolysis.

Organs affected. In the dog the organ most obviously affected is the intestine, and haemorrhagic infarction results. In the human the situation is less clear, but renal, cardiac, pulmonary, hepatic, and intestinal damage may all ensue. Death from shock may occur for one of many reasons, either directly related to a particular organ (e.g. myocardial infarction) or as an indirect consequence of organ damage, e.g. metabolic acidosis or electrolyte imbalance. From a practical point of view the efficiency of treatment is of overriding importance, because many of the potentially lethal effects of shock can be counteracted. Irreversible shock may be regarded as being almost always due to inefficient treatment.

The types of treatment will therefore be summarised:[22]

Restoration of Blood Volume

The importance of restoring the blood volume as soon as

---

*This is known as *Rheomacrodex*, and has an average molecular weight of about 40 000 daltons.

possible in hypovolaemic shock is widely recognised. So long as the cardiac output is low, there is compensatory peripheral vasoconstriction. This has the effect of maintaining the blood pressure. At first this is advantageous, but if it persists it may lead ultimately to damage in vital organs.[23]

1. **Blood transfusion.** In severe haemorrhage it is often not appreciated that blood must be given rapidly. Several units must be administered by the fastest means available. Some workers have used intra-arterial transfusions, and it is claimed that these give better results, as the blood is immediately available to support the coronary and cerebral circulations. The use of slow intravenous transfusions after a severe haemorrhage merely induces a false sense of security in both patient and doctor. One of the curious features of human traumatic shock is the response to treatment by transfusion. In wartime this was found to be very effective both in preventing and treating shock. In civilian life, however, the results of such treatment are not nearly so dramatic or effective. This may be related to the fact that in wartime the casualties are usually young, previously healthy people, whereas in civilian practice it is the elderly and sick who are most frequently affected. It is known that shock tends to be more severe in such subjects.[24]

2. **Administration of fluid and electrolytes.** Although some workers have found 'irreversible shock' to be quite unresponsive to fluid therapy, others have been more successful. Thus, hypertonic saline has been reported to be beneficial in severe haemorrhagic shock in dogs,[25] and vigorous fluid replacement is of value in experimental shock due to burns, haemorrhage, and trauma. It is often taught that the body is defenceless against an overdosage of sodium in shock, but this is by no means universally accepted. In the management of patients, the measurement of the blood volume is of much greater value than that of blood pressure. The *Volemetron*,[26] a machine using an isotope dilution technique and incorporating a built-in computer, is invaluable in this respect.

Unfortunately the measurement of blood volume in a shocked patient produces a value which is not easy to interpret. The capacity of the venous reservoir is dependent on the venous tone (p. 413), and furthermore large quantities of blood can be sequestered in the splanchnic area and to all intents and purposes be lost so far as the maintenance of an efficient circulation is concerned. Hence the measurement of the *central venous pressure* has been used as a guide to the quantity of fluid which can be administered intravenously to fill up the vascular system, without at the same time causing pulmonary oedema.

However, this measurement has proved to be less useful than was at first hoped.[27] An estimation of the *left atrial pressure* is now regarded as a more useful guide. This is carried out by inserting a balloon-tipped catheter (Swan and Ganz) into the right ventricle *via* an arm vein. On inflating the balloon, the catheter passes into the pulmonary artery and wedges into a branch of the vessel. A measurement of the wedged pulmonary artery pressure is an accurate guide to the pressure in the left atrium. The catheter can be modified to measure the right ventricular output.

Maintenance of Renal Function

The administration of adequate fluids can do much to maintain the urine output, and some authorities advocate the intravenous administration of an osmotic diuretic, e.g. mannitol. This appears to increase glomerular filtration by causing vasodilatation. Renal damage is a potent cause of death if shock is prolonged. The tubules are most severely affected, and the damage is generally attributable to ischaemia. This, however, is not accepted by all authorities.

Reversal of Sludging

Adequate fluid administration and intravenous Rheomacrodex can do much to reverse the sludging in shock.

Correction of Metabolic Acidosis

Sodium bicarbonate can be given intravenously in sufficient quantity to correct the acidosis.

Maintenance of Adequate Pulmonary Ventilation

Because of the increase in dead-space ventilation, any interference with the hyperpnoea may cause arterial desaturation and respiratory acidosis. Avoidance of airways obstruction is life-saving, and the inhalation of 30 per cent oxygen is helpful.

The Administration of Drugs

It is worth remembering that in any form of shock drugs administered by the intramuscular or subcutaneous routes are slowly absorbed owing to the poor state of the circulation. Failure to get a satisfactory clinical response may necessitate a repetition of the dose. In this way a large depot, e.g. of morphine, may accumulate in the tissues, only to be absorbed later; poisoning then results.

Patients in shock are particularly sensitive to depressant drugs like barbiturates and anaesthetic agents. Furthermore, these drugs decrease venous tone and their injudicious use may be detrimental. Halothane is especially dangerous. The place of morphine in shock is very limited. It is useful in alleviating severe pain, and it may allay the apprehension that follows severe haemorrhage, e.g. haematemesis, but on the whole it is best avoided.

Vasoactive drugs.[13] The administration of adrenergic drugs with a predominant α-receptor stimulating effect (see p. 450), e.g. noradrenaline and metaraminol (aramine), raises the blood pressure in shock, but far from being beneficial tends to worsen the prognosis, because the vasoconstriction which is induced further compromises the already inadequate blood supply to various vital organs, e.g. the kidneys and intestine. An alternative approach, stressed by Lillehei, is therefore to administer vasodilator drugs, e.g. phenoxybenzamine (dibenyline), which has a powerful α-adrenergic blocking action. Experimentally it counters traumatic, haemorrhagic, and endotoxic shock as well as the shock that follows the administration of toxic doses of adrenaline. Drugs with a β-adrenergic receptor stimulating effect, such as isoprenaline (isoproterenol), have also been used. Pharmacological or massive doses of glucocorticoids have also been advocated in the treatment of shock[17] and there is experimental evidence that they protect against endotoxic shock. The mode of action is not clear, but one suggestion is that in pharmacological doses (e.g. 15 to 30 mg per kg of hydrocortisone every 24 hours) they block the action of adrenaline. The logical drug treatment of shock is therefore to administer agents which produce vasodilatation in the vital organs, and at the same time to give adequate intravenous fluids to guard against the development of dangerous hypotension.

Temperature

If the patient is actively warmed, the skin vessels dilate and the effective circulating blood volume is further diminished. The administration of alcohol has a similar effect, and both of these time-honoured treatments of shock should be avoided.

Treatment of Infection

Although obvious enough in diseases like gas-gangrene or diphtheria, infection may sometimes pass unnoticed and untreated.

Treatment of Mechanical Complications

The development of raised intracranial pressure, pneumothorax, haemopericardium, etc. may cause a rapid deterioration in the patient's condition, which is liable to be misdiagnosed as shock and left untreated.

Even with efficient treatment the blood pressure may continue to fall, and the patient dies. This is seen under the following circumstances:

(*a*) With very severe injuries.
(*b*) When the shock has been present for some time.
(*c*) In patients already ill with some disease.
(*d*) In the presence of severe infection.

It is evident that the treatment of shock is often complicated and costly. The more intensive the treatment, the less likely is the patient to die. 'Irreversible shock' should not be accepted as a diagnosis except *post mortem*: there are some surgeons who feel that the term 'shock' itself should be abandoned, as its use tends to result in remediable conditions being overlooked. Nevertheless, there can be little doubt that the condition of shock does exist, and that in spite of even the best treatment some patients die. This may be as a result of the initial injury involving some vital organ, or else through damage sustained during the period of shock. As pointed out previously, there is considerable uncertainty as to which organ is most affected: the intestine, heart, kidney, liver, and brain have all been suggested. Undoubtedly under particular circumstances failure of one of these organs can cause death, and it is naïve to expect the pathogenesis of all types of shock to be identical.

SUMMARY

The changes that occur in a wounded animal from the time of injury to return to complete health are thus highly complex.

During the first few hours the response is concerned largely with circulatory adjustments, the aim of which appears to be to maintain an adequate blood supply to the vital organs. It is only when these mechanisms fail to keep pace with the load placed upon them that the clinical state of shock occurs. During this phase there is reduced energy production associated with changes in carbohydrate metabolism, the nature of which is poorly understood. The only obvious advantage that this confers would seem to be a reduction in the amount of food required during a phase when the injured animal is unlikely to be able to hunt.

Following the successful circulatory adjustment, the animal enters the state of *convalescence*. This consists of two phases:

A catabolic phase, in which protein breakdown is the most conspicuous feature, and is accompanied by sodium and water retention.

An anabolic phase, in which protein is laid down, weight is gained, and the electrolyte balance returns to normal.

It is difficult to explain these changes other than on a teleological basis. During the early phase, the retained sodium and water is required for the inflammatory exudate as well as to help maintain the circulation. A little later the body proteins are broken down and converted into amino acids and glucose. The purpose of this catabolism appears to be twofold. In the first place it provides a source of energy during the early phase of convalescence; for this reason glucose administration reduces the rate of protein breakdown. There is, however, a second reason: when healing commences, the products of protein breakdown provide the raw materials from which are built the new tissues required for repair and regeneration. In the formation of collagen, the sulphur-containing amino acids are essential, and it has been suggested that the catabolism of protein is largely designed to meet this local need in the wounded area. Vitamin C is also required, and this may explain why it also is so carefully conserved.

The duration of the catabolic phase is related to the severity of the injury, and rarely exceeds 10 to 14 days in the absence of further haemorrhage or secondary infection. Considerable loss of weight is to be expected during this phase. As convalescence proceeds and the wounded area heals, so the animal becomes fit enough to resume its search for nourishment. Protein catabolism ceases, and energy is produced from ingested food; the depleted stores are replaced and health is restored.

It would be foolish to imagine that the above account explains the changes that occur in the wounded animal. It is, however, not unreasonable to assume that the complex reactions, while not designed to aid in the restoration of health, have nevertheless been evolved by a process of selection as a means of attaining that same end. John Hunter nearly two centuries ago appreciated this, for in his treatise on the blood, inflammation, and gun-shot wounds, which was published in 1794, a year after his death, he wrote: 'There is a circumstance attending accidental injury which does not belong to disease, viz., that the injury done has in all cases a tendency to produce both the disposition and the means of cure.'

REFERENCES

1. RYAN, N. T. (1976) Metabolic adaptations for energy production during trauma and sepsis. *Surgical Clinics of North America*, **56**, 1073.
2. DICKINSON, C. J. & PENTECOST, B. L. (1974) In *Clinical Physiology*, ed. Campbell, E. J. M., Dickinson, C. J. & Slater, J. D. H., 4th edn, p. 69. Oxford: Blackwell.

3. RODDIE, I. C. & SHEPHERD, J. T. (1963) Nervous control of the circulation in skeletal muscle. *British Medical Bulletin*, **19**, 115.
4. PEKKARINEN, A. (1960) In *Biochemical Response to Injury*: a C.I.O.M.S. Symposium, ed. Stoner, H. B. & Threlfall, C. J., p. 217. Oxford: Blackwell.
5. GULLIVER, G. (Ed.) (1846) *The Works of William Hewson, F.R.S.*, p. 46. London: Sydenham Society.
6. ROBERTS, K. B. (1970) In *General Pathology*, ed. Florey, H. W., 4th edn, p. 319. London: Lloyd-Luke.
7. GELIN, L.-E. (1963) In *Proceedings of a Conference on the Evaluation of Low Molecular Weight Dextran in Shock: Pharmacology and Pertinent Rheology*, ed. Eiseman, B. & Bosomworth, P., p. 6. Washington, D.C.: National Research Council Division of Medical Sciences.
8. SHIRES, G. T., CARRICO, C. J. & CANIZARO, P. C. (1973) *Shock*. Philadelphia: Saunders.
9. MUSTARD, J. F. & PACKHAM, M. A. (1970) Platelet aggregation and the platelet release reaction in thromboembolism. *Canadian Medical Association Journal*, **103**, 859.
10. FONG, J. S. C. & GOOD, R. A. (1971) Prevention of the localized and generalized Shwartzman reactions by an anticomplementary agent, cobra venom factor. *Journal of Experimental Medicine*, **134**, 642.
11. Leading Article (1972) Endotoxaemia in man. *Lancet*, **1**, 1377.
12. ELIN, R. J. *et al.* (1975) Lack of clinical usefulness of the Limulus test in the diagnosis of endotoxemia. *New England Journal of Medicine*, **293**, 521.
13. Leading Article (1970) Septic shock. *British Medical Journal*, **1**, 3.
14. HACKEL, D. B., RATLIFF, N. B. & MIKAT, E. (1974) The heart in shock. *Circulation Research*, **35**, 805.
15. SKILLMAN, J. J. & SILEN, W. (1972) Stress ulcers. *Lancet*, **2**, 1303.
16. Leading Article (1971) Haemorrhagic ulceration of gut. *British Medical Journal*, **3**, 132.
17. WILSON, J. W. (1972) Treatment or prevention of pulmonary cellular damage with pharmacologic doses of corticosteroid. *Surgery, Gynecology and Obstetrics*, **134**, 675.
18. KWAAN, H. M. & WEIL, M. H. (1969) Differences in the mechanism of shock caused by bacterial infections. *Surgery, Gynecology and Obstetrics*, **128**, 37.
19. Leading Article (1977) The Jarisch-Herxheimer reaction. *Lancet*, **1**, 340.
20. WARLOW, C. P. & HINTON, P. (1969) Early neurological disturbances following relatively minor burns in children. *Lancet*, **2**, 978.
21. Baue, A.E. (1976) Metabolic abnormalities of shock. *Surgical Clinics of North America*, **56,** 1059.
22. WALT, A. J. & WILSON, R. F. (1975) Treatment of shock. *Advances in Surgery*, **9**, 1.
23. Leading Article (1963) The reversibility of irreversible shock. *Lancet*, **2**, 1365.
24. SMITH, L. L: & MOORE, F. D. (1962) Refractory hypotension in man—is this irreversible shock? *New England Journal of Medicine*, **267**, 733.
25. Leading Article (1963) Hypertonic sodium for 'irreversible' oligaemic shock. *Lancet*, **1**, 539.
26. WILLIAMS, J. A. & FINE, J. (1961) Measurement of blood volume with a new apparatus. *New England Journal of Medicine*, **264**, 842.
27. IRVIN, T. T. *et al.* (1972) Clinical assessment of postoperative blood volume. *Lancet*, **2**, 446.

Chapter 33. Some Disorders of Metabolism

GLUCOSE METABOLISM

The most important upset in glucose metabolism is diabetes mellitus. It is the great frequency of this disease, which affects about 3 per cent of the population, that has stimulated a vast amount of research into the metabolism of glucose, yet even today there are many aspects that are incompletely understood.

Glucose is used as a fuel by many of the body's cells, and is the only substance used by the brain under normal circumstances. Hence the maintenance of a blood-glucose level within narrow limits (3·0 to 5·0 mmol per litre, or 55 to 90 mg per dl in the fasting subject) is an important homeostatic mechanism. The blood level is mainly regulated by the balanced production of insulin, which lowers the blood-glucose level, and the activity of the liver, which can either store glucose as glycogen or produce glucose from glycogen or non-carbohydrate sources (*gluconeogenesis*) (see Fig. 33.1).

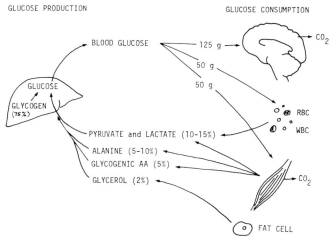

Figure 33.1
Glucose balance in normal man in the postabsorptive, overnight-fasted state. Alanine forms the principal amino acid released from muscle, and is utilised by the liver to form glucose. The muscle can utilise glucose to form alanine, and this constitutes the glucose-alanine cycle analogous to the Cori cycle. In the latter, lactate and pyruvate formed from glucose in the muscle are released into the blood, taken up by the liver, and there converted into glucose. (*From Felig, P. (1975) The liver in glucose homeostasis in normal man and diabetes. In Diabetes, ed. by Vallance-Owen, J. Baltimore: University Park Press.*)

Glucose Homeostasis[1]

It is best to consider glucose homeostasis under the three headings:
1. Following glucose administration
2. In the postabsorptive state—following an overnight fast
3. During exercise.

Following glucose administration. Following the oral administration of glucose there is an increase in the amount of insulin released from the pancreas. This promotes the storage and utilisation of glucose and prevents an undue rise in the blood-glucose level. The oral administration of glucose evokes more insulin release than does a comparable intravenous loading with glucose. This may be due to the stimulation of the islets by a nervous reflex *via* the vagi, but of greater importance is the release into the bloodstream of an *intestinal factor or hormone* that promotes the pancreatic release of insulin. The nature of this factor is unknown, but secretin, gastrin, cholecystokinin-pancreozymin, vasoactive intestinal polypeptide, and gastric inhibitory peptide have all been proposed as likely candidates.

Following the absorption of glucose from the intestine, the rise in blood-glucose level stimulates the secretion of insulin from the pancreatic islets by a direct action. Insulin aids the entry of glucose into resting muscle and fat cells: these are the insulin-dependent tissues. Following the ingestion of 100 g of glucose, however, only about 15 per cent enters these tissues along insulin-dependent pathways. An additional 25 per cent escapes from the splanchnic bed and is utilised to meet the ongoing glucose needs of insulin-independent tissues, especially the brain. From 55 to 60 per cent is retained in the liver, for there is no barrier to the entry of glucose into liver cells, and this organ is well situated anatomically to intercept glucose from the portal vein and prevent it entering the systemic circulation. In the liver the glucose is utilised in the synthesis of glycogen and triglycerides. Two enzymes are involved in the phosphorylation of glucose occurring prior to glycogen synthesis: hexokinase, which is insulin independent, and glucokinase, which is insulin dependent.

It follows that in the normal person, even after a carbohydrate meal, the blood glucose does not rise above 9 mmol per litre (160 mg per dl); this forms the basis of the glucose tolerance test.*

In the postabsorptive state. If an individual fasts overnight, the liver and the insulin-dependent tissues (resting muscle and fat) show little glucose uptake. The insulin-independent tissues (brain, blood cells, and renal medulla) show a continued glucose uptake at a rate of 150 to 200 g per day; the blood-glucose level is maintained by

---

*In this test a fasting subject, previously on an adequate carbohydrate diet, is given 100 g of glucose by mouth. The blood glucose should not exceed 5 mmol per litre (90 mg per dl) at the start of the test nor 9 mmol per litre (160 mg per dl) an hour later; it should have returned to 5 mmol per litre after 2 hours. At a blood-glucose level of 10 mmol per litre (180 mg per dl) glycosuria may be expected.

It should be noted that the normal levels of blood glucose cited in this chapter are somewhat lower than those found in older textbooks. This is because current biochemical methods measure the glucose content of blood specifically and not merely the content of reducing substances, of which glucose is the predominant component.

the release of glucose from the liver (Fig. 33.1). The liver contains about 70 g of glycogen which provides an immediate source of glucose by glycogenolysis. The supply, however, lasts less than 1 day, and gluconeogenesis is stimulated; pyruvate, lactate, and alanine are used as the main raw materials for this. After 2 or 3 days gluconeogenesis is more important than glycogenolytic activity. Protein provides the ultimate source for this, a fact reflected in the brisk rate of nitrogen excretion that occurs early in starvation.

During exercise. In the resting state the major source of energy for muscular contraction is provided by the oxidation of fatty acids. During exercise the uptake of fatty acid is increased, but in addition there is a marked (up to 20-fold) increase in glucose uptake and oxidation. To compensate for this peripheral utilisation, the liver releases glucose into the blood stream, and the blood-glucose level shows little change. During short-term exercise the major source of this glucose is liver glycogen (glycogenolysis). During prolonged exercise gluconeogenesis plays an increasingly important role, because the liver's supply of glycogen is limited. The mechanisms involved in these changes are not well understood. A reduction in blood-insulin level or an increase in blood-glucagon level play some part, but the release of catecholamines is probably of greater importance; these agents stimulate glycogenolysis in the liver (p. 411).

Secretion and Actions of Insulin

Insulin is synthesised in the beta cells of the islets of Langerhans as proinsulin, a polypeptide containing 81 to 86 amino-acid residues. The tail and head of this long polypeptide are joined by two disulphide bonds. By the action of peptidases the middle segment (termed the *C peptide*) is excised, leaving the two ends of the molecule to form the A and the B chains of the insulin molecule; these remain united by the original disulphide bonds.[2] The formation and excretion of C peptide has been used as a measure of the rate of insulin synthesis.[3]

Insulin is formed in the rough endoplasmic reticulum; the product passes into the Golgi complex and is subsequently released as membrane-bound secretory granules. These mature to a crystalline form in the presence of zinc ions, and are finally released by a process of exocytosis. The actual movement and release of these granules is guided by microtubules and effected by the contractile proteins of the microfilaments. Calcium ions are required for this.

The major stimulus for both insulin synthesis and release is hyperglycaemia. ACTH, glucagon, gastrin, and other intestinal hormones also increase insulin secretion, an effect accompanied by a rise in the intracellular level of cyclic-AMP. A number of amino acids, particularly leucine, have a similar effect, as does parasympathetic stimulation. It is unlikely, however, that these mechanisms play a major role in normal glucose homeostasis.

Sulphonylurea compounds also cause a release of insulin from the islet cells, but unlike the other agents mentioned above, they do not stimulate insulin synthesis.

The target cells of insulin are those of the adipose tissue and muscle, both of which have specific receptors: glucose transport into the cell is enhanced, and glycogen synthesis is increased. Insulin promotes the synthesis of protein from amino acids; it inhibits the breakdown of neutral fat (lipolysis).

Furthermore, insulin has two important effects on the liver: *glycogenolysis is inhibited* by small increments in insulin secretion. Larger increments *inhibit gluconeogenesis*. The net effect of insulin is to lower the blood-glucose level; since the half-life of the hormone is from 3 to 4 minutes, the continuous and varying secretion of insulin is the main regulatory mechanism whereby the blood-glucose level is normally maintained within narrow limits.

Other hormones affecting glucose metabolism. Four other hormones have important effects on glucose metabolism:

Glucagon.[4] This hormone is the secretion of the alpha cells of the islets of Langerhans. It is released whenever the blood-glucose level drops below 4·5 mmol per litre (80 mg per dl), and its main action is stimulating the liver to break down glycogen into glucose, which is then released into the blood. In the adipose tissue lipolysis is stimulated. It is evident that glucagon opposes the action of insulin.

Adrenaline. This raises the blood-glucose level by promoting glycogenolysis in the liver and muscles.

Pituitary growth hormone. This opposes the actions of insulin, thereby raising the blood-glucose level.

Adrenal glucocorticoids. These decrease glucose utilisation in muscle and fat. Gluconeogenesis in the liver is stimulated, and the blood-glucose level rises.

DIABETES MELLITUS[5]

The discovery of insulin by Banting and Best appeared to provide both an explanation of the pathogenesis of diabetes mellitus and an effective treatment. Ironically, this outstanding discovery retarded further research into the true nature of the disease, so that even today its precise pathogenesis is not understood. It has become evident that insulin deficiency is only one factor in the disease. Many diabetic subjects need insulin in quantities far in excess of those required by a totally pancreatectomised individual. Some diabetics have a blood-insulin level that is normal or even above normal. Finally, insulin therapy can prolong the life of some diabetic subjects, but it fails to prevent premature death from the cardiovascular complications or the onset of blindness. The life expectancy of a diabetic patient is still below that of the normal individual.

Aetiology of Diabetes Mellitus

Diabetes mellitus may be regarded as a syndrome characterised by a relative or absolute deficiency of insulin. Several types of the disease probably occur and have different causes. Hereditary factors are most important (see below), but damage to the islets by a viral infection has been suggested as a possible cause. There is experimental evidence that Coxsackie-B virus can damage islet tissue in mice.

Three major types of diabetes have been recognised:

1. Hereditary diabetes mellitus.[6,7] This is by far the commonest type, but although the disease is clearly familial, the precise mode of inheritance is not decided. It was at one time thought to be an autosomal recessive trait, but the current trend is to incriminate a dominant gene which renders the individual liable to develop diabetes, but is not itself the only cause. It is possible that about 25 per cent of the population possess this gene, but only 2 to 3 per cent actually develop the disease. The hereditary factor is more marked in the maturity-onset type of diabetes than in the juvenile-onset type. Nevertheless, heredity plays a part in the juvenile-onset type also, since the disease is more common in subjects who possess certain HLA antigens, e.g. HLA-B8 and HLA-Dw3. As noted previously, the genetic factor may act in concert with other events, e.g viral infection, the effects of an abnormal diet or simply overeating, or the liability to produce autoantibodies.

2. Diabetes mellitus associated with other endocrine disorders. Diabetes is encountered in Cushing's syndrome (and following glucocorticoid therapy), acromegaly, and phaeochromocytoma. Under these circumstances the disease is due to the overabundance of hormones that antagonise insulin. To this is probably added the hereditary factor, since ultimately the islet cells may become exhausted or unresponsive.

3. Diabetes associated with pancreatic disease. Diabetes is occasionally encountered as a complication of chronic pancreatitis, cystic fibrosis, and total pancreatectomy. Its occurrence in haemochromatosis is also due to pancreatic involvement.

Clinical Types of Diabetes Mellitus[8]

The disease occurs in two main clinical forms:

Growth-onset diabetes. This form affects children and young adults, and appears to be due to an absolute failure of the pancreas to secrete insulin. Polyuria (due to the osmotic diuresis promoted by the glycosuria) (see p. 551), polydipsia, and polyphagia are characteristic symptoms. The disease is severe, wasting is marked, and without treatment the patients die in diabetic coma. Insulin is particularly valuable in saving the lives of these patients.

Maturity-onset diabetes. This form occurs typically in middle-aged and elderly subjects, and is usually associated with obesity. The amount of insulin in the blood may be normal or reduced, but it is not absent. The disease is generally mild, there is no great risk from ketosis, and treatment by diet alone is often successful particularly if this leads to weight loss. Since this type of diabetes can occur in younger patients also, the name is somewhat misleading.

Pathogenesis of Diabetes Mellitus

The fundamental error in the common types of diabetes is not understood. It appears that the pancreas is unresponsive to an increase in the blood-glucose level. Thus in the early diabetic, after the ingestion of glucose, there is no early burst of insulin production, and a transient *hyperglycaemia* develops. This is due to an impaired hepatic uptake of glucose and a consequent entry of an abnormal quantity into the systemic circulation. A later release of insulin may be so excessive that the patient next develops *hypoglycaemia*. An abnormality in the release of the intestinal factor (p. 425) or an insensitivity on the part of the pancreas to it might play a part in the pathogenesis of diabetes, but this at present remains speculative.

The hyperglycaemia of diabetes leads to an increased peripheral utilisation of glucose, an effect particularly evident in the mild, maturity-onset disease. There is enough insulin present to prevent lipolysis, so that fat continues to accumulate and the patient becomes obese. In the severe diabetic there is hyperglycaemia even in the fasting state; peripheral utilisation by the insulin-independent tissues continues unabated, and the accumulation of glucose in the blood is due to overproduction by the liver. This continues despite the hyperglycaemia. The raw materials for this gluconeogenesis are amino acids (particularly alanine) released from the peripheral tissues, especially the muscles. The liver extracts these glycogenic substrates from the blood at a much higher rate than normal. The virtual absence of insulin leads to augmented lipolysis in the adipose tissues, so that free fatty acid is released and transported to the liver. The glycerol component contributes to the formation of glucose, while the remainder is used in the production of ketone bodies. Ketosis and diabetic coma are, therefore, common. An increase in the secretion of glucagon may potentiate the effect of insulin lack.

Effect of obesity. There is little doubt that people who are overweight are especially liable to diabetes. The obese person tends to have an increased secretion of insulin, and the fat and muscle cells show a decreased response to this hormone. The liver also appears to be resistant to the action of insulin, and gluconeogenesis is increased. It is not clear whether obesity *per se* predisposes to the development of diabetes, or whether those persons who are genetically predisposed to develop diabetes also become obese.

There is evidence that the genetically affected individual is liable to show exhaustion of the islets of Langerhans under the influence of some stress—whether obesity, pregnancy, infection, or an excess of one of the hormones that antagonises insulin. In the early-onset type of diabetes the islets of Langerhans may actually be hypertrophied in the very early stages, and following the acute development of the disease the insulin requirements of the patient may then diminish for a few months. Nevertheless, the patient soon appears to become absolutely dependent on an external source of insulin if diabetic ketosis and coma are to be prevented.

In the obese diabetic, on the other hand, insulin secretion may actually be in excess of normal or only slightly reduced. It has been suggested that an important factor in this type of the disease is the presence of an insulin antagonist. One such substance is associated with the albumin component of plasma, and is called *sinalbumin*; it appears to be manufactured in the liver, and is probably a component of the B chain of insulin itself.

Although injections of insulin greatly diminish the characteristic hyperglycaemia of diabetes, and prevent the onset of ketosis and coma, it is not known whether the control of this metabolic defect has any effect on the other manifestations of diabetes. The retinopathy and nephropathy, both manifestations of microangiopathy, appear to continue unabated; indeed, their development is not obviously related to the severity of the diabetes as gauged by glucose intolerance. Precisely how these complications arise is not understood. One possible mechanism by which hyperglycaemia could cause damage is by the formation of sorbitol;[9] this is a polyol, or sugar alcohol, derived from D-glucose. In diabetes mellitus the hyperglycaemia leads to an increased formation of sorbitol in certain cells. This substance cannot readily escape from the cells, which therefore tend to swell and die. This mechanism has been evoked to explain the damage to the lens of the eye, the nerves, and the arterial intimal tissues.

Diagnosis of Diabetes Mellitus

Four stages of the disease are recognised:

Prediabetes. The subject has the inherited tendency to develop the disease, but is asymptomatic and has no detectable biochemical abnormality. Since no genetic marker is at present known for diabetes, a diagnosis at this stage is impossible except in retrospect when the subject has already progressed to chemical or clinical diabetes.

Chemical diabetes. There are no symptoms, and the fasting blood sugar is normal. The glucose tolerance test, however, is abnormal. A random blood-glucose determination is of little value in diagnosis at this stage, since it may well be normal. Hyperglycaemia develops only in response to a good carbohydrate meal. To avoid the tedious glucose tolerance test, an examination of a single blood sample taken 2 hours after a carbohydrate meal may be used as a simple screening test.

Latent or stress diabetes. Some patients who are known to have been diabetic previously when under some form of stress, e.g. pregnancy, may be found to have a normal glucose tolerance test. This latent diabetic state may be detected by providing an additional stress in the form of glucocorticoid administration when performing the glucose tolerance test. This is called the *augmented glucose tolerance test*. If positive, it is an indication that the subject should be examined periodically for the development of frank chemical or overt clinical diabetes.

Overt or clinical diabetes. Symptoms are present, the fasting blood sugar is generally raised, and glycosuria is present at least at some time during the day.

The Anatomical Lesions of Diabetes Mellitus

Patients with diabetes mellitus exhibit a wide range of pathological lesions. Thus, the small blood vessels, the kidneys, and the retina often show characteristic changes, but whether these should be regarded as typical of the disease or merely complications is a moot point. These are described below under the heading of complications.

The islets of Langerhans. These show a variety of changes, but in about one-third of cases no abnormality can be detected. In early-onset diabetes a lymphocytic infiltrate ('insulitis') may be present. If the patient had marked hyperglycaemia before death, the beta cells show vacuolation due to an accumulation of glycogen. Longstanding diabetics may show atrophy of the islets with replacement by amyloid or fibrous tissue (see Fig. 5.5, p. 68).

Islet-cell hyperplasia in the child of a diabetic mother.[10] In this condition the fetus is subjected to a high blood-glucose level, and the beta cells of its islets respond by hypersecretion and hyperplasia (Fig. 33.2 (a) and 33.2 (b)). At birth these continue to secrete insulin, and the infant may rapidly develop severe hypoglycaemia unless glucose is given; treatment of this rare condition may be life-saving.

(a)   (b)

Figure 33.2
Hyperplasia of the islet of Langerhans. (*a*) This is a section of the pancreas of a newborn infant, whose mother was a diabetic. The greatly increased size of the islet of Langerhans is very obvious when compared with an islet of a normal newborn child, which is quite inconspicuous amid the acinar tissue (*b*). The enlargement is due to a proliferation of the constituent cells. × 120.

It is important to note that the children of prediabetic women are also endangered. Normally there is an increase in maternal insulin resistance in pregnancy, which puts extra demands on the beta cells. A normal woman can cope with this, but one who is prediabetic has a marginal insulin deficiency when not pregnant. The stress of pregnancy leads to chemical diabetes with hyperglycaemia and glycosuria, and the fetus is subjected to a high level of blood glucose even though the mother may appear quite well clinically.

A mild, but more common effect of maternal diabetes on the fetus is an increase in its weight; indeed, the birth of an overweight child should alert the obstetrician to the possibility of diabetes in the mother.

Complications of Diabetes Mellitus

Diabetic ketosis and coma. This is most common in the growth-onset type of the disease, and may be precipitated by the patient's failure to administer his insulin. Vomiting and abdominal pain may be severe enough to simulate an abdominal emergency.

Hyperosmolar non-ketogenic coma.[11] This condition is generally encountered in patients with maturity-onset diabetes, and may be precipitated by an acute illness, such as an infection or a myocardial infarct. The plasma glucose level is over 33 mmol per litre (600 mg per dl), and may exceed 55 mmol per litre (1000 mg per dl). The osmotic diuresis that this engenders leads to hypernatraemia, an increase in plasma osmolality,* and hypovolaemic shock. The effect of the dehydration is most marked on the central nervous system—coma is characteristic, and fits occur in about one-third of cases. Ketosis is not a feature of this condition, the precise pathogenesis of which is not known.

Cardiovascular disease.[12] There is good evidence that diabetics are more prone than normal people of the same age-group to develop atheroma, peripheral vascular disease, gangrene of the toes and feet,[13] and ischaemic heart disease. This tendency does not seem to be related to the severity of the diabetes nor to the efficiency of the treatment; indeed, treatment with tolbutamide and phenformin may actually increase the mortality from cardiovascular disease. The pathogenesis of the arterial disease in diabetes is poorly understood; a greater incidence of systemic hypertension, microangiopathy of the vasa vasorum, obesity, and hypertriglyceridaemia (particularly an elevated very low-density lipoprotein level, see p. 583) may all be relevant factors. The hypoxia that these vascular lesions engender may be aggravated by changes in the chemistry of the haemoglobin that occurs in severe diabetes mellitus (see p. 604).

Diabetic microangiopathy. A thickening of the basement membrane of capillaries has been described in the skin, muscles, kidney, retina, and other parts of the body. This change may be present before the onset of clinical diabetes, and it has been suggested that this is the primary lesion of the common type of the disease. However, it is more probably an effect of the low insulin level or the hyperglycaemia, since the changes have also been described in the diabetes secondary to pancreatic destruction. The effects of the microangiopathy are

*A simple guide to the plasma osmolality is to multiply the plasma sodium (in mmol per litre) by two and add 5·5 for each 100 mg per dl of blood glucose and 3·6 for each 10 mg per dl of blood urea nitrogen. The normal range is 290 to 310 milliosmoles per litre.

particularly important in the kidney, the retina, and the nerves.

Diabetic nephropathy.[14] The common *diffuse glomerulosclerosis* involves thickening of the basement membrane of the glomerular vessels together with mesangial proliferation and an increase in the amount of basement-membrane-like material in the mesangium (Fig. 33.3 (a)).

The most characteristic change is, however, *nodular glomerulosclerosis*, described by Kimmelstiel and Wilson. In this there are focal depositions of basement-membrane-like material in the peripheral parts of the glomeruli, thereby forming nodules of varying size (Fig. 33.3(b)). These nodules stain strongly by the PAS method. They contain collagen in which there is an abnormally high degree of glycosylation of hydroxylysine residues as compared with normal basement-membrane collagen[15] (p. 64).

The kidney in diabetes mellitus shows other changes. There is often well-marked hyaline, PAS-positive thickening of the afferent arterioles with ischaemic glomerular changes (Fig. 33.3 (c)). The *exudative lesion* consists of deposits of fibrin on the glomeruli beneath the podocytes (*fibrin caps*) as well as beneath the epithelial lining of the parietal layer of Bowman's capsule (the *capsule drop*, Fig. 33.3 (d)).

If glycosuria is present, the cytoplasm of the cells of the proximal convoluted tubules may be vacuolated due to the **accumulation of glycogen in them** (the *Armanni-Ebstein lesion*).

Urinary-tract infection is common in diabetic subjects, especially women, and papillary necrosis may occur; clinically this is characterised by haematuria and the rapid onset of renal failure.

Glomerulosclerosis itself leads to proteinuria which may be of sufficient intensity to produce the nephrotic syndrome. In the terminal stages nitrogen retention and renal failure occur.

Changes in the eye. The small retinal vessels show thickening of their basement membranes and luminal narrowing, which leads to ischaemic changes in the retina. Focal dilatations of the vessels lead to the formation of microaneurysms, which completes the picture of *diabetic retinopathy*.

Bleeding may occur into the vitreous, and when the haematoma organises, the fibrous tissue that forms undergoes contracture. This condition is called *retinitis proliferans*, and results in retinal detachment. Vascularisation of the iris occurs by a similar mechanism (*rubeosis iridis*).

Cataract formation is another important complication of diabetes; it is little wonder that the disease is one of the leading causes of blindness in the world.

Changes in the nerves. The microangiopathy causes ischaemic changes in the peripheral nerves, thus producing the common peripheral neuropathy of diabetics. The diarrhoea that plagues the patient with severe diabetes is attributed to autonomic neuropathy. A malabsorption syndrome may also occur.

Liability to infection. Diabetic patients are susceptible to bacterial infections, especially of the skin, lungs, and urinary tract. The mechanism is incompletely understood, but abnormal polymorph function (chemotaxis and bactericidal action) may be of importance (p. 163). Vaginal candidiasis is a troublesome complication in diabetic women.

Skin changes. Apart from the effects of infection and ischaemia, several characteristic lesions may occur: necrobiosis

Figure 33.3

Diabetic nephropathy. (*a*) Diffuse glomerulosclerosis. There is considerable mesangial proliferation and thickening. Note the hyalinised afferent arteriole entering the glomerular tuft. × 250.

(*b*) Nodular glomerulosclerosis. There are focal accumulations of hyaline material disposed especially in the peripheries of the glomerulus. × 100.

(*c*) Hyaline change of the afferent arteriole. This is more marked than in (*a*). × 250.

(*d*) Capsular drop. This is an exudative lesion consisting of a deposit of fibrin beneath the epithelial lining of Bowman's capsule. × 250.

lipoidica, widespread granuloma annulare, and eruptive xanthomata are characteristic. Diabetic dermopathy consists of atrophic brown lesions, generally on the lower leg; they are probably of ischaemic origin.

GLYCOGEN-STORAGE DISEASES[16]

There are a number of inherited disorders in which there is an excessive accumulation of glycogen in various tissues due to an abnormality of glucose metabolism. These may be divided into eight main groups according to the enzyme defect present and the type of glycogen deposited. Their pathogenesis can be

Figure 33.4
Synthesis and degradation of glycogen. Roman numerals indicate the different types of glycogenosis and the underlying enzyme deficiencies. (To avoid a too intricate scheme, liver phosphorylase and muscle phosphorylase, although controlled by different genes, have been represented by a single arrow.)
Key: 1. UDP-glucose-pyrophosphorylase. 2. Glycogen synthetase.
3. Amylo(1,4→1,6)transglycosylase (branching enzyme).
4. Phosphorylase. 5. α(1→4)glucosidase (acid maltase).
6. Amylo(1→6)glucosidase (debranching enzyme).
7. Phosphoglucomutase. 8. Glucose-6-phosphatase.
9. Glucose-ATP-phosphotransferase (hexokinase-glucokinase).
10. Phosphoglucoisomerase. 11. Phosphofructokinase.
12. Diphosphofructose phosphatase. 13. Lactic dehydrogenase.
14. Phosphorylase kinase.
ATP = Adenosine triphosphate; ADP = Adenosine diphosphate;
P = Phosphate radical; P_i = Inorganic orthophosphate;
P-P = Inorganic pyrophosphate; UTP = Uridine triphosphate;
UDP = Uridine diphosphate.

Figure 33.5
Schematic representation of a part of a glycogen molecule.

understood only in relation to the normal metabolic pathways involving glucose and glycogen. These are outlined in Figures 33.4 and 33.5.

Type I glycogen-storage disease (von Gierke's disease). This is inherited as an autosomal recessive trait, and is due to glucose 6-phosphatase deficiency. As described on page 425, about 60 per cent of the glucose absorbed from a carbohydrate meal is normally retained by the liver; it is phosphorylated to glucose 6-phosphate and subsequently stored as glycogen. Hours later this glycogen is broken down again to glucose 6-phosphate, and subsequently free glucose is released into the blood stream to maintain the blood-glucose level. In the absence of glucose 6-phosphatase, glucose 6-phosphate is not broken down, glucose is not released, and hypoglycaemia results. In this way a normal type of glycogen is retained in the liver and to a lesser extent the kidneys. Fat is metabolised for energy requirements (as in diabetes mellitus), and hyperlipoproteinaemia and ketosis develop. Furthermore, the accumulated glucose 6-phosphate is disposed of by increasing anaerobic glycolysis. Lactic acid and pyruvic acid accumulate, thereby accentuating the acidosis. Hyperuricaemia is not uncommon, and appears to be due to impaired renal excretion of uric acid. It is suggested that competitive inhibition occurs by lactate excretion.

The disease shows itself in infancy, enormous hepatomegaly (due to the deposition of glycogen) being the most prominent feature. The kidneys are also enlarged. Hypoglycaemic fits are common, but as the child grows these become less frequent. The chronic acidaemia appears to be responsible for the stunted growth and the osteoporosis that these children exhibit. There is a high incidence of cutaneous xanthomata and gouty tophi, from which the xanthomata must be distinguished.

Type II glycogen-storage disease (Pompe's disease). This is inherited as an autosomal recessive trait, and is due to a deficiency of the lysosomal enzyme α(1→4)glucosidase. The disease is generally detected at about 2 months of age, and is characterised by pronounced hypotonia and enormous cardiomegaly. The child usually dies by about the age of 2 years.

There is an increased amount of normal glycogen deposited in the heart, tongue, and other skeletal muscles. Electron microscopy shows many glycogen-stuffed lysosomes; this disease can be regarded as a type of lysosomal disease. The biochemical defect is a deficiency of α-1,4-glucosidase (acid maltase), a lysosomal enzyme that is responsible for the degradation of glycogen.

Type III glycogen-storage disease (Cori's disease, or limit dextrinosis). Clinically this resembles the type-I disease, but is less severe. There may be splenomegaly, and the hepatic enlargement tends to diminish at the age of puberty. Gout does not occur in this type of disease.

The disease is inherited as an autosomal recessive trait, and is due to a defect in the debranching enzyme amylo($1 \rightarrow 6$) glucosidase, in the absence of which glycogen cannot be broken down completely. The tissues accumulate an abnormal form of glycogen, which resembles the limit dextrin that is produced by the degradation of glycogen by phosphorylase in the absence of the debranching enzyme.

Type IV glycogen-storage disease (Andersen's disease). This rare condition is characterised by failure to thrive, progressive hepatic cirrhosis, and death within the first two years of life. An abnormal, less soluble form of glycogen is laid down in the tissues due to a deficiency of the branching enzyme amylo($1,4 \rightarrow 1,6$) transglucosidase.

Type V glycogen-storage disease. (McArdle's disease). In this uncommon disease there is an inability to perform strenuous exercise because of the development of cramps. Myoglobinuria occurs in about half the patients. These symptoms generally commence between the ages of 20 and 40 years, and are later followed by muscular wasting and weakness. The defect is in the muscle phosphorylase, an enzyme which is essential for sustained, vigorous exercise.

Type VI glycogen-storage disease (Hers's disease). This is described as resembling the type-I disease but being much milder. Some cases have been reported as having a low liver phosphorylase activity, but the condition is probably a heterogeneous group of different diseases temporarily assembled together pending their further classification.

Type VII glycogen-storage disease. This very rare condition resembles the type-V disease. It is due to a deficiency of muscle phosphofructokinase, and glycogen accumulates in many muscles.

Type VIII glycogen-storage disease. In this condition there is a deficiency of hepatic phosphorylase *b* kinase, an enzyme required to activate phosphorylase. Since the phosphorylase is itself normal, the disease has now been removed from type VI and placed in this separate group.

Clinically the disease is mild, being characterised by mild hypoglycaemia and hepatomegaly due to glycogen deposition. It is inherited as an X-linked trait, and is fully manifest only in males.

Summary

There are many examples of inherited defects in the enzymes involved in the synthesis and degradation of glycogen. Well-recognised syndromes have been labelled I to VIII, but other types are also encountered in individual families. Sometimes several enzyme defects appear to be involved.

PURINE METABOLISM

GOUT[17]

Gout is a disease of great antiquity. It is characterised by hyperuricaemia, recurrent attacks of a characteristic acute arthritis, and the development of tophi. Deposits of urates in the cartilages of joints lead to chronic arthritis. The clinical features of gout were well recognised by Hippocrates, and the classical condition was described by Thomas Sydenham, who was himself a sufferer. The disease is commoner in times of plenty than during wars and famines; it is a malady of the affluent rather than the poor. Among its famous victims were Martin Luther, Isaac Newton, Samuel Johnson, and the Pitts. Gout responds well to colchicine, a drug still in current use and introduced into North America by Benjamin Franklin, yet another famous person afflicted by the disease.

Gout is now regarded as a symptom complex of multiple aetiology. In some cases, labelled *primary gout*, there is often a strong hereditary factor. In others, labelled *secondary gout*, there is an obvious associated disease that is the primary cause. In both types there is an upset of purine metabolism, which should first be understood before the disease is considered in detail.

Purine Metabolism

The purines (adenine and guanine) together with the pyrimidines (uracil, thymine, and cytosine) are the common bases present in the nucleic acids. A base combined with a ribose sugar (either D-ribose or 2-deoxy-D-ribose) forms a *nucleoside* (either a ribonucleoside or a deoxyribonucleoside). Ribonucleosides can occur free, but are often present as 5'-phosphates, and are called *nucleotides*, for example adenosine 5'-monophosphate (AMP or adenylic acid), adenosine 5'-diphosphate (ADP), and adenosine 5'-triphosphate (ATP).

The starting point in purine biosynthesis is α-D-ribose 5-phosphate, on to which molecule a purine ring is built step by step so that a nucleotide is formed directly. An intermediate in this synthetic pathway is 5-phospho-α-D-ribose 1-pyrophosphate (PRPP), also called 5-phosphoribosyl-1-pyrophosphate, or PP-ribose-P. This substance next reacts with glutamine, and ultimately the ribonucleotide *inosinic acid* is formed. This is the precursor substance of adenosine 5'-monophosphate (AMP) and guanosine 5'-monophosphate (GMP).

Degradation of purines. The degradation of nucleic acids by nucleases results in the formation of the free purine and pyrimidine bases. Adenine and guanine are converted to hypoxanthine, which is acted upon by xanthine oxidase to form xanthine. In the human this is converted into uric acid and excreted.

The drug allopurinol acts as a xanthine-oxidase inhibitor, therefore reducing the amount of uric acid that is formed; it is of value in preventing hyperuricaemia and its effects in patients in renal failure and in those being treated with cytotoxic drugs.

Under normal circumstances up to 5 g of free purine are formed daily, but only 0.5 g are excreted; the remainder is salvaged and recycled. Thus adenine and guanine react with PRPP to form AMP and GMP respectively. An important element in this salvage of purines is the enzyme hypoxanthine-guanine phosphoribosyltransferase.

Pyrimidine Metabolism[18]

Although pyrimidine metabolism is not concerned in the pathogenesis of gout, it is convenient to consider the subject at this stage. The pyrimidines are synthesised by a pathway that differs from that involved in purine synthesis. It results in the formation of orotic acid, which reacts with PRPP to form the nucleotide orotidine 5'-phosphate (orotidylic acid), which is the precursor of nucleotides containing the pyrimidines. When these nucleotides are degraded, the bases are further broken down to urea and ammonia. They may also be utilised as precursors in the biosynthesis of β-alanine. Uric acid is not an end-product in pyrimidine metabolism.

Pathogenesis of Primary Gout

Overproduction of uric acid is a feature of many patients with primary gout, but in most of these the precise biochemical error is not known. In a few families there is a low level of the enzyme hypoxanthine-guanine phosphoribosyltransferase, and purines are excreted as uric acid rather than being recycled. These patients exhibit neurological signs as well as gouty arthritis and renal stones. A complete absence of the enzyme is characteristic of the Lesch-Nyhan syndrome (p. 37).

In several families variants of the enzyme phosphoribosyl-pyrophosphate synthetase have been found. These abnormal forms of the enzyme have an increased activity; presumably there is an overproduction of PRPP and hence also of uric acid. Abnormalities of glutathione metabolism, e.g. glutathione reductase variants with increased activity, have been incriminated in other families.

A deficiency of a urate-binding α_1-α_2-globulin has been described, and this may favour the deposition of urates in the tissues.

Gout also occurs in type I glycogen-storage disease (p. 431).

Renal handling of uric acid. Uric acid passes freely into the glomerular filtrate, and most of it is reabsorbed by the tubules; 80 per cent of the uric acid excreted in the urine is derived from tubular secretion. A reduction in the normal secretion of urate per nephron has been demonstrated in some patients with gout, and is prominent in those in whom there is no evidence of uric-acid overproduction.

It is evident that many defects in the metabolism of purines can result in the clinical state of gout. There may be an overproduction of purines, with or without impaired renal excretion of uric acid. In some patients diminished excretion appears to be the major, if not the sole, explanation of the hyperuricaemia. A familial tendency is well established in primary gout, but its reported incidence varies from 6 to 75 per cent of cases. In a few families the mode of inheritance is known. Thus in hypoxanthine-guanine phosphoribosyltransferase deficiency the inheritance is that of an X-linked recessive trait. In the majority of families the exact mode of inheritance is more erratic. The situation is comparable to that encountered in diabetes mellitus; it is probable that the tendency to develop gout is inherited but that other factors are of importance in actually precipitating the onset of the disease. The development of obesity and overindulgence in alcohol are important factors in this regard.

Clinical Features of Gout

Gout may be divided into three phases.

1. Asymptomatic hyperuricaemia. The normal plasma uric acid (usually reported as urate) is 0·1 to 0·4 mmol per litre (2·2 to 7·5 mg per dl in men and 2·1 to 6·6 mg per dl in women). The normal daily excretion ranges from 250 mg to 600 mg. Hyperuricaemia may persist throughout the patient's entire life asymptomatically, or it may progress to the next stage after a variable period.

2. Acute gouty arthritis.[19] This generally affects a joint of the lower extremity, usually the first metatarso-phalangeal joint; occasionally it is bilateral. There is a sudden onset of severe pain with fever and rigors. The pain becomes intolerable, but without treatment it slowly subsides over a period of days or even weeks. Further acute attacks may occur affecting either the same or other joints. Over 50 per cent of untreated cases develop permanent joint damage and tophi (deposits of urates).

Attacks of acute gouty arthritis may be precipitated by trauma, stress, fatigue, or alcoholic excess. The mechanism is obscure, since there is no constant change in the plasma-urate level either in the phase preceding or during the acute attack. Precipitation of monosodium urate in the joint cavity appears to be the immediate cause of the attack: activation of Factor XII, the kinin system, and complement by the crystals has been postulated. Of more importance probably are the lysosomal enzymes released by polymorphs that are damaged during the process of phagocytosis of the crystals. The presence of urate crystals in the synovial fluid is of diagnostic value in gouty arthritis.

3. Chronic gouty arthritis. The progressive deposition of monosodium urate in the articular cartilage leads to the degeneration of the cartilage, pannus formation, and eventual fibrous or bony ankylosis. Similar deposits of urate in the adjacent bone, synovium, and soft tissues complete the picture of chronic gouty arthritis. As the chronic changes advance, so renal insufficiency develops and acute attacks occur less frequently and are more mild. No joint is exempt, but the legs are affected more often than the arms; distal joints are affected more frequently than the proximal ones. Tophi also occur in the cartilages of the ears, and in bursae (especially the olecranon and prepatellar), tendons, and soft tissues generally. There may be much deformity (Fig. 33.6).

Microscopically a tophus consists of sheaves of urate crystals and a surrounding granulomatous reaction with numerous foreign-body giant cells (Fig. 33.7). Since the crystals are soluble in water, they are liable to be washed out during routine formalin fixation; they are best preserved in alcohol-fixed material.

Renal Lesions of Gout[14]

Between 20 and 40 per cent of patients with gout develop uric-acid stones; in about 20 per cent the urolithiasis is the first indication of the disease. Stones are most common in patients with high uric-acid excretion rates and in those who

Figure 33.6
Gout. This left hand shows the effects of severe, chronic gout. There are irregular swellings on the dorsum corresponding with the position of the metacarpo-phalangeal joints. Similar swellings are present over the interphalangeal joints, where opaque, chalky deposits are visible through the atrophic skin. (S88.1, *Reproduced by permission of the President and Council of the R.C.S. Eng.*)

Figure 33.7
Gout tophus. There are deposits of crystalline sodium urate surrounded by exuberant foreign-body giant-cell systems. × 100.

have a tendency to secrete an acid urine. Uric acid is much less soluble than monosodium urate, and is therefore the predominant component of the stones.

Apart from the changes secondary to urolithiasis (obstruction and infection), the kidneys often show a glomerulosclerosis which is probably secondary to ischaemia. It is accompanied by an interstitial inflammation. There may be deposits of urates both in the interstitial tissues and in the tubules themselves. Systemic hypertension is present in about one-third of the patients.

Secondary Gout

Hyperuricaemia and secondary gout can occur under two circumstances:

(*a*) *Overproduction of uric acid due to increased cellular turnover*, as in the myeloproliferative diseases (see p. 631) and leukaemias especially after treatment with cytotoxic drugs. Chronic haemolytic anaemia (e.g. sickle-cell anaemia) and psoriasis are other examples of conditions in which there is an increased cellular turnover.

(*b*) *Impaired renal excretion*. This is encountered as a complication of certain drugs, chiefly the thiazide diuretics, and with renal damage. Lead poisoning in particular causes chronic renal damage that may be complicated by gout. In most patients with chronic renal disease gout is uncommon. This may be because the patients rarely survive long enough for gout to develop. The clinical picture of gout may be seen

in patients on chronic haemodialysis, but this may be due to the deposition of calcium phosphates rather than urates. (See p. 464.)

PORPHYRIN METABOLISM

The porphyrins are cyclic tetrapyrroles which exist in nature in three forms, each combined with a different metal: *haem* contains iron, *chlorophyll* contains magnesium, and *cobalamin* (vitamin B_{12}) contains cobalt.

Haem is the important component of haemoglobin, and is also present in several enzymes, including catalases, peroxidases, and cytochromes. Abnormal quantities of porphyrin are formed under two circumstances: in the *porphyrias* and in the *porphyrinurias*.

In the *porphyrinurias* there is an increased excretion of coproporphyrin in the urine secondary to haemolytic anaemia or lead poisoning. The latter may simulate acute intermittent porphyria, but the increased porphyrin metabolism is not thought to be related to the symptoms.

THE PORPHYRIAS[20—22]

The *porphyrias* are an uncommon group of diseases in which there is a primary abnormality in porphyrin metabolism. The metabolic pathways involved in porphyrin syn-

Figure 33.8
Diagram to illustrate the metabolic pathways involved in the synthesis of haem. The condensation of glycine and succinyl coenzyme A in the presence of ALA synthetase results in the formation of α-aminolaevulinic acid (ALA). Two molecules of this condense to form porphobilinogen (PBG). This is the rate-limiting step in haem synthesis, and is controlled by a feedback mechanism involving haem. Abnormalities in this feedback mechanism, sometimes initiated by drugs, is a proposed mechanism in the excessive formation of porphyrins encountered in certain of the porphyrias. Normally about 99 per cent of porphobilinogen is converted into uroporphyrinogen III by the combined activity of two enzymes porphobilinogen deaminase and uroporphyrinogen III cosynthetase (also called porphobilinogenisomerase). Porphobilinogen deaminase acting alone leads to the production of series-I products. These together with uroporphyrin III and coproporphyrin III cannot be used in the synthesis of haem, and are excreted.

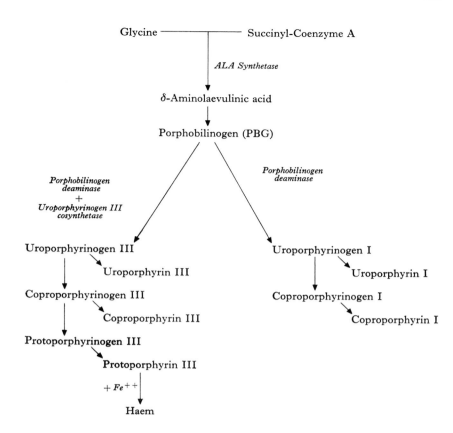

thesis are outlined in Figure 33.8. It should be noted that the porphyrins of series I are by-products, and are not utilised. Series III, on the other hand, are intermediates in the production of haem in the red-cell precursors, and in other cells (predominantly in the liver) for the synthesis of enzymes such as catalase, cytochromes, and peroxidase. Abnormalities in porphyrin metabolism may therefore be divided into two main groups: (*a*) *erythropoietic porphyria*, in which the abnormality is in the red-cell precursors of the bone marrow, and (*b*) *hepatic porphyria*, in which the erythroid cells are normal, but the liver contains and produces excess quantities of porphyrins.

A remarkable feature of some of the porphyrins is that their presence in the skin causes a sensitivity to light and trauma. This is most marked with uroporphyrin, less so with coproorphyrin, and least with protoporphyrin. Finally it should be noted that delta-aminolaevulinic acid (ALA), porphobilinogen (PBG), and uroporphyrin are excreted mainly in the urine, coproporphyrin is excreted preferentially in the bile but may overflow into the urine in liver disease, while protoporphyrin is excreted entirely in the bile.

Erythropoietic porphyrias. *Congenital erythropoietic porphyria.* This is a rare inborn error of metabolism, probably inherited as an autosomal recessive trait, which first manifests itself in infancy, and is characterised by mutilating skin lesions and haemolytic anaemia. The urine is Burgundy-red in colour and contains an excess of uroporphyrin I and coproporphyrin I. There appears to be a defect in uroporphyrinogen III cosynthetase activity, so that an excessive amount of PBG is converted into the photosensitising uroporphyrin I. The skin exhibits marked photosensitivity: bullae followed by infection and scarring occur both after trauma and exposure to light (*hydroa aestivale*). Deposits of porphyrin impart a red-brown discoloration to the bones and teeth. A chronic haemolytic anaemia of variable severity is the rule.

Erythropoietic protoporphyria. The red cells and faeces contain a great excess of protoporphyrin, but there is no excess of porphyrin in the urine. Urticaria and chronic eczema develop in areas of skin exposed to light, but the bullae and sensitivity to trauma so characteristic of congenital erythropoietic porphyria are not present.

Erythropoietic coproporphyria has also been described, and is associated with light sensitivity.

Hepatic porphyria. *Acute intermittent porphyria.* This disease is the most common of the porphyrias and is inherited as an autosomal dominant trait. It is associated with increased delta-aminolaevulinic acid synthetase activity, which results in an overproduction of ALA in the liver. Excess ALA and porphobilinogen are present in the urine. The disease becomes manifest after puberty, and is characterised by acute episodes which may be of three patterns, either singly or in combination:

1. Abdominal—the symptoms closely resemble those of an 'acute abdomen', and are thought to be due to autonomic neuropathy.

2. Neurological—a polyneuritis, predominantly paralytic in effect.

3. Psychotic—acute delirium. This may be caused by hypothalamic damage leading to the inappropriate secretion of antidiuretic hormone and water retention.

Photosensitisation of the skin does not occur. The disease may be latent, and acute attacks can be precipitated by various factors, e.g. pregnancy, infection, and drugs—especially the barbiturates.

Variegate porphyria (porphyria cutanea tarda hereditaria). Many cases of this disease have been reported from South Africa, and most of them can be traced to a Dutch couple who married at the Cape of Good Hope in 1688. As in acute intermittent porphyria, there are acute abdominal and nervous manifestations which may be precipitated by drugs. There is a persistent elevation in the amount of protoporphyrin and coproporphyrin in the faeces, and during the attacks there is in addition an excess excretion of porphobilinogen in the urine. Photosensitivity of the skin occurs, and the disease is usually first noted during the third decade.

This mixed, or variegate, porphyria is of historical interst, for many members of the Royal Houses of Hanover, Prussia, and Stuart are thought by some authorities to have been its victims. Frederick the Great's hemiplegia at the age of 35 years, George III's periods of madness, and Mary Queen of Scot's attacks of colic and fits which earned her the unenviable title of one of the great invalids of history, may all have been manifestations of this unusual disease.

Hereditary coproporphyria is very rare, and is characterised by an increased excretion of coproporphyrin in the urine. Clinically the disease resembles variegate porphyria.

Porphyria cutanea tarda symptomatica. During attacks of this type, the urine contains an excess of uroporphyrin and appears red. Photosensitisation and skin fragility are the presenting symptoms. The repeated formation of subepidermal bullae leads ultimately to considerable scarring of the sun-exposed parts. Hyperpigmentation is common, and so also is an increased growth of hair (hypertrichosis)—an unexplained feature which is also found in other types of porphyria. The patients usually have obvious liver disease, and many of them are alcoholics.

Although the metabolism of the porphyrins is well understood, the precise defect in the various types of porphyria is not known. There appears to be an overproduction of porphyrins, either in the bone marrow or in the liver. Photosensitivity can usually be explained by the presence of porphyrins in the skin, and the wave length of light that produces the greatest damage is around 400 nm.* This is the same region (the Soret band) where absorption by the porphyrin molecule is the strongest. The pathogenesis of the abdominal and nervous manifestations is not known. In some types there is a genetic basis, but even in these the disease may be precipitated by other factors like liver disease or the administration of drugs; sometimes indeed a toxic substance appears to be the major factor. This is well illustrated by the outbreak of porphyria that occurred in Turkey in 1956 due to the accidental ingestion of hexachlorbenzene used as a fungicide in wheat. The present classification of the porphyrias must therefore be regarded as tentative and subject to future change.

---

*This wave length is in the visible spectrum and can pass through ordinary sunlight barrier preparations, glass, and even light clothing. This is in contrast to the 300 nm region of the spectrum that causes normal sunburn.

REFERENCES

1. LEVINE, R. & HAFT, D. E. (1970) Carbohydrate homeostasis. *New England Journal of Medicine*, **283**, 175 and 237.
2. STEINER, D. F. *et al.* (1974) Proteolytic processing in the biosynthesis of insulin and other proteins. *Federation Proceedings*, **33**, 2105.
3. CAHILL, G. F. (1973) C-peptide: a new method of assessing pancreatic beta-cell function. *New England Journal of Medicine*, **288**, 1181.
4. FELIG, P. (1970) Glucagon: physiologic and diabetogenic role. *New England Journal of Medicine*, **283**, 149.
5. VALLANCE-OWEN, J. (Ed.) (1975) *Diabetes*, 208 pp. Baltimore: University Park Press.
6. Leading Article (1975) Heritability of diabetes. *British Medical Journal*, **4**, 127.
7. ZONANA, J. & RIMOIN, D. L. (1976) Inheritance of diabetes mellitus. *New England Journal of Medicine*, **295**, 603.
8. IRVINE, W. J. (1977) Classification of idiopathic diabetes. *Lancet*, **1**, 638.
9. GABBAY, K. H. (1973) The sorbitol pathway and the complications of diabetes. *New England Journal of Medicine*, **288**, 831.
10. Leading Article (1975) Diabetes and the fetus. *Lancet*, **1**, 669.
11. McCURDY, D. K. (1970) Hyperosmolar hyperglycemic nonketotic diabetic coma. *Medical Clinics of North America*, **54**, 683.
12. STOUT, R. W., BIERMAN, E. L. & BRUNZELL, J. D. (1975) In *Diabetes*, pp. 125–169 (Atherosclerosis and disorders of lipid metabolism in diabetes), *loc. cit.*
13. Leading Article (1977) Diabetic foot ulcers. *Lancet*, **1**, 232.
14. HEPTINSTALL, R. H. (1974) *Pathology of the Kidney*, 2nd edn, Ch. 25. Boston: Little Brown.
15. SPIRO, R. G. (1973) Biochemistry of the renal glomerular basement membrane and its alterations in diabetes mellitus. *New England Journal of Medicine*, **288**, 1337.
16. HOWELL, R. R. (1972) In *The Metabolic Basis of Inherited Disease*, Ed. Stanbury, J. B., Wyngaarden, J. B., & Fredrickson, D. S. 3rd edn, pp. 149–173. New York: McGraw-Hill.
17. WYNGAARDEN, J. B. & KELLEY, W. N. (1972) In *The Metabolic Basis of Inherited Disease*, 3rd edn, pp. 889–968, *loc cit*.
18. SMITH, L. H. (1973) Pyrimidine metabolism in man. *New England Journal of Medicine*, **288**, 764.
19. Leading Article (1973) Mechanism of gouty inflammation. *British Medical Journal*, **4**, 125.
20. MARVER, H. S. & SCHMID, R. (1972) In *The Metabolic Basis of Inherited Disease*, 3rd edn, pp. 1087–1140, *loc cit*.
21. HARVER, L. C. & BICKERS, D. R. (1975) *The Porphyrias: Basic Science Aspects, Clinical Diagnosis and Management*, ed. Malkinson, F. D. & Pearson, R. W. Chicago: Year Book Medical Publishers.
22. TSCHUDY, D. P., MAGNUS, A. I. & KALIVAS, J. (1971) In *Dermatology in General Medicine*, ed. Fitzpatrick, T. B. *et al.*, p. 1143. New York: McGraw-Hill.

Chapter 34. Disorders of Nutrition

With the world population expanding at an estimated rate of 70 million each year, it is likely that starvation and malnutrition will become increasingly common. The effects of total starvation will first be described.

STARVATION

Metabolic Changes During Starvation[1-3]

The body's stores of glucose and glycogen are sufficient for only 1 day's metabolic needs. The protein supply and the triacylglycerols (triglycerides) of adipose tissue provide enough energy for an additional 3 months in the average individual. For a fat person there are enough energy reserves for about 1 year's survival. After an overnight fast (the post-absorptive state) the insulin-dependent tissues (resting muscle and fat) cease to take up glucose. Insulin-independent tissues (brain, blood cells, and renal medulla), on the other hand, continue to utilise glucose at a rate of 150 g per day. The liver releases glucose at a similar rate in order to maintain a normal blood-glucose level. The initial source of this glucose is the glycogen store of the liver, but as starvation proceeds, so other sources of fuel for gluconeogenesis are required.

Immediate changes in starvation. The brain normally uses only glucose as fuel; after the first day of starvation the blood glucose level is maintained by new glucose formation in the liver, in which amino acids, particularly alanine, are used as fuel. The amino acids are provided by the breakdown of protein. Because the nitrogen component is excreted as urea, the body is in negative nitrogen balance.

The triacylglycerols of adipose tissue are broken down to glycerol and fatty acids. Fatty acids are converted into ketone bodies in the liver, and these are used directly by most organs of the body instead of glucose.

Later changes in starvation. After the first week of starvation the breakdown of protein declines rapidly, and gluconeogenesis continues at a reduced rate. A change occurs in the brain's metabolism such that it is able to utilise ketone bodies, particularly beta-hydroxybutyrate, instead of glucose. Starvation can now continue until all the stores of body fat are utilised. When the supply of fat has been exhausted, only protein remains. The muscle masses decline and death soon follows.

During starvation the body conserves energy by reducing energy output. The starved individual is apathetic, lacking interest in life. Hypothermia is a danger in cold climates. This picture of starvation differs from that of the patient with anorexia nervosa, who is usually restless (see Ch. 35).

Loss of water is a characteristic feature of early starvation. Its cause is unknown. For individuals who try weight-reducing diets this loss provides false encouragement during the first few days of the regimen. In starvation the kidney is unable to concentrate urine, and polyuria results.

The oedema of starvation affects the dependent parts and appears to be due to the laxity of the subcutaneous tissues as well as to hypoalbuminaemia.

The wasted appearance of the starving person is all too familiar. The lax dry skin and wasted muscles are matched by wasting of the internal organs. In particular, with advanced starvation the intestine becomes increasingly thin; hence, when treating a starving patient one must give frequent small feeds if the person's life is to be saved.

Protein-Calorie Malnutrition in Childhood

Protein-calorie malnutrition is regarded as a spectrum of disease with marasmus at one end and kwashiorkor at the other end.

Nutritional marasmus. Marasmus is the name given to starvation in infants. It is due to deficiency of both protein and calories, and is encountered in infants under 1 year of age. It is a common condition in the developing countries of the world, and is usually due to cessation of breast feeding when the mother again becomes pregnant. The child exhibits the wasted appearance of starvation and in addition shows lack of growth. In those who survive, dwarfism is a frequent complication. As with starvation in adults, the marasmic child is very susceptible to infection; tuberculosis and dysentery often complete the lethal process initiated by starvation.

Kwashiorkor. This is a syndrome observed in children between the ages of 1 and 3 years. Its name is derived from a local African word denoting illness in a child displaced from the breast by a subsequent pregnancy.

Kwashiorkor is due to a low protein intake in the presence of an adequate carbohydrate supply. It is characterised by a fatty liver and marked oedema of the subcutaneous tissues. The inadequate protein supply leads to defective pigment formation: the hair becomes pale and even red in Black African children, and the skin is often depigmented and shows hyperkeratosis and flaking.

THE VITAMINS[1,3]

Definition and Classification

Vitamins are organic substances that the body cannot manufacture and that are necessary for normal metabolism; only 10 such substances are known in the human being. If these substances are present in insufficient quantity, disease results. The 10 vitamins essential for good health are listed below in Table 34.1.

TABLE 34.1 The essential vitamins

Fat-soluble	Water-soluble
Vitamin A	Vitamin C
Vitamin D	Vitamin B complex:
Vitamin K	Thiamine
	Riboflavin
	Niacin
	Pyridoxine
	Cobalamin (B_{12})
	Folate

CAUSES AND EFFECTS OF INDIVIDUAL VITAMIN DEFICIENCIES AND EXCESSES

Vitamin A (Retinol)

Vitamin A is one of the fat-soluble vitamins. In herbivorous animals the carotenoid pigments, such as the carotenes of plants and vegetables, are converted into vitamin A in the intestine, absorbed, and subsequently stored in the liver. Human beings acquire their supply either directly from the carotenoids in vegetable matter (e.g. carrots, beetroot, and green vegetables in general) or indirectly from animal or dairy produce. The concurrent absorption of fat and the presence of bile salts in the intestine favour vitamin-A absorption.

Causes of vitamin A deficiency. This is usually due to a deficient diet. This nutritional problem usually occurs in Indonesia, parts of Asia, India, the Middle East, and Latin America; it is almost unknown in North America and Europe. Vitamin-A deficiency does, however, occur as a complication of the malabsorption syndrome; indeed, the blood level of carotene or vitamin A is used as a measure of the severity of the malabsorption.

Effects of vitamin A deficiency. *The eye.* Vitamin A forms an essential component of rhodopsin, a pigment in the rods of the retina. By absorbing light, rhodopsin initiates an electrical impulse that is transmitted to the brain and is interpreted as light. The first sign of vitamin-A deficiency, therefore, is night blindness. Apart from this one known biochemical action of vitamin A, its other functions remain a mystery in spite of much research. It is known that vitamin A regulates the structure of certain epithelial cells. In vitamin A deficiency the epithelia of the genito-urinary tract, the trachea, the nose, and the conjunctiva tend to undergo squamous metaplasia. The most important effect is in the eye. The conjunctival epithelium loses its mucus-secreting goblet cells and becomes keratinised, thereby taking on the characteristics of epidermis. An early sign is the formation of desquamating hyperkeratotic plaques on the conjunctiva at the lateral margin of the cornea. These are triangular in shape, and appear as areas of dry foam. They are known as *Bitôt's spots*. The lacrimal ducts show hyperkeratosis, so that the eye becomes dry and subject to cracking and infection. The condition is called *xerophthalmia*. In due course the cornea becomes cloudy; with infection it can soften (*keratomalacia*), so that the globe may become perforated. The lens is then extruded, and blindness results. Indeed, vitamin-A deficiency is a leading cause of blindness in the world.*

*Other common causes are trachoma, diabetes mellitus, smallpox, (now likely to become extinct), onchocerciasis, gonococcal ophthalmia, injury through accidents, cataract, and glaucoma.

The skin. The skin shows dryness and follicular plugging, but whether these changes are specific for vitamin-A deficiency is not clear.

Other effects. The replacement of respiratory-type epithelium (with its goblet cells and cilia) by keratinised squamous epithelium is a factor in the production of respiratory infections. Nevertheless, in the presence of a normal amount of vitamin A there is no evidence that an excessive intake can prevent respiratory infections. The time-honoured practice of giving children large quantities of vitamin A (in cod-liver oil) in order to prevent colds and respiratory infections appears to be quite ill-founded. Indeed, such a practice can cause toxic effects (see below).

In spite of the dramatic changes seen in epithelium in vitamin-A deficiency, the biochemical nature of the defect is unknown. If a small piece of skin is grown in organ culture and subjected to vitamin-A deficiency, it soon shows hyperkeratosis. If an excess quantity of vitamin A is now added to the medium, the epithelium changes to a goblet-cell, mucus-secreting type. There is no evidence, however, that excess vitamin A in the human can convert normal keratinised epidermis into mucus-secreting epithelium.

Toxicity of vitamin A. Very large doses of vitamin A are toxic and can cause an increase in intracranial pressure with headache, blurring of vision, vomiting, and drowsiness. This effect has been described by Arctic explorers when they ate polar bear liver, which is a very rich source of vitamin A. Chronic poisoning can cause loss of hair, bone pains, calcification of ligaments and tendons, hyperpigmentation of the skin, liver damage, and psychiatric symptoms.

Vitamin D

Vitamin D is present in all fat-containing animal products, but its richest source is cod-liver oil. Vitamin D is also formed in the skin by the action of ultraviolet light on 7-dehydrocholesterol.

The main action of the vitamin is the maintenance of calcium balance by facilitating the absorption of calcium from the intestine. The effects of *hypovitaminosis D* are rickets and osteomalacia, and these are considered in Chapter 36.

Hypervitaminosis D due to toxic doses of the vitamin or to an increased response to its action is also considered in Chapter 36; there is hypercalcaemia and metastatic calcification. Vomiting, anorexia, nausea, constipation, and renal failure are the main clinical features.

Vitamin K

Vitamin K is widely distributed in vegetable and animal foods. It is also synthesised by bacteria in the gut. Vitamin-K deficiency is considered in Chapter 54.

Vitamin E[4]

Vitamin E includes a group of fat-soluble substances that act as antioxidants. The vitamin's more formal name is *tocopherol*; this derives from the Greek 'tocos' meaning childbirth and 'phero' meaning bring forth, and alludes to the original belief that the vitamin was essential for reproduction. Its antioxidant activity might prevent the oxidative degradation of cell membranes, which contain phospholipids, and thus maintain the integrity of the cell. In fact, little is known about the natural function of vitamin E or the effects of its deficiency. Sterility in rats, cerebellar disorders in chicks, and myopathy in ducklings have all been reported as accompaniments of vitamin-E deficiency in animals.

In the human, tocopherols are not actively transported from the maternal to the fetal circulation and are poorly absorbed by infants of gestational age less than 36 weeks. Vitamin-E deficiency in premature infants has been associated with haemolytic anaemia and widespread oedema; the haemolysis is aggravated by iron. Cystic fibrosis is invariably associated with vitamin-E deficiency when there is pancreatogenic steatorrhoea.

Vitamin E has been regarded as a panacea by some enthusiasts, but unfortunately it cannot delay the effects of senility nor decrease the incidence of coronary-artery disease. It is said to be beneficial in abetalipoproteinaemia, where it may delay the progress of the neurological and retinal lesions. It is also recommended for muscle cramps. In rats tocopherol enhances drug hydroxylation; it would be of interest if it had a similar role in the human subject, for instance in neonatal jaundice where phenobarbitone is sometimes used (see p. 562).

Vitamin C (Ascorbic Acid)

Human beings share with other primates, the guinea-pig, and certain birds the inability to synthesise vitamin C. The main dietary sources of this vitamin are citrus fruit, currants, berries, green vegetables, and potatoes. Vitamin C is necessary for the synthesis of collagen (Chapter 5), and a deficiency leads to *scurvy*. The main clinical effect is a bleeding tendency, the cause of which is probably poor anchorage of the smaller blood vessels in a thin, watery intercellular substance devoid of adequate collagen fibres. The site of bleeding varies according to the age of the patient.

Adult scurvy. Bleeding often first takes place into the skin, being first detected around the hair follicles, which also show follicular hyperkeratosis. There may be a characteristic 'saddle' distribution of petechiae on the medial surface of the thighs and buttocks. Cutaneous ecchymoses may follow minor trauma. There is also bleeding into muscles and along fascial planes, particularly at points of mechanical stress. A very characteristic finding is gingival haemorrhage, which occurs only in those who have teeth: the gingivae become spongy, swollen, and ultimately ulcerated. There may be severe bleeding with later superimposed infection.

Anaemia is common in scorbutic subjects, but this is probably due, when it cannot be explained in terms of blood loss, to multiple nutritional deficiencies. The vitamin probably does not have a direct role in haematopoiesis (p. 605). A very important effect of vitamin-C deficiency is delayed wound healing, which is dealt with in Chapter 9. Death occurs in untreated cases, usually from severe infection.

In the past scurvy plagued sailors on long sea voyages, since the disease first becomes manifest about two months after commencing a deficient diet. For example, Vasco da Gama is reported to have lost 100 men of his 160-man crew on his journey around the Cape of Good Hope in 1497. James Lind (1716–1794), a British naval surgeon, introduced oranges, lemons, and limes into his sailors' diet in 1747, thereby preventing the lethal effects of scurvy and earning the name 'limey' for his countrymen.

Scurvy in infants and children. Milk and milk products are often a poor source of vitamin C, especially if the milk has been stored or processed. Consequently scurvy can develop in infants at about the age of 8 months.

In infantile scurvy the outstanding feature is subperiosteal haemorrhages, which are very painful; these are rare in adults. On the other hand, although bleeding can occur elsewhere, gingival lesions are not seen in infants unless the teeth have erupted.

Osseous lesions are also seen in infantile and early childhood scurvy, since there is an impaired formation of osteoid. An X-ray of a scorbutic bone shows generalised rarefaction due to osteoporosis, which is particularly well marked at the metaphyseal ends of the shaft. By contrast, the zones of provisional calcification are very dense; in the long bones this density appears as a transverse line at the junction between the epiphysis and the end of the shaft. There is heavy calcification of the cartilage with foci of fragmented spicules of calcified cartilage forming during the period of retarded longitudinal growth. The epiphysis may be fractured at the line of junction and undergo displacement and dislocation. Microscopically there is little evidence of bone formation either beneath the periosteum or at the margins of the calcified spicules of cartilage in the metaphyseal zone. Instead there is an accumulation of cells of fibroblast type embedded in a loose-textured, oedematous ground substance. These cells are in fact osteoblasts, and they start to lay down osteoid as soon as ascorbic acid is administered. The subperiosteal haemorrhages follow the disruption of the collagenous attachments (Sharpey's fibres) from the cortex of the bone. There is also an impairment in the formation of dentine, and the teeth may be loosened from the alveolar bone.

Vitamin B Complex

Thiamine

Thiamine is a coenzyme necessary for several steps in carbohydrate metabolism. In the absence of this vitamin, lactic acid and pyruvic acid accumulate in the blood instead of entering the Krebs cycle. The vitamin is widely distributed in foodstuffs. Thiamine deficiency was once prevalent in the Far East, where polished (highly milled) rice formed the staple diet (the process of milling removes most of the thiamine from the rice). Thiamine deficiency is now much less common in the world generally, but is still encountered in the Far East, particularly in persons of all ages living in isolated communities, in infants, and in pregnant women. In North America it is sometimes encountered in chronic alcoholics.

Effects of thiamine deficiency. The early symptoms of thiamine deficiency, which is called *beriberi*, are vague: weakness, ankle oedema, and paraesthesiae and numbness of the legs. At any time one of the two major forms may develop.

Wet beriberi. In this form it is postulated that the accumulation of lactic acid and other vasodilator chemical agents causes so much vasodilatation that high-output heart failure develops. The outstanding feature is extensive oedema with an accumulation of fluid in the serous sacs. Sudden death from heart failure is not uncommon.

Dry beriberi. The outstanding feature of this form is peripheral neuropathy. Numbness and anaesthesia are the result of sensory-nerve damage, whereas weakness and muscle wasting are the effects of motor-nerve involvement. The patient eventually becomes bedridden.

Two other effects of thiamine deficiency are noteworthy:

Infantile beriberi. Infants with a low thiamine intake may develop acute beriberi between the ages of 2 and 6 months. The sudden development of heart failure, which is often fatal, is characteristic.

Wernicke's encephalopathy and Korsakoff's psychosis. These conditions may occur with other forms of beriberi, but in Europe and North America they are invariably encountered in alcoholics. *Wernicke's encephalopathy* manifests itself by disturbances of consciousness, ataxia, and nystagmus, and in fatal cases lesions are found in the regions of the third and fourth ventricles and the aqueduct. The mammillary bodies are consistently involved, and often show conspicuous petechial haemorrhages. Histologically there is dilatation and proliferation of capillaries and also some astrocytic and microglial proliferation; there may be degenerative changes in the neurons. The experimental model is provided by thiamine-deficient pigeons; in them death may occur so quickly that there are no microscopical lesions (see p. 47).

In less severe and acute cases the mental changes of *Korsakoff's psychosis* are noted: spatial disorientation and a gross defect in memory for recent events. The patient fills in the gaps by giving imaginary accounts of his activities, a symptom called confabulation.

Treatment of beriberi. Beriberi responds promptly to thiamine administration; with the wet form early treatment is essential, since sudden death is common. Likewise, in Wernicke's encephalopathy delay may lead to irreparable brain damage.

Riboflavin[5]

Riboflavin is a constituent of many foods, and is a component of several enzymes that play a vital role in metabolism. Yet the lesions associated with riboflavin deficiency are ill-defined. A sore mouth is an early symptom: the angles of the mouth become macerated and later develop cracks (*angular stomatitis* or *perlèche*), the lips become sore, dry, and cracked (*cheilosis*), and the tongue becomes smooth and sore (*glossitis*). A scaly dermatitis, resembling seborrhoeic dermatitis, develops later, and affects the face and the scrotum or vulva.

Niacin

As with thiamine and riboflavin, niacin (nicotinic acid) is widely distributed in plant and animal food and is also a component of important enzymes. A deficiency of niacin causes *pellagra*, a disease so named because of the rough skin (from the Italian *pelle agra*, or 'rough skin') that is present. Pellagra is a disease of poor peasants who subsist chiefly on maize (American corn). Although this cereal contains niacin, the vitamin is in a bound form. Furthermore, maize is deficient in tryptophan, an amino acid from which the body can manufacture niacin.

Pellagra was once common in Spain and Italy. It became widespread in the USA in the early years of the present century, but has been largely eliminated by improved economic conditions. Nevertheless, it is still sometimes encountered in chronic alcoholics.

Pellagra may develop in patients with the carcinoid syndrome, presumably because tryptophan and nicotinic-acid precursors are deviated to the 5-HT pathway. Likewise, pellagra develops in Hartnup disease[6] a rare, inherited disorder in which there is a defect in the absorption of amino acids (including tryptophan) from the intestine; this leads to tryptophan deficiency.* A failure of reabsorption from the renal tubules results in aminoaciduria, which aggravates the tryptophan deficiency. Episodes of cerebellar ataxia are an unexplained feature of this rare disease.

The symptoms of pellagra are most easily remembered as the *three Ds.*

Dermatitis. Erythema, superficially resembling a sunburn, develops on the sun-exposed areas. This may progress to blistering and a chronic type of dermatitis.

Diarrhoea. This is one of the principal gastrointestinal symptoms. A smooth, sore tongue of 'raw-beef' appearance is another common finding.

Dementia. Mental changes are common; they may take the form of acute delirium, or a more chronic manic-depressive state followed by progressive dementia. There may also be neurological accompaniments, such as peripheral neuritis, ataxia, and visual and auditory disturbances.

Death (the fourth D) was a common end-result of pellagra before the advent of vitamin therapy.

The modern view is that pellagra results from a diet that is poor in protein and reduced in nicotinic acid, riboflavin, and haematopoietic factors; toxic or antivitamin substances may also be involved.

Pyridoxine (Vitamin B₆)

Pyridoxine is also a component of important coenzymes. Dietary deficiencies are unusual, but pyridoxine deficiency has been reported as a complication of drug therapy, particularly isoniazid. It has also been reported as a complication of the oral contraceptive. The effects of pyridoxine deficiency are vague; dermatitis, cheilosis, angular stomatitis, and glossitis have all been noted. A sideroblastic anaemia has been described (p. 616).

It is evident from this short account that thiamine, riboflavin, niacin, and pyridoxine are widely distributed in food and that deficiencies are due to an unbalanced or inadequate diet. Such dietary deficiencies are generally the effect of poverty, ignorance, or alcoholism. It follows therefore that multiple deficiencies are often present in the same patient, and it is proper practice to prescribe a mixture of these members of the vitamin B complex.

Cobalamin (Vitamin B₁₂) and Folate

These vitamins are necessary for red-cell maturation. Their absence leads to a megaloblastic anaemia (Ch. 52).

THE MALABSORPTION SYNDROME

The small intestine has two main functions, (*a*) the intraluminal digestion of food, mainly by the action of pancreatic enzymes

---

*The intestinal tryptophan is broken down by bacterial action to indol derivatives, absorbed, and excreted in the urine as indican. See also the rare 'blue-diaper syndrome' (p. 15).

aided by the bile salts, and (*b*) the absorption of nutrients, which is often aided by enzymes in the brush border of the absorptive cells that complete the process of digestion. An abnormality of the function of the small intestine may lead to a failure in digestion or absorption. This failure may involve a single substance or it may be of a more general nature, involving the absorption of many components of the diet, in which case the effects are far-reaching, if severe constituting the malabsorption syndrome. It is useful first to consider the normal mechanisms involved in the digestion and absorption of nutrients.

Carbohydrates.[7] Starch, which constitutes a major component of the diet, is hydrolysed by salivary and pancreatic amylase to oligosaccharides and then to disaccharides, mostly maltose. The oligosaccharides together with maltose and other disaccharides, such as sucrose and lactose, are hydrolysed by specific disaccharidases, e.g. maltase, β-galactosidase (lactase), and sucrase, that are an integral part of the intestinal luminal surface. These enzymes are situated in the brush border of the intestinal cell, being probably a component of the glycocalyx. Monosaccharides (glucose, galactose, and fructose) are the end-result of carbohydrate digestion, and are absorbed by two specific and separate mechanisms: glucose and galactose are actively absorbed by a common mechanism, while fructose utilises a separate mechanism. The hydrolysis of disaccharides is a rapid process, absorption being the rate-limiting factor; lactose provides the only exception to this rule, since it is only slowly hydrolysed. This relative lack of lactase activity in the human intestine is the explanation of the lactose intolerance so frequently encountered clinically. The absorbed monosaccharides are passed into the portal blood stream and thence to the liver.

Proteins. After the partial hydrolysis of protein by the pepsin of the gastric secretion, the pancreatic trypsin, chymotrypsin, and carboxypeptidases continue the process of digestion; polypeptides, dipeptides, and finally amino acids are produced. Dipeptidases and tripeptidases associated with the mucosal cells complete the process of hydrolysis, and the dipeptides and amino acids so produced are absorbed by an active transport mechanism. Some amino acids share a common mechanism, and it is therefore understandable that in certain genetic defects there is an impaired absorption of a specific group of amino acids, for example cystine, arginine, ornithine, and lysine in cystinuria (p. 559) and the neutral amino acids (tryptophan, phenylalanine, and histidine) in Hartnup disease (p. 440). In these genetic defects the uptake and absorption of dipeptides is normal.

Fat. Bile salts play an important part in fat absorption, since they have an emulsifying, detergent action which aids the action of pancreatic lipase. The bile salts also aid fat absorption by forming micelles with fatty acids and monoglycerides. About 25 per cent of ingested lipid is hydrolysed to glycerol and fatty acid, while the remaining 75 per cent remains at the monoglyceride stage. Fatty acids and monoglycerides are absorbed into the intestinal cells, after which they follow one of two pathways depending upon the chain length of the fatty-acid component. Fatty acids (and their associated monoglycerides) of long chain length (C16 to C18 fatty acids) are esterified to triglyceride and very low-density lipids. These, in combination with apoproteins (p. 582), form chylomicrons and very low-density lipoproteins, which enter the lacteals. In contrast to this, fatty acids of medium chain length (C8 to C10 fatty acids) are not esterified, and pass directly to the portal circulation where they are bound to

albumin.[8] On reaching the liver, the medium-chain fatty acids are mostly metabolised to CO_2, acetate, or ketones. Any medium-chain fatty acids not metabolised thus are converted into long-chain fatty acids and then esterified to triglyceride. It follows that a patient with impaired fat absorption due to lymphatic blockage will fare better on a diet containing medium-chain fatty acids than on one containing the long-chain fatty acids.

Even in the absence of pancreatic enzymes a considerable portion (60 to 80 per cent) of ingested fat is absorbed by mechanisms that are not clearly understood. The faecal fat is partly of endogenous origin, being derived from desquamated epithelial cells, and partly the residue of undigested food. The composition of the fat is modified by bacterial action in the colon. An increase in the amount of fat in the faeces is a common finding in the malabsorption syndrome, and is called *steatorrhoea*.

DISORDERS OF INTESTINAL ABSORPTION

A failure in the absorption of nutrients may be due to a derangement of either digestion or absorption. Three classes of disorder may be recognised:

1. The defect may be specific for a particular food component; this is usually associated with an enzyme defect, e.g. lactose intolerance and Hartnup disease.

2. There may be a lack of a major digestive fluid, e.g. the gastric juice following total gastrectomy, the pancreatic juice in pancreatic disease, or the bile in bile-duct obstruction.

The gastric juice is not essential for digestion, apart from the secretion of intrinsic factor and its vital part in the absorption of vitamin B_{12}. Nevertheless, even a partial gastric resection leads to a degree of general malabsorption,[9] because the stomach provides a place of temporary arrest so that food is admitted into the intestine in a slow, controlled manner. After gastrectomy there is a much more hurried passage of food in the intestine, and digestion is rendered less complete. Both pancreatic and biliary secretions are reduced after partial gastrectomy, the reason for which is probably that diminished gastric digestion and acid secretion provide inadequate stimulation of pancreatic secretion by way of pancreozymin and secretin. Protein digestion is particularly severely affected due to the combined effects of reduced pancreatic trypsin, poor mixing with the enzyme as a result of intestinal hurry, and a greater bacterial decomposition of protein in the lower reaches of the small bowel—this bacterial flora is more prominent after gastrectomy because the disinfectant activity of the hydrochloric acid is lost. Fat absorption is also impaired, but the digestion of carbohydrate is only slightly affected. It is not surprising that there is a considerable loss of weight after gastrectomy, due more to defective intestinal absorption than to decreased intake. Another common result of gastrectomy is iron-deficiency anaemia, which is due to the combined effects of intestinal hurry and reduced hydrochloric-acid secretion.

3. There may be a gross abnormality of the small intestine itself such that many processes are affected.

In the last two groups there is a defective absorption of many food components, that of fat being particularly severely affected. The clinical state is that of the *malabsorption syndrome*.

Specific Defects of Absorption

Carbohydrate maldigestion and malabsorption. The

effects of a failure to digest and absorb carbohydrate are mainly attributable to the osmotic pressure exerted by the unabsorbed oligosaccharides or monosaccharides. Soon after ingesting the offending carbohydrate the patient feels bloated and the abdomen becomes distended. Furthermore, bacteria convert the carbohydrate to fatty acids, which appear to irritate the intestine; abdominal colic and diarrhoea may result.

Idiopathic lactase deficiency in adults. This is a common condition, its prevalence showing a racial incidence. It is commonest in the Oriental groups (100 per cent in some groups), frequent in the Black population (over 50 per cent), and least common in White people. The individual experiences no trouble during infancy or childhood, but only later exhibits intolerance to milk, which is eliminated from the diet in order to avoid symptoms. There may sometimes be a preceding intestinal disease or a resection of bowel; presumably these can precipitate lactose intolerance in a susceptible person. The most reliable method of laboratory diagnosis is a jejunal biopsy with an estimation of the lactase content of the specimen.

The condition must not be confused with *lactose intolerance in children* without lactase deficiency. This is a separate entity; it is rare, and severe inanition, dehydration, and even death may follow the ingestion of lactose in the form of milk. The pathogenesis is unknown, and a directly toxic effect of lactose is postulated.

Selective sucrase deficiency and the *malabsorption of glucose and galactose* due to a defective transport mechanism are two other known, but rare conditions.

Protein malabsorption. There are a number of inherited diseases in which there is a defective absorption of specific amino acids or groups of amino acids. Hartnup disease and cystinuria are examples that have already been noted.

GENERAL MALABSORPTION SYNDROME

If the functions of the small intestine are markedly impaired a state of severe undernutrition results. The digestion and absorption of protein, carbohydrate, and fat are variably affected, and in addition there may be defective absorption of vitamins and minerals.

Causes of the Malabsorption Syndrome[10]

These may be either extrinsic or intrinsic.

Extrinsic causes of malabsorption may be gastric, pancreatic, or biliary, and are related to impaired digestion of food products or intestinal hurry.

Intrinsic causes are due primarily to defective intestinal function, and are related both to impaired absorption and disturbed enzyme action in the mucosal cells themselves. These will now be considered.

(1) Intrinsic disease of the intestine itself. A good example of such a condition that leads to severe malabsorption is the *sprue syndrome.* It is typified by atrophy of the intestinal villi, the cause of which is not known (Fig. 34.1). Two types of sprue syndrome are recognised:

(*a*) *Tropical sprue*, which is seen extensively in the Far East. It is not related to gluten sensitivity, but it often responds to oral antibiotics.

(*b*) *Gluten-sensitive enteropathy*, which in children is called

Figure 34.1
Gluten-sensitive enteropathy (coeliac disease, or non-tropical sprue). This section from a jejunal biopsy shows the typical flat surface and absence of villi. The lamina propria is heavily infiltrated by lymphocytes and plasma cells. × 150.

coeliac disease and in adults *non-tropical sprue.* The intestinal lesions and symptoms can be relieved by a diet that is low in gluten, a protein contained in flour. There is a marked familial incidence, the condition probably being inherited as an autosomal dominant trait with incomplete penetrance. Whether the gluten damages the small intestine by a directly toxic action or indirectly by an immunological reaction is not known.

Malabsorption may also follow infiltration of the intestine with *lymphoma, Whipple's disease,** *progressive systemic sclerosis,* and *amyloid.* Lymphatic obstruction is not an important factor in malabsorption, except in *intestinal lymphangiectasia,* which is probably a congenital lesion in which the mucosal lymphatics are abnormal and extremely dilated.

Ischaemia of the intestine (p. 517) can lead to malabsorption. Malabsorption can also be part of a systemic disease of

---

*This strange disease occurs most often in middle-aged men, who present with steatorrhoea, wasting, and migratory polyarthritis. The lamina propria of the small bowel contains many macrophages filled with PAS-positive material and also various bacteria. Similar cells are found in the lymph nodes, synovial membrane, and other sites. The nature of the disease is obscure, but what was previously a uniformly fatal condition can now be cured by broad-spectrum antibiotics. It may be that the disease represents an immunological deficiency on the part of the host to organisms resident in the bowel.

endocrine origin, e.g. *diabetes mellitus* and the *Zollinger-Ellison syndrome*. Certain drugs, notably *neomycin* and the *folic-acid antagonists*, can have a similar effect.

(2) **The blind loop syndrome,** also called *the stagnant bowel syndrome*, may complicate extensive diverticulosis of the small intestine (an uncommon condition, seen most often in the jejunum), blind loops of bowel between surgical anastomoses, fistulae between coils of small bowel, and strictures of the small bowel (these last two were seen in intestinal tuberculosis in the past, but nowadays are nearly always due to Crohn's disease, at least in the developed countries). It is generally accepted that the mechanism of malabsorption in this syndrome is an upset in the intestinal bacterial flora. Normally the small bowel is virtually sterile (p. 89), but blind loops, abnormalities in peristalsis, and gastro-colic fistulae all allow bacterial proliferation to occur. One effect of this is the deconjugation of the bile salts, which leads to impaired fat absorption. Impaired vitamin B_{12} absorption is another effect, which follows the bacterial metabolism of the vitamin (p. 609).

(3) **Surgical resection of the small intestine.** This, if extensive, leads to a serious reduction of the absorptive area. Such a resection may be necessitated by abdominal gunshot wounds, recurrent Crohn's disease, or massive intestinal infarction.

Effects of Malabsorption

The effects of malabsorption may vary from subclinical disturbances to fatal malnutrition, depending on the portion of small bowel affected and the extent of the disease. The lack of absorption of essential nutrients may produce some effects similar to those of starvation, such as *weight loss* and *generalised body atrophy*.

Fat absorption is usually severely affected. If much fat— some of it undigested—is passed in the faeces, these will be pale and bulky. An estimation of the fat passed in the stools is an important investigation in a case of malabsorption. The classical fat balance, in which the patient is fed a known quantity of fat for several days and the fat content of the faeces passed during that time is estimated (normally 95 per cent of fat is absorbed, whereas in steatorrhoea there is less than 90 per-cent absorption) is cumbersome and very unpleasant to conduct. A more acceptable method is to estimate the fat content of a patient's stools when a standard ward diet is fed. A normal person excretes less than 5 g a day (5 to 7 g is borderline).[11] About 20 per cent of cases of coeliac disease have faecal fats within the normal range.

Carbohydrate absorption is often affected, and the excess carbohydrate in the bowel is fermented by resident bacteria. The resulting gas renders the stool frothy and offensive. When the malabsorption is due to intestinal disease, especially the sprue syndrome, the *glucose tolerance test* often shows a flat curve; in pancreatic steatorrhoea there is little disturbance of carbohydrate absorption, and the test is normal or even diabetic if there is severe pancreatic destruction.

Another useful test in intestinal malabsorption is the *xylose absorption test*:[11] a known amount of xylose is given orally after an overnight fast, and urine is collected over the subsequent 5 hours. Normally at least 20 per cent of the total amount is excreted, but in intestinal malabsorption less than 10 per cent escapes into the urine. The test is normal in pancreatic steatorrhoea.

Protein absorption is affected in intestinal and pancreatic steatorrhoea. If the hypoproteinaemia is severe enough to produce generalised oedema, an additional protein-losing gastroenteropathy should be suspected (p. 579).

Vitamin absorption. The vitamin-B complex may be inadequately absorbed, producing effects already described. Vitamin-C absorption is rarely impaired. The fat-soluble vitamins tend to be more severely affected, the lack of vitamins A and K producing characteristic effects. The malabsorption of vitamin D is aggravated by a concomitant binding of calcium to fatty acids in the bowel. Important effects of this dual interference with calcium absorption are a negative calcium balance, mild hypocalcaemia, a tendency to tetany, and in more prolonged cases osteomalacia. There may also be osteoporosis due to protein deficiency. Malabsorption of folic acid and vitamin B_{12} produces a megaloblastic type of anaemia (see Ch. 52).

Mineral absorption. An impaired absorption of iron is common, and this leads to a characteristic anaemia (Ch. 52). Other minerals that may be poorly absorbed are sodium, potassium, magnesium, and chloride (as well as calcium previously noted). Malabsorption may therefore be accompanied by symptoms of dehydration and muscular weakness.

Many of these substances are absorbed normally from the proximal part of the small bowel; this applies especially to the minerals, carbohydrates, fats, proteins, and most of the vitamins. Vitamin B_{12}, however, is absorbed exclusively from the terminal ileum, and the enterohepatic circulation of bile salts is also mediated by an active transport mechanism in the lower ileum. Therefore disease of this part of the small bowel is particularly liable to lead to megaloblastic anaemia and a tendency to gallstones (see pp. 609 and 596).

It is evident that the effects of intestinal malabsorption are diverse, producing widespread disorder on many of the body's organs. This emphasises the importance of the small intestine in the economy of the whole body.

REFERENCES

1. LEHNINGER, A. L. (1975) *Biochemistry*, 2nd edn. New York: Worth Publishers. See Chapter 13 (pp. 335–360) for a description of the vitamins and pp. 840–845 for a description of starvation.
2. CAHILL, G. F. (1970) Starvation in man. *New England Journal of Medicine*, **282**, 668.
3. TRUSWELL, A. S. & WRIGHT, F. J. (1974) In *Davidson's Principles and Practice of Medicine*, ed. Macleod, J., 11th edn, pp. 111–172 (Nutritional factors in disease). Edinburgh: Churchill-Livingstone.
4. Leading Article (1977) Vitamin E for babies. *Lancet*, **2**, 1268.
5. RIVLIN, R. S. (1970) Riboflavine metabolism. *New England Journal of Medicine*, **283**, 463.

6. JEPSON, J. B. (1972) In *The Metabolic Basis of Inherited Disease*, ed. Stanbury, J. B., Wyngaarden, J. B. & Fredrickson, D. S., 3rd edn, pp. 1486–1503 (Hartnup disease). New York: McGraw-Hill.

7. GRAY, G. M. (1975) Carbohydrate digestion and absorption. *New England Journal of Medicine*, **292**, 1225.

8. GREENBERGER, N. J. & SKILLMAN, T. G. (1969) Medium-chain triglycerides. *New England Journal of Medicine*, **280**, 1045.

9. DAVENPORT, H. W. (1971) *Physiology of the Digestive Tract*, 3rd edn, p. 170. Chicago: Year Book Medical Publishers.

10. MORSON, B. C. & DAWSON, I. M. P. (1972) *Gastrointestinal Pathology*, pp. 299–335. Oxford: Blackwell.

11. CREAMER, B., HELLIER, M. D. & PIERCE, J. W. (1974) In *The Small Intestine*, ed. Creamer, B., pp. 47–64. London: Heinemann.

Chapter 35. *Disturbances of Endocrine Function*

Introduction

Although the nervous system exerts the major controlling influence over the activities of the higher animals, there is an additional mechanism by which one type of cell can influence another: by the secretion of potent chemicals into the blood stream cells can exert an influence at a distant site. That the secretions be called hormones (from the Greek root *hormaein*, which means to excite, arouse, or set in motion) was proposed by Starling. Secreting cells that perform this endocrine function may be grouped together to form a compact organ, such as the thyroid gland, or they may be scattered more diffusely in the tissues. This latter tendency is well shown by the APUD cells. This chapter concentrates on the functional aspects of endocrine disorders, particularly those of a hyperplastic nature.

Mode of action of hormones. Hormones have an extremely potent and highly specific action on their target cells. This selective action is due to the binding of the hormone to specific cell receptors. The water-soluble hormones, such as adrenaline and glucagon, act on receptors situated in the cell membrane; cyclic AMP is formed, acting as a second messenger to stimulate or depress a characteristic biochemical activity (see Fig. 2.3, p. 14). In the case of insulin, cyclic GMP appears to be the second messenger. The lipid-soluble steroid hormones act on receptors in the cytoplasm, and the hormone-receptor complex, after modification, enters the nucleus and then acts by influencing the expression of the cell's genetic material.

THE HYPOTHALAMUS

Although the pituitary gland has been called the 'leader of the endocrine orchestra', it is now clear that it plays second fiddle to the hypothalamus, for many of the pituitary's activities are themselves controlled by hormones secreted in the hypothalamus (Fig. 35.1).

The hypothalamus consists of a complex collection of nerve cells and fibre tracts that participate in, and help regulate, many functions of the body. These include the autonomic nervous system, temperature, blood pressure, plasma osmolality, hunger, thirst, emotions, sexual drive, and sleep. The hypothalamus controls the body rhythms; a specific cycling centre is responsible for regulating the menstrual cycle. The development of this cycling centre is itself under hormonal control. Thus, if newborn female rats are given a single injection of testosterone, there is a permanent inhibition of the centre such that the cyclic release of LH-releasing factor does not occur, and the animals fail to ovulate spontaneously in later life.

The hypothalamus may be regarded as an endocrine organ because its cells synthesise two groups of hormones (Fig. 35.1):

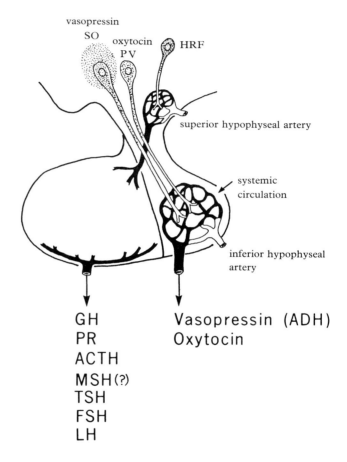

HYPOTHALAMUS

GH
PR
ACTH
MSH(?)
TSH
FSH
LH

Vasopressin (ADH)
Oxytocin

Figure 35.1

The relationship between the hypothalamus and the pituitary gland. Vasopressin (antidiuretic hormone, or ADH) and oxytocin are manufactured in nerve cells in the supraoptic (SO) and paraventricular (PV) nuclei of the hypothalamus. These hormones are not released into the circulation until they have reached the neurohypophysis. The shaded area surrounding the SO cell body represents the 'osmoreceptor' that is responsive to changes in osmolality of the fluid perfusing it. HRF represents an ill-defined group of cells that secrete a series of releasing factors into the primary capillary network of a portal vein. This vein passes in the pituitary stalk to the adenohypophysis, where cells manufacture the 7 hormones of this lobe of the pituitary: growth hormone (GH); prolactin (PR); adrenocorticotrophic hormone (ACTH); melanocyte-stimulating hormone (MSH), which is present in some species; thyroid-stimulating hormone (TSH); follicle-stimulating hormone (FSH); and luteinising hormone (LH). (*Drawn by Margot Mackay, Department of Art as Applied to Medicine, University of Toronto. After a drawing by E. Blackstock in Ezrin, C., Godden, J. O., Volpé, R. and Wilson, R. (Eds) (1973) Systematic Endocrinology. New York: Harper & Row.*)

1. *Oxytocin and vasopressin.* These are discussed later in this chapter.

2. *Releasing and inhibiting factors or hormones.* These are polypeptides of low molecular weight that pass to the adenohypophysis *via* a short portal vein, and stimulate or inhibit it. The following releasing hormones are recognised:

Corticotrophin-releasing factor (CRF).

Thyrotrophin-releasing factor (TRF); this also acts as a prolactin-releasing factor.

Gonadotrophin-releasing factor (GRF); this causes the release of both follicle-stimulating hormone and luteinising hormone.

Growth hormone-releasing factor (GHRF).

Prolactin-releasing hormone, which is distinct from TRF.

The action of these hormones can be understood by considering the action of CRF. This hormone leads to the release of corticotrophin (also known as adrenocorticotrophic hormone or ACTH) from the adenohypophysis. ACTH acts on the adrenal cortex to cause the release of cortisol (hydrocortisone). Cortisol inhibits the release of both CRF and ACTH. This inhibition is an example of negative feedback, which is a mechanism encountered in the regulation of other hormone secretions. The releasing factors are produced in picogram (10^{-12} gram) quantities, the pituitary hormones in nanogram (10^{-9} gram) quantities, and the target cells, e.g. the thyroid, produce hormone in microgram (10^{-6} gram) quantities. Thus the chain reaction shows a considerable amplification effect.

In addition to forming release factors, the hypothalamus forms three inhibiting factors:

Gonadotrophin-inhibiting factor.

Prolactin-inhibiting factor.

Growth-hormone-release-inhibiting hormone (GRIH or somatostatin). In addition to inhibiting the release of growth hormone by the pituitary, this polypeptide also blocks TRF-stimulated TSH release. It also inhibits insulin and glucagon release by the pancreatic islet cells.

DISEASES OF THE HYPOTHALAMUS

Many pathological processes affect the hypothalamus; these include meningitis, encephalitis, vascular lesions, head injury, hamartoma, histiocytosis X, and tumour. The effects differ widely depending on which function is predominantly deranged. These effects include the following:

(*a*) Obesity due to overeating.

(*b*) Somnolence, or alternatively restless hyperactivity.

(*c*) A failure of maintenance of body temperature. There may be hypothermia or alternatively hyperpyrexia.

(*d*) Diabetes insipidus due to a deficiency of vasopressin (antidiuretic hormone).

(*e*) Delayed puberty due to a failure of formation of GRF. When combined with obesity the condition is known as *Fröhlich's syndrome.*

(*f*) Precocious, or premature, puberty due to a failure of formation of gonadotrophin-inhibiting factor.

(*g*) Visual disturbances due to pressure on the optic chiasma.

(*h*) Hypothyroidism (rare).

The regulation of hypothalamic-pituitary function is complex, for apart from the gross lesions mentioned above, hypothalamic function can be influenced by impulses emanating from other parts of the brain. For example, the assumption of the erect posture affects baroreceptors which relay impulses to the hypothalamus and lead to a secretion of vasopressin, which produces water retention and an increase in blood volume. Other examples are more intricate; for instance, stress can inhibit pituitary growth-hormone release in children so that growth is delayed, and there may also be amenorrhoea in young girls. Another example is impaired production of prolactin-inhibiting factor, which can lead to an overproduction of pituitary prolactin that in turn causes galactorrhoea. This may be the mechanism of persistent lactation either following pregnancy (*Chiari-Frommel syndrome*) or spontaneously (*Forbes-Albright syndrome*).

THE PITUITARY GLAND (HYPOPHYSIS)

Although small, the pituitary gland, or hypophysis, secretes an amazing variety and number of hormones. The gland and its stalk consist of two parts: the neurohypophysis, which develops as an outpouching from the primitive brain, and the adenohypophysis, which originates as a diverticulum from the primitive foregut. Both are probably derived entirely from neuroectoderm.[1]

THE ADENOHYPOPHYSIS

The adenohypophysis consists of the pars anterior (anterior lobe), the pars intermedia (which barely exists in the human), and the pars tuberalis in the pituitary stalk. It consists of several cell types (probably seven), and secretes seven hormones:

1. *Adrenocorticotrophin* (also called *adrenocorticotrophic hormone* or *ACTH*), which stimulates the adrenal cortex to produce cortisol.

2. *Melanocyte-stimulating hormone (MSH)* This is a definite entity in some animals, where it causes darkening of the skin. It is closely related to ACTH. Its existence in the human is problematic (see p. 586).

3. *Thyroid-stimulating hormone (TSH)*, which stimulates the thyroid gland to form its hormone.

4. *Growth hormone (GH)*. This is necessary for the growth of many tissues, particularly the skeleton.

5. *Follicle-stimulating hormone (FSH)*, which stimulates the growth of the Graafian follicle and consequent ovarian oestrogen production; in the male it stimulates spermatogenesis.

6. *Luteinising hormone (LH)*, which initiates ovulation and stimulates luteinisation of the mature follicle with consequent progesterone production. In the male it stimulates the interstitial cells of the testis to secrete testosterone.

7. *Prolactin, or lactogenic hormone*, which is responsible for milk secretion in the properly prepared breast. At least in rodents prolactin plays a part in the maintenance of the corpus luteum of pregnancy.

FSH, LH, and prolactin act on the ovary, and are often grouped together as the pituitary gonadotrophins.

DISORDERS OF THE ADENOHYPOPHYSIS

Hyperplasia or neoplasia of the anterior lobe of the pituitary gland may be associated with hypersecretion of one or several of its hormones. On the other hand, non-hormone-secreting pituitary tumours, or tumours arising in the neighbourhood, may press on and destroy the parenchyma so that there is a diminished hormonal secretion. The same effect may follow pituitary destruction by some other process, such as infarction or inflammation. In view of the possibly complicated clinical picture, only the common types will be described. In addition to these, tumours in the region of the pituitary may give rise to two additional effects by virtue of their anatomical situation: compression of the optic chiasma, which causes a loss of the temporal visual fields of both eyes (*bitemporal hemianopia*), and enlargement of the sella turcica, which is demonstrable radiologically.

Hyperpituitarism. The cells that form growth hormone are usually involved, so that the effects of excessive growth hormone are predominant. If the condition arises in childhood, the result is *gigantism*: a well-proportioned but very large individual. If the condition occurs in adult life after the epiphyses have fused, *acromegaly* results, in which the hands, feet, and lower jaw are considerably enlarged (the acral, or distal parts of the body). All the viscera are increased in size (splanchnomegaly), the facial features are coarsened, and the glucose tolerance is often impaired (see Ch. 33). Clinical diabetes mellitus occurs in from 10 to 15 per cent of patients. There may also be systemic hypertension.

Hypopituitarism. In children a deficiency of growth hormone leads to severe retardation of growth; the result is a midget. The unopposed action of insulin can lead to attacks of hypoglycaemia (see Ch. 33).

Hypopituitarism with a lack of gonadotrophins impairs gonadal maturation. Puberty does not take place, and fusion of the epiphyses, normally under the control of the sex hormones, is delayed. If the production of growth hormone is normal, these eunuchoid patients develop abnormally long limbs—their span exceeds their height (normally the two are equal). Gonadotrophin deficiency can also occur in adults: males show testicular atrophy and loss of libido, whereas in females there is amenorrhoea and a regression of the secondary sexual characteristics. In adults insufficiency of the anterior pituitary can manifest itself as hypothyroidism; often this is combined with evidence of adrenal cortical and gonadotrophic deficiency.

Acute pituitary insufficiency sometimes follows parturition, and is due to infarction of the gland. The condition is then called *Sheehan's syndrome*. When there is complete destruction of the adenohypophysis, the condition is characterised by extreme wasting. The patient is apathetic, and without treatment death will ultimately occur as a result of adrenal insufficiency (see later). The condition is called *Simmonds's disease* when there is extreme wasting.

Conditions simulating hypopituitarism. *Anorexia nervosa.* This is encountered usually in emotionally disturbed adolescent girls who develop an obsessive aversion to food. Extreme wasting and amenorrhoea, which are the main features, are due to starvation. The patients are restless and hostile.

Adiposogenital dystrophy. This is the male counterpart of anorexia nervosa. It occurs in emotionally disturbed boys who overeat; they are fat and show delayed onset of puberty. The condition resembles Fröhlich's syndrome, which is also sometimes called adiposogenital dystrophy.

THE NEUROHYPOPHYSIS

The neurohypophysis consists of the posterior lobe of the pituitary, part of the pituitary stalk (the *infundibular stem*), and part of the brain adjacent to the hypothalamus (the *median eminence of the tuber cinereum*). Two peptide hormones, oxytocin and vasopressin, are manufactured by cells in the hypothalamus (particularly the supraoptic and paraventricular nuclei), and pass *via* the cells' axons into the neurohypophysis, where they are stored and subsequently released when needed.

Oxytocin. This hormone causes uterine contraction during labour, and is responsible for milk ejection when an infant is breastfed; the act of suckling initiates a reflex that causes the release of oxytocin.

Vasopressin (antidiuretic hormone or ADH). This hormone acts on the distal and collecting tubules of the kidney, causing water to be retained (see pp. 477 and 551).

Disorders of the Neurohypophysis

Diabetes insipidus. This disease is caused by a failure in the development of the neurohypophysis or its destruction by inflammation, ionising radiation (during pituitary ablation), or a tumour. There is the passage of enormous quantities of very dilute urine (polyuria), with consequent thirst and voracious water drinking (polydipsia).

The syndrome of inappropriate ADH secretion. In this syndrome the secretion of ADH is unrelated to plasma osmolality. The retention of water leads to hyponatraemia; the urinary osmolality exceeds that of the plasma. Lung tissue has the capacity to synthesise ADH, and the syndrome occasionally complicates chronic lung disease, but by far the commonest cause is oat-cell carcinoma of the lung. Occasionally organic lesions of the hypothalamus are responsible for this syndrome, or else ADH secretion is stimulated by a drug, such as chlorpropamide, vincristine, or cyclophosphamide.

ADRENAL CORTEX

Introduction

With the exception of the gonads and the placenta, the adrenal cortex is the source of all the steroid hormones. These are responsible for regulating salt, water, carbohydrate, and protein metabolism. They also play an important role in the body's resistance to stress and infection.

The cortical steroids may be defined in terms of their main actions or according to the number of carbon atoms present in the molecule. The hormones are all derived from cholesterol, itself synthesised in the cortex from simple substrates, such as acetate. The basic formula is a reduced cyclopentophenanthrene ring. By the progressive loss of carbon atoms three groups may be recognised. The *C21 group* includes hydrocortisone (cortisol) and aldosterone, the *C19 group* are androgenic, and the *C18 group* are oestrogenic. As indicated above, there are three functional groups: the glucocorticoids typified by cortisol, the mineralocorticoids (namely aldosterone), and the sex hormones (namely androgens). Each of these groups will be described separately, but it should be noted that some hormones, e.g. corticosterone, have both glucocorticoid and mineralocorticoid activity.

The glucocorticoids. Cortisol is released from the adrenal cortex under the influence of adrenocorticotrophic hormone (ACTH) secreted by the adenohypophysis. ACTH release is controlled by the corticotrophin-releasing factor (CRF) formed in the hypothalamus. The release of CRF is controlled by a number of factors:

(*a*) There is an important *diurnal* fluctuation with a peak of secretion occurring just before the subject awakens; the lowest activity for those who are daytime workers is at about 6 p.m.

(*b*) *Nervous influences*, such as stress, can act on the hypothalamus to cause a release of CRF; this is an important mechanism in the body's response to trauma.

(*c*) *The cortisol circulating in the plasma (the free-cortisol of the plasma)* acts directly on the hypothalamus, constituting a feedback mechanism. An elevation of the cortisol level also acts on the pituitary, rendering it less responsive to CRF. Cortisol is partly bound to cortisol-binding globulin and partly to plasma albumin; about 5 per cent is normally free in the plasma.

Actions of glucocorticoids. (*a*) *Metabolic effects.* Glucocorticoids promote gluconeogenesis from protein in the liver, and inhibit the peripheral utilisation of glucose by antagonising the action of insulin. The blood sugar therefore tends to rise. There is increased glycogen deposition in the liver.

Glucocorticoids stimulate the release of fatty acids from the fat depots, mobilise amino acids from the peripheral tissues, and increase amino-acid uptake by the liver. Thus the over-all effect of glucocorticoids is catabolic, except in the liver where the action is anabolic. Indeed, in the liver there is an increased synthesis of RNA, and this might be the primary effect, for on it depends the increased protein synthesis necessary for the production of the enzymes involved in the metabolism of amino acids and fatty acids.

(*b*) *Anti-inflammatory effect.* Glucocorticoids have an important anti-inflammatory action. They appear to decrease vascular permeability, thus counteracting the action of the chemical mediators of inflammation, which increase vascular permeability.

(*c*) *Effect on lymphocytes.* Glucocorticoids appear to cause the destruction of T lymphocytes; thus lymphopenia is a feature of glucocorticoid administration, and there is an inhibition of the T-cell-mediated immune response. B-cell functions are much less severely affected.

(*d*) *Stabilisation of the lysosomal membrane.*

(*e*) *Decreased calcium absorption from the intestine.*

(*f*) *Eosinopenia.*

(*g*) *A weak effect on sodium and potassium metabolism*, tending to cause sodium retention and potassium loss with a rise in the systemic blood pressure. The mechanism of these varied and diverse actions is not well understood.

The corticosteroids are excreted in the urine, mainly as *17-hydroxysteroids* and *17-ketogenic steroids*.

The mineralocorticoids. The chief mineralocorticoid is aldosterone, a C21 steroid hormone. It is formed in the zona glomerulosa of the adrenal cortex under the influence of angiotensin II. The kidney plays a vital part in this control mechanism through the secretion of renin. This is described on page 556. The control of renin secretion is complex. It is related to the blood volume, and its secretion is stimulated by a reduction in the blood pressure of the renal arterioles. It is also influenced by a feedback mechanism from the cells of the macula densa of the juxtaglomerular apparatus that monitor the sodium concentration in the fluid of the distal renal tubule. About 50 per cent of the plasma renin is free, the remainder being bound to albumin.

Actions of mineralocorticoids. The mineralocorticoids influence the rate of sodium and potassium transport across cell membranes. They promote the entry of sodium into cells and the exclusion of potassium. These effects are most obvious in the cells of the distal renal tubule, where the mineralocorticoids promote potassium loss and sodium retention.

They indirectly regulate the volume of the extracellular fluids. Nevertheless, an excessive amount of aldosterone does not lead to oedema formation, because the body can escape from this activity.

The sex hormones. The main androgen secreted by the adrenal cortex is dehydroepiandrosterone. Its secretion is stimulated by ACTH. It is the source of two-thirds of the urinary 17-ketosteroids* (the other third is derived from testicular androgen).

Oestrogens are probably not produced in the adrenal cortex, but androgen-precursor steroids produced in the gland can be converted into oestrogens by the liver, fat cells, and the placenta.

DISEASES OF THE ADRENAL CORTEX

Cushing's Syndrome

Cushing's syndrome is found more commonly in women than in men. It is characterised by abdominal striae, polycythaemia, systemic hypertension, glycosuria, osteoporosis, acne vulgaris, and in women hypertrichosis and amenorrhoea. There is a striking redistribution of fat, which results in obesity confined to the trunk, neck, and face. The characteristic moon face is partly attributable to this, but there is also fluid retention (see p. 524). All the signs and symptoms of Cushing's syndrome can be reproduced by the prolonged, excessive administration of glucocorticoids or ACTH.

The adrenal glands may be the seat of a simple adenoma, a carcinoma, or bilateral hyperplasia, the cause of which is undecided. The hyperplasia might be the result of excessive ACTH production by the pituitary, perhaps secondary to hypothalamic overactivity, but this is unproven. The normal diurnal rhythm is absent, and it may be that the hypothalamic set-point is changed and excess CRF is produced. The usual pituitary change in Cushing's syndrome is hyalinisation of the basophil cells. It may be that the adrenals are unduly sensitive to the effects of a normal amount of ACTH.

Sometimes a pituitary tumour is present or becomes apparent at a later period after adrenalectomy. The tumour may produce visual-field defects and enlargement of the sella

---

*17-ketosteroids are also called 17-oxosteroids.

turcica; its secretion of ACTH (and perhaps MSH) can lead to marked hyperpigmentation of the skin (*Nelson's syndrome*, see p. 586). It is noteworthy that the original description of the condition by Harvey Cushing in 1932 concerned cases in which there was an accompanying basophil tumour of the pituitary, a variant that has been designated *Cushing's disease.*

Cushing's syndrome is sometimes caused by ectopic ACTH secretion from a malignant tumour, generally an oat-cell carcinoma of the lung (see p. 339).

Biochemical findings. Although cortisol has some mineralocorticoid activity, the sodium and water retention of Cushing's syndrome is generally due to an increased secretion of deoxycorticosterone by the adrenals. In simple adrenal hyperplasia the plasma cortisol, urine free cortisol, and 17-hydrocorticoids are all elevated. Low-dose dexamethasone fails to suppress the adrenal activity, probably because the hypothalamic-pituitary mechanism is relatively insensitive, or else the adrenal glands are hyper-reactive to ACTH. High-dose dexamethasone does cause suppression. A complete absence of suppression indicates adrenal hyperplasia due to an ectopic source of ACTH, or else an adrenal tumour.

The metyrapone test helps to distinguish between hyperplasia and neoplasia. With hyperplasia cortisol production is blocked and pituitary over-secretion of ACTH occurs; hence the urinary secretion of 17-hydroxycorticoids is increased. In Cushing's syndrome due to an adrenal adenoma metyrapone depresses cortisol production by the tumour and the secretion of ACTH by the pituitary increases, but the adenoma does not respond to this. Neither can the atrophic adrenal tissue that remains respond. Hence there is no rise in the 24-hour urinary output of 17-hydroxycorticoids. In cases of adenoma the pituitary ACTH production is already depressed and the dexamethasone test is negative, since the pituitary ACTH output cannot be further lowered.

In functional adrenal carcinoma the tumour is completely autonomous, and neither ACTH, dexamethasone, nor metyrapone affects steroid excretion. In addition, there is often an increased androgen secretion, which is manifest as virilism in the female. There is an increase in urinary 17-ketosteroids as well as in 17-hydroxycorticoids. There is also an increase in the excretion of intermediates of steroid biosynthesis, indicating a disordered or inefficient conversion to the final products.

In the ectopic ACTH syndrome the plasma ACTH level is extremely high, and no additional ACTH or change in pituitary function can make any appreciable difference to adrenal activity. Abnormal forms of ACTH may be detected in the plasma.

Hyperaldosteronism

Primary hyperaldosteronism (Conn's syndrome). Most cases of Conn's syndrome are due to a small adrenal cortical adenoma, but sometimes there is bilateral cortical hyperplasia. There is systemic hypertension, increased urinary potassium loss, and hypokalaemia, which causes muscular cramps and weakness. Severe hypokalaemia damages the kidney (see p. 480). Despite salt retention, there is no oedema (see p. 524). Possibly the hypokalaemic nephropathy, by causing polyuria, also plays a part in causing sodium loss and preventing oedema.

Biochemical findings. The urinary 17-ketosteroids and 17-

hydroxycorticoids are normal. Plasma aldosterone levels are raised, but to be of any value in diagnosis the measurements must be made under standardised conditions. The plasma renin level is decreased, and fails to rise during blood-volume-reduction or sodium-depletion tests.

Secondary hyperaldosteronism. This is a feature of malignant hypertension, and is probably due to renal ischaemia. It also occurs in cirrhosis of the liver, the nephrotic syndrome, and congestive heart failure (see pp. 523 and 524). A rare renin-producing tumour of the kidney has been described as well as *Bartter's syndrome*, in which there is hyperplasia of the juxtaglomerular cells; hypokalaemic alkalosis without oedema or systemic hypertension are the main features (see p. 556).

Adrenogenital Syndrome

This syndrome is characterised by masculinisation in the female and precocious puberty in the male. Adrenal cortical hyperplasia, adenoma, or carcinoma may be the cause.

The adrenogenital syndrome is most easily recognised in the female. Acne vulgaris, deepening of the voice, hirsutism, male-pattern baldness, and a redistribution of fat to male proportions are the main features of *adrenal virilism.* Enlargement of the clitoris is characteristic.

The main androgen secreted is a dehydroepiandrosterone which has about 5 per cent of the masculinising effect of testosterone. Hence in cases of adrenal virilism the urinary output of 17-ketosteroids is very high. In cases of adrenal hyperplasia (ths most common cause) the administration of glucocorticoids (the low-dose dexamethasone test) decreases the output of ketosteroids due to an inhibiting effect on pituitary ACTH production. If the cause of the virilism is an adrenal tumour, no such suppression occurs. Likewise in those rare cases of virilism due to testosterone-producing ovarian tumours the dexamethasone test is negative. Indeed, so potent is testosterone that the 17-ketosteroid output in the urine is not raised above normal.

The adrenogenital syndrome is less easily recognised in males. In boys there is an increased rate of growth, particularly of the muscles, and an 'infantile Hercules' results. Nevertheless, the epiphyses fuse prematurely, and the individual ultimately shows stunted growth. There is a failure of testicular development.

Congenital adrenal hyperplasia also produces effects on the sex organs, but it is a separate entity and is described on page 41.

Adrenal feminisation in the male is a rare condition, and is nearly always due to a carcinoma which secretes oestrogen or a steroid (androstenedione) which is converted into oestrogen peripherally.

Adrenal Insufficiency

Acute adrenal insufficiency is generally encountered when patients who are unable to increase their corticosteroid production are exposed to sudden stress, such as trauma, haemorrhage, or severe infection. This is seen most often in patients with Addison's disease or panhypopituitarism who are on a maintenance dose of glucocorticoids, and is called an addisonian crisis. The stress may itself cause damage to the adrenals, e.g. the haemorrhage encountered in meningococcal septicaemia (Waterhouse-Friderichsen syndrome) or in diphtheria. Acute adrenal insufficiency is characterised by shock, hypotension, collapse, and sometimes fever. It superficially resembles the effects of sodium and water depletion, but the administration of sodium and water alone will not relieve it.

Chronic adrenal insufficiency (Addison's disease). Over half the cases of Addison's disease are due to an idiopathic atrophy, possibly of an autoimmune type, since anti-adrenal antibodies can be demonstrated. Tuberculosis, histoplasmosis, coccidioidomycosis, blastomycosis, sarcoidosis, leukaemia, and haemochromatosis account for the remainder.

The disease is characterised by the features of cortisol lack: weakness, anorexia, weight loss, hypotension, abdominal pain, and hypoglycaemia. The impaired renal blood flow causes a rise in the plasma urea, and the impaired power of water concentration by the tubules (see p. 552) leads to polyuria, dehydration, and thirst. Hyperkalaemia is a characteristic early finding, and hyponatraemia occurs later in the course of the disease.

The cortisol lack causes an increased pituitary secretion of ACTH (and possibly MSH). There is a typical hyperpigmentation of the skin, especially those areas exposed to trauma or sunlight. There is also mucosal pigmentation.

The urinary output of 17-ketosteroids and 17-hydroxycorticoids is low. The ACTH stimulation test evokes a poor response; indeed, it may lead to adrenal exhaustion and even precipitate an addisonian crisis. Therefore dexamethasone (1 mg) should be given to protect the patient (in this dose it does not interfere with the test).

Secondary adrenal insufficiency. A deficiency of ACTH leads to adrenal atrophy and secondary insufficiency. There is weakness and gastrointestinal symptoms. The condition resembles Addison's disease, but the plasma electrolytes and blood pressure remain normal until late in the disease. There is cutaneous pallor due to the lack of ACTH, and also evidence of hypofunction of other endocrine glands, e.g. the thyroid.

Tests of Pituitary and Adrenal Cortical Function

Many tests of adrenocortical function have been devised, but only those that are commonly available will be described.

Static tests: blood hormone levels. *Plasma levels* of many hormones, e.g. ACTH, cortisol, testosterone, aldosterone, renin, and angiotensin II, can be estimated (mainly by radioimmunoassay) in specialised laboratories.

Urinary excretion rates. The excretion rates of *17-hydroxycorticoids* and *17-ketogenic steroids* give an indication of the C21 steroid hormone production, i.e. cortisol. The *17-ketosteroids* are derived mainly from the C18 and C19 adrenal steroids. These are predominantly the adrenal androgens and, to a lesser extent, testicular androgen.

Dynamic tests. *Stimulation tests.* In the *ACTH stimulation test* the ability of the adrenal glands to respond to a test dose of ACTH is assessed by measuring either plasma hormone levels or the urinary output of 17-hydroxycorticoids or 17-ketogenic steroids.

Stimulation of the adrenal cortex by sodium depletion, blood-volume depletion, or the administration of angiotensin II is used to assess mineralocorticoid function. Hypoglycaemia induced by the administration of insulin stimulates ACTH production; this manoeuvre assesses the degree of pituitary response.

Suppression tests. Dexamethasone suppression test. A low dose of dexamethasone (e.g. 2 mg in 24 hours) normally suppresses pituitary ACTH production, and hence the adrenal cortex. The urinary output of 17-hydroxycorticoids and 17-ketogenic steroids is therefore reduced. A high dose of dexamethasone (e.g. 8 mg in 24 hours) is necessary to bring about the suppression of hyperplastic adrenal glands.

In the *aldosterone suppression test*, sodium loading or the administration of DOCA normally causes a decrease in the production of aldosterone and renin.

Metyrapone (Metopirone) test. Metyrapone inhibits adrenocortical 11-β-hydrolase. Hence it inhibits cortisol production, and the pituitary responds by increasing the output of ACTH. The adrenal cortex is in turn stimulated, and the immediate precursor of cortisol (11-deoxyhydrocortisone) is produced in increased amount. This is reflected in an increased urinary output of 17-hydroxycorticoids and 17-ketogenic steroids. The test thus assesses both pituitary and adrenal function.

ADRENAL MEDULLA

The cells of the adrenal medulla convert tyrosine into the two catecholamines adrenaline and noradrenaline. These are continuously secreted into the blood stream in small amounts; larger quantities are secreted under the influence of preganglionic cholinergic fibres or the stimulation of other hormones, such as insulin and histamine. The release of adrenaline and noradrenaline into the circulation as a response to trauma is described on page 411.

Adrenaline is synthesised almost exclusively in the adrenals. It affects both the α-receptors (which cause vasoconstriction in the skin and viscera and also mydriasis) and the β-receptors (which act on the heart as well as producing vasodilatation in the muscles and dilatation of the bronchi). Most of the body's noradrenaline is synthesised by the cells of the sympathetic ganglia. Its action is predominantly on the α-receptors.

The most important lesion of the adrenal medulla is the *phaeochromocytoma*. This tumour arises most commonly in the adrenal medulla, but can occur elsewhere in relation to other chromaffin tissues in the neck, thorax, bladder, and in other sites. Ninety-five per cent of the tumours are benign. Bilateral adrenal tumours are a feature of familial cases (p. 452). The characteristic feature of this condition is systemic hypertension, which is characteristically paroxysmal. However, intermittent hypertension is found in only about half the cases; in the remainder it is persistent. The hypertension is due to the excessive release of adrenaline and noradrenaline. If the tumour secretes adrenaline there may also be hyperglycaemia (noradrenaline does not have this effect).

The diagnosis of phaeochromocytoma is assisted by finding an increased excretion of catecholamines or their metabolites in the urine, e.g. vanillylmandelic acid or metadrenaline and normetadrenaline. If metadrenaline constitutes a considerable component, the tumour is almost certainly in the adrenal medulla or else is derived from the organ of Zückerkandl (the only extra-adrenal site where adrenaline is normally made).

THE APUD SYSTEM[1,2]

The APUD cells derive their name from the initial letters associated with their three most important properties.

1. A high content of *a*mines.
2. The capacity for amine *p*recursor *u*ptake.
3. The presence of amino acid *d*ecarboxylase.

This enzyme converts amino acids, such as 5-hydroxytryptophan and DOPA, into amines. The associated cells contain characteristic granules in their cytoplasm on electron microscopy, and are believed to be of neuroectodermal origin (derived from the neural crest, see Fig. 35.2). The APUD cells secrete polypeptides, or amines, or both of these. There is general agreement that cells of neuroectodermal origin migrate widely throughout the body, but it is technically difficult to trace their migration, because, at the time of their travelling, they are poorly differentiated. As at present conceived, the following cells are included amongst this group:[2-5]

1. *The chromaffin cell system.* These cells are characterised by granules that have an affinity for chromium salts due to their content of catecholamines. When fixed in formalin vapour, the cells exhibit fluorescence under ultraviolet light. The cells are found in the adrenal medulla and in relationship to the paravertebral sympathetic plexuses.

Figure 35.2
Argentaffin cell of the small intestine. The characteristic granules (arrow) are well shown in the cytoplasm between the nucleus (Nuc) and the basement membrane. The appearances are typical of a cell of the APUD system. × 15 000 (*Photograph by courtesy of Dr. Y. C. Bedard.*)

2. *The non-chromaffin paraganglia*, notably the carotid body, aortic body, glomus jugulare, and similar structures.

3. *The argentaffin cells.* The argentaffin cells of the intestine (Kultschitzky cells) have cytoplasmic granules containing 5-hydroxytryptamine and its precursors. When combined with formalin, these granules have the ability to reduce alkaline silver salts to metallic silver. The intestinal argentaffin cells also exhibit the chromaffin reaction, and are sometimes called the *enterochromaffin cells.* Similar cells occur in many other areas, e.g. salivary glands, bronchial mucosa, and pancreas.

4. *The argyrophil cells.* These cells also have an affinity for alkaline silver salts, but an additional reducing agent must be added before metallic silver is deposited. These cells are widely distributed in the intestine and in organs that arise by endodermal outpouching.

5. *Other neuroectodermal cells of the gastrointestinal tract.* Many other types of cells are present in the stomach and small intestine. Together with the argentaffin and argyrophil cells they are responsible for secreting a number of polypeptide hormones, including 5-hydroxytryptamine, gastrin, secretin, enteroglucagon, vasoactive intestinal peptide (VIP), and cholecystokinin.

6. *Pancreatic islet cells.* These constitute several types of cells.

7. *Thyroid C cells*, which secrete calcitonin.

8. *Melanocytes.*

9. *Hypothalamic neuroendocrine cells.*

10. *Some cells of the adenohypophysis*, notably those secreting ACTH, MSH in some species, growth hormone, and prolactin. The cells that secrete TSH, FSH, and LH are not included; these hormones are glycoproteins.

11. *The autonomic neurons.*[1] Tumours of these, e.g. neuroblastomata, secrete catecholamines.

The APUD cells associated with the gastrointestinal tract and the pancreas have attracted special attention because they secrete polypeptide hormones that exert powerful effects. Thus the beta cells of the pancreatic islets secrete insulin, and a tumour of these cells, an *insulinoma*, leads to hyperinsulinism with attacks of hypoglycaemia. It would be expected that tumours of other APUD cells would also be recognised and be associated with effects of an excess of the appropriate hormone; indeed, such has been the case. However, in many neoplasms of one type of APUD cell, the abnormal cells secrete hormones and amines that are normally produced by other members of the APUD series. Thus insulin is sometimes produced by carcinoid tumours, and Cushing's syndrome can occur as a result of inappropriate ACTH secretion by a carcinoid tumour or an oat-cell carcinoma of the lung (both of these cell types are of APUD cell origin). Furthermore, a particular syndrome may be associated with hyperplasia, adenoma (not infrequently multiple), or carcinoma of a particular APUD cell type.

It follows then that the APUD cell tumours, or *apudomas*, may be described either in terms of morphological pathology or in biological terms. Tumours that secrete the normal hormone of their presumptive cell of origin may be termed *orthoendocrine*, as opposed to the *paraendocrine* tumours, which secrete hormones or humoral agents that are characteristic of other APUD cells. Indeed, they may secrete substances such as prostaglandins, histamine, and erythropoietin that are characteristic products of non-APUD cells.

SYNDROMES ACCOMPANIED BY APUDOMAS

Hypoglycaemia

Attacks of hypoglycaemia are generally caused by adenomata of the beta cells of the pancreatic islets. Sometimes the tumours are multiple; a carcinoma is rarely responsible.

The Glucagonoma Syndrome[6,7]

The association of diabetes mellitus with necrotic, migratory erythema, angular stomatitis, glossitis, and weight loss is characteristic of this syndrome. The skin eruption is widespread, erythematous, and shows epidermal necrosis. The lesions tend to heal in the centre while they extend peripherally, thereby producing an annular or figurate pattern. There is usually an adenoma of the alpha cells of the pancreatic islets.

The Zollinger-Ellison Syndrome

The outstanding feature is intractable, recurrent peptic ulceration; the duodenum is often involved, and sometimes multiple ulcers are present in the jejunum. There is marked gastric hypersection, which may lead to diarrhoea. This follows flooding of the intestine by excessive gastric secretion which tends to neutralise the alkalinity of the pancreatic secretion, so that steatorrhoea may also occur. The syndrome was originally described in association with a non-beta cell islet tumour of the pancreas, which is called a *gastrinoma*.[8] In more than 50 per cent of cases the tumour is malignant. The syndrome is due to an oversecretion of gastrin, and has also been described in association with hyperplasia of the G cells of the pyloric antrum, and even in parathyroid adenoma.

The Verner-Morrison Syndrome (Pancreatic Cholera)[9,10]

This is also known as the WDHA syndrome, since it is characterised by profuse *w*atery *d*iarrhoea, *h*ypokalaemia, and *a*chlorhydria (or hypochlorhydria). A non-beta islet-cell tumour is the usual cause, but the syndrome has been described in oat-cell carcinoma of the lung and neuroblastoma. Excessive secretion of vasoactive intestinal peptide (VIP) appears to be the mechanism of production of this syndrome.

Cushing's Syndrome (Ectopic ACTH Syndrome)

The onset of symptoms is usually acute. Hypokalaemic alkalosis, diabetes mellitus, and hyperpigmentation of the skin are prominent. Muscle wasting with weakness may be severe. The usual cause is an oat-cell carcinoma of the lung, but the syndrome can also be seen in association with bronchial carcinoid tumour, carcinoid tumour of the thymus, pancreatic islet-cell tumour, medullary carcinoma of the thyroid, phaeochromocytoma, and ovarian carcinoma.

The Carcinoid Syndrome

Most carcinoid tumours are derived from the enterochromaffin cells, and those arising in the midgut produce 5-hydroxytryptamine and kallikrein. If the tumour is small, as with the common carcinoid tumour of the appendix, or confined to the area of portal-venous drainage, no systemic symptoms are evident, because the tumour secretes only a little hormone in the one instance or the hormone is inactivated during its passage through the liver in the other instance. However, if the tumour has metastasised to the liver or has arisen outside the portal tract, e.g. carcinoid tumour of the thyroid as part of the medullary carcinoma syndrome or carcinoid tumour of the ovary arising in a teratoma, the appropriate hormones escape into the systemic circulation. The carcinoid syndrome may then develop: attacks of facial flushing, persistent telangiectasia, diarrhoea, asthmatic attacks, and thickening of the endocardium of the right side of the heart. This last tends to produce tricuspid regurgitation and pulmonary stenosis (see also pp. 332–333).

Carcinoid tumours of the foregut region (the stomach and the lung) tend to produce 5-hydroxytryptamine and histamine; the syndrome associated with them is often severe. By contrast, carcinoid tumours derived from the hindgut are usually functionless.

The Multiple Endocrine Adenopathy Syndromes

Although hyperplasia or neoplasia of an endocrine gland can occur as an isolated event, it is not uncommon for several endocrine tissues to be affected at the same time. Two syndromes, both familial (autosomal dominant), are recognised.[5]

The multiple endocrine adenopathy syndrome type I (Wermer's syndrome.) The parathyroid glands are most commonly involved in this syndrome, and there are signs of hyperparathyroidism in 90 per cent of cases; chief-cell hyperplasia is the usual lesion. Islet-cell tumours occur in 80 per cent of cases; they exhibit a typical ribbon pattern. The Zollinger-Ellison syndrome, hyperinsulinism, or the Verner-Morrison syndrome may be the main feature. The adenohypophysis is included in 65 per cent of cases, and adrenal hyperplasia and carcinoid tumours are not uncommon.

The multiple endocrine adenopathy syndrome type II (Sipple's syndrome). The main features are hyperparathyroidism, medullary carcinoma of the thyroid gland, and phaeochromocytoma. Other lesions that may be present include neurofibromatosis, megacolon, and subcutaneous and submucous fibromata. The occurrence of this syndrome lends strong support for the concept that the APUD cells and nerve tissue have a common origin.

The occurrence of hyperparathyroidism in both syndromes is surprising, since the parathyroid gland does not appear to be a member of the APUD system.[1] It may be that the parathyroid gland arises from an area of neuroectoderm. Another possible explanation is that the parathyroid overactivity is secondary to the secretion of calcitonin in cases of medullary carcinoma of the thyroid (type II syndrome). In the type I syndrome it may be that the various other hormones secreted stimulate the secretion of calcitonin, which once again leads to the compensatory outpouring of parathyroid hormone.[5]

Conclusion

The two concepts of the APUD cell and the neuroendocrine cell appear to be merging. The concept of the APUD cell was initially a grouping of normal and neoplastic cells with shared biochemical properties, especially the capacity for amine-precursor uptake and decarboxylation. The similarity of these properties to those possessed by cells derived from the neural crest led to the hypothesis that APUD cells had a neural origin. This has been demonstrated by transplantation experiments in respect of some cells, e.g. the thyroid C cells, the carotid-body cells, and the cells of the adenohypophysis.[1] A neural origin is also supported by data that suggest a neuron-like mechanism for excitation-secretion coupling in APUD cells.[1]

THE THYROID GLAND

The thyroid gland was the first endocrine organ to evolve in the vertebrates; it is derived from an invagination of the pharyngeal epithelium. It commences activity by the tenth week of gestation under the influence of fetal TSH. The role of the human chorionic thyrotrophin (HCT) formed by the placenta is unknown.

Iodides are selectively trapped by the thyroid gland; iodide is also excreted in the urine, the kidney thereby competing passively with the thyroid. In the thyroid iodide is pumped into the follicles by an active mechanism that can be inhibited by perchlorate and thiocyanate ions. In the follicles the iodide is oxidised under the influence of iodide peroxidase, being converted to a form that is capable of iodinating tyrosine to monoiodotyrosine (MIT) and diiodotyrosine (DIT). The tyrosine is in fact present as a tyrosyl residue in the large globulin molecule called thyroglobulin. MIT and DIT undergo oxidative condensation, and by a coupling reaction yield *3,5,3'-triiodo-L-thyronine (T3)* and *L-thyroxine (T4)*. These thyroid hormones are retained in the gland bound to thyroglobulin. The hormones T3 and T4 are released from the colloid by a process of pinocytosis. The thyroglobulin in pinocytotic vesicles is hydrolysed by lysosomal enzymes so that free hormone is released by the thyroid gland into the blood stream. During this process any inactive MIT or DIT that is formed is deiodinated by the action of the enzyme iodotyrosine dehalogenase. The iodine released is recycled within the thyroid gland.

Control of thyroid hormone secretion. The adenohypophysis secretes thyroid-stimulating hormone (TSH) under the influence of thyrotrophin-releasing hormone (TRH) formed in the hypothalamus. A high blood level of thyroid hormone inhibits TSH release, whereas a low level stimulates it. There is thus a negative feedback mechanism which acts mainly on the pituitary and possibly also on the hypothalamus.

Transport of thyroid hormones. T4 is avidly bound to a thyroxine-binding globulin (TBG); this protein is the primary carrier of T4, and is normally about one-third saturated. T4 is also bound, but less firmly, to thyroxine-binding prealbumin (TBPA) and also to albumin. The amount of free T4 in the blood is less that 0·05 per cent of the total.

T3 is not bound to TBPA, and it binds less firmly than T4 to TBG. There is therefore eight to ten times more free T3 in the blood than free T4. Moreover, in the non-thyroid cells of the body about 30 per cent of T4 is broken down to T3. T3 is, in many respects, about three times as potent as T4. Therefore the major functional thyroid hormone is T3.

Action of thyroid hormone. Despite much research the precise mode of action of thyroid hormone is unknown. It has a characteristic effect on amphibian metamorphosis, for without it tadpoles do not develop legs nor do they become frogs. In the human thyroid hormone is necessary for the normal development of the body, particularly the central nervous system. It reduces the tissues' sensitivity to insulin, therefore hyperthyroidism aggravates diabetes mellitus. At a cellular level thyroid hormone stimulates metabolism so that oxygen consumption and heat production are increased.

At one time it was believed that this was achieved by uncoupling oxidative phosphorylation, so that heat could be produced without useful energy conservation or ATP synthesis. This hypothesis has not been confirmed. Since 20 to 45 per cent of the total energy produced in the cell is utilised to maintain the sodium pump (p. 22), it has been suggested that overactivity of this pumping mechanism could explain the increased metabolic rate of cells induced by the action of thyroid hormone. This too remains a hypothesis. However, much has been learned by comparing the normal individual, who is described as *euthyroid*, with those who suffer from excessive or deficient thyroid secretion (*hyperthyroid* and *hypothyroid* respectively).

DISEASES OF THE THYROID GLAND

Hyperthyroidism

In hyperthyroidism, also called thyrotoxicosis, there is a raised metabolic rate. The common causes are *Graves's disease* and *toxic nodular goitre*, which are described later. Occasionally hyperthyroidism is encountered in the course of hydatidiform mole and choriocarcinoma, when it is due to chorionic TSH-like substance (p. 340). Hyperthyroidism due to excessive pituitary secretion is extremely rare.

Hypothyroidism

The effects in the child differ from those in the adult.

Cretinism. An insufficiency of thyroid hormone in the infant, due to a failure of development of the thyroid gland, leads to cretinism: the child has a bloated face, protruding tongue, vacant expression, and becomes mentally defective. The milestones of development are reached late, and there is a retardation of growth which results in dwarfism.

Myxoedema. This condition, which is the manifestation of hypothyroidism in the adult, is usually idiopathic. In fact there is probably an autoimmune basis, the thyroid atrophy often following burnt-out Hashimoto's disease. The gland shows atrophy of the epithelial elements and a lymphocytic infiltrate. Another cause of thyroid atrophy leading to myxoedema is damage produced by the radioactive-iodine therapy of hyperthyroidism. Hypothalamic lesions and pituitary hypofunction can also lead to thyroid atrophy and myxoedema. Myxoedema can also follow a too-radical thyroidectomy for hyperthyroidism.

In myxoedema there is a depression of mental and physical activity, and the patient exhibits a characteristic bloated appearance which is produced by the deposition of glucosaminoglycan in the dermis. Intolerance to the cold is typical, and in untreated cases of myxoedema the lethargic state may proceed to coma. There is also often terminal heart failure and hypothermia.

HYPERPLASIA OF THE THYROID GLAND

Simple Non-Toxic Goitre

Any enlargement of the thyroid gland is called a goitre. Amongst the causes of the simple, non-toxic variety are:

(*a*) *Stress.* This causes a minor degree of thyroid enlargement; it is seen during puberty and pregnancy. Indeed, it is reported that in ancient Egypt the rupture of a thread tied around the neck of a bride was used as an indication of pregnancy.

(*b*) *Iodine deficiency.* This is a much more potent cause of goitre, the reason being that the thyroid, rendered incapable of manufacturing its hormone, cannot check the secretion of TSH that stimulates it to activity. Before iodine was added to table salt, goitres were common in many parts of the world, e.g. the Great Lakes area of North America, the Andes, the Himalayas, and in the county of Derbyshire in England. In these areas the soil carries insufficient iodine for food-stuffs to contain even the minute quantities of the element that are required for the body's metabolism. Repeated phases of hyperplasia followed by involution lead to the formation of large goitres containing many nodular, colloid-filled areas, the so-called nodular colloid goitre. In the larger goitres there may be areas of necrosis, haemorrhage, and later dystrophic calcification.

(*c*) *Conditions that inhibit the secretion of thyroid hormone.* These cause a similar type of goitre. Thus perchlorate and thiocyanate ions inhibit iodine transport. Thiourea has a more complex action, and appears to block the coupling of the iodotyrosines to form T3 and T4. It also inhibits the oxidation and organic binding of iodide.

Iodides, or iodine itself in large doses, can also block organic binding, but usually only for a short while; there is also inhibition of proteolysis and hormone release. These actions are of value in the temporary alleviation of thyrotoxicosis, and have been used in the pre-operative treatment of this condition. In some individuals, particularly children, this iodine effect can be prolonged, so that excessive iodine administration can lead to hypothyroidism and goitre formation. Other goitrogenic agents have been identified, for example in cabbages, and these may contribute to goitre formation under particular circumstances.

(*d*) *Inherited enzyme defects.* An uncommon cause of goitre is an inherited defect or absence of one of the enzymes involved in the various stages of iodine uptake and thyroid-hormone production. These 'dyshormogenetic goitres' are generally manifest in children, and are associated with hypothyroidism, whereas in the common type of simple nodular goitre the patient is euthyroid.

Graves's Disease (Primary Thyrotoxicosis)

This disease is characterised by a diffuse, uniform enlargement of the thyroid gland due to a marked hyperplasia of its epithelial elements with a patchy lymphocytic infiltrate amid the acini (Fig. 35.4 as compared with Fig. 35.3, a normal thyroid). There is a raised metabolic rate that manifests itself as a persistent increase in the heart rate and an intolerance to heat.

The patient is typically jumpy and nervous. The hands are warm and moist; they are seldom at rest, and exhibit a fine tremor when the fingers are outstretched. Muscular weakness is a common symptom, and can be severe (*thyrotoxic myopathy*). The eyes have a characteristic appearance: the eyelids are retracted, giving the patient a staring expression, while in severe cases the globe is actually pushed forward. If these changes are severe, the eye muscles can become paralysed and sight can be lost. This is called *malignant exophthalmos*. The skin overlying the tibia may show a focal accumulation of glucosaminoglycan (mucopolysaccharide), a condition called *pretibial myxoedema*.

A dangerous complication is the *thyrotoxic crisis* (*thyroid storm*), in which there is a sudden exacerbation of the symptoms with hyperkinesis, tachycardia, hyperpyrexia, vomiting, and shock. Dehydration and coma precede death, which is common even with therapy. A crisis may occur spontaneously, or else follow an infection, trauma, or surgery.

Histologically there are accumulations of lymphocytes, called lymphorrhages, in the muscles; in the ocular muscles this lymphoid component contributes to the exophthalmos which is due primarily to the marked oedema consequent on the

Figure 35.3
Normal thyroid gland. The gland consists of follicles of varying size, lined by a simple flattened or cuboidal epithelium, and filled with homogeneous colloid. The colloid contains thyroglobulin. × 175.

Figure 35.4
Graves's disease. The thyroid gland is hyperplastic. The epithelium is columnar, and in some small follicles where colloid is deficient, the epithelium encroaches on the acinar spaces. In the large follicles the colloid shows vacuolation where it abuts on the epithelium. × 175.

accumulation of glucosaminoglycan. Not only are there lymphoid accumulations in the muscles and thyroid gland, but there is also enlargement of the lymph nodes, thymus, and spleen. Indeed, the cause of Graves's disease, while still obscure, appears to have an autoimmune element.

The actual stimulus to thyroid hyperplasia is an agent present in the blood. The first thyroid stimulating factor to be isolated differs from TSH in having a much longer stimulating effect on the gland. It is called *LATS (long-acting thyroid stimulator)*, and is an autoantibody; how it acts and the nature of the corresponding antigen are still not clear. Since it is quite often absent in cases of primary thyrotoxicosis and is in highest concentration in cases where there is pretibial myxoedema, LATS is unlikely to be the only factor in the pathogenesis of the disease. A more likely contender for the role is a second IgG which has more recently been discovered. This is called *human thyroid stimulating immunoglobulin (HTSI)*, is present in the serum of most, and possibly all patients with primary thyrotoxicosis, and appears to displace TSH from its binding site on the human thyroid cell membrane. This suggests that HTSI is capable of binding to the thyrotrophin receptor sites and that the receptor is itself the antigen.[11]

Toxic Nodular Goitre (Secondary Thyrotoxicosis)

This occurs as a secondary phenomenon in a patient who is already suffering from a goitre from some other cause, such as iodine deficiency. The administration of iodine may precipitate the condition. The disease is less severe than Graves's disease, and there are no ocular manifestations. The condition tends to occur in an older age group than that affected by Graves's disease, and the hypermetabolic state is particularly liable to affect the heart. Atrial fibrillation and heart failure occurring in a patient who has no pre-existing cardiac lesion should always arouse the suspicion of thyrotoxicosis.

It is noteworthy that all acquired thyroid disease affects women much more often than men. This applies to Hashimoto's disease, primary myxoedema, simple nodular goitre, Graves's disease, and also carcinoma.

Tests of Thyroid Function

Many tests are available to assess thyroid function; these will be considered under five headings:

Direct tests of thyroid function. *The thyroid radioactive iodine uptake (RAIU).* A dose of ^{131}I is administered, and its accumulation in the thyroid is measured. An increased uptake is found in thyrotoxicosis.

Thyroid hormone levels in the blood. The serum protein-bound iodine (PBI) concentration is commonly used as a method of estimating serum T4, since in the normal state all the iodine bound to protein is present in thyroxine. The PBI is raised in thyrotoxicosis and lowered in hypothyroidism, but unfortunately a raised level follows the administration of iodine-containing dyes that are used in radiology; this state may persist for life. Furthermore, abnormal iodoproteins may be produced in some conditions, e.g. Hashimoto's disease, in which case a raised PBI does not indicate thyrotoxicosis.

More precise estimates of thyroid hormone have been introduced. The serum T4 concentration, known as T4 (D), can be measured by assessing the ability of T4 extracted from the patient's serum to *displace* labelled T4 from a protein mixture containing TBG. The serum T3 concentration can be measured by radioimmunoassay, and is abbreviated T3 (RIA). Both these measurements include the bound hormone. Measurements of free hormone (FT3 and FT4) can be made, but the techniques are difficult and not generally available. Measurements of bound hormone are complicated by variations in the concentrations of the carrier protein. In particular, the TBG concentration is affected by many factors; thus it is increased in pregnancy, liver disease, and in women on oral contraceptives. Since the protein readily binds thyroid hormone, an increase in the TBG will give an increased PBI and T4 (D). These elevated levels are misleading, since the amount of free hormone remains normal when the patient is euthyroid.

The resin-T3 uptake (RT3U) is a useful, simple test which indirectly measures free hormone. The resin used binds T3 and T4. The patient's serum mixed with resin is incubated with labelled T3. The uptake of the labelled hormone by the resin is in competition with the uptake of labelled hormone by the patient's TBG. Hence, if the TBG is fully saturated, as in thyrotoxicosis, the resin uptake will be high. Conversely, when unsaturated binding sites of TBG are available, as in myxoedema, pregnancy, or oestrogen therapy, the resin T3 uptake is low. The normal range is 25 to 35 per cent. The results of the resin uptake can be expressed as a quotient of the RT3U of the patient to that obtained in a normal control specimen (RT3U ratio). The product of this ratio and T4 (D) is called the T4-RT3 index, and provides an index of the free T4. This is a useful figure, since alterations in TBG produce reciprocal alterations in the RT3U and the T4 (D). Hence the index remains normal. Alterations in T4 secretion produce changes of both RT3U and T4 (D) which are in the same direction; hence the index changes, and provides a useful measure of thyroid function.

Metabolic measurements. Measurements of the basal metabolic rate (BMR) were widely used as a test of thyroid function, but they are open to many errors and in practice detect only gross abnormalities.

Tests of homeostatic control. TSH can be measured by radioimmunoassay methods. The level is high in untreated myxoedema of thyroid origin, but low in the hypothyroidism of hypothalamic or pituitary origin.

The THS stimulation test measures the ability of the thyroid to respond to the hormone. The response is measured by the radioactive iodine uptake of the gland and the serum T4 (D). The test distinguishes between hypothyroidism of pituitary origin (when the gland responds to stimulation) and that of primary thyroid origin.

The thyrotrophin-releasing hormone (TRH) stimulation test is performed by estimating the serum TSH levels following a dose of TRH. The test is greatly influenced by the level of thyroid hormone in the blood, since this hormone inhibits the response of the pituitary to TRH stimulation. Thus in hypothyroidism of thyroid origin the response is brisk, while in thyrotoxicosis the pituitary does not respond to TRH stimulation.

The Werner suppression test is of value in diagnosing thyrotoxicosis. If triiodothyronine is administered to a normal subject, there is suppression of pituitary TSH production. Hence the thyroid itself becomes underactive, and the radioactive iodine uptake falls. In hyperthyroidism the thyroid function cannot be suppressed by the administration of T3, and the radioactive uptake remains at its previous level. This indicates that the thyroid is either functioning autonomously or that it is under the influence of an abnormal stimulator.

Other tests. The identification of *antithyroid antibodies* is mentioned in Chapter 16.

Radioactive scanning is a useful aid in the diagnosis of nodules in the thyroid; either radioactive iodine or technetium may be used. Nodules that take up radioactivity avidly are suggestive as causes of thyrotoxicosis. 'Cold' nodules, on the other hand, are likely to be tumours, cysts, or areas of degeneration.

GENERAL READING

EZRIN, C., GODDEN, J. O., VOLPÉ, R. & WILSON, R. (1973) *Systematic Endocrinology*, 509 pp. Hagerstown: Harper and Row.

REFERENCES

1. TISCHLER, A. S. *et al.* (1977) Neuroendocrine neoplasms and their cells of origin. *New England Journal of Medicine*, **296**, 919.
2. PEARSE, A. G. E. (1974) The APUD cell concept and its implications in pathology. *Pathology Annual*, **9**, 27.
3. WEICHERT, R. F. (1970) The neural ectodermal origin of the peptide-secreting endocrine glands. *American Journal of Medicine*, **49**, 232.
4. BOLANDE, R. P. (1974) The neurocristopathies. *Human Pathology*, **5**, 409.
5. WELBOURN, R. B. (1977) Current status of the apudomas. *Annals of Surgery*, **185**, 1.
6. SWEET, R. D. (1974) A dermatosis specifically associated with a tumour of pancreatic alpha cells. *British Journal of Dermatology*, **90**, 301.
7. MALLINSON, C. N. *et al.* (1974) A glucagonoma syndrome. *Lancet*, **2**, 1.
8. WALSH, J. H. & GROSSMAN, M. I. (1975) Gastrin. *New England Journal of Medicine*, **292**, 1324 and 1377.
9. SOERGEL, K. H. (1975) Hormonally mediated diarrhoea. *New England Journal of Medicine*, **292**, 970.
10. Leading Article (1975) VIP and watery diarrhoea. *British Medical Journal*, **4**, 3.
11. Leading Article (1975) Hyperthyroidism and Graves's disease. *British Medical Journal*, **2**, 457.

Chapter 36. Calcium Metabolism and Heterotopic Calcification

Introduction

In addition to providing rigidity to the bones, calcium ions play an important role in many physiological functions. The permeability of cell membranes is affected by the calcium-ion concentration of the extracellular fluids: elevation of the calcium concentration reduces permeability. The calcium ion is important in regulating the electrical properties of membranes; thus, hypocalcaemia increases excitability (see tetany). Calcium plays an essential role in muscle contraction. It is involved in the release of preformed hormones from the endocrine glands, as well as playing a part in the formation of the cyclic AMP that is generated in target cells when acted upon by the relevant non-steroid hormones. Finally it will be recalled that calcium is important in many steps of blood clotting as well as in the activation of complement.

The total body content of calcium is about 1 kilogram. The average North-American diet involves an intake of 600 to 1000 mg, and a rather similar quantity (about 600 mg) enters the gastrointestinal tract in the various digestive secretions. In all, about 800 mg of calcium is absorbed per day, and this involves a net gain of about 200 mg. This is approximately equal to the urinary loss, so that the individual is in calcium balance. Calcium is absorbed in the duodenum by an active transport mechanism, but the greatest amount is absorbed in the remainder of the small intestine. Its absorption is reduced in vitamin-D deficiency, uraemia, and in the malabsorption syndrome. The presence of phytic acid[1] and an excess of unabsorbed fatty acids inhibit absorption.

The concentration of calcium in the glomerular filtrate is equal to that of the plasma diffusible calcium (1·4 mmol per litre, or 5·5 mg per dl). Approximately 98 per cent of this is reabsorbed in much the same manner as sodium. Metabolic acidosis decreases the tubular absorption of calcium, whereas parathyroid hormone increases it. In chronic renal failure the reduced volume of glomerular filtrate leads to a reduced excretion of calcium.

Role of Bone

Since bone constitutes the main repository for calcium, it is not surprising that it plays a vital part in calcium metabolism and that upsets in calcium balance can cause severe bone disease.

The osteoid tissue of bone is manufactured by osteoblasts, and after a 5 to 10-day period of extracellular maturation this osteoid undergoes mineralisation with the deposition of calcium salts in the form of hydroxyapatite. Bone salts are deposited first in the region of the gap between tropocollagen molecules; their composition is not fixed since ions other than calcium and phosphate are involved in their formation, e.g. magnesium, sodium, potassium, and fluoride. Initial mineralisation of bone is a rapid process, about 70 per cent of the total salts being deposited within a few hours. The remaining 30 per cent are deposited slowly over a period of several weeks. The mechanism of normal mineralisation of osteoid is not well understood. If the calcium-phosphate ion product of extracellular fluids is reduced, osteoid calcification does not take place normally and large amounts of osteoid remain unmineralised. This is the defect found in rickets and osteomalacia. As bone matures, the osteoblasts become trapped within it and form osteocytes. These cells are not inactive, and are in communication with each other by means of delicate processes that lie in the canaliculi. The osteocytes are bathed in a fluid which is in equilibrium with the bone, but is separated from the general extracellular tissue fluids. The osteocytes play an important, though ill-defined, role in bone homeostasis: thus if they die the bone crumbles and is removed. There is considerable evidence that osteocytes are able to demineralise the bone adjacent to them and also remove its osteoid matrix. This process is called *osteolysis*, and is probably of great importance in the hour-to-hour regulation of the plasma calcium level. Having mobilised calcium by the process of osteolysis, the same cell can subsequently lay down more bone. It is generally agreed that the multinucleate osteoclast is capable of mobilising calcium from bone by removing both the salts and the protein matrix. This destructive osteoclastic activity is probably of great importance in the general remodelling of bone that is continually taking place.

It is evident that the processes of osteolysis and osteoclastic resorption both involve the simultaneous removal of bone salts and bone matrix. The bone salts presumably enter the fluid surrounding the osteocytes and osteoclasts, but are not immediately able to diffuse into the plasma. Nevertheless, diffusion between this pericellular fluid and that of the extravascular extracellular space ultimately occurs, and the interchange of salts between bone and plasma is of vital importance in the regulation of plasma calcium levels. The mechanism involved is not well understood, but is governed by three factors: parathyroid hormone, vitamin D, and calcitonin. The actions of these substances is considered after a review of the normal plasma calcium levels.

Plasma Calcium

The normal plasma calcium is remarkably constant and is about 2·4 mmol per litre (9·5 mg per dl). It exists in three forms:

1. *Ionised calcium.* This component is diffusible and constitutes about 1·1 mmol per litre (4·5 mg per dl). It is the most important fraction, and it is maintained at a constant level by the regulatory mechanisms to be described.

2. *Nonionised, diffusible calcium.* This is the smallest fraction (0·25 mmol per litre, or 1 mg per dl), and is present for the most part as citrate.

3. *Protein-bound calcium.* This component (1 mmol per

litre, or 4 mg per dl) is bound mostly to albumin and is therefore nondiffusible.

It is the total plasma calcium that is usually measured in clinical practice, and in the absence of a marked alteration of plasma proteins, it is a good guide to the level to the ionised fraction. The normal concentration lies between 2·3 and 2·6 mmol per litre (9·2 and 10·4 mg per dl), the precise figures varying from one laboratory to another. The plasma calcium remains remarkably constant in health due to the efficiency of the regulating mechanisms. Even drastic attempts to alter the plasma calcium level fail. Presumably the vast area (estimated at about 100 acres) of bone salts is in equilibrium with tissue-fluid calcium and indirectly with the plasma calcium. As noted previously, the precise relationship of this equilibrium is ill defined.

CALCIUM BALANCE

In spite of a varying diet, the amount of calcium absorbed from the intestine, the amount excreted in the urine, and the amount deposited or withdrawn from bone are so regulated that the level of plasma ionised calcium remains constant. The actions of parathyroid hormone, vitamin D, and calcitonin are vitally concerned in this homeostatic mechanism.

Parathyroid Hormone

There is a continuous secretion of hormone from the parathyroid glands, but the rate of secretion is influenced by the plasma ionic calcium level: a fall in calcium level stimulates parathyroid secretion, and a rise in calcium level inhibits it. The parathyroid hormone is a polypeptide containing 84 amino-acid residues; it acts on its target organs by activating cyclic AMP. Its major targets are bone, kidney, and intestine.

The effects of parathyroid hormone on bone. Parathyroid hormone promotes the resorption of bone by osteoclasts as well as promoting osteolysis by osteocytes. Thus the bone minerals are mobilised, and osteoid is removed. Osteoclasts appear to be directly stimulated so that their number increases. This has been shown experimentally by transplanting parathyroid tissue heterotopically into bone, where it causes localised osteoclastic proliferation and bone destruction. Likewise, in hyperparathyroidism osteoclastic masses are characteristic (see later). The initial action of parathyroid hormone on osteoblasts is to inhibit their action, but there is evidence that it can later stimulate them to produce bone. Hence the action of parathyroid hormone on bone is somewhat complex, although the over-all picture is that of resorption.

Effects of parathyroid hormone on kidney. A characteristic effect of the hormone is to increase phosphate excretion. The result of this is that the plasma phosphate decreases in spite of the continued release of phosphate from the bone. The hormone, on the other hand, increases calcium reabsorption from the kidney, and this, together with the calcium released from the skeleton, results in a rise of plasma calcium. The increased level of ionised calcium leads to an increased glomerular load of calcium; the result is an increased quantity of calcium passed in the urine (*hypercalciuria*). Thus hyperparathyroidism is characterised by hypercalcaemia and an over-all calcium loss from the body. Another important action of parathyroid hormone on the kidney is related to its

effect on the synthesis of 1,25-dihydroxycholecalciferol: it is one of the regulators of the synthesis of this powerful form of vitamin D. Its presence increases the formation of the substance.

Effects of parathyroid hormone on intestine. The hormone tends to increase the absorption of calcium from the intestine and augment the activity of vitamin D.

Parathyroid hormone thus appears to be the major factor regulating the level of plasma ionised calcium. By its action it mobilises calcium from the bone and retards its excretion by the kidney. The regulation of parathyroid hormone secretion is determined by the plasma ionic calcium level by a simple feed-back mechanism.

Vitamin D[2-4]

Various forms of vitamin D exist. The first apparently pure compound was called D1, but was in fact a mixture. The radiation of ergosterol produces an active substance called vitamin D2, or ergocalciferol, and this is present in a diet containing artificially fortified foods. Natural vitamin D is produced in the skin by the ultraviolet radiation of 7-dehydrocholesterol, and is called D3, or cholecalciferol. This substance has been regarded as a hormone by some authorities, and indeed the effects of vitamin D on the body have features in common with those of the hormone of the parathyroids. Both vitamins D2 and D3 are hydroxylated in the liver to 25-hydroxy compounds (25-hydroxycholecalciferol, 25-HCC, or 25-OHD_3 in the case of vitamin D3) and these are the forms in which they circulate in the blood, being carried by a specific binding protein. 25-HCC is further hydroxylated to 1,25-dihydroxycholecalciferol (1,25-DHCC or $1,25\text{-}(OH)_2D_3$) in the kidney, and this is currently believed to be the final active metabolite. This final hydroxylation is promoted by a low blood calcium or phosphate level, parathyroid hormone, prolactin, and possibly growth hormone.[5]

The main action of vitamin D is to aid the absorption of calcium from the gut. There are several suggestions as to how this is mediated. It may be that the vitamin stimulates an active transport mechanism or that it promotes the formation of a calcium-binding protein in the intestinal wall. There is considerable confusion regarding the action of vitamin D on bone. In physiological concentrations vitamin D probably has no direct effect on bone, but in pharmacological doses it exhibits a parathyroid-hormone-like action. There is increased calcium mobilisation from bone, a rise in plasma-calcium level, and hypercalciuria. This action of vitamin D is utilised in the treatment of hypoparathyroidism.

A deficiency of vitamin D results in an impaired absorption of calcium from the intestine and consequent hypocalcaemia. There is a diminution, or even a complete cessation, of calcification; in the growing child calcification of the epiphyseal cartilage does not occur at the growing ends of the bones. The cartilage therefore does not die and instead continues to proliferate, so that the epiphyses undergo enlargement with greatly delayed ossification. The result is *rickets*. In the normal adult, bone is being continuously removed by osteoclastic activity, and is replaced by osteoid which promptly calcifies to form bone. If this calcification fails, the bones gradually become replaced by osteoid, which forms characteristically wide seams, and the result is *osteomalacia*.

Although parathyroid hormone and vitamin D both play important roles in maintaining calcium homeostasis, the action of vitamin D is the more vital. Patients with hypoparathyroidism can be maintained on vitamin-D therapy and additional calcium. On the other hand, the absence of vitamin D leads to severe skeletal disease, and no substitute for the vitamin will prevent it.

An analogue of 1,25-hydroxyvitamin D, or 1,25-$(OH)_2D_3$, called 1α-hydroxyvitamin D, or 1αOHD$_3$, has been produced. It is converted to 1α25$(OH)_2D_3$ in the liver, but since it possesses a 1α-hydroxyl group, the need for renal hydroxylation is bypassed. It could therefore be of use in renal osteodystrophy and possibly in hypoparathyroidism, where there is impaired production of 1,25-hydroxyvitamin D.[6]

Calcitonin

This hormone is a polypeptide containing 32 amino-acid residues and has the effect of lowering the plasma calcium level. It is secreted by cells of the ultimobranchial body, which is itself derived from the last branchial pouch. The calcitonin-secreting cells, however, are not of endodermal origin, but are derived from the neural crest and form part of the APUD system of cells (see p. 451). In some species the ultimobranchial cells form a separate body, but in mammals they are incorporated into the thyroid gland. In the human they exist as the parafollicular, or C, cells which lie on the basement membrane of the thyroid acini and are separated from the colloid by the follicular cells. They contain characteristic granules on electron microscopy.

The existence of calcitonin was indicated by experiments in which the perfusion of the thyroid-parathyroid region with a high-calcium-containing fluid produced a more rapid reduction in plasma calcium than did total parathyroidectomy. Hence, the effects could not have been due to a reduction of parathyroid hormone secretion, but could be attributed to a new calcium-lowering hormone.

The action of calcitonin is on the bone: it causes a reduction of bone resorption by inhibiting osteoclastic activity. Since in young animals there is active osteoclastic activity owing to extensive bone remodelling, the effects of calcitonin are more marked in the young than in the older animal. This is in contradistinction to the effect of parathyroid hormone. The effect of calcitonin administration is to lower the plasma-calcium level. The precise role of this hormone in calcium homeostasis has not yet been delineated, but it could clearly complement parathyroid hormone, since the stimulus for its secretion is hypercalcaemia. Calcitonin has been used with some success in the treatment of hypercalcaemia and in diseases which are characterised by excessive bone resorption, e.g. Paget's disease.[7]

Medullary carcinoma of the thyroid is a tumour of the C cells. It contains large quantities of calcitonin, but produces no outstanding change in plasma-calcium levels. Indeed, no effects of excess calcitonin secretion have so far been recorded in any tumours of the APUD series.

DISORDERS OF CALCIUM METABOLISM

Disorders of calcium metabolism form a complex group of topics, and will be described under four headings: hypocalcaemia, hypercalcaemia, hypoparathyroidism, and hyperparathyroidism. Some interrelationships between these conditions are depicted in Figure 36.1.

Figure 36.1
Diagrammatic representation of the important effects of disturbed calcium metabolism. The effects of parathyroid hormone and dietary calcium intake on vitamin D are not shown (see pp. 458 and 555).

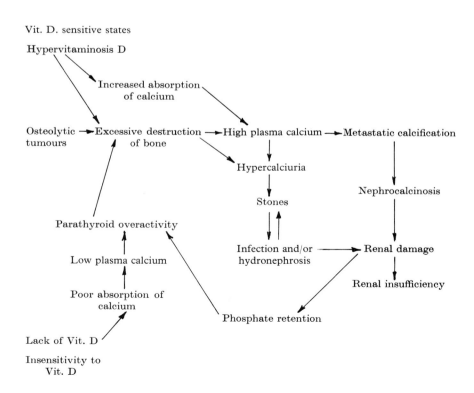

HYPOCALCAEMIA

Causes

The following are important causes of hypocalcaemia.

In association with hypoalbuminaemia. A low plasma calcium is found in hypoalbuminaemia, for example that found in liver failure and the nephrotic syndrome. Since the ionised, diffusible calcium level is normal, tetany does not occur.

Hypoparathyroidism. This is described on page 461.

Renal failure. The mechanism of this is described on page 555. It is in part due to the raised level of plasma phosphate which induces a reciprocal lowering of the plasma calcium; sometimes the calcium salts precipitate out in the tissues (metastatic calcification). Another important factor is deficient formation of 1,25-hydroxyvitamin D with a consequent impairment in the intestinal absorption of calcium.

Vitamin-D deficiency. This may occur as a result of dietary deficiency, the malabsorption syndrome, or the administration of anticonvulsant drugs.

Widespread osteoplastic metastases. These may utilise so much calcium that hypocalcaemia results. The usual primary source of the tumour is the prostate.

Infantile hypocalcaemia. Neonatal tetany is well recognised and is due to functional immaturity of the parathyroid glands during the first 2 days of life. Prematurity, twin birth, birth by caesarian section, and diabetes mellitus in the mother are other contributing factors. Maternal hyperparathyroidism has been known to be associated with neonatal tetany.

Tetany with hypocalcaemia can occur in the first or second weeks of life, and has been attributed to the high intake of phosphate provided by cow's milk and poorly tolerated because of the reduced glomerular filtration rate at this age.

The tetany of vitamin-D deficiency may be seen at the age of 4 months, but it usually manifests itself from the age of 6 to 18 months.

Acute pancreatitis. Hypocalcaemia in this condition can be attributed partly to the deposition of calcium salts in the foci of fat necrosis (dystrophic calcification), and partly to the release of glucagon from the damaged pancreas. This stimulates the release of calcitonin from the thyroid; experimentally the hypocalcaemia of pancreatitis can be prevented by previous thyroidectomy.

Magnesium deficiency. This magnesium deficiency may be dietary in origin or else due to chronic alcoholism. The explanation of the hypocalcaemia is uncertain; impaired function of the parathyroid glands is one suggestion. It may also be that magnesium deficiency inhibits the action of parathyroid hormone on its target organs.

Excessive transfusion of citrated blood. This is rare, but has been described following exchange transfusions in infants.

Effects of Hypocalcaemia

(*a*) Tetany and epileptiform convulsions. There may also be mental disturbances, especially states of depression and anxiety.

In milder hypocalcaemia, where there are no clinical symptoms, there are 2 simple manoeuvres which may elicit latent tetany: (1) *Trousseau's sign*, which is a spasm of the interossei and of the adductor and opponens muscles of the thumb following the inflation of a sphygmomanometer cuff on the upper arm to above the systolic blood pressure for up to 3 minutes, and (2) *Chvostek's sign*, which is a twitching of the muscles of that side of the face when the branches of the facial nerve in the parotid gland at the angle of the jaw are tapped. If Trousseau's sign takes more than 2 minutes to elicit, it is of doubtful significance. Chvostek's sign has been found in from 5 to 20 per cent of normal people.

The actual manifestations of tetany usually commence with paraesthesiae of the hands and feet, and these are followed by classical carpopedal spasms. In severe cases there may also be spasms of the diaphragm, abdominal muscles, and back. Spasm of the glottis in children leads to the alarming manifestation of *laryngismus stridulus*.

(*b*) Abdominal pain of obscure origin. It may be due to smooth-muscle spasm.

(*c*) Electrocardiographic changes: a prolonged QT interval principally in the ST segment.

(*d*) A predisposition to eczema in chronic cases. There is also an increased incidence of *Candida albicans* infections of the skin.

(*e*) Cataract, a well-known complication of chronic hypocalcaemia. The cause is uncertain.

HYPERCALCAEMIA

An increase in the level of plasma calcium occurs in the following conditions:

Primary hyperparathyroidism. This important condition is described on page 461.

Hypervitaminosis D. Excessive administration of vitamin D leads to hypercalcaemia and generalised metastatic calcification. The parathyroid-hormone-like activity of vitamin D is responsible for this action.

Vitamin-D-sensitive states. There are several conditions which resemble hypervitaminosis D, but in which there is little or no evidence of excessive dietary intake. An increased susceptibility to the actions of the vitamin is postulated, but this theory cannot be regarded as proven. Two conditions are worth noting:

Sarcoidosis. The hypercalcaemia that is occasionally seen in this condition is due to increased calcium absorption rather than bone destruction. Exposure to sunlight appears to increase the hypercalcaemia.

Infantile hypercalcaemia. This condition, first described in 1952, is seen in infants between the ages of 6 weeks and 8 months. Two types are recognised:

THE BENIGN FORM is characterised by anorexia, vomiting, constipation, and marked hypotonia of the limbs. The plasma level of calcium is over 3 mmol per litre (12 mg per dl), and the plasma urea is raised. After some months of illness recovery generally ensues.

Although the condition closely resembles hypervitaminosis D, the evidence for excessive intake is not conclusive. Some infants were receiving 1000 to 3000 units daily, a dose not generally regarded as toxic. However, the disease has been prominent in Great Britain, where milk and foods are artificially fortified, whereas it is unknown in North America. Furthermore, it has not been reported in breast-fed babies; cows' milk contains four times as much calcium as does human milk. An alternative suggestion that the disease is due to an abnormal sensitivity to vitamin D has not been convincingly substantiated. The high plasma cholesterol level often present has led to the suggestion that faulty steroid metabolism may be a factor.

THE MALIGNANT FORM of the disease is accompanied by marked physical and mental retardation. The face shows a characteristic 'elfin' appearance which can be detected at birth. Severe nephrocalcinosis is reflected in nitrogen retention. Hypertension may be present. The bones may show sclerosis of an intensity reminiscent of Albers-Schönberg disease. Extensive metastatic calcification occurs. The disease appears to be a separate entity from the benign form. The pathogenesis is not known, but extreme sensitivity to vitamin D has been postulated.

Destructive bone lesions. Extensive destruction of the skeleton by osteolytic metastases of carcinoma, multiple myeloma, or Hodgkin's disease may lead to the release of excessive amounts of calcium. The resulting hypercalcaemia is often fatal, and can be precipitated by oestrogen therapy in cases of breast cancer.[8] Metastatic calcification can also occur, but it is usually not very marked because of the fairly short duration of the hypercalcaemia before death occurs.

Hypercalcaemia in immobilisation. Mechanical stresses exert an influence on both bone formation and resorption. In a patient confined to bed there is both increased bone resorption and diminished formation. In childhood, adolescence, and in patients with Paget's disease, the amount of calcium released may occasionally be sufficient to cause hypercalcaemia.

Compulsive milk drinking. Subjects with this neurosis absorb excess calcium from the bowel, and the consequent hypercalcaemia leads to nephrocalcinosis. The most severe examples are met with in patients suffering from peptic ulceration, in whom the situation is aggravated by concomitant alkali administration (*milk-alkali syndrome*). The ensuing alkalosis aggravates the nephrocalcinosis, and severe renal failure may result.

Hyperthyroidism. The increased metabolic activity in bone in hyperthyroidism is occasionally sufficient to produce hypercalcaemia. Paradoxically, hypercalcaemia sometimes complicates hypothyroidism.

Thiazide therapy. The thiazide diuretics reduce the urinary output of calcium and may lead to hypercalcaemia, particularly if there is also present some other disorder tending to cause an increase in plasma calcium, e.g. hyperparathyroidism.

Miscellaneous causes. Hypercalcaemia may occur in *congenital hypophosphatasia*. This is inherited as an autosomal recessive trait; both the plasma and tissues have a low level of alkaline phosphatase. Bone formation is abnormal, and a condition resembling rickets develops. An excess of phosphorylethanolamine is found in the plasma and urine, the precise significance of which is not understood. The abnormality in bone formation suggests that alkaline phosphatase is of great importance in the normal formation of bone. Hypercalcaemia and hypercalciuria may result in nephrocalcinosis.

Hypercalcaemia may be the presenting feature of *Addison's disease* on rare occasions.[9]

Effects of Hypercalcaemia

(*a*) Fatigue, lethargy, and muscle asthenia.

(*b*) Anorexia, nausea, and vomiting. Constipation is prominent, possibly due to the muscular hypotonia.

(*c*) Pruritus, an unexplained symptom (see also page 557).

(*d*) Psychotic manifestations.

(*e*) Symptoms of progressive renal dysfunction starting with polyuria due to an unresponsiveness of the distal and collecting tubules to antidiuretic hormone. There is an accompanying thirst, which may also be due to the high plasma calcium directly stimulating the hypothalamus. This is followed by disturbances in pH regulation and glomerular function, which terminate rapidly in renal failure. Indeed, the renal effects of hypercalcaemia are the most lethal aspects of the condition.

(*f*) Electrocardiographic changes: a shortened QT interval and depressed T waves. These are seldom of diagnostic value.

(*g*) Metastatic calcification.

(*h*) Peptic ulceration. This is particularly common in primary hyperparathyroidism, but can occur in other types of hypercalcaemia also. The excess plasma calcium releases gastrin.[10]

(*i*) Pancreatitis, both acute and chronic. This again is seen most often in association with primary hyperparathyroidism, but can occur in other types of hypercalcaemia also. The mechanism is unknown (as indeed is that of pancreatitis generally); suggested factors include stones forming in the pancreatic ducts and the ionised calcium favouring the conversion of trypsinogen to trypsin in the pancreatic ducts.

HYPOPARATHYROIDISM

The most common cause of hypoparathyroidism is damage to the glands or their blood supply sustained during thyroid surgery. Hereditary hypoparathyroidism may become manifest during the first year of life, but more commonly it occurs during childhood when it may be accompanied by cutaneous candidiasis, adrenal insufficiency, or pernicious anaemia. Hypoparathyroidism is a component of the Di George syndrome (p. 171).

Hypoparathyroidism is characterised by hypocalcaemia which causes tetany and convulsions and the other effects noted on page 460. Hyperphosphataemia is also present. These changes are also found in pseudohypoparathyroidism, in which condition the parathyroids are normal but there is end-organ unresponsiveness to parathyroid hormone; this is described on page 305 and page 559.

Surprisingly, in view of the severe hypocalcaemia, there is a tendency to soft-tissue calcification (especially of the basal ganglia of the brain). This calcification appears to be metastatic rather than dystrophic, and is probably related to the raised level of plasma phosphate.

HYPERPARATHYROIDISM

Excessive secretion of the parathyroid glands may occur as a primary or a secondary condition.

Primary hyperparathyroidism. The first account of this disease was published in 1743 by a Welshman, Sylvanus Bevan. It is generally due to an idiopathic hyperplasia of the parathyroid glands, but sometimes a simple adenoma is responsible; rarely the tumour is malignant. Adenoma of the parathyroids is a component of the multiple endocrine adenopathy syndromes (p. 452).

Primary hyperparathyroidism can present in a variety of ways. The best known is classical *osteitis fibrosa cystica*, or *von Recklinghausen's disease of bone*, in which intense osteoclastic resorption leads to destructive cystic changes involving many bones. Bone pain is a prominent symptom, pathological fractures are common, and sometimes tumour-like masses ('brown tumours') may simulate giant-cell tumours (see p. 321).

More commonly the resorption is generalised, and the bone disorder is inconspicuous. In these cases the hypercalcaemia causes the characteristic effects already noted. Death is due to renal failure. If the plasma calcium reaches very high levels (above 5 mmol per litre, or 20 mg per dl), there may be a *hypercalcaemic crisis*. There is shock, haemoconcentration, anuria, and death preceded by confusion and coma.

Another well-known presentation of hyperparathyroidism is recurrent renal-calculus formation. These cases are usually of long standing, bone lesions may be absent, and the systemic effects of hypercalcaemia are often mild.

The biochemical changes of hyperparathyroidism are a raised level of plasma calcium (it may rise to 5·5 mmol per litre, or 22 mg per dl),* a lowered level of plasma phosphate, and an increased urinary output of calcium. The hypercalcaemia is not lowered by the administration of glucocorticoids (unlike the hypercalcaemia of sarcoidosis, the milk-alkali syndrome, and most cases of multiple myeloma).

As the disease progresses, so the plasma phosphate level may rise owing to secondary renal failure, and the urinary calcium may fall as the result of the reduced glomerular filtration rate (in addition parathyroid hormone aids calcium reabsorption—see p. 458). Metastatic calcification in the usual sites is common, and is aggravated when renal failure develops.

Secondary hyperparathyroidism. Hyperplasia of the parathyroids occurs in many types of osteomalacia and rickets; probably there is an associated increased parathyroid-hormone secretion, but this is difficult to prove as there is no simple assay method available. It is the hypocalcaemia that stimulates the glands into activity. In some cases this is sufficiently marked to initiate osteoclastic activity in the bones, and therefore in addition to the changes of rickets or osteomalacia there develop those of osteitis fibrosa cystica. This type of response occurs only occasionally, and renal disease is the usual antecedent.

Renal osteodystrophy (renal rickets). Chronic renal disease, especially in young people, is sometimes attended by skeletal lesions which comprise a mixture of calcification defects—osteomalacia (or rickets according to age) and osteitis fibrosa

---

*Normocalcaemia occasionally occurs in hyperparathyroidism, especially in cases that show themselves with renal calculi.[11]

cystica. Metastatic calcification affecting principally the kidneys, arteries, and subcutaneous tissues sometimes occurs, and may be worsened by dialysis unless hyperphosphataemia is controlled.[12] Corneal and conjunctival deposits can be detected by slit-lamp examination in patients who complain of conjunctivitis. In addition, there may also be osteosclerosis, which in the vertebral bodies tends to occur in the areas adjacent to the intervertebral discs. The central parts of the bodies are osteoporotic, and therefore a radiograph of the spine presents a banded appearance, the so-called rugger-jersey spine. The pathogenesis of the condition is discussed on page 555.

Tertiary hyperparathyroidism. It is now recognised that some cases of long-standing parathyroid hyperplasia secondary to malabsorption or chronic renal failure may undergo adenomatous change. Hypercalcaemia then develops (p. 555).

Ectopic parathyroid-hormone syndrome. A number of patients with malignant disease have hypercalcaemia without evidence of metastatic bone disease. This syndrome is due to the elaboration by the tumour of a substance resembling parathyroid hormone. Squamous-cell carcinoma of the lung and carcinoma of the kidney are the usual culprits.

Table 36.1 below summarises the usual changes in the plasma levels of calcium, inorganic phosphate, and alkaline phosphatase found in some of the conditions described in this chapter. It should be noted that the normal plasma level of inorganic phosphate is 0·8 to 1·4 mmol per litre (2·5 to 4·5 mg per dl), being slightly higher in children than in adults. The normal plasma level of alkaline phosphatase is 3 to 13 King-Armstrong units.

HETEROTOPIC CALCIFICATION

It is convenient to conclude this account of calcium metabolism with a description of *heterotopic calcification*. This is defined as the deposition of calcium salts in tissues other than osteoid or enamel. Because calcium salts are radiopaque, their deposition is conspicuous on X-ray examination, and heterotopic calcification has therefore come to assume an importance in diagnostic radiology which far outweighs its pathological significance (Fig. 36.2).

Two quite distinct types of heterotopic calcification are recognised:

Dystrophic calcification, which is the deposition of calcium salts in dead or degenerate tissue. The plasma levels of calcium and

TABLE 36.1

	Calcium	Phosphate	Alkaline Phosphatase
Osteoporosis	Normal	Normal	Normal
Primary hyperparathyroidism	Raised (greatly)	Lowered, except with renal failure	Raised (moderately)
Hypoparathyroidism	Lowered (greatly)	Raised (greatly)	Normal
Osteomalacia, dietary and malabsorption	Normal or lowered	Lowered	Raised (moderately)
Renal tubular acidosis	Normal or lowered	Lowered	Normal or raised
Hypophosphataemia	Normal	Lowered	Normal or raised
Renal rickets (uraemia)	Lowered	Raised (greatly)	Normal or raised
Hypophosphatasia	Normal or raised	Normal	Lowered
Paget's disease of bone	Normal	Normal	Raised (greatly)
Osteolytic metastases	Normal or raised	Normal	Normal
Osteosclerotic metastases	Normal or lowered	Normal	Normal or raised

Figure 36.2
Calcified gallbladder. The patient had had a history of gallbladder dyspepsia for many years. There was a palpable tumour in the right hypochondrium, and X-rays showed a calcified gallbladder with a calculus impacted in the neck. The specimen was X-rayed after excision, and the patchy calcification of the walls of the fundus is well shown. (EA 117.2, *Reproduced by permission of the President and Council of the R.C.S. Eng.*)

phosphate are normal, and local conditions are presumably of overriding importance. The calcium deposits are localised.

Metastatic calcification, which is the precipitation of calcium salts in apparently normal tissues as the result of a generalised upset in calcium-phosphate metabolism. There is usually hypercalcaemia.

The deposition of calcium salts in calculi is a special example of pathological calcification and is considered in Chapter 51.

Appearance of heterotopic calcification. Microscopically calcium salts appear as granular deposits which stain a very deep blue colour with haematoxylin. They simulate bacterial colonies, which are also deeply basophilic, but lack the uniformity in size and shape exhibited by micro-organisms. Calcium deposits typically form an incrustation on such surfaces as the elastic fibres of the lung and arteries, and on ova. Calcium deposits can be identified by their red staining with alizarin red S. The more commonly used silver-impregnation method of von Kóssa in fact stains phosphate and carbonate. Nevertheless, these ions are almost always associated with calcium when in particulate, insoluble form.

The amount of calcium revealed by staining methods does not correlate well with the amount present as estimated chemically. Electron-probe analysis promises to be more useful. In this a beam of electrons is focused on a small spot of tissue in a vacuum, and the emitted X-rays are analysed by a spectroscope. The presence of a given element is recognised by its characteristic spectrum, and its concentration is determined by the intensity of the emission.

DYSTROPHIC CALCIFICATION

The cause of dystrophic calcification can be considered under two headings: (*a*) calcification in dead tissue, and (*b*) calcification in degenerate tissue. Though the distinction between the two may be somewhat arbitrary, this forms a convenient division.

Calcification in Dead Tissue

Caseous material. Calcification is of frequent occurrence in caseous material, and remains as a permanent landmark of previous tuberculous infection. It is seen in healed Ghon foci and the associated lymph nodes, and also in the mesenteric nodes of a primary intestinal infection. Calcification is not confined to childhood infection, nor indeed need the lesion be healed, for it is also seen in chronic adult tuberculosis, e.g. in the wall of a psoas abscess. It should furthermore not be forgotten that well-calcified tuberculous lesions sometimes contain living bacilli, which may cause future disease. Calcification is also seen in the healed lesions of histoplasmosis and coccidioidomycosis.

Dead parasites. Many parasites undergo calcification, but this occurs only after their death (Fig. 36.3). *Trichinella spiralis*, hydatid cysts, schistosome ova, and the lesions of cysticercosis are common examples. The dead fetus may also be included under this heading. In the rare occurrence of ruptured tubal pregnancy in which the fetus survives for a while, its subsequent calcification converts it into a *lithopaedion*.

Fat necrosis. This is seen after acute pancreatitis as well as in traumatic lesions of the breast (see p. 56).

Infarcts. Some infarcts have a peculiar liability to undergo calcification. Experimentally, infarcts in the rat kidney invariably calcify.

Thrombi. Thrombi in veins may calcify to produce *phleboliths*; these are quite commonly seen radiologically in the pelvic veins. Arterial thrombi are less liable to calcification, unless, of course, atheroma is included under this heading (see p. 497).

Haematomata. Although collections of blood in any situation may undergo calcification, this is particularly common when the haematoma is in close association with bone. It is seen in the traumatic subdural haematoma. In traumatic myositis ossificans there is calcification and subsequent ossification of the haematoma in a muscle. The bone-forming cells have presumably been derived from the periosteum.

Calcification in Degenerate Tissue

Scars. The fibrous tissue of scars may undergo hyaline degeneration and subsequent calcification. Some individuals show a definite predisposition to this.

Chronic inflammatory granulation tissue. Dystrophic calcification is quite common in the degenerate tissue of chronic

Figure 36.3
Dystrophic calcification of schistosome ova.
In this section of pancreas there are a number
of deeply-staining, calcified ova of
Schistosoma haematobium. They stain deeply
with haematoxylin owing to their calcium
content. Although these ova are dead, they can
still excite a chronic inflammatory reaction.
× 200.

inflammatory lesions. It is seen in the walls of chronic abscesses. It is important in constrictive pericarditis, and is prominent in the scarred valves of rheumatic heart disease and healed infective endocarditis.

Atheroma. Calcification in the degenerate tissue of atheroma is of very frequent occurrence in the aorta and coronary vessels. This intimal calcification must be clearly distinguished from the medial lesions of Mönckeberg's sclerosis.

Mönckeberg's sclerosis. The hyalinised tunica media in this condition regularly becomes calcified, thereby converting the artery into a rigid tube. The calcified tissue is disposed in the form of rings, as it has the same distribution as the muscle coat that it replaces.

Senile degenerate tissue. Calcification occurs normally in the costal cartilages of elderly people, and is not uncommon in the pineal gland after middle age; indeed, it forms a useful landmark in X-ray examinations of the brain. The dura mater may calcify in old age. Degeneration and calcification in the supraspinatus tendon is possibly a senile change, but previous traumatic vascular damage probably also plays a part. The lone calcareous aortic stenosis seen in the middle-aged and elderly is the end-result of a congenital valvular malformation.

Degenerate colloid goitres and so-called adenomata of the thyroid. Flecks of calcification are present in many nodular goitres; this may be of value in the detection of retrosternal goitres.

Cysts. Many cysts of long-standing show calcification of their walls. Good examples are afforded by epidermoid and pilar cysts of the skin.

Degenerate tumours. Large uterine fibroids often undergo extensive calcification, usually after the muscle element has undergone necrosis and become replaced by hyaline fibrous tissue. Some tumours show circumscribed spherules of calcification (calcospherites); the psammoma bodies of meningiomata are outstanding examples, and similar structures are seen in some cystadenocarcinomata, especially of the ovary. Many tumours show foci of calcification which may well have followed necrosis;

this has been put to practical use in the diagnosis of breast cancer[13] (Figs. 36.4 and 36.5).

Electron-microscopic studies of breast cancer have shown that the calcification starts within the cytoplasm of the cancer cells in the intraluminal spaces of duct-like structures. This luminal calcification appears to be the consequence of an active secretory process and not simply dystrophic calcification in cellular debris.[14]

Sundry lesions. Pulmonary alveolar microlithiasis is a remarkable condition in which calcified laminated structures are found in the alveoli. Presumably they are formed by the calcification of successive accumulations of secretion, so as to produce the typical laminated structures reminiscent of starch granules. A similar condition occurs in the prostate (corpora amylacea), and again calcification may occur.

Calcinosis. In this rare condition abnormal deposits of calcium salts are laid down in skin, subcutaneous tissues, muscles, and tendons. The cause is unknown, and the condition should not be confused with fibrodysplasia ossificans progressiva (see p. 305). Calcinosis of the finger pulps is a common feature of scleroderma.

An interesting variant is *tumoural calcinosis*, also called *tumoural lipocalcinosis*, in which there are large calcareous swellings in the subcutaneous tissue near the larger joints, e.g. the elbows, shoulders, hips, and knees. This condition is seen most often in Black Africans. It may be precipitated by minor trauma, but its pathogenesis is obscure.[15]

Chondrocalcinosis.[16] This is characterised by the deposition of calcium pyrophosphate crystals in cartilage. Fibrocartilage is most commonly involved, particularly the menisci of the knee and the triangular cartilage of the wrist, but articular hyaline cartilage may also calcify. A chronic arthritis results, and its course is sometimes aggravated by attacks of acute synovitis during which crystals of calcium pyrophosphate are present in the joint fluid. The condition is also called *pseudogout*, and as in gout, the crystals in the joint fluid are phagocytosed by polymorphs. A release of damaging lysosomal enzymes is the probable pathogenesis of the

Figure 36.4
Typical radiographic appearance of a benign lesion in a breast. This patient, a 66-year-old woman, had a very hard mass which was discovered on routine examination. It proved to be a fibroadenoma. (*From Egan, R. L.* (1964), 'Mammography', *Springfield, Ill.: Thomas*)

Figure 36.5
This patient presented with a vague nodularity of the breast. Mammograms revealed no mass, but showed a fine stippled calcification which is characteristic of many intraduct carcinomata. The lesion was removed, and study revealed a 2·5 cm adenocarcinoma of the breast with no axillary lymph-node metastases. (*From Egan, R. L.* (1964), 'Mammography', *Springfield, Ill.: Thomas*)

synovitis in both conditions. Chondrocalcinosis may occur as a complication of other diseases, e.g. ochronosis, haemochromatosis, hyperparathyroidism, and gout, or it may appear as an idiopathic isolated condition.

Heterotopic bone formation may occur at any site of dystrophic calcification, and is considered in Chapter 24.

METASTATIC CALCIFICATION

Metastatic calcification is caused by a disordered metabolism of calcium and phosphate, and although in the common type (following hyperparathyroidism) the calcium salts are truly metastatic, being derived from bone, there are other conditions in which the excess calcium is absorbed from the gut. Nevertheless, it is convenient in practice to use the term 'metastatic calcification' to cover both these varieties, and it will be used in this context in the account that follows.

Generalised metastatic calcification is usually due to hypercalcaemia, but occasionally, as in renal osteodystrophy, a high plasma phosphate appears to be the precipitating factor. The bone salts are deposited in certain sites of election:

Kidney. This is the most frequent and important site. Deposition occurs especially around the tubules, where severe damage is produced. The condition is called *nephrocalcinosis*, and it may lead to renal failure (see Ch. 46). In addition calculi often form in the pelvis and ureter, where they may predispose to infection and cause further renal damage. *Renal failure is therefore a prominent feature of generalised metastatic calcification whatever may be the primary cause* (Fig. 36.1).

An important factor in the causation of nephrocalcinosis is hypercalciuria. While this is usually caused by hypercalcaemia, e.g. in primary hyperparathyroidism, it may on occasion be found with low plasma levels, e.g. in renal tubular acidosis, see page 559. Nephrocalcinosis may therefore occur as an isolated event.

Lung. Calcium is deposited in the alveolar walls, where it forms an incrustation on the elastic fibres. These are thereby prominently outlined in blue on routine H. and E. staining.

Stomach. Calcification occurs around the fundal glands. It has been suggested that as these glands secrete hydrochloric acid, the

tissues are left relatively alkaline, and that this favours calcification.

Blood vessels. The coronary vessels (and even the heart) may be affected. Sometimes the internal elastic lamina is incrusted as has already been described with regard to the lungs.

Cornea. A site frequently affected is the cornea of the eye, and the condition can be discovered by slit-lamp examination during life.

Causes of Metastatic Calcification

It must be acknowledged that the actual basis of metastatic calcification is not understood. Although it is usually associated with hypercalcaemia, a normal or low plasma calcium level may be found in certain syndromes. In these the site of calcification may be atypical, e.g. the basal ganglia in hypoparathyroidism, or confined to the kidney in renal tubular acidosis. In renal osteodystrophy calcification occurs in the subcutaneous tissues as well as in the arteries, kidneys, and other more usual sites.

The following causes of metastatic calcification can be recognised:

Hyperparathyroidism—Hyperplasia—primary or secondary.
Neoplasia.
Excessive absorption of calcium from the bowel
Hypervitaminosis D.

Vitamin-D sensitive states, e.g. idiopathic hypercalcaemia of infants and sarcoidosis.

Compulsive milk drinking.

Hypophosphatasia

Destructive bone lesions, especially widespread osteolytic cancer metastases.

Hypoparathyroidism

Renal tubular acidosis, where there is only nephrocalcinosis.

GENERAL REFERENCES

FOURMAN, P. & ROYER, P. (1968) *Calcium Metabolism and the Bone*, 2nd edn, 656 pp. Oxford: Blackwell.

NORDIN, B. E. C. (1973) *Metabolic Bone and Stone Disease*. Edinburgh: Churchill Livingstone.

PATERSON, C. R. (1974) *Metabolic Disorders of Bone*, 373 pp. Oxford: Blackwell.

VAUGHAN, J. M. (1975) *The Physiology of Bone*, 2nd edn, 306 pp. Oxford: Clarendon Press.

REFERENCES

1. WILLS, M. R. *et al.* (1972) Phytic acid and nutritional rickets in immigrants. *Lancet*, **1**, 771.
2. RAISZ, L. G. (1972) A confusion of vitamin D's. *New England Journal of Medicine*, **287**, 926.
3. KODICEK, E. (1974) The story of vitamin D from vitamin to hormone. *Lancet*, **1**, 325.
4. Leading Article (1974) Cholecalciferol metabolism. *Lancet*, **1**, 492.
5. Leading Article (1977) Vitamin D and the pituitary. *Lancet*, **1**, 840.
6. Leading Article (1978) 'One-alpha'. *Lancet*, **1**, 973.
7. Leading Article (1973) Treatment with calcitonin. *British Medical Journal*, **1**, 371.
8. CORNBLEET, M., BONDY, P. K. & POWLES, T. J. (1977) Fatal irreversible hypercalcaemia in breast cancer. *British Medical Journal*, **1**, 145.
9. DOWNIE, W. W. *et al.* (1977) Hypercalcaemic crisis as presentation of Addison's disease. *British Medical Journal*, **1**, 145.
10. WALSH, J. H. & GROSSMAN, M. I. (1975) Gastrin. *New England Journal of Medicine*, **292**, 1324 and 1377.
11. WILLS, M. R. (1971) Normocalcaemic primary hyperparathyroidism. *Lancet*, **1**, 849.
12. Leading Article (1972) Metastatic calcification and dialysis. *British Medical Journal*, **1**, 762.
13. KOEHL, R. H. *et al.* (1970) The incidence and significance of calcifications within operative breast specimens. *American Journal of Clinical Pathology*, **53**, 3.
14. AHMED, A. (1975) Calcification in human breast carcinomas: ultrastructural observations. *Journal of Pathology*, **117**, 247.
15. VERESS, B., MALIK, M. O. A. & HASSAN, A. M. E. (1976) Tumoural lipocalcinosis: a clinicopathological study of 20 cases. *Journal of Pathology*, **119**, 113.
16. RUSSELL, R. G. G. *et al.* (1970) Inorganic pyrophosphate in plasma, urine, and synovial fluid of patients with pyrophosphate arthropathy (chondrocalcinosis or pseudogout). *Lancet*, **2**, 899.

Chapter 37.   Temperature Regulation: Fever and Hypothermia

One of the most important developments in the higher animal is the evolution of mechanisms whereby a constant environment is maintained for its constituent cells. This fixity of the internal environment has been well recognised since the time of Claude Bernard. Temperature regulation is an important aspect of homeostasis, which in humans and other warm-blooded mammals has attained a high degree of efficiency. Cellular activity, involving as it does numerous chemical reactions largely dependent upon enzymatic activity, is very susceptible to changes in temperature. On the other hand, some of the energy produced during cell respiration is emitted as heat. Indeed, the temperature of highly active organs, like the brain and heart, would rise were it not for the cooling effect of the blood stream which carries away the excess heat and distributes it to those areas where it can be dissipated to the atmosphere, viz. the skin and the mucosa of the upper respiratory tract.

It is probable that the development of a reliable temperature-regulating mechanism has contributed considerably to the biological supremacy of the warm-blooded group of animals.

The Normal Body Temperature

It is curious that, although fever has been recognised since ancient times, actual measurements of body temperature were not made till comparatively recently. Reliable clinical thermometers became available in the seventeenth century, but it was not until the nineteenth century that they were used to any extent.

Body temperature is usually measured with the thermometer placed under the tongue, or else in the axilla, groin, or rectum. Of these, readings obtained from the axilla and groin show the widest variation, and are generally regarded as being least reliable. This is hardly surprising, since the surface skin temperature fluctuates widely, and may approximate to that of the external environment. The rectal temperature is highest, being about 0·3°C higher than the arterial temperature. Measuring the urine temperature has also been advocated, and it approximates to the rectal temperature .[1] The rectal temperature is said to be the least responsive to changes in the arterial temperature. Thus, if warm saline is infused into a vein, the rise in blood temperature is reflected in an elevation of the sublingual temperature but not that of the rectum. The sublingual temperature taken with the lips closed is therefore held to be the most reliable guide to the arterial temperature; in addition the mouth is near the hypothalamus (see p. 468).

The normal temperature taken in this way is 36·8°C with a range of 36·1 to 37·4°C (97–99·3°F). The maximum temperature is generally attained at about 6 p.m., while it is at its lowest at about 3 a.m. In women there is an elevation of the temperature during the middle of the menstrual cycle; its onset is thought to herald ovulation.

TEMPERATURE REGULATION[2]

The constancy of the body's temperature is maintained by balancing the amount of heat produced in the body with that which is lost.

Sources of Heat

From the environment. Whenever the external temperature exceeds that of the body, heat will be gained by radiation, conduction, and convection. It is a remarkable fact that under such conditions the body's temperature can be maintained at its correct level. The regulating mechanisms are not, however, working under favourable conditions, and it is not surprising that they may break down under these circumstances (see heatstroke, p. 469).

From metabolic activity. The major source of heat is the body's metabolic activity. Heat production under fasting conditions with the individual at complete mental and physical rest is called the *basal metabolic rate* (*BMR*), which ranges from 1400 to 1800 calories per day. Under normal active conditions additional heat is produced by exercise, which can be quite modest with sedentery workers (e.g. 1000 calories) or rather high in those engaged in heavy manual labour (e.g. 6000 calories). The BMR is increased by thyroxine; this effect is seen in individuals exposed to cold and in thyrotoxicosis. Fever also affects the BMR, a rise of 1°C in body temperature increasing it by about 10 per cent.

The metabolic rate of a normal active individual is the summation of the BMR and the additional metabolism needed to sustain exercise. Involuntary muscular activity, e.g. contraction of the arrector pili muscles and shivering, further increases heat production. The ingestion of food also increases the metabolic rate, the effect of protein being particularly marked (specific dynamic action of protein).

The heat produced by metabolism raises the temperature of the blood through the relevant organs. Thus, the blood leaving the brain and the liver is warmer than that entering it. Likewise, during manual work blood leaving the skeletal muscles is heated. The warm blood from these centres of heat production is distributed to the organs of heat loss. Of these the skin is the most important.

Areas of Heat Loss

Heat loss occurs in three main ways:

Heat required to warm inspired air and ingested food. In the human the amount of heat lost in this way is to a large extent governed by factors beyond the control of the heat-regulating mechanism. The heat lost in the breath is dependent not only upon the temperature of the inspired air, but also upon the rate of breathing. In the dog the amount of heat lost can be increased by panting, but in the human this is of little importance.

Heat lost by convection, conduction, and radiation from the body surface. The amount of heat lost depends on three factors:

(*a*) The temperature of the skin.
(*b*) The temperature of the environment.
(*c*) The movement of air over the skin.

The temperature of the skin is dependent on its blood supply, which is under the control of the autonomic nervous system. Heat is lost from the skin surface by conduction to the adjacent air, which is then carried away by convection currents. Clothing hinders the removal of this layer of warm air.

Heat loss by evaporation of water. There is a constant insensible water loss from the skin surface and the respiratory tract. In the respiratory passages the amount lost depends on the temperature and humidity of the air. This heat loss is obligatory, but can be increased in dogs by panting. It comes into its own during strenuous exercise.

In the skin there is also the sweating mechanism which is under control. In temperate climates the amount of sweat secreted is. negligible, but in the tropics it is a very important source of water loss.

The Temperature Regulating Mechanism

Mechanisms are present for both increasing and decreasing the body's temperature. These come into play in response to impulses from the temperature-sensitive receptors. These receptors are situated both centrally within the nervous system and peripherally, mainly in the skin. A change of as little as 0·2°C can activate the compensatory mechanisms.

The central receptor. Situated in the anterior part of the hypothalamus, in the *preoptic area*, is a group of nerve cells that are sensitive to the temperature of the arterial blood reaching them. When the temperature of the blood changes, impulses pass from this area to other parts of the hypothalamus. There are two main areas: (1) an anterior *heat-losing centre*, which when stimulated leads to changes in the remainder of the body, causing increased heat loss, and (2) a posterior *heat-promoting centre*, which when stimulated leads to increased heat production and conservation (Fig. 37.1).

Peripheral temperature receptors. The heat-regulating mechanism is also influenced by impulses received from the peripheral receptors mainly in the skin. This influence can be demonstrated by an experiment in which the blood to one arm is occluded by a cuff and the arm is then immersed in cold water. Within seconds the skin of the opposite arm undergoes vasoconstriction, indicating that a nervous reflex is involved rather than a change in blood temperature. After a while this vasoconstriction wanes, but on restoration of the circulation, a more prolonged period of vasoconstriction ensues as the cooled blood of the limb reaches the hypothalamus and activates the central mechanism directly.

The peripheral receptors are of greatest importance when the body's temperature falls. Impulses then pass to the posterior centre in the hypothalamus and lead to conservation of heat.

Mechanism of decreasing body temperature. When the body's temperature tends to rise, there is a withdrawal of sympathetic vasoconstriction activity, the skin becomes warm, and heat is lost. The subject feels hot and may remove clothing, retire to the shade, or take other appropriate action. If this regulating mechanism does not suffice, the heat-losing centre initiates sweating from the eccrine glands. Evaporation of this fluid requires heat, but an additional effect of sweating is the local release of bradykinin from the glands. This induces further vasodilatation and heat loss.

It should be noted that the eccrine sweat ducts reabsorb sodium in a manner similar to that of the renal tubules. If the rate of sweat production increases, the ducts reabsorb less

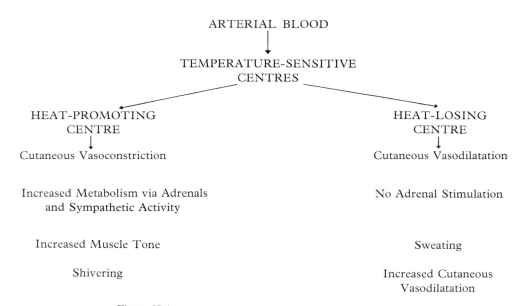

Figure 37.1
Diagram to illustrate the principal heat-regulating mechanisms.

sodium; hence excessive sweating, if prolonged, can lead to sodium depletion (see heat exhaustion, p. 478).

Mechanism for increasing body temperature. The heat-promoting centre acts mainly through the sympathetic division of the autonomic nervous system. Cutaneous vaso-constriction reduces the amount of heat lost from the skin, and blood diverted to the internal organs is insulated from the exterior by the subcutaneous fat. Furthermore, as the skin becomes cooler, the subject feels cold and may take appropriate voluntary action such as putting on extra clothing.

An important effect of increased sympathetic activity is a generalised *increase in muscle tone*. This alone can increase heat production by 50 per cent; the mechanism appears to be related to a partial uncoupling of oxidative phosphorylation. The increased sympathetic outflow causes an increased output of adrenaline and noradrenaline from the adrenal glands. Together with the increased sympathetic tone, these hormones increase the metabolic rate of all cells by a mechanism that is not well understood. This combined effect can raise the metabolic rate of children by 100 per cent, but it is less effective in the adult, in whom the increase is 15 to 25 per cent. Sympathetic impulses cause contraction of the arrector pili muscles; in animals this leads to the hair standing on end, and by increasing the thickness of the fur, decreases the amount of heat lost.

If these mechanisms are inadequate, muscle tone increases to the extent that stretch reflexes are elicited and *shivering* commences. As one group of muscles contracts, a stretch reflex of the antagonistic group is set in motion and initiates a fresh stretch reflex of the first group. This continuous shaking can increase the rate of heat production severalfold.

FEVER[2,3]

Fever, or pyrexia, may be defined as an elevation of the body's temperature consequent upon a disturbance of the regulating mechanism. When the temperature reaches or exceeds 40·5°C (105°F) the condition is called *hyperpyrexia*. Fever occurs under the following conditions:

Heatstroke.[4] Some rise in body temperature normally occurs during severe exercise when the heat-eliminating mechanisms cannot keep pace with the excessive heat production in the muscles. When the environment is hot and humid, even mild exercise may cause a marked rise in body temperature.* When the temperature rises unduly, the heat-regulating centre becomes depressed and the temperature rises further. This increases the metabolic rate so that a vicious circle is established, and the temperature rises to 41°C or more. This is 'heatstroke', or 'sunstroke', and unless treated promptly the temperature may continue to rise, reaching 43°C or more, a level at which the patient becomes comatose. Cerebral, hepatic, and renal damage is prominent. Convulsions are common, and permanent brain damage may be evident if the patient survives.

Infection. Fever is a frequent accompaniment of infection by viruses, bacteria, and larger parasites. The pattern of the pyrexia is often characteristic of particular diseases, e.g. the

intermittent fever of benign malaria and the relapsing course of brucellosis.

Infarction. This is of use in the diagnosis of myocardial infarction.

Tumours. Some tumours are particularly liable to produce pyrexia, e.g. Ewing's tumour of bone and clear-cell renal cancer. The cyclical Pel-Ebstein fever is characteristic of deep-seated Hodgkin's disease.

Haemorrhage. Fever may follow haemorrhage, especially into the gastrointestinal tract or coelomic cavities, e.g. after a ruptured ectopic pregnancy.

Brain damage. Cerebral haemorrhage, especially in the region of the pons, and other intracranial lesions may disturb the central regulating mechanism. This leads to a rise in temperature.

Following injury during the catabolic phase of convalescence.

In severe anaemia, and following acute haemolysis.

Miscellaneous conditions. Fever is a prominent feature of acute gout and some of the collagen diseases, e.g. acute rheumatic fever. A slight rise may occur in thyrotoxicosis (especially during a crisis) and in congestive heart failure.

Of all the causes of pyrexia infection is by far the most important. The development of fever in acute illnesses like lobar pneumonia or malaria has been the object of most study. Three stages are described:

The cold stage. At the onset of the illness there is a feeling of intense cold, peripheral vasoconstriction is manifested by pallor, and the patient starts to shiver. Chattering of the teeth completes this picture of the familiar rigor. Heat production is thereby increased, and heat loss reduced; the temperature rises, as does also the blood pressure. There is usually a rise in pulse rate of 18 beats per minute for each 1°C rise of temperature (10 per 1°F).

The hot stage. As the temperature approaches its peak, the peripheral vasoconstriction relaxes and the patient feels dry and warm. Heat loss now balances heat gain, and the temperature remains constant. The heat-regulating mechanism is still in control, but is geared to maintain the temperature at a level higher than normal. The extra heat produced is due to the raised metabolic rate caused by the fever. Should hyperpyrexia occur, this regulation may fail. During this phase the blood pressure falls. The RQ* is low, and there is a tendency to ketosis. Wasting of fat and muscle occurs together with an increased excretion of nitrogen in the urine.

The sweating phase. The temperature begins to fall, and the patient soon experiences a sensation of intense heat. Bedclothes are thrown off, sweating becomes profuse, and the temperature returns to normal. This is described as termination by *crisis*.

The Cause of Fever

The fact that fever often accompanies necrosis, e.g. in tumours and infarcts, suggests that dead tissue contains a pyrogenic substance, and pyrogens similar to those of bacteria have been isolated.

---

*Heatstroke was the largest single cause of death amongst the pilgrims to Mecca in 1959 and 1960.

*Respiratory quotient (RQ) is the ratio

$$\frac{\text{Volume of } CO_2 \text{ produced}}{\text{Volume of } O_2 \text{ consumed}}$$

Intravenous injections of Gram-negative organisms produce a sharp rise in temperature. This is due to lipopolysaccharide or polysaccharide substances which are called *bacterial pyrogens*. These have the following properties.

(*a*) On injection they produce fever after a latent period.

(*b*) Leucopenia also occurs.

(*c*) Repeated injections lead to a state of refractoriness.

This tolerance is not due to antibody production. It can be abolished by the prior injection of thorotrast, and appears to be due to the heightened ability of the RE system to remove endotoxin.

These bacterial pyrogens are of importance because they can produce febrile reactions by polluting the fluids and apparatus used in intravenous therapy.

The pyrogens act indirectly. They cause the polymorphs to release an *endogenous pyrogen*, which acts on the central regulating mechanism. Pyrogens are also released by polymorphs during phagocytosis and in response to antigen-antibody complexes. This explains the pyrexia of non-infective inflammatory conditions (such as gout) as well as the fever of diseases with an autoimmune component, e.g. systemic lupus erythematosus.

In the human being there is evidence that a similar pyrogen can be released from monocytes as well as polymorphs. This helps to explain the pyrexia which occurs in infections with organisms that excite a mononuclear response and also the fever in patients with agranulocytosis.

This endogenous pyrogen differs from the bacterial pyrogens in several respects. The fever which it causes is more rapid in onset, but also more transient. There is no leucopenia, and tolerance does not develop. Animals made resistant to bacterial pyrogen remain sensitive to endogenous pyrogen. It appears therefore that fever is produced by an endogenous chemical mediator.

Certain *steroid hormones* can produce a rise of body temperature. Progesterone is an example, and is probably responsible for the elevated temperature that occurs at the time of ovulation during the menstrual cycle. Another steroid, *aetiocholanolone*, which arises from the metabolism of adrenocortical and gonadal hormones and is found in the ketosteroid fraction of the urine, causes a marked rise in temperature after injection. There is a latent period of 4 to 8 hours, and the fever abates after 18 hours.

Disturbances of the central nervous system also affect the body's temperature.[5] Emotion can raise it, and *periodic fever*, a cyclical pyrexia of unknown origin, is perhaps related to cerebral dysfunction, but some authorities blame excessive aetiocholanolone production. General anaesthesia impairs the heat regulating mechanism—the fully anaesthetised patient is poikilothermic.

Fulminating, or malignant, hyperpyrexia.[6–8] This newly recognised syndrome is characterised by a rapid rise in temperature during the administration of a general anaesthetic; in most cases either halothane or suxamethonium has been given. Tachypnoea, tachycardia, hypotension, cyanosis, and metabolic acidosis develop, and the pyrexia may go unrecognised until by chance the patient is noted to be very hot. The progress of the pyrexia is extremely rapid, and unless vigorous cooling is employed the temperature rises to very high levels, e.g. 43 to 44°C (110 to 112°F), and death occurs from cardiac arrest. In the majority of cases the skeletal muscles develop an increase in tone and show fasciculation. It is believed that this is responsible for the sudden increase in heat production, but in a minority of cases rigidity is absent and some other mechanism must be postulated. In some cases of malignant hyperpyrexia, particularly those which develop rigidity, an inherited abnormality has been suggested; in some families the predisposition towards malignant hyperpyrexia is inherited as an autosomal dominant trait. In some families a type of myopathy has been demonstrated, and if subclinical this may be detected by an elevation in the plasma levels of creatine phosphokinase (CPK) and aldolase. A preoperative estimation of the CPK level will indeed help to prevent some cases of malignant hyperpyrexia.

Although recent work has shed some light on the mystery of fever, much has yet to be learned. It would be satisfying to believe that a rise in temperature in infection was a beneficial reaction designed to aid the body's defences. There is, however, little evidence that this is so. As yet we must regard the maintenance of body temperature as an important homeostatic mechanism for the proper functioning of the body. Any marked departure from the normal appears to be at the best, of no value, and at the worst, deleterious to well-being.

Attention has been drawn to the possibly beneficial effect of fever on viral infections. There is considerable evidence to indicate that viruses, especially those of poor virulence, stimulate the production of larger amounts of interferon at higher temperatures, e.g. up to 42°C (107·6°F). It may be that fever stimulates greater interferon production by the infected cells, and so limits the course of viral disease.

HYPOTHERMIA

Hypothermia may be defined as a body temperature below 35°C (95°F). It is an important cause of death in cold climates especially at the extremes of life, and it has therapeutic implications.

Three grades of lowered body temperature can be recognised.

(*a*) 37 to 32·2°C (98·4 to 90°F), in which the body reacts vigorously (maximally at 35°C or 95°F) against the chilling. There is violent shivering, cutaneous vasoconstriction, tachycardia, and a raised blood pressure. Breathing is increased, and a diuresis is common.

(*b*) 32.2 to 24°C (90 to 75°F), in which the tissue metabolism throughout the body is depressed. There is a progressive decrease in the pulse rate, respiration, and blood pressure. This is the range generally employed in surgery.

(*c*) Below 24°C (75°F), in which the temperature-regulating centre ceases to function, and heat is lost from the body as from an inanimate object.

THE BODY'S RESPONSE TO HYPOTHERMIA[9]

Much experimental work has been done on the physiological response to hypothermia, but as this depends on such diverse factors as the species, age, and size of the animal used, the duration of chilling, the temperature reached, the season of the year, and the anaesthetic used, it is hardly surprising that a mass of conflicting data has accumulated, and complete correlation is not yet possible.

Effect on the Circulatory System

There is general depression. The heart rate, cardiac output, and regional blood flow to the organs are decreased. The blood pressure falls despite an increased peripheral resistance—sometimes there is vasodilatation at very low temperatures. The renal blood flow is reduced due to vasoconstriction and the low blood pressure.

The effect on the blood volume varies according to the species, but in general there is haemoconcentration due to a shift of fluid to the interstitial tissues. The increased viscosity of the blood is an important factor in causing vascular stasis. Sludging is also a common finding.

A great danger is ventricular fibrillation. It is related to the degree of chilling and the anaesthetic used. Its cause is not known; hypoxia cannot usually be blamed, but it is possible that it is related to local electrolyte imbalance involving potassium, calcium, and hydrogen ions.

Effect on the Metabolism

There is a reduced oxygen consumption. As already explained, less oxygen reaches the tissues due to circulatory depression and vasoconstriction, but in addition the oxygen requirements of the tissues drop almost proportionately to the decreased blood flow. Therefore there is little oxygen debt when the temperature is raised once more. This applies even to the brain (it is estimated that 8 minutes' occlusion of the cerebral circulation at 30°C (86°F) or 45 minutes' occlusion at 15°C (59°F) is safe). Oxygen dissociation is retarded as the temperature falls, and the curve shifts to the left (see p. 541).

As hypothermia proceeds, there is a mounting retention of CO_2, for although CO_2 production drops, there is an even greater impairment of ventilation. Furthermore, the solubility of CO_2 in plasma increases at lower temperatures. There is therefore a respiratory acidosis, which is easily reversed by controlled respiration. There is usually also a metabolic acidosis due to hypoxia during the stage of induction (associated with shivering and possibly hypovolaemic shock) causing anaerobic glycolysis. It is much reduced if these factors are corrected by proper technique.

Glucose consumption is reduced to a greater extent than oxygen consumption, and the RQ falls. Hepatic and renal function are severely depressed.

Effect on the Nervous System

There is progressive depression of function. There is probably little interference with enzyme activity and synaptic conduction until 28°C (82·4°F). In mild hypothermia the nervous system may be hyper-reactive, and convulsions are not uncommon. Nervous tissue can tolerate severe cooling for limited periods of time.

Effect on the Endocrine Glands

There is no clear-cut pattern, as the response depends on the species, age, and size of the animal. In general, the effect is explicable in terms of ischaemia secondary to vasoconstriction and sludging rather than to any primary effect on the glands themselves.

HYPOTHERMIA IN INFANCY

Newborn infants are particularly susceptible to cold because of the relatively high ratio of surface area to body mass, the paucity of subcutaneous fat, and the low production of heat by physical means because of the inability to take exercise or to shiver. Furthermore, the thermoregulatory mechanism is relatively inefficient at birth, at least for several hours.

The effects are somewhat offset by the action of the collection of *brown fat*.[10,11] This tissue is composed of special fat cells in which there are numerous small lipid droplets, as against the large droplet which characterises the common white-fat cell. A further difference is the presence of numerous mitochondria; indeed, the brown colour is due to the high concentration of iron-containing cytochromes, an essential part of the oxidising enzyme apparatus in the mitochondria. Brown fat is an important tissue in relation to heat production in the very young of some species, in animals during hibernation, and during cold adaptation. Under the influence of noradrenaline released at the sympathetic nerve endings lipid turnover in the brown fat is increased, and the cells split triglyceride molecules into glycerol and fatty acids. The fatty acids are metabolised locally, and this triggers the cycle of heat production. Much of the energy released is converted into heat, and is not stored as ATP.[12] In this way the brown fat helps to increase metabolism and heat production without shivering.

In the human infant there are deposits of brown fat between the shoulder blades and around the neck, with smaller foci behind the sternum and along the spinal column. The part it plays in thermogenesis is uncertain.

In the first few weeks of life infants need constant warmth, especially when ill. In cold countries there is a danger of neglect as coal fires go out and electric and gas heaters are extinguished because of power cuts. Open windows are another hazard. Lukewarm baths in cold surroundings are dangerous as is also the use of tight wrappings which restrict movement.

The early signs of cold injury are lethargy and difficulty in feeding. Indeed, the child has a still, serene appearance, and the cheeks, nose, and extremities have a flush that deludes the onlooker into believing that all is well. The cry is whimpering, and the body feels very cold. The rectal temperature may fall to 32·2°C (90°F). Later there is bradycardia and oedema of the eyelids and extremities.[13] There may be hardening of the subcutaneous tissues in the worst cases.

Oliguria is a common accompaniment, and infection and haemorrhage from the respiratory tract are important complications. Indeed, diffuse pulmonary haemorrhage is an invariable *post-mortem* finding; its cause is obscure, since there is usually little bleeding elsewhere.

The infants should be gradually warmed up for a period of days in a hospital. Prophylaxis is important: the domiciliary midwife should be instructed, and clinical thermometers that record to 24°C (75°F) should be provided.

HYPOTHERMIA IN ADULTS

Hypothermia can occur in adults in a number of circumstances. *Immersion hypothermia* is one of the lethal factors in shipwreck.[14] Hypothermia is an important complication of severe *myxoedema* and *hypopituitarism*, and it occurs also in patients with *widespread eczema* and *generalised erythroderma*. In such skin diseases the passive diffusion of water through the epidermis is greatly increased, and heat is lost by evaporation.

The most important example is the *spontaneous hypothermia* that occurs in old people, usually women, who live alone in poorly-heated rooms and are poorly clothed. Undernutrition is sometimes an additional factor; in both caloric and protein deficient states the basal metabolic rate is decreased.[15] There is often senile dementia, or else depressant drugs like alcohol and chlorpromazine have dulled the mind. There is sometimes a severe precipitating infection such as pneumonia.

Patients in hypothermia look ill; there is a corpse-like chill of the body, and the rectal temperature may drop as low as 21°C (70°F). The skin is pale and the subcutaneous tissues are pliant and doughy. The limbs are still, the muscles rigid, and shivering is rare. The tendon reflexes are sluggish and delayed, and the pupils react sluggishly to light. There is bradycardia, often with atrial fibrillation, and characteristic ECG changes are seen.[16] Peripheral oedema and puffy eyelids are common, so that myxoedema may be simulated in euthyroid individuals. The blood pressure is low, and breathing slow with a prolonged expiratory phase.

Renal function is depressed, and oliguria is a common complication. Pancreatic damage is particularly frequent,[17] and raised serum amylase levels are often noted. Hyperglycaemia is common, and hypoglycaemia may occur as the condition improves. Hypoxia and CO_2 retention due to respiratory depression are other effects of hypothermia. Death occurs from cardiac arrest.[18]

Post-mortem findings include micro-infarcts of many organs (bowel, heart, lung, spleen, kidney, and brain), due probably to stagnation of blood as a result of haemoconcentration and sludging. Pancreatitis and gastric erosions are also frequent findings. Their cause is unknown, but vascular occlusion is the most likely explanation.

The patient should be immersed in warm water and returned expeditiously to a warm atmosphere while general supportive treatment is given.[18] The prognosis is, on the whole, bad. In one series of cases only 7 out of 23 survived. Death usually occurs at a temperature of about 25°C (77°F). It has been found that survivors do not respond to cold with as much increase in heat production and decrease in heat loss as would be expected in normal people. There may be a fundamental abnormality in temperature regulation in these people.[19]

INDUCED HYPOTHERMIA

Hypothermia has played an important part in the development of cardiac surgery, for at a low temperature the body's metabolism is so reduced that cardiac standstill can be tolerated for about an hour. In the early days surface cooling (by immersion in cold water) and venovenous cooling (by removing blood from the body, passing it through a cooling system, and returning it to the body) were used. These procedures are unsatisfactory because ventricular fibrillation occurs at a temperature of about 28°C (82·4°F).

The development of extracorporeal circulatory systems has allowed profound hypothermia to be used in open-heart surgery. In one method the blood is cooled rapidly by passage through a heat-exchanger, and the circulation maintained extracorporeally. At a temperature of 13 to 15°C (55·4 to 59°F) this circulation is stopped, and the heart opened in a bloodless field. When the operation is finished, the blood is rewarmed, the heart defibrillated, and a normal circulation restored. Nowadays extracorporeal circulations are so efficient that hypothermia is not used at all or else merely as an adjunct during the period when the extracorporeal circulation is being discontinued and the patient's own circulation restored.

Experimental hypothermia in animals has revealed remarkable survival patterns.[20] Small animals, like mice, rats, and hamsters, can be cooled to temperatures below 0°C (32°F). They are first made to ingest propylene glycol, and are precooled to 15°C (59°F) under CO_2 narcosis. They are finally immersed in a refrigerant solution until the colonic temperature reaches −3°C (26·6°F) to −5°C (23°F). They can be kept in suspended animation for about an hour and then be re-animated by artificial respiration and microwave diathermy. Larger animals do not tolerate this treatment so well. Although there may be initial survival, death invariably occurs within a few days: gastric haemorrhage and heart failure are common findings.

LOCAL HYPOTHERMIA

When the extremities are exposed to a low temperature there is intense vasoconstriction and the blood flow is reduced. If the immersion is continued, there is a period of vasodilatation. This is short lived, but has the effect of raising the surface temperature temporarily. The phases of vasodilatation are repeated at 5 to 20 minute intervals, thereby producing a 'hunting phenomenon'. During phases of vasoconstriction the blood flow passes through the arteriovenous anastomoses,[21] but the mechanism is still debated; it can occur even after sympathectomy, but is often abnormal in patients with digital vasospasm.[21] The response is best in those who are habitually exposed to the cold. The muscular vessels also dilate when the forearm is immersed in ice-cold water.

Extreme examples of cold injury occur in explorers, soldiers, and mountaineers, in whom there is direct damage to the capillary bed. In severe cases the vascular occlusion leads to infarction and gangrene. This condition of 'frost-bite', or 'trench-foot', is considered further on page 510. It is important to note that local cold injury is due to vascular occlusion and not intracellular ice-crystal formation. This occurs only at extremely low temperatures. A milder cold injury is the common chilblain (*erythema pernio*). It is an inflammation of the subcutaneous fat, i.e. a panniculitis, and appears as a tender, red, pruritic swelling.

There are a number of pathological conditions aggravated by cold: (*a*) *Raynaud's phenomenon*, where even minor degrees of cold can cause vascular spasm and digital ischaemia; (*b*) *cold-antibody syndromes* due to haemagglutinins or haemolysins leading to peripheral vascular occlusion or paroxysmal cold haemoglobinuria (p. 613); (*c*) *cryoglobulinaemia* causing vascular occlusion; (*d*) *cold hypersensitivity*,[22,23] in which local or generalised urticaria appears during the rewarming that follows exposure to cold. There may be oropharyngeal oedema after eating cold foods or even a systemic reaction resembling anaphylaxis following extensive exposure to the cold, as after entering a swimming pool.

The condition is usually acquired in adult life, but a rarer *familial cold urticaria*, inherited as an autosomal dominant trait, is also recognised. It is associated with attacks of urticaria during which there is also malaise, fever, and arthralgia.

In the acquired type the patient usually has a factor in his serum which will transfer the urticaria to a normal person. If the person is given an intradermal injection of the patient's serum, a localised urticarial lesion develops when the area is exposed to cold. The factor is IgE.[24] The actual mediator of the urticarial reaction is still not certain. Histamine is probably not important, and current research favours the kinins and complement cleavage products, possibly anaphylatoxins C3a and C5a. It is, however, strange that an immunoglobulin can be activated by an external physical agent, and not an obvious antigen, to produce an immediate type of hypersensitivity reaction.

Local hypothermia is also used therapeutically. Skin freezing with ethyl chloride spray is an old-fashioned method of local anaesthesia.

Extreme cold is being used in surgical practice (*cryosurgery*).[25] Probes of various shapes refrigerated by liquid nitrogen and other liquefied gases, or by thermo-electric devices, are used. The applications include the destruction of tumours both benign and malignant, ophthalmological procedures, especially the fixation of detached retinae, and destructive intracranial surgery. Gastric hypothermia for controlling peptic ulceration has proved disappointing. At present, the use of cold in surgery is confined to specialist centres, and the late effects are still being assessed.

REFERENCES

1. Fox, R. H. *et al.* (1971) Diagnosis of accidental hypothermia of the elderly. *Lancet,* **1,** 424.
2. Atkins, E. & Bodel, P. (1972) Fever. *New England Journal of Medicine,* **286,** 27.
3. Wood, W. B. (1970) In *Infectious Agents and Host Reactions,* ed. Mudd, S., pp. 146–162. (The pathogenesis of fever). Philadelphia: Saunders.
4. Leading Article (1968) Heat stroke. *Lancet,* **2,** 31.
5. Leading Article (1900) Body-temperature and the emotions. *Lancet,* **2,** 475.
6. Leading Article (1971) Malignant hyperpyrexia. *British Medical Journal,* **3,** 441.
7. Kalow, W. *et al.* (1970) Metabolic error of muscle metabolism after recovery from malignant hyperthermia. *Lancet,* **2,** 895.
8. Gordon, R. A., Britt, B. A. & Kalow, W. (1973) *International Symposium on Malignant Hyperthermia.* Springfield: Thomas.
9. Various Authors (1961) Hypothermia and the effects of cold. *British Medical Bulletin,* **17,** 1–73.
10. Lindberg, O. (1970) *Brown Adipose Tissue.* New York: Elsevier.
11. Hollenberg, C. H., Angel, A. & Steiner, G. (1970) The metabolism of white and brown adipose tissue. *Canadian Medical Association Journal,* **103,** 843.
12. Hochachka, P. W. (1974) Regulation of heat production at the cellular level. *Federation Proceedings,* **33,** 2162.
13. Bower, B. D., Jones, L. F. & Weeks, M. M. (1960) Cold injury in the newborn: a study of 70 cases. *British Medical Journal,* **1,** 303.
14. Keatinge, W. R. (1969) *Survival in Cold Water.* Oxford: Blackwell.
15. Ablett, J. G. & McCance, R. A. (1971) Energy expenditure of children with kwashiorkor. *Lancet,* **2,** 517.
16. Emslie-Smith, D. (1958) Accidental hypothermia: a common condition with a pathognomonic electrocardiogram. *Lancet,* **2,** 492.
17. Read, A. E. *et al.* (1961) Pancreatitis and accidental hypothermia. *Lancet,* **2,** 1219.
18. Leading Article (1972) Severe accidental hypothermia. *Lancet,* **1,** 237.
19. Macmillan, A. L. *et al.* (1967) Temperature regulation in survivors of accidental hypothermia of the elderly. *Lancet,* **2,** 165.
20. Kenyon, J. R. (1961) Experimental deep hypothermia. *British Medical Bulletin,* **17,** 43.
21. Fox, R. H. (1968) Effects of cold on the extremities. *Proceedings of the Royal Society of Medicine,* **61,** 785.
22. Leading Article (1975) Cold hypersensitivity. *Lancet,* **1,** 207.
23. Leading Article (1975) Cold hypersensitivity. *British Medical Journal,* **1,** 643.
24. Houser, D. D. *et al.* (1970) Cold urticaria; immunologic studies. *American Journal of Medicine,* **49,** 23.
25. Leading Article (1968) Surgical cold. *British Medical Journal,* **4,** 342.

Chapter 38. Disturbances in the Body's Fluid and Electrolyte Balance

Water is the principal constituent of the body. It forms the bulk of the cellular protoplasm, and is the vehicle of transport of essential metabolic factors to the cell and of waste products to the exterior. In this aqueous medium the electrolytes of the body are held in solution. Some of these, like potassium, calcium, and magnesium, are necessary for normal cell function, whereas others, like sodium and chloride, maintain an adequate osmotic pressure for the extracellular water. Cells can survive only within a very narrow range of hydrogen ion concentration, and the pH of the extracellular water is regulated to a great extent by the bicarbonate ion.

Any serious deficiency of extracellular water soon interferes with the circulation of the blood, and death rapidly ensues. This circulating fluid is sustained osmotically by those electrolytes which are normally present in the greatest concentration, namely sodium and chloride. A depletion of salt rapidly leads to circulatory failure. For this reason it is necessary always to relate disturbances in water metabolism to the state of salt balance in the body. In the clinical condition of 'dehydration' there is usually a combined salt and water depletion, but even if there is a pure water deficiency, the ensuing manifestations are related to a secondary alteration in salt balance as well as to the primary water lack.

THE NORMAL DISTRIBUTION OF WATER AND ELECTROLYTES IN THE BODY WATER[1]

About 72 per cent of the lean body weight consists of water. As the water content of adipose tissue is very low, the actual water content of the body is somewhat less than this; it is about 60 per cent in the normal adult male, and about 5 per cent less in the female. This water is contained in two compartments, an intracellular and an extracellular one. The extracellular compartment is further subdivided into an intravascular and extravascular (interstitial) space. There is a constant interchange of fluid between the intracellular and extracellular compartments, and the methods used to determine the body's fluid spaces depend on the principle of administering a known amount of a substance whose distribution is accurately confined to one or more spaces, and then determining its final concentration in the plasma. Thus, tritiated water or urea is used to measure the *total body water*, inulin or radioactive sodium the *extracellular fluid volume*, and dye-dilution techniques (using Evans blue) or radio-iodinated plasma proteins the *plasma volume*.

The following figures provide a guide for the volumes in a normal male adult weighing 70 kg:

Total body water: 42 litres.

Intracellular water: 28 litres (two-thirds of total body water, or 40 per cent of the body's weight). It is obtained by subtracting the extracellular volume from the total body water.

Extracellular water: 14 litres (one-third of total body water, or 20 per cent of the body's weight). It has two components:

Interstitial water: 11·2 litres are present in the extracellular extravascular space. This is obtained by subtracting the plasma volume from the extracellular water.

Plasma volume: 2·8 litres.

Blood volume: 5 litres. This is obtained by adding the red-cell mass, as measured directly or calculated from the haematocrit reading, to the plasma volume.

In practice it is difficult to define the boundary between the extracellular and intracellular water, because some of the extracellular water is sequestered in dense connective tissue, cartilage, and especially bone, and cannot equilibrate rapidly with the other portions of the extracellular fluid, viz. the plasma, interstitial fluid, and lymph. About 15 per cent of the body's water is present in dense connective tissue and bone, and is liable to be included in the intracellular moiety in equilibration measurements. Nevertheless, the concept of separate tissue spaces is helpful so long as the difficulties in absolute measurement are borne in mind.

Electrolytes[1]

The electrolyte composition of the intracellular and extracellular fluids is quite distinct:

(a) In the intracellular fluid the principal cations are *potassium* and *magnesium*, and the principal anions are *phosphate* and *protein*.

(b) In the extracellular fluid the predominant cation is *sodium*, and the principal anions are *chloride* and *bicarbonate*.

The electrolytes perform two main functions:

1. They are the principal *solutes* in the body fluids, and therefore account for most of their osmotic pressure.

2. The concentration of individual *ions* influences the properties and behaviour of excitable membranes, e.g. of nerve cells, and the performance of many intracellular enzymes.

Electrolytes as solutes. The osmotic effect of substances in solution is determined by the number of particles present, i.e. ions and unionised molecules. For dilute solutions, the osmotic activity is very nearly equal to the actual concentration of particles: a solute concentration of 1 millimole per litre has an osmotic activity of 1 milliosmole per litre. A millimole is one thousandth of a mole, or gram-molecular weight. Thus, 1 millimole of glucose (MW 180) is 180 mg, and 1 millimole of urea (MW 60) is 60 mg. The same terminology can be used for ions, so that 1 millimole of Na^+ is 23 mg, 1 millimole of Cl^- is 35·5 mg, and 1 millimole of Ca^{2+} is 40 mg. The osmotic activity of electrolytes depends on the number of ions. Thus 58·5 mg NaCl in 1 litre of water becomes 23 mg Na^+ and 35·5 mg of Cl^-; the concentration of each ion is 1 millimole per litre, but the osmotic activity of the solution is due to both ions, and will be 2 milliosmoles per litre. Again, 111 mg of $CaCl_2$ in a litre of water becomes 40 mg of Ca^{2+} and 71 mg of Cl^-; the concentration of Ca^{2+} is 1 millimole per litre, that of Cl^- is 2 millimoles per litre, and the osmotic activity of the solution is 3 milliosmoles per litre.

The total osmotic activity of plasma (measured by depression of freezing point) is about 300 milliosmoles per kg water. Expressing each solute in the same terms (millimoles per litre), Na^+ (140) and Cl^- (100) are clearly the predominant contributors, followed by HCO_3^- (27), K^+, urea, and glucose (about 5 each), with much smaller contributions from Ca^{2+}, protein, phosphate, Mg^{2+}, etc. *The concentration of sodium is the best indication of the osmolality* of the plasma, i.e. the concentration of particles in solution.*

The osmotic pressure of the interstitial fluid (extravascular extracellular fluid) differs from that of plasma only by the small contribution of plasma protein. This is about 1·5 milliosmoles per litre, which corresponds to a hydrostatic pressure of about 25 mm Hg.

The osmotic pressure of intracellular fluid is thought to be equal to that of interstitial fluid because measurements of the depression of freezing point show no difference. However, since the concentrations, and indeed the effective molecular weights, of many of the intracellular constituents are still unknown, one cannot draw up an exact table of their respective contributions to the total intracellular osmotic pressure. The principal solutes are K^+, Mg^{2+}, protein, and organic phosphates.

Electrolytes as ions. Ions are charged particles, either atoms (e.g. Na^+ and Cl^-), or larger radicals (e.g. HCO_3^- and SO_4^{2-}), or molecules (e.g. protein, which carries a net negative charge at the pH of body fluids). *Cations* are positively charged, and *anions* negatively charged. Any one positive charge is equivalent to any one negative charge. Thus, 1 Na (monovalent) ion is equivalent to 1 Cl (monovalent) ion, but 1 Ca (divalent) ion is equivalent to 2 Cl ions. The equivalent weight of an ion is its atomic or molecular weight in grams divided by its valency, and a milliequivalent is one thousandth part of an equivalent. A milliequivalent of Na^+ (atomic weight 23) is 23 mg, of Cl^- 35·5 mg, and of Ca^{2+} (atomic weight 40) 20 mg.

The biological effect of an electrolyte depends to a considerable extent on its equivalent concentration, i.e. the number of particles present and the number of charges carried by each. It is therefore appropriate to describe the concentration of electrolytes in milliequivalents per litre.† Not only is this a more

logical description of electrolytes than one in grams or milligrams per dl, but it also allows the relative importance of each ion to be seen. Moreover, since any solution must contain the same concentration of cations as of anions, a balance can be struck between the two categories of electrolytes. This is shown in the following table of the composition of plasma:

Cations (in mEq per litre)			*Anions* (in mEq per litre)		
Na^+	142	(range 137–148)	Cl^-	103	(range 99–108)
K^+	5	(range 4.0–5.5)	HCO_3^-	24	(range 21–27)
Ca^{2+}	3	(ionised fraction)	Other	8	(includes HPO_4^-,
Mg^{2+}	1·5	(ionised fraction)	anions		SO_4^{2-}, and
					organic acids, e.g.
					keto acids)
			Protein	16	(range 15–20)
Total:	150	(approx)	Total	150	(approx)

In this table the values for calcium and magnesium are less than their normal plasma levels, because only the ionised fraction can be accurately expressed in mEq per litre. Now that Système International (SI) units are used in many countries, it is better to express the concentrations of electrolytes in millimoles per litre, as described above. The following table gives the concentration of some of the more important electrolytes; it will be noted that the figures for sodium, potassium, chloride, and bicarbonate remain unchanged in mmol per litre as compared with mEq per litre.

Plasma sodium	137–148 mmol per litre
Plasma potassium	4·0–5·5 mmol per litre
Plasma chloride	99–108 mmol per litre
Plasma bicarbonate	21–27 mmol per litre
Plasma calcium	2.3–2.6 mmol per litre
Plasma magnesium	0.7–1.0 mmol per litre

Plasma proteins are not measured in mmol per litre but in grams per litre.

It is clear from the table that sodium is all-important in sustaining the cationic level of the extracellular fluid, and that it is balanced on the anionic side by the combined concentrations of chloride and bicarbonate. This combined level is normally about 12 mmol per litre less than that of sodium. In practice the level of plasma chloride follows the level of plasma sodium quite closely, provided the plasma bicarbonate level remains constant. An alteration of plasma bicarbonate in response to an acidosis or alkalosis is usually attended by an opposite alteration in the chloride level, and the combined concentration of the two anions remains fairly constant. If, however, the acidosis is due to an excess of keto acids, as in diabetic coma, the plasma bicarbonate falls, the chloride is unchanged, and the anions of the keto acids rise.

The anion gap.[2] With the electrolyte concentrations expressed in mEq (or mmol) per litre, the anion gap is defined as the difference between the sum of the major plasma cations and the major anions:

$$\text{Anion gap} = (Na^+ + K^+) - (Cl^- + HCO_3^-)\text{*}$$

* Some clinicians omit the potassium from this calculation, and the anion gap is lowered. The normal figure is then about 12. If the biochemical profile obtained by the use of the SMA-12 AutoAnalyzer is available, there is no virtue in introducing an additional error due to variations in the potassium level.

---

*Osmolality = solute concentration per kg water.
Osmolarity = solute concentration per litre solution.
In most biological fluids the two are very similar, but the procedures used (determinations of freezing point and vapour pressure) measure osmolality (in milliosmoles per kg water) rather than osmolarity.

†In order to convert concentrations of ions from mg per dl to mEq per litre, a simple formula is used:

$$\frac{\text{mg per 100 ml}}{\text{equivalent weight of element}} \times 10$$

In practice the value in mg per dl is divided by 2·3 for sodium, 3·9 for potassium, 2·24 for bicarbonate (as ml CO_2 per dl), and 3·55 for chloride.

To convert concentrations of substances (including ions) from mg per dl to mmol per litre, a similar formula is used, except that the molecular weight of the substance is substituted for the equivalent weight of the element.

The normal value is about 16 mEq (or mmol) per litre, but the range varies among individual laboratories. Calculating the anion gap is simple; a raised level indicates an increase in the anions excluded from the calculation: e.g. phosphate, sulphate, lactate, hydroxybutyrate, or acetoacetate. Common causes are renal failure, lactic acidosis, and diabetic ketoacidosis. It also occurs following poisoning with methanol, ethylene glycol, and paraldehyde, and in the acidotic phase of salicylate poisoning.

A low anion gap is uncommon but occurs in hypoalbuminaemia, since albumin contributes a major fraction to the gap. The gap is also low in monoclonal gammopathies with a high level of M protein. This is probably because the increased viscosity of the serum produces errors in the automatic analysers in common use. A low anion gap is also a feature of *bromism*. Although bromide replaces chloride, the common AutoAnalyzer method for chloride cannot distinguish between the two halides and, in fact, is more sensitive to bromide than chloride. Hence the 'plasma chloride' estimation is greater than the actual halide concentration, and the estimated anion gap is low or even negative.

Figure 38.1
Diagrammatic representation of the three compartments in which the body's water is accommodated. An excess or deficiency of water, which is freely diffusible, produces the greatest effects in the largest compartment, the intracellular one, whereas changes in sodium affect mainly the volume of the interstitial fluid.

The mode of transport of water and electrolytes from one compartment to another is still imperfectly understood. It is generally accepted that the three compartments (see Fig. 38.1) are in osmotic equilibrium with one another, and that shifts from one to another are always secondary to changes in electrolyte concentration, so that the movement of water in or out of compartments depends on the balance of ions on either side of the dividing membrane.

DISTURBANCES IN WATER AND SODIUM METABOLISM[1]

Normal Water Balance

The loss of water from the body is of two types: uncontrolled, or inevitable, as from the skin and lungs, and controlled as from the sweat glands and kidneys. The inevitable skin loss is due to diffusion of water from the deeper layers, which is evaporated from the surface. It is called transpiration and in temperate climates is from 300 to 500 ml per day. It plays only a small part in the regulation of the body's temperature, and can, if necessary, be supplemented by the active secretion of sweat. This is not pure water, like the fluid of transpiration, but contains actively secreted sodium chloride in a concentration rather less than half that of plasma. The secretion of sweat is normally less than 100 ml per day in temperate climates.

The loss of water from the lungs is about 700 ml per day, and is due to the humidification of air in the respiratory tract. About 200 ml of water are lost in the faeces each day; the remainder of the 8 litres secreted in the alimentary tract is reabsorbed. Finally there is the obligatory loss in the urine. This varies according to the fluid intake; the kidney can concentrate urine to 1400 milliosmoles per kg (this represents a specific gravity of 1·035), and dilute it down to 30 milliosmoles per kg.

The precise fluid intake varies with the climate and personal habits of the individual. A minimum in temperate climates is from 500 to 1000 ml per day. Some of this is consumed as food, for from 200 to 300 ml are provided from the water of oxidation of the food.

Normal Sodium Balance

The sodium content of a normal adult is about 4000 mmol (90 g). Only about 3 per cent is present in the intracellular fluid. Forty per cent is stored in the bones, and the remainder circulates in the extracellular fluid. All the sodium present in the soft tissues is freely exchangeable, but only about 45 per cent of that in the bones is available for exchange. About 70 per cent of the total sodium is exchangeable.

The average daily intake of sodium in a temperate climate is probably 100 to 300 mmol (2·3 to 6·9 g). In hot climates, where sweating is profuse, it is much greater than this. An amount almost equal to the intake of sodium is excreted in the urine each day, and a much smaller quantity is lost in the faeces. The amount lost by sweating is negligible in temperate climates.

The balance of sodium (and chloride) is finely adjusted by the kidney. Two mechanisms are known:

The glomerular filtration rate. About 80 per cent of the sodium is normally reabsorbed by the proximal convoluted tubule. While some authorities believe that this is under hormonal control, the more important factor is the rate of glomerular filtration. If this is reduced, the amount of sodium excreted in the urine is decreased, and sodium is retained. This occurs promptly whenever the cardiac output is decreased, e.g. following haemorrhage. The afferent part of this response is believed to be the arterial baroreceptors, e.g. in the carotid sinus and aortic arch. They are susceptible to changes in blood volume. The efferent part of the response is probably *via* the vasomotor centre and the sympathetic outflow. In this way the renal blood flow is reduced whenever the blood volume is reduced; glomerular filtration is decreased and sodium is retained.

There is a rapid fall in the urinary output of sodium on standing. This may be due to a higher proportion of the filtered sodium being reabsorbed by the proximal tubule. The mechanism is not known.

Proximal tubular sodium reabsorption may be influenced by the volume of the blood or extracellular fluid space in another way, when an expansion of the volume causes an increased excretion of sodium that is independent of an increased glomerular filtration rate or a diminished secretion of aldosterone. The mechanism concerned is still unknown; the secretion of a sodium-losing hormone has been postulated but not proven.[3–5]

The completeness of reabsorption of sodium by the distal tubule. This is controlled by *aldosterone*, secreted by the zona glomerulosa of the adrenal cortex. It is the principal mineralocorticoid, and has an important influence on the exchanges of sodium, potassium, and hydrogen in the distal tubule. The secretion of aldosterone is related to the volume of the extracellular fluid and the concentration of sodium in it. The most important stimulator of aldosterone is angiotensin, which itself is produced when the renal blood flow is decreased. Angiotensin also has a direct effect on sodium excretion by the kidney—slow infusions cause its retention and more rapid ones may lead to a diuresis of sodium and water.[1] ACTH has little effect on aldosterone secretion.

Cortisol has mild mineralocorticoid activity. It is important for sustaining the normal rate of glomerular filtration and allowing the normal response to a water load (see p. 552).

It therefore follows that a reduction of blood volume, in addition to reducing the glomerular filtration rate, also leads to the secretion of aldosterone and the further retention of sodium (Fig. 38.2). Expansion of the blood volume has the converse effect.

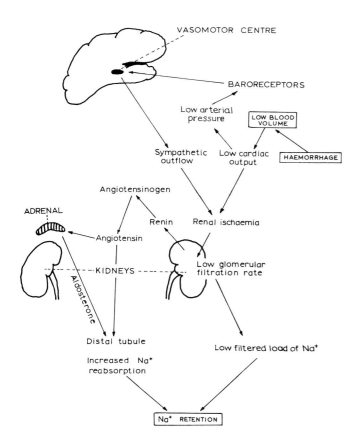

Figure 38.2
Diagrammatic representation of the means whereby the body retains sodium after a sudden reduction in blood volume, e.g. following severe haemorrhage.

Fluid balance is controlled by three factors:

1. Indirectly by the mechanisms that regulate sodium balance. Sodium is not retained without water provided thirst and antidiuretic hormone are active.

2. The mechanisms that regulate the output of water by the kidney—the antidiuretic hormone of the pituitary is important.

3. Regulation of water intake by the sensation of thirst.

Antidiuretic hormone (ADH), or *vasopressin*, is secreted by the posterior lobe of the pituitary, which is closely connected to the hypothalamus. It conserves water by increasing reabsorption from the distal tubules and collecting ducts (p. 551). Its secretion is regulated by the following factors:

The osmotic concentration of the extracellular fluid in the hypothalamus. If this is diluted, there is a diuresis of hypotonic urine, whereas if it is concentrated through fluid deprivation, a scanty hypertonic urine is secreted. This response is mediated by osmoreceptors, which lie close to the supraoptic nuclei of the hypothalamus.

The baroreceptors sensitive to blood volume. A reduction of blood volume stimulates ADH secretion. On the other hand, left atrial distension simulates an increase in blood volume and inhibits its secretion. The baroreceptor effect on ADH secretion is less sensitive than the osmoreceptor effect. Thus, the rapid ingestion of a litre of water so decreases the osmolality of the plasma and interstitial fluids that a diuresis ensues within 15 to 30 minutes, and the whole volume is excreted in a few hours. If the fluid is isotonic saline, the diuresis is much slower and more prolonged; 12 to 24 hours may elapse before the litre is eliminated. Thus a change in osmolality affects ADH secretion more rapidly than does an alteration in blood volume.

Pain, fear, and *certain pharmacological agents,* e.g. nicotine, anaesthetics, adrenaline, and histamine, all stimulate ADH secretion, while alcohol inhibits it and causes a diuresis.

Thirst.[6] The sensation of dryness in the mouth and throat that accompanies thirst is of great importance in motivating fluid intake, but its mechanism is not well understood. It is experienced both after a reduction in extracellular fluid volume, e.g. haemorrhage, and when there is intracellular dehydration, e.g. after salt ingestion. Presumably impulses from the baroreceptors and osmoreceptors are integrated centrally in the hypothalamus, where fresh impulses control the secretions of the mouth and throat. However, the thirst is quenched long before the water is absorbed from the intestine. Perhaps a central mechanism receives afferent impulses directly from the oesophagus and stomach.

DISTURBANCES OF WATER AND SODIUM BALANCE

Pure Water Deficiency

There is a direct deprivation or loss of water without a corresponding depletion of electrolytes. It is uncommon, but may occur under the following circumstances:

(*a*) Following deprivation of water, e.g. in people who cannot swallow because of oesophageal obstruction or coma, during enforced starvation, and after shipwreck.

(*b*) In diabetes insipidus, where there is defective reabsorption of water from the collecting tubules of the kidney.

Effects. There is an increased osmolality of the extracellular fluid. This leads to a transfer of intracellular water to the extracellular compartment and a consequent cellular dehydration. As the water leaves the cells, it is accompanied by potassium ions. The water excretion in the urine is reduced to a minimum (in diabetes insipidus there can be no spontaneous decrease in urinary volume) as a result of an increased secretion of ADH. Sodium excretion is unchanged at first, but later on, when there is a shrinkage of the extracellular fluid volume, aldosterone is secreted, and this reduces sodium excretion. This effect is accentuated in those cases where the water deprivation is part of a general starvation. Loss of potassium in the urine continues, and is indeed augmented by the increased secretion of aldosterone. This type of dehydration affects the intracellular fluid *par excellence*, and is associated especially with water and potassium loss.

Clinical and Biochemical Manifestations

Intense Thirst.

Oliguria. The urine is concentrated and of very high specific gravity. It contains much sodium chloride at first, but later on the level drops. In diabetes insipidus there is a continued polyuria.

Plasma changes. The plasma constituents, e.g. sodium and proteins, rise in concentration, but the haemoglobin concentration and packed cell volume are unchanged because of a loss of water from the red cells. The plasma urea level rises early because of the increased urea reabsorption from the tubules, and not through renal failure.

Fever. This is important in infants.

Results. There are no immediate ill-effects, but eventually hypotension and coma occur due to intracellular dehydration of vital organs.

Treatment. Non-saline fluids are given orally or parenterally.

Combined Sodium and Water Deficiency

This is a combined deficiency, but sodium depletion often predominates. It is often called salt depletion, for sodium and chloride are usually lost in equal proportions. But in vomiting due to gastric disease and in the diuresis that follows the use of some diuretics, the chloride loss exceeds that of sodium. This does not in itself affect the volume of the extracellular fluid appreciably, as the chloride is replaced by bicarbonate (see p. 475). Thus the level of chloride in the plasma or urine is an unsatisfactory index of sodium balance.

The deficiency is due to a loss of sodium and water:

From the gastrointestinal tract. The commonest examples are encountered in gastrointestinal disorders associated with severe vomiting or diarrhoea, e.g. intestinal obstruction, pyloric stenosis, acute dilatation of the stomach, ulcerative colitis, and cholera. Intestinal and biliary fistulae have a similar effect.

From the sweat. A single large sweat produces the picture of pure water depletion with severe thirst and oliguria, but repeated sweating leads to sodium depletion as well. If the water loss is remedied without giving adequate additional salt, the picture becomes one of predominant sodium deficiency, and the state of *heat exhaustion* follows.

From the urine. One of the commonest examples of severe sodium loss from the kidneys is seen in patients with chronic heart failure who are fed on a low-salt diet and given thiazide diuretics. Other conditions associated with increased sodium loss in the urine are Addison's disease, salt-losing nephritis, and diabetes mellitus with its osmotic diuresis. Acute pathological processes involving the brain, e.g. bulbar poliomyelitis, acute encephalitis, and cerebrovascular disease are sometimes accompanied by an increased excretion of salt in the urine and hyponatraemia, though occasionally the converse condition of decreased urinary salt excretion and hypernatraemia is encountered. The mechanism is obscure: possibly a nervous connexion between the brain and the kidneys is destroyed by the disease. There are some authorities who deny the existence of a specific syndrome, and attribute the disturbances to the effects of starvation and dehydration.[7]

From the blood and plasma. Severe haemorrhage and the great plasma loss following extensive burns lead to sodium deficiency.

Effects. When sodium depletion predominates, the osmotic support of the extracellular fluid is undermined. In order to maintain its tonicity, the extracellular fluid transfers its water to the cells which become relatively overhydrated. In the early stages there may even be a similar tendency to excrete water in the urine, so that oliguria is not necessarily an immediate manifestation. Later, however, the volume of extracellular fluid becomes seriously reduced.

With a combined loss in which there is an equal depletion of both sodium and water, there is a rapid reduction in the volume of extracellular fluid without at first any fall in the level of sodium, although it may later fall as ADH secretion is stimulated and water is retained.

The reduction in volume of the extracellular fluid leads to a state of shock. This is manifested particularly in the renal circulation, the arterioles of which undergo vasoconstriction. This type of dehydration affects the extracellular fluid *par excellence*, and is associated with severe water and sodium loss.

Clinical and biochemical manifestations. '*Dehydration*'. The eyeballs are sunken, the skin wrinkled, the tongue dry, and the face haggard. Thirst is often absent. Despite a compensatory vasoconstriction, the blood pressure is low and the veins are poorly filled. There is tachycardia.

Muscle cramps in the legs and abdomen are a feature of predominant sodium deficiency.

The urine contains very little sodium and chloride. Early on there may be no reduction in volume, and the concentrating power of the kidneys is good. Later there is severe oliguria due to renal failure.

Plasma changes. There is a reduced plasma volume evidenced by raised levels of proteins, packed cell volume, and haemoglobin. The viscosity of the blood is increased, and its specific gravity—normally 1·050 to 1·060—rises. The plasma sodium level drops as the condition progresses. A rising plasma urea indicates renal failure.

Results. Death due to circulatory failure rapidly follows. In patients who survive there is a danger of subsequent renal tubular necrosis.

Treatment. Remedy the cause and administer saline solutions.

Pure Water Excess

This is called *water intoxication* and it is encountered under the following circumstances:

(*a*) In the early postoperative period when patients are given large infusions of glucose solution. This cannot be excreted rapidly because of the tendency to water and salt retention after traumatic incidents.

(*b*) The administration of water to patients suffering from sodium depletion, e.g. in cardiac disease being treated with diuretics and a low-sodium diet, in Addison's disease where there is an inability to excrete a water load as well as a salt deficiency, and in heatstroke.

(*c*) The administration of injudiciously large amounts of water in renal failure, especially the acute type.

(*d*) Where there is excessive secretion of ADH. This may occur in lesions near the supraoptic nuclei. ADH is produced in some cases of oat-cell lung cancer (see p. 340).

Effects. The extracellular compartment is distended and its osmolality is reduced. The excess water moves freely into the cells, and the resulting intracellular oedema causes damage. There may be an early diuresis, but soon the renal cells also are damaged, and oliguria or even anuria may follow.

Clinical and biochemical manifestations. *Nausea, Vomiting, and Weakness.*

Cerebral symptoms, e.g. headache, drowsiness, apathy, stupor, epileptiform convulsions, and coma.

Plasma changes. There is a reduction in the concentration of all the plasma electrolytes, and the plasma osmolality is decreased. The packed cell volume and plasma protein level are also reduced.

Results. Death due to widespread cellular damage occurs if the condition persists.

Treatment. Hypertonic saline may be given intravenously, but caution should be observed. It is usually safer to wait for water loss.

Combined Sodium and Water Excess

This is an artificially-induced condition in which patients with defective renal function are given excessive amounts of saline solutions, e.g. during the early postoperative period or during the course of acute renal failure. The fluid is distributed evenly throughout the extracellular compartment which becomes expanded. There is no alteration in the level of plasma electrolytes, but the packed cell volume and plasma protein level are decreased. The manifestations are an increased venous pressure and systemic oedema. In due course pulmonary oedema will kill the patient.

DISTURBANCES OF POTASSIUM BALANCE[1]

Normal Potassium Balance

The potassium content of a normal adult is about 133 g (3400 mmol). Over 95 per cent of it is intracellular, and less than 5 per cent extracellular. About three-quarters of the intracellular potassium is present in the skeletal musculature.

The normal daily consumption of potassium is 2 to 3 g (52 to 78 mmol), and a similar amount is excreted in the urine, together with small quantities in the faeces and sweat. There is an active secretion of potassium from the colonic mucosa.

The concentration of potassium in the extracellular fluid is very low (4 to 5·5 mmol per litre); it is predominantly a cellular electrolyte, forming over two-thirds of the intracellular cations. When it leaves the cells, it is rapidly excreted by the kidneys. A plasma level above 7·5 mmol per litre produces clinical symptoms, and over 10 mmol per litre it is rapidly fatal. The body possesses no means of intensive potassium retention comparable with those for sodium.

An unobtrusive loss of potassium from the cells into the plasma and then into the urine occurs under the following circumstances:

Whenever water is mobilised from the cells, e.g. during water deprivation.

Whenever cell protein is broken down, e.g. as a normal response to trauma or following starvation. It is estimated that 100 to 120 mg potassium are liberated with every gram of nitrogen (about 2·5 to 3·0 mmol per gram).

Conversely, the administration of glucose and insulin diverts the extracellular potassium into the cells where it aids in the deposition of glycogen.

Potassium is actively secreted by the distal tubules of the kidney, and this is potentiated by aldosterone, and to a lesser extent by cortisol and deoxycorticosterone.

The concentration of potassium in the plasma is an inadequate indication of potassium balance, because a high level may be merely an indication of its effective mobilisation from the cells prior to its excretion by the kidneys. Only in the later stages of potassium loss does the plasma concentration fall appreciably. In the same way a low concentration may be merely an indication of a diversion of potassium ions into the cells, as after glucose and insulin administration. In the commonest type of the rare disorder *familial periodic paralysis* there are paroxysms of generalised muscular weakness associated with a dramatic fall in the level of plasma potassium

TABLE 38.1 The main metabolic changes in the various types of sodium and water disturbance

	Plasma sodium	Plasma urea	Plasma proteins	Packed Cell volume	Urine
Pure Water Deficiency	Raised	Raised	Raised	Normal	Oliguria[a] (concentrated)
Sodium and Water Deficiency	Reduced[b]	Raised later	Raised	Raised	Variable at first; soon severely reduced
Water Excess	Reduced	Raised terminally	Reduced	Reduced	Variable. Reduced terminally
Water and Sodium Excess—No specific changes apart from expansion of extracellular compartment. There is a lowering of plasma proteins and packed cell volume.					

[a]This does not apply to diabetes insipidus.

[b]In predominant sodium deficiency this occurs early, but in a combined deficiency with equal depletion of sodium and water the plasma sodium is reduced later.

and a decrease in its urinary excretion. It appears that there is a shift of potassium to the intracellular phase, and that attacks may be precipitated by agencies that potentiate this shift, e.g. adrenaline, emotion, carbohydrate ingestion, and insulin. The condition is relieved by the administration of potassium salts.

Potassium Depletion

The loss of potassium may take place either in the gastrointestinal secretions or in the urine.

From the gastrointestinal tract. The gastric juice contains about twice the concentration of potassium of plasma, but severe vomiting is not an important cause of hypokalaemia unless there are secondary renal changes as in pyloric stenosis (see p. 485). The faecal excretion of potassium is high (twice that of sodium), and chronic diarrhoea, as in ulcerative colitis and the malabsorption syndrome, leads to serious potassium deficiency. Potassium-secreting villous adenomata of the colon have the same effect. Obsessional purgative-users may develop extreme hypokalaemia.

From the urine. The osmotic diuresis of diabetes mellitus is a potent cause of potassium loss. Diuretics, e.g. chlorothiazide, may have the same effect. Primary hyperaldosteronism (Conn's syndrome) leads to very severe potassium loss, and is easily mistaken for potassium-losing nephritis. Cushing's syndrome produces a milder effect, but the Cushing-like disorder associated with oat-cell lung cancers that secrete ACTH may lead to severe hypokalaemic alkalosis (see p. 452).

Finally, intrinsic renal disease may lead to serious potassium loss. This is uncommon, and is always associated with an impaired excretion of hydrogen ions by the distal tubules (see Ch. 46). Uretero-colic anastomosis leads to hypokalaemia by a combined colonic and renal loss.

Effects. Potassium deprivation impairs cellular function; muscular weakness is a feature of this. The kidneys are damaged by severe potassium depletion. Histologically there appears to be vacuolation of the cells of the proximal tubules, but in fact this is due to the accumulation of fluid outside the cells (p. 52). Potassium deficiency probably also predisposes the kidney to pyelonephritis.

Hypokalaemia leads to metabolic alkalosis. Hydrogen ions and sodium ions enter the intracellular fluid to replace the lost potassium ions.[8] Thus there is a cellular acidosis and sodium retention with an extracellular alkalosis and sodium depletion. However, chloride depletion, if it occurs simultaneously, may be more important in producing both the alkalosis and the potassium depletion (see p. 485).

In true potassium-losing nephritis there is severe acidosis because the primary defect is a failure of urine acidification.

Clinical manifestations. *Intense muscular asthenia.* This is not confined to the skeletal musculature, but affects the smooth muscle of the gut also, and may lead to paralytic ileus. Paradoxically enough, potassium depletion occasionally causes tetany.

Mental changes. Apathy, confusion, and amnesia may be prominent. Coma eventually follows.

Renal dysfunction is particularly important in chronic potassium deficiency. There is an early failure of concentration, for the tubules do not respond to antidiuretic hormone. Polyuria and nocturia are prominent symptoms, and later on

clinical pyelonephritis may supervene. There may also be a failure to acidify the urine.

Cardiac changes. These are particularly common in elderly people. There is irregularity of the heart rate, hypotension, and cardiac dilatation; the toxic effects of digitalis are potentiated. The electrocardiograph shows flattened T waves with ST segment depression and prominent U waves.

Death is generally due to respiratory failure caused by weakness of the muscles of respiration, though it may also be attributable to cardiac failure and renal damage.

Potassium Excess

Hyperkalaemia is due to renal inadequacy in excreting potassium. The most important cause of severe potassium retention is acute renal failure with anuria. In the terminal uraemia of chronic renal failure there is also considerable potassium retention.

In Addison's disease there is moderate hyperkalaemia due to a deficiency of adrenal cortical hormones, but the raised potassium concentration in the plasma is seldom sufficient to produce ill-effects.

A third cause of hyperkalaemia is the rapid infusion of potassium salts in conditions of hypokalaemia. Sudden death has followed the injudicious parenteral administration of potassium salts.

The clinical manifestations of potassium retention are somewhat vague. Confusion, apathy, and sensory disturbances (paraesthesiae) are often present and, rather unexpectedly, there may also be severe muscular weakness as in potassium depletion. Indeed, there is a very rare form of familial periodic paralysis due to hyperkalaemia.[9] Cardiac dysfunction is important. There are characteristically high, peaked T waves on the electrocardiograph. Ventricular fibrillation may follow, and cause death.

DISTURBANCES IN MAGNESIUM BALANCE[1,10]

The magnesium content of a normal adult is about 25 g (1000 mmol), about half being in the bones and the other half in the cells, where it is the second most important cation, forming rather less than a third of the cationic content. It is an essential component of many enzymes, including the phosphoglucomutase in the mitochondria. The daily intake varies, usually being in the range of 0·2 to 0·42 g (8 to 17 mmol).

The plasma level (which is the same as that of the gastrointestinal secretions) is low, 0·7 to 1·0 mmol per litre (1·8 to 2·4 mg per dl). About 55 per cent of the plasma magnesium is ionised. Magnesium is filtered by the glomeruli, and some is reabsorbed in the tubules. In some respects its renal metabolism resembles that of potassium, and aldosterone promotes its urinary excretion, but there is no active tubular secretion as is seen in connexion with potassium.

Magnesium excess. This is seen in chronic renal failure, especially if magnesium sulphate is given to the patient. There is drowsiness at a plasma level of 4 mmol per litre, and coma at 7 mmol per litre. Peripheral vasodilatation, hypotension, and muscular flaccidity like that produced by curare are other features. Death is preceded by cardiac arrest.

Magnesium depletion. It is difficult to produce hypomagnesaemia experimentally in the human subject because there is good renal conservation of the mineral when the plasma level drops. In addition, magnesium is abundant in a normal diet, especially in green vegetables and cereals. Magnesium deficiency is seen clinically in renal tubular defects, chronic alcoholism, hyperaldosteronism, hepatic cirrhosis, and the malabsorption syndrome. It gives rise to severe psychotic symptoms (delirium, delusions, and hallucinations), tremor, muscular twitching, athetoid movements, and convulsions. There is, however, often a poor correlation between plasma levels and clinical effects.

When it occurs in the malabsorption syndrome there is also hypocalcaemia, but hypomagnesaemia is sometimes found in hyperparathyroidism in association with hypercalcaemia; the magnesium level may fall further after parathyroidectomy due probably to its sequestration in bone. Hypomagnesaemia furthermore tends to depress the plasma level of calcium (see p. 460).

ACID-BASE BALANCE—THE BICARBONATE ION[11-14]

During the course of normal metabolic activity various acids are produced, e.g. phosphoric, sulphuric, lactic, and hydrochloric acid. In addition, the keto acids β-hydroxybutyric and acetoacetic acid are formed in considerable quantities during starvation and especially in uncontrolled diabetes mellitus. The acid produced in the largest amount, however, is carbonic acid, for it is an inevitable product of aerobic tissue activity. Despite this acidifying tendency the pH of the blood remains constantly at about 7·4 in health, and this is due to the buffering capacity of the body and the disposal of acid from the body, which limit any change.

It is accepted that *an acid is a molecule or an ion which is capable of yielding a hydrogen ion (i.e. a proton)*, while *a base is a molecule or an ion which is capable of taking up a hydrogen ion to form an acid*. This is called the *Bronsted-Lowry proposition*. The strength of an acid or a base depends on its ability to give up or receive a hydrogen ion. In the equation $HB \rightleftharpoons H^+ + B^-$, which symbolises the dissociation and formation of an acid, B^- is the base, and is called the *conjugate base* of the acid HB, just as HB is the *conjugate acid* of the base B^-. HB and B^- together are the *conjugate pair*. The more readily the acid gives up its hydrogen ion, the less readily does the conjugate base accept it, i.e. the stronger the acid, the weaker is its conjugate base. In the equation $HCl \rightleftharpoons H^+ + Cl^-$, the conjugate base Cl^- is very weak, because HCl is a very strong acid; on the other hand, in the equation $H_2CO_3 \rightleftharpoons H^+ + HCO_3^-$, the conjugate base HCO_3^- is strong, because H_2CO_3 is a weak acid. When sodium hydroxide is added to water, it contributes equal quantities of Na^+ ions (which are neither acidic nor basic) and OH^- ions, which are strongly basic. As the product $[H^+]$. $[OH^-]$ has to remain constant, H^+ ions are removed from the solution by reacting with the OH^- ions, according to the equation $H^+ + OH^- \rightleftharpoons H_2O$. At 25°C the product of the molar concentrations of hydrogen and hydroxyl ions in pure water is 10^{-14}, i.e. $[H^+] = [OH^-] = 10^{-7}$. A pH*

*The pH is the negative logarithm of the hydrogen ion concentration of a solution. The form $[H^+]$ = hydrogen ion concentration. At 37 C the product $[H^+]$. $[OH^-] = 10^{-13\cdot6}$. This means that at body temperature a pH of 6·8 corresponds to neutrality.

of 7 corresponds to neutrality. If H^+ ions are removed the pH rises, and if H^+ ions are added the pH falls. According to this the solution becomes alkaline or acid. In fact, a proton cannot exist free in aqueous solution, and it at once combines with a molecule of water to form an OH_3^+ ion (hydroxonium ion), but by convention it is referred to as a hydrogen ion.

Buffers

In order to limit the change in hydrogen ion concentration to the range (pH about 6·9 to 7·7) within which survival is possible, the body is provided with certain *buffer* systems. These are capable of mopping up H^+ ions, and are also able to contribute H^+ ions. The essential feature of a buffer is that it consists of a strong base and a weak conjugate acid. In the dissociation equation of such a weak acid, $HB \rightleftharpoons H^+ + B^-$, it is found that if there is an excess of H^+ ions, these are removed from solution by combining with the strong base, B^-, to form more of the weak acid. On the other hand, if the pH rises too much, there is an increased dissociation of the acid with the production of more H^+ ions. In other words, the conjugate pairs take up H^+ ions when the pH falls, and supply them when the pH rises.

By far the most important buffer in extracellular fluid is the bicarbonate ion, the normal concentration of which in plasma is 21 to 27 mmol per litre. It is aided by two other bases, monohydrogen phosphate and the plasma proteins (which carry a negative charge at the pH of the blood). Intracellularly, haemoglobin is extremely important as a buffer, and so probably are the other cell proteins. The following equations illustrate the buffering of an acid in the circulation:

$$H^+ + HCO_3^- \rightarrow H_2CO_3$$
$$H^+ + HPO_4^{2-} \rightarrow H_2PO_4^-$$
$$H^+ + Protein^{n-} \rightarrow H\ Protein^{(n-1)-}$$

The carbonic acid produced in the first reaction is removed by its diffusion as CO_2 into the alveolar air of the lungs. *The great importance of the bicarbonate ion lies not only in its buffering capacity, but also in the extreme volatility of carbonic acid and its ease of elimination by the lungs.*

The only other route whereby H^+ ions can be excreted from the body is in the urine. The cells of the tubules secrete H^+ ions which are buffered in the glomerular filtrate partly by phosphate, but also by combination with ammonia to form ammonium ions. Filtered bicarbonate ions combine with secreted H^+ ions to form carbonic acid, which dissociates so that CO_2 diffuses back into the blood, where it can reform bicarbonate ions. The whole process amounts to a reabsorption of the filtered bicarbonate ions.

The handling of the carbonic acid produced during tissue activity is a supreme tribute to the red cells which contain both haemoglobin, the most important buffer in the blood after bicarbonate, and a high content of carbonic anhydrase, which accelerates the following reversible reaction:

$$CO_2 + H_2O \rightleftharpoons H_2CO_3$$

The carbonic acid then dissociates into bicarbonate and hydrogen ions:

$$H_2CO_3 \rightarrow HCO_3^- + H^+$$

The hydrogen ions are largely buffered by the haemoglobin:

$$H^+ + Hb^- \rightleftharpoons HHb$$

The excess bicarbonate ions then diffuse into the plasma in exchange for chloride ions, which diffuse into the red cells. This is called the *chloride shift*. In this way the bicarbonate level of the plasma rises. There is no cation exchange between the red cells and the plasma comparable with this shift of anions.

In the lungs, as CO_2 diffuses into the alveolar air, these reactions are reversed. The reversal is assisted by the oxygenation of the Hb, because oxyhaemoglobin is a stronger acid than reduced haemoglobin, i.e. it gives off H^+ ions more readily. The carbonic anhydrase converts carbonic acid into its anhydride, CO_2.

There is a second method of CO_2 transport in the blood: a direct reversible combination with Hb to form a carbamino compound.

In general the body copes with an influx of strong acid firstly by the effect of dilution with the copious tissue fluids, and secondly by buffering. Finally the pulmonary and renal mechanisms come into play to restore equilibrium once more. Of these the lungs act more immediately than do the kidneys.

The Maintenance of the pH of the Blood

According to the Henderson-Hasselbalch equation

$$pH = pK + \log \frac{[salt]}{[acid]},$$

where pK is the negative logarithm of the dissociation constant of an acid. The pK is equal to the pH of a dilute solution in which a weak acid is half neutralised, so that the concentrations of the acid and its conjugate base are equal. The stronger the acid, the smaller is its pK.

Applying this equation to the pH of the blood,

$$pH = pK + \log \frac{[conjugate\ base]}{[conjugate\ acid]},$$

it is found that the pK for carbonic acid is 6·1, the concentration of bicarbonate is about 24 mmol per litre, and the concentration of H_2CO_3 in solution, at a partial pressure of CO_2 of 40 mm Hg (the normal alveolar tension), is about 1·2 millimole per litre. Therefore

$$pH = 6·1 + \log \frac{24}{1·2} = 6·1 + \log 20 = 6·1 + 1·3 = 7·4.$$

The equation can also be written as follows:

$$pH = 6·1 + \log \frac{[HCO_3^-]}{\alpha . P_{CO_2}},$$

where α is the 'solubility coefficient' per mm Hg, and P_{CO_2} is the partial pressure of CO_2 in mm Hg. This at once demonstrates that the pH of the plasma depends principally on two factors: (*a*) the concentration of bicarbonate, and (*b*) the partial pressure of CO_2, which determines the concentration of carbonic acid. If the pH is to be maintained at 7·4, the ratio $\frac{[HCO_3^-]}{[H_2CO_3]}$ has to remain at 20.

ABNORMALITIES OF THE pH OF THE BLOOD

An increase in the hydrogen ion concentration of the blood (pH less than 7·36) is called an *acidaemia* and a decrease (pH

over 7·44) an *alkalaemia* (or *basaemia*). The terms *acidosis* and *alkalosis* are sometimes used synonymously with acidaemia and alkalaemia, but it is preferable to restrict them to describing conditions in which there would be a corresponding change in pH were there no compensation.

Respiratory Acidosis and Alkalosis

If the P_{CO_2} changes, the pH moves in the opposite direction, whereas a change in the concentration of bicarbonate moves the pH in the same direction. The P_{CO_2} is closely dependent on the removal of CO_2 from the lungs. If ventilation is inadequate, the P_{CO_2} rises. This is called *respiratory acidosis*, because the retained CO_2 forms carbonic acid, which is a source of H^+. $[HCO_3^-]$ rises too, but by a lesser amount; the ratio of $[HCO_3^-]$ to $[H_2CO_3]$ falls, as does the pH. In the opposite state of hyperventilation, the P_{CO_2} falls. So does $[HCO_3^-]$, but by a lesser amount. The ratio of $[HCO_3^-]$ to $[H_2CO_3]$ rises, as does the pH. This is *respiratory alkalosis*.

It is evident that respiratory acidosis is directly related to underventilation of the lungs with a resulting rise in the arterial P_{CO_2}. Likewise in respiratory alkalosis there is overventilation with a drop in arterial P_{CO_2}. A measurement of the arterial P_{CO_2} is therefore an accurate and useful method of assessing the respiratory component of acid-base balance.

Respiratory acidosis. This is due to underventilation of the lungs leading to CO_2 retention and a rise in arterial P_{CO_2} (see Ch. 45). The blood pH falls and the plasma bicarbonate level rises. The standard bicarbonate remains normal (p. 483).

Clinical and biological effects. *There is peripheral vasodilatation*, which is the direct effect of raised P_{CO_2}. Such vasodilatation may raise the intracranial pressure. Other effects of acidosis are described under metabolic acidosis (see below).

Excretion of hydrogen ions and ammonia by the distal tubules of the kidney with a concomitant reabsorption of bicarbonate. In acute respiratory acidosis the renal excretion of sodium and potassium is decreased, whereas chloride is excreted in proportionately greater amounts.

The level of the plasma chloride drops in step with the rise in the plasma bicarbonate level. This is particularly marked in chronic respiratory acidosis.

Respiratory alkalosis. There is a rise in blood pH and a fall in the plasma bicarbonate level. It is due to hyperventilation removing so much carbon dioxide that its tension in the blood is reduced. Hyperventilation is ventilation in excess of that required to remove CO_2 as fast as it is produced. It is encountered:

During hysteria, working at high temperatures or at great altitudes, or following salicylate intoxication. Salicylates in toxic doses have a directly stimulating effect on the respiratory centre. The effects of salicylate poisoning are complex, because there is also a tendency towards metabolic acidosis.

During anaesthesia, when muscular relaxants are being used and excessively vigorous artificial respiration is applied.

Clinical and biochemical effects. *Pallor* due to peripheral vasoconstriction, a direct effect of the low tension of CO_2 in the blood.

Light-headedness.

Tetany. This, like the light-headedness, can be reversed by the inhalation of CO_2, e.g. rebreathing.

The renal changes described in metabolic alkalosis. There is a great bicarbonate excretion, while the secretion of hydrogen ions is much reduced.

A corresponding rise in the level of plasma chloride.

Non-Respiratory, or Metabolic, Acidosis and Alkalosis

If there is an excess of H^+ ions in the blood as a result of the ingestion or production of acid substances, the bicarbonate of the plasma is replaced by the anion of the acid involved; the $[HCO_3^-]$ drops. This is a *metabolic acidosis*. On the other hand, the ingestion of sodium bicarbonate leads to a rise of $[HCO_3^-]$ and pH of the plasma. This is a *metabolic alkalosis*.

Metabolic acidosis. There is a fall in both the pH of the blood and the bicarbonate level of the plasma. It is encountered in the following conditions:

Lactic acidosis.[15] Lactic acidosis commonly occurs in shock when there is underperfusion of the tissues and consequent anaerobic metabolism with the production of lactic acid (see p. 421).

Lactic acidosis can also occur in the absence of shock, and is ascribed to a failure of the liver and kidneys to metabolise the lactic acid normally produced elsewhere, e.g. in the skeletal muscles. This occurs in liver and kidney disease and especially in patients on phenformin therapy. The sudden onset of hyperpnoea, abdominal pain, and coma accompanied by a neutrophil leucocytosis may be the first manifestation. An increase in the anion gap may be the first diagnostic clue.

In severe diarrhoea, where the fluid lost has a higher pH than that of plasma due to the increased bicarbonate present in the colonic secretion. The same effect may occur with pancreatic and biliary fistulae.

In starvation, and especially in uncontrolled diabetes mellitus, where there is a ketosis. The acetoacetic and β-hydroxybutyric acids produce extra H^+ ions.

Following the administration of ammonium chloride. The ammonia is converted into urea by the liver, while hydrogen ions are left behind with chloride ions.

$$Cl^- + NH_4^+ \rightarrow NH_3(removed) + H^+ + Cl^-$$

In renal disease, due either to impaired filtration as in anuria and terminal uraemia, or else to a failure of acidification by the distal tubules as in renal tubular acidosis. In this type of condition H^+ ions are retained and not secreted.

After uretero-colic anastomosis. This is described later.

Clinical and biochemical effects. *The classical symptom of air-hunger* (deep, sighing, rapid respiration). It is a compensatory mechanism because it lowers the P_{CO_2}, and thereby causes a respiratory alkalosis which tends to reverse the fall of the blood pH. It is believed that the lowered blood pH stimulates the respiratory centre.

Excretion of hydrogen ions and ammonia by the distal tubules of the kidney with a concomitant reabsorption of bicarbonate. This mechanism is impaired in an acidosis of renal origin.

As the plasma bicarbonate falls, there is a corresponding rise in some of the other plasma anions. If the plasma chloride concentration rises there will be a *hyperchloraemic acidosis*. In diabetic acidosis the keto acid level increases considerably.

Severe metabolic acidosis may cause various neurological symptoms culminating in coma and death. It impairs cardiac contraction, and a state of shock with low cardiac output and hypotension may result. Acidosis seems to potentiate the effects of trauma and haemorrhage, and has been considered an important cause of irreversible shock. Cardiac dysrhythmias, cardiac arrest, and sudden death have also been attributed to severe acidosis even when there has been no preceding evidence of failure.

Metabolic alkalosis. There is a rise both in the blood pH and the bicarbonate level of the plasma. It is encountered in the following conditions:

Following the administration of an alkaline salt like sodium bicarbonate. Salts with organic anions, e.g. potassium citrate and sodium lactate, are also alkalinising, presumably because the anion is metabolised to form bicarbonate.

In a condition of persistent vomiting, e.g. pyloric stenosis. There is a loss of hydrogen ions in excess of hydroxyl ions.

In severe hypokalaemia as in primary hyperaldosteronism and Cushing's syndrome. The mechanism of the ensuing alkalosis has already been described.

Clinical and biological effects. *Depression of respiration*, which would, by causing retention of CO_2, tend to reverse the rise of pH of the blood, is inconspicuous. It is probably limited by the effect of hypoxia on the chemoreceptors.

Tetany may occur due to a decrease in the ionised fraction of plasma calcium as well as by a direct effect of the lowered H^+ ion concentration.

There is an increased glomerular filtration rate with corresponding increase in the amount of bicarbonate in the filtrate. The tubules respond by reabsorbing less bicarbonate than normally. There is also a decreased secretion of hydrogen ions, and a tendency towards increased potassium secretion. There may be a diminished reabsorption of sodium.

There is a fall in the level of plasma chloride, corresponding to the rise in plasma bicarbonate.

Assessment of the Metabolic Component of Acid-Base Balance

The assessment of the metabolic, or nonrespiratory, component of acid-base balance is a subject of considerable difficulty and controversy. Merely measuring the plasma bicarbonate is of limited value, for although the level is raised in metabolic alkalosis and reduced in metabolic acidosis, it is also influenced by respiratory function. Thus in respiratory alkalosis it is *reduced*, and in respiratory acidosis it is *raised*. Several methods can be used to eliminate this respiratory component.

The alkali reserve. This is the bicarbonate content of plasma after it has been separated from the blood cells and equilibrated at 38°C with a gas mixture containing CO_2 at a partial pressure of 40 mm Hg.

Standard bicarbonate. This is the bicarbonate content of plasma after a sample of *whole blood* has been equilibrated at P_{CO_2} of 40 mm Hg (and P_{O_2} of at least 100 mm Hg) at 38°C. It is thought to be more useful than the alkali reserve. It is raised in metabolic alkalosis and reduced in metabolic acidosis. The normal range is 22 to 26 mmol per litre.

Buffer base. This is the sum effect of the buffer anions in the blood. The normal range is 44 to 48 mmol per litre.

The most logical measurement of the metabolic component of the acid-base balance is probably the *standard bicarbonate*. The effect of any abnormality in P_{CO_2} in life is corrected by equilibrating the blood at P_{CO_2} 40 mm Hg *in vitro*. The hydrogen ion concentration is then related to the metabolic

TABLE 38.2 The main metabolic changes in different types of acidosis and alkalosis (uncompensated)

	Blood pH	Plasma bicarbonate	Plasma chloride	Urine
Metabolic acidosis	Low	Low	Usually raised	Much hydrogen ions and ammonia. Little bicarbonate
Respiratory acidosis	Low	Raised	Low	As above
Metabolic alkalosis	High	Raised	Low	Much bicarbonate. Little ammonia and hydrogen ions
Respiratory alkalosis	High	Low	Raised	As above

component and is expressed in the bicarbonate content. The buffer base determinations include other buffers, e.g. protein, also present in the plasma. However, these buffers are largely confined to the plasma, while bicarbonate is present in the extracellular, extravascular fluids as well—a volume about four times that of the plasma.

It must be stressed that isolated measurements of pH are of limited value in elucidating the cause of the change. A low level may occur in either respiratory or metabolic acidosis, and furthermore an only slightly abnormal pH can occur in the presence of severe acid-base derangements. Thus a patient with severe respiratory failure and respiratory acidosis, by secreting excess hydrogen ions in the urine (perhaps aided by diuretics), may develop a compensating metabolic alkalosis, so that a pH only a little off the normal range results. It is indeed usual for an acidosis or alkalosis of one type to be adjusted by an appropriate metabolic or respiratory compensation. However, this does not always occur, for both components may work in the same direction, as is commonly seen in the postoperative period when respiratory complications cause respiratory acidosis and shock leads to an additional metabolic acidosis.

ABNORMALITIES IN ELECTROLYTE BALANCE IN VARIOUS CONDITIONS

It is instructive to conclude this discussion of electrolyte balance by briefly considering a few clinical conditions in which disturbances of the balance are important.

Postoperative Alterations in Electrolyte Balance[1]

From the time of operation until nearly a week afterwards there is a consistent alteration in electrolyte and water balance. The response described below is the classical account of electrolyte changes following trauma, but it can be altered by the use of intensive intravenous therapy, as mentioned in Chapter 32, where the changes in nitrogen metabolism are also considered (see pp. 411–412).

The main feature of the postoperative response is a marked oliguria which normally persists for 24 to 48 hours. During this period there is an almost complete retention of sodium and chloride ions. After the first 2 days the urinary volume gradually increases, until it reaches a full amount after the first week, by which time there is a normal excretion of sodium and chloride ions. Within 24 hours of operation there is an increased urinary excretion of potassium, which persists for about 4 days.

These changes are associated with an increased secretion of

glucocorticoids. They can be explained teleologically in terms of the extensive inflammatory exudate that forms around any traumatised area. This exudate is rich in water, sodium, chloride, and protein, all of which are necessary for the healing process. There is therefore a decreased loss of water and sodium chloride in the urine. The protein (and also extra water) is derived from the protoplasmic breakdown of other body tissues, especially skeletal muscle, and in this process of catabolism there is a release of potassium ions which are excreted in the urine.

During the early postoperative period there may be a very slight rise in the levels of plasma urea and potassium, because they are being produced in such great quantities that they may not be excreted by the kidneys with sufficient speed. This explains the paradox of increased plasma level despite a negative metabolic balance.

On the other hand, the plasma levels of sodium and chloride are low despite their retention in the body. This 'sodium paradox' has been attributed to a dilution effect secondary to an even greater water retention, the water having been extracted from the cells during their breakdown. Another suggestion is the intracellular deviation of sodium and chloride following the extrusion of potassium, phosphate, and sulphate into the extracellular fluid.

The inability to secrete a water load is the result of an excessive secretion of ADH. This occurs postoperatively as a result of pain, trauma, and anaesthetic and analgesic drugs.

It is important to be aware of these minor changes in blood chemistry, lest patients be given intravenous fluids at a time when they cannot excrete an extra water and salt load in the urine.

Likewise the passage of a small volume of urine low in sodium and chloride content need occasion no alarm during the first few days after an operation. Such urine should, however, be highly concentrated. A low specific gravity of around 1·010 is ominous, and may be the first indication of tubular necrosis.

Conditions of Gastrointestinal Fluid Loss

The secretions of the gastrointestinal tract are not only copious in amount, but they also contain high concentrations of electrolytes. The intestinal juice, for example, has roughly the same concentrations of sodium, chloride, and bicarbonate as the plasma, but twice as much potassium. Normally about 3000 ml are secreted each day.

The gastric juice, the normal daily volume of which is about 2500 ml, being strongly acid has a high concentration of hydrogen ions and no free bicarbonate. The more acid the gastric juice, the lower is the sodium concentration compared with plasma. Thus at a pH of 1 the concentration of H^+ ions is 100 mmol per litre and the concentration of sodium is only a third that of the plasma. But at a pH of 2 the concentration of H^+ ions is only 10 mmol per litre, and the concentration of sodium is the same as that of the plasma (140 mmol per litre) Furthermore, the gastric juice has a potassium concentration twice that of plasma and one-and-a-half times as much chloride.[16]

The biliary secretion, normally 500 ml a day, resembles the plasma closely in its electrolyte content, though it has a slightly increased concentration of bicarbonate. The pancreatic juice, normally 700 ml a day, though similar in sodium concentration to plasma, has a lower chloride and a much higher bicarbonate concentration. Both biliary and pancreatic secretions have a slightly higher concentration of potassium than is found in the plasma.

Normally all these secretions are reabsorbed, but when they are lost there are serious disturbances in the body's electrolyte balance.

Acute intestinal obstruction. In any *mechanical obstruction* there is a dilatation of the loops of bowel proximal to it. These become distended with secretion, and the greater the distension, the greater the stimulus to further secretion. In addition there is also a loss of fluid into the wall of the bowel and into the peritoneal cavity. The higher up the obstruction, the more marked is the fluid loss and the earlier is the advent of severe vomiting. A high jejunal obstruction may lead to the loss of several litres of fluid in a day, whereas an obstruction involving the rectum may persist for several weeks and cause little fluid loss.

A high intestinal obstruction is always accompanied by great sodium and water depletion, and this rapidly produces severe dehydration. In the event of extensive strangulation there is also an extravasation of blood into the devitalised loop and its mesentery. As fluid is replaced by infusion, so more secretion enters the distended loops above an obstruction. It therefore follows that the obstruction should be relieved as soon as possible.

Ileus secondary to *generalised peritonitis* presents special problems. In addition to the secretion of much fluid into the distended loops of bowel, there is also a considerable plasma loss in the extensive inflammatory exudate filling the peritoneal cavity. The combined loss of fluid in the intestinal secretion and inflammatory exudate produces a characteristically intractable dehydration.

Severe shock is characteristic of acute peritonitis, and it may be unresponsive to intravenous infusions of blood and plasma as well as saline. There is an important bacteraemic element in this shock and also in that of acute intestinal obstruction, where intestinal organisms penetrate the devitalised bowel wall and enter the circulation.

Primary *paralytic ileus* presents a somewhat similar picture, but here the atony is due to an intrinsic impairment of muscular motility and co-ordination. There is some evidence that this may be precipitated by a fall in the concentration of plasma potassium. Another important cause is the use of ganglion-blocking agents.

Pyloric stenosis. Of all the disturbances of electrolyte balance pyloric stenosis is the most complex. Unlike acute intestinal obstruction it runs a more protracted course, so that there is time for a depletion of potassium and a disturbance of acid-base equilibrium to complicate the picture of sodium and water depletion. It has already been noted that pure gastric juice has a high concentration of potassium and hydrogen ions. On the other hand, the intrinsic disease of the stomach responsible for the stenosis may alter this composition, e.g. gastric carcinoma is usually accompanied by an achlorhydria. The three common causes of pyloric stenosis are a cicatrising or oedematous peptic ulcer, pyloric cancer, and hypertrophy of the pyloric muscle in infants. In adults the picture is often complicated by a previous overdose of sodium bicarbonate. The following sequence of events follows the persistent vomiting of pyloric stenosis:

(*a*) There is a primary depletion of sodium, chloride, and water which leads to dehydration with oliguria.

(*b*) Soon the loss of hydrogen ions leads to a metabolic alkalosis. The kidney responds at first by secreting an alkaline urine rich in bicarbonate. The urinary excretion of potassium is also increased because the loss of sodium and water in the vomitus, by decreasing the extracellular fluid volume, powerfully stimulates the secretion of aldosterone. The excretion of sodium in the urine is almost entirely in abeyance.

(*c*) There is a progressive depletion of potassium as a result of its loss both in the vomitus and the urine. The urinary loss is due to the hyperaldosteronism mentioned above, but, in addition, chloride depletion, also due to the vomiting, plays an important part. It has been found experimentally that chloride depletion leads to the secretion of considerable amounts of hydrogen and potassium ions in the urine, an effect arrested by the administration of chloride.[17] The mechanism of this effect is not clear, but one suggestion is that a lack of chloride in the glomerular filtrate prevents the proximal tubule reabsorbing sodium properly; as a result, the sodium reaches the distal tubule, where the high sodium content of the filtrate stimulates the secretion of aldosterone with its effect on potassium excretion.

If the potassium depletion persists for a long time it may impair renal function by interfering with the normal concentration of the urine. Under these circumstances polyuria may develop and increase the dehydration.

(*d*) In due course the sodium loss may become very severe as a result of the vomiting. If both the sodium and potassium depletion become marked, the condition of 'paradoxical aciduria' may occur. This remarkable state of affairs is brought about by the almost complete reabsorption of sodium by the distal tubule. As there is virtually no potassium to be excreted in exchange, the place of this cation is taken by hydrogen ions, which are then secreted into the urine. The high concentration of hydrogen ions in the cells secondary to potassium depletion may assist this process, but chloride depletion is the important factor in 'paradoxical aciduria'.

There is therefore no single pattern of electrolyte disturbance in pyloric stenosis. There may be oliguria or polyuria, and the urine may be alkaline or acid. A fall in plasma chloride level is inevitable, and with it there is a rise in the level of plasma bicarbonate. The plasma potassium level may be deceptively high due to its mobilisation from the cells prior to its loss in the vomitus and the urine. Despite the sodium depletion, the level of sodium in the plasma is sometimes raised in the early stages, possibly due to the continuous loss of water by insensible routes and in the urine. Sodium bicarbonate administration aggravates the alkalosis and all the effects accruing from it.

It is noteworthy that the administration of isotonic saline not only corrects the dehydration and restores the circulation to normal, but it will also raise the chloride concentration of the plasma and therefore correct the effects of chloride depletion on the kidney mentioned above.

Uretero-Colic Anastomosis

Following the transplantation of both ureters into the colon, an operation that is performed after total cystectomy for carcinoma of the bladder, a complex derangement of electrolyte balance follows.[8] It is due to the absorption of chloride and sodium from the colon and the secretion of bicarbonate and potassium. In addition urea is allowed to diffuse back into the blood. The mechanism of the disturbance is as follows:

(a) The colonic secretion of bicarbonate ions produces a metabolic acidosis (p. 483). The increased reabsorption of chloride ions makes it a hyperchloraemic acidosis, which can be severe.

(b) Urea diffuses back into the blood so that there is a corresponding rise in its plasma concentration. In addition some of the urea is split up by the bacteria of the colon, and ammonia is produced. The pH of the urine, low when it was secreted by the kidney, rises when the colon adds bicarbonate to the urine. This will favour the diffusion of ammonia into the blood.

(c) There is a tendency towards potassium depletion. This is due mainly to an increased colonic loss. In addition there may possibly be a renal basis for the potassium loss, as progressive pyelonephritis is inevitable. This is an example of potassium depletion due to a combined faecal and urinary loss.

(d) There is also sodium absorption which may occasionally be sufficient to lead to oedema. The plasma sodium concentration is sometimes slightly raised.

Until they suffer structural damage, the kidneys can adjust their output of sodium, chloride, hydrogen ions, and ammonia to moderate the disturbance. But there is always the danger of pyelonephritis and ureteric obstruction; these complications will further impair renal function.

The intricate pattern of electrolyte disturbance that complicates uretero-colic transplantation is a fine example of the baneful effects that may follow interference with a normal anatomical pathway. Even before any damage occurs to the renal or alimentary system, each can contribute to the metabolic disorder.

REFERENCES

1. COHEN, R. D. (1974) In *Clinical Physiology*, ed. Campbell, E. J. M., Dickinson, C. J. & Slater, J. D. H., 4th edn, p. 1. Oxford: Blackwell.
2. Leading Article (1977) The anion gap. *Lancet*, **1**, 785.
3. Leading Article (1968) The fate of sodium in the renal tubules. *New England Journal of Medicine*, **279**, 381.
4. EARLEY, L. E. & DAUGHARTY, T. M. (1969) Sodium metabolism. *New England Journal of Medicine*, **281**, 72.
5. Leading Article (1977) Natriuretic hormone. *Lancet*, **2**, 537.
6. KLEEMAN, C. R. & FICHMAN, M. P. (1967) The clinical physiology of water metabolism. *New England Journal of Medicine*, **277**, 1300.
7. Leading Article (1962) Hypernatraemia and the brain. *Lancet*, **2**, 438.
8. COOKE, R. E. *et al.* (1952) The extrarenal correction of alkalosis associated with potassium deficiency. *Journal of Clinical Physiology*, **31**, 798.
9. FRENCH, F. F. & SOLER, N. G. (1968) Hyperkalaemic periodic paralysis starting at age of 48. *British Medical Journal*, **2**, 472.
10. BELL, G. H., EMSLIE-SMITH, D. & PATERSON, C. R. (1976) *Textbook of Physiology and Biochemistry*, 9th edn, p. 81. Edinburgh: Churchill. Livingstone.
11. ROBINSON, J. R. (1967) *Fundamentals of Acid-Base Regulation*, 3rd edn. Oxford: Blackwell.
12. CAMPBELL, E. J. M. (1974) In *Clinical Physiology*, p. 232, *loc. cit.*
13. NUNN, J. F. (1965) In *General Anaesthesia*, ed. Evans, F. T. & Gray, T. C., 2nd edn, Vol. 1, p. 300. London: Butterworth.
14. SIGGAARD-ANDERSEN, O. (1965) *The Acid-Base Status of the Blood*, 3rd edn. Baltimore: Williams and Wilkins. Also (1963) *The Scandinavian Journal of Clinical and Laboratory Investigation*, **15**, Supplement 70.
15. Leading Article (1973) Lactic acidosis. *Lancet*, **2**, 27.
16. DAVENPORT, H. W. (1971) *Physiology of the Digestive Tract*, 3rd edn, pp. 100–101. Chicago: Year Book Medical Publishers.
17. SCHWARTZ, W. B., DE STRIHOU, C. VAN Y. & KASSIRER, J. P. (1968) Role of anions in metabolic alkalosis and potassium deficiency. *New England Journal of Medicine*, **279**, 630.

Chapter 39. *General Features of Thrombosis and its Occurrence in the Venous System*

Two obvious prerequisites of any circulation are the presence of fluid and a means whereby this can be retained in the vessels should they be damaged. In the blood vascular system the clotting mechanism guards against the danger of haemorrhage, while vascular damage is remedied by the deposition of platelets and fibrin on the vessel wall. If this deposition becomes excessive, the circulation is progressively obstructed and eventually completely occluded by *thrombus*. It is evident that there must be a balance between platelet deposition and clotting on the one hand and the fluidity of blood on the other. This homeostatic mechanism guards the body against the two hazards of thrombosis and haemorrhage.

The clotting mechanism. Clotting, or coagulation, is the conversion of the plasma fibrinogen into a solid mass of fibrin. The mechanism is described in Chapter 54. At this stage it is sufficient to note that the clotting is initiated by prothrombinase derived from either the blood (intrinsic) or the tissues (extrinsic). The intrinsic system is activated by a lipid factor liberated by platelets which adhere to a surface, and by a clotting factor in the plasma (Factor XII) which is activated by an abnormal surface also.

Platelets.[1] Platelets are 1·5 μm in diameter and from 0·5 to 1 μm in thickness. They have no nucleus, and their cytoplasm has many azurophil granules which in blood films tend to be concentrated in the centre. On electron microscopy platelets are seen to be bounded by a plasma membrane, and in their cytoplasm there are prominent dense granules which correspond to the azurophil ones seen on light microscopy. These contain hydrolytic enzymes, and also lipoprotein which is important in blood clotting. They are probably the main site at which 5-HT is bound. They also bind histamine and catecholamines. Platelets contain microtubules, a few mitochondria, and some vesicular elements which may be derived from the endoplasmic reticulum or the Golgi complex of the megakaryocyte from which they originated. Further details of platelet development and disorder are discussed in Chapter 54.

The deposition of platelets on to the intimal surface of a blood vessel is the first step in the formation of a thrombus, and it is important to understand the mechanisms whereby platelets adhere to surfaces (*adhesiveness*) and stick to each other (*aggregation*).[2]

Platelet aggregation. Platelets aggregate immediately in the presence of *adenosine diphosphate (ADP)*. This may be demonstrated *in vitro* by the addition of ADP to a platelet-rich preparation of plasma which is kept agitated. The aggregation can be detected by measuring the ensuing decrease in optical density.[2] Adrenaline, noradrenaline, and 5-HT have a similar effect. *Thrombin* leads to aggregation, but only after a delay of 5 to 10 seconds. It probably acts by converting adenosine triphosphate (ATP) in the platelets to ADP.

Platelet adhesiveness.[2] Platelets adhere to a variety of foreign surfaces, and the drop in platelet count when blood is passed through a column of glass beads has been used as an *in-vitro* method of measuring platelet adhesiveness. Platelets will also adhere to vascular endothelium if it is damaged mechanically, and to *collagen* and basement membrane, but not to fully polymerised fibrin.

When platelets adhere to collagen they swell and release a variety of chemicals, including phospholipid (platelet factor 3), heparin neutralising substance (platelet factor 4), 5-HT, and ADP. This is called the *platelet release reaction*. The ADP causes platelet aggregation, and a small platelet thrombus is built up. This is unstable, and *in vivo* the platelets may break off and be released into the circulation as small emboli. Though clotting is not involved in the mechanism of platelet adhesiveness, the clotting system is soon activated by factor 3 released from the platelets and by the activation of Factor XII. Fibrin is formed, and this is thought to stabilise the platelet thrombus. In addition, the thrombin-coated fibrin leads to the further deposition of platelets. Prostaglandins are formed together with thromboxane A_2 (see p. 488).

Platelet adhesion is stimulated by ADP and inhibited by ATP. Both aggregation and adhesion take place only in the presence of ionic calcium, but whereas aggregation does not occur at low temperatures, adhesion can still take place. It is noteworthy that aspirin affects the function of platelets by preventing the release of ADP from them.[3, 4]

The healing of vascular damage. Minor degrees of injury are being constantly sustained by blood vessels, and a layer of platelets is soon laid down to restore the integrity of the wall and prevent haemorrhage. A small amount of fibrin is also formed. The process has been studied in detail under the electron microscope.[5] Initially the platelets adhere in loose masses to the area of damage, and then these become compact. At first there is little morphological change in the platelets, and there is no tendency to fusion, since the plasma membrane remains intact. Later the platelets tend to apply themselves to the neighbouring cells, and close packing and distortion of shape become evident.[6] These morphological changes are most prominent at the edges of the aggregations, where the platelets lose their dense granules, adhere to leucocytes, and become entangled in meshes of fibrin. Then the internal structure of the platelet disintegrates, probably due to the release of autolytic enzymes, but the plasma membrane remains intact for a long time. Ultimately the platelets are found widely spread amid much fibrin. The close aggregation of platelets is traditionally called *viscous metamorphosis* as seen under the light microscope, but the illusion of fusion of platelets to form an amorphous mass is refuted electron-microscopically.

This deposit of platelets and fibrin is rapidly covered by endothelial cells, so that the smooth lining of the vessel is restored and further deposition ceases. The platelet deposit is removed by phagocytosis as well as by autolysis, and the fibrin is dissolved by fibrinolysins. The factors that limit the clotting tendency of circulating blood, confronted so frequently with vascular damage, are (a) naturally occurring anticoagulant substances, like heparin and antithrombin III, (b) the fibrinolytic mechanism, which removes fibrin by the action of the enzyme plasmin (see p. 636), and (c) the rapid endothelialisation of damaged areas, which limits the amount of clotting factors liberated into the circulation whether from aggregated platelets or damaged tissue.

Platelets do not adhere to a normal, intact endothelium. Although this may be due to the active blood flow sweeping them along, there is also a possibility that a chemical mechanism is involved.[7] There is a powerful platelet aggregator called *thromboxane A_2* which is formed from prostaglandins G_2 and H_2. It seems likely that the aggregation of platelets on the damaged vessel wall involves the formation of free arachidonate, presumably from membrane phospholipid. The arachidonate is the precursor of prostaglandin endoperoxides, which can be converted into other prostaglandins and thromboxane A_2 by enzymes that are present in the platelets.

In addition, another compound can also be formed from prostaglandins G_2 and H_2. It is unstable and a powerful inhibitor of platelet aggregation; it is called *prostaglandin X*. An enzyme has been isolated from the aortas of pigs and rabbits that can transform the two prostaglandins into prostaglandin X.

It is possible that a dynamic balance exists between thromboxane A_2 formed by the platelets and prostaglandin X formed by the blood vessels, and that the maintenance of this balance is important in preventing thrombus formation. Platelets attempting to stick to vessel walls might release prostaglandin G_2 or H_2, which is then used by the vessel wall to generate prostaglandin X, which prevents the build-up of a platelet thrombus.

THROMBOSIS[8]

Thrombosis is the formation of a solid mass in the circulation from the constituents of the streaming blood. The mass itself is called a *thrombus*, and as can be appreciated from the preceding description, consists of aggregated platelets and fibrin in which the red and white cells are trapped.

The initial stage of thrombosis is the deposition of platelets on a vascular surface. This occurs under three circumstances: (a) When the endothelial lining is damaged or removed. Exposure of the collagen in the vessel wall may be of importance. (b) When there is vascular stasis; the platelets fall out of the axial stream and impinge on the wall. (c) When the streamline of the blood is disrupted and eddy currents are produced; these deflect the platelets on to the wall of the vessel. It will be recalled that ADP causes aggregation of platelets *in vitro* only if the mixture is agitated. Eddy currents probably act in this way. If a number of platelets adhere to a damaged surface they release ADP, and a thrombus is steadily built up as more platelets impinge on the surface.

The resulting thrombus is called a *pale*, or *platelet*, *thrombus*. It is, as already described, composed of a small amount of fibrin as well as the platelets, but if it is not speedily endothelialised, or if there is stasis, the fibrin in-

Figure 39.1
Portion of a thrombus. Strands of fibrin are seen radiating from clumps of platelets. Intermingled among these there are red cells and a few white cells. × 300.

creases in amount and in its meshes there are trapped red cells and leucocytes (Fig. 39.1). Furthermore, the irregular fibrin surface and the released thrombin encourages more platelet deposition, and so the thrombus increases markedly in size. At this stage it is the blood clot which is the major component, and the mass is called a *red*, or *coagulation*, *thrombus*. Most thrombi have both pale platelet and red clot components, and are then called *mixed thrombi*.

Since the process starts with platelet deposition on a vascular surface, it can occur only in a flowing stream and is therefore encountered spontaneously only in a living animal. The clotting is a secondary phenomenon, and can occur in any column of static blood whether in the living animal or in a test-tube. Therefore a clot is not the same as a thrombus; the important feature of the latter is the platelet scaffold which is lacking in a clot.

Normally thrombosis is obviated by the smooth endothelial lining of the vessels and the streamline of blood in the complex circulatory pathways, which results in the formed elements being restricted to the central axial stream. This streamline of blood can be disturbed by obstruction of the vascular lumen through *rigid valves*, *spasm*, *intrinsic disease of the wall*, and *adjacent cicatrisation*. *Diffuse dilatation*, e.g. in an aneurysm, also disturbs the flow. All these lesions lead to stasis as well as to eddy currents, and the deposition of platelets performs a remedial function in that it smooths out the contour of the wall and restores the streamline of blood in the vessel (Fig. 39.2). The small amount of prothrombinase that is generated is dissipated in the flowing blood. It is when this dissipation is retarded that the thrombus increases in size.

Figure 39.2
This diagram shows seven different causes of a disruption of the normal streamlining of the blood flow, and the manner whereby platelets (shown in black) are laid down to restore the architecture.
(*a*) Bulging due to external pressure and spasm.
(*b*) Endothelial swelling and damage due to inflammation, a plaque of intimal thickening, e.g. atheroma, and corrugation due to adjacent cicatrisation.
(*c*) Aneurysm and a sclerotic, rigid valve.
(*From Hadfield, G.* (1950), Annals of the Royal College of Surgeons, England, **6,** 219)

Causes of Thrombosis

There are three factors concerned in the causation of thrombosis:

1. **The vessel wall,** especially its endothelial lining.
2. **The flow of blood.**
3. **The constituents of the blood,** notably the platelets and clotting factors.

Derangements of these constitute *Virchow's triad* of factors which determine the occurrence of thrombosis.

Changes in the vessel wall. These various anatomical changes have already been considered. In general, they are especially important in the pathogenesis of arterial and cardiac thrombosis. In the veins and atria of the heart these factors are less important with the exception of thrombophlebitis, where the inflamed vein wall is the cause of the thrombosis.

Changes in the blood flow. The most important is *stasis*, which is the usual cause of venous and atrial thrombosis. It also plays a part in the thrombus occurring in aneurysmal sacs. Where the viscosity of the blood is increased, whether locally in acute inflammation or systemically in polycythaemia vera and dehydration, there is a tendency to thrombosis. Thrombi in which stasis plays a prominent part are red or mixed.

The other alteration in blood flow is *eddy-current* formation, which is important in fast-flowing streams in the arteries and heart. The thrombus is mixed, the pale component predominating.

Changes in the composition of the blood. *Platelets.* Conditions associated with an increased platelet count (thrombocytosis) are not infrequently complicated by thrombosis. This increased count may be transient, as after parturition,

trauma, and severe haemorrhage, or it may be persistent as in polycythaemia vera. Splenectomy is followed by a considerable thrombocytosis which may last some time.

The tendency to thrombosis is also related to platelet adhesiveness. There is evidence that during the early postoperative period the platelets are more adhesive, and aggregate more strongly in the presence of ADP and noradrenaline.[2] Increased aggregation has also been noted in patients with brain tumours and multiple sclerosis, conditions in which thrombosis is not unusually frequent.[9] Hyperlipidaemia increases platelet adhesiveness and aggregation in both humans and animals.

Clotting factors. The clotting time is shortened after severe haemorrhage, and to a lesser extent after trauma and during the course of severe infections, e.g. typhoid fever. Glucocorticoids and oestrogen also cause a decreased clotting time. Thrombosis sometimes complicates these conditions or follows the administration of these drugs. The oral contraceptive may lead to venous and cerebral thrombosis; its oestrogen component is responsible. Hyperlipidaemia both shortens the clotting time and inhibits fibrinolysis. Heparin, in addition to being an anticoagulant, clears the chylomicrons which appear in the blood after a fatty meal.

Patients with an inherited deficiency of *antithrombin III*,[10] which interferes especially with the actions of thrombin and activated factor X, are highly susceptible to venous thrombosis. Heparin in low concentrations dramatically increases the rate at which activated factor X is neutralised by antithrombin III.*

VENOUS THROMBOSIS

Though the veins are apparently less commonly subject to disease than the arteries, thrombosis is commoner in them than in arteries. The venous system is capacious, and of low pressure and velocity; it is therefore particularly liable to bear the brunt of stasis. There are two types of venous thrombosis: *phlebothrombosis*, which is due to stasis of blood in uninflamed veins, usually in the calves of the legs, and *thrombophlebitis*, in which the vein wall is inflamed. Though some types of thrombosis are difficult to classify, the distinction is useful both theoretically and clinically.

PHLEBOTHROMBOSIS

This condition is the most important of all the complications that follow major surgery. Modern methods of detection have revealed that deep vein thrombosis of the leg occurs in about 35 per cent of patients after major surgery, and it is even more frequent in cases of recent myocardial infarction.[11] It is a particularly common postoperative hazard of splenectomy, surgery on the hip joint, and retropubic prostatectomy.[12] The incidence is greatest in the older age group, but young people who are immobolised for any length of time are also prone to this non-infective thrombosis of the leg veins.

*Low levels of antithrombin III are often found in patients liable to deep vein thrombosis after surgery, but the method of assay is still too arbitrary to make this a useful clinical procedure. The basis for this low level is presumably an increased concentration of clotting factors binding the antithrombin.

Figure 39.4
Diagram showing the structure of the coralline thrombus and the underlying platelet thrombus.
(*From Hadfield*, G. (1950), Annals of the Royal College of Surgeons of England, **6**, 219)

Figure 39.3
The pathogenesis of phlebothrombosis.
  A. Primary platelet thrombus.
  B. Coralline thrombus.
  C. Occluding thrombus.
  D. Consecutive clot to the next venous tributary.
(*From Hadfield*, G. (1950), Annals of the Royal College of Surgeons, England, **6**, 219)

The Pathogenesis of Phlebothrombosis

Five stages can be recognised (Fig. 39.3 and Fig. 39.6).

Primary platelet thrombus. Due perhaps to some trivial intimal damage platelets adhere to the vein wall and aggregate to form a pale thrombus, as has already been described. The process has been likened to the formation of a snowdrift during a snowstorm. This would not proceed further were it not for the stasis which allows clotting factors to accumulate in the area. These promote an increase in the fibrin element which stabilises the mass of platelets and leads to the next stage.

The coralline thrombus. The fibrin deposition on the primary platelet thrombus encourages further platelet accumulations, which take the form of upstanding laminae growing across the stream. They are bent in the direction of the blood flow by the force of the stream. These laminae anastomose to form an intricate structure which resembles coral (Fig. 39.4). Between the laminae there is complete stasis, and fibrin is deposited; in it there are trapped numerous red and white blood cells. This is an example of a mixed thrombus, as it is composed of both platelet masses and blood clot. In a paraffin section it is seen to consist of alternate layers of fused platelets and fibrin with entrapped blood cells (Fig. 39.5). The retraction of the fibrin layers leads to the characteristically ribbed ('ripple') appearance seen when the surface of the thrombus is examined. The elevated platelet ridges are called the *lines of Zahn*, and they are best seen with the aid of a hand-lens. They are often conspicuous in thrombi formed in a fairly rapid stream of blood, e.g. in the aorta (Fig. 40.1, p. 497). Up to this stage it is possible for the process to cease, and for endothelialisation of the thrombus to occur.

Figure 39.5
Coralline thrombus. Photomicrograph of vertical section including free surface of a coralline thrombus adherent to the wall of a large artery. Pale platelet laminae are seen projecting from the surface. Coagulated plasma containing leucocytes lies between them. Many leucocytes are adherent to the platelet laminae.
(*From Hadfield*, G. (1950), Annals of the Royal College of Surgeons of England, **6**, 219)

Occluding thrombus. The growth of the coralline thrombus progressively occludes the lumen of the vein, and the ensuing stasis rapidly leads to the formation of more thrombus which completely occludes the lumen and trails away from the coralline thrombus in the direction of the blood flow. In this way there is formed an occluding thrombus which is composed of blood clot with a smaller platelet element. It is therefore red.

Consecutive clot. Once the vein is occluded, blood flow stops; with it stops thrombosis, which by definition can occur only in streaming blood. The stationary column of blood beyond the occluding thrombus clots to form a *consecutive clot*, which extends up to the entrance of the next venous tributary. At this point the edge of the clot may become endothelialised, in which case spread, or *propagation*, is halted, but otherwise more thrombus or clot develops.

Propagated clot. Propagation can occur by two methods (Fig. 39.6):

(a)   (b)

Figure 39.6
Methods of propagation in phlebothrombosis.
(*a*) With thrombus formation at each entering tributary.
(*b*) Clotting *en masse* in an extensive length of vein.
(*From Hadfield, G. (1950), Annals of the Royal College of Surgeons of England, 6, 219*)

(*a*) The clot which reaches to the entrance of the venous tributary may lead to the formation of another platelet and coralline thrombus, so that there is occlusion of the ostium of the tributary (Fig. 39.6(*a*)). Consecutive clot will then form up to the ostium of the next venous tributary. Eventually a long piece of propagated clot may be produced, which is well anchored at each successive ostium.

(*b*) Sometimes the column of blood above the consecutive clot is so stagnant, due to stasis of the venous circulation of the whole limb, that it clots *en masse*, forming one long cord of clotted blood, anchored only at the original site of thrombus formation. This length of clot retracts, and lies loose in the vein except at its one point of anchorage. It is easy to imagine how it might break off, and be carried to the heart as a massive pulmonary embolus. It is this type of propagation which is particularly dangerous to life (Fig. 39.6(*b*)).

This account of propagation is necessarily simplified, and in practice it is probably a complex process in which both mechanisms described above play their part. It is quite likely that part of the propagated clot may be well attached to the points of entry of venous ostia, and that higher up it may be unattached. A great deal depends on the vigour of the circulation. A complicating factor is the retraction of the propagated clot, so that the circulation becomes re-established. This may lead to the deposition of a coating of thrombus over the original clot.

CAUSES OF PHLEBOTHROMBOSIS

Changes in the Vessel Wall

Frequently there is no evidence of damage at all, but a possible factor is pressure on the veins exerted by the heavy calf tissues themselves when the patient is immobilised in bed. This may be aggravated by the effect of local hypoxia due to pressure on the arteries. Sometimes, of course, there are more obvious precipitating factors, e.g. direct trauma by fracture edges, and the effects of ill-applied tourniquets and plasters.

Changes in Blood Flow

Stasis is without doubt the most important factor. It is most likely to occur in the leg veins; whenever the cardiac output is reduced, it is here that the effects of stasis are most marked, and thrombosis is most likely to occur. In addition, local factors may be responsible for regional venous stasis, and again it is the leg veins that are most vulnerable. The causes of venous stasis may be classified under the following headings:

I. GENERAL CONDITIONS

Reduced cardiac output, due to

(i) Heart failure.
(ii) Shock following haemorrhage, trauma, burns, and dehydration.
(iii) Low metabolic rate, e.g. during rest in bed.

Impaired venous return due to shallow respiration.

II. LOCAL CAUSES

Lack of muscular activity. The venous return from the legs is greatly facilitated by the squeezing action of the surrounding muscles. This important mechanism is in abeyance in the bedridden patient. The arms are less likely to be affected, being in constant use in all conscious patients.

Incompetent valves. The effect is somewhat debatable.

Pressure from outside, e.g. tumours, ascites, plasters, and bandages. A particularly good example of this was seen in England during the Second World War in 1940. Many people retired to their air-raid shelters to spend the night in a deck-chair. While sheltering from the bombs, they exposed their popliteal veins to the pressure of the wooden bar, with the result that phlebothrombosis developed. The pressure of the calves on the mattress may be a factor in the bedridden and after an operation.

Changes in the Composition of the Blood

The decreased clotting time, increased platelet count, and the tendency to increased platelet adhesiveness and aggregation are important contributory factors in postoperative and post-traumatic phlebothrombosis.[2]

It is evident that although venous stasis is the most important aetiological factor in phlebothrombosis, there are also many contributory causes.

Merely confining a patient to bed is liable to jeopardise the venous flow in the legs both by reducing the cardiac output and inhibiting muscular activity. If in addition to this there is cardiac failure or shock, conditions are ideal for the occurrence of thrombosis. The dangers of the postoperative period are obvious, especially when respiration is painful as after chest and upper abdominal surgery. In recent years the incidence of clinically significant phlebothrombosis has diminished due to the practice of early ambulation and teaching the patient to exercise the legs in bed. But there is abundant evidence that venous thrombosis usually starts during the course of the operation, especially if it is of long duration. Indeed, studies of the incidence of thrombosis using more refined modern methods of detection indicate that most of it is present very early in the postoperative period, and the use of electrical stimulation of the leg muscles during the course of the operation has been found to decrease the incidence of the condition considerably. Low-dosage heparin therapy is of value.[13,14]

A certain amount of venous thrombosis starts preoperatively, especially in patients with cancer and those receiving intravenous nutrition.[15]

Sites Affected and Naked-Eye Appearances

Phlebothrombosis commonly starts in the deep veins of the calf, and then spreads to the posterior tibial vein (Fig. 39.7). From here it may extend to involve the popliteal, femoral, and iliac veins, and even the inferior vena cava. Careful dissections have, however, shown that thrombosis sometimes starts at points higher up, e.g. at the beginning of the femoral vein or even in the external iliac vein just above the inguinal ligament. Indeed, it is not rare for thrombus to arise independently at several sites in the venous system of the lower limb. The pressure of the right common iliac artery on the left common iliac vein probably explains why iliac venous thrombosis is more common on the left side.

The most obvious feature of the affected veins is the long propagated clot, or *tail*, which may extend up to 45 cm (18 in.). This is deep red in colour, but following retraction some blood may pass around it giving it a thin, pale covering of platelets. The *head* (platelet and coralline thrombus) is small and firmly attached to the vein wall. By contrast, the tail is loosely attached.

Clinical Features

Clinically phlebothrombosis is remarkably silent. There is little spasm of the vessel walls and little pain. Direct pressure produced by squeezing the calf muscles may elicit tenderness, while forced passive dorsiflexion of the foot may produce pain by stretching the veins (*Homans's sign*). Oedema may develop distal to the obstructed veins, but this is neither invariable nor marked. Indeed, all the clinical signs of phlebothrombosis are unreliable, and frequently the first indication of the condition is the occurrence of pulmonary embolism.

Specialised diagnostic procedures.[16–19] As already noted, modern methods of detection have indicated that deep vein thrombosis of the legs is much more common than is clinically evident. Furthermore, some cases in which there are signs suggestive of thrombosis prove negative to specialised tests. The most important diagnostic procedures are:

(*a*) *Phlebography*, in which a contrast medium is injected into a foot vein, and the venous circulation of the leg and thigh studied.

(*b*) *Radio-active iodine-labelled fibrinogen test*. In this test

Figure 39.7
Phlebothrombosis. The muscles of the calf have been dissected to show extensive thrombosis of the main veins and their muscular branches. Several thrombi removed from the pulmonary artery are also displayed. Their calibre and branching reveal their origin from the leg. (C 40.3, *Reproduced by permission of the President and Council of the R.C.S. Eng.*)

[125]I-labelled human fibrinogen is administered intravenously (after giving suitable doses of potassium iodide to block any uptake of the radio-active iodine by the thyroid gland). The labelled fibrinogen is incorporated into forming thrombi, and the concentration of the isotope in the local area is detected and assessed by an external counter.

(*c*) *Doppler ultrasound*, using a special apparatus that detects a flow of blood by the production of ultrasound that is heard from a loudspeaker. If there is thrombosis there is complete silence. The method is useful, but false positives and false negatives must be expected.[20]

Complications

(*a*) Massive pulmonary embolism.

(*b*) Smaller pulmonary emboli, with or without pulmonary infarction.

(*c*) Repeated episodes of silent embolisation leading to a syndrome of progressive pulmonary hypertension. This is occasionally seen as a complication of pregnancy.

THROMBOPHLEBITIS

Inflammation of a vein wall causes damage to the endothelial lining, and on this platelets are deposited. The blood flow is either normal or accelerated because of the inflammation, so that if thrombosis proceeds to complete obstruction, there is much less tendency for propagation to occur; if it does, the clot is well anchored to the vein wall. The thrombus is so firmly adherent to the wall that the danger of embolism is negligible, except when the inflammation is due to pyogenic bacteria.

Sterile inflammation may be produced by direct trauma, ionising radiations, and chemicals. It is induced deliberately in varicose veins and haemorrhoids by the injection of 'sclerosing solutions'. Strong dextrose solutions given intravenously rapidly induce thrombosis. They are therefore delivered directly into the superior vena cava through a long catheter introduced into a forearm vein. Thrombosis of the vena cava does not occur, as the solution is immediately diluted with a large volume of blood. It has been found that when rubber tubing is used in intravenous transfusion sets, the incidence of thrombosis is greater than when plastic tubing is used.[21]

A rare disorder sometimes associated with thrombophlebitis, not infrequently affecting the venae cavae, is *Behçet's disease*.[22] The classical features are a triad of relapsing uveitis, oral ulceration of aphthous type, and ulceration of the genital area. There may also be pyoderma, erythema nodosum, polyarthritis (which is seronegative), and various central-nervous lesions, which may eventually cause death. The aetiology of the condition is unknown, but the basic pathological process is a vasculitis of venules and arterioles with frequent thrombosis.

Bacterial inflammation. Veins in the region of an infected area may become inflamed and undergo thrombosis. In pyogenic infections the organisms may invade the thrombus, soften it, and cause its disintegration. This suppurative thrombophlebitis results in the release into the circulation of numerous infected emboli, i.e. pyaemia. It is occasionally seen in the appendicular veins in acute appendicitis, and can complicate infected haemorrhoids; *portal pyaemia* results, and this may be accompanied by suppurative thrombophlebitis of the portal vein itself (*pylephlebitis suppurativa*). Suppurative mastoiditis similarly leads to thrombophlebitis of the lateral sinus. It must be noted that the emboli of pyaemia are tiny as compared with the massive ones frequently seen in phlebothrombosis.

Clinical Aspects of Thrombophlebitis

Spasm of the affected vein occurs, and pain is a marked feature. There are signs of acute inflammation if the vein is superficial. The condition is therefore clinically obvious. Embolism is rare when the thrombus is sterile.

Complications

(*a*) Pyaemic embolisation in infective cases.

(*b*) Venous engorgement. This is liable to occur when a large extent of venous drainage has been obliterated. It leads to residual oedema, and under some circumstances to infarction, e.g. mesenteric thrombosis (p. 518). After iliofemoral thrombophlebitis the superficial leg veins become varicose, and it is important to test the patency of the deep veins before varicose veins are ligated or stripped.

Other Types of Venous Thrombosis

There are some examples of venous thrombosis which cannot readily be classified as either phlebothrombosis or thrombophlebitis, and these are best considered separately.

Iliofemoral thrombosis occurs from time to time in debilitated, bedridden patients. It was a well-recognised late complication of typhoid fever in days gone by. Two important variants are:

(*a*) *Phlegmasia alba dolens*, which is the 'white leg' of late pregnancy and the puerperium. Its cause is unknown. In addition to the venous involvement, there is apparently some arterial spasm causing the pallor. It is possible that there is also lymphangitis. The condition is very painful. Massive pulmonary embolism sometimes occurs, but it probably arises from an unsuspected phlebothrombosis in the other leg in some cases. On the other hand, residual oedema and varicose leg veins are common sequelae.

(*b*) *Phlegmasia caerulea dolens* (see p. 509).

Thrombophlebitis migrans. In this condition there are recurrent thrombotic episodes in the superficial and deep veins, especially of the extremities. Many cases are idiopathic, or form a part of Buerger's disease, and these show a diffuse inflammatory reaction.

The condition is also a well-known complication of deep-seated cancer—this was first noted by Trousseau in 1865. The usual sites of the primary tumour are the pancreas (tail and body), lung, stomach, and female genital tract.[23] There is sometimes little inflammatory reaction in the vein wall, and the condition may be due to an increased coagulability of the blood. High levels of various clotting factors are sometimes found in these cases, and the blood may be unusually resistant to the action of heparin.[24]

Primary mesenteric vein thrombosis is an important cause of infarction of the bowel; its aetiology is unknown.

The inferior and superior venae cavae may undergo

TABLE 39.1 Comparison between phlebothrombosis and thrombophlebitis

	Phlebothrombosis	*Thrombophlebitis*
Major cause	Stasis	Inflammation of vein wall
Size of primary thrombus	Small	Larger—depending upon the extent of the phlebitis
Size of propagated clot	Long and often poorly anchored	Usually none; if present, short and well anchored
Emboli	Common and massive. Sterile	Rare except in infective cases. Pyaemic
Site	Usually calf veins	Anywhere
Clinical picture	Silent—few signs or symptoms	Obvious—pain and signs of acute inflammation

thrombosis in the course of disease involving the retroperitoneal and mediastinal regions. The symptoms are those of venous obstruction (see Ch. 43); embolism does not occur.

THROMBOSIS IN THE ATRIA OF THE HEART

Atrial thrombosis is generally due to stasis, the condition being analogous to phlebothrombosis. The atrial appendages are usually involved, because it is here that stasis is most marked. Mitral stenosis is a common cause of thrombosis in the left atrium, especially when complicated by fibrillation. It may occur in either atrium in heart failure. With valvular regurgitation there are also eddy currents.

The thrombi may become detached and lead to embolism. Precautions must be taken to prevent this when operating on the heart, e.g. when performing a valve replacement. Rarely the thrombus remains in the atrium after becoming detached: this leads to the classical *ball-thrombus* that is occasionally encountered in the enormously dilated left atrium of long-standing mitral disease with combined regurgitation and stenosis. It remains free in the chamber, increases in size, and may finally block the atrioventricular orifice and cause sudden death.

Thrombi on the valves (vegetations) and in the ventricles are considered in the next chapter, because they are not associated with stasis.

GENERAL READING

HUDSON, R. E. B. (1965). *Cardiovascular Pathology*. London: Arnold. This book now in three volumes is useful for reference.

REFERENCES

1. WEISS, H. J. (1975) Platelet physiology and abnormalities of platelet function. *New England Journal of Medicine*, **293**, 531 and 580.
2. Leading Article (1968) Platelet function. *Lancet*, **1**, 285.
3. O'BRIEN, J. R. (1968) Effects of salicylates on human platelets. *Lancet*, **1**, 779, and Effects of anti-inflammatory agents on platelets (1968) *Lancet*, **1**, 894.
4. Leading Article (1969) Platelets and aspirin. *British Medical Journal*, **3**, 371.
5. FRENCH, J. E. (1967) *In Modern Trends in Pathology*, ed. Crawford, T. Vol. 2, p. 208. London: Butterworth.
6. STEHBENS, W. E. & BISCOE, T. J. (1967) The ultrastructure of early platelet aggregation *in vivo. American Journal of Pathology*, **50**, 219.
7. Leading Article (1976) P.G.X.: a natural antithrombic substance? *Lancet*, **2**, 1005.
8. MUSTARD, J. F. (1975) Function of blood platelets and their role in thrombosis. *Transactions of the American Clinical and Climatological Association*, **87**, 104.
9. Annotation (1968) Plasma phospholipids and platelet stickiness in multiple sclerosis. *Lancet*, **1**, 134.
10. Leading Article (1976) Antithrombin. *Lancet*, **1**, 1333
11. Leading Article (1971) Prophylaxis of venous thrombosis. *British Medical Journal*, **1**, 305.
12. KEMBLE, J. V. H. (1971) Incidence of deep vein thrombosis. *British Journal of Hospital Medicine*, **6**, 721.
13. Leading Article (1971) Prevention of deep-vein thrombosis: the way ahead? *Lancet*, **2**, 693.
14. Leading Article (1975) Prevention of postoperative thromboembolism. *Lancet*, **2**, 63.
15. HEATLEY, R. V. *et al.* (1976) Preoperative or postoperative deep-vein thrombosis? *Lancet*, **1**, 437.
16. EVANS, D. S. & COCKETT, F. B. (1969) Diagnosis of deep-vein thrombosis with an ultrasonic Doppler technique. *British Medical Journal*, **2**, 802.
17. O'BRIEN, J. R. (1970) Detection of thrombosis with iodine-125 fibrinogen. *Lancet*, **2**, 396.
18. EVANS, D. S. & NEGUS, D. (1971) Diagnosis of deep vein thrombosis. *British Journal of Hospital Medicine*, **6**, 729.
19. THOMAS, M. L. (1971) Radiology of deep vein thrombosis. *British Journal of Hospital Medicine*, **6**, 735.
20. MEADWAY, J. *et al.* (1975) Value of Doppler ultrasound in diagnosis of clinically suspected deep vein thrombosis. *British Medical Journal*, **4**, 552.
21. MOLLISON, P. L. (1972) *Blood Transfusion in Clinical Medicine*, 5th edn, p. 592. Oxford: Blackwell.
22. Leading Article (1978) Behçet's disease. *British Medical Journal*, **1**, 234.
23. AZZOPARDI, J. G. (1966) In *Recent Advances in Pathology*, ed. Harrison, C. V., 8th edn, p. 115. London: Churchill.
24. WINTROBE, M. M. et al. (1974) *Clinical Hematology*, 7th edn, p. 1237. Philadelphia: Lea & Febiger.

Chapter 40. *Thrombosis in Arteries and in the Heart*

SOME COMMON ARTERIAL DISEASES

In the previous chapter the general features of thrombus formation have been described. In the high-velocity arterial system the most important cause of thrombosis is disease of the arterial wall itself. This acts in three ways:

1. Eddy-current formation leads to platelet aggregation and deposition.

2. Ulceration of the endothelial lining contributes to platelet aggregation.

3. Disease of the arterial wall may so weaken it that aneurysmal dilatation occurs; this leads to stasis which favours thrombosis and clotting.

The causes of arterial thrombosis are those of arterial damage. Spasm, which may also initiate thrombosis, is considered in Chapter 42.

CAUSES OF ARTERIAL DAMAGE

Inflammation

1. **Trauma.** The arterial wall may be damaged by sharp spicules of bone in fractures, by adjacent missiles, or by operative procedures. The continual rubbing of the subclavian artery over a cervical rib may lead to thrombosis. In arterial injuries there is an important additional factor of vascular spasm.

2. **Infective and chemical lesions.** Infected emboli, during the course of a pyaemia, can cause an arteritis when they become impacted in the lumen of a small artery or in one of the vasa vasorum of a large vessel. The weakening of the arterial wall leads to the formation of a *mycotic aneurysm.** Arteritis can also occur following the spread of an infection from an adjacent lesion, e.g. a carbuncle, but it is of much less importance and frequency than similar damage to veins. It is of much greater importance in chronic infective diseases, where it leads to *endarteritis obliterans.* This may be complicated by thrombosis, e.g. the cerebral vessels in syphilis and the arteries in the wall of a tuberculous cavity in a lung. It is of great importance in preventing massive haemorrhage, e.g. in peptic ulcers.

3. **Idiopathic inflammatory conditions.** *Thromboangiitis obliterans (Buerger's disease).* The disease, originally described by Buerger in 1908, is characterised by a diffuse inflammation involving segments of arteries, veins, and surrounding connective tissue. It was originally described in Jews, but there is in fact no definite racial incidence. It affects males almost exclusively. The highest incidence is during the third and fourth decades. A viral infection and (more probably) hyper-

*The origin of the term mycotic is obscure. It is not used in the sense that fungi are involved. Perhaps it indicates that the aneurysmal bulges are mushroom shaped. It is used in this context in mycosis fungoides.

sensitivity to tobacco have both been suggested as aetiological agents.

Arterial thrombosis occurs in the course of the disease, and it is the medium-sized arteries (with their venae comitantes) of the leg which are most frequently affected. Intermittent claudication and gangrene are the usual clinical manifestations. The visceral vessels are seldom involved.

There is considerable controversy as to whether Buerger's disease is a distinct entity or merely the end-result of atheroma occurring in young men. Most pathologists believe that it is a specific disease of blood vessels, and its distinguishing features are the age and sex of its victims, its relationship to smoking (though atheroma is also aggravated by smoking[1]), and the tendency to attacks of superficial thrombophlebitis migrans. Histologically the diffuse inflammation, the highly cellular thrombus, and the absence of lipid material in the wall do not suggest atheroma.

Polyarteritis nodosa. This disease is described in Chapter 16. There is an acute necrotising inflammation of a segment of the wall of an artery. Thrombosis is a common sequel. Thrombosis occasionally occurs in the related 'collagen diseases', systemic lupus erythematosus and the arteritis associated with acute rheumatic fever and rheumatoid disease.

Giant-cell arteritis. This disease occurs in elderly subjects, and affects the arteries of the scalp, eyes, and brain predominantly, but on occasion it involves the aorta and its branches also. There is an inflammatory reaction involving the intima and the inner part of the media. The internal elastic lamina is fragmented, and there is a conspicuous giant-cell reaction around it. Thrombosis is a common sequel, and in the ophthalmic artery it leads to retinal infarction and blindness. The nature of the disease is unknown.

Primary aortic arteritis,[2,3] also called *Takayasu's disease,* is an idiopathic inflammatory condition of the aorta and its branches. There is massive intimal fibrosis, inflammatory destruction of the media, and fibrosis of the adventitia. The condition has many histological features in common with syphilitic aortitis, but the lesions are more severe, and the aorta is remarkably hard. There is an abrupt edge between the end of the thickened intima and the adjacent healthy aorta. Clinically there is an absence of pulses and cranial ischaemia, and also hypertension due to narrowing of the renal arteries. The condition has been called 'pulseless disease'. It occurs predominantly in young adults, and although it is commoner in Japan and Korea, it is encountered in other parts of the world also.

Aortitis can be associated with ankylosing spondylitis. It has many of the features of syphilitic aortitis.

Neoplastic Infiltration

Tumours which invade arteries (and veins) are soon covered

by thrombus. This is quite often seen in cancer of the lung, which is a notorious invader of blood vessels.

Arteriosclerosis

This term is used loosely to described any condition in which the arterial wall is thickened and hardened. It includes atheroma as well as a number of conditions associated with hypertension and the ageing process. Inflammatory disease, e.g. polyarteritis, and that of known aetiology, e.g. syphilitic arteritis, are by convention excluded.

Arteriosclerosis obliterans.[4] Progressive thickening of the intima by fibrous tissue appears to be a feature of the ageing process in many vessels. It is found frequently in the leg arteries of patients with peripheral vascular disease. It is often accompanied by atheroma, but whereas the atheromatous element is well marked in the proximal arteries (femoral and iliac), the more distal ones show fibrosis and hyalinisation of the intima. It is not known whether this is related to atheroma, or indeed whether arteriosclerosis obliterans represents a distinct entity. Probably some of the lesions described under this heading are organised thrombi or thrombo-emboli.

Fibrous thickening of the intima of the coronary arteries is common in heavy cigarette smokers.[1]

Mönckeberg's medial sclerosis. This affects the large arteries of the lower limbs predominantly, and it is characterised by isolated rings of calcification in the media. The intima is normal. It is considered in relation to calcification in Chapter 36. It produces dramatic radiological appearances, but it does not cause ill-effects. Although commoner in elderly people, it is sometimes discovered accidentally in comparatively young adults who are otherwise healthy.

Diffuse hyperplastic sclerosis. This occurs in the small, muscular arteries, e.g. in the kidney and spleen, and in its fully-developed form it is typical of benign systemic hypertension. There is muscular hypertrophy of the media, thickening of the intima due to fibrous and elastic overgrowth, and reduplication of the internal elastic lamina.

In malignant hypertension there is intimal thickening with cellular fibrous tissue which produces an onion-skin appearance. Frequently there is an excess of acid mucopolysaccharide, so that the intima has a distinctly mucoid appearance. Similar changes are found in arterioles, particularly of the kidney. Similar changes occur in the renal lesions of progressive systemic sclerosis (see p. 212).

Arteriolosclerosis

It is convenient at this point to consider also the arteriolar changes which lead to ischaemia.

Hyaline arteriolosclerosis. In this condition the wall is thickened, and converted into a uniform hyaline ring. Hyalinisation of some arterioles, e.g. of the white pulp of the spleen and the ovary, is part of the normal ageing process, but when it affects the *afferent renal arterioles*, it is pathognomonic of benign systemic hypertension whether essential or secondary. Hyaline thickening of the myocardial arterioles is often found in heavy cigarette smokers.[1]

Diabetic angiopathy. The arteriolar lesion of diabetes mellitus is very similar to that described as hyaline arteriolosclerosis. However, the hyaline intimal material has a high glycoprotein content, and therefore stains strongly with the PAS method.

Arteriolar necrosis. This is a fibrinoid necrosis of part or the whole of an arteriolar wall, and it leads to diffuse haemorrhage in the vicinity. It is seen in malignant hypertension of whatever cause, and it can affect many viscera, being especially prominent in the kidney. The necrosis is apparently due to the tension of an extremely raised blood pressure on the arteriolar wall. A similar lesion has been noted in the mesenteric arterioles after the successful surgical repair of a coarctation of the aorta. In this instance the previous hypotension of the lower part of the body has been suddenly replaced by a normal blood pressure, which is too high for the unprepared arterioles of the gut.[5] Extensive arteriolar necrosis may also lead to thrombosis and infarction; the condition resembles polyarteritis in its effects, and indeed arteriolar necrosis is a feature of some types of arteritis (see p. 210).

Atheroma

Without doubt this is the commonest cause of arterial thrombosis. It is the commonest killing disease in Britain (next in frequency come cancer and chronic respiratory disease), and is present to some degree in almost all adult members of the community. Indeed, its early lesions are said to commence at birth. Although of such importance and frequency, exact definition of the disease presents extreme difficulty, the reasons for which will shortly become apparent.

It is important to note that the intima of the normal aorta contains occasional smooth muscle cells and the various components of extracellular connective-tissue matrix. Both the cells and the matrix gradually increase in amount with age.

The media consists predominantly of smooth-muscle cells surrounded by variable amounts of collagen, elastic fibres, and mucoproteins (alternatively called proteoglycans). Neither the intima nor the media contains fibroblasts. It has been found that arterial smooth-muscle cells in tissue culture can form collagen, elastic fibres, and proteoglycans.

Atheroma characteristically affects the large systemic arteries like the aorta and its main branches. Of the medium-sized vessels the coronary and cerebral vessels are the most commonly involved. This is extremely unfortunate in view of the vital nature of the organs they supply, and it accounts for the lethal effects of atheroma. Atheroma may be considered as consisting of two types of condition:

TYPE 1. **Yellow plaques in the tunica intima (fatty streaking or simple atheroma).** There is an accumulation of smooth muscle cells containing and surrounded by deposits of lipid in the intima. There are also some lipid-containing macrophages. In this way there are produced the yellow plaques or streaks which are a common *post-mortem* finding in the aorta at all ages. Although they may also be found in smaller arteries, they do not produce narrowing of the lumen. When the vessels are examined in their contracted state at necropsy, the plaques appear to be elevated. However, if the arteries are distended with fixative, the plaques more closely resemble their form in the living state: they become flattened, and far from causing narrowing of the lumen, the wall may be sufficiently weakened to allow a degree of dilatation to take place. There is some indirect evidence to suggest that the yellow plaques can be removed.

TYPE 2. **The accumulation of fatty material in the intima with additional fibrosis.** This is the common type of lesion seen in middle and old age. It is sometimes referred to as *atherosclerosis*, and may cause varying degrees of stenosis when smaller vessels are affected. Characteristic lesions are seen in the aorta.

The plaques consist principally of an accumulation of lipid-laden smooth-muscle cells in the intima, the lipid being primarily cholesterol and its esters. The cells are also surrounded by lipid and by collagen, elastic fibres, and proteoglycans. Together, the cells and the extracellular components of the matrix form a fibrous covering for a large deeper deposit of free extracellular lipid intermixed with cell debris. This occurs later in the course of evolution of the lesion, which then is composed macroscopically of a central mass of fatty, yellow, porridge-like material (*athere* is Greek for porridge), surrounded by dense fibrous tissue which gives the plaque a white pearly appearance. In advanced, or *complicated, lesions* the fibrous plaques are altered as a result of *haemorrhage, calcification, ulceration,* and *thrombosis* (Fig. 40.1).

Atheroma of this type often has a capricious distribution. Sometimes the coronary vessels are severely affected, while the cerebral ones show minimal change. The thoracic aorta is less severely affected than the abdominal part. It always tends to be particularly severe in areas of vascular stress, e.g. over syphilitic aortitis. It is more marked in hypertensive than normotensive subjects of the same age, and it tends to occur in the pulmonary arteries when there is pulmonary hypertension.

Aetiology

It is evident that the two types of atheroma described above are distinct. It is not known for certain whether the first leads on to the second, or even whether the causative factors are the same.

Figure 40.1

Thrombosis of aorta. This specimen was removed from an aged woman who died of hypostatic pneumonia. The aorta shows advanced atheroma, on the basis of which there are two areas of thrombosis. These thrombi probably formed shortly before death, when the circulation was unduly sluggish. The lines of Zahn on the surfaces of the thrombi are unusually well-marked.

There are two classical theories regarding the aetiology of atheroma:

The imbibition theory proposes that atheroma is due to accumulation of fats in the intima which are derived from the circulating lipoproteins.

The evidence for this depends on (*a*) the production of arterial lesions resembling atheroma in rabbits fed on excessive doses of cholesterol (carnivorous animals respond less obligingly to this regime), (*b*) the presence of severe atheroma in patients with a few conditions accompanied by hypercholesterolaemia, notably myxoedema and hyperlipoproteinaemia (p. 583), and possibly diabetes mellitus, which is associated with a raised level of plasma lipids when the control is poor but not when the patient is well controlled (a more probable explanation of the tendency to atheroma in diabetics is an angiopathy affecting the vasa vasorum of the large arteries with subsequent arterial damage), and (*c*) many people who suffer from severe atheroma have an abnormal lipid pattern in their plasma.

The subject is complex and controversial, but most authorities recognise that the β-lipoproteins (which include cholesterol) are elevated. Since the diet influences the plasma lipids, much work has been done on this subject. It has been found that unsaturated fats of vegetable origin lower the plasma cholesterol level. This may be due to the fats themselves or to the steroid content, for it is known that some steroids, e.g. oestrogens, lower the plasma cholesterol level. Choline has the same effect.

While it may be accepted that diet influences the plasma lipid level, it should not be forgotten that the body manufactures about 2 g of cholesterol daily, whereas only about 400 mg is derived from the diet. The plasma cholesterol level in fact appears to be dependent more upon the total quantity and type of fats ingested than upon their actual cholesterol content.

If atheroma is to be explained on a lipid basis, it must be assumed that the β-lipoproteins in some way pass through the endothelial barrier to the intimal tissue. It is known that the passage of macromolecules is restricted through the endothelium except in certain focal areas such as arterial branch points or sites of endothelial injury or desquamation. Exactly how this imbibed lipoprotein stimulated a fibrous reaction around itself was never adequately explained by this theory, since there are no fibroblasts in the intima nor any evidence of an inflammatory reaction such as cholesterol induces when injected experimentally into an animal's tissues.

The thrombosis (incrustation) theory. Rokitansky in 1842 regarded atheroma as an incrustation of fibrin, which had become organised on the vessel walls. Virchow, however, disagreed, and the theory remained unpopular till 1946 when it was revived by Duguid.[6] He noted that an artery, which in one place contained a recanalised thrombus, showed typical 'atheroma' in an immediately adjacent area.

Thrombosis can be induced in an artery by transfixing its lumen with a piece of silk; the thrombus so produced undergoes organisation and then resembles atheroma. The fatty material is presumably derived from plasma components in the thrombus.

The thrombotic theory has much to recommend it. The obstructive nature of the lesions is easily understood.

Thrombosis causing complete obstruction would then no longer be considered a complication of atheroma, but merely a continuation of the same process which produced the plaque. A powerful objection to the theory is that, since thrombosis is more common in veins, atheroma ought also to be found in these vessels. A possible explanation of this paradox may lie in the disposition of the vasa vasorum in the two types of vessel. In veins these small vessels, which supply the wall itself, penetrate its whole thickness. A thrombus can therefore be easily invaded by capillaries from the media as well as the surface endothelium. In the larger arteries the vasa vasorum from the adventitia penetrate only as far as the outer half of the media. A thrombus can therefore be organised only from the surface endothelium. Presumably this process is slow, with the result that the deeper parts of the thrombus tend to break down. The production of the avascular fatty material characteristic of atheroma is the result.

A considerable amount of fibrin can be demonstrated immunologically even in a small fatty plaque.[7] It is possible that it is derived from fibrinogen that leaks through the endothelium. In the fully developed lesion platelet debris can also be shown immunologically.[7]

A significant advance in research into atherogenesis has been the discovery of the important role smooth-muscle cells play in the structure of the atheromatous plaque. It has been found that a factor derived from platelets causes a proliferation of these cells in tissue culture, and that low-density lipoproteins have a supportive role. On the basis of this a third theory regarding the aetiology of atheroma has been tentatively put forward.[8]

It is known that a number of factors can cause endothelial damage in experimental animals, for example the monkey. Amongst these are mechanical trauma, prolonged intravenous infusions of homocystine (see p. 66), and more significantly induced hypercholesterolaemia. Injury to the endothelium causes an immediate platelet response; the platelets adhere to the subendothelial connective tissue, aggregate, and lose their granules (the release reaction). The platelet factor together with the plasma lipoproteins leads to focal proliferation of arterial smooth-muscle cells, which form large amounts of connective-tissue matrix. At the same time lipid is deposited both in these cells and in the surrounding connective tissue laid down by them.

This theory explains how conditions that cause endothelial damage, e.g. hypertension, syphilitic aortitis, and probably tobacco smoking, predispose to atheroma. It also makes the role of the plasma lipoproteins clearer in atherogenesis. It is to be seen as an extension of the imbibition theory in that it explains the smooth-muscle proliferation that is a central feature of atheroma. At the same time it does not deny the importance of platelet thrombus either in the early stages of atheroma or in the later lesions, which grow by a combination of smooth-muscle proliferation and superimposed thrombosis.

It is believed that atheromatous lesions produced experimentally by endothelial trauma tend to regress as the endothelial barrier is restored. If, however, there is repeated or continuous injury, the progressive lesion of atheroma develops.

At the present time much research is being devoted to the smooth-muscle element of atheroma. One school of thought likens the proliferation of smooth-muscle cells to a benign tumour, and claims that, using the cell-marker technique for glucose-6-phosphate dehydrogenase mentioned on page 367, each lesion of atheroma is derived from a single smooth-muscle cell.[9] It is evident that a new field of research into atheroma has been opened up, but that for the present it is best considered as a broad category of arterial disease which may have many different manifestations in different sites in different arteries. The common features appear to be smooth-muscle proliferation, the laying-down of connective tissue, and the deposition of lipid in the intimal layer following damage to the endothelium.

Effects of atheroma. *Gradual obstruction*: this is most frequent in the coronary and cerebral vessels.

Sudden complete obstruction: this may be due either to *thrombosis* or to *haemorrhage into a plaque*. Rupture of the vasa vasorum in the degenerate central region of the plaque will lead to haematoma formation. This may completely block the vessel, and is thought by some authorities to be an important factor in acute coronary occlusion. The bleeding vessels may be the high pressure capillaries coming straight off the lumen.

Dilatation and aneurysm formation. Though atherosclerosis is regarded as the prime cause of obstruction in the arterial circulation, it is common, especially in elderly women, to find coronary arteries diffusely affected and yet widely dilated. Indeed, this type of lesion may be related to the longevity of the patient. Atheroma uncomplicated by thrombotic episodes is prone to cause dilatation due to atrophy of the media. This again indicates the multiformity of the factors in the causation of atherosclerosis. In the abdominal aorta there is such severe weakening of the tunica media that the dilatation often progresses to aneurysm formation (Fig. 40.2 and Fig. 40.3).

Embolism. Atheromatous and thrombotic material from the aorta and its major branches sometimes becomes detached and embolises distally. The effects of this are considered on pages 507 and 518.

ANEURYSMS

An aneurysm is a local dilatation of an artery or a chamber of the heart due to a weakening of its wall. It may be localised and saccular or diffuse and fusiform. The commonest site is the aorta, and then follow the arteries of the leg (especially the popliteals), the carotids, the subclavians, and the innominate.

Causes of Aneurysm Formation

Trauma, especially of the leg arteries. Subclavian aneurysm may be related to a cervical rib.

Inflammation. Syphilitic aortitis (see p. 250) was the commonest cause, but is now very rare. Polyarteritis nodosa and pyogenic arteritis (causing a mycotic aneurysm) are other examples. Primary aortic arteritis and the aortitis associated with ankylosing spondylitis can both be complicated by aneurysm formation.

Atheroma. This is the commonest cause of aortic aneurysms (both abdominal and thoracic), and is discussed above.

Congenital defects in the wall. The most important example is the berry aneurysm of the circle of Willis. Aneurysm of the aorta may occur proximal to a coarctation, and Marfan's syndrome may lead to dissecting aneurysm of the aorta.

Two different lesions, misleadingly called aneurysms,

Figure 40.2
Atheromatous aneurysm of abdominal aorta. The abdominal aorta is the seat of advanced atheromatous ulceration, and just above its bifurcation there is a saccular aneurysm. It is almost completely occluded with alternate layers of white and red thrombus; this is laminated thrombus. (C 31b.7, *Reproduced by permission of the President and Council of the R.C.S. Eng.*)

should be noted: (*a*) *arteriovenous aneurysm*, a sac of connective tissue surrounding an arteriovenous fistula, and (*b*) *cirsoid aneurysm*, a leash of dilated, intercommunicating arteries and veins, usually on the scalp; it is congenital and a type of vascular hamartoma.

Effects. Aneurysms cause harm in the following ways:

Pressure. A good example is pressure of an aortic aneurysm on the oesophagus and the recurrent laryngeal nerve causing dysphagia and aphonia. Likewise pressure atrophy of the spinal column or sternum may occur.

Thrombosis. The main factors involved are eddy currents following the disruption of the streamline of blood entering a dilated sac, irregularity of the diseased wall, and stasis in the sac which favours clotting. Eventually a classical *laminated thrombus* develops, consisting of alternate layers of pale platelet thrombus and red blood clot. The parallel laminae result from the expansile force of the arterial pulse compressing the layers against the vessel wall (Fig. 40.3). The process is slow, but eventually the sac becomes filled with thrombus.

Haemorrhage. Unfortunately repair of an aneurysm is not effective because of the avascularity of the vessel wall. Rupture frequently follows, not so much at the apex of the aneurysm which is full of thrombus as at the sides. External

Figure 40.3
Laminated thrombus in an aneurysmal sac. This is a cross-section of an atheromatous aneurysm of the abdominal aorta, and it is almost completely filled with laminated thrombus. This specimen was removed *post-mortem* from an old man who died of an intercurrent disease. (C 31b.4, *Reproduced by permission of the President and Council of the R.C.S. Eng.*)

haemorrhage may be impeded by the thrombus, and it is not uncommon for some small leaks to precede the final fatal gush. A good example is the recurrent haemoptysis produced by a syphilitic aortic aneurysm eroding the trachea. A ruptured aortic aneurysm is now a common cause of death.

Ischaemia. This is produced by pressure of the aneurysm on nearby branches and by the contained thrombus occluding the ostia of emerging vessels.

Dissecting Aneurysms of the Aorta [10, 11]

This is the second most frequent type of aortic aneurysm, and is due to haemorrhage occurring in the media which is thereby split, or dissected, for a variable distance. The two usual sites of dissection are just above the aortic valve and just beyond the origin of the left subclavian artery.

The most important precursor condition is *idiopathic cystic medionecrosis*, in which there are accumulations of mucoid material in the media with associated destruction of smooth muscle fibres and elastic tissue and subsequent cyst formation. A similar condition is sometimes found in *Marfan's syndrome*, except that cysts are less common. Hypertension is a frequent association, especially in the distal type of dissecting aneurysm (in the proximal type medionecrosis is especially common), but atheromatous ulceration is not important in the pathogenesis of this condition.

The initial bleeding is thought to be due to a rupture of one of the vasa vasorum in the media. A small dissection results, and this eventually leads to a rupture of the intima through into the lumen, generally 2 to 3 cm above the aortic valve. The aneurysmal sac is then subjected to the full force of the arterial blood pressure. Rapid dissection occurs in all directions between the inner two-thirds and the outer third of the media. It extends down the aorta and into the origins of its large branches. Sometimes there is a rupture back into the lumen, and in this way a double-barrelled aorta results. However, it is much more usual for the aneurysmal sac to rupture externally—often into the pericardial sac causing acute cardiac tamponade. Clinically the disease usually starts as a sudden rending pain in the chest, followed by shock and the effects of obstruction of the various branches of the aorta. The blood pressure is often unequal in the two arms, as are the pulses. Ischaemia in the distribution of any branch may produce a characteristic syndrome. Involvement of the spinal arteries can cause necrosis of the spinal cord and paraplegia, involvement of the coronary arteries angina and myocardial infarction, and involvement of the renal arteries renal failure.

THROMBOSIS IN THE HEART

Thrombosis in the Atrium

This has already been described (see p. 494).

Thrombosis in the Ventricles

Thrombosis occurring on the ventricular wall is generally associated with some underlying damage to the myocardium, e.g. myocardial infarction, especially if this has progressed to aneurysm formation. It is the left ventricle that is almost always affected. Mural thrombosis is common in both ventricles in congestive cardiomyopathy (p. 530). Myocarditis is occasionally complicated by thrombosis.

In the right ventricle a thrombus composed largely of clot is sometimes found loosely adherent to the wall. It is formed as a terminal event, presumably as the result of slowing of the blood stream, and is called an *agonal thrombus*.

At other times the blood in the right ventricle clots to form a *post-mortem clot*. In conditions accompanied by a high ESR its upper part may consist largely of plasma, when it is called 'chicken-fat clot'. The post-mortem clot and the agonal thrombus are of no functional significance, and should not be confused with a massive pulmonary embolus (see p. 504).

Thrombosis on the Valves

This occurs only when their endothelial covering is damaged, usually as the result of inflammation. The resulting thrombi are by tradition called *vegetations*.

Acute rheumatic fever (see Ch. 16). This affects the heart as a whole, and the oedematous endocardium is liable to be damaged along the line of contact of the valve cusps. The mitral valve is most often affected. The vegetations are of pin's-head size, and are pinkish-grey in colour. They are firmly attached to the endocardium, and never undergo embolisation. Microscopically they consist of aggregations of platelets with an admixture of fibrin, and they are invariably sterile (Fig. 40.4).

There is often mitral regurgitation in the acute stage, and the jet of regurgitated blood may damage the endocardium

Figure 40.4
Organising rheumatic vegetation. The mass is surmounted by a layer of fibrin, in which no doubt there are are aggregated platelets. The base of the thrombus consists of granulation tissue, which is invading the thrombus from below. × 110.

lining the posterior wall of the left atrium, which is already the seat of severe rheumatic inflammation. This area, 1 to 2 cm above the mitral ring, is called *MacCallum's patch*, and is a common site of thrombus formation. It is particularly liable to be implicated in subacute infective endocarditis.

The vegetations are eventually organised (Fig. 40.4), and the valve may be rendered stenotic or incompetent.

Non-bacterial thrombotic endocarditis. Small, warty or friable vegetations along the line of closure of the mitral or aortic valves are not uncommon as a *post-mortem* finding. The vegetations are sterile, and the valves may be normal or deformed by disease, generally rheumatic. The condition is also termed *terminal*, *marantic*, or *cachectic* endocarditis, and has been described in association with cancer, particularly of the stomach, pancreas, and lung. It is probable that the vegetations are more common than is generally assumed, and are only regarded as terminal because they can be found only at necropsy. Occasionally the vegetations become detached: cerebral embolism may result. Organisation can lead to the formation of a papillary tumour-like nodule called a *Lambl's excrescence*.[12] The vegetations may form the site of infection for infective endocarditis. Usually, however, the vegetations of non-bacterial thrombotic endocarditis are of no significance and are removed, probably by lysis.

Subacute infective (bacterial) endocarditis (and endarteritis). The adjective 'subacute', hallowed by tradition, is meaningless; the course of the disease is chronic. It is much more helpful to describe the condition in terms of the causative organism than its course.[13] The usual organism is *Strept. viridans*, but sometimes other bacteria, e.g. *Staph. albus*, *Strept. faecalis*, anaerobic streptococci, *H. influenzae*, and coliform organisms, are responsible. The organism involved is one of relatively low virulence. The adjective infective is more appropriate than bacterial, since fungal cases (due especially to *Candida albicans*) are now recognised, and a special rickettsial and chlamydial endocarditis may occur in Q-fever and psittacosis[14] respectively.

The disease occurs typically on vascular endothelium which has been previously abnormal, usually as the result of rheumatic fever. Sometimes a congenital lesion, e.g. a bicuspid aortic valve, coarctation of the aorta, or patent ductus arteriosus, is the seat of trouble, indicating that the condition need not always be an endocarditis. The disease is being encountered more frequently in the elderly than it was previously, and usually there is no obvious preceding valvular disease to account for its localisation. Perhaps minor degenerative lesions are present in the affected valve.

The organisms reach the heart by the blood stream. *Strept. viridans* is a commensal organism in the mouth. A transient bacteraemia is frequent after dental extraction, and it is possible that it occurs after vigorous mastication in those who have infective oral disease. However, *Strept. viridans* endocarditis has been reported on a number of occasions in edentulous people as well as in those without dental disease, and it seems probable that in these cases the source of the organism has been the nose, throat, or gastrointestinal tract. It is not understood why the other members of the copious bacterial flora of these areas do not colonise the heart valves.[15,16]

At any rate, this bacteraemia is of no consequence in a healthy person, but in a patient with organic valvular disease there is a distinct danger of the organism colonising the valve and setting up endocarditis. The mechanism whereby this happens is not known, but the coincidental presence of non-bacterial thrombotic endocarditis is a possibility. As a prophylactic measure any patient known to have a valvular lesion should be given antibiotic cover before being subjected to dental extraction or other manipulation of a potentially infected area, e.g. the urinary tract. It should be given immediately before the operation—if given too early, there will be a chance of more resistant organisms replacing those eliminated. A recurrence of the endocarditis can occur in edentulous patients, and the wholesale extraction of sound teeth is not recommended for the prophylaxis of this disease.[17,18]

Valve lesions. The vegetations are much larger and redder than those of acute rheumatic fever. They are friable and are liable to break off and embolise. Histologically they consist of thrombus containing numerous bacterial colonies which are well protected from the blood stream. The vegetations are attached to the valve by means of granulation tissue, but this is neither profuse nor does it penetrate far into the vegetation. The organisms are once more beyond the reach of the blood. The poor vascularity of the valve cusps is the explanation of this inadequate organisation. It is a good example of frustrated repair, and as such is typical chronic inflammation. The vegetations spread on to the mural endocardium, and are often found on MacCallum's patch.

Features of the condition. The disease pursues a chronic course in which a persistent low-grade pyrexia is typical. Multiple embolic phenomena are characteristic. Large emboli may cause infarction of the brain, intestine, kidney, or spleen; smaller ones may possibly be responsible for the splinter haemorrhages of the nails, the Osler nodes, and the haematuria, but immune-complex vasculitis is a more satisfactory explanation. *It is important to note that the emboli behave as if they were sterile.* The organisms which they contain are exposed to the bactericidal action of the blood when once they break off from the valves. It is known that the patient's blood contains a high content of antibodies against the causative organisms. As a result of the bacteraemia there is considerable reticuloendothelial hyperplasia which is reflected in the splenomegaly usually present.

One of the curious features of this disease is that organisms of relatively low virulence are able to survive in the presence of a high degree of immunity. Their inaccessiblity in the thrombus appears to be the explanation.

Final diagnosis is dependent upon a positive blood culture. Frequent episodes of bacteraemia occur, but the organism is often difficult to isolate, and grows slowly (see Appendix 2).

Prior to the days of antibiotics the disease was invariably fatal. With modern treatment cure is possible, but the healed valves are often grossly distorted and show calcification. The usual cause of death is heart failure due not only to progressive valvular destruction, but also to a concomitant myocarditis. Other modes of death are embolism causing infarction of vital organs, and uraemia due to progressive glomerulonephritis in which there is a characteristic focal necrosis of the glomerular tufts. This 'flea-bitten' kidney is believed to be of immune-complex origin.[19]

Acute bacterial endocarditis. In this variety of bacterial endocarditis the organism is virulent, and it usually colonises the valve during a septicaemia.

The vegetations are large and friable, and embolism is invariable. Often the disease is masked by the accompanying septicaemia and is discovered *post mortem*. The infected emboli become impacted in arteries where they lead to acute arteritis with weakening of the wall and the formation of mycotic aneurysms. Rupture may follow. The organs show septic infarcts and pyaemic abscesses. There is great destruction of the affected valve which may undergo rapid perforation. Thus the diagnosis may be suggested by changing heart murmurs in a desperately ill patient.

Chronic verrucous endocarditis. This is the Libman-Sacks lesion of systemic lupus erythematosus (see Ch. 16).

Thrombi in the Coronary Arteries

These almost invariably occur on the basis of pre-existing atheromatous plaques, although rarely other arterial diseases, like polyarteritis nodosa, are responsible. Ischaemic heart disease is less common in women before the menopause than amongst men of comparable age—an effect generally attributed to the protective action of oestrogens.

FATE OF THROMBI

Figure 40.5 summarises the possible fate of thrombi.

(*a*) Some thrombi undoubtedly undergo lysis and leave no trace of their previous existence; plasmin may be of importance in this process, and it is of interest that there is a fibrinolytic enzyme, an activator of plasminogen, in the intima of large veins. With venous stasis there is an increase in blood fibrinolytic activity, probably because of a release of this enzyme. In the superficial veins the fibrinolytic activity is confined to the vasa vasorum, and it is higher in the arms than in the legs both in normal subjects and in those with venous thrombosis.[20-22] The enzyme is kallikrein (see p. 636).

(*b*) If an occluding thrombus in an artery or vein contains much clot, it may retract sufficiently for blood to pass by, forming a new channel. Endothelium quickly lines the passage; this is one way in which recanalisation can occur.

(*c*) In arteries the thrombus may become converted into an atheromatous plaque (see incrustation theory of atheroma, p. 497).

(*d*) A thrombus which is not removed becomes organised. In veins the granulation tissue invades it from the mural aspect, and endothelium grows over the thrombus from the adjacent uncovered intima.

It has been suggested that arterial thrombi are not vascularised from the vasa vasorum, as these extend only as far as the tunica media and do not penetrate the internal elastic lamina. Instead there may be retraction of the clot with the formation of channels, which become lined by endothelium derived either from the adjacent vessel wall or else deposited from the circulation, in which endothelial cells may normally be present. Whatever their origin, these endothelial cells also contribute to the vascularisation of the thrombus. The granulation

Figure 40.6
Recanalisation of a small thrombosed artery. Note the muscular arteriole in the centre of the old vessel. The diffuse cellular infiltration is due to surrounding infection. The section was taken from a bronchiectatic lung. × 130.

tissue is at first vascular, but later becomes dense and avascular. The blood vessels link up longitudinally, and by opening on to the luminal surface constitute another method of recanalisation (Fig. 40.6). There is no significant circulation of blood through these newly-formed channels.

(*e*) The fibrosed thrombus may undergo hyalinisation and calcification. This occurs in the pelvic veins, where the calcified thrombi are known as *phleboliths*. They may be seen during radiological examinations of the pelvic area.

(*f*) Thrombi may become detached to form emboli. This depends on their anchorage, which is poor in phlebothrombosis and atrial thrombosis. The emboli produced are *bland*, or *non-infective*.

Embolisation may also follow invasion of a thrombus by bacteria. These are usually pyogenic, the emboli are *septic*, and the condition is one of pyaemia. If the organisms are of low virulence, the emboli are 'bland' in behaviour (as in *Strept. viridans* endocarditis).

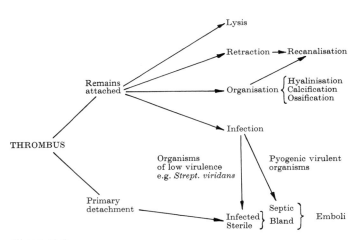

Figure 40.5

GENERAL READING

HUDSON, R. E. B. (1965) *Cardiovascular Pathology*, 3 vols. London: Arnold.

REFERENCES

1. AUERBACH, O. *et al.* (1977) Smoker's heart. *Archives of Internal Medicine*, **137**, 435.
2. HARRISON, C. V. (1966) In *Recent Advances in Pathology*, ed. Harrison, C. V., 8th edn, p. 237. London: Churchill.

3. Leading Article (1977) Takayasu's arteritis. *British Medical Journal*, **1**, 667.

4. ALLEN, E. V., BARKER, N. W. & HINES, E. A. (1962) *Peripheral Vascular Diseases*, 3rd edn, p. 293. Philadelphia: Saunders.

5. TRUMMER, M. J. & MANNIX, E. P. (1963) Abdominal pain and necrotising mesenteric arteritis following resection of coarctation of the aorta. *Journal of Thoracic and Cardiovascular Surgery*, **45**, 198.

6. DUGUID, J. B. (1949) Pathogenesis of atherosclerosis. *Lancet*, **2**, 925.

7. CRAWFORD, T. (1967) In *Modern Trends in Pathology*, ed. Crawford, T. **2**, p. 238. London: Butterworth.

8. ROSS, R. & GLOMSET, J. A. (1976) The pathogenesis of atherosclerosis. *New England Journal of Medicine*, **295**, 369 and 420.

9. Leading Article (1977) Monoclonal theory of atheroma. *British Medical Journal*, **1**, 1371.

10. OLSEN, E. J. G. (1975) In *Recent Advances in Pathology*, ed. Harrison, C. V. & Weinbren, K. 9th edn, p. 1, Edinburgh: Churchill Livingstone.

11. Leading Article (1976) Diagnosis of dissecting aneurysm of the aorta. *Lancet*, **2**, 299.

12. POMERANCE, A. (1961) Papillary 'tumours' of the heart valves. *Journal of Pathology and Bacteriology*, **81**, 135.

13. VOGLER, W. R., DORNEY, E. R. & BRIDGES, H. A. (1962) Bacterial endocarditis: a review of 148 cases. *American Journal of Medicine*, **32**, 910.

14. LEVISON, D. A. *et al.* (1971) Infective endocarditis as part of psittacosis. *Lancet*, **2**, 844.

15. Leading Article (1971) Prevention of infective endocarditis. *Lancet*, **2**, 589.

16. HILSON, G. R. F. (1970) Is chemoprophylaxis necessary? *Proceedings of the Royal Society of Medicine*, **63**, 267.

17. CROXSON, M. S., ALTMANN, M. M. & O'BRIEN, K. P. (1971) Dental status and recurrence of streptococcus viridans endocarditis. *Lancet*, **1**, 1205.

18. SIMON, D. S. & GOODWIN, J. F. (1971) Should good teeth be extracted to prevent streptococcus viridans endocarditis? *Lancet*, **1**, 1207.

19. GUTMAN, R. A. *et al.* (1972) The immune complex glomerulonephritis of bacterial endocarditis. *Medicine (Baltimore)*, **51**, 1.

20. ASTRUP, T. (1966) Tissue activators of plasminogen. *Federation Proceedings*, **25**, 42.

21. FEARNLEY, G. R. (1965) *Fibrinolysis*, p. 56. London: Arnold.

22. PANDOLFI, M. *et al.* (1967) Fibrinolytic activity of human veins. *Lancet*, **2**, 127.

Chapter 41. *Embolism*

An *embolus* is an abnormal mass of undissolved material which is transported from one part of the circulation to another. The most satisfactory classification is based upon its composition.

Types. Five categories may be recognised.

1. THROMBI AND CLOT. This may be bland or infected ('septic').

2. GAS: Air and nitrogen.

3. FAT.

4. TUMOUR.

5. MISCELLANEOUS.

1. Emboli Composed of Thrombus or Clot

Pulmonary embolism. Thrombi most frequently become detached in the veins, and are then carried to the pulmonary circulation. The effects are largely related to the size of the embolus: the long, loosely-attached, propagated clot of phlebothrombosis frequently becomes detached and produces the syndrome of *massive pulmonary embolism.*

In this condition a clot 20 to 45 cm long is detached from the femoral or popliteal vein, and is carried to the heart where it reaches the right ventricle. There is often sudden death, and the embolus may then be found coiled in the right ventricle with part of its length projecting into the main pulmonary artery. The embolus may be found straddled across the bifurcation of the pulmonary trunk, or forced into one of its two branches. It is important to distinguish between such an embolus and an *agonal thrombus* or *post-mortem clot*. The latter is moist, shiny, and gelatinous. It is loosely inserted into the pulmonary trunk, and its shape conforms to that of the situation where it is found. The clot may extend into the pulmonary vessels, and on withdrawal a cast of the pulmonary tree is obtained. Massive embolic clot, on the other hand, is dry, friable, and granular, as it has already retracted in the leg veins; ripples of platelets may be visible on its surface. The shape of the embolus does not conform to that of its surroundings, and it is so tightly inserted into the pulmonary tree that removal is difficult. The coiled mass is usually bound together by recent thrombus (Fig. 41.1).

The *cause of death* in massive pulmonary embolism is obvious enough when the main trunk is obstructed. Not infrequently, however, only one of its branches is blocked, and death under these circumstances is more difficult to explain, because it is known that a pulmonary artery can be occluded suddenly without apparent untoward effects, e.g. during pneumonectomy. Some form of reflex 'shock' or pulmonary vasoconstriction has been suggested, but never substantiated. The symptoms (dyspnoea, substernal pain, and cough) may be due to underventilation of the underperfused lung (see also p. 515).

Experimentally, death from pulmonary embolism occurs only when there is *extensive mechanical obstruction*, caused either by the emboli themselves or by superadded thrombosis. It is possible that in the human the final lethal embolus is merely one of many which have produced increasing arterial obstruction. Even in a patient who has died from a massive embolus, smaller pieces of clot may be found in branches of the pulmonary tree.

An alternative to this theory of mechanical blockage is the suggestion that the embolus, or associated thrombus, liberates 5-hydroxytryptamine, which causes *spasm* of the remainder of the pulmonary tree.[1] It must be admitted that the cause of death in many cases of this important condition is not understood.

It should be noted that pulmonary embolism does not always produce the clinical picture regarded as characteristic of the condition. Emboli, frequently unsuspected during life, were found in one series of cases in about 25 per cent of elderly folk dying of various causes.[2] Such 'quiet' pulmonary embolism is easily mistaken for bronchopneumonia, heart failure, etc., especially in elderly, obese, bedridden patients in whom clinical and X-ray examination is difficult.

Smaller pulmonary emboli also arise from the calf veins and the right atrial appendage, and these may lead to pulmonary infarction, as is described in the next chapter. Recurrent episodes of minor pulmonary embolism may so damage the lungs as to lead to progressive pulmonary hypertension.[3] Persistent hypertension is rare after a single episode of pulmonary embolism.[4]

Small septic pulmonary emboli may arise in the course of suppurative thrombophlebitis.

In severe pulmonary hypertension emboli in the right side of the heart may traverse a patent foramen ovale, or an atrial or ventricular septal defect, to enter the systemic circulation. Such an event is called 'paradoxical embolism'. It is extremely rare, though apparently a few authentic cases have been reported.[5] Usually, however, the thrombosis has in fact occurred either in the left atrium or else in the pulmonary veins. It is possible that pulmonary embolism may cause sufficient stasis in the pulmonary veins to produce thrombosis. Detachment of these thrombi would result in systemic embolism. Since pulmonary embolism also produces pulmonary hypertension, the conditions are ideal for the syndrome of 'paradoxical embolism'.

Fate of pulmonary emboli.[4] In those who survive, the thrombus is either lysed or organised. Bands or webs may be the only residua of previous occlusive emboli, and as with thrombi in systemic arteries, their organisation and incorporation into the vessel wall can produce plaques of atheroma.

Systemic embolism. Emboli arising in the heart are generally systemic. They may arise in the left atrium, e.g. in mitral stenosis, on the mitral or aortic valves, e.g. in infective endocarditis, or in the left ventricle, e.g. following infarction. The

Figure 41.1

Massive pulmonary embolism. These thrombi were removed as one large coiled mass from the pulmonary arteries of a man who died a week after operation. There was extensive phlebothrombosis in both calves. It is apparent that the calibre of the unfolded thrombi corresponds with the lumina of the leg veins. (C 40.5, *Reproduced by permission of the President and Council of the R.C.S. Eng.*)

possibility of pulmonary-vein thrombosis has already been mentioned.

Emboli arise from the larger arteries from time to time. The importance of thrombotic embolism from atheromatous plaques is described later in this chapter. More occasionally, atheromatous material from the aorta and its major branches becomes detached and embolises distally. The kidney, pancreas, intestine, spleen, heart, brain, and limbs are all sites where this has been described.

Effects of systemic emboli. The effects of impaction of any embolus are those of obstruction. It may be broken up by the pounding of the arterial pressure, and in this way move on to more distant branches; thrombosis or clotting beyond the block usually occurs.

In the peripheral vasculature severe local pain may occur, and is generally attributed to spasm of the vessel wall. Pain, however, is not a feature of embolisation in internal organs, e.g. kidney and brain. The effects of ischaemia on various tissues are considered in Chapter 42.

Bland emboli produce no other effects, whereas *septic emboli* set up secondary foci of suppuration. According to local anatomical circumstances, pyaemic abscesses, septic infarcts, or mycotic aneurysms are produced.

2. Gaseous Emboli

Air.[6] Air may be introduced into a systemic vein under the following conditions:

Operations on the head and neck. The accidental opening of a large vein, like the jugular, may allow air to be sucked in.

A mismanaged blood transfusion. This is likely to be of serious consequence only when positive pressure is being employed with old-fashioned equipment.

During haemodialysis for renal failure.[7]

Insufflation of the uterine tubes.

Interference with the placental site during criminal abortion.

During the procedure of artificial pneumoperitoneum.

The air enters the right side of the heart, and is churned up into a froth. During systole the heart merely compresses this froth, but scarcely any blood actually enters the pulmonary artery. The effects are therefore very similar to massive pulmonary embolism. The characteristic churning noise, which may be heard without the aid of a stethoscope, serves to distinguish the two conditions clinically. It will be readily appreciated that in order to produce this effect, large quantities of air must be introduced suddenly. In dogs about 9 ml per kg is regarded as a lethal amount.[8] In humans it is probably considerably less (see p. 653). Small quantities are unimportant, because they pass through the heart and become impacted in a branch of the pulmonary artery. Air, however, is readily absorbed, and the effects of the block are not usually long-lasting enough to be serious.

Air may be introduced into a pulmonary vein during the induction of a pneumothorax. This may block the ostium of a vital coronary or cerebral artery, so that only a few ml are necessary to cause serious, even fatal, effects.[8] This is one of the causes of the clinician's 'pleural shock'. Air may also reach the systemic circulation from the venous side in the air embolism that complicates haemodialysis.[7]

Nitrogen. The important example is *decompression sickness*, also called *caisson disease*.[9] This occurs in people who have been exposed to a high pressure, e.g. divers, tunnellers, and those encased in a caisson (diving-bell), and then return to a normal atmospheric pressure too rapidly, or in those exposed to a low pressure after having been at a normal atmospheric pressure, e.g. airmen. As the pressure is reduced, bubbles of air come out of solution from the blood and interstitial fluid; whereas oxygen and CO_2 are readily absorbed and removed, the inert nitrogen remains in the tissues for some time and causes damage. As it is fairly soluble in fat, much is present in the subcutaneous tissues and the central nervous system. When it comes out of solution, it leads to tissue disruption, particularly in areas of poor blood supply where absorption is delayed. This effect is most important in the lower thoracic region of the spinal cord and the peripheral nerves. Considerable damage may be done, causing severe pain (the 'bends') and sometimes permanent paraplegia or death. Damage is marked around the ends of long bones; aseptic necrosis occurs, and this leads to severe osteoarthritis.

Several cases of decompression sickness have been reported in which there were large air cysts in the lungs. It has been suggested that these cysts discharge bubbles of air into the pulmonary veins during decompression, and so aggravate the condition.[10] Caisson disease can be averted by slow decompression or by using a helium and oxygen mixture instead of air.

3. Fat Emboli[11]

Globules of fat may enter small veins after a fracture, and in the case of multiple injuries this embolisation may be quite extensive. Actual fragments of bone marrow may be found in the pulmonary arterioles. This is commonly seen in patients who have sustained multiple fractures of the ribs as a result of vigorous external cardiac massage. A similar event has been reported in sickle-cell anaemia as a rare complication of the patchy infarction of the bone marrow which is seen quite often in this condition (Fig. 41.2). Interosseous phlebography (using the pertrochanteric route) may be complicated by fat embolism. This is nearly always subclinical, and only rarely causes symptoms.[12] Cerebral fat and silicone emboli are commonly found in patients who have recently undergone unsuccessful cardio-bypass operations.

The clinical features vary as to whether or not the emboli pass through the lung barrier.

Pulmonary fat embolism. The presence of fat globules in the capillaries of the lung is a frequent *post-mortem* finding in fracture patients, but the tremendous vascular bed of the lung is not likely to be appreciably obstructed by these small droplets of fat. Occasionally, however, pulmonary fat embolism may be extensive enough to be the immediate cause of death.[11] In the investigation of accidents like air crashes the presence of fat emboli provides evidence of survival after the injury.

Systemic fat embolism. Sometimes the emboli pass through the pulmonary bed, and become lodged in the capillaries of the brain, kidney, skin, and other organs. This is a serious event, and constitutes the fat-embolism syndrome.

In severe cases the patient becomes comatose within a few hours of injury, and dies within 1 to 2 days. More usually symptoms occur 24 to 48 hours after injury: these include fever, restlessness, respiratory distress, cyanosis, and cerebral symptoms. If the brain damage is severe, coma results and death follows. A petechial skin eruption is helpful diagnostically, but is not usually manifest until the second or third day. There may be subconjunctival and retinal haemorrhages also.

The important effect of systemic fat embolism is cerebral damage; this dominates the clinical picture, and is the cause of death. It is blamed also for the respiratory symptoms, which may be severe and associated with multiple areas of pulmonary haemorrhage and oedema. At necropsy the brain shows striking changes: numerous petechial haemorrhages are present in the white matter (the grey matter is also severely affected by the fat emboli, but perhaps because of better anastomosis does not show many petechiae).[13] Fat emboli are found in the glomeruli and in the skin petechiae. Pulmonary involvement is always marked, and opinions are divided on whether this is secondary to brain damage or a direct effect of the pulmonary fat emboli.

During life fat may be found in the sputum, but its presence only indicates pulmonary involvement. Examination of the urine may reveal fat, but the test is unreliable. Renal

Figure 41.2
Bone-marrow embolism. This small pulmonary artery contains a fragment of fatty bone marrow. Around the fat spaces haematopoietic tissue is recognisable. The remainder of the lumen is occluded by blood clot. The patient was a Jamaican who had sickle-cell anaemia. She died suddenly in a state simulating massive pulmonary embolism, and at necropsy many of the pulmonary arterioles were found to contain fat and bone-marrow emboli. The latter occluded so much of the pulmonary vascular bed that death ensued. There were no systemic emboli, such as are encountered in post-traumatic fat embolism. × 130.

involvement has also been detected by needle biopsy. The plasma calcium level is sometimes reduced, possibly due to the affinity of calcium ions for the free fatty acid released as the fat emboli are hydrolysed. The platelet count is invariably lowered; indeed, this may be a factor in the production of the petechial skin lesions.[11]

The mechanism of fat embolism is imperfectly understood. While there can be little doubt that mechanical entry of fatty tissue into the veins is of great importance, it sometimes seems inadequate to explain the extent of the lesion in comparison with the mildness of the trauma. It has been suggested that there is also an alteration in the emulsion stability of the circulating blood lipids, so that the chylomicrons aggregate and form composite globules of fat emboli. Nevertheless, emboli recovered from the lungs of dogs with fractured legs have a triglyceride composition similar to that of bone marrow and depot fat but quite unlike that of the circulating chylomicrons.[11]

It has been suggested that the effects of fat embolism are due not so much to ischaemia as to the toxic action on the vascular endothelium of the fatty acids which are derived from the broken-down fat. Such a mechanism would explain the delay in onset of symptoms and the severity of the lung lesions, which are an outstanding necropsy feature of the fat-embolism syndrome. They produce a 'snow-storm' appearance in the chest radiograph, and are the cause of the hypoxaemia, itself the major precipitating cause of death.

Soft-tissue injuries unassociated with fractures are said to cause fat embolism occasionally, but it may be that a fracture was missed in these cases. If, however, a fatty liver is injured, fat embolism may certainly ensue; indeed, it has occurred spontaneously in cases of fatty liver.

4. Tumour Emboli

It is probable that all malignant tumours invade the local blood vessels at an early stage of the disease, and that isolated malignant cells are of frequent occurrence in the circulation. The tumour cells are covered by thrombus, and the majority of these emboli are destroyed, leaving only a small percentage to develop into metastatic deposits. Multiple small tumour emboli, by leading to fibrin deposition, may initiate a consumptive coagulopathy (see p. 643).

Some tumours, notably clear-cell carcinoma of the kidney and carcinoma of the lung, tend to invade larger blood vessels, and occasionally a mass of tumour becomes detached to produce a large embolus (see p. 363).

5. Miscellaneous Emboli

Foreign bodies. Bullets,[14] silk, talc, etc., are all reported to have been carried from one part of the body to another by the blood stream. Drug addicts who inject themselves intravenously with crushed tablets, designed for oral use and containing talc, can develop extensive non-caseating granulomata in the lungs, eyes,[15] and other organs.

Polythene tubing may embolise during intravenous therapy and cardiac catheterisation.[16,17] There is a great danger of it acting as a nidus for infection and thrombosis.

Fibre embolism, consisting of cotton or cellulose, has been reported as a common post-mortem finding in patients who have died after cardiac operations or cardiac catheterisation.[18]

Parasites. Various parasites and their ova are carried by the blood stream. Schistosomes and their ova may lodge in the branches of the portal vein in the liver, and induce a fibrosis of 'pipe-stem' type (Fig. 41.3). They may pass on to the lung and produce an inflammatory reaction around the pulmonary arterioles, which may lead to pulmonary hypertension.[19]

Red-cell aggregates. Blockage of small vessels by aggregates of red cells is commonly seen in infections and following trauma. The condition is generally called *sludging*, and is considered in detail on page 421.

Red-cell aggregations also occur in the exposed limbs when cold autohaemagglutinins are present. This is the cause of the Raynaud-like phenomenon seen in patients with acquired haemolytic anaemia of the cold antibody type.

Microemboli.[20] White bodies can sometimes be seen in the retinal vessels, and by plugging them produce microinfarcts. Some of these bodies appear to consist of atheromatous material probably derived from plaques in the carotid arteries. Others are platelet aggregates or fibrin derived perhaps from

Figure 41.3
Parasitic embolus. This is a cross-section of a portal vein in which there is the parasitic trematode *Schistosoma haematobium*. Surrounding the vein there is a wide zone of small round cells, and at the periphery liver tissue is recognisable. The perivascular infiltration is the precursor of the later 'pipe-stem' fibrosis. × 110.

the heart in cases of rheumatic heart disease. During open-heart surgery emboli may consist of calcium (from calcified valves), silicone, or fat.[21] The role of these emboli in disease is conjectural. In the *eye* they have been blamed for transient attacks of unilateral blindness (amaurosis fugax), but it appears more likely that the sudden onset of blindness is due to a reduced perfusion and flow in the retinal vessels from other causes and that platelet aggregation is a secondary phenomenon.[21] Platelet emboli have also been blamed for *transient strokes*, and progressive obliteration of the microcirculation of the lower limbs is probably an important contributory factor in the pathogenesis of peripheral vascular disease. It is difficult to prove this because examination of the vasculature of the legs is tedious and time consuming. However, it is quite common to find small arterioles in the kidney obstructed by atheromatous material. Often there is a foreign-body giant-cell reaction to this cholesterol-containing material, and since the vessels are small it is reasonable to assume that the atheromatous material is embolic, for atheroma does not affect such small vessels.

Amniotic fluid. Amniotic fluid containing meconium and squamous cells may enter the uterine veins and travel to the lungs. The condition usually occurs during labour and abruptio placentae, and is characterised by shock and a generalised bleeding tendency. The plasmin system is activated, and since this enzyme digests fibrinogen as well as fibrin, acute afibrinogenaemia occurs. It is possible that the symptoms are due to a type of anaphylactic shock rather than a direct effect of the amniotic emboli themselves.

REFERENCES

1. THOMAS, D. P. *et al.* (1965) In *Pulmonary Embolic Disease*, ed. Sasahara, A. A. & Stein, M., p. 59. New York: Grune and Stratton.
2. TOWBIN, A. (1954) Pulmonary embolism; incidence and significance. *Journal of the American Medical Association*, **156**, 209.
3. FLEISCHNER, F. G. (1967) Recurrent pulmonary embolism and cor pulmonale. *New England Journal of Medicine*, **276**, 1213.
4. Annotation (1967) Sequelae to pulmonary embolism. *Lancet*, **2**, 1291.
5. Leading Article (1973) Paradoxical embolism. *British Medical Journal*, **1**, 630.
6. Annotation (1963) Air embolism. *Lancet*, **1**, 96.
7. WARD, M. K. *et al.* (1971) Air embolism during haemodialysis. *British Medical Journal*, **3**, 74.
8. KENT, E. M. & BLADES, B. (1942) Experimental observations upon certain intracranial complications of particular interest to thoracic surgeons. *Journal of Thoracic Surgery*, **11**, 434.
9. DEWEY, A. W. (1962) Decompression sickness, an emergency recreational hazard. *New England Journal of Medicine*, **267**, 759 and 812.
10. COLLINS, J. J. (1962) An unusual case of air embolism precipitated by decompression. *New England Journal of Medicine*, **266**, 595.
11. Leading Article (1972) Fat embolism. *Lancet*, **1**, 672.
12. YOUNG, A. E., THOMAS, M. L. & BROWSE, N. L. (1976) Interosseous phlebography and fat embolism. *British Medical Journal*, **2**, 89.
13. SEVITT, S. (1972) Fat embolism. *Lancet*, **1**, 848.
14. KINMONTH, J. B. *et al.* (1961) Gunshot wounds of the heart with embolism. *British Medical Journal*, **2**, 1666.
15. ATLEE, W. E. (1972) Talc and cornstarch emboli in eyes of drug abusers. *Journal of American Medical Association*, **219**, 49.
16. UDWADIA, T. E. & EDWARDS, A. E. (1963) Accidental loss of plastic tube into venous system. *British Medical Journal*, **2**, 1251.
17. BENNETT, P. J. (1963) Use of intravenous plastic catheters. *British Medical Journal*, **2**, 1252.
18. DIMMICK, J. E. *et al.* (1975) Fiber embolisation—a hazard of cardiac surgery and catheterisation. *New England Journal of Medicine*, **292**, 685.
19. SPENCER, H. (1977) *Pathology of the Lung*, 3rd edn, Vol. 1, p. 341. Oxford: Pergamon Press.
20. Leading Article (1972) Platelet embolism. *British Medical Journal*, **3**, 67.
21. WILLIAMS, I. M. (1971) Intravascular changes in the retina during open-heart surgery. *Lancet*, **2**, 688.

Chapter 42. *Ischaemia and Infarction*

Ischaemia is defined as a condition of inadequate blood supply to an area of tissue. It produces harmful effects in three ways:

1. Hypoxia. Oxygen deprivation is by far the most important factor producing damage in ischaemic tissue. It is especially so when considering the effect on very active cells, e.g. muscle. On the other hand, it plays no part in the lesions produced by pulmonary arterial obstruction, because the alveolar walls derive their oxygen supply directly from the alveolar gas.

2. Malnutrition. This is probably of little importance, because the blood contains much more glucose and amino acids than could be metabolised by the amount of oxygen which it contains.

3. Failure to remove waste products. The accumulation of metabolites is the most probable explanation of pain in muscle ischaemia. The presence of waste products or the failure to maintain important electrolyte (or other) balances is the probable cause of necrosis in pulmonary infarction.

Hypoxia is a state of impaired oxygenation. Four types are described:

Hypoxic, due to a low oxygen tension in the arterial blood, as in lung disease and cyanotic congenital heart disease with a right-to-left shunt.

Anaemic, due to a low level of haemoglobin, which carries the oxygen in the blood.

Stagnant or *ischaemic*, due to an inadequate blood supply to the tissues. This, as will be seen, is due either to heart failure or some local vascular obstruction.

Histotoxic, due to cellular intoxication, which prevents the uptake of oxygen, e.g. cyanide poisoning.

The subject of hypoxia is dealt with in standard physiology textbooks, and will not be considered further.

CAUSES OF ISCHAEMIA

General

Ischaemia may be caused by an inadequate cardiac output; not all tissues are equally affected because of the redistribution of the available blood. Symmetrical gangrene of the extremities is an occasional manifestation of myocardial infarction (see p. 534).[1]

In the *Stokes-Adams syndrome* of complete heart block, and during ventricular arrest or fibrillation the blood supply to the whole body is stopped. The manifestations are confined to a single organ, the brain, which is particularly sensitive to hypoxia. If the arrest continues for 15 seconds consciousness is lost, and if the condition lasts more than about 4 minutes itreparable damage is done.[2] The neurons degenerate and replacement gliosis occurs, which is exactly similar to that produced by the acute hypoxic hypoxia that may occur as the result of a poorly administered anaesthetic. If cardiac arrest lasts for more than 8 minutes death is inevitable.

Local Causes of Ischaemia

By far the most important cause of ischaemia is obstruction to the arterial flow. It should not, however, be forgotten that extensive venous and capillary damage can also produce ischaemia.

Arterial obstruction. Most of the causes of obstruction have already been described in Chapter 40. They will therefore only be summarised:

Thrombosis.

Embolism. The effects of the embolus are potentiated by the reflex spasm of the arterial wall, and completed by the rapid development of thrombus over the embolus.

Spasm. This includes not only local spastic conditions, but also states of generalised vasoconstriction that follow haemorrhage and dehydration.

Atheroma produces partial obstruction in medium-sized vessels, e.g. cerebral, coronary, and renal.

Occlusive pressure from without, e.g. tourniquets and tightly-fitting plasters.

Venous disease. Extensive venous obstruction leads to engorgement of the areas drained by the affected veins. This may reach such an intensity that blood flow is impeded and ischaemia results. There are many good examples of this:

Mesenteric venous thrombosis, leading to intestinal infarction.

Strangulation of a hernia. The venous obstruction at the neck of a hernia leads to damage long before the arterial blood flow is implicated. The same mechanism applies to volvulus and intussusception (see p. 522).

Phlegmasia caerulea dolens. This is a rare variant of iliofemoral thrombosis, in which there is sudden intense venous engorgement followed by gangrene of the limb. It has been proved by subsequent dissection that the main arteries are not affected, but that there is almost complete venous obstruction by thrombosis.[3–5]

Cavernous-sinus thrombosis leads to retinal-vein thrombosis and retinal changes resulting in blindness.

Varicose veins of the leg. Venous stasis secondary to varicose veins of the leg leads to ischaemic changes of the skin (stasis dermatitis). Ultimately indolent ulcers develop, often being precipitated by local trauma.

Small-vessel damage. When vascular disease is considered, the vessels of microscopic size are often forgotten. There are nevertheless many conditions in which so many arterioles, capillaries, or venules in an area are occluded that ischaemia results. An additional effect is bleeding; haemorrhage is a common feature of damage even when the extent of the vascular occlusion is not enough to lead to local ischaemia.

Vasculitis. The necrosis, polymorph infiltration, and thrombosis that follows damage to the walls of small vessels is commonly called vasculitis, since arterioles, capillaries, and venules are often involved together, and it is difficult to distinguish the one from the other when there is damage. Vasculitis can follow the deposition of damaging immune complexes in the vessel walls; a typical example is seen in the lesions of the Arthus reaction, and similar lesions are encountered in many drug eruptions and in Henoch-Schönlein purpura. The same is true of the vasculitis of small-vessel polyarteritis nodosa and probably also of the petechial haemorrhages and renal lesions of subacute infective endocarditis.

Acute vasculitis is also a feature of gonococcal and meningococcal septicaemia (Figs. 42.1 and 42.2). Organisms are scanty and difficult to find. By contrast, the vasculitis of *Pseudomonas* septicaemia shows extensive necrosis, little inflammatory reaction, and is teeming with bacteria.

Frost-bite. The harmful effect of cold on exposed parts is due in large measure to damage to the small blood vessels. There is initial arteriolar spasm, and the ischaemia is aggravated by stasis of blood in the damaged capillaries. In the most severe cases extensive intracapillary blockage causes infarction of the area. Even if necrosis does not occur, the capillary damage leads to the development of large bullae when the circulation is restored after the part is warmed. Pain may be severe. Severe freezing injury promotes ice-crystal formation in the cells, and this causes further damage.[6-8]

Occlusion of capillaries by red cells, e.g. in sickle-cell anaemia, cerebral malaria, and conditions associated with severe autohaemagglutination, e.g. acquired haemolytic anaemia due to cold antibodies. Sludging of the blood may also cause capillary obstruction (p. 421).

Occlusion by fibrin. This occurs in the defibrination syndrome, see page 643.

Occlusion by precipitated cryoglobulins. (See p. 580.)

Occlusion of capillaries by white cells. Clumping of the abnormal white cells in chronic myeloid leukaemia may be responsible for the infarcts that occur in this condition, e.g. of spleen.

Fat embolism.

Decompression sickness.

External pressure, e.g. bedsores.

Figure 42.1

Gonococcal septicaemia. The patient, a woman aged 24 years, complained of flitting polyarthralgia for 5 days starting from the onset of her last menstrual period. The right knee was particularly painful; on examination it was tender and swollen. A day or two after the onset of the joint pains she developed a skin eruption consisting of scattered lesions on the distal parts of the arms and legs. Some of these lesions were small erythematous papules, but others enlarged and developed haemorrhagic pustules in their centres. The figure shows one of these lesions on a finger. There was also malaise, anorexia, and a mild pyrexia in the evenings. A biopsy of one of the skin lesions showed an acute vasculitis. This finding, together with the history and the clinical findings, strongly suggested a diagnosis of gonococcal septicaemia. A slight vaginal discharge was noted, and a swab of the cervix subsequently grew gonococci. The condition recovered on penicillin therapy.

The patient had been on a holiday 2 weeks before the onset of the disease. During that time she had had intercourse with a new acquaintance. Prior to this she was not aware of having had intercourse with anyone who had a discharge.

Figure 42.2

Acute gonococcal vasculitis. This is a biopsy from the case described in Fig. 42.1. The dermis, with its thick collagen fibres (COL), shows an arteriole that is obstructed by thrombus rich in fibrin (FIBRIN). The vessel wall has undergone necrosis, and there is a heavy infiltration of polymorphs (POLYS). The presence of many red cells (RBC) in the interstitial tissues indicates that the vessel has ruptured. × 300.

The Effects of Arterial and Capillary Obstruction

The effects depend largely upon the degree of ischaemia produced, and may range from sudden death to virtually no damage at all. The following are the possibilities:

1. There may be *no effects* on the tissue supplied by the vessel, if ischaemia is obviated by collateral channels.

2. There may be *functional disturbances*. The collaterals supply sufficient blood during inactivity, but cannot sustain normal exercise, e.g. angina pectoris and intermittent claudication. In sudden coronary arterial occlusion there may be ventricular fibrillation; this can follow quite small occlusions, and if death is averted by defibrillation, the resulting infarct may not be large.

3. There may be *cellular degeneration* affecting the parenchyma, e.g. cloudy swelling and fatty change which may proceed to necrosis. This is a patchy affair, and leads to atrophy. It is accompanied by *replacement fibrosis* (Fig. 42.3) or, in the central nervous system, *gliosis*. This is seen under a variety of conditions: sudden, complete arterial obstruction of short duration, e.g. of brain, and partial arterial obstruction of gradual onset, e.g. atheroma affecting the cerebral vessels.

Pressure atrophy is an example of this type of lesion; it is due to gradual ischaemia at capillary level in which there is time for atrophy to occur. The affected cells not only become smaller, but also ultimately undergo necrosis. The connective tissue framework is left behind, e.g. in the capsule of a benign tumour, because it is more resistant to the effects of ischaemia. This is not replacement fibrosis, because the expanding lesion that has caused the pressure atrophy provides the extra tissue.

Figure 42.3
Myocardial fibrosis. There is a patchy replacement of myocardial fibres by dense, acellular fibrous tissue. There is no inflammatory reaction. × 80.

It is doubtful whether ischaemia of the heart ever leads to atrophy; if ischaemic myocardium is examined microscopically it is seen to consist of foci of avascular fibrous tissue, interspersed amongst which there are surviving muscle cells. These, on the whole, are hypertrophied, no doubt a compensatory phenomenon.

4. Both arterial and venous obstruction may lead to a circumscribed necrosis of tissue; this is called *infarction*, and will be described in detail later. Complete occlusion of the capillary bed either by frost-bite or pressure produces a similar result. The latter is well illustrated by the formation of bedsores.

Factors Determining the Extent of Ischaemia in Arterial Obstruction

There are three crucial factors:

1. Speed of Onset

If the obstruction is sudden the effects are more severe than if it is gradual, because there is less time for an effective collateral circulation to develop.

2. The Extent of Obstruction

A complete obstruction is obviously much more serious than a partial one. This is well illustrated in the heart: partial coronary occlusion due to atheroma may be well tolerated, while complete obstruction usually causes infarction and sometimes death.

3. The Anatomy of the Collateral Circulation

Some arteries have no anastomotic channels. These are called *end arteries*; the central artery of the retina is a classical example, as are also the smaller vessels of the cerebral cortex. Others, like the larger cerebral vessels, the coronary arteries, the interlobular arteries of the kidney, and the splenic arteries, have so inadequate an anastomosis that, should they be blocked, some degree of infarction would be inevitable. They are indeed functional end arteries. The branches of the superior mesenteric artery have an extensive arcade of vessels emerging from them, but even here the anastomosis between each branch is poor. The inferior mesenteric artery is much more effectively arrayed with anastomotic branches, and infarction is less common in the distal colon than in the small intestine and proximal colon. The stomach has the benefit of three separate arterial supplies all derived from the coeliac axis, and it is not surprising that it is the least frequently infarcted part of the gastrointestinal tract.

The lungs and liver are peculiar in having a double blood supply, and this modifies the effect of occlusion of one set of vessels to these organs.

The precise anatomy of the collateral circulation can have some curious effects, as demonstrated by the various *steal syndromes*.[9] For example, obstruction of the first part of the subclavian artery can cause blood (from the carotid arteries or the opposite vertebral artery) to be diverted down the vertebral artery to the arm; brain-stem ischaemia can be precipitated by arm exercises. The stealing of blood from one area may thus be confusing diagnostically, leading to the false localisation of an arterial obstruction.

Another example is the reno-splanchnic steal: if the coeliac artery is obstructed, blood can be diverted from the renal artery *via* its suprarenal branch anastomosing with branches of the coeliac artery distal to the obstruction of its main stem. Renal-artery stenosis can be mimicked, and hypertension ensues.[9]

Four other subsidiary factors modify the effects of arterial blockage:

(*a*) **The pathology of the collateral circulation.** A collateral circulation severely affected with spasm, atheroma, or other condition is of little value in maintaining a good alternative blood supply.

(*b*) **The state of oxygenation of the blood**, in respect of arterial Po_2 and haemoglobin level.

(*c*) **The efficiency of the heart.**

(*d*) **The nature of the affected tissue.** Brain and heart are more vulnerable to ischaemia than are any other organs. Connective tissue survives much better than does the parenchyma of an organ.

THE PROCESS OF INFARCTION

Infarction usually leads to a circumscribed area of coagulative necrosis, which is subsequently organised into scar tissue. The process is as follows:

(*a*) There is death of the cells in the area deprived of its blood supply. Blood usually continues to seep into the devitalised area for a short time due to three possible processes:

(i) An opening-up of peripheral anastomotic channels. This is particularly well marked in the lung because of its double blood supply.

(ii) Blood may continue to trickle in through the occluded artery (which is atonic distally), because the obstruction is not complete initially. The aperture between the obstruction and the vessel wall, however, soon becomes occluded by thrombus.

(iii) There may be venous reflux.

At all events most infarcts contain a great deal of blood in the early stages, and are swollen and red in colour. The red cells entering the affected area escape through the damaged capillaries, and lie free in the dead tissue. There is also a great deal of fibrin derived from the blood (*infarcire* = to stuff). Infarcts of lax structures, e.g. lung and intestine, are much more engorged than those of compact organs, e.g. kidney and heart.

(*b*) The dead tissue undergoes necrosis; in solid organs the associated swelling of the cells may squeeze the blood out of the infarct. In this way it becomes paler. It is very important to note that until necrosis is visible, the ischaemic area cannot be called an infarct. Histochemical or electron-microscopic changes may be detected very shortly after cardiac muscle has been rendered ischaemic, but these very closely resemble the changes of autolysis. Hence in human material it is not possible to distinguish *post-mortem* changes from those of early infarction. In practice it takes from 12 to 24 hours for a myocardial infarct to become macroscopically recognisable, while the first microscopical changes of necrosis can be seen only from 6 to 12 hours after the ischaemic episode. Unless the patient survives the ischaemic episode for a number of hours, infarction cannot be diagnosed morphologically or histochemically.

(*c*) There is progressive autolysis of necrotic tissue and haemolysis of the red cells.

(*d*) At the same time the surrounding tissue undergoes an acute inflammatory reaction, stimulated presumably by products of autolysis. The initial polymorph response, which is quite marked (Fig. 42.4), is followed after a few days by a macrophage infiltration.

(*e*) There is an outward diffusion of tissue breakdown products and free haemoglobin, which are ingested by macrophages. Bilirubin and haemosiderin are produced locally. By this stage, approximately a week after occlusion, the infarct is firm and dull yellow in colour, and is surrounded by a red zone of inflammation.

(*f*) This phase of demolition is followed by a shrinkage of the infarct, which becomes white in colour. In some organs, notably the kidney, the necrotic tissue is so well preserved that its outlines are recognisable as ghosts without nuclei for many months (Fig. 42.5). There is a slow but progressive ingrowth of granulation tissue from the periphery, and eventually the infarct is organised into a fibrous scar which later undergoes hyaline change. Dystrophic calcification may occur in the midst of the infarct, and also in the area of scarring. Around many infarcts there is a residual zone of pigmentation. This consists mostly of haemosiderin, but there may also be lipofuscin derived from broken-down parenchymatous cells, especially heart muscle.

The process is somewhat different in infarcts of the central nervous system:

Figure 42.4
Myocardial infarction. The muscle fibres are necrotic, but their structure is easily recognisable. There is a profuse cellular infiltration, including many polymorphs, around the necrotic tissue. × 150.

Figure 42.5
Renal infarct. The renal tubules and glomerulus are necrotic but their structure is well preserved. On the left-hand side there is a polymorph infiltration. × 100.

(*a*) The necrotic tissue undergoes rapid colliquative necrosis.

(*b*) There is an infiltration of macrophages, derived from the monocytes and the microglia, which demolish the debris and ingest the disintegrated myelin. These swell up, and in their cytoplasm there is lipid material and some pigment which consists of variable amounts of haemosiderin derived from the small amount of blood in the infarct and lipofuscin from the disintegrated neurons. These macrophages are called *compound granular corpuscles* (Fig. 30.2, p. 393). Polymorphs are absent unless the meninges are involved.

(*c*) Repair by gliosis ensues, but sometimes a cyst surrounded by a layer of glial tissue remains.

The Morbid Anatomy of Infarcts

Infarcts of solid organs are usually wedge-shaped, with the apex directed internally in relation to the occluded artery and the base on the surface of the organ. Cerebral infarcts are ill-defined, soft, and pulpy; this is called *cerebral softening*.

Infarcts have been classified according to their colour, but this is of limited value. It is apparent that most start by being red, and become white as blood is squeezed out and as the free haemoglobin is later removed. Cerebral infarcts are usually initially white because there is virtually no anastomosis, and the vessels occluded are often so small that obstruction is usually complete right from the beginning. On the other hand, pulmonary infarcts seldom become white because of the enor-

mous amount of blood trapped in the necrotic alveolar sacs. They are organised in the red stage.

Infarcts secondary to venous obstruction are haemorrhagic.

Infarcts may be classified as *bland* and *septic* (or *infected*), according to whether they are sterile or contain organisms. As explained in Chapter 40, the infarcts of *Strept. viridans* endocarditis behave in a bland way, because the organisms in the emboli are rapidly destroyed at the site of impaction. In septic infarction there is a rapid transition from the stage of necrosis to one of suppuration, and the result is a large ragged abscess. Septic emboli which become impacted in vessels supplying tissue which does not normally show infarction, lead to a local acute inflammatory reaction terminating in suppuration. In this way multiple pyaemic abscesses are formed in the liver (portal pyaemia) and lung.

General Effects of Infarction

It should finally be noted that infarction of any significant extent is accompanied by constitutional effects. There is fever, a neutrophil leucocytosis, and a raised ESR. These effects are presumably caused by products of autolysis (see p. 56). In addition the necrotic tissue may release its enzymes into the circulation, and these may be of diagnostic help. In myocardial infarction the plasma glutamate-oxaloacetate transaminase (aspartate aminotransferase) rises from a normal level of 5 to 17 units to over 200 units per litre (see p. 569). This is useful diagnostically in the first few days, but then the level drops.

Other enzymes that are liberated include creatine phosphokinase (CPK) and lactate dehydrogenase (LDH). The creatine phosphokinase, like the SGOT, rises early and returns to normal within 3 days. The LDH, on the other hand, begins to rise by 12 hours, reaches a maximum at 48 hours, and returns to normal by the eleventh day. There are five isoenzyme bands of LDH as revealed by electrophoresis. The fast-moving components LDH_1 and LDH_2 are found in heart, kidney, and red cells. A rise in LDH_1 is a useful indicator of myocardial infarction. The slow-moving band LDH_5 is present in liver and muscle, and its level is a useful gauge of the extent of liver necrosis. $LDH_{2,3,4}$ are present in lung and, together with LDH_1 from broken-down red cells, are found in increased quantities in pulmonary infarction. Alpha-hydroxybutyrate -dehydrogenase (HBD) measures the same enzymatic activity as does LDH_1, and its plasma level has the same significance as that of LDH_1.[10]

THE EFFECTS OF ISCHAEMIA ON VARIOUS ORGANS

It is instructive to conclude by considering the effects of ischaemia on a few tissues.

Heart

Myocardial ischaemia and infarction can occur in hearts with normal coronary arteries when the coronary perfusion is impaired by extreme tachycardia, shock, or severe aortic stenosis. Nevertheless, in most cases there is an organic stenosis of the vessels. Syphilitic occlusion of the ostia, polyarteritis nodosa, coronary embolism, and dissecting aneurysm of the aorta are occasional causes, but atheroma and the intimal thickening that is part of the ageing process are by far the most common and important. Gradual occlusion of a coronary artery may be symptomless for a long time, and is accompanied by the development of considerable anastomotic channels between branches of the coronary system. Eventually the occlusion may become severe enough to lead to functional insufficiency during exercise and cause angina pectoris. If the patient dies at this stage the heart will show appreciable areas of fibrous replacement of myocardium. In addition microscopic areas of myocardial necrosis may be present; and it is noteworthy that these do not show the acute inflammatory reaction which is so marked in large infarcts. The anginal pain has not been adequately explained. A 'factor P' produced by ischaemic muscle was suggested by Lewis, but it has never been isolated. Pain-producing substances are produced by ischaemic muscle, e.g. K^+ ions leaking out of cells, lactic acid, and phosphates, and perhaps these are responsible. It is possible that vasodilator metabolites released from ischaemic muscle open up anastomotic channels, but hypoxia is more important.

In classical, effort-induced Heberden's angina, the myocardial ischaemia is thought to be induced by increased myocardial contraction acting in the face of the relatively constant coronary blood flow prescribed by structural coronary stenosis produced by atherosclerosis. Factors that raise the blood pressure (such as emotion and exposure to cold),[11] the cardiac output, or the pulse rate induce angina and electrocardiographic changes indicative of subendocardial ischaemia. The drugs that provide relief, for instance nitroglycerine, do so by lowering the systemic blood pressure and therefore the cardiac oxygen requirement. There is a rare type of angina, described by Prinzmetal and before him by Osler, in which pain occurs not on exercise but at rest.[12,13] Angiography reveals coronary narrowing during attacks but not in the intervals of freedom from pain. Spasm is thought to be the cause of this type of angina.[14]

Two major patterns of myocardial infarction are seen:

Regional infarction. This is the usual finding in patients who die of acute heart attacks after surviving for more than 12 hours. If the anterior descending branch of the left coronary artery is occluded the anterior wall and septum of the left ventricle are affected, while blockage of the circumflex branch involves the posterior wall. Occlusion of the right artery also implicates the postero-inferior and postero-septal wall of the left ventricle, and may spread to the posterior wall of the right ventricle. Regional infarction is often accompanied by thrombosis of the associated artery, and it is generally assumed to be secondary to the occlusion. However, this is by no means proven. In one series it was found that patients who survived an acute attack of myocardial ischaemia showed a thrombosis in 16 per cent of cases if they lived for 1 hour, in 37 per cent if they lived from 1 to 24 hours, and in 54 per cent if they lived for over 24 hours.[15] Such a finding leads to the unorthodox view that myocardial ischaemia and infarction occur first, and that the thrombosis is secondary. A possible explanation is that showers of small platelet thrombi are shed into the coronary circulation. They might have been formed on atheromatous plaques and released into the fast coronary flow before fibrin formation stabilised them (p. 487). Experimentally, infusion of ADP into the coronary artery of a

pig leads to the formation of small platelet thrombi and the subsequent development of myocardial infarction.[16] Whatever the mechanism, there seems little doubt that infarction can occur in the human without large occlusive arterial thrombi. Indeed, angina and myocardial infarction have been described in young adults with no coronary-arterial occlusion or other apparent cause.[17]

Papillary muscle infarction.[18] Ischaemia of the papillary muscles can lead to infarction, fibrosis, and atrophy. Muscle dysfunction can interfere with the associated valve and cause mitral insufficiency. Occasionally the muscle ruptures, and the sudden onset of mitral regurgitation is heralded by the rapid development of acute pulmonary oedema.

Subendocardial infarction.[19] The subendocardial muscle is prone to ischaemic damage, and subendocardial infarction followed by fibrosis is a common result of an impaired coronary blood flow such as occurs in coronary-artery disease, tachycardia, anaemia, hypotension, and the complications of cardiac surgery. When all the major coronary arteries are severely stenosed but not completely obstructed by thrombus, a wide zone of subendocardial muscle may show infarction.[20]

Myocardial infarcts are coagulative in type and heal to form a fibrous scar. Pericarditis, either localised to the infarcted area or else generalised, is common, and so also is endocardial involvement leading to mural thrombosis and embolism. If the scar is extensive and thin, as occurs after infarction of the whole thickness of the wall, the lesion may proceed to aneurysmal dilatation of the ventricle. The wall becomes heavily calcified and the sac filled with laminated thrombus. Rupture of the aneurysm is uncommon. Recent infarcts sometimes rupture, and the process is usually called colliquative necrosis (*myomalacia cordis*). In fact, the muscle is friable rather than liquefied. It is occasionally seen in elderly people, usually women, and may be virtually symptomless until sudden rupture leads to a fatal haemopericardium.

Sudden death is common in occlusive coronary disease and is most common during the first 24 hours after the onset of the pain; sometimes a thrombus is found but often there is only generalised stenosis. The muscle may show little abnormality, and death is attributed to ventricular fibrillation. Patients who experience an episode of ventricular fibrillation and are successfully resuscitated have as good a prognosis as those who do not.[21]

NERVOUS TISSUE

The nervous tissue has a high rate of metabolism and cannot tolerate oxygen lack for long. With complete ischaemia, functional changes occur within seconds and cell death within a few minutes. The peripheral nerves and the nerve tracts within the central nervous system survive ischaemia for a very much longer period than does the neuron itself. Thus a lesion of the cervical cord may cause permanent lower-motor-neuron paralysis of the arms while sparing the long tracts to the legs.

Cerebral infarction. The two important causes of cerebral infarction are cerebral thrombosis and embolism from the heart. Thrombosis of the cerebral arteries most often occurs as a complication of atheroma, and is particularly common in hypertensive subjects. As already noted, there is colliquative necrosis, which may in the most severe cases implicate much of a hemisphere. The infarct usually remains pale, but with cerebral embolism it sometimes becomes haemorrhagic. This is ascribed to the restoration of some blood flow when the embolus breaks up or is pushed further down the vascular tree.

Generalised cerebral ischaemia follows cardiac arrest and severe haemorrhage; in fatal cases there is no obvious infarction, but the neurons may show degenerative changes. Some cases of infarction do not show particularly severe cerebral arterial disease, and in these the ischaemia is often produced by marked extracerebral arterial atheroma.[22] In addition, there may be hypotension and sludging. The possible importance of thrombotic embolism from atheromatous plaques in causing transient ischaemic attacks ('encephalopathies') has been noted on page 507.

Haemorrhagic infarction of the brain follows extensive venous-sinus thrombosis. A good example is the superior-sagittal-sinus thrombosis (marantic thrombosis) that occasionally occurs in weakly newborn infants. At necropsy much of the cerebral cortex is found to be infarcted.

Kidney

Renal infarction is also due either to local renal arterial disease, or more commonly, to embolism. The infarcts are wedge-shaped areas of coagulative necrosis, and heal to form depressed scars.

Renal-artery atherosclerosis is an important cause of progressive hypertension in young adults, and this is due to the ischaemia that follows a fall in the afferent arteriolar pressure (p. 556). Renal ischaemia of gradual onset leads to renal atrophy, and it is surprising that even when the renal artery becomes completely obstructed, some renal function is maintained. This is due to the development of anastomoses from adjacent lumbar, adrenal, and other arteries. These can be demonstrated radiographically in both the human subject and the experimental animal.[23]

Renal ischaemia of a more generalised type occurs after the arterial vasoconstriction which complicates states of shock, haemorrhage, incompatible blood transfusion, and abruptio placentae. This last condition occasionally proceeds to bilateral symmetrical cortical necrosis, a fatal condition in which the outer two-thirds of the cortex of both kidneys is infarcted (see Fig. 32.4, p. 418). A similar effect is seen in the experimentally-produced generalised Sanarelli (Shwartzman) phenomenon. The mechanism of this appears to be generalised renal arterial vasoconstriction involving especially the outer part of the cortex.

In the *crush syndrome* tubular necrosis is probably caused by ischaemia. The condition arises when a casualty has sustained a continuous compression to one or more limbs. On being released, there is a temporary improvement in the clinical state, but this is followed by progressive renal impairment which culminates in acute renal failure and death. It resembles tourniquet shock (see p. 419).

Selective spasm of the renal vessels has also been suggested as the explanation of 'reflex anuria' in the following conditions: hysteria; passage of a ureteric stone; handling of the ureters during operation; following catheterisation.

Spleen

Infarction of the spleen is usually postembolic, but any enlarged spleen is liable to undergo infarction, possibly because its blood supply becomes inadequate. Localised infarcts are especially common in the enormous spleen of chronic myeloid leukaemia.

Splenic infarction is coagulative, and the base of the infarct often impinges on the peritoneal surface (Fig. 42.6). The focal perisplenitis so caused leads to severe pain in the left hypochondrium. Sometimes the infarct undergoes later softening. Healing is accompanied by fibrosis and shrinkage.

Lung

Effects of pulmonary-artery obstruction.[24] The syndrome of massive pulmonary embolism due to clot has been described on page 504. Surprisingly enough, occlusion of the right or left pulmonary artery in an unanaesthetised man (by inflating a balloon at the tip of a cardiac catheter) produces neither pain nor discomfort. An immediate increase in airways resistance occurs, and this results in a decrease in ventilation of the affected lung.[25, 26] The underventilation of the underperfused lung is partly mediated by the alterations in gas tensions. Thus it can be prevented by supplying 5 per cent CO_2 in air to the lung through the bronchospirometry tube. The local release of 5-hydroxytryptamine may also be a factor in causing collapse, because this agent produces bronchospasm which impedes ventilation by increasing airways resistance. The administration of heparin reduces bronchospasm, presumably by preventing further platelet deposition.

Poor ventilation of the affected lung accounts for the elevated diaphragm seen radiographically, and it sometimes leads to collapse. Nevertheless, collapse is neither invariable nor complete, and it follows that a lung scan using macro-aggregated ^{131}I-labelled human albumin shows an ischaemic lung field whereas a ^{133}Xe-ventilatory lung scan reveals a relatively normal field.[27] (Fig. 42.7 and 42.8).

In the experimental animal occlusion of one branch of the pulmonary artery is followed by collapse of that lung. Recovery commences within a week or two, but the lung always remains smaller than normal and shows some scarring. It has been suggested that the collapse is due to a deficiency of surfactant. Furthermore, a reduction in the amount of this layer, or the presence of an inhibitor, may also be a factor in causing the collapse which follows open-heart surgery, when the lungs are not perfused for an hour or more.

Pulmonary infarction.[24] Infarction does not occur in healthy people even if a main pulmonary artery is occluded. This is because of the additional bronchial arterial supply, which provides well-aerated blood. It is in heart failure, and especially mitral stenosis, that pulmonary infarction occurs, since there is an inadequate cardiac output due to left ventricular failure or inadequate filling of the left ventricle in mitral stenosis. The bronchial arterial supply is thus reduced, and blockage of a pulmonary artery may lead to infarction of the lung.

The usual cause of pulmonary infarction is an embolus arising from the leg veins in phlebothrombosis. About 90 per cent of pulmonary emboli arise in this way, and the other 10 per cent come from the right atrial appendage in the course of heart disease, especially mitral stenosis. Pulmonary infarction may also follow a primary thrombosis of the pulmonary

Figure 42.6
Infarct of spleen. This specimen was removed during the necropsy on a patient who died of subacute infective endocarditis. A section through the spleen shows a pale, circumscribed, wedge-shaped infarct under the capsule. The lymphoid follicles are unduly prominent. (H 26.1, *Reproduced by permission of the President and Council of the R.C.S. Eng.*)

arteries, which occasionally occurs in severe pulmonary hypertension.

Pulmonary infarcts are generally described as being conical in shape and deep red in colour (Fig. 42.9). The broad base is certainly on the pleural surface, but the apex of the lesion is often not infarcted so that the infarct has the shape of a truncated cone; pleural effusions of a haemorrhagic character sometimes complicate pulmonary infarction. The engorgement of pulmonary infarcts is due to the pre-existing chronic venous congestion of the lungs which is the result of heart failure. Blood pours into the alveoli through the damaged walls, and some of it is expectorated from the bronchioles; haemoptysis is a frequent accompaniment of pulmonary infarction. Organisation proceeds rapidly because of the comparatively good vascularity of the surrounding lung. The infarct is eventually converted into an insignificant pigmented scar, concealed by surrounding lung tissue which shows compensatory overdistension. Large infarcts can become pale with the passage of time, and the centre occasionally breaks down to form a cavity.

It is not uncommon for a patient to develop the symptoms of pulmonary infarction together with an X-ray shadow that lasts for a few days and then disappears. Pathologically this consists of oedema and bleeding into the alveoli, as in an early infarct, but there is no progression to necrosis of the alveolar walls. Resolution can therefore be rapid. Technically this lesion cannot be called an infarct since there is no necrosis.

The lung is the first site for pyaemic abscesses resulting from suppurative thrombophlebitis of the systemic veins. They usually cause empyema because of their close proximity to the pleural surface.

Liver

Hepatic infarction is very uncommon, presumably because spontaneous occlusion of the hepatic artery is rare. Nevertheless, it has been proved both experimentally and clinically (following the accidental ligation of the vessel during cholecystectomy) that occlusion of the hepatic artery can lead to extensive white infarction of the liver.[28] Likewise, patchy infarction can occur if the branches of the hepatic artery are involved in polyarteritis nodosa. It would therefore appear that the portal vein contributes blood of so low an oxygen tension as to be inadequate for the survival of the parenchyma.

It is not surprising that thrombosis of the portal vein, while having serious effects on the abdominal viscera, does not lead to hepatic infarction. Pyaemic abscesses occur in the liver secondary to suppurative thrombophlebitis of the portal vein (portal pyaemia).

Focal acute congestion and haemorrhagic infarction is seen after thrombosis of the hepatic vein, which is a rare complication of polycythaemia vera and tumour invasion. It should be noted that the so-called *infarcts of Zahn* are not infarcts but focal, well-delineated areas of congestion. They are usually multiple and their pathogenesis is obscure.

Figure 42.7
Pulmonary embolism. This is a straight chest radiograph in a patient whose right pulmonary artery has been occluded. Note the relatively normal appearance of the right lung field.

Intestine[29, 30]

The usual cause of intestinal ischaemia is an obvious mechanical obstruction to the blood supply in such regional

Figure 42.8
Pulmonary embolism. This is a lung scan (on the same patient as Fig. 42.5) using macro-aggregated radioactive-iodine labelled human albumin. Note the ischaemic right lung field.

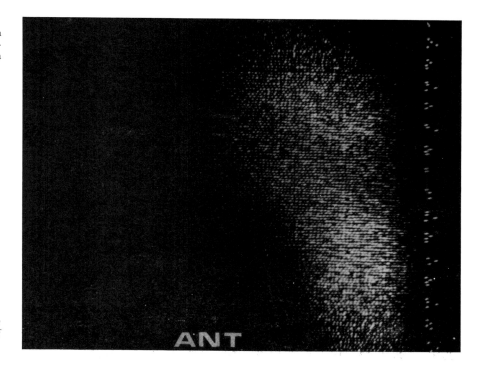

Figures 42.7 and 42.8 are from photographs by courtesy of Dr. H. P. Demshar, Department of Nuclear Medicine, Toronto General Hospital.

Figure 42.9
Pulmonary infarct. This vertical section through the left upper lobe shows a typical dark, wedge-shaped infarct. (R 27.2, *Reproduced by permission of the President and Council of the R.C.S. Eng.*)

conditions as hernial strangulation, volvulus, and intussusception, and the changes in an affected loop of bowel are considered on page 522. Sometimes the primary lesion is in the mesenteric artery, and the effects vary according to the acuteness and severity of the ischaemia.

Thrombosis or embolism of the superior mesenteric artery leads to infarction of the intestine.

Stenosis of the artery, usually atheromatous, leads to chronic ischaemia which may cause *intestinal angina*, a syndrome in which abdominal pain occurs shortly after meals due to the increased peristalsis accentuating the effects of ischaemia. Diarrhoea, weight loss, and a frank malabsorption syndrome may occur. The condition may progress to infarction.

Acute intestinal ischaemia insufficient to cause massive infarction may nevertheless lead to *pseudomembranous enterocolitis.** In this condition the bowel wall becomes congested and oedematous, and the mucosa undergoes necrosis, hanging from the wall as a characteristic white or greenish membrane. The lesions are patchy and may affect both the small intestine and the colon, but the rectum is usually spared, presumably because of its good blood supply. Acute ischaemic colitis can closely simulate acute ulcerative colitis or toxic megacolon. As an acute transient condition

*Pseudomembranous enterocolitis[31] has also been described as a complication of broad-spectrum antibiotic therapy with superinfection of the intestine; *Staph. aureus*, clostridia, and *Candida* species are incriminated. Such cases are rare compared with the ischaemic type. It has been suggested that pseudomembranous enterocolitis is mediated by a Shwartzman-type reaction involving the bowel rather than the skin (p. 95). Unfortunately this suggestion is not very helpful, as the Shwartzman reaction itself is poorly understood.

ischaemic damage to the bowel is not uncommon in shocked patients, and is therefore an important complication of major surgery.

Complete healing can occur, or alternatively repair and chronic ischaemia can lead to an *ischaemic stricture*. The affected bowel shows patchy ulceration, and the intervening mucosa is atrophic. Granulation tissue containing macrophages full of haemosiderin is laid down in the submucosa and also in areas of more severe damage in the muscle layers. The scarring leads to stricture formation; strictures may be found in the small intestine or in the colon where the splenic flexure and descending colon are most commonly affected.

Mesenteric venous thrombosis is another important cause of ischaemia. The process starts distally in the small venous radicles and spreads proximally to implicate the main mesenteric veins. The bowel is engorged, and fresh blood may be passed *per rectum* or vomited, and the condition may simulate acute ulcerative colitis or peptic ulceration. As in all bowel infarction there is early intestinal obstruction due to paralysis of the affected portion.

Once the whole wall is infarcted the bowel becomes stiff, plum-red in colour, and covered with a fibrinous peritoneal exudate. It is rapidly colonised by saprophytes from the faeces, and gangrene ensues. Death soon follows due to the following three factors:

(*a*) *Acute intestinal obstruction.*
(*b*) *Haemorrhage into the bowel wall and lumen.*
(*c*) *Perforation and generalised peritonitis.*

Immediate resection alone can save the patient's life.

Skeletal Muscle[32,33]

Ischaemia of skeletal muscle results in necrosis. When this is due to arterial obstruction, the resulting fibrous replacement is not marked. When the ischaemia is produced by or accompanied by venous obstruction, the necrotic muscle is haemorrhagic and a brisk fibrosis results in contracture. This is the basis of *Volkmann's ischaemic contracture*, which generally affects the forearm but it is described also in the legs. The basic lesion is arterial occlusion, either due to pressure from fracture edges (e.g. a supracondylar fracture of the humerus), ill-applied plasters, or a haematoma, or to spasm complicating such arterial damage or pressure. The importance of venous obstruction is noted above. The result of the ischaemia is infarction of the muscles of the forearm.

In the mildest cases there is slight residual fibrosis with an attempt at regeneration of partly destroyed muscle fibres at the edge. In the worst cases, however, the muscle is replaced by dense fibrous tissue, and the patient develops a severe contracture. Sometimes there is an area of calcareous, putty-like debris in the midst. The nerves and tendons are often also involved, but the skin is left intact, and there is no gangrene.[33]

The blood supply to skeletal muscle varies considerably from one muscle to another.[32] Thus there may be only one nutrient artery, and if it is obstructed severe damage results, e.g. in gastrocnemius and biceps brachii. Some muscles have multiple nutrient arteries—either from one source (tibialis anterior from the anterior tibial artery) or from several sources (extensor digitorum longus from anterior tibial and the perfor-

ating vessels). It is obvious that muscles with the latter type of blood supply are the least likely to be rendered ischaemic following injuries.

Extremities

Infarction of the limbs, most commonly the legs, is often due to a combination of disorders which are grouped together as *peripheral vascular disease*. Atherosclerosis of the large arteries is often a major component, and it may also lead to atheromatous or thrombotic material embolising to small peripheral vessels. Alternatively the main artery may be blocked by thrombus or by a large embolus. Medium-sized arteries may show arteriosclerosis obliterans, while peripheral arterioles may be occluded by the arteriolosclerosis associated with hypertension and especially diabetes mellitus. Other causes of ischaemia are Raynaud's phenomenon, trauma with spasm, ergotism, cold autohaemagglutinins blocking capillaries, frost-bite (trench-foot), iliofemoral thrombosis, and Buerger's disease. Heart failure following coronary-artery disease often aggravates the ischaemia.

There may be no effect of vascular occlusion for a long time if the collateral circulation is adequate. Eventually the blood supply becomes inadequate to sustain muscular exercise, in which case intermittent claudication occurs. At this stage the skin of the legs begins to show trophic changes: glossiness, loss of hair, and a tendency towards ulceration with colonisation by extraneous organisms which would normally be eradicated by the decontaminating mechanisms of the area. Any ulcers that form tend to persist and spread, as ischaemia weakens the tissue's response to infection (see Ch. 8).

In due course ischaemia may become severe enough to lead to infarction, affecting primarily the toes and feet. This is usually precipitated by thrombosis (or else embolism from the heart). The infarcted area becomes dry, shrivelled, and black (due to an alteration in the haemoglobin consequent on desiccation and perhaps putrefaction). A red *line of demarcation*, the equivalent of the inflammatory zone of an internal infarct, develops around the area of union of dead and living. The dead area undergoes mummification (loosely called 'dry gangrene'), and is amputated spontaneously at the line of demarcation if it is not resected surgically beforehand.

In many cases, however, the dead tissue is colonised by saprophytes, and putrefaction occurs; this is 'wet gangrene'. There is concomitant infection by organisms of low virulence around the line of demarcation, and the stump is implicated. The progressive infection of the stump accentuates the effects of ischaemia, and is itself augmented by the ischaemia; thus the necrosis and gangrene spread rapidly. It is for this reason that amputation should be carried out as soon as possible in the presence of gangrene. The question of 'wet' and 'dry' gangrene is considered in Chapter 4.

There is a marked contrast between the natural history of an infarct of an internal organ and one of an extremity. In one there is organisation to form a scar, and the free haemoglobin is metabolised in the RE cells to haemosiderin and bilirubin. In an extremity the infarcted area is spontaneously amputated, and there is no attempt at replacement. The haemoglobin remains *in situ*, and undergoes changes due to desiccation or putrefaction.

VASCULAR SPASM

Although vascular occlusion is generally caused by an organic lesion, there are a number of conditions in which spasm of the vessel wall plays a most important part. Spasm may occur in both veins and arteries, but it is debatable whether the capillaries are capable of independent contraction.

Venous Spasm

Trauma applied directly to the vessel wall can cause marked spasm; this may be a source of great difficulty during an inexpert venepuncture, e.g. for transfusion purposes.

Generalised venospasm has been postulated as occurring during heart failure, and is a feature of hypovolaemic shock.

Arterial Spasm

The thick wall of the muscular arteries and arterioles is admirably designed for reducing the size of the lumen of these vessels. This property is of immense value in the regulation of blood flow to the various organs. In this way, blood is diverted to the muscles and heart during exercise, to the skin when heat has to be lost, and to glands when secretion is required. Following haemorrhage, arterial spasm is an important factor in maintaining the blood pressure.

Local trauma to arteries frequently causes local spasm, a function which may be of life-saving importance. Cases of avulsion of a limb are on record in which, due to spasm of the main artery, the patient did not die of massive haemorrhage. The contraction of the vessel may in part be mediated by 5-hydroxytryptamine liberated from platelets (see p. 633).

The ability of arteries to contract can be utilised by the surgeon who is inadvertently faced with a large haemorrhage during the course of an operation. It is a wise policy to pack the wound and await the onset of spasm, rather than make heroic though blind efforts with a pair of haemostats.[34]

Certain syndromes or diseases are recognised as being due to arterial spasm:

Raynaud's phenomenon.[35] The digital arteries appear to be unduly sensitive to cold. Measurements of blood flow show that it is decreased: dry gangrene may develop.

Ergot poisoning. Arterial spasm may lead to gangrene of the extremities.

Traumatic damage. Spasm may occur not only when an artery is severed, but also when it is subjected to relatively trivial injury. Thus, a missile or a fractured bone end may cause sufficient damage to an artery to be a precipitating factor. Even pressure from a plaster or a tourniquet can cause spasm which may last for many hours. Clinical and experimental work has indicated that this spasm is produced by a nervous reflex, and that it can spread to vessels not directly damaged.

In the rabbit the application of a tourniquet to a leg can cause spasm not only at the site of application but also of the arteries distally and proximally. It may extend to the aorta and even to the opposite limb. Similar extensive arterial spasm can be produced by electrical stimulation of the proximal end of the divided sciatic nerve or the distal end of the severed splanchnic nerve. This spasm also affects the kidney, and in the rabbit the outer two-thirds of the cortex becomes pale.

In the human there seems little doubt that arterial spasm can occur in response to trauma, and that it can spread to involve vessels not primarily damaged.

Generalised arteriolar spasm has been suggested as the primary factor in the causation of essential hypertension, but as yet the pathogenesis of this common condition is not known.

REFERENCES

1. COHEN, H. (1961) Peripheral gangrene in a case of myocardial infarction. *British Medical Journal*, **2**, 1615.
2. DICKINSON, C. J. & PENTECOST, B. L. (1974) In *Clinical Physiology*, ed. Campbell, E. J. M., Dickinson, C. J. & Slater, J. D. H., 4th edn, p. 69. Oxford: Blackwell.
3. BOYD, D. P. & CLARKE, F. M. (1962) Phlegmasia cerulea dolens. *Surgery*, **51**, 19.
4. GILLENWATER, J. Y., BRESLOW, I. H. & LISKER, S. (1962) Phlegmasia cerulea dolens. *Circulation*, **25**, 39.
5. FOGARTY, T. J. *et al.* (1963) Surgical management of phlegmasia cerulea dolens. *Archives of Surgery*, **86**, 256.
6. WASHBURN, B. (1962) Frostbite. *New England Journal of Medicine*, **266**, 974.
7. BIGELOW, D. R. & RITCHIE, G. W. (1963) The effects of frostbite in childhood. *Journal of Bone and Joint Surgery*, **45B**, 122.
8. GOLDING, M. R. *et al.* (1963) Protection from early and late sequelae of frostbite by regional sympathectomy: mechanism of 'cold sensitivity' following frostbite. *Surgery*, **53**, 303.
9. Leading Article (1973) 'Steal' syndromes and hypertension. *British Medical Journal*, **1**, 438.
10. Various Authors (1970) *Journal of Clinical Pathology*, **24**, suppl. (Association of Clinical Pathology), 4, 1 *et seq*. Enzyme Assays in Medicine.
11. Leading Article (1974) Cold and the heart. *British Medical Journal*, **3**, 430.
12. MACALPIN, R. (1976) Provoking variant angina. *New England Journal of Medicine*, **294**, 277.
13. Leading Article (1975) Prinzmetal's variant angina. *British Medical Journal*, **2**, 298.
14. Leading Article (1977) Coronary artery spasm. *British Medical Journal*, **1**, 1176.
15. SPAIN, D. M. & BRADESS, V. A. (1960) The relationship of coronary thrombosis to coronary atherosclerosis and ischemic heart disease. *American Journal of Medical Science*, **240**, 701.
16. JØRGENSEN, L. *et al.* (1967) Adenosine diphosphate-induced platelet aggregation and myocardial infarction in swine. *Laboratory Investigation*, **17**, 616.
17. GLANCY, D. L., MARCUS, M. L. & EPSTEIN, S. E. (1971) Myocardial infarction in young women with normal coronary arteriograms. *Circulation*, **44**, 495.
18. Leading Article (1974) Problems with the papillary muscles. *British Medical Journal*, **1**, 3.
19. HOFFMAN, J. I. E. & BUCKBERG, G. D. (1975) Pathophysiology of subendocardial ischaemia. *British Medical Journal*, **1**, 76.
20. DAVIES, M. J., WOOLF, N. & ROBERTSON, W. B. (1976) Pathology of acute myocardial infarction with particular reference to occlusive coronary thrombi. *British Heart Journal*, **38**, 659.
21. LAWRIE, D. M. (1969) Long-term survival after ventricular fibrillation complicating acute myocardial infarction. *Lancet*, **2**, 1085.

22. Leading Article (1971) New studies of strokes. *British Medical Journal*, **3**, 723.
23. ABRAMS, H. L. & CORNELL, S. H. (1965) Patterns of collateral flow in renal ischemia. *Radiology*, **84**, 1001.
24. SASAHARA, A. A. & STEIN, M. (Eds.) (1965) *Pulmonary Embolic Disease*, 312 pp. New York: Grune and Stratton.
25. SEVERINGHAUS, J. W. *et al.* (1961) Unilateral hypoventilation produced in dogs by occluding one pulmonary artery. *Journal of Applied Physiology*, **16**, 53.
26. SWENSON, E. W., FINLEY, T. N. & GUZMAN, S. V. (1961) Unilateral hypoventilation in man during temporary occlusion of one pulmonary artery. *Journal of Clinical Investigation*, **40**, 828.
27. DENARDO, G. L. *et al.* (1970) The ventilatory lung scan in the diagnosis of pulmonary embolism. *New England Journal of Medicine*, **282**, 1334.
28. CARROLL, R. (1963) Infarction of the human liver. *Journal of Clinical Pathology*, **16**, 133. The extent and distribution of experimental hepatic infarcts. (1963) *Journal of Pathology and Bacteriology*, **85**, 349.
29. BOLEY, S. J., SCHWARTZ, S. S. & WILLIAMS, L. F. (Eds.) (1971) *Vascular Disorders of the Intestine*, p. 657. New York: Appleton-Century-Crofts. In particular see chapter 6, Histopathology of Intestinal Ischemia, by B. C. Morson.
30. Leading Article (1972) Ischaemia of the intestinal tract. *British Medical Journal*, **4**, 566.
31. Leading Article (1977) Pseudomembranous enterocolitis. *Lancet*, **2**, 839.
32. ADAMS, R. D., DENNY-BROWN, D. & PEARSON, C. M. (1974) *Diseases of Muscle*, 3rd edn. New York: Harper and Row.
33. SEDDON, H. (1964) Volkmann's ischaemia. *British Medical Journal*, **1**, 1587.
34. WATSON-JONES, R. (1952) In *Fractures and Joint Injuries*, 4th edn, Vol. 1, p. 105. Edinburgh: Livingstone.
35. Leading Article (1972) Raynaud's disease. *British Medical Journal*, **3**, 782.

Chapter 43. *Oedema*

Oedema may be defined as an excessive extravascular accumulation of fluid. In its usual context it is applied to the morbid accumulation of fluid in the interstitial tissues. It is particularly liable to occur in the various preformed serous sacs, giving rise to ascites, hydrothorax, and hydropericardium, as effusions into the peritoneal, pleural, and pericardial cavities are specifically called. When generalised it is called *anasarca*. It is, of course, also possible to have intracellular oedema, as in hydropic degeneration (see Ch. 4), but for the remainder of the discussion only the interstitial type will be considered. It is necessary first to understand the normal mechanisms which regulate the distribution of fluid in the body.

MECHANISMS OF NORMAL CONTROL IN THE SYSTEMIC CIRCULATION

Local

Starling postulated that the movement of fluid between the vessels and the extravascular spaces was determined by the balance of the hydrostatic and osmotic forces acting upon it.

THE FORCES TENDING TO DRIVE FLUID OUT OF THE BLOOD VESSELS ARE:

The hydrostatic pressure in the vessel. This is generally accepted as 32 mm Hg at the arterial end of the capillary and 12 mm Hg at the venous end, in the skin of the human subject at heart level.

The colloidal osmotic pressure, also called the oncotic pressure, of the interstitial fluid. Since the vascular wall is completely permeable to water and crystalloids, the only effective osmotic forces are those due to the colloids (very largely proteins). The interstitial fluids normally have a low protein content, and this is therefore not an important factor in the formation of the extravascular fluids under normal conditions. Furthermore, those proteins which do escape into the tissue spaces are normally removed by the lymphatics.

THE FORCES DRAWING FLUID INTO THE BLOOD VESSELS ARE:

The tissue tension. This is low (3 to 4 mm Hg). It is of importance in relation to the distribution of the oedema. For instance, lax areas, like the eyelids, ankles, scrotum, and the tissues over the sacrum, tend to accumulate fluid, while tense areas, like the palms and soles, are never the site of marked oedema. A rise in tissue tension is probably an important factor in limiting interstitial-tissue fluid formation in the legs under normal conditions, and also in acutely inflamed parts.

The colloidal osmotic pressure (oncotic pressure) of the plasma. As in the case of the interstitial fluid, this is due very largely to the protein content. The osmotic pressure of a substance in solution is determined by the number of molecules present. Albumin, with its higher concentration and lower molecular weight (65 000 daltons), therefore exerts a much greater osmotic force than do the other plasma proteins, such as the globulins with a molecular weight varying from 90 000 to 10^6 daltons. The plasma proteins exert a force of about 25 mm Hg. The importance of the normal vascular permeability in regulating the distribution of fluid between the intravascular and extravascular compartments cannot be over-emphasised. In the event of increased permeability there is the formation of an exudate rich in protein, e.g. in acute inflammation.

Oedema can indeed be placed in one of two categories:

Exudates, which are morbid accumulations of fluid due to an increased vascular permeability, and *transudates*, which are morbid accumulations of fluid due to a hydrostatic imbalance between the intravascular and extravascular compartments, despite normal vascular permeability.

The basis of an exudate is the free passage of plasma proteins to the extravascular compartment, so that there is a balance between the osmotic pressures of the plasma and the interstitial fluid. There is virtually nothing, except the mounting tissue tension, to hinder the outward flow of plasma.

Table 43.1 indicates the main differences between exudates and transudates.

The mode of passage of crystalloids and water through the wall of a capillary is discussed in Chapter 6.

The importance of the lymphatics should not be forgotten. They form an elaborate network in most tissues, and their function is to drain away fluid and protein. The fluid in the lymphatics has a considerably higher protein content than that of the interstitial fluid itself.

The various factors involved in Starling's hypothesis are depicted in Fig. 6.5 (p. 75). It must be realised, however, that this merely represents an average state of affairs found in many capillaries at the level of the heart. Pressures in individual vessels show considerable variation.

Over-all Fluid Balance

The total amount of fluid in the body is governed by a balance between the amount ingested and produced by metabolic activity on the one hand, and that lost in the urine, sweat, etc. on the other. The regulating mechanisms involve the sensation of thirst, secretion of antidiuretic hormone from the posterior pituitary, and the secretion of aldosterone from the adrenal cortex (see Ch. 38).

In the causation of any type of oedema there are usually a combination of factors. Starling himself recognised that dropsy was probably never due to the derangement of a single mechanism only.

TYPES OF OEDEMA

Oedema may be local or generalised (widespread). The local

TABLE 43.1

	Exudate	Transudate
Total protein content	High as in plasma	Less than 10 g per l
Distribution of proteins	As in plasma	Nearly all albumin (smallest molecule)
Fibrinogen	Present. It clots spontaneously	Not present. No tendency to coagulation
Specific gravity[a]	High	Low
Cells	Plentiful; those of inflammation, e.g. polymorphs or lymphocytes depending on the cause	Few present; nearly all mesothelial cells

[a]The specific gravity of plasma is normally about 1·027, and it is related to its protein content. A protein-free filtrate of plasma has an SG of 1·010, and this is also the SG of the urine secreted by a failing kidney which has lost its power of concentration (see Chapter 46). A transudate with its low content of protein will have an SG of about 1·012, whereas an exudate will have an SG of over 1·018.

oedemas are simpler to understand, because there are usually fewer factors involved.

Local Oedema

Acute inflammatory oedema. The formation of an exudate due to an increased vascular permeability to proteins is basic to the inflammatory response. The causes have been fully considered in Chapter 6, and will merely be summarised at this point:

(a) Increased vascular permeability.

(b) Increased osmotic pressure of interstitial fluid due to the protein of the exudate, and its breakdown into osmotically-active smaller molecules.

(c) Increased hydrostatic pressure in the capillaries.

(d) Increased fluidity of ground substance.

The extent of the oedema is related to the tissue tension.

Hypersensitivity (allergic oedema). Oedema due to an increase in vascular permeability is present in the lesions of anaphylactic and immune-complex hypersensitivity. It is a true exudate. The oedema of anaphylaxis is widespread.

Oedema is also seen in the acute inflammatory response of delayed-type hypersensitivity reactions.

Oedema of venous obstruction. A rise in venous pressure leads to an increase in the capillary pressure. The result is the formation of a transudate. This is seen even in normal people whose work entails long periods of standing, and is particularly evident after thrombophlebitis, e.g. pregnancy 'white leg', when there is often much residual oedema.

Oedema of a limb may be produced experimentally by applying a cuff or tourniquet; under these circumstances there is an additional factor of lymphatic obstruction. If the venous pressure is maintained at 40 mm Hg or more, the vascular permeability alters, allowing protein to leak through. Hypoxia has a similar effect.

By enclosing a limb, or part of a limb, in a plethysmograph the rate of accumulation of transudate in response to a given increase in venous pressure can be measured. A coefficient of vascular permeability can be expressed in ml increase in volume/min/mm Hg increase in pressure/100 ml of tissue. Such measurements have shown an increased value in patients with rheumatoid arthritis, especially those who develop oedema of the legs. In many cases the fluid has a low protein content, and presumably the oedema is produced by an increase in filtration rate rather than an increase in vascular permeability.[1] It is apparent therefore that the oedema following venous obstruction depends on a number of factors: the venous pressure, the presence of hypoxia, and the degree of lymphatic obstruction.

This is illustrated by the changes in a loop of bowel which is undergoing volvulus or strangulation. The first effect is venous obstruction causing congestion of the gut wall, and there is considerable haemorrhage into the lumen. The turgid tissue increases the pressure around the constricted neck and so progressively aggravates the venous obstruction. The oedema first has the character of a transudate, but its protein content soon rises as the pressure increases. Lymphatic obstruction, increased venous pressure, hypoxia, and infection with inflammation all contribute to its formation. Finally venous thrombosis may occur. In due course the arterial supply is occluded either by direct pressure or thrombosis. Infarction results, and the necrotic bowel is at once colonised by putrefactive saprophytes native to the faeces; gangrene follows, and the bowel ruptures.

Lymphatic oedema. Extensive lymphatic obstruction can produce an oedema of rather high protein content (though not as high as that of an exudate). If it persists it stimulates an overgrowth of fibrous tissue, and therefore has a brawny consistency and does not pit easily on pressure. In due course the fibrous-tissue and epithelial overgrowth may become so pronounced that *elephantiasis* results. A good example of this is the tropical disease filariasis due to the nematode *Wuchereria bancrofti*, which in its adult stage lives in the lymphatics of the groin. While alive the worm causes little disability to its host, but when it dies it stimulates an inflammatory reaction. The lymphangitis leads to lymphatic obstruction, and elephantiasis of the legs and external genitalia is a common result. A similar effect is produced by recurrent bacterial lymphangitis, and in lymphogranuloma· venereum there is vulval elephantiasis.

The lymphatic oedema of the arm and the *peau d'orange* appearance of the breast are the results of obstruction to the axillary and mammary lymphatics through permeation by a breast carcinoma. The arm oedema is often aggravated by postoperative radiotherapy.

Oedema is sometimes seen in patients with hemiplegia. It usually affects the arm rather than the leg, and it may be confined to a hand. The fluid has a high protein content, and it may be that the oedema is due to impaired lymphatic drainage resulting from reduced muscular activity. It is interesting that in heart failure, oedema is sometimes especially marked and persistent in a paralysed limb. Patients with acute nephritis have more peri-orbital oedema on awaking in the morning than they do later in the day; the oedema is dispersed by constant blinking.

Primary lymphoedema[2] is a special variety of lymphatic oedema due to a malformation of the lymphatics of the lower limbs—hypoplasia, varicose dilatation, and obstruction have all been reported. If the condition is hereditary and congenital it is called *Milroy's disease*; this is inherited as an autosomal dominant trait of variable penetrance. Usually the oedema is not hereditary and appears in childhood or adult life. It may be unilateral, but frequently it affects both legs, which become greatly disfigured. The condition persists throughout life.

There is an association between primary lymphoedema, recurrent pleural effusions (due to lymphatic oedema), and yellow finger and toe nails. The explanation of this last feature is not understood, but it is probably due to poor lymphatic drainage.[3]

Mild lymphatic oedema of the hands and feet is common in newborn infants with Turner's syndrome, but this usually disappears in childhood.

Generalised Oedema

Cardiac oedema. Although the oedema of congestive cardiac failure is familiar enough, the mechanisms involved are by no means simple or clearly understood. In right-sided and congestive cardiac failure the oedema is accompanied by a general retention of fluid, as is shown by an increase in body weight. Its distribution is influenced by gravity: when the patient is ambulant, the legs are first involved, and swelling of the ankles is often the first symptom. In the recumbent posture, however, the oedema appears in the sacral and genital areas. Oedema may occasionally also develop in the upper limbs and jaw. The oedema pits readily on pressure.

The mechanism of cardiac failure is described in Chapter 44. If the back-pressure hypothesis is accepted, it would seem that the main factor leading to oedema is a *rise in the central venous pressure*, which is transmitted backwards to the venous end of the capillaries. This would have the effect of causing a transudation, as already described. Generalised oedema of any type should lead to a decrease in blood volume because of the diversion of a large amount of fluid to the extravascular compartment. This in turn stimulates antidiuretic hormone and aldosterone secretion (see Ch. 38), and there is water and salt retention. In this way the oliguria and salt retention of heart failure could be explained, as well as the increase in body weight. Unfortunately, the facts do not fit the case. There is an increased blood volume in heart failure,[4] and it may occur before there is any rise in central venous pressure. Furthermore, oedema itself may occur before there is any rise in venous pressure, and it is manifested by an increase in body weight. In addition, the amount of oedema is not proportional to the height of the venous pressure.[4] Oedema of the legs is not necessarily produced after the ligation of the inferior vena cava below the renal veins.[4] It seems that the increased venous pressure acting together with gravity determines the situation rather than the formation of cardiac oedema.

If the theory of forward-failure is accepted, it would appear that the vascular endothelium suffers from *stagnant hypoxia*. This leads to an increased permeability. If this were the case,

the oedema would have the protein content of an exudate. In fact it is a typical transudate, though it is worth qualifying this objection by remembering the lymphatics could be responsible for removing some of the protein that might be present. In heart failure there is mild proteinuria, which is presumably due to a slight increase in permeability of the glomerular capillaries.

It is obvious that neither of these two theories can explain all the features of cardiac oedema satisfactorily.

Hypoproteinaemia is not a factor, because the plasma proteins are well maintained and do not fall to that level (about 50 g per l) at which oedema might be expected.

It has been suggested that there is an element of *lymphatic obstruction*, because dyes injected into the subcutaneous tissue of oedematous legs do not stream up the lymphatics as they do normally. In fact, lymphatic drainage is dependent on muscular activity, which is poor in such patients, and also on the venous pressure, in that all lymphatics finally drain into the veins. The low protein content of cardiac oedema does not point to any important degree of lymphatic obstruction.

Finally, the question of *altered tissue tension* has to be considered. One of the limiting factors in oedema formation is the rise in tissue tension. In a cardiac patient, once oedema has developed and stretched the tissues sufficiently, there is an increased tendency for the oedema to recur.

As none of the local conditions explains the oedema satisfactorily, much attention has been focused on the renal changes of heart failure: *oliguria* and *salt retention*. If salt is withheld, cardiac oedema lessens; it recurs when salt is administered. The daily glomerular filtrate amounts to nearly 180 litres, which contains about 1200 g of salt. Ninety-nine per cent of this is reabsorbed by the tubules, and even a slight upset in this absorption mechanism could cause a marked change in salt balance.

In congestive cardiac failure there is renal vasoconstriction due to sympathetic overactivity. In addition, the renal vasoconstriction diverts the blood away from the superficial part of the cortex, and the juxtamedullary glomeruli filter most of the urine. There is evidence to suggest that there is more complete reabsorption of sodium in these nephrons than in those whose glomeruli lie in the superficial cortex.[5] The renal blood flow may be reduced to about a half of normal, and the glomerular filtration rate from 120 to about 70 ml per minute. Normally about 80 per cent of the sodium in the glomerular filtrate is reabsorbed by the proximal tubule, and if the filtration rate were reduced the amount of sodium excreted in the urine would be decreased, and sodium would be retained. Therefore some of the sodium retention could be explained in terms of a reduced glomerular filtration rate. Furthermore, the vasoconstriction mobilises the renin-angiotensin system, and this leads to the secretion of aldosterone, the urinary excretion of which is raised in most patients with right-sided heart failure, but not usually in those with left-sided failure. The plasma level of aldosterone is often somewhat raised in heart failure, but not to the heights found in the nephrotic syndrome or hepatic cirrhosis. Normally the continuous administration of mineralocorticoids leads to only a transient retention of sodium and water, and after a few days there is an escape from the control of the hormones. The nature of this escape is unknown, and it appears to be in abeyance in cases of heart failure. Perhaps it is related to the shift in action to the juxtamedullary glomeruli.[5]

The factors concerned in cardiac oedema are obscure, but a possible mechanism is as follows: the reduction in cardiac output leads to renal vasoconstriction which in turn aids the retention of sodium; it also facilitates the reabsorption of sodium by diverting blood to the juxtamedullary glomeruli and by increasing the secretion of aldosterone. The resulting salt and water retention produces an expansion of the extracellular fluid compartment. Conditions are therefore propitious for the development of oedema, and local factors act to precipitate its actual occurrence, e.g. raised venous pressure and local tissue overstretching.

Renal oedema. *Acute glomerulonephritis.* Oedema is often the first symptom of the disease. It affects the face and eyelids predominantly; the ankles and genitalia are also often affected, but the oedema is seldom severe. There is no entirely satisfactory explanation for the facial distribution of the oedema; it can hardly be postural, since it is often first noticed when the patient is still ambulant. Its cause is equally obscure. At one time an allergic effect on the capillaries was blamed, but the protein content of the fluid is low (about 4 g per l) and not in keeping with vascular damage. It is not due to hypoproteinaemia, because it occurs at a time when the plasma proteins are not appreciably reduced. An important factor is probably heart failure produced by the sudden systemic hypertension, and aggravated by a raised blood volume due to fluid retention. This is a result of oliguria, which may be quite severe, and is due to glomerular damage. It is noteworthy that the anuria caused by tubular necrosis is not usually accompanied by peripheral oedema.

Nephrotic syndrome. The outstanding feature here is a heavy proteinuria. This results in a low plasma protein level affecting especially the albumin fraction. On Starling's hypothesis the diminished osmotic pressure of the plasma proteins can easily explain the generalised oedema, and this is undoubtedly the most important factor. However, once again there are other considerations. A salt-free diet reduces the oedema, especially if combined with diuretics. In the nephrotic syndrome there is a reduced blood volume.[6] This in turn stimulates the secretion of aldosterone (which is found in considerable amounts in the urine) and ADH. There is ensuing water retention, as already described, and oliguria is present as the oedema accumulates. If the plasma volume is expanded with albumin or dextran, the oedema is checked and a considerable diuresis occurs. There may also be spontaneous diureses during the course of the disease, in which the oedema is cleared though the level of plasma proteins remains unaltered. The syndrome is described on pages 557 to 558.

Chronic glomerulonephritis. This is almost invariably associated with hypertension. The oedema is due to heart failure. The pulmonary oedema of uraemia is considered on page 557.

Famine oedema (nutritional oedema). The oedema that is seen after prolonged starvation is usually confined to the legs, but sometimes it is more generalised. At first sight it would appear to be explicable in terms of hypoproteinaemia, but in fact there is no close correlation between the level of plasma proteins and the presence of oedema; it is sometimes extensive when the plasma proteins are normal. The true explanation of famine oedema is unknown. An important factor appears to be a loss of compact tissue (mostly fat) and its replacement by a loose connective tissue which can accumulate fluid without a rise in tissue tension. When the patient is confined to bed, there is a diuresis and the oedema decreases rapidly, even if the diet is unaltered. It is noteworthy that cachectic patients with cancer do not generally exhibit oedema, therefore a mere loss of tissue mass cannot be the whole answer. In some of the victims of starvation there is heart failure due to thiamine deficiency (beriberi), and perhaps this is an additional factor in some cases of famine oedema.

An interesting type of malnutrition that is accompanied by marked oedema is *kwashiorkor*. This condition is considered in Chapter 34. The oedema is presumably related to hypoproteinaemia but in addition there are multiple dietary deficiencies in many cases.

Protein-losing enteropathy. Oedema is a prominent feature of this rare condition (see p. 579).

Hepatic oedema (see Ch. 47). Its main manifestation is ascites, and in a way it falls midway between the local and generalised oedemas. However, there may sometimes be a more widespread oedema affecting the legs also. The factors involved are lymphatic obstruction, a fall in the level of plasma proteins, an increase in the regional venous pressure due to portal hypertension, and a failure in the hepatic inactivation of aldosterone.

Oedema due to adrenal hormones. Salt retention occurs during the therapeutic administration of glucocorticoids or ACTH. There is an increase in weight, and oedema may develop. Hypertension is another common effect. These manifestations are also seen in Cushing's syndrome. The cause of the oedema is complex, being due to several mechanisms.

(*a*) There may be an increased blood volume due to sodium retention. As mentioned in Chapter 38, cortisol has a mild mineralocorticoid action.

(*b*) There may be a change in the ground substance of the connective tissue, rendering it more water-soluble. The typical 'moon face' might well be due to a local oedema of this type.

(*c*) There may sometimes be heart failure secondary to hypertension.

Primary hyperaldosteronism (Conn's syndrome) does not cause oedema despite considerable sodium retention. It seems that aldosterone secretion aggravates the tendency to oedema rather than producing it initially.

Myxoedema.[7,8] Effusions into the body cavities are an uncommon manifestation of myxoedema, but may on occasion be the presenting feature. In addition to ascites and pleural and pericardial effusions there may also be hydrocele. The fluid has the protein content of an exudate, and it is believed that the extravasation of hygroscopic mucopolysaccharides into the body cavities is largely responsible for the effusions.

Pregnancy. Retention of fluid over and above that required for the uterine contents is normal in pregnancy, and in some women is manifest as oedema of the ankles and occasionally of a more generalised distribution. Oedema is also a feature of pre-eclampsia, and is accompanied by hypertension and proteinuria.

Unexplained oedema. Generalised oedema sometimes occurs in the absence of any known cause, and although such

TABLE 43.2

	Increased venous pressure	Low plasma proteins	Lymphatic obstruction	Sodium and water retention
Cardiac oedema	+ +	−	±	+ + + +
Acute nephritis	+	±	−	+ + + +
Nephrotic syndrome	−	+ + + +	−	+ + + +
Hepatic oedema (ascites)	+ (portal hypertension)	+ +	+ + +	+ + + +
Famine oedema	−	+ +	−	+ +
Adrenal steroids	±	−	−	+ + +

cases are uncommon, they indicate that factors other than those already discussed may operate even in the common types of oedema.

A well-recognised condition is *cyclical*, or *periodic, oedema*,* in which there are recurrent attacks of oedema involving skin, mucous membranes, joints, or even internal organs, e.g. the brain. In some cases the oedema is widespread and the attacks so severe that the loss of fluid and plasma proteins from the circulation can lead to hypovolaemic shock and death. Usually, however, the area involved is more localised. Thus, one patient is recorded as having pain and swelling of the left hand on alternate Wednesdays, lasting one week, for 18 years. The immediate cause of the oedema appears to be an increase in vascular permeability, and both hereditary factors and allergy have been blamed. Cyclical oedema is more common in women and is often related to the menstrual cycle; attacks may cease after the menopause.

In the familial variety of *angio-oedema* the Cl esterase inhibitor is either absent or present in an abnormal and inert form. The inhibitor is present in normal people, and is presumably important in preventing the unwanted activation of the complement system with the production of permeability factors (p. 161). Another consideration is that the Cl esterase inhibitor also inhibits the capacity of activated Clotting Factor XII to convert prekallikrein to kallikrein. It also directly inhibits kallikrein, plasmin, and plasma thromboplastin antecedent (Factor XI). The acute attacks are probably related to activation of Factor XII, but the precipitating cause remains obscure.[10]

It is normal for there to be some salt and water retention during the premenstrual phase, but this is not associated with a change in vascular permeability, nor is there a marked gain in weight. This contrasts with the syndrome of *idiopathic oedema of women*,[11] which affects women between the ages of 30 and 45. During attacks there is obvious swelling of the face, hands, and legs. The oedema develops during the day, and diminishes during the night. An abnormal leakage of fluid from the circulation when the patient is in the upright position is the essential abnormality. Although the condition is associated with stress and strain, its pathogenesis is quite obscure. It is also found that psychological factors may influence electrolyte and water balance both in the normal individual[12] and in those with congestive heart failure.[13] Hypnosis has been used to treat 'allergic' diseases, like asthma,

*Other periodic syndromes are also described, e.g. fever, arthrosis, neutropenia, paralysis (familial periodic paralysis), purpura, peritonitis, vomiting, and headaches.[9]

and has also been shown to influence the exudative component of the Mantoux test and the P-K reaction.[14] It is evident that the complex relationships between allergy, vascular permeability, and the nervous system are poorly understood at the present time.

Table 43.2 summarises the main factors in the causation of generalised oedema.

PULMONARY OEDEMA[15]

The hydrostatic balance of the lung capillaries is somewhat different from that of the systemic circulation.

The blood pressure in the pulmonary circuit is about 15 to 25 mm Hg systolic and 6 to 12 mm Hg diastolic. The mean capillary pressure is 7 mm Hg, being highest at the base and lowest at the apex.

The interstitial fluid pressure is negative, and may be as low as -16 mm Hg. Both these forces tend to drive fluid out of the capillaries into the interstitial tissue, which consists of the mucopolysaccharide gel of the shared basement membrane (see Fig. 45.1, p. 538).

The plasma and interstitial fluid osmotic pressures are like those elsewhere in the body. Normally the plasma colloid osmotic pressure (25 to 28 mm Hg) is adequate to prevent fluid escaping into the interstitial tissue. The lungs are 'dry'; saline introduced into them is soon absorbed, though serum is removed more slowly.

If excess fluid does enter the interstitial tissue, there is a copious system of lymphatics which not only drain it away but are also able to remove any large molecules which might leak from the vascular compartment. There are no lymphatics in the alveolar walls, but they commence in the ducts and form large channels in the peri-bronchial tissue. Once the lymphatic drainage is overwhelmed, the volume of interstitial fluid increases and its pressure rises to zero. It eventually exceeds the pressure of the thin film of liquid lining the alveolar epithelium, which is itself slightly negative because of surface tension. At this juncture the lung is poised for the onset of alveolar flooding. There is some argument as to whether this takes place by direct leakage through the alveolar epithelium or whether it occurs in the terminal bronchioles with the fluid then running back into the alveoli.

The capillaries derive their oxygen supply from the alveolar gas, and if the alveoli are full of fluid the cells become hypoxic. The vascular permeability increases, and a protein-rich fluid accumulates and spreads to adjacent alveoli both through the pores of Kohn and *via* the alveolar ducts. In this way pulmonary oedema, once formed, spreads rapidly and asphyxiates the patient. Furthermore, the protein-containing fluid favours bacterial proliferation.

Acute fulminating pulmonary oedema is quite common, and whatever the cause, increased vascular permeability increases its extent. The following are important conditions leading to its production:

Causes of Pulmonary Oedema[16]

Heart failure. In left ventricular failure there is a rise in pulmonary venous pressure which presumably leads to the formation of a transudate. Acute pulmonary oedema is a frequent complication of left ventricular failure, and is also common in mitral stenosis. It may occur prior to the fluid retention which is so important in peripheral cardiac oedema. This suggests that a local redistribution of fluid is the basis of acute pulmonary oedema. The back-pressure theory, while intellectually satisfying, is not the whole explanation.

It is probable that peripheral vasoconstriction also plays an important role in precipitating the pulmonary oedema of heart disease.[17] In mitral stenosis and the 'low output' failures there is widespread vasoconstriction (see p. 529). It is to be expected that this will lead to the displacement of blood from the systemic to the pulmonary circulations. Support for this contention is provided by the finding that adrenaline has a considerable effect on the pulmonary circulation: there is a moderate rise in pulmonary arterial pressure, and the pulmonary blood flow is greatly increased.[17] Acute pulmonary oedema is a well-known hazard of adrenaline administration, and it is relieved by the ganglion-blocking drugs which cause systemic vasodilatation.

In the dramatic paroxysmal dyspnoea, which is described on page 533, there is a rise in blood pressure and systemic vasoconstriction. It may well be that the attack is precipitated by a raised pulmonary venous pressure accentuated during recumbency (the pulmonary blood flow is greater in the horizonal than in the upright position), and that it is continued by the adrenaline secreted as the result of fear and anxiety. This would explain the ameliorative effects of cerebral depressants like morphine and anaesthetics, and the lethal effect of adrenaline. Once the acute stage is survived, the oedema is rapidly removed *via* the pulmonary lymphatics. In due course the situation is further remedied by constriction of the pulmonary arterioles, which limits the pulmonary blood flow, and by a thickening of the connective tissue around the alveolar capillaries, which impedes the outward flow of plasma to the alveoli.

The oedema of the lungs that follows overloading of the circulation with intravenous saline solutions is no doubt attributable to left ventricular failure. Clinically the danger of blood transfusions and other intravenous therapy in patients with heart failure is well known.

Withdrawal of effusions.[18] Pulmonary oedema may follow the aspiration of fluid or air from a pleural cavity. This hazard is most likely to follow the rapid removal of a large amount of fluid or air that has been present for at least a few days. The oedema is often confined to the lobe rendered airless by the compression of the fluid, and it usually resolves

quite rapidly. Less often it becomes widespread and may cause death. The mechanism of this pulmonary oedema is obscure. It may be that the prolonged collapse and airlessness leads to a deficiency of surfactant, and when there is a sudden increase in negative intrathoracic pressure following the aspiration, the lungs re-expand less easily. The trauma incurred may engender leakage of fluid from the pulmonary capillaries into the connective tissue and the alveolar spaces. A similar effect may follow the removal of a massive ascites. Clearly all large effusions should be drained slowly, especially if they are chronic.

Cerebral damage.[19] It is apparent from the above discussion that neurogenic factors play an important part in pulmonary oedema. A fulminating oedema, rich in protein, occurs in rats and rabbits when a fibrin-forming mixture is injected into the basal cisternae. If the animal is vagotomised beforehand no pulmonary oedema forms, and it appears that the permeability of the lung capillaries is affected by an outflow of stimuli from the brain stem *via* the vagus nerves. The nature of the reflex is obscure.

Pulmonary oedema is seen occasionally in patients with head injuries and lesions involving the hind-brain. It is also a dangerous complication of neurosurgery. These conditions are attended by peripheral vasoconstriction (the animals mentioned above also have systemic hypertension and a raised right atrial pressure), and it is probable that sympathetic overaction is an important factor. As already described, it leads to pulmonary displacement of blood.

Experimentally pulmonary oedema can be produced by the administration of large doses of adrenaline, the induction of prolonged hypoglycaemia (which probably acts by adrenaline release), and the infliction of cerebral trauma of various kinds. Cerebral depressant drugs and sympathetic inhibitors ameliorate the effects of these experiments. Even in phosgene poisoning, where there is a primary action on the vascular endothelium of the lung, these drugs are helpful; this suggests an additional neurogenic factor in phosgene poisoning.

Infections. Acute pulmonary oedema was a notorious feature of the 1918 influenza pandemic, during which over 15 million people died of this dread complication. It is also encountered from time to time in fulminating bronchopneumonia due to *Strept. pyogenes*, *B. anthracis*, and *Y. pestis*.

Toxic irritants. Many irritant gases are capable of causing pulmonary oedema; these include nitrogen peroxide (which is responsible for silo-filler's disease, an obliterative bronchiolitis which also follows the inhalation of nitrous fumes in manufacturers of nitrocellulose), ozone, chlorine, phosgene, and paraquat (which is used as a herbicide).

Oxygen toxicity. High concentrations of oxygen, when inhaled for long periods especially under pressure, may precipitate pulmonary oedema. Even at a partial pressure of one atmosphere, an exposure to pure oxygen for from 6 to 30 hours can produce toxic effects in some individuals. The lungs become inelastic, congested, oedematous, and haemorrhagic, and they show hyaline-membrane formation. These acute changes may be followed by a focal or diffuse overgrowth of fibrous tissue into the alveoli.[20]

It is evident that an increased partial pressure of oxygen is toxic to the lung and can add to the respiratory difficulties of a chronically ill patient, especially if on a respirator.

Aspiration pneumonia. The acid contents of the stomach are acutely irritant when inhaled, and they lead to severe pulmonary oedema.

Drowning and near drowning. The inhalation of either fresh or salt water leads to lung damage such that pulmonary oedema develops immediately or sometimes after a latent interval.

Circulating toxins. Some chemicals after absorption, e.g. α-naphthyl thiourea (used as a rat poison), produce pulmonary oedema. Circulating bacterial endotoxins can have a similar effect. Pulmonary oedema is also seen as an idiosyncratic reaction to some drugs, such as methotrexate, busulphan, nitrofurantoin, and hexamethonium. The oedema may be interstitial and lead to progressive fibrosis, or the fluid may accumulate in the alveolar spaces.

Radiation pneumonia. High doses of ionising radiation applied to the chest lead to pulmonary oedema.

Uraemia. Pulmonary oedema is also seen in uraemia, where it has a peculiar fibrinous consistency.

Other conditions. Pulmonary oedema is a common event in many severe conditions. It has been reported after blast injury to the lung, severe hypoxaemia after burns or other injuries, renal failure, septicaemia, fat embolism, drug overdosage (particularly with heroin and barbiturates), and after cardio-pulmonary bypass operations. It is also a feature of amniotic-fluid embolism and disseminated intravascular coagulation. It is evident that many factors play a part in the production of the oedema under these varying circumstances, but presumably a common factor is increased permeability of the pulmonary capillaries following damage to the alveolar-capillary membrane.

Clinically there is a shock, dyspnoea, cyanosis, and severe hypoxaemia. This pulmonary manifestation occurring in a patient with previously normal lungs and without cardiac disease is collectively called the *adult respiratory distress syndrome*.[21]

Acute pulmonary oedema is an occasional complication of 'mountain fever'[22,23] and is seen in mountaineers, often the young and healthy members of a party, who climb too high too fast. It occurs between 12 and 72 hours after going above 9000 feet. The pathogenesis is uncertain. Hypoxia is certainly involved, and it may cause capillary damage in the lungs directly. It also leads to a lowering of the arterial PCO_2, which induces peripheral vasoconstriction causing deviation of blood from the peripheral circulation to the pulmonary bed. Exposure to cold has a similar effect.

High-altitude cerebral oedema is another manifestation of acute mountain sickness, and it may be that the associated pulmonary oedema also has a neurogenic basis. High-altitude pulmonary oedema is becoming more common in these days of rapid, cheap air travel, and is seen in tourists as well as soldiers engaged in manoeuvres in mountainous areas.

Conclusions

Pulmonary oedema may accumulate as a transudate following increased pulmonary venous pressure, as in heart failure. The low protein content of the transudate is soon added to as the mounting oedema deprives the alveolar capillaries of their oxygen supply and consequently increases their permeability. Hence there is no clear-cut distinction between transudation and exudation as there is in the pathogenesis of much oedema in the systemic circulation (this does not apply to the oedema of venous obstruction). Although the explanation of pulmonary oedema may sometimes appear obvious, as in phosgene poisoning, in other cases the mechanism is obscure. A nervous reflex causing peripheral vasoconstriction may well be of great importance. When once oedema formation has commenced, the resulting changes in the lung explain its rapid spread and high protein content. Under some circumstances the fluid contains much fibrinogen which clots to form fibrin. This may line the alveolar walls and lead to the formation of a hyaline membrane (Fig. 43.1). This feature is particularly common in the primary atypical pneumonia of certain infective agents (see p. 226), in oxygen toxicity (particularly in patients on a respirator), and in the 'busulphan lung'.

Figure 43.1
Oedema of the lung. The alveoli are filled with a lightly-staining coagulum of oedema fluid which has condensed on the walls to form a much more darkly-staining exudate, which is called a hyaline membrane. The alveolar walls are thicker than normal and contain an inflammatory exudate, the cells of which are mostly lymphocytes and macrophages. This patient had a primary atypical pneumonia of viral origin. × 100.

REFERENCES

1. JAYSON, M. I. V. & BARKS, J. S. (1971) Oedema in rheumatoid arthritis: changes in the coefficient of capillary filtration. *British Medical Journal*, **2**, 555.
2. Leading Article (1963) Milroy's disease and lymphoedema. *British Medical Journal*, **2**, 1483.
3. Leading Article (1972) Yellow nails and oedema. *British Medical Journal*, **4**, 130.
4. WOOD, P. (1968) *Diseases of the Heart and Circulation*, 3rd edn, p. 319. London: Eyre and Spottiswoode.
5. BROD, J. (1972) Pathogenesis of cardiac oedema. *British Medical Journal*, **1**, 222.
6. GARNETT, E. S. & WEBBER, C. E. (1967) Changes in blood-volume produced by treatment in the nephrotic syndrome. *Lancet*, **2**, 798.
7. SACHDEV, Y. & HALL, R. (1975) Effusions into body cavities in hypothyroidism. *Lancet*, **1**, 564.
8. ISAACS, A. J. & HAVARD, C. W. H. (1976) Myxoedema and hydrocele. *British Medical Journal*, **1**, 322.
9. Leading Article (1963) Periodic syndromes. *Lancet*, **2**, 563.
10. ROSEN, F. S. & AUSTEN, K. F. (1969) The 'neurotic edema' (hereditary angioedema). *New England Journal of Medicine*, **280**, 1356.
11. Leading Article (1976) Idiopathic oedema of women. *British Medical Journal*, **1**, 979.
12. SCHOTTSTAEDT, W. W. *et al.* (1958) Sociologic, psychologic and metabolic observations on patients in the community of a metabolic ward. *American Journal of Medicine*, **25**, 248.
13. BARNES, R. & SCHOTTSTAEDT, W. W. (1960) The relation of emotional state to renal excretion of water and electrolytes in patients with congestive heart failure. *American Journal of Medicine*, **29**, 217.
14. Annotation (1963) Hypnosis and allergy. *British Medical Journal*, **1**, 968.
15. Leading Article (1976) Pulmonary oedema. *Lancet*, **2**, 350.
16. ROBIN, E. D., CROSS, C. E. & ZELIS, R. (1973) Pulmonary edema. *New England Journal of Medicine*, **288**, 239 and 292.
17. HARRIS, P. & HEATH, D. (1977) *The Human Pulmonary Circulation*, 2nd edn, pp. 185 and 362. Edinburgh: Churchill Livingstone.
18. SAINI, G. S. (1974) Unilateral pulmonary oedema after drainage of spontaneous pneumothorax. *British Medical Journal*, **1**, 615.
19. THEODORE, J. & ROBIN, E. D. (1975) Pathogenesis of neurogenic pulmonary oedema. *Lancet*, **2**, 749.
20. SEVITT, S. (1974) Diffuse and focal oxygen pneumonitis. *Journal of Clinical Pathology*, **27**, 21.
21. Leading Article (1975) Adult respiratory-distress syndrome. *British Medical Journal*, **2**, 523.
22. Leading Article (1976) See Nuptse and die. *Lancet*, **2**, 1177.
23. Leading Article (1972) Pulmonary oedema of mountains. *British Medical Journal*, **3**, 65.

Chapter 44. Heart Failure

Heart failure may be defined as a condition where the output of the heart is insufficient to meet the demands of the tissues, despite satisfactory venous filling.[1] This definition serves to eliminate extracardiac circulatory failure due to haemorrhage and vasovagal syncope. It also excludes constrictive pericarditis and cardiac tamponade, conditions in which the failure in the circulation is due to impaired atrial filling as the result of external compression.

The normal cardiac output at rest is 4·5 to 5 litres per minute. Since the heart can normally expel all the venous blood reaching it, it follows that the cardiac output is determined by the venous return. This is the volume of blood draining all the tissues and organs of the body, and is itself directly related to their arterial blood supply. The blood supply of a tissue is determined mainly by the local autoregulatory mechanisms.[2] The cardiac output is therefore governed by extracardiac factors, namely the metabolic requirements of the body as a whole. Thus the cardiac output can be increased four-fold during strenuous exercise. Indeed, a young man can increase his cardiac output to about 30 litres per minute in steady, severe exertion.

The range of the normal systemic blood pressure at rest is

$$\frac{120 \text{ to } 150 \text{ mm Hg systolic}}{60 \text{ to } 90 \text{ mm Hg diastolic}},$$

and a reading above 150/90 is suggestive of systemic hypertension, especially in a young person. The range of 'normal' blood pressures is, however, wide, and a figure above 180/110 would be considered indicative of systemic hypertension in an elderly subject.

By the time the blood reaches the capillaries the pressure has dropped to 32 mm Hg, and on the venous side it is about 12 mm Hg (these figures refer to a capillary at heart level). There is a steady drop in the venous circulation. Measurements of blood pressure in the chambers of the right side of the heart and the pulmonary circulation are obtained during cardiac catheterisation.[3] Cardiologists measure these pressures at a point somewhere near the centre of the heart, e.g. 5 cm below the sternal angle with the patient lying recumbent. Under these conditions the right atrial pressure averages 0 mm Hg, and the right ventricular pressure 22/0 mm Hg. The pulmonary arterial pressure averages 22/10 mm Hg, and a figure over 30/15 mm Hg indicates pulmonary hypertension. The left atrial pressure averages 5 mm Hg, which is about 10 mm Hg lower than the pulmonary arterial pressure.

The normal heart rate is about 70 beats per minute, and the normal stroke volume about 70 ml per beat. The ventricles do not empty completely with each beat, and there is a residual volume of about 50 ml; the ventricular end-diastolic volume is therefore about 120 ml.[4]

THE MECHANISM OF HEART FAILURE[1]

There are two classical approaches to heart failure:

The back-pressure theory of James Hope (1832), which attributes failure to an inadequate discharge of blood from the ventricles. The accumulation of blood behind them leads to atrial and venous engorgement.

The forward-failure theory of James Mackenzie (1913), which states that the heart fails as a whole, so that there is insufficient propulsion of blood from behind.

In fact there is a great deal of truth in both these concepts, which can usefully be combined. Most of the pathological effects of heart failure are due to forward failure, which is the basis of *stagnant hypoxia*, i.e. hypoxia due to an inadequate blood supply consequent on a poor cardiac output, while most of the signs and symptoms of heart failure, e.g. engorged jugular veins, hepatomegaly, and peripheral oedema, are due in no small measure to the effects of venous back-pressure.

THE CAUSES OF HEART FAILURE

An inadequate cardiac output occurs under the following three circumstances:

Overburdening due to a sustained increase in ventricular pressure. This occurs in systemic (and pulmonary) hypertension and in aortic or pulmonary valvular stenosis. In these conditions the heart has progressively greater difficulty in maintaining a normal output, and eventually a state of *low output failure* results. In order to conserve the blood as efficiently as possible, there is peripheral vasoconstriction with a small thready pulse.

Overburdening due to a sustained increase in cardiac output. There is a group of widely diverse conditions which have one feature in common: the necessity for an increased cardiac output to supply the demands of the tissues. The cardiac output may rise to 10 litres per minute at rest, and eventually the heart fails under the strain. Such conditions are:

Anaemia, where under the stress of anaemic hypoxia the tissues need more blood.

Thyrotoxicosis, where the metabolic needs of the tissues are increased.

Arteriovenous fistulae, which shunt so much blood that only a greater cardiac output can meet the demands of the remainder of the body.

Chronic pulmonary heart disease ('cor pulmonale') where there is hypoxic hypoxia, and also possibly a pulmonary-bronchial arterial anastomosis that acts as a shunt.

Extensive Paget's disease of bone, where there are innumerable arteriovenous shunts in the affected bones, which are extremely vascular.

Generalised erythrodermas, e.g. exfoliative dermatitis and erythrodermic psoriasis.[5, 6]

Advanced liver disease. Anastomoses between the portal and pulmonary veins *via* the azygos and bronchial veins have been demonstrated. The failure of detoxification of a vasodepressor substance has also been suggested.[7]

Beriberi. See Chapter 34.

All these conditions are associated with a hyperkinetic circulatory state: the hands are warm, the pulses throbbing, and the forearm veins distended. This is *high output failure*. Though the cardiac output is raised relative to the normal, it is still insufficient to meet the demands of the body.

Although it is often easy enough to explain the vasodilatation on a teleological basis, i.e. in terms of an increased demand for blood due to hypoxia or greater tissue metabolism, it must be admitted that there is considerable ignorance about the actual reflexes brought into action to produce it.

Myocardial disease. This may be *hypoxic*, as in anaemia and ischaemia due to coronary-artery disease, or hypotension occurring in shock, *metabolic*, as in amyloidosis, myxoedema, and glycogen-storage disease, *toxic*, as in diphtheria, or due to a *specific myocardial lesion*, e.g. acute rheumatic fever, viral myocarditis,[8] systemic lupus erythematosus, and tumours of the heart. Into this last group fall the *cardiomyopathies*, in which there is cardiac enlargement and eventual failure in the absence of valvular or coronary arterial disease.

Two groups have been recognised. In *primary cardiomyopathy* the heart is considered to be the only organ involved, whereas in *secondary cardiomyopathy* the heart lesion is part of a systemic disease, or has a known cause.[9] This latter group includes the myocardial diseases caused by numerous physical, chemical, and infective agents.

A useful clinical classification of the cardiomyopathies is into the four groups: congestive, hypertrophic, constrictive (restrictive), and obliterative.[10, 11] *Congestive cardiomyopathy* is the commonest type: the heart is hypertrophied, but this is masked by the concomitant dilatation. The myocardium is soft, and there is often endocardial thrombosis. Some cases are due to viral infection, and others are the result of poisoning or are idiopathic. Congestive cardiomyopathy occurs in chronic alcoholics; its pathogenesis may be related to the cardiac effects of beri-beri. Some cases have been attributed to cobalt poisoning following the addition of cobalt salts to beer during its manufacture.[12] But there is, in addition, both clinical and experimental evidence that alcohol has a directly damaging effect on the myocardium. Most of these cases are well nourished, and respond to bed rest with abstinence from alcohol.[13]

The second most common type of cardiomyopathy is the *hypertrophic* variety. The left ventricular wall is massively thickened by hypertrophic fibres, which tend to be arranged in irregular whorls. In many cases the hypertrophy in the region of the septum causes obstruction to the outflow tract of the left ventricle. This type is also called hypertrophic obstructive cardiomyopathy or idiopathic hypertrophic subaortic stenosis. In some cases there is a familial incidence, and in others there is an association with Friedreich's ataxia or a myopathy. *Constrictive cardiomyopathy* resembles constrictive pericarditis in its effects. The commonest type is due to amyloid infiltration. *Obliterative cardiomyopathy* includes endomyocardial fibrosis, a disease that is common in East Africa and of unknown aetiology. Löffler's eosinophilic cardiomyopathy is a similar condition morphologically but occurs in temperate zones, and as its name implies, is associated with marked blood eosinophilia.

Myocardial disease is by far the most important cause of heart failure. It often acts with the other two factors, e.g. in syphilitic aortic regurgitation there may be myocardial ischaemia due to occlusion of the coronary ostia, and in hypertensive heart disease there is often ischaemia due to coronary-artery disease.

The contributory factors to a state of heart failure include *anxiety*, which raises the heart rate and blood pressure, *exertion* and *infection*, which increase the cardiac output, and *pregnancy*, which increases the strain on the heart as the result of an increased blood volume. *Dysrhythmias* are also important. Those that cause tachycardia interfere with diastolic filling and the coronary blood flow, while those that cause marked bradycardia decrease the cardiac output directly.

Sometimes the brunt falls on the left side of the heart, e.g. in systemic hypertension and aortic-valve disease, and then the condition is called *left ventricular failure*. Less often the right side is first affected, e.g. in pulmonary stenosis and pulmonary hypertension, and this is called *right ventricular failure*. Most commonly the heart fails as a whole (this occurs in myocardial disease), and *congestive cardiac failure* ensues. Left ventricular failure eventually progresses to congestive cardiac failure if the patient survives long enough.

THE EFFECTS OF HEART FAILURE[1]

The effect of forward-failure, i.e. an inadequate cardiac output, is that some organs obtain an insufficient blood supply. The arteriovenous oxygen difference (normally 50 ml per litre) is increased, as more oxygen is extracted by the tissues in order to obtain their necessary supply. This leads to a reduction of the tissue oxygen tension, and the resulting hypoxia is called 'stagnant hypoxia'. If the blood supply is further diminished, the actual amount of oxygen available to the tissues becomes so inadequate that its quantity as well as its tension is reduced. Degenerative changes culminating in necrosis then occur.

Not all organs suffer equally.

The cerebral circulation is maintained at a volume near normal. Normally it is 54 ml/100 g brain/minute, or 750 ml/minute for a brain weighing 1400 g. Terminally the cerebral circulation may decrease enough to cause symptoms. Consciousness is lost when the cerebral blood flow is sustained at less than about 32 ml/100 g/min, and irreversible damage occurs at values less than 10 ml/100 g/min.

The coronary blood flow (normally 250 ml/min) is also well maintained until terminally. Severe dysrhythmias, e.g. paroxysmal atrial or ventricular tachycardia, endanger this circulation. Severe systemic hypotension has the same effect.

The renal blood flow can drop from 1·1 litre to about 0·5 litre per minute, and the glomerular filtration rate from 120 ml to 70 ml per minute. These effects are the result of arteriolar vasoconstriction. Diuresis is preceded by an increase in the renal flow, which may be independent of any change in cardiac output.

The hepatic blood flow is normally about 1·5 litre per minute, and is reduced in proportion to the reduction of cardiac output. The stagnant hypoxia is most severe in the peripheral areas of the acini of the liver, and it is here that the most marked changes occur (see p. 534).

Blood flow to the extremities. Peripheral vasoconstriction causes a reduction in blood flow; the skin then becomes pale and cold. In vascular areas like the lips and face the effect of stagnant hypoxia on the dammed-up venous blood often produces visible cyanosis (of the peripheral type).

As has already been noted, these changes are seen in the low output type of heart failure but not in the high output type. Here there is generalised vasodilatation, which is still insufficient to meet the tissues' demands.

The effects of back-pressure. The rise in ventricular diastolic pressure causes a corresponding rise in the left atrial and pulmonary venous pressures in left ventricular failure. Similarly the rise in right ventricular pressure raises the systemic venous pressure, and leads to liver engorgement.

The pulmonary symptoms of left ventricular failure are due largely to venous engorgement, and the peripheral oedema of congestive cardiac failure owes its situation to the effects of an increased venous pressure.

A very important factor in heart failure is the early rise in blood volume discussed in Chapter 43. It is related to increased salt and water retention by the kidneys.

THE CARDIAC RESERVES[1]

Despite an organic lesion of the heart, the individual may not only have a normal cardiac output at rest, but also be able to undertake moderate exercise with ease. This is the state of *compensation*, when with the aid of the cardiac reserves, a damaged heart can supply an output of blood which is sufficient to meet the tissues' needs even during exercise. In due course the reserves may fail and exercise tolerance becomes poorer and poorer. Eventually with all the reserves utilised the cardiac output is only just adequate at rest. This is the state of total *decompensation*, and the patient is in the terminal stages of heart failure.

There are four cardiac reserves:

The strength of the cardiac contraction. Despite the *all-or-none law* of cardiac contraction, the heart as a whole can nevertheless beat more vigorously to meet an extra load. The intrinsic state of the muscle may change from beat to beat, e.g. increased sympathetic tone strengthens the cardiac contraction and increased vagal tone weakens it. This adrenergic activity is the first reserve, and it comes into play at once during exercise to increase the ventricular emptying. The direct stimulation of the myocardium producing increased contractility is termed a positive *inotropic effect*.[14] It is an important action of digitalis, a drug that is a mainstay in the treatment of heart failure.

Cardiac hypertrophy. This is a long-term method of increasing the strength of contraction. The muscle fibres increase in size, but not in number. Unfortunately, there is no increase in the number of capillaries supplying each muscle fibre, and the enlarged heart eventually suffers from ischaemia.

Increased heart rate. The cardiac output rises with an increase in rate until a critical speed is reached (180 beats per minute). As most of the ventricular filling occurs in early diastole, a moderate tachycardia interferes little with the stroke volume. At great rates, however, the shortness of diastole does interfere with ventricular filling, and furthermore, the coronary blood flow, which is mostly diastolic, is impaired. Finally, the mechanical efficiency of the heart itself declines. Acting together with increased adrenergic activity, which strengthens the cardiac contraction, an increased heart rate is the main mechanism whereby the cardiac output is increased in exercise. It also comes into play in most cardiac conditions.

Increased filling pressure and cardiac dilatation. According to *Starling's 'Law of the Heart'*, the energy of contraction is proportional to the initial length of the cardiac muscle fibres.[15] This means that the increase in stroke volume that follows an increased filling pressure depends on the degree to which the ventricular muscle is stretched at the end of diastole. There is a critical point beyond which any further dilatation of the ventricles results in a fall of output. In a classical graph (Starling) the resting cardiac output is plotted against the central venous filling pressure (this is the right atrial pressure minus the negative intrathoracic pressure). Ascent represents compensation, and descent decompensation (Fig. 44.1).

Starling's Law has been accepted as a significant factor in the normal heart. Refined radiographic techniques have demonstrated an increase in the end-diastolic volume of the exercising heart. In exercise the stroke volume can double itself—this is due both to the increased end-diastolic volume and to a reduction of the residual volume. The effects of exercise are an increased heart rate (to about $2\frac{1}{2}$ times the normal) and a 6-fold rise in cardiac output.[4]

But it is in heart failure that Starling's Law is especially important. The failing heart resembles a heart-lung preparation more closely inasmuch as the reserves of rate and autonomic stimulation are already in operation and are proving inadequate. It is at this point that an increased central venous pressure becomes vitally important (see Fig. 44.2).

The central venous pressure may rise under the following conditions:

(*a*) When there is an increased back-pressure behind a raised ventricular diastolic pressure, as previously described. The obstruction behind a stenosed mitral valve has a similar effect.

(*b*) When the blood volume is increased. This occurs in heart failure.

(*c*) A primary reflex venoconstriction stimulated as a compensatory mechanism has been suggested, but as yet there is no direct evidence to support it.

Beyond a critical point, the ventricle cannot respond to an increase in filling pressure by an increase in output; distension actually decreases the cardiac output. The diastolic volume and pressure rise, and the venous pressure increases. This is decompensation, and it may be precipitated by sodium and water retention. It is easy to understand how a therapeutic venesection could relieve congestive failure at this stage.

To summarise, the main reserve of a failing heart is a raised central venous filling pressure acting to increase the stroke volume. Autonomic influences on the strength of contraction and tachycardia are important at first, but as these mechanisms fail to be effective, they later play only a subsidiary

Figure 44.1
Relationship of cardiac output to venous filling pressure (Starling's curve). (*From Paul Wood* (1956), Diseases of the Heart and Circulation, *2nd ed. London: Eyre and Spottiswoode*)

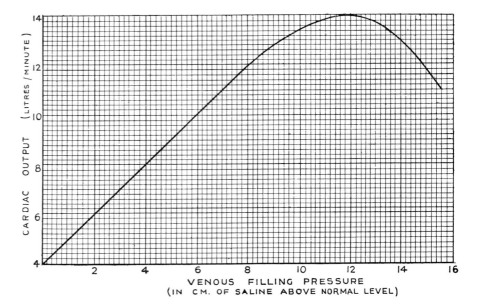

part. Hypertrophy is a long-term matter. It is worth noting that an increased central venous pressure leads to tachycardia due to the atrial reflex of Bainbridge. Figure 44.2, summarises the cardiac reserves during exercise and in states of high and low output.

LEFT VENTRICULAR FAILURE

The most important causes are:
Systemic hypertension.
Aortic stenosis or regurgitation.
Mitral regurgitation.
Myocardial ischaemia (including infarction, which nearly always involves the left ventricle).
Coarctation of the aorta.
Finally, it occurs as a part of *congestive cardiac failure.*

Morbid Physiology

When the left ventricle fails to discharge its contents adequately, the cardiac output tends to fall. The diastolic pressure rises, and this is followed by an increase of pressure in the left atrium and pulmonary veins. A similar rise in pressure occurs in mitral stenosis, where the cause is an obstruction at the entrance of the left ventricle, and not a failure of the ventricle itself. The rise in pulmonary venous pressure is extremely serious because of the imminent danger of acute pulmonary oedema (see Ch. 43): a pressure above 35 mm Hg is dangerous to life. It is not uncommon for patients with mitral stenosis to experience attacks of pulmonary oedema quite early in the course of the malady. These are usually precipitated by exertion and emotion, and may be fatal. Later on, both in left ventricular failure and mitral

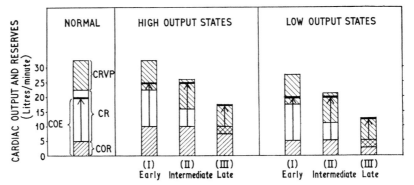

Figure 44.2
In the normal individual the resting cardiac output (COR) is shown as 5 litres/min. Severe exercise, depicted by the arrow, increases this to 20 litres/min. (COE) by utilising especially those cardiac reserves not involving an increase in venous pressure (CR). The reserve of increased venous pressure (CRVP) is not greatly used under physiological conditions.

In a high output state, the cardiac output at rest is shown as 10 litres/min., and on severe exercise the reserve of increased venous pressure must be utilised (I); this causes symptoms. The other cardiac reserves fail, and symptoms occur on even modest exercise (II). Finally, the venous pressure is raised even at rest and severe exercise is no longer possible (III).

In low output states the reduction in those cardiac reserves not involving a venous pressure rise (e.g. due to myocardial damage) necessitates the increase in venous pressure to attain a satisfactory cardiac output. At first this occurs only on severe exercise (I), but later as the reserves fail, symptoms occur on modest exercise (II), and finally at rest (III).

stenosis the pulmonary circulation is made more capable of accommodating the dammed-up blood. This appears to be brought about by a redistribution of the total blood volume, more of which is held in the lungs, and less in the systemic circulation than before.[16] In left ventricular failure the increased diastolic stretch engendered by the raised pulmonary venous and ventricular diastolic pressures may increase the left ventricular output for a time, and so balance the outputs of the two ventricles. This balance is always precarious, and as the left ventricle fails, the danger of pulmonary oedema increases.

In due course more far-reaching mechanisms come into play, whereby the amount of blood entering the lung is reduced:

(*a*) There is a rise in pulmonary arterial pressure due to active arteriolar vasoconstriction. In this way the amount of blood entering the lungs is decreased, the venous pressure tends to fall, and the risk of oedema is obviated.

(*b*) There may be a shift of the interventricular septum, so that the right ventricle is somewhat occluded. In this way less blood enters it. This is called the *Bernheim effect*, and although it is sometimes a prominent *post-mortem* finding, opinions vary as to its importance in reducing the pulmonary blood flow.

The first mechanism leads to secondary pulmonary hypertension; in mitral stenosis high pressures are common. Although this succeeds in protecting the patient from the immediate danger of pulmonary oedema, it soon leads to right ventricular failure. Systemic venous congestion ensues. But it is worth noting that the increased central venous filling pressure acts to increase the cardiac output to near normal levels.

Clinical Features of Left Ventricular Failure

Undue breathlessness on effort. This is not due to carbon dioxide retention or arterial hypoxia, but is a direct effect of the pulmonary congestion which decreases the compliance of the lungs. Breathing is therefore rendered more arduous: the resulting dyspnoea is the commonest symptom of heart failure. The pulmonary congestion has an additional effect: the Hering-Breuer reflex which inhibits inspiration is enhanced, and this results in rapid, shallow breathing. This type of respiration is inefficient because it involves excessive movement of dead-space air (p. 539). Furthermore, the increased metabolic activity that it demands is a factor in increasing the BMR (see p. 467).

Orthopnoea. The patient breathes most comfortably in the upright position; when recumbent, the vital capacity is reduced due to the elevation of the diaphragm. Furthermore, the right atrial pressure is increased by the inflow of blood from the lower parts of the body, because the effect of gravity is minimised in the recumbent posture. There is a corresponding increase in the output of the right ventricle, and more blood reaches the left atrium. The left atrial pressure rises accordingly. The inadequate left ventricle does not respond properly by increasing its output. Pulmonary engorgement and dyspnoea, which are already present, are further aggravated.

Paroxysmal (nocturnal) dyspnoea. The patient wakes up breathless in the early hours of the morning with a sense of oppression in the chest. Sitting up is of no help, for the dyspnoea

increases. Growing restlessness drives the patient out of bed to seek the fresh air at the window. The sense of suffocation becomes unbearable and is accompanied by profound distress. The skin has an ashen cyanosis; sweat breaks out and is profuse. Blood-stained sputum may be coughed up, and in severe cases profuse pulmonary oedema develops with dramatic suddenness. The blood pressure is raised at first, but as pulmonary oedema develops both the breathing and the pulse weaken, and death finally ensues.

The complete explanation of this paroxysmal dyspnoea is not known. During the attack the jugular venous pressure, the systemic blood pressure, and the cardiac output are all raised. One possible explanation is that the ambulant cardiac patient already has oedema of the legs; on retiring to bed the fluid is absorbed. The pulmonary oedema might therefore be due to a sudden increase in blood volume, similar to that seen after the administration of excessive saline infusions. Dependent oedema is not, however, a feature of left ventricular failure. Another explanation is sudden imbalance between the outputs of the two ventricles. This is rather begging the question, since the cause of the hypothetical imbalance is unknown.

It is very probable that a neurogenic factor is involved, because there is usually dramatic relief after the administration of morphine, which is an important component in the treatment of this emergency (see p. 526).

Finally, bronchospasm is often a marked feature of left ventricular failure, and when this element of spasm is prominent, the condition is called *cardiac asthma*. It is important to distinguish it clinically from bronchial asthma, because morphine is detrimental in the bronchial type, whereas adrenaline is often lethal in the cardiac type.

X-ray signs. The hilar fan-shaped shadow of pulmonary congestion and oedema is characteristic. Bilateral hydrothorax is common, and usually more marked on the left side.

Other signs. There is a prolongation of the pulmonary circulation time. The arm-tongue time (normally 9 to 18 seconds) is increased to about 30 seconds in left heart failure. This test is performed by injecting saccharin into an arm vein, and noting the time taken before the substance is tasted in the tongue.

The other manifestations of left ventricular failure, e.g. Cheyne–Stokes respiration, gallop rhythm, and pulsus alternans, are dealt with in physiology text-books. Indeed, there is no satisfactory explanation of the various types of gallop rhythm.

RIGHT VENTRICULAR FAILURE

There is a rise of pressure in the right atrium and the venae cavae. This is manifested by general venous engorgement and an enlarged, tender liver.

Sometimes the failure is primarily right-sided as in pulmonary hypertension secondary to *lung disease*, e.g. pulmonary fibrosis due to tuberculosis, pneumoconiosis, or bronchopneumonia, and also chronic bronchitis and emphysema; *massive pulmonary embolism; multiple emboli* composed of blood clot, tumour, or schistosomal parasites; *post-pneumonectomy*; and finally as an idiopathic condition called *primary pulmonary hypertension.*

It may also be due to certain *congenital heart lesions*, notably pulmonary stenosis and atrial septal defect.

The commonest cause, however, is as a secondary event in *left ventricular failure* and *mitral stenosis*.

In conditions in which the heart fails as a whole, e.g. high output failure and myocarditis, there is a prominent right-sided element.

Where there is a combined left-sided and right-sided failure, the condition is called *congestive cardiac failure*. In fact, pure right-sided failure is uncommon; in most chronic lung diseases there is high output failure as well as pulmonary hypertension.

Features

Elevated venous pressure is a most important sign. The pressure may be normal at rest, but with exercise it rises. Normally the jugular venous pressure falls on exertion, because there is a lowered mean intrathoracic pressure due to the increased ventilation.

Enlargement and tenderness of the liver. This is due to chronic venous congestion. Liver function tests show no abnormality other than a slight rise in plasma bilirubin. The spleen is slightly enlarged in congestive cardiac failure, but it is rarely clinically palpable. Jaundice occasionally occurs in heart failure complicated by extensive pulmonary infarction, when there is a vigorous breakdown of haemolysed red cells in the lung.

Oedema. The extent of cardiac oedema is very variable. As noted in Chapter 43, the important factor in its production is fluid retention, and its site is related to the raised venous pressure acting with gravity. Hydrothorax, often right-sided, is a frequent accompaniment; ascites is rare except in tricuspid valve lesions and constrictive pericarditis.

Other Features include:

Cerebral effects, e.g. fatigue, confusion, and impaired ability to concentrate. These are terminal features due to an impaired cerebral blood flow.

Renal effects. There is moderate oliguria. The urine is of high specific gravity, since the concentrating ability of the kidney is good. The plasma urea is seldom raised except terminally. There is often slight proteinuria.

Venous thrombosis is a common complication of heart failure (see Ch. 39). Pulmonary infarction is the result of subsequent embolism.

Haematological effects. There is a depression of the ESR, the cause of which is unknown. This occurs even during the course of an inflammatory condition, e.g. acute rheumatic fever. The peripheral blood sometimes contains nucleated red cells, perhaps due to the effect of hypoxia on the bone marrow.

Metabolic effects. The BMR is raised by about 20 per cent; the cause of this is unknown, but it may be related to inefficient breathing. Some patients with long-standing cardiac disease develop 'cardiac cachexia'. This may be due to the combined effects of a raised BMR and a poor dietary intake due to anorexia.

MORBID ANATOMY OF HEART FAILURE

Acute Left Ventricular Failure

The lungs are deeply congested and the alveoli contain a variable amount of serous fluid. Sometimes this oedema is so marked that the lungs have a solid consistency resembling the consolidation of pneumonia, but usually they are bulky and crepitant, and on pressure exude an abundant blood-stained, frothy fluid. The basal parts of the lung show the severest change. Bronchopneumonia may be superadded at a later stage (see p. 225). The mechanism of pulmonary oedema is considered in Chapter 43.

Chronic Venous Congestion of Lung

This occurs in chronic left ventricular failure and especially in mitral stenosis. The lungs are tougher in consistency than normal, and have a brownish colour. The condition is known as *brown induration of the lungs*. Histologically there are three features:

(1) The alveolar septa are widened as the result of distension of the capillaries with blood.

(2) The septa show a mild increase in connective tissue which contributes to the thickening, and is the cause of the toughness of the lung. It is possible that this fibrous thickening may prevent fluid entering the alveoli, and so diminish the tendency to oedema.

(3) Small haemorrhages are present within the alveoli. Clinically these can be correlated with the frequently occurring haemoptyses that are a feature of the condition. The lungs also show abundant evidence of previous haemorrhage. The alveoli are filled with macrophages containing haemosiderin; it is these 'heart-failure cells' which give the lung its brown colour.

It must not be thought that the presence of heart-failure cells is pathognomonic of cardiac disease. They are found wherever haemorrhage has occurred, e.g. around infarcts and tumours. In mitral stenosis the haemosiderosis is sometimes especially well marked, and its focal distribution in groups of alveoli gives a characteristic mottled appearance radiologically.

Finally, the frequent occurrence of pulmonary infarcts in heart failure (especially in mitral stenosis) must be borne in mind.

Congestive Cardiac Failure

The clinical onset of congestive heart failure is a serious event: about 50 per cent of patients will have died within 5 years.[17] The changes seen in the various organs in congestive cardiac failure are classically described as those of *chronic venous congestion*. However, the decreased blood supply to many of the tissues is of even greater importance than the congestion.

Skin and extremities. The vasoconstriction of low output failure may rarely produce sufficient ischaemia to cause necrosis. 'Dry gangrene' may then affect the nose and ears. This complication is occasionally seen in severe myocardial infarction.

Liver. The *acinus of the liver*, as described by Rappaport,[18] has an arteriole in its centre, and it is the *peripheral zone* which is most hypoxic and shows the most severe damage (Fig. 44.3). The cells undergo degenerative changes and finally die, so that the area is composed of capacious, blood-filled vascular channels, among which there is often brown pigment derived from the liver cells. An element of venous back-pressure contributes to the congestion. The central area of the

Figure 44.3

The liver acinus. The liver acinus is depicted as an area supplied by a terminal branch of the hepatic artery arising in a portal triad (labelled P.S.). The cells in zone 1 are closest to their blood supply, whereas those in zone 3 are most remote. Note that the acinus contains cells belonging to 2 adjacent, classical, hexagonal lobules. The latter are pictured as being centred on a terminal hepatic venule (T.h.V.). When the blood supply of the liver is impaired (as in congestive heart failure), the cells in zone 3 first undergo necrosis. The damaged area therefore assumes the shape of a starfish (designated by heavy crosshatching). (*Photograph by courtesy of Dr. A. M. Rappaport. From Rappaport, A. M. (1976) The microcirculatory acinar concept of normal and pathological hepatic structure.* Beitraege Pathologie (Stuttgart), **157**, 215.)

Figure 44.4

Nutmeg liver. The alternating pattern of dark congestion and pale fatty change is apparent. (A 95.1, *Reproduced by permission of the President and Council of the R.C.S. Eng.*)

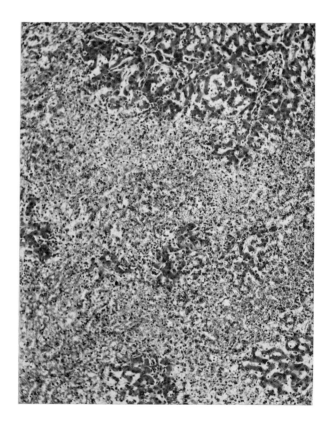

Figure 44.5

Nutmeg liver. In this section many liver cells have disappeared and are replaced by dilated sinusoids filled with blood. The periportal liver cells show marked degenerative changes. × 90.

acinus is less affected, and merely shows the yellow coloration of fatty change. This red and yellow mottling produces the characteristic *nutmeg liver* (Figs. 44.4 and 44.5). It is often debated whether it is the venous back-pressure or the hypoxia which is responsible for the changes of 'chronic venous congestion' in the liver. Probably both play a part, since a similar picture can be produced by venous obstruction, e.g. following hepatic-vein thrombosis. The term chronic is not always appropriate, for the appearances of a nutmeg liver can be produced in a few days, e.g. when a patient dies shortly after a myocardial infarct. It should be noted that if the liver is pictured in terms of the classical *lobule*, it is the *central zone* which shows the congestion. However, the concept of the acinus is more helpful in understanding the features of nutmeg liver.

With long-standing disease the liver may show fine fibrosis and even some evidence of regeneration (cardiac cirrhosis), but this is of no great functional significance.

The spleen is slightly enlarged, deeply congested, and resilient (*cyanotic induration of the spleen*). The sinuses are dilated, and their walls somewhat thickened. The congestion is greater, and the fibrosis less, than in the congestive splenomegaly of hepatic cirrhosis.

Kidney. Although changes in renal function appear to play an important part in the causation of cardiac oedema, there is remarkably little to be seen in the way of structural damage. The organ is congested (cyanotic induration), and the tubules may show degenerative changes like cloudy swelling and fatty change. The glomeruli may show mesangial proliferation.

William Harvey, in his grandiloquent dedication of 'De Motu Cordis' to King Charles I, describes the heart of animals as 'the foundation of their life, the sovereign of everything within them, the sun of their microcosm, that upon which all growth depends, from which all power proceeds' (translated by Robert Willis in 1847).

The pathologist is certainly humiliated when called upon to explain the manifold clinical features of heart failure in terms of the meagre findings noted at necropsy. In few other conditions is the inadequacy of current pathological techniques so apparent. The mysterious feature of heart failure is the progressive nature of the process. There is no satisfactory explanation of why an overburdened heart fails.[19] Until more accurate methods are in hand to investigate cellular dysfunction at a biochemical level, the nature of heart failure will elude exact explanation.

REFERENCES

1. WOOD, P. (1968) *Diseases of the Heart and Circulation*, 3rd edn, p. 291. London: Eyre and Spottiswoode.
2. GUYTON, A. C. (1976) Regulation of cardiac output. *New England Journal of Medicine*, **277**, 805.
3. HARRIS, P. & HEATH, D. (1977) *The Human Pulmonary Circulation*, 2nd edn, p. 58. Edinburgh: Churchill Livingstone.
4. DICKINSON, C. J. & PENTECOST, B. L. (1974) In *Clinical Physiology*, ed. Campbell, E. J. M., Dickinson, C. J. & Slater, J. D. H., 4th edn, p. 43. Oxford: Blackwell.
5. SHUSTER, S. (1963) High-output cardiac failure from skin disease. *Lancet*, **1**, 1338.
6. FOX, R. H. *et al.* (1965) Cardiovascular, metabolic, and thermoregulatory disturbances in patients with erythrodermic skin diseases. *British Medical Journal*, **1**, 619.
7. HUDSON, R. E. B. (1965) *Cardiovascular Pathology*, p. 262. London: Arnold.
8. Leading Article (1974) Viruses and heart disease. *Lancet*, **2**, 991.
9. BURCH, G. E. & DEPASQUALE, N. P. (1970) Recognition and prevention of cardiomyopathy. *Circulation*, **42**, A−47.
10. GOODWIN, J. F. (1974) Prospects and predictions for the cardiomyopathies. *Circulation*, **50**, 210.
11. GOODWIN, J. F. (1966) The cardiomyopathies. *Royal College of Physicians Symposium, Edinburgh*, p. 76.
12. HALL, L. J. & SMITH, E. B. (1968) Cobalt heart disease. *Archives of Pathology*, **86**, 403.
13. Leading Article (1972) Alcoholic cardiomyopathy. *British Medical Journal*, **2**, 247.
14. KOCH-WESER, J. (1967) Mechanism of digitalis action on the heart. *New England Journal of Medicine*, **277**, 417 and 469.
15. Leading Article (1974) Starling's Law survives. *Lancet*, **2**, 818.
16. WOOD, P. (1954) An appreciation of mitral stenosis. *British Medical Journal*, **1**, 1051 and 1113.
17. MCKEE, P. A. *et al.* (1971) The natural history of congestive heart failure: the Framingham study. *New England Journal of Medicine*, **285**, 1441.
18. RAPPAPORT, A. M. (1976) The microcirculatory acinar concept of normal and pathological hepatic structure. *Beitraege Pathologie (Stuttgart)*, **157**, 215.
19. BRAUNWALD, E., ROSS, J. & SONNENBLICK, E. H. (1967) Mechanisms of contraction of the normal and failing heart. *New England Journal of Medicine*, **277**, 794, 853, 910, 962, and 1012.

Chapter 45. Respiratory Failure

The cells of the higher animals show considerable diversity in their specialisation, but insofar as energy production is concerned each cell is self-sufficient. Energy is produced by the oxidation of substances derived from the food and brought to the cell by the blood stream. Although the oxidative process, centred around the Krebs cycle, is referred to as intracellular respiration, respiration in its broadest context involves four other processes. Gases are *transported* to and from the tissues by the blood stream, while in the capillaries actual *exchange* occurs between blood and cells. In the lungs the gases exchange with the alveolar air by *diffusion* across the alveolar walls. The final act of respiration is the exchange between alveolar air and the atmosphere mediated by the *ventilation* produced by the lungs. Respiration in its clinical sense is restricted to these aspects which directly concern the lungs, and *respiratory failure* is defined as a condition in which there is a fall in arterial blood Po_2* (below 60 mm Hg or 8 kPa) or a rise in arterial blood Pco_2* (above 49 mm Hg or 6.5 kPa) due to dysfunction of the lungs.[1] The causes are nearly always to be found in the lungs themselves, and it is therefore necessary to consider their normal structure and function.

STRUCTURE OF THE LUNG AND AIR PASSAGES

The trachea is lined by a pseudostratified columnar ciliated epithelium containing in addition numerous goblet cells. How the secretion of these cells is regulated is not known, but local 'irritation', e.g. trauma and chemicals, leads to an increased discharge of mucus. Opening on to the surface are the ducts of compound mucous and seromucous glands. Vagal stimulation produces secretions from these glands, an action blocked by atropine. The wall of the trachea contains hoops of cartilage, incomplete posteriorly; this allows considerable change in size of the lumen. Thus, on inspiration there is an increase, and on expiration a decrease in size. During coughing the trachea can be occluded almost completely, and foreign bodies and accumulations of mucus can be speedily ejected. Muscle and elastic fibres complete the wall, together with a small amount of collagenous connective tissue.

The bronchi, as they enter the substance of the lung, divide into smaller branches and ultimately into bronchioles. The structure of the bronchial wall is very similar to that of the trachea except that the cartilage rings are replaced by irregular

*The following abbreviations are used in this chapter:

Po_2 — partial pressure of oxygen; Pco_2 — partial pressure of carbon dioxide. In each case the site will be designated, e.g. in arterial or venous blood or in alveolar gas.

The SI unit for measuring pressure is the pascal (Pa). The kilopascal (kPa), which is 1000 times the pascal, is used for measuring pressures in human physiology. To bring mm Hg to kPa, divide by a factor of 7.5.

plates that completely surround the bronchus. These prevent collapse of the bronchi, but nevertheless, as in the trachea, some alteration in size does occur with respiration. It follows therefore that a mass nearly occluding a bronchus will not prevent air entering the affected lung, but will effectively block its escape on expiration. The lung, therefore, becomes overdistended. Contraction of the bronchial muscle on expiration helps to reduce the anatomical dead-space to a minimum (see p. 539).

As the bronchi decrease in size their walls become thinner, and at about 1 mm in diameter the bronchioles lose their cartilage. At this point the glands also disappear. The smallest bronchiole that is found without alveoli budding from its wall is called the *terminal bronchiole*. It is the last part of the bronchial tree to receive an oxygenated bronchial arterial supply and also the last part to act purely in a conducting capacity.

That part of the lung distal to the terminal bronchiole is called the *acinus*, or the *unit of the lung*. Several units are together grouped to form the lobules which can be seen on the lung surface, when outlined by carbon deposits. Each terminal bronchiole divides into a number of *respiratory bronchioles*, of which there are usually three generations. They are about 0.5 mm in diameter, and are lined at their commencement by ciliated columnar epithelium devoid of goblet cells. Lower down the cilia disappear, and the epithelium becomes low cuboidal. In the wall there is muscle, collagen, and elastic fibres. A few alveoli bud off directly from the respiratory bronchiole (hence its name). The respiratory bronchioles themselves branch into 2 to 11 *alveolar ducts* which follow a long, tortuous course, and finally divide into *air sacs*. The alveolar ducts and sacs have no mucosal lining, and their walls consist of the orifices of the numerous alveoli which open into them. Elastic fibres are disposed in the walls at the entrances of the alveoli.

The alveoli are polygonal in shape, like soap bubbles packed closely together, and it is in their walls that gaseous exchanges take place between blood and air. Electron microscopy reveals that they are lined by a complete layer of flattened cells which is separated from the capillary endothelial cells by a thin space containing basement membrane, reticulin, and an occasional elastic fibre (Fig. 45.1). The alveolar surface is covered by a layer of lipoprotein, rich in dipalmitoyl lecithin,[2] which has important surface-active ('surfactant') properties.[3,4] Two types of epithelial cell are described (Fig. 45.2). Type I pneumocytes are more abundant, and the lateral extension of their cytoplasm forms the major part of the continuous epithelial lining. Type II pneumocytes usually occur singly, are larger, and on electron microscopy are seen to contain characteristic osmophilic granules, or inclusions. These cells are thought to secrete surfactant, since fetal lung shows a simultaneous

Figure 45.1
Blood-air pathway of the normal human lung. The alveolar air space (Alv) is separated from the basement membrane (Bm) by an alveolar epithelial cell (Ep). On the other side of the basement membrane there are two endothelial cells (End), the cell membranes of which overlap (Cm). The space internal to the endothelial cells is the pulmonary capillary (Cap). ×42 000. (*From Schulz, H.* (1962), *In 'Pulmonary Structure and Function', a Ciba Foundation Symposium, Fig.* 2(*a*), *p.* 205. *London: Churchill*)

Figure 45.2
Electron micrograph of normal mouse lung. The red cell lies in a capillary (Cap), which is bounded on each side by an alveolus. A type II pneumocyte lines part of one alveolus. The cytoplasm contains several mitochondria (m) and osmophilic inclusions (Inc), and the free border of the cell has numerous microvilli (mv) extending into the alveolar space. The remainder of the alveolar surface is covered by the thin lateral extensions of Type I cells. One such extension partially covers the Type II cell, and forms a junctional complex (jc) at the luminal surface. Uranyl acetate and lead hydroxide stain. ×13 000. (*From Curry, R. H.* (1968), 'A Morphologic Study of Mouse Lung, the Adenomatous Tumours of Mice', M.Sc. Thesis, *University of Toronto. Reproduced by permission of the Director, School of Graduate Studies*)

appearance of surfactant and inclusions. Furthermore, animals exposed to a high concentration of oxygen or subjected to bilateral vagotomy show a loss of both surfactant and inclusions.[2]

Although each respiratory unit has a separate anatomical integrity, defects of the walls between adjacent alveoli (forming the pores of Kohn) result in an air communication with neighbouring units. Furthermore, there are channels, described by Lambert, connecting bronchioles directly with alveoli. It therefore follows that the only complete separation of lung tissue occurs at the anatomically distinct septa, and it is for this reason that collapse due to bronchial obstruction is frequently lobar in distribution. Blockage of smaller bronchi does not always produce collapse.

In the alveoli there are free macrophages. In tissue cultures of lung inconspicuous cells in the septa (*septal cells*) assume a typical macrophage appearance and function, and these probably are a reservoir of macrophages (see Fig. 7.2, p. 90).

THE CONTROL OF BREATHING[5]

Breathing is accomplished by the contraction of the respiratory muscles, which causes expansion of the thorax and overcomes the elastic resistance (elastance) of the lungs and also the resistance of the airways to the flow of air through them. The rate, depth, and rhythm of breathing are determined by nerve cells in the reticular system. There is no anatomically localised respiratory centre, but rather a diffuse system of neurons in the brain-stem. It appears to have an intrinsic rhythmicity of its own, but is influenced by a variety of extramedullary functions:

The cortex. Impulses from the higher centres are probably an important factor in the causation of the increased ventilation of voluntary exercise.

Proprioceptive impulses from the muscles of respiration.[6] The tension developed in the inspiratory muscles is integrated with the movement produced. Any decrease in the volume of inspired air produced by an additional load, e.g.

airways obstruction, therefore produces an abnormal sensation. This stimulates an increase in inspiratory effort to overcome the obstruction.

Blood Pco$_2$ and pH. The volume of respiration is finely regulated by arterial Pco$_2$, an increase stimulating and a decrease depressing it. A fall in blood pH also stimulates ventilation.

Blood Po$_2$. Hypoxia stimulates breathing, not through a direct effect on the chemoreceptors of the reticular formation, but indirectly *via* the aortic and carotid-body receptors. If pure oxygen is given to a normal subject, ventilation is depressed, indicating that the control of breathing is influenced by the Po$_2$ level. However, this response is less sensitive than that to changes in Pco$_2$. At high altitudes the hypoxia stimulates breathing so much that the Pco$_2$ of the blood is permanently lowered and the central chemoreceptors have their sensitivity adjusted to a lower level. In chronic lung disease the hypoxia acts as a spur to respiration, and if it is relieved by oxygen administration, the drop in ventilation may cause so great a rise in arterial Pco$_2$ that coma ensues (CO$_2$ narcosis).

Factors Governing Respiratory Gas Exchange in the Lungs

The primary function of the lung is to arterialise the mixed venous blood. This involves the controlled elimination of CO$_2$ and absorption of O$_2$ such that the blood-gas tensions are maintained at their correct levels. The exchange of gas depends upon three factors:

Ventilation. This includes both the *volume* and the *distribution* of the inspired air which ventilates the alveoli.

Diffusion. The passage of gases between the alveoli and blood in the alveolar capillaries.

Pulmonary capillary blood flow (perfusion). This involves the total *volume* of blood and its *distribution* to all the ventilated alveoli.

Control of the Volume of Ventilation[5]

Ventilation involves two phases: inspiration and expiration.

Inspiration is carried out by the contraction of the diaphragm and intercostal muscles, assisted if necessary by the accessory muscles of inspiration. The result is an increase in the negative intrathoracic pressure,* which is about -5 cm H$_2$O (about -4 mm Hg or -0.53 kPa) when the muscles are inactive and there is no airflow. The inspiratory muscles are opposed by two forces:

The elastic force, which has two approximately equal components.

(*a*) The elastic properties of the lung substance.

(*b*) The surface tension of the fluids lining the airways (see below).

The non-elastic or resistive load. This is chiefly due to the frictional resistance of the respiratory passages to airflow.

The elastic load is commonly measured as the *compliance of the lung*, i.e. the increase in lung volume per unit increase in

---

*This is the pressure outside the lung but inside the thoracic cage, and is measured intrapleurally or intra-oesophageally. It must be distinguished from the alveolar pressure, which is equal to the mouth pressure when there is no airflow.

distending pressure, and is measured by dividing the volume of air inspired by the change in negative intrathoracic pressure. It is normally 0.12 to 0.25 litres per cm H$_2$O.

An alternative concept is *elastance of the lung*, which is the pressure required to distend it by a given volume.

Expiration is achieved by the elastic recoil of the lungs, during which the inspiratory muscles relax. During forced expiration there is contraction of the accessory muscles of expiration, e.g. those of the abdominal wall.

The elastic properties of the lung are obviously of great moment in allowing the lung both to be inflated and emptied. It was noticed nearly 40 years ago that for a given distending pressure, a cat's lung would inflate to twice the volume when filled with water as opposed to air. This is due to the water abolishing the surface-tension effect of the fluid-gas interface that normally exists in the lungs, and which provides half the elastic resistance to inflation.

The surface-tension resistance of the lung is less than would be expected were the alveoli lined by either saline or plasma. The surface tension of the film lining the alveoli is lowered by the lipoprotein surfactant agent. Its presence thus decreases the work needed to expand the lungs in each inspiration, and its absence leads to stiffness and loss of compliance.

In addition this lipoprotein lowers the surface tension of a saline film, *especially when the film is compressed*. During expiration the lining of the alveoli is compressed and its surface tension is rapidly lowered. It is thus of importance in preventing the collapse of alveoli following their emptying during expiration. A loss of this surfactant property of the lung lining is recognised in the respiratory distress syndrome of the newborn (hyaline-membrane disease) and in the 'post-perfusion lung' syndrome that follows open-heart surgery (see p. 515), but it is not certain whether it causes or merely follows these conditions. It is also found in lung damage from prolonged positive pressure breathing or high inspired oxygen concentrations, and in some cases of collapse, pulmonary oedema, and pulmonary vascular obstruction.[5]

The *tidal volume* (the volume of air which enters and leaves the lungs during normal quiet breathing) is normally 500 ml, and at a rate of 15 respirations per minute, 7.5 litres are inspired and expired each minute. The *amount* of air that is inspired depends on the compliance of the lungs. The *rate* of airflow is related to the calibre of the airways. This forms the principal part of the non-elastic resistance to ventilation, the other factor being the displacement of tissues and blood in the lungs themselves. The last 100 ml to 170 ml of each breath (500 ml) is expended in filling the conducting airways, and does not reach the alveoli—it is called the *anatomical dead-space*.

It is obvious that the compliance and the non-elastic resistance are important factors in influencing the depth and rate of respiration. With a low compliance or a high non-elastic resistance a greater pressure difference or a longer time is required for proportional ventilation as compared with a high compliance or a low non-elastic resistance. When compliance is low, the work of breathing is increased, and it is most advantageous to take frequent, shallow respirations. The rate and depth of respiration are optimally adjusted in relation to dead-space volume, compliance, and non-elastic resistance. Exactly how this is brought about is not known, but it appears to be a function of the reticular centres.

Figure 45.3
Diagrammatic representation of the lung showing two alveoli with ideal ventilation/blood flow relationships. The
oxygen tensions are in mm Hg, and the figure in brackets
are the percentage oxygen saturation of the blood. (*After
Comroe, J. H. et al.* (1962), 'The Lung: Clinical Physiology
and Pulmonary Function Tests', *2nd ed., Fig. 26, p. 88.
Chicago: Year Book Medical Publishers*)

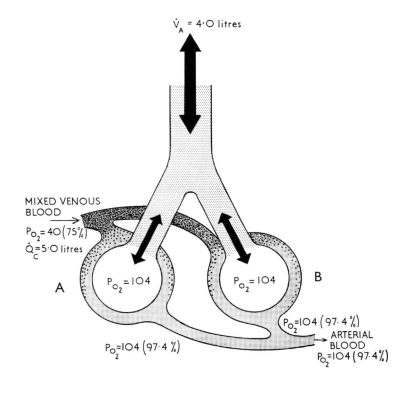

Distribution of Ventilation in Relation to Perfusion[5]

From the point of view of maintaining the normal gaseous
composition of the arterial blood, the distribution of ventilation relative to pulmonary capillary blood flow (*perfusion*) is
very important. Considering the lung as a whole, under
normal conditions the ratio

$$\frac{\text{Alveolar ventilation}}{\text{Perfusion of capillaries}}*\text{ is approximately unity.}$$

The situation in an ideal lung is shown in Fig. 45.3.
Although in the normal lung the alveolar ventilation and
perfusion are closely coordinated, there are areas where ventilation exceeds perfusion. Thus, in the erect position the apices
of the upper lobes receive relatively little blood in comparision
with the volume of air ventilating them.

Some effects of badly correlated ventilation and perfusion
are shown in Fig. 45.4. The following points are noteworthy:

1. There is a rise in the P_{O_2} of the blood leaving alveolus
A, but because of the nature of the oxygen dissociation curve
(Fig. 45.5) this does not appreciably raise the oxygen saturation. Hence it does not compensate for the desaturated blood
leaving alveolus B. The excess ventilation of alveolus A is
therefore wasted, and when added to the anatomical dead-
space constitutes the *physiological dead-space*. This in itself
leads to an increase in ventilation.

*Generally written $\dfrac{\dot{V}_A}{\dot{Q}_C}$ the dot indicating that the volumes are in

unit time. Thus, in a normal subject at rest

$$\frac{\dot{V}_A}{\dot{Q}_C} = \frac{4 \text{ litres per min}}{5 \text{ litres per min}} = 0.8$$

2. The mixed venous blood reaching alveolus B is not as
fully arterialised as in the 'ideal lung'. This wasted blood
produces the same effect as a direct *right-to-left shunt*.

3. The increased ventilation of alveolus A has the effect of
washing out an excessive quantity of CO_2 from the blood
perfusing it. This tends to compensate for the raised P_{CO_2} of
the blood leaving the under-ventilated alveolus B.

4. The mixed arterial blood is desaturated (P_{O_2} 84 mm Hg),
while the P_{O_2} of the mixed alveolar gas is raised (106 mm
Hg). This difference therefore appears as a *diffusion defect*.

5. The desaturated, mixed, arterial blood causes an increase
in the total ventilation as a compensatory mechanism. This
reduces the P_{CO_2} to near normal levels, and also increases the
arterial saturation because alveolus B is better ventilated.
However, the alveolar P_{O_2} is also raised, and the alveolar-
arterial P_{O_2} difference remains.

A similar situation arises if the ventilation of alveoli is
uniform but the perfusion is non-uniform. In the alveolus
receiving little blood there is wasted ventilation, but the blood
leaving it is fully oxygenated. In the alveolus receiving the
excess blood there is not enough ventilation to oxygenate the
blood fully or to reduce the P_{CO_2} to normal. Arterial desaturation and an increase in the physiological dead-space
bring about similar compensatory changes to those described
above.

Imbalance between distribution of perfusion and ventilation
thus introduces great inefficiency in the act of respiration, and
it is not surprising that there are mechanisms for co-ordinating
these two parameters. These mechanisms are not well understood. If one lung is ventilated with gas of a low P_{O_2} or a high
P_{CO_2}, or if there is bronchial obstruction, the blood flow
through that lung is dramatically reduced. The gas tensions
therefore regulate blood flow. Furthermore, a reduced blood

Figure 45.4
Diagrammatic representation of the lung showing two al-
veoli which are unevenly ventilated but uniformly perfused.
Note how the over-ventilation of one alveolus does not
compensate for the under-ventilation of the other, with the
result that some arterial desaturation occurs and the P_{O_2} is
considerably reduced. (*After Comroe, J. H. et al. (1962),
'The Lung: Clinical Physiology and Pulmonary Function
Tests', 2nd ed., Fig. 28, p. 94. Chicago: Year Book Medical
Publishers*)

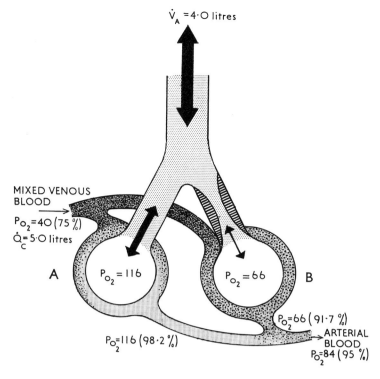

Figure 45.5
Oxygen dissociation curve of blood. (*After Starling and Lovatt Evans
(1962), 'Principles of Human Physiology', 13th ed., p. 79. Edrs.
Davson, H. and Eggleton. M. G. London: Churchill*)

flow, e.g. due to arterial obstruction, is followed by reduced
ventilation, probably as a result of increased airways resistance
and reduced compliance.

Diffusion[5]

In the normal lung the barrier between the alveolar gas and
the blood consists of the alveolar cell, the endothelial cell, and
the thin layer of intervening connective tissue. In addition to
this membrane barrier there is also the red-cell envelope,
which constitutes a further barrier. Diffusion depends on the
difference between the partial pressures of the gas in the
alveolar air and the interior of the red cell, the solubility and
molecular weight of the gas, the thickness of the barriers
mentioned above, and the speed of the physico-chemical
processes in the red cell. Apart from these conditions, diffusion also depends upon the area over which the blood gases
and alveolar gas can interchange. This is related to the total
volume of functioning lung and the balance between perfusion
and ventilation.

CO_2 is much more soluble than O_2, and diffuses 20 times as
readily through the pulmonary membranes. The arterial P_{CO_2}
is therefore the same as that of the alveolar gas, both in health
and when there are defects of diffusion. The arterial P_{O_2}, on
the other hand, is slightly lower than the alveolar gas P_{O_2} even
in the normal individual, due to the fact that his lungs are not
'ideal'. Arterial desaturation is characteristic of diffusion
defects.

The pulmonary diffusion capacity can be estimated clinically, being measured in ml of oxygen or carbon-monoxide
transfer each minute for each mm Hg pressure difference of
oxygen or carbon monoxide across the lung. The diffusing
capacity is impaired under the following circumstances:

1. When there is a decrease in the anatomical area available
for diffusion, e.g. following lung destruction or resection.

2. When there is a decrease in the *functional* alveolar-
capillary surface due to *impaired distribution*. It therefore
follows that *distribution and diffusion defects produce the same
functional end-results, and respiratory failure due to these causes
may be considered together.*

Figure 45.6
Carbon-dioxide dissociation curve of blood.
(*After Starling and Lovatt Evans (1962),
'Principles of Human Physiology', 13th ed.,
p. 89. Edrs. Davson, H. and Eggleton, M. G.
London: Churchill*)

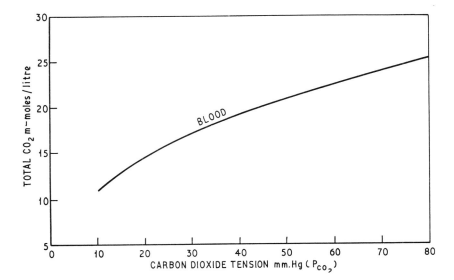

It was formerly believed that the diffusing capacity could be decreased when there was an increase in the distance between the alveolar gas and the red cell. This was called the 'alveolar-capillary block syndrome', and was described in many fibrotic conditions of the lung (see p. 543). It is now believed that the diffusion defect in these conditions is due either to destruction of lung tissue or an impaired ventilation-perfusion ratio.

Blood-gas Transport[5]

The relation between the P_{O_2} of the arterial blood and the volume of O_2 carried in the blood is demonstrated by the classical S-shaped dissociation curve (Fig. 45.5). The normal arterial P_{O_2} is 80 to 110 mm Hg (10·6 to 14·6 kPa) and the arterial saturation 93 to 98 per cent. A considerable reduction of arterial P_{O_2} causes no significant change in the oxygenation of the arterial blood, e.g. an arterial saturation reduction below 90 per cent does not occur until the P_{O_2} is less than 60 mm Hg (8 kPa).

It is evident that a fall of ventilation by almost half causes little decrease in the arterial saturation, but below 60 mm Hg a further drop produces disproportionate desaturation. Overventilation of parts of the lung to compensate for the underventilation elsewhere cannot alter the arterial saturation much, for a raised P_{O_2} above normal leads to only a negligible increase in arterial O_2 saturation.

The normal arterial P_{CO_2} is 34 to 46 mm Hg (4·5 to 6·1 kPa). The CO_2 dissociation curve in the physiological range is much steeper, and greater changes in saturation occur for a change in partial pressure that would have little effect on O_2 saturation (Fig. 45.6).

Therefore overventilation of the lungs can remove CO_2 not properly eliminated by areas of underventilated alveoli.

TYPES OF RESPIRATORY FAILURE[1]

Two main types are recognised:
1. Ventilatory failure due to an inadequate volume of inspired air available for exchange.
2. Impaired alveolar-arterial gas exchange due to failure of distribution or diffusion.

Ventilatory Failure (Hypoxia with Hypercapnia)[1]

This is caused by (a) *airways obstruction** due usually to chronic bronchitis, emphysema, and asthma, which are considered on p. 544, (b) *restriction of thoracic movement*, e.g. in severe kyphoscoliosis, progressive systemic sclerosis, pneumothorax, pleural effusion, ascites, and pregnancy, (c) *neuromuscular impairment*, e.g. in poliomyelitis, polyneuritis, or curare poisoning, and (d) *disturbances of the reticular centres*, e.g. due to organic disease or depressant drugs such as an overdosage of barbiturates.

Effects. Since arterial $P_{CO_2} \propto \dfrac{CO_2 \text{ production}}{\text{alveolar ventilation}}$

and at rest the CO_2 production is constant, it follows that when alveolar ventilation is reduced, the arterial P_{CO_2} is increased, and there is an arithmetically equivalent fall in P_{O_2}. Thus, if the P_{CO_2} rises from 40 to 60 mm Hg, then the P_{O_2} falls from 100 to 80 mm Hg. As already explained above, a drop of P_{O_2} of this order does not greatly affect the oxygen saturation of the arterial blood; desaturation, with cyanosis, is a late event in ventilatory failure.

The main effect is a raised arterial P_{CO_2} (*hypercapnia*), and the symptoms are referable to this. The pulse is rapid and bounding, the hands moist and warm, the pupils small, and the blood pressure raised. If there is severe CO_2 retention, confusion, drowsiness, coarse tremors, and coma may ensue. The reflexes are depressed, and the plantar response is extensor. Papilloedema is an uncommon, though well recognised, effect of prolonged, very severe hypercapnia, and it is a manifestation of the cerebral vasodilation caused by CO_2 excess. Dyspnoea is often absent.

The plasma bicarbonate level is high. There is a raised arterial P_{CO_2}, and a respiratory acidosis ensues. As the difference between arterial and venous P_{CO_2} at rest is slight (6 mm Hg in a normal person), the mixed venous P_{CO_2} is often measured. The *rebreathing method* is very easy: the patient

*This is defined as persistent, widespread narrowing of intrapulmonary airways, at least on expiration, causing increased resistance to airflow.[7]

rebreathes from a bag containing a CO_2 mixture. The contents of the bag and lungs mix, and the CO_2 mixture equilibrates with the pulmonary blood. This equilibrium persists until the blood recirculates around the body and returns to the lungs with an increased CO_2 tension, and therefore after 20 seconds the CO_2 content in the bag is ascertained and the CO_2 tension calculated.

Impaired Alveolar-Arterial Gas Exchange (Hypoxia without Hypercapnia)[1]

In this type of failure there is a reduction of alveolar-capillary surface available for gas exchange. This may occur as a result of either lung destruction or resection or of an imbalance between the distribution of perfusion and ventilation. Frequently these factors are combined, and of the two maldistribution is much more important and becomes prominent in all progressive lung disease. It is indeed the usual cause of cyanosis in lung disease.

Impaired alveolar-arterial gas exchange occurs in emphysema and severe chronic bronchitis, especially postoperatively (see p. 544). It is a feature of pulmonary embolism and chronic obstructive pulmonary vascular disease. It is also seen in such diffuse fibrotic lung conditions as asbestosis, berylliosis, rheumatoid disease, progressive systemic sclerosis, radiation damage to the lung, and allergic reactions in the alveoli following the inhalation of organic dusts—a good example is farmer's lung due to actinomycetes in mouldy hay. If the fibrosis is idiopathic the condition is called *diffuse fibrosing alveolitis*, or the *Hamman-Rich syndrome*. In a number of cases of idiopathic fibrosing alveolitis there is also a tendency to polyarthritis, chronic active hepatitis, Sjφgren's syndrome, and thyroid disease, conditions with a background of immunological abnormality. Non-organ-specific antibodies are sometimes present, and sometimes deposits of immune complexes have been found in alveolar walls. But other cases have no immunological basis, and may be related to infection or extrinsic inhaled agents.[8]

Effects. There is an interference with O_2 uptake, and, as on exercise the venous blood becomes more desaturated, increasing arterial desaturation also occurs. A useful clinical sign of this is *central cyanosis*. Cyanosis is taken to indicate the presence of more than 5 g of reduced Hb per dl blood in the capillaries. It is best detected in the mucosa of the mouth, where the blood flow is always good; in this situation *peripheral cyanosis* (due to stasis) does not occur. When destructive lung disease is a major factor there is little unsaturation at rest, but a dramatic fall in saturation accompanies exercise, and cyanosis rapidly develops.[5]

Mild hypoxia causes little damage; it leads to adaptive responses such as an increase in ventilation, blood-flow, and red-cell formation. Neurological damage starts at an arterial saturation of 50 per cent (arterial Po_2 of 30 mm Hg, or 4 kPa), and is manifested initially by intellectual impairment. At lower saturations there will be convulsions and irreversible cerebral damage.

Although in impaired alveolar-arterial gas exchange there is a severe interference with O_2 uptake, CO_2 elimination, on the other hand, is little impaired. In the distribution-failure group some alveoli are underventilated relative to alveolar perfusion. This is remedied by overventilation of the remainder of the lung. This serves to eliminate more CO_2 from the blood, but it cannot compensate for an unequal O_2 uptake, for, as has been shown, overventilation does not produce an appreciable increase in the amount of O_2 taken up by the blood above the normal level.

In some cases of distribution failure where some alveoli are poorly ventilated, an increased respiratory effort may so improve the ventilation of the affected areas that oxygenation of the blood is corrected. The Pco_2 is, however, lowered. The administration of 30 per cent O_2 produces the same effect, and this may be used as a diagnostic measure.

Other Manifestations of Lung Disease

Tachypnoea,[5] an increased rate of respiration, is seen when pain restricts respiratory movements, as in pleurisy and Bornholm disease, and when the lung compliance is decreased; rapid, shallow respiration results. It is also seen when there is an increased need for ventilation, due to exercise or to chemical changes in the blood, e.g. hypercapnia, hypoxia (hypoxic or anaemic), and metabolic acidosis. High external temperatures may have a similar effect. Usually it is accompanied by an increase in depth of breathing, and the term *hyperpnoea* embraces both conditions. *Hyperventilation* means breathing in excess of the metabolic need, and is seen occasionally in hysterical people.

Dyspnoea is best restricted to a condition in which the act of breathing causes distress. It occurs under two main conditions:

1. When tachypnoea or hyperpnoea are of marked degree.
2. When the ventilatory effect produced on inspiration is small in comparison with the muscular effort needed to produce that effect. This occurs in any disease interfering with the respiratory excursions of the lung. It is seen when there is decreased compliance due to fibrosis, pneumonia, or venous congestion. Airways obstruction, whether due to pulmonary disease like chronic bronchitis or to strangulation, has a similar effect and produces severe dyspnoea. However, this is not invariable, for sometimes airways obstruction does not produce severe dyspnoea; instead the changes in blood-gas tensions are tolerated, and polycythaemia develops (see 'blue bloaters', p. 545).

Although dyspnoea is a common symptom, there is little precise information about the mechanisms involved in its production. Conditions which apparently cause severe dyspnoea in one patient may be found in another who suffers little discomfort. Psychological factors certainly play a part. Thus, the sudden blockage of a tube through which a person is breathing occasions intense dyspnoea. However, if the subject is asked to block the tube himself, the manoeuvre causes no immediate discomfort.

Right-sided heart failure. This is due to a variety of causes of which pulmonary hypertension is the most obvious, and probably the most important. Pulmonary hypertension is due to the destruction of the pulmonary capillary bed (as in emphysema), and also to functional vasoconstriction secondary to hypoxia. The increased tension in the right ventricular myocardium which develops during systole has the effect of reducing the coronary blood flow. Myocardial ischaemia therefore contributes to the right ventricular failure.

An aggravating factor is the secondary polycythaemia which

not only increases the load on the heart, but also predisposes to pulmonary arterial and systemic venous thrombosis (with subsequent embolism).

When there is respiratory acidosis due to CO_2 retention, the reabsorption of sodium and bicarbonate ions from the glomerular filtrate increases. This sodium retention increases the blood volume, thus causing an additional strain on the heart. Peripheral oedema is not uncommon in chronic lung disease and may in part be due to right-sided heart failure. Patients with chronic obstructive airways disease have an impaired ability to excrete water in response to a standard water load (20 ml/kg body weight).[9]

RESPIRATORY EFFECTS OF VARIOUS CONDITIONS

General Surgical Procedures

The use of general anaesthesia produces important changes in carbon dioxide excretion. During the operation the P_{CO_2} of the blood rises due to the depressant effect of the anaesthetic agent on the brain. If respiration is actively assisted by the anaesthetist, the P_{CO_2} may actually be lower than normal. In either event the arterial P_{CO_2} remains above normal after the operation for a few hours as a result of the continued action of the anaesthetic agent. This is particularly important in cura-rised patients whose breathing is completely controlled by the anaesthetist; if the curare-effect is not promptly counteracted after the operation, there may be a dangerous rise in the blood P_{CO_2}.

There is also a danger of hypoxia. This is not usually due in any great measure to poor ventilation except in unusual circumstances, but rather to an error of distribution. This is not important in healthy people, but is of great moment in patients predisposed to airways obstruction through chronic bronchitis. The cause is probably partial collapse of some air-spaces, resulting in a reduced ventilation-perfusion ratio. There is a danger of massive segmental collapse ensuing. The predisposing factors are the increased amount of sputum (which is said to be very viscous after operations), impaired cough reflex and ciliary action due to the anaesthetic, the aspiration of vomitus and blood during the induction of anaesthesia, and later a decreased power of coughing after thoracic and abdominal surgery. It is advisable to administer oxygen for some time after an operation on chronic bronchitic subjects.

Conditions associated with Abnormal Blood-Gas Transport

In *anaemia* (and also methaemoglobinaemia and sul-phaemoglobinaemia) the volume of O_2 taken up is reduced, but the arterial P_{O_2} and P_{CO_2} are normal. If the anaemic hypoxia is severe, it stimulates breathing *via* the aortic and carotid chemoreceptors, and the P_{CO_2} falls below the normal. The hyperpnoea does not usually cause much distress.

In *metabolic acidosis* the increased hydrogen-ion concentration of the blood stimulates breathing and reduces the blood P_{CO_2}. *Metabolic alkalosis* has the opposite effect—in fact, the depression of respiration is usually not very marked (see p. 483).

Left-Sided Heart Failure and Mitral Stenosis

Pulmonary venous engorgement decreases the compliance of the lungs; it leads to brown induration which aggravates this effect. Engorgement of the bronchi causes a ventilatory impairment comparable with that of chronic bronchitis; indeed, recurrent 'chronic bronchitis' is a frequent complaint of victims of mitral stenosis. The tendency to pulmonary oedema interferes with the distribution of the gases. Finally, the increased pulmonary arterial pressure leads to vascular changes which interfere with the perfusion of the lungs. It is the lungs that bear the brunt of left-sided heart disease, and their dysfunction is an important cause of death.

CHRONIC NON-SPECIFIC LUNG DISEASE[10]

This collective title includes chronic bronchitis, emphysema, and asthma, so frequently diagnosed together though often in fact found separately. Their aetiology is unknown, and it is advisable to consider each as a separate condition.

Chronic Bronchitis

This is defined as a condition in which there is a chronic or recurrent increase in the volume of mucoid bronchial secretion, sufficient to cause expectoration, and which is not due to localised broncho-pulmonary disease.[11] At first the expectoration is intermittent, and worse on rising in the morning, but eventually it becomes continuous. It is much commoner in tobacco-smokers than in non-smokers, but chronic bronchitis may occur in those who do not smoke at all. Atmospheric pollution is another contributory factor, but much less important than tobacco smoking.[12] Morphologically the bronchial mucosa is thickened due to hyperplasia of the mucous glands, and there is an increase in the number of goblet cells in the lining epithelium. Chronic inflammation is not a constant feature, and Laennec's term 'bronchial catarrh' is peculiarly apt. At this stage there is little interference with respiratory function and the condition is called *simple chronic bronchitis*.[13,14]

Recurrent inflammation is a common complication, especially in urban areas. It is due to infection with respiratory-tract viruses, pneumococci, and *H. influenzae*, and is aggravated by atmospheric pollution—smoke and sulphur dioxide are particularly dangerous. The clear mucoid sputum with its predominance of macrophages becomes purulent. In the acute stage of infection there may be constitutional symptoms, but these wane as chronicity follows. This is called *chronic or recurrent muco-purulent bronchitis*.[14]

The main effect of progressive chronic bronchitis is obstruction of the airways due to such factors as mucous-gland hyperplasia, mucosal oedema, and fibrosis following localised bronchopneumonia. The excess mucus in the lumen also plays a part, and together with bronchospasm produces acute episodes which can be reversed by treatment. The airways obstruction leads to progressive ventilatory failure, and the condition is called *chronic obstructive bronchitis*.[13,14]

In some patients with chronic bronchitis there is, despite the airways obstruction, little dyspnoea; in fact there is hypoventilation with progressive hypercapnia. There is also arterial desaturation due to poor distribution of ventilation. It is not known why these patients tolerate the changes in blood-gas tensions with so little discomfort. However, there is cyanosis, and later the low Po_2 leads to secondary polycythaemia. There is sodium retention and right-sided heart failure. These cyanosed, oedematous people have been called 'blue bloaters'.* A similar picture is found in some patients with brain damage who do not breathe normally (*primary alveolar hypoventilation*).[1]

If the hypoxia is relieved by oxygen administration, the ventilation can sometimes become so depressed that CO_2 retention occurs, leading to the effects described on p. 542. On the other hand, the vasodilator effect of CO_2 excess ensures that the brain receives an adequate blood supply,[16] and vigorous artificial ventilation of the lungs to relieve the hypercapnia may produce such a fall in the blood Pco_2 that generalised vasoconstriction results. This leads to cerebral ischaemia, and serious sequelae may occur.[16] In the treatment of respiratory failure it is the hypoxia and acidosis rather than the hypercapnia which demand the most attention.

Emphysema[10]

The word, introduced by Laennec, is derived from the Greek, meaning an inflation. It is defined as a condition in which there is an increase beyond the normal size of the acini, due either to dilatation or destruction of the walls. Such emphysema used to be called 'vesicular' in contrast to the interstitial variety in which air was present in the connective tissues of the lung, but nowadays this adjective is regarded as redundant. Though emphysema is suspected clinically by signs of hyperinflation and decreased vascularity of the lung, the final diagnosis is made by the pathologist on the properly-fixed, inflated lung. This is prepared by distending the organ by controlled intrabronchial infusion of fixative prior to sectioning.

Dilatatory emphysema. Emphysema due to dilatation of the air passages occurs as a compensatory phenomenon following removal or collapse of adjacent lung. It also follows a partial bronchial block. If the dilatation affects mainly the larger respiratory bronchioles the emphysema is *centrilobular* (or *centriacinar*), while if third-generation respiratory bronchioles and alveolar ducts are also involved, the whole acinus is affected and the emphysema is called *panacinar*. Centrilobular emphysema is also described in coal-miner's lung, in which it appears to be related to the deposits of carbon around the respiratory bronchioles, and is called 'focal dust emphysema'. Neither type is of any great importance as a cause of respiratory failure.

Destructive emphysema. This is of great moment, so much so that the WHO Committee on Chronic Cor Pulmonale has defined emphysema simply as an increase in the size of the air spaces distal to the terminal bronchioles with destruction of their walls.[11]

There are two main varieties of destructive emphysema (Figs. 45.7–45.9):

(*a*) Panacinar (or *panlobular*), in which there is a uniform enlargement of air spaces throughout the acini comprising the

Figure 45.7
Centrilobular emphysema of destructive type. In this section of lung (prepared by barium-sulphate impregnation) the lesions are severe enough to transmit light through the slice, and there are bullae at the top. In view of the strictly centrilobular emphysema in the lower part of the field and its continuity and apparent grading into the severe upper lesions, all the lesions are regarded as centrilobular emphysema. However, some observers would term this bullous emphysema. (*Photograph by courtesy of Dr B.E. Heard.*)

lobules—it is the alveolar ducts that are principally enlarged due to destruction of the alveoli comprising their walls; (*b*) *centrilobular* (or *centriacinar*), in which there is a large air space in the centre of each lobule—this is the enlarged respiratory bronchiole. The terminal bronchioles may show chronic inflammatory changes, and some authorities have maintained that bronchiolitis and adjacent bronchopneumonia are major aetiological factors in centrilobular emphysema. This, however, is debatable, and the true cause is unknown. Both types of destructive emphysema may be *localised* to a few lobules, or else be *widespread* (a better term than generalised, which could be confused with panacinar).

There is probably a spectrum of clinical types with pure chronic bronchitis at one end and pure emphysema at the other, while most patients have a mixture of both conditions. Emphysema, particularly the centrilobular type, may be accompanied by airways obstruction, but this is probably the result rather than the cause of the condition. The obstruction is probably brought about by a collapse of the bronchioles deprived of their support by the destruction of the walls of the surrounding air spaces. The absence of emphysema in asthma

*The concept of pink puffers and blue bloaters has apparently been derived from the teaching of Professor A. C. Dornhorst, who pointed out the distinction between those patients with chronic respiratory difficulty that were 'pink and puffing' and those that were 'blue and bloated'.[15]

Figure 45.8
Centrilobular emphysema of destructive type. This is a higher power magnification (× 12) of the centre of the upper lobe of Fig. 45.7. The appearances are interpreted as advanced centrilobular emphysema in which much of the peripheral parenchyma of the lobule has been encroached upon. (*Photograph by courtesy of Dr B.E. Heard.*)

of long duration is further evidence that obstruction is not a factor in its pathogenesis.

An inherited factor in the aetiology of emphysema is likely. Homozygous subjects with α_1-antitrypsin deficiency tend to develop emphysema, and so, but to a lesser extent, may the heterozygotes with a low enzyme level. The precise relationship between enzyme deficiency and emphysema is still not clear, but one suggestion is that proteolytic enzymes, especially those contained in leucocytes, can cause emphysema. The emphysema of α_1-antitrypsin deficiency is panacinar with a predominantly basal distribution, which is in

keeping with the greater tendency for bronchopneumonia to affect the lower lobes of the lungs.[17,18]*

The effects of emphysema vary. A widespread panacinar type is quite common in the aged, and it produces little functional impairment.[21] Likewise there may be widespread centrilobular emphysema in symptomless people.[21] On the other hand, there can be a variety of functional effects. Airways obstruction has already been referred to, and in addition there may be impaired alveolar-arterial gas exchange due to diffusion failure following the loss of capillary surface. Another important factor is an increase in the physiological dead-space due to the ventilation of large avascular bullae.

All these effects cause dyspnoea, which is often severe. As ventilation is maintained, the P_{CO_2} is normal or even rather below normal, and these patients remain pink in spite of the difficulty they have in maintaining this ventilation. They are called 'pink puffers' (see footnote, p. 545). The blood-gas tensions are kept normal, and there is no right-sided heart failure until terminally. Despite their bright appearance these patients are the victims of a relentlessly progressive disease, and little can be done to help them. On the other hand, the 'blue bloater', despite the alarming appearance, can usually be tided over the attack of acute infection with antibiotics. 'Pink puffers' can be given oxygen without the danger of CO_2 retention.

Chronic bronchitis is said to be more common in Britain— the 'English disease'—than in the USA, where emphysema is said to predominate, but the difference may lie more in terminology than in incidence.[22]

Asthma[23]

This is a condition of widespread narrowing of the bronchial airways, which changes its severity over short periods of time either spontaneously or under treatment, and is not due

*α_1-antitrypsin deficiency is also associated with neonatal hepatitis which progresses to cirrhosis,[19] and with cirrhosis of the liver in adults.[20] In both age-groups the liver cells contain PAS-positive globules which are characteristic.

Figure 45.9
Panlobular emphysema of destructive type. This is a severe grade, and the alveoli are absent as well as the respiratory bronchioles and alveolar ducts. The confluent, large air-spaces are traversed by thin strands which consist of pulmonary vessels, remnants of air-space walls, and connective tissue. Barium-sulphate impregnation, × 11. (*Photograph by courtesy of Dr B. E. Heard.*)

to cardiovascular disease. It is characterised clinically by paroxysms of wheezing dyspnoea, relieved by bronchodilator drugs. The airways obstruction is caused by contraction of the bronchial muscle which is hypertrophied, mucosal oedema, and partly by plugging with thick viscid mucus.

A considerable amount of asthma is *extrinsic* and associated with hypersensitivity reactions to inhaled agents. This usually starts in childhood and is often associated with atopic eczema and hay-fever. It is due to IgE antibodies against inhaled antigens such as pollens, animal danders, and house dust containing mite antigens, particularly of the species *Dermatophagoides*.[24] The reaction is immediate and transient, and eosinophilia is prominent.

Extrinsic asthma should not be confused with *extrinsic allergic alveolitis*, which is an immune-complex reaction mediated by sensitising IgG and is not characterised by asthmatic symptoms (see p. 182).

Asthma with pulmonary infiltrates and eosinophilia and *bronchopulmonary aspergillosis* are described on page 182. Asthmatic attacks are also characteristic of *progressive allergic granulomatosis* (p. 211). An *intrinsic* asthma often complicates chronic bronchitis in later life, but sometimes it arises *de novo*. It may sometimes also have an allergic basis, e.g. to an infecting organism. The pathogenesis of asthma is complicated by strong hereditary and psychological factors.

The disease can terminate fatally in status asthmaticus, and it is interesting that the lungs seldom show emphysema even if the condition has persisted for many years. Indeed, if status asthmaticus can be prevented, the ultimate prognosis is much better than in chronic bronchitis and emphysema.

ASSESSMENT OF RESPIRATORY FUNCTION[5]

Respiratory function may be assessed under the following headings:

Clinical examination in respect of symptoms, e.g. cough, dyspnoea, expectoration, and cyanosis, and physical examination of the chest.

Radiographic appearances of the lungs. The diagnosis of chronic bronchitis and emphysema is notoriously difficult.

Blood-gas analysis is desirable, since respiratory failure is defined in terms of arterial P_{O_2} and P_{CO_2}.

Tests of ventilation, distribution, and gas diffusion.[5] Many of these are highly complicated, and involve knowledge and apparatus which are available only at certain specialised centres. Detailed monographs should be consulted.

Three simple tests will be described here:

Vital capacity. This is the volume of air expelled by a maximum voluntary expiration after a maximum voluntary inspiration (normally 4·5 to 5 litres in a man). The amount of air left is called the *residual volume* (normally 1200 ml.). As maximum inspiration depends on the chest volume, the bony cage, the muscles of respiration, and the compliance of the lungs, and maximum expiration on the patency of the airways,

it is evident that the vital capacity is reduced in nearly all the conditions mentioned in this chapter. Its main use is as a measure of progress in any condition.

Forced expiratory volume and time. Normally about 75 per cent of the vital capacity can be expelled in one second, and the other 25 per cent in another 2 to 3 seconds. In airways obstruction less than 40 per cent is expelled in the first second, and the remainder takes much longer, in fact it may be incompletely removed before the next inspiration is made. A spirometer and kymograph are used to measure the amount of expired air. The forced expiratory volume in one second is reduced in all conditions, obstructive and non-obstructive, which reduce the vital capacity. It is a more sensitive index of the severity of airways obstruction than the vital capacity, but it does not distinguish between the various causes.

The ratio:

$$\frac{\text{forced expiratory volume in one second}}{\text{vital capacity}} \text{ or } \frac{FEV_1}{VC},$$

is a useful measurement of the degree of airways obstruction. Normally it exceeds 70 per cent. In restrictive lung disease the vital capacity is low because of the limited chest expansion. The FEV_1 is much less affected, and therefore the ratio

$$\frac{FEV_1}{VC}$$

is either normal or high.

A useful clinical test on the same lines is the 'match test'. The patient is asked to blow out a lighted match after taking a deep breath. Normally this can be done at a distance of 3 to 4 inches, but with obstructive disease the distance is much less.

Maximum Breathing Capacity. The patient breathes as rapidly and deeply as possible for about 15 seconds. The volume is collected in a bag or recorded with a spirometer, and the result expressed as litres per minute.

Results of all these tests are abnormal in airways obstruction; in ventilatory failure due to restriction, e.g kyphoscoliosis, the match test is relatively normal; the forced expiratory volume in one second is reduced, but it remains normal in proportion to the vital capacity, i.e. over 75 per cent.

CONCLUSIONS

The advances in respiratory physiology over the last 20 years have been most impressive and have revolutionised our understanding of the clinical and functional aspects of lung disease. There has also been a mounting knowledge of the morbid anatomy of common pulmonary disease, such as chronic bronchitis, emphysema, and asthma.[21] The mortality figures for chronic respiratory disease are nevertheless still extremely high. In 1973 over 27 000 people in England and Wales died of this group of diseases, and 1280 of them succumbed to asthma.

GENERAL READING

COMROE, J. H., FORSTER, R. E., DUBOIS, A. B., BRISCOE, W. A. & CARLSEN, E. (1962) *The Lung: Clinical Physiology and Pulmonary Function Tests*, 2nd edn, 390 pp. Chicago: Year Book Medical Publishers, Inc.
SPENCER, H. (1977) *Pathology of the Lung*, 3rd edn, Vols. 1–2, 1099 pp. Oxford: Pergamon Press.

REFERENCES

1. CAMPBELL, E. J. M. (1965) Respiratory failure. *British Medical Journal*, **1**, 1451.
2. ASKIN, F. B. & KUHN, C. (1971) The cellular origin of pulmonary surfactant. *Laboratory Investigation*, **25**, 260.
3. SCARPELLI, E. M. (1968) *The Surfactant System of the Lung*. Philadelphia: Lea and Febiger.
4. MORGAN, T. E. (1971) Pulmonary surfactant. *New England Journal of Medicine*, **284**, 1185.
5. CAMPBELL, E. J. M. & CADE, J. F. (1974) In *Clinical Physiology*, ed. Campbell, E. J. M., Dickinson, C. J. & Slater, J. H. 4th edn, p. 100. Oxford: Blackwell.
6. CAMPBELL, E. J. M. & HOWELL, J. B. L. (1962) In *Ciba Foundation Symposium on Pulmonary Structure and Function*. p. 29, ed. de Reuck, A. V. S. & O'Connor, M. London: Churchill.
7. Medical Research Council Committee on Aetiology of Chronic Bronchitis (1965): Definition and classification of chronic bronchitis for clinical and epidemiological purposes. *Lancet*, **1**, 775.
8. TURNER-WARWICK, M. (1974) A perspective view on widespread pulmonary fibrosis. *British Medical Journal*, **2**, 371.
9. WHITE, R. J. & WOODINGS, D. F. (1971) Impaired water handling in chronic obstructive airways disease. *British Medical Journal*, **2**, 561.
10. HEARD, B. E. (1969) *Pathology of Chronic Bronchitis and Emphysema*, 136 pp. London: Churchill.
11. Report on an Expert Committee on Chronic Cor Pulmonale (1961) *World Health Organisation Technical Report Series*, **213**, 15.
12. LOWE, C. R. (1969) Industrial bronchitis. *British Medical Journal*, **1**, 463.
13. STUART-HARRIS, C. (1972) Chronic bronchitis. *British Journal of Hospital Medicine*, **7**, 719.
14. Leading Article (1976) Natural history of chronic bronchitis. *British Medical Journal*, **1**, 1297.
15. SCADDING, J. G. (1963) Meaning of diagnostic terms in broncho-pulmonary disease. *British Medical Journal*, **2**, 1425.
16. Leading Article (1965) Convulsions during treatment of pulmonary insufficiency. *Lancet*, **1**, 94.
17. Leading Article (1973) Enzymes and emphysema. *British Medical Journal*, **1**, 1.
18. Leading Article (1974) Pathogenesis of emphysema. *British Medical Journal*, **1**, 527.
19. PORTER, C. A. *et al.* (1972) α_1-Antitrypsin deficiency and neonatal hepatitis. *British Medical Journal*, **3**, 435.
20. BERG, N. O. & ERIKSSON, S. (1972) Liver disease in adults with alpha$_1$-antitrypsin deficiency. *New England Journal of Medicine*, **287**, 1264.
21. REID, L. (1967) *The Pathology of Emphysema*. London: Lloyd-Luke.
22. Leading Article (1967) Obstructive airways disease. *British Medical Journal*, **4**, 436.
23. PEPYS, J. (1972) Asthma. *British Journal of Hospital Medicine*, **7**, 709.
24. Leading Article (1971) Mites and house dust allergy. *British Medical Journal*, **2**, 601.

Chapter 46. *Renal Failure*

Renal failure is a state in which the body's metabolism is deranged as a consequence of dysfunction of the kidneys. There are numerous manifestations of metabolic disturbance. Most of these are attributable to a failure of excretion or conservation of various chemical substances by the kidney. The kidney is the most important regulator of the extracellular fluid; it controls the concentration of its various electrolytes, it is essential for acid-base balance, and it is responsible for the excretion of nitrogenous waste products. In addition the kidney may play a part in the maintenance of the blood pressure, and it is concerned in erythropoiesis and vitamin-D metabolism.

From a clinical point of view renal failure is a common and very serious condition, in which the retention of nitrogenous substances like urea and creatinine is the most conspicuous biochemical finding. The condition is called *uraemia* (which originally meant urine in the blood); in fact, few of its clinical manifestations can be directly attributed to urea retention. The failure in acid-base regulation and the disordered handling of electrolytes are of much greater importance. A true conception of renal failure demands a much broader scope than this, since there are many renal lesions which produce metabolic disturbances in which neither nitrogenous retention nor uraemic symptoms are present. Examples of such conditions are the nephrotic syndrome, in which the kidney excretes large amounts of plasma proteins, and certain tubular defects, in which there is a selective loss of amino acids and various electrolytes. In order to comprehend the diverse manifestations of renal failure, it is important first to consider certain aspects of urine formation.

PHYSIOLOGICAL ASPECTS OF URINE FORMATION[1]

The secretion of urine by the kidney entails two distinct processes: (*a*) the passive filtration of plasma through the glomeruli with the formation of a fluid identical with plasma except that it contains only a trace of protein, and (*b*) the passage of this glomerular filtrate through a complex system of tubules in which much of the water and many of its solutes are absorbed back into the blood stream, while some substances are secreted directly into the tubules from the blood. The resulting urine differs very considerably from the glomerular filtrate from which it was derived, not only in the concentration of its solutes but also in its hydrogen-ion concentration.

Glomerular Filtration[2]

The glomerular capillary wall consists of an endothelial cell layer, an epithelial cell layer, and a basement membrane, 50 to 100 nm thick, lying between them. The epithelial cells are called *podocytes*; they are suspended in the fluid of Bowman's capsule and make contact with the basement membrane by innumerable terminal foot processes, or *pedicels*.

The hydrostatic pressure of the blood forces a 'protein-free' filtrate from the plasma through the walls of the glomerular capillaries, which act as if they were ultrafilters perforated by pores 7·5 to 10 nm in diameter. In fact, such pores have never been demonstrated by electron microscopy. The structural basis of the impermeability to colloids may bear a relation to the 'slit pores' lying between the pedicels of the epithelial cells, but the essential factor is the basement membrane which allows small molecules in the aqueous phase to pass through, but restricts larger proteins (see Figs. 46.1 and 46.2).

The rate of glomerular filtration is about 120 ml per minute, and it is intimately influenced by the renal blood flow. The concept of *clearance* is used in assessing the glomerular filtration rate, because it measures the volume of plasma 'cleared' of any substance by the kidney in a given time. It is calculated by the formula (UV)/P, where U and P are the concentrations in mg per dl of the substance in the urine and plasma respectively, and V is the volume of urine excreted in ml per minute. In the human inulin is neither absorbed nor secreted by the tubules, therefore its clearance provides a good estimate of the glomerular filtration rate. In the dog the creatinine and inulin clearances are identical, indicating that both substances are treated similarly by the kidney. However, in the human there is also some tubular secretion of creatinine, so that its clearance value is somewhat higher than that of inulin. The inulin clearance test is technically difficult and time consuming, and the creatinine clearance is often used clinically as a measure of glomerular filtration. The normal range is 90 to 130 ml per minute. In a diseased kidney, however, the creatinine clearance sometimes greatly overestimates the glomerular rate, so that a single normal value does not necessarily indicate normal renal function.[3]

In practice, urea is more often used, because it is more easily measured. In the urea clearance test the patient is often given a dose of 15 g of urea, though this may be simplified (and improved) by omitting the urea, and merely measuring the excretion of endogenous urea. In this case there is no alteration in the plasma urea. The clearance of urea is less than that of inulin, because some of it is reabsorbed by the tubules. If the urine flow is greater than 2 ml per minute, the urea clearance is five-eighths of the normal glomerular filtration rate, i.e. 75 ml per minute (range 60 to 100 ml per minute). This is called the 'maximal urea clearance'. If the urine flow is less than 2 ml per minute, the factor of tubular reabsorption becomes even more important, as more urea is absorbed at a slower rate of flow. An estimation called 'standard urea clearance' is often calculated, using a revised

Figure 46.1
Normal kidney surveyed by electron micro-scopy. This is a survey electron micrograph of a portion of a normal human glomerulus. The capillaries (CAP) are lined by attenuated endothelial cells; the nucleus of one of these is labelled 'END'. Red cells are easily identified (rbc). A mesangial cell (MES) is situated between several capillary loops. The capillaries possess a well-marked basement membrane (bm), and are covered by endothelial cells, or podocytes (POD), of the visceral layer of Bowman's capsule. These cells are attached to the basement membrane of the capillaries by numerous foot processes, or pedicels. × 2000. (*Photograph by courtesy of Dr. Susan Ritchie.*)

Figure 46.2
Electron-micrograph of a glomerular capillary loop of the rat. In the centre there is the capillary lumen, which is bounded by flattened endothelial cells supported on a dense, amorphous basement membrane. On the other side of this basement membrane there are the epithelial cells, or podocytes. They are suspended in the fluid of Bowman's capsule, and make contact with the basement membrane by numerous terminal foot processes, or pedicels. The spaces between the pedicels are called slit pores. × 20 000. (*From Farquhar, M. G., Wissig, S. L. and Palade, G. E.* (1961), Journal of Experimental Medicine, **113**, 47)

formula $(U\sqrt{V})/P$, but the adequacy of this is open to doubt. It is better not to employ the test if the flow is less than 2 ml per minute, but rather to give enough water beforehand to make sure that the urine exceeds 2 ml per minute.

The simplest, though crudest and most imprecise, method of assessing glomerular filtration is by estimating the plasma concentration of urea (normally 2·5 to 6 mmol per litre or 15 to 35 mg per dl; if expressed as blood urea nitrogen (BUN), it is 2·9 to 8·9 mmol per litre or 8 to 25 mg per dl). A more accurate measurement of glomerular filtration is the plasma creatinine, which is 60 to 120 μmol per litre or 0·7 to 1·4 mg per dl. The production is creatinine in the body is almost constant.

These concentrations depend on two factors: the rate of production in the body and the rate of excretion through the glomeruli. A drop in filtration to half the normal rate will lead to a corresponding rise in the plasma levels of these substances, e.g. the plasma urea will rise from 20 to 40 mg per dl, which is just outside the 'normal' range. With greater drops in rate the rise in level becomes much more obvious, e.g. a four-fold drop in rate results in a plasma urea of 80 mg per dl. When filtration drops to 10 to 15 per cent of normal, uraemic manifestations are imminent.

It is important to understand that, though an estimation of the plasma urea is the first step to be taken in assessing renal efficiency, a normal value is compatible with a considerably decreased filtration rate. Even a small rise in the level of the plasma urea is evidence of a serious decrease in glomerular filtration. Furthermore, the concentration of urea is related to the diet. It is low in patients on a low protein diet. On the other hand, it is raised after gastrointestinal haemorrhage. This is in part due to the digestion of free blood in the bowel, but there is also often acute renal failure.

If the plasma urea is normal, other tests may yet reveal renal dysfunction. A high plasma urea, on the other hand, might simply be due to a great production of urea with normal renal function.

Tubular Function

Tubular reabsorption starts in the proximal convoluted tubule where about 80 per cent of the water of the glomerular filtrate is returned to the blood stream. The reabsorption of water is the passive result of active reabsorption of much of the filtered sodium (accompanied by chloride). Thus the reabsorption of electrolytes is such that the luminal fluid is isotonic with the plasma; this is called isosmotic absorption. The glucose, amino acids, and the trace of protein that passed the glomerular filter are completely reabsorbed. On the other hand, most of the filtered urea remains in the lumen, passing on through the proximal tubule, because little escapes by diffusion through the wall back into the blood.

In the ascending limb of the loop of Henle there is a considerable transfer of sodium chloride from the lumen to the interstitial fluid of the medulla. As this part of the loop of Henle is impermeable to water, it follows that the filtrate within it becomes progressively more hypotonic as compared with the plasma, whilst the interstitial fluid becomes hypertonic.

In the distal tubule the pH of the filtrate and its electrolyte composition are finally adjusted, and in the collecting tubule a certain amount of its water and urea is absorbed from the lumen to the medullary interstitial fluid. At this stage the luminal fluid has the full composition of urine.

Water excretion. When the hypotonic filtrate leaves the loop of Henle and enters the distal tubule, it becomes isotonic with plasma once more, as this part of the nephron is fully permeable to water in the presence of ADH. In its course through the collecting tubules the filtrate, being surrounded by the hypertonic interstitial fluid of the medulla, tends to attain osmotic equilibrium by transferring some of its water to the interstitial tissue. In this way the filtrate attains the final hypertonicity characteristic of urine as compared with plasma. The permeability of the distal and collecting tubules is related to the circulating level of ADH, which renders these tubules permeable to the passage of water from the lumen to the interstitial fluid. Large amounts of the hormone therefore produce a highly concentrated urine, whereas its deficiency leads to a hypotonic polyuria. This passive absorption of water

is said to be accompanied by a similar passage of urea to the interstitial fluid of the medulla.

This rather detailed discussion of water excretion is relevant, because one of the most widely employed tests of renal function, the tubular ability to concentrate urine (the *water concentration test*), is based on an application of its mechanism. It is well known that when a patient is deprived of fluid for about 24 hours, or alternatively given ADH in the form of an injection of vasopressin tannate in oil, a highly concentrated urine is passed. The degree of concentration of the urine reflects its osmolality (i.e. its concentration of particles in solution), and can to some extent be correlated with its specific gravity. The specific gravity of the urine is, however, related also to the weight of the dissolved particles. In the absence of abnormal solutes like albumin or glucose, the specific gravity of the urine is determined by its urea concentration. After water deprivation or vasopressin administration it should exceed 1·025 on at least one occasion, and should certainly be higher than 1·020.

The ability to concentrate depends upon three factors:

(*a*) *The secretion of ADH* (see p. 477). This is reduced in diabetes insipidus, which may complicate hypothalamic and pituitary lesions.

(*b*) *The capacity of the tubules to respond to the hormone*, which is defective in congenital nephrogenic diabetes insipidus. A similar defect may occur in acquired renal disorders like those associated with hypercalcaemia and hypokalaemia.

(*c*) *The solute load.* If there is an increased amount of solute to be removed by the kidneys, an increased amount of water is excreted in order to contain it. This is called *osmotic diuresis*,[4] and it occurs even in the presence of ADH. An osmotic diuresis is induced by glycosuria, and this accounts for the polyuria so typical of diabetes mellitus. It is noteworthy that the specific gravity of the urine in this condition is high, because the abnormal solute glucose is a heavy molecule. An osmotic diuresis following the administration of urea will be attended by the production of a urine of much lower specific gravity, because urea has a much lower molecular weight.

If three-quarters of the functioning renal tissue of an animal is removed, the remaining quarter has to cope with the entire endogenous solute load, i.e. the nitrogenous products, which are mostly urea, produced in the course of the body's metabolism. This renal tissue, even if functionally normal, cannot produce a concentrated urine because of the large solute load relative to the amount of renal tissue. The blood urea rises four-fold, because the glomerular filtration rate is reduced to a quarter. An osmotic diuresis in the remaining tubules is essential to remove all the normal waste products of the body: it is the increased urea in the glomerular filtrate that stimulates the diuresis. In due course there is an enlargement of the remaining nephrons due to a proliferation of the cells of the glomeruli and tubules, and the blood urea level drops.

A similar sequence is seen in all morbid conditions in which there is a great destruction of nephrons. Eventually so few survive that renal failure is inevitable. In clinical practice a failure of urine concentration is more often due to extensive renal destruction than to tubular dysfunction.

Another test often used, the *water dilution test*, measures the kidney's ability to produce a dilute urine after the patient has been loaded with water. Three-quarters of such a load should be excreted within 4 hours, and the specific gravity of the urine should fall below 1·004. This test is unpredictable, because the water diuresis is sometimes unaccountably delayed or else precipitously accelerated by nervous factors. There is an inability to secrete a water load properly in both renal failure and Addison's disease.

The cause of this failure in Addison's disease is unknown; it is reversed with cortisol. In renal failure it is possibly related to the destruction of nephrons and a consequent water retention. The inability to produce a urine of very low specific gravity is in part explicable in terms of the poor water diuresis, but the most important factor is the persistent osmotic diuresis. Just as the presence of much urea prevents the formation of a urine of high specific gravity by its diuretic effect, so its continual presence during the water dilution test serves to prevent the production of a very hypotonic urine. It is this osmotic diuretic effect of urea that causes the fixity of the urine's specific gravity in progressive renal disease.

A state of affairs eventually comes about in which the kidneys can produce neither a hypertonic nor a hypotonic urine. Usually the failure of concentration precedes that of dilution. A stage is finally reached in which the kidney produces a urine of fixed specific gravity (about 1·010), a condition called *isosthenuria*. At this stage the osmolality of the urine is similar to that of plasma.

It is also well known that there is a normal diurnal rhythm of urine formation. During the night there is a diminished excretion of water and electrolytes, the pH falls, and the concentration rises. The nature of this phasic pattern of urine formation is ill understood. An abolition of the diurnal rhythm is an early manifestation of renal failure, but it also occurs in many other conditions, especially those associated with the production of generalised oedema, e.g. cardiac failure, cirrhosis of the liver, malnutrition, and the nephrotic syndrome.

Control of acid-base equilibrium. The kidney plays a vital part in the control of the acid-base balance of the body by varying the rate of secretion of hydrogen ions.

Secretion of hydrogen ions occurs throughout the whole tubular system including the collecting ducts, but is greatest in the distal convoluted tubules. As the hydrogen ions enter the lumen, there is a return into the blood of bicarbonate ions (see p. 481). The hydrogen ions in the filtrate also combine with buffer base radicals, particularly phosphate, and with ammonia to form ammonium ions. These are then excreted in the urine. Ammonia formation follows the enzymatic breakdown of glutamine by glutaminase and α-amino acids by α-amino oxidases, all of which are present in the cells of the tubules.

In acidosis, whether metabolic or respiratory, there is an increased excretion of hydrogen ions into the tubular fluid and an increased reabsorption of bicarbonate ions into the plasma. There is a concomitant formation of large amounts of ammonia to combine with the hydrogen ions.

The handling of electrolytes. *Sodium.* About 80 per cent of the sodium contained in the glomerular filtrate is reabsorbed together with chloride and bicarbonate ions in the proximal tubules. A variable amount of the remaining sodium is reabsorbed in the distal and collecting tubules, where the process appears to be a selective one, as compared with the isosmotic absorption of electrolytes that takes place in the

proximal tubule. Chloride ions follow the actively absorbed sodium ions, while hydrogen and potassium ions travel in the opposite direction into the filtrate. The absorption of sodium ions in the distal tubules is influenced by aldosterone (see p. 477).

Potassium. Some of the potassium in the glomerular filtrate is reabsorbed in the proximal tubule, but there is an active secretion from the distal tubule which, as noted above, follows the reabsorption of sodium into the cells of the distal tubule. Aldosterone increases potassium excretion, apparently secondarily to its effect on sodium absorption. Potassium ions compete with hydrogen ions for the available transport systems in the distal tubule; it follows that an alteration in the secretion of one of them affects that of the other also.

Calcium. There is reabsorption of calcium from the proximal tubules, and if an excessive amount is present, from the distal and collecting tubules also. Parathyroid hormone actually increases calcium absorption, but as it also mobilises calcium from the bones, the total effect is one of increased calcium excretion in the urine (*hypercalciuria*). Hypercalcaemia damages the tubular cells (see p. 461).

Phosphate. The excretion of phosphate, like that of urea, is closely related to the glomerular filtration rate. Parathyroid hormone increases phosphate excretion in the urine, probably by depressing its reabsorption in the proximal tubules. Whenever there is nitrogenous retention due to renal disease, there is always an associated rise in the plasma phosphate level. This in turn induces a fall in the plasma calcium level which stimulates parathyroid hormone secretion. Nevertheless, although there may be a considerable hyperplasia of the parathyroid glands, the parathyroid hormone secreted cannot lower the phosphate to a normal level.

SYNDROMES OF RENAL INSUFFICIENCY

The two most characteristic syndromes of renal insufficiency, *acute renal failure* and *chronic renal failure*, are both associated with a retention of nitrogenous waste products in the blood. In both of them clinical uraemia is encountered. Though many of the manifestations of uraemia are still unexplained, it is possible to correlate some of its symptoms with known disturbances in renal function. Both the mechanisms and the manifestations of acute and chronic renal failure are so distinct that it is better to consider them separately, while always remembering that many cases of chronic failure are complicated by acute exacerbations during their course.

ACUTE RENAL FAILURE

In this condition there is a sudden drop in the urinary output of the kidneys to below 400 ml per day. It must be clearly distinguished from urinary retention in the bladder secondary to prostatic enlargement or urethral obstruction.

Causes of Acute Renal Failure

Renal vasoconstriction. A fall in arterial pressure will usually reduce the glomerular filtration rate and renal blood flow (which is normally about 1200 ml per minute). Often, for example after haemorrhage, it will be accompanied by constriction of the renal vessels, which have a sympathetic (vaso-constrictor) innervation and also respond to circulating adrenaline. Nervous or hormonal vasoconstriction may even cause renal ischaemia without any fall in arterial pressure, and if it persists after restoration of normal arterial pressure, ischaemic damage is likely to follow (see acute tubular necrosis, below).

Transient reduction of renal blood flow produces 'extra-renal' uraemia. If it persists long enough to cause cellular damage in the kidney, the acute renal failure that follows may yet be reversible if the damage is reparable. Examples of conditions in which vasoconstriction is thought to be an important cause of acute renal failure are:

(i) *Following a sudden decrease in blood volume* due to haemorrhage, or severe plasma loss as in burns, or a great decrease in extracellular fluid due to prolonged vomiting, diarrhoea, or even profuse diuresis as in diabetic coma. These conditions all fall into the category of 'shock'.

(ii) *Cardiac failure* is attended by a fall in renal blood flow sometimes to less than 500 ml per minute. Renal effects are seldom marked except occasionally in myocardial infarction, where there may be sudden severe vasoconstriction with anuria.

(iii) *The presence of free haemoglobin and myoglobin in the circulation*, especially when they are suddenly released in large quantities, leads to a degree of vasoconstriction. If it is associated with antibodies against red cells, e.g. in incompatible blood transfusions, the effect of haemoglobinaemia is more severe.

The renal failure of the *crush syndrome*, in which there is extensive contusion of the muscles of the leg, is due to free myoglobin in the circulation and also to fluid loss into the damaged muscles causing a decrease in blood volume.

(iv) *Certain complications of pregnancy*, notably eclampsia, abruptio placentae (concealed accidental haemorrhage), and abortion may be accompanied by severe renal vasoconstriction. An extreme example of this is the rare, fatal, bilateral symmetrical cortical necrosis which occasionally complicates abruptio placentae. The renal vasoconstriction may be entirely attributable to sudden, severe blood loss, but some authorities believe that in addition an acute rise in intra-uterine pressure reflexly decreases the renal blood flow.

(v) *Acute renal failure is sometimes seen postoperatively*, and is particularly common in patients who are jaundiced. The explanation is not known, but it is claimed that the administration of mannitol helps to prevent this complication.[5]

Acute bilateral renal artery obstruction. The commonest cause of this is dissecting aneurysm of the aorta.

Acute tubular necrosis.[6] This may be toxic or ischaemic. Nephrotoxic agents include the heavy metals, carbon tetrachloride, and sulphonamides; they lead characteristically to necrosis of the proximal part of the tubules. The damage is widespread, but the basement membrane is not destroyed.

The effects of ischaemia depend on its severity and duration—if transient or mild there are no obvious microscopic changes in the tubules. More severe ischaemia leads to patchy tubular necrosis, affecting particularly the terminal portions of the proximal convoluted tubules and the distal convoluted tubules, and characteristically the basement membrane is disrupted.[7] There is oedema of the interstitial tissue and sometimes an inflammatory infiltrate. The oedema is a useful histological sign of tubular necrosis, because the separation of tubules which it causes helps to distinguish tubular necrosis from *post-mortem* autolysis. Functionally the interstitial oedema probably aggravates the anuria by occluding nephrons. Severe ischaemia leads to massive cortical necrosis, which involves destruction of glomeruli and therefore precludes recovery of renal function.

Acute renal diseases, e.g. polyarteritis nodosa, acute glomerulonephritis, acute interstitial nephritis, and pyelonephritis with papillary necrosis, may occasionally be so fulminating that they lead to complete anuria. The prognosis is extremely grave in such cases. Certain infections, e.g. Weil's disease, yellow fever, and epidemic haemorrhagic fever, are characterised by renal damage which may progress rapidly to cause death from renal failure.

Acute urinary-tract obstruction. This may be due to a stone in the pelvis or ureter, and sometimes a calculus in one ureter causes a reflex 'calculous anuria' on the other side; the cause of this is unknown, but it might be vascular in origin. Sometimes the obstructing agents are intrarenal, e.g. sulphonamide crystals in the tubules or uric-acid obstruction in leukaemia or polycythaemia vera, especially after cytotoxic drugs have been given. It has been suggested that the oliguria of acute renal failure is in part due to tubular blockage by casts composed of Tamm-Horsfall urinary mucoprotein,[8] which is probably derived from the tubular epithelium.[9]

Acute renal failure may be superimposed on chronic renal failure following the uraemic manifestations of profuse vomiting and diarrhoea.

Effects of Acute Renal Failure

The most important type of acute renal failure is that following tubular necrosis. The functional effects are divided into an oliguric phase which corresponds to the period of necrosis, and a diuretic phase (provided the patient survives) in which there is epithelial regeneration.

The oliguric phase is associated with the necrosis already mentioned. Histologically the glomeruli appear normal, and it is possible that the filtrate is entirely reabsorbed through the damaged tubules. The effective glomerular filtration may be zero. A very common finding is the presence of blood-stained casts in the tubules. These are called *pigment casts* and contain haemoglobin; they were originally thought to be peculiar to cases of incompatible blood transfusion, but are in fact encountered in ischaemic tubular necrosis from whatever cause. They are more likely to be the result of the tubular damage than the cause of the oliguria, though, as mentioned above, casts of mucoprotein may aggravate the oliguria by obstructing the tubules.

The functional changes are:

(i) *The passage of small amounts of dark urine* containing protein, blood products, and cell debris. Its specific gravity is about 1·010.

(ii) *The extreme retention of nitrogenous substances* (like urea and creatinine), potassium, magnesium, phosphate, and other anions in the blood. There is also a mounting metabolic acidosis. The main source of these substances is from the endogenous breakdown of muscle protein. The rise in plasma potassium is particularly serious, and is the main indication for dialysis. The plasma calcium is somewhat lowered secondarily to the raised plasma phosphate. These changes are aggravated by the administration of protein to the patient.

(iii) *A possible increase in extracellular water* with a decrease in the plasma concentrations of sodium and chloride. This occurs only if too much water is given.

(iv) *A rapidly developing anaemia.* This may be accentuated by the diluting effect of an increased blood volume secondary to water retention, but there is a severe haemolytic process in uraemia. There is also a neutrophil leucocytosis.

The usual modes of death in this phase are (i) potassium intoxication causing cardiac arrest. Its effect is potentiated by the lowered level of plasma calcium; (ii) overhydration leading either to water intoxication or else to an overexpansion of the extracellular compartment with pulmonary oedema; (iii) concomitant infection, much of which is due to hospital cross-infection; (iv) a gradual clouding of consciousness which terminates in coma. It seems that waste-products of unidentified nature are responsible. There is often a dramatic relief of symptoms following dialysis even if the dialysing fluid has the same urea and electrolyte concentrations as the patient's plasma; (v) haemorrhagic manifestations.

Hypertension is not usual in acute renal failure.

This phase of oliguria may last for many days even if the cause of the tubular necrosis has been successfully remedied. The oliguria is accompanied by persistent renal ischaemia, the explanation of which is unknown. One possibility is vasoconstrictor substances liberated from the damaged tubular cells.

The diuretic phase is the functional counterpart of the epithelial regeneration. This is particularly satisfactory in toxic necrosis, because the basement membrane remains intact and complete recovery can be expected. In ischaemic necrosis there is some destruction of the basement membrane with a tendency to the ingrowth of granulation tissue, so that a complete restoration of all the tubules may be impossible. However, the lesions are usually patchy, and a considerable degree of recovery can be expected. The regenerating cells are flattened and atypical, and lack a brush border; the tubule is merely a channel for the filtrate. Soon, however, the cells differentiate, and normal function is acquired.

The diuretic phase occurs quite dramatically. The urinary output rises rapidly and soon exceeds a litre a day. The urine at first is little more than a protein-free plasma filtrate, since its other constituents are present in concentrations similar to those found in plasma. The regenerating tubules soon start to conserve sodium and to concentrate urea, yet the urine remains isotonic with the plasma for quite a long time. There is a similar delay in the recovery of the acidifying function of the tubule.

It is interesting that, despite dramatic clinical improvement, the plasma urea often shows no fall whatsoever for at least a week after the commencement of the diuresis. This demonstrates the minor role played by urea retention in the production of uraemic symptoms.

The diuresis is principally attributable to the excretion of accumulated fluid and waste products by the newly-functioning nephrons. It is accentuated by the osmotic effect of a high plasma urea and the poor concentrating capacity of the nephrons. The patient's life is now in jeopardy because of dehydration, which is apt to be complicated by acute sodium and potassium loss.

In due course renal function tends to be restored to a satisfactory extent, but perfect recovery is unusual.

CHRONIC RENAL FAILURE

The causes of chronic renal failure are extremely numerous:

Chronic destructive renal disease. This is the most important group, and it includes such conditions as chronic pyelonephritis (which is the commonest cause of chronic renal failure), chronic glomerulonephritis, systemic lupus erythematosus, polyarteritis nodosa, progressive systemic sclerosis, bilateral renal tuberculosis, and radiation nephritis.

Chronic renal vascular disease. Malignant hypertension, renal-vein thrombosis, and bilateral occlusion of the renal arteries with infarction of the kidneys are all associated with progressive renal failure. Non-malignant ('benign') hypertension causes only minor impairment of renal function; death is due either to heart failure or to cerebral haemorrhage.

Obstruction to the outflow of urine. This is manifested by bilateral hydronephrosis, and occurs secondarily to urethral obstruction following a stricture, prostatic enlargement, or carcinoma of the cervix (often complicated by radiation fibrosis), which may also occlude both ureters.

Congenital lesions like polycystic disease and certain tubular defects may eventually lead to severe renal failure.

Metabolic conditions, e.g. hypercalcaemia, multiple myeloma, hypokalaemia, amyloidosis, gout, and diabetic nephropathy, may all lead to serious renal dysfunction, especially if they are of long duration.

Effects of Chronic Renal Failure[10,11]

The metabolic disturbances that may occur in chronic renal failure are diverse and very complex. They result from a primary inadequacy of the kidney to regulate the internal environment of the body. It is not surprising that there may be rapid fluctuations from dangerous excesses to severe depletions of water and various electrolytes consequent on dietary indiscretions or gastrointestinal disturbances, which may be either primary, or else secondary to the renal condition itself.

Disturbances in water metabolism. The inability of the failing kidney to concentrate urine adequately or to cope with an increased load of water has already been discussed. Nocturia and moderate polyuria are early symptoms of renal failure. The polyuria is due to the effect of osmotic diuresis, and it is not severe because of the decreased number of functioning renal elements. It is especially marked in chronic pyelonephritis, as the concentrating part of the medulla is affected early. There is usually a mild degree of dehydration which is manifested by thirst. As soon as the patient ceases to maintain an adequate fluid intake, or if there is persistent 'uraemic' diarrhoea and vomiting, dehydration becomes severe. This in its turn by decreasing the blood volume causes renal vasoconstriction and leads to acute renal failure.

On the other hand, injudicious administration of fluids, especially those given intravenously, may precipitate the very serious syndrome of water intoxication (see p. 478).

Disturbances in sodium balance. An adequate excretion of sodium is compatible with even a severely decreased glomerular filtration rate, and sodium retention is not a feature of chronic renal failure. On the other hand, there is a persistent tendency towards sodium depletion, due primarily to the inevitable loss of sodium that attends the osmotic diuresis already mentioned. There is a compensatory secretion of aldosterone in order to retain sodium, but eventually the distal tubules may become less responsive to this hormone. There is a rare condition of *salt-losing nephritis*, almost always a late result of chronic pyelonephritis, in which the tubules are completely unresponsive to aldosterone. The clinical picture is very similar to Addison's disease, but in salt-losing nephritis there is a functional hyperplasia of the adrenals with an increased aldosterone production, whereas in Addison's disease there is adrenal destruction or atrophy with a diminished production of aldosterone. Obviously any gastrointestinal upset leads to further sodium depletion.

Disturbances in potassium balance. The loss of potassium is not altogether dependent on the glomerular filtration rate, because some that passes into the filtrate is reabsorbed by the proximal tubules. The excretion of potassium by the distal tubules is an active process, and is accompanied by an active reabsorption of sodium ions into the cells. In chronic renal failure there is commonly a mild retention of potassium which may become severe terminally.

Potassium depletion is very unusual in chronic renal failure. A primary *potassium-losing nephritis* is almost invariably associated with a failure of the tubules to acidify the urine due to their inability to secrete hydrogen ions. As a consequence the tubules secrete more potassium ions in place of hydrogen ions, in order to counterbalance the opposing movement of sodium ions into the tubular cells. The loss of potassium during the diuretic phase of acute tubular necrosis is explained by the inability of the newly-regenerated cells to acidify the urine in this way.

Any tendency to potassium retention is aggravated by the administration of potassium citrate, whereas diarrhoea and vomiting lead to potassium depletion.

Disturbances in acid-base balance. Progressive renal failure is attended by a metabolic acidosis due to a relative failure of acidification of the urine. There is predominantly an impairment in ammonia production; the ability to secrete hydrogen ions is less severely impaired. Dietary or therapeutic indiscretions, like the administration of ammonium chloride, aggravate the acidosis, as also does diarrhoea with its inevitable excessive excretion of bicarbonate ions.

Alkalosis is very rare in uncomplicated renal failure. Potassium depletion leads to alkalosis, because there is an intracellular deviation of hydrogen ions to replace the lost potassium ions. It therefore comes about that renal failure secondary to potassium depletion in Conn's syndrome is accompanied by an alkalosis (see p. 480).

Disturbances in calcium and phosphate metabolism. In chronic renal disease where there is a persistent retention of phosphate, the plasma phosphate is raised and the plasma calcium often reduced. A raised plasma phosphate itself induces a fall in plasma calcium, the reason for which is not clear. But, in addition, the metabolism of vitamin D is impaired in chronic renal failure. As explained in greater detail on page 458, before the vitamin D in the diet, or that formed in the skin, can exert its effect, it has to undergo two metabolic steps, the first in the liver and gut, and the second in the kidney, where 1,25 dihydroxycholecalciferol, or 1,25 $(OH)_2D_3$, is formed. This is the most potent humoral agent regulating calcium metabolism.[12] Very low levels are found in the plasma of patients with chronic renal failure. The result is defective absorption of calcium from the gut, an effect relatively resistant to the administration of vitamin D, since this too cannot be properly metabolised by the kidneys. The patient shows the lesions of osteomalacia, to which rickets will be added if the epiphyses have not yet fused (renal rickets).

Chronic renal disease is often associated with secondary hyperparathyroidism, which may be so severe as to lead to osteitis fibrosa cystica. The most reasonable explanation is the lowered plasma calcium stimulating the parathyroids directly; the increased amount of parathyroid hormone secreted acts to mobilise calcium from the bones to restore the level of plasma calcium. Indeed, in those cases of renal bone disease in which osteitis fibrosa cystica predominates, the plasma calcium is usually normal. But this sequence is not necessarily always the case, since in the evolution of renal osteodystrophy the lesions of osteitis fibrosa cystica usually appear early, whereas those of osteomalacia (and rickets) develop later as the disease progresses.[13]

Indeed, *renal osteodystrophy* is a complex condition, because there may also be osteosclerosis associated with the lesions of osteomalacia and osteitis fibrosa cystica. This formation of dense bone, like the widespread metastatic calcification that may sometimes occur, is probably due to the very high level of plasma phosphate.

The bone lesions cannot be directly correlated with the plasma levels of calcium and phosphate. They are commoner in children than in adults. Widespread metastatic calcification is usually a terminal manifestation.

The parathyroid hyperplasia is not always relieved by successful renal transplantation. Symptoms of hyperparathyroidism may persist, necessitating a parathyroidectomy, when adenomatous change may be found. This 'tertiary hyperparathyroidism' indicates an autonomous change in the hyperplastic parathyroids, and demonstrates how a hyperplasia can develop neoplastic potentialities. Sometimes there is only a generalised hyperplasia similar to that found in some cases of primary hyperparathyroidism.[14]

It is noteworthy that patients on dialysis may have an osteodystrophy rather similar to that associated with renal failure.[15] Osteomalacia, however, predominates. The mechanism is not certain, but two possible factors are the inadequate formation of 1,25 dihydroxycholecalciferol by the damaged kidneys and phosphate deficiency. This might be due to a poor dietary intake of phosphate as part of the therapy, intestinal malabsorption, and loss by dialysis.

Disturbance of carbohydrate metabolism. Impaired glucose tolerance is common and may lead to diagnostic confusion with diabetes mellitus. It rarely causes clinical symptoms and its pathogenesis is not understood.

Retention of waste products. These include urea, uric acid, creatinine, phenol derivatives, various ill-defined anions ('the anuric anions'), and urochromogen.

Hypertension.[16,17] Many chronic renal diseases are complicated by hypertension which may progress to a malignant phase, i.e. one in which there is frank necrosis of arterioles. Examples of such diseases are chronic pyelonephritis, chronic glomerulonephritis, polyarteritis nodosa, polycystic disease, and diabetic nephropathy. Stenosis of the renal arteries is particularly liable to be complicated by severe, rapidly progressive hypertension. Furthermore, unilateral renal disease, e.g. hydronephrosis or the stenosis of one renal artery, also tends to produce hypertension, which may be reversed if the kidney (or the arterial obstruction) is removed in time. Renal compression by a haematoma is another cause of reversible hypertension.

When the renal artery of a dog is partially occluded, hypertension develops, and will persist if the other kidney is removed; in some other animals the mere constriction of one renal artery leads to permanent hypertension. The kidney liberates a proteolytic enzyme called *renin*. This acts on an α_2-globulin called *angiotensinogen*, which is present in the plasma and acts as a substrate. The product *angiotensin I* is a decapeptide with feeble pressor activity, but it is converted into *angiotensin II*, a powerfully pressor octapeptide, by another plasma enzyme. Angiotensin is degraded by *angiotensinase*, which is present in many tissues, including the kidney. There is histochemical evidence that renin is formed in the juxta-glomerular complex, possibly in the cells of the afferent arterioles. The two important stimuli leading to the release of renin are a reduction in afferent arteriolar pressure and sodium depletion.

Angiotensin in the human is not only a powerful vasoconstrictor but it also stimulates aldosterone secretion from the adrenal. This leads to sodium retention by the tubules, an effect potentiated by angiotensin which has a direct action on the tubules as well. It is noteworthy that the hypertension of Conn's syndrome is relieved by spironolactone, thus proving that the changes in sodium metabolism brought about by aldosterone can be important in causing hypertension.

There is mounting evidence that the hypersecretion of renin is important in the genesis of hypertension produced by renal ischaemia. This evidence is based largely on the use of compounds which block the renin system, either by interfering with the formation of angiotensin II or by inhibiting its action. Compounds with an inhibitory action are antibody to angiotensin II and competitive peptide inhibitors of the sarcosyl[1]–ala[8] type. The infusion of these substances into rats made hypertensive by unilateral renal ischaemia lowers the blood pressure as long as the opposite kidney is not removed. Where the blood pressure is not reduced to normal by these compounds, as in long standing hypertension, nephrectomy also fails, suggesting that extrarenal factors have taken over the role of blood-pressure elevation. Fewer investigations have been performed upon human beings, but the data available are comparable with those in rats. In all these situations the renin level is highest where there is sodium deprivation.

The purest form of high-renin state is that associated with a small renal cortical tumour, usually a haemangiopericytoma, rich in renin, and the resulting hypertension is associated with a high plasma renin and aldosterone level and a low level of plasma potassium. Once the tumour, or the kidney, is removed these effects are all reversed.

There is another condition in which hyperplasia of the juxta-glomerular apparatus is associated with hypokalaemic alkalosis, and raised plasma levels of renin, angiotensin II, and aldosterone, and yet the blood pressure is normal or even low.

It is called *Bartter's syndrome*,[18] and the resistance to angiotensin II is extremely high—even saline loading to expand the extracellular space does not raise the blood pressure. In this syndrome there seems to be an intrarenal defect in sodium metabolism. There is also an abnormally high plasma level of prostaglandin A, which is a vasodepressor agent that inhibits the action of angiotensin II. Indomethacin, which lowers plasma prostaglandin A to normal, also lowers the plasma renin and aldosterone, raises the plasma potassium, and partly restores the blood-pressure response to infused angiotensin II. The full nature of this fascinating condition is still obscure, but it demonstrates the complexity of factors involved in renal hypertension.

Bilaterally nephrectomised patients do not develop hypertension provided the sodium and water balance is kept perfect by dialysis, but they are extremely susceptible to alterations in this balance, and hypertension can easily develop. This susceptibility to hypertension may be due to the absence of a normal renal mechanism for inactivating some extrarenal pressor agent; certainly the tendency to hypertension is remedied as soon as a fresh kidney is transplanted.

There is no evidence that essential hypertension has a renal basis, but plasma renin levels may be raised when it has produced serious renal damage, as, for instance, in the malignant phase. On other occasions it is lowered.

Haematological effects. A severe normocytic, normochromic *anaemia* is common in the later stages of renal failure.[19] It may be related to an impaired production of erythropoietin, which is normally formed in the kidney (see p. 605).

Another frequent feature of renal failure is *purpura*, which is probably due to a qualitative deficiency in the platelets (see p. 640).

URAEMIA[11]

Uraemia is a clinical syndrome which is associated with a retention of nitrogenous waste products in the blood. Its manifestations are protean, and most of them cannot be explained in terms of recognisable renal dysfunction. It is instructive to consider those features which may be related to known biochemical abnormalities:

Symptoms related to disturbances of sodium and water metabolism. There may be dehydration or water intoxication. These are discussed in detail in Chapter 38. Water intoxication (cellular overhydration) may be responsible for the nausea, vomiting, headache, convulsions, and stupor seen in terminal uraemia especially in acute renal failure. If the extracellular compartment is overexpanded, symptoms of pulmonary oedema may develop.

Symptoms related to disturbances of potassium metabolism. In acute renal failure there may be hypotension and paraesthesiae due to hyperkalaemia, and death from cardiac arrest and ventricular fibrillation may ensue.

Symptoms related to disturbances in acid-base balance. The deep, sighing respiration so typical of uraemia can be attributed to metabolic acidosis. It may also account for the clouding of consciousness, coma, and the cardiovascular complications which may cause sudden death.

Disturbances in calcium metabolism. The hypocalcaemia is seldom severe enough to cause tetany especially while there is an acidosis, which maintains the ionised fraction of the plasma calcium near normal levels. If the acidosis is suddenly corrected, attacks of tetany may ensue. Likewise any tendency towards alkalosis leads to severe tetany by diminishing the plasma level of the ionised fraction of calcium. It is possible that the irregular muscle twitchings seen in uraemic coma may be indirectly related to a lowered level of plasma calcium, since intravenous calcium salts often abolish them.

The retention of waste products. It has been suggested that the raised plasma urea plays a part in producing the severe gastritis and colitis sometimes seen in uraemia. The urea diffuses into the gastric and colonic secretions where it is converted into ammonia by the resident organisms of the bowel, and also by the enzyme urease which is present in the gastric mucosa. The ammonia so produced is absorbed and used in the synthesis of amino acids in the liver.[20] An excess might irritate the mucosa, and lead to persistent vomiting and diarrhoea. Rarely the urea excretion in the sweat may be so great that it crystallises out as 'urea frost'. The excretion of urea in the saliva and its breakdown into ammonia gives rise to an unpleasant taste in the mouth and an ammoniacal odour in the breath.

Some of the other retained waste products, e.g. the phenol derivatives and the 'anuric anions', are possibly responsible for the deepening coma of uraemia, but there is no certain evidence of this.

A retention of the normal pigment of the urine, urochromogen, may explain the pale colour of the urine, and this has even been postulated as the cause of the earthy pigmentation of the skin so characteristic of chronic renal disease.

There are many features of uraemia which elude explanation. These include hiccup, pruritus, and a terminal sterile fibrinous pericarditis which is often clinically silent. It is possible that these manifestations are due to toxic waste products circulating in the blood stream and damaging nerve endings and endothelial surfaces, but at present no such substances have been isolated. Of the various substances implicated, certain derivatives of the guanidines appear to be most liable to reproduce some of the symptoms of uraemia, e.g. nerve damage, convulsions, red-cell destruction, and gastric ulceration. The pruritus is usually relieved by dialysis, but sometimes even this is ineffective. In such cases relief has sometimes followed parathyroidectomy, suggesting that the secondary hyperparathyroidism of renal disease may be a factor.[21]

The associated hypertension may lead to heart failure. An interesting condition occasionally seen in uraemic, hypertensive patients is *uraemic lung*. There are dense radiological opacities extending from the hila of the lungs out to the midzones. Although the condition is usually seen in association with left ventricular failure, the diagnosis is made on radiological, not clinical, grounds. Histologically there is much fibrinous exudate (unassociated with infection) as well as oedema fluid in the affected alveoli. It has been suggested that there is a failure of the normal fibrinolytic mechanism in uraemic lungs.[22]

Acute exacerbations of hypertension may be yet another factor in the causation of the cerebral manifestations of uraemia. The so-called hypertensive encephalopathy may lead to epileptiform convulsions. The retinal changes typical of renal disease are all due to the associated hypertension.

Many patients with chronic renal disease ultimately succumbing to uraemia remain normotensive throughout the course of their illness. Indeed, the presence of mounting hypertension is of particularly bad omen.

THE PROTEIN-LOSING KIDNEY

Normally only a trace of protein passes through the glomerular filter, and all this should be reabsorbed by the proximal tubule. The urine contains less than 150 mg in a 24-hour specimen, and this small amount is not detected by the routine clinical tests. In nearly all renal disease of clinical significance there is some degree of proteinuria due to an increased permeability of the glomerular filter and perhaps accentuated by tubular dysfunction. The degree of proteinuria is no indication of the severity of the disease, because in progressive renal failure the glomerular filtration rate may fall so much that with the onset of uraemia the urine may contain only a trace of protein.

There is, however, a syndrome in which massive proteinuria is the main feature. This is the *nephrotic syndrome*. It sometimes arises idiopathically, and several types are described.

In *idiopathic membranous glomerulonephritis* the glomeruli show, on light microscopy, a thickening of the basement membrane—a change described as 'membranous'. Electron microscopy reveals that this membranous change is due to the deposition of material on one or other side of the lamina densa of the true basement membrane (p. 66). In the adult type of idiopathic membranous glomerulonephritis the deposits are on the epithelial side of the basement membrane, while in the childhood type they are on the endothelial side. In addition there are striking changes in the foot processes of the podocytes, described as 'fusion of the foot processes', because the basement membrane is covered by a continuous layer of epithelial-cell cytoplasm. Some authorities maintain that this appearance is not due to actual fusion of the processes but rather to the retraction of some of them and the spreading-out of the others.[23]

In *minimal change glomerulonephritis (lipoid nephrosis)* which generally occurs in childhood, the glomeruli appear normal on light microscopy. Electron microscopy reveals some thickening of the basement membrane and fusion of the foot processes as described above (Fig. 46.3). The latter change is in fact a concomitant of marked proteinuria irrespective of cause, and is probably the effect of protein leakage; the fundamental cause of proteinuria is a defect in the basement membrane.

The nephrotic syndrome may also appear during the course of other renal disease, e.g. chronic glomerulonephritis particularly of the lobular type (p. 202), systemic lupus erythematosus, diabetic glomerulosclerosis, amyloidosis, and as an occasional complication of benign quartan (*P. malariae*) malaria and a rare one of secondary syphilis; in these last two conditions it appears to be related to the deposition of immune complexes in the glomeruli.[24,25] It is a common feature of renal-vein thrombosis, which occasionally complicates renal tumours and amyloidosis.

Finally, it can also be produced by drugs, e.g. troxidone and mercury. Mercurial preparations used as teething powders or diuretics are dangerous, and the nephrotic syndrome has also been reported as an occupational hazard in those using mercury.[26]

Figure 46.3
Electron micrograph of glomerulus in systemic lupus erythematosus. The capillaries (CAP) are lined by attenuated endothelial cells; the nucleus of one of these is labelled 'END'. In some areas the foot processes (FP₁) of the prodocytes appear relatively normal, but elsewhere they are swollen and spread over the basement membrane (bm) of the capillary (FP₂). This change is commonly described as 'fusion of the foot processes'. Prominent subendothelial deposits are present (DEP₁). Subepithelial deposits are smaller and less obvious (DEP₂). In this patient the deposits were shown by immunofluorescence to contain IgG and components of complement. × 14 000. (*Photograph by courtesy of Dr. Y. Bedard.*)

Effects of the Protein-Losing Kidney

Gross proteinuria. The loss is usually 10 to 15 g a day, but it may be much greater than this. Albumin, the smallest of the protein molecules, is lost in greatest bulk, but the globulins are also excreted; α_2-globulin is retained because of its greater molecular size. The cells of the proximal tubules often contain large 'hyaline droplets' composed of protein material absorbed from the glomerular filtrate (see p. 53 and Fig. 48.4, p. 574).

Hypoproteinaemia. There is a large fall in the total protein content of the plasma, and the albumin level commonly drops below 10 g per litre. There is a fall in the globulin fractions also, except for α_2-globulin, the level of which rises considerably.

Oedema (see Ch. 43). The lowered plasma protein level causing a decrease in the plasma osmotic pressure is largely responsible for the anasarca so typical of nephrosis, and the fluid retention is aggravated by an increased secretion of aldosterone.

Increased plasma lipids. This is constantly present, and the plasma cholesterol may sometimes exceed 26 mmol per litre (1000 mg per dl). The cause of this hyperlipoproteinaemia, which is also sometimes present in other cases of chronic renal disease, is unknown.[27]

Increased susceptibility to infection. Death from pneumonia, peritonitis, and other pyogenic infections is very common, and is probably related to the low level of immunoglobulin in the plasma, which results from its loss in the urine.

Renal function is usually very good, and often the glo-

merular filtration rate is raised in the early stages. The plasma urea may be abnormally low, due to the combined effects of a raised filtration rate and a negative nitrogen balance. Sometimes there is a degree of potassium depletion as a result of endogenous aldosterone secretion, exogenous cortisone administration, and the use of diuretics.

In due course nitrogen retention usually supervenes. The glomerular filtration rate falls, and the protein content of the urine may drop quite considerably. Death from uraemia is the usual outcome, though in the idiopathic group spontaneous remissions and even permanent cure may sometimes occur.

The blood pressure is normal, but it may rise as renal function fails. In amyloid disease a normal blood pressure usually persists to the end.

DEFECTS OF TUBULAR FUNCTION

There is an uncommon, though very interesting, group of renal conditions in which the defect is primarily one of tubular dysfunction. This may be either an inability to reabsorb certain constituents of the glomerular filtrate, or more rarely, an excessive reabsorption of such constituents. Most of these conditions are congenital, but occasionally they may be acquired in later life.

Impaired water reabsorption—nephrogenic diabetes insipidus. It is an example of a disease often inherited as a sex-linked recessive characteristic.* It manifests itself in infancy with symptoms of pyrexia, dehydration, vomiting, and collapse. There is severe polyuria, as the kidney does not respond to antidiuretic hormone.

Impaired glucose reabsorption—renal glycosuria.

Impaired phosphate reabsorption—familial hypophosphataemia, or vitamin-D resistant rickets. This condition is interesting in being inherited as a sex-linked dominant characteristic. There is an increased renal excretion of phosphate and also an impaired absorption of calcium from the bowel. The plasma calcium is usually normal, but the plasma phosphate is very low. This is a disease of childhood; between the ages of 2 and 5 years growth is retarded and the signs of rickets appear. The severity of the disease, and the age at which it commences, varies greatly among families and within a single family. The pathogenesis of the bony lesions is not understood, since there appears to be no lack of vitamin D or any detectable defect in its metabolism.

An adult type of hypophosphataemia is also described: it affects both sexes equally, and there is also muscle weakness which is not found in the familial type of hypophosphataemia.[29]

Impaired reabsorption of amino acids, glucose, and phosphate. This is usually called the *Fanconi syndrome*. When congenital, it appears to be inherited as an autosomal recessive characteristic. Such cases have widespread deposits of cystine crystals in their tissues, hence the alternative names 'cystinosis' and 'cystine-storage disease' that are sometimes

---

*It is of interest that the 'water drinker's curse' which affects certain families in the Maritime provinces of Canada and in New England was known in the folklore to affect males but be passed on by the females for more than a hundred years before Mendel proposed his laws of heredity.[28]

used. The amino-aciduria is more extensive in variety, but much less copious than in cystinuria, and only small amounts of cystine are present in the urine. The condition is frequently attended by other renal defects as well: (*a*) proteinuria; (*b*) an inability to secrete hydrogen ions, so that the urine is imperfectly acidified. This in turn is accompanied by excessive potassium excretion and symptoms of hypokalaemia; (*c*) impaired glomerular filtration leading to renal failure, which is the usual cause of death.

As with familial hypophosphataemia, lesions of rickets or osteomalacia appear, and their pathogenesis is likewise obscure.

Impaired amino-acid reabsorption[30]**—cystinuria.** There are small amounts of certain amino acids like glycine, taurine, and alanine normally present in the urine, but in some conditions there are much larger amounts of other amino acids in addition. In cystinuria there is much cystine in the urine, while small amounts of arginine, lysine, and ornithine are also present. The danger is the formation of cystine calculi, which are very insoluble in acid solution. The condition is inherited as an autosomal recessive trait. About a third of heterozygotes excrete small quantities of cystine and lysine in their urine (the excretion of arginine and ornithine is usually normal), while the other two-thirds have a normal urinary amino-acid excretion.[31]

Impaired xanthine reabsorption—xanthinuria.[32] There is a defect in the conversion of xanthine to uric acid due to the absence of xanthine oxidase in the tissues—especially the liver and the mucosa of the small bowel. The plasma uric acid is therefore very low. The xanthine is excreted by the kidney, and xanthine stones may be formed. The condition is inherited as an autosomal recessive trait.

Some patients, usually adults, form xanthine stones, and have a normal or even a raised plasma uric acid. In them there is clearly no defect in xanthine oxidase activity, and it must be assumed that there is an increased urinary excretion of xanthine.

Inability to secrete hydrogen ions—renal tubular acidosis. In this condition the distal tubules cannot transfer hydrogen ions to the filtrate. Whereas the normal kidney can acidify the urine to a pH of 4·4, in renal tubular acidosis the pH remains at a higher level (over 6) despite a severe metabolic acidosis. The plasma bicarbonate concentration is low, while the plasma chloride is raised. Hyperchloraemic acidosis is produced. As in the Fanconi syndrome there is an associated hypokalaemia.

In addition, calcium is lost in the urine; this has been ascribed to the chronic acidosis bringing calcium and phosphate out of the bones. The loss is increased as the result of inadequate tubular reabsorption. Nephrocalcinosis and stone formation frequently ensue; perhaps the relative alkalinity of the urine facilitates the precipitation of the calcium and phosphate. Osteomalacia and calcium deficiency are common findings.

There is no abnormality in the absorption of amino acids, glucose, or phosphate as seen in the Fanconi syndrome. The disease is most common in early childhood, but an adult type is also described. Its aetiology is uncertain; it is familial in some cases.

Excessive reabsorption of phosphate—pseudohypoparathyroidism. In this very rare condition the renal tubules are congenitally unresponsive to parathyroid hormone. The plasma phosphate is raised and the plasma calcium is low. The patient suffers from severe tetany which does not respond to parathyroid hormone. Other features of this condition are a flat, round face, stumpy hands, and mental retardation (see also p. 305).

The above conditions are all congenital, but similar defects of tubular reabsorption may occur during the course of other diseases. Galactosaemia and Wilson's disease, for example, damage the tubules and lead to amino-aciduria, while chronic pyelonephritis may be associated with defective hydrogen-ion production by the distal tubule.[30] An acquired Fanconi syndrome may follow the toxic action on the tubules of heavy metals like mercury and lead, and may complicate the copper intoxication of Wilson's disease. The acquired syndrome is not accompanied by cystinosis.

These tubular defects are of the greatest theoretical interest, because they throw fresh light on the more obscure aspects of renal function.

GENERAL READING

BLACK, D. A. K. (1972) *Renal Disease*, 3rd edn, 871 pp. Oxford: Blackwell.
DE WARDENER, H. E. (1973) *The Kidney*, 4th edn, 432 pp. London: Churchill.
PITTS, R. F. (1968) *Physiology of the Kidney and Body Fluids*, 2nd edn, 266 pp. Chicago: Year Book Medical Publishers.

REFERENCES

1. BRITTON, K. E. (1974) In *Clinical Physiology*, ed. Campbell, E. J. M., Dickinson, C. J. & Slater, J. D. H., 4th edn, p. 166. Oxford: Blackwell.
2. RENKIN, E. M. & ROBINSON, R. R. (1974) Glomerular filtration. *New England Journal of Medicine*, **290**, 785.
3. KIM, K. E. *et al.* (1969) Creatinine clearance in renal disease. A reappraisal. *British Medical Journal*, **4**, 11.
4. GENNARI, F. J. & KASSIRER, J. P. (1974) Osmotic diuresis. *New England Journal of Medicine*, **291**, 714.
5. Leading Article (1968) Mannitol and renal function. *Lancet*, **1**, 1183.
6. DUNNILL, M. S. (1974) A review of the pathology and pathogenesis of acute renal failure due to acute tubular necrosis. *Journal of Clinical Pathology*, **27**, 2.
7. OLIVER, J., MACDOWELL, M. & TRACY, A. (1951) The pathogenesis of acute renal failure associated with traumatic and toxic injury, renal ischemia, nephrotoxic damage and the ischemuric episode. *Journal of Clinical Investigation*, **30**, 1305.
8. PATEL, R., MCKENZIE, J. K. & MCQUEEN, E. G. (1964) Tamm-Horsfall urinary mucoprotein and tubular obstruction by casts in acute renal failure. *Lancet*, **1**, 457.
9. GRANT, G. H. (1959) The proteins of normal urine. *Journal of Clinical Pathology*, **12**, 510.
10. MERRILL, J. P. & HAMPERS, C. L. (1970) Uremia. *New England Journal of Medicine*, **282**, 953 and 1014.

11. MERRILL, J. P. & HAMPERS, C. L. (1971) Uremia. 115 pp. New York: Grune and Stratton. This book represents an enlargement and updating of the previous reference.

12. Leading Article (1977) Vitamin D and the pituitary. *Lancet*, **1**, 840.

13. ELLIS, H. A. & PEART, K. M. (1973) Azotaemic osteodystrophy: a quantitative study on iliac bone. *Journal of Clinical Pathology*, **26**, 83.

14. ANDERSON, T. J. & BOYLE, I. T. (1971) Autonomous nodular hyperplasia of the parathyroid glands. *Journal of Pathology*, **105**, 211.

15. Leading Article (1976) Dialysis osteodystrophy. *Lancet*, **2**, 451.

16. PEART, W. S. (1975) Renin-angiotensin system. *New England Journal of Medicine*, **292**, 302.

17. Leading Article (1975) When to measure renin. *Lancet*, **1**, 783.

18. Leading Article (1976) Bartter's syndrome. *Lancet*, **2**, 721.

19. Leading Article (1975) Anaemia in chronic renal failure. *Lancet*, **1**, 959.

20. Leading Article (1971) Urea metabolism in man. *Lancet*, **2**, 1407.

21. HAMPERS, C. L. *et al.* (1968) Disappearance of 'uremic' itching after subtotal parathyroidectomy. *New England Journal of Medicine*, **279**, 695.

22. MacLEOD, M., STALKER, A. L. & OGSTON, D. (1962) Fibrinolytic activity of lung tissue in renal failure. *Lancet*, **1**, 191.

23. SIMON, G. T. & CHATELANAT, F. (1969) In *The Kidney*, ed. Rouiller, C. & Muller, A. F., Vol. 1, p. 261. New York: Academic Press.

24. Memorandum on Immunology of Nephritis in Africa (1972) *Bulletin of the World Health Organization*, **46**, 387.

25. BRAUNSTEIN, G. D. *et al.* (1970) The nephrotic syndrome associated with secondary syphilis. *American Journal of Medicine*, **48**, 643.

26. KAZANTZIS, G. *et al.* (1962) Albuminuria and the nephrotic syndrome following exposure to mercury and its compounds. *Quarterly Journal of Medicine*, **31**, 403.

27. CRAMP, D. G., MOORHEAD, J. F. & WILLS, M. R. (1975) Disorders of blood-lipids in renal disease. *Lancet*, **1**, 672.

28. BODE, H. H. & CRAWFORD, J. D. (1969) Nephrogenic diabetes insipidus in North America—the Hopewell hypothesis. *New England Journal of Medicine*, **280**, 750.

29. Leading Article (1971) Hypophosphataemic osteomalacia in adults. *Lancet*, **1**, 1343.

30. MILNE, M. D. (1964) Disorders of amino-acid transport. *British Medical Journal*, **1**, 327.

31. WOOLF, L. I. (1961) Aminoaciduria. *British Medical Bulletin*, **17**, 224.

32. WYNGAARDEN, J. B. (1972) In *The Metabolic Basis of Inherited Disease*, ed. Stanbury, J. B., Wyngaarden, J. B. & Fredrickson, D. S., 3rd edn, p. 992. New York: McGraw-Hill.

Chapter 47. Hepatic Failure and Jaundice

Hepatic failure is a condition in which there is a disturbance of the body's metabolism due to a derangement in the function of the liver. The functions of the liver are manifold: amongst those that immediately come to mind are bile excretion, protein, carbohydrate, and fat metabolism, vitamin storage, and detoxification. In its widest application the concept of hepatic failure includes conditions in which any of these functions is impaired.

In its clinical connotation, however, liver failure is a very serious condition indeed. It is the result of severe structural damage to the liver, and is attended by such characteristic manifestations as jaundice, ascites, bleeding tendencies, and neuro-psychiatric disturbances. The syndrome is called *cholaemia*, and it is often fatal. Much of the ensuing account will be devoted to an analysis of the principal manifestations of cholaemia, and an attempt will be made to assess which of them is attributable directly to hepatocellular failure, and which to extraneous factors like biliary obstruction and portal venous hypertension.

CAUSES OF LIVER FAILURE

The functional reserve capacity of the liver is remarkable. It is a commonly observed clinical finding that, though the liver may be extensively infiltrated with metastatic cancer, there is seldom any obvious failure of its function. Likewise, large amoebic abscesses and hydatid cysts are not attended by symptoms of liver dysfunction, and jaundice is seldom encountered during their course. The remarkable regenerative capacity of the hepatocytes is an additional safeguard against hepatic failure secondary to such relatively localised lesions. The presence of very extensive lesions is an exception. Thus the rare alveolar type of hydatid disease, in which the entire liver is permeated by cystic spaces, kills as a result of liver failure.

Liver failure is the result of *hepatocellular necrosis* causing widespread destruction of parenchymatous tissue or of *cirrhosis*.

Necrosis. The question of hepatic *necrosis* and its relationship to cirrhosis has already been discussed in Chapter 10. Focal necrosis need not be attended by any evidence of liver dysfunction, although the widespread lesions of viral hepatitis do cause biochemical changes. Zonal necrosis also causes dysfunction, and massive necrosis is a very important antecedent of cholaemia.

Cirrhosis. Hepatic failure is an important complication of cirrhosis, whether macronodular or micronodular. It may be precipitated by bleeding from oesophageal varices or episodes of hepatocellular necrosis. Cardiac cirrhosis causes no disturbance other than a mild hyperbilirubinaemia. Biliary cirrhosis is attended by the symptoms of obstructive jaundice; liver failure occurs only terminally.

Vascular lesions. Infarction of the liver is uncommon and is considered on page 516. If extensive it leads to rapidly developing liver failure. A slow idiopathic occlusion of the hepatic veins leads to the *Budd–Chiari syndrome*, in which there is marked hepatic congestion, ascites, and progressive liver failure. A rather similar effect is seen in *veno-occlusive disease*, in which the small radicles of the hepatic vein undergo progressive intimal fibrosis. The result is a reverse-type cirrhosis similar to that of cardiac disease, but unlike cardiac cirrhosis it leads to liver failure. The condition was common in Jamaica due to the ingestion of 'bush-tea'. This is an infusion prepared from various *Crotalaria* species.

ACCOMPANIMENTS OF LIVER DISEASE[1]

JAUNDICE (ICTERUS)

Of all the symptoms of liver disease icterus is the most immediately apparent. It is due to an excessive amount of bilirubin in the plasma, the normal range being 5 to 17 μmol per litre (0.3 to 1.0 mg per dl). When the level reaches about 51 μmol per litre (3·0 mg per dl), jaundice becomes clinically obvious, and is especially noticeable in the sclerae, skin, and palatal mucosa.

Bilirubin is demonstrated qualitatively and estimated quantitatively by means of the *diazo reagent*. This is diazotised sulphanilic acid (sulphanilic acid treated with a mixture of sodium nitrite and hydrochloric acid), and in the presence of bilirubin a red compound, azobilirubin, is formed. It has been known for some time that bilirubin which has passed through the liver cells gives an immediate reaction with the diazo reagent, and this is called a *direct van den Bergh reaction*. On the other hand, there is no reaction between the diazo reagent and bilirubin which has not passed through the liver, until alcohol has been added to the mixture, when an immediate red colour appears. This is called an *indirect van den Bergh reaction*. In order to understand the different types of jaundice, it is necessary to consider the metabolism of the bile pigments.

Bilirubin Metabolism[2,3]

By far the largest amount of the body's bilirubin is derived from the haem moiety of the haemoglobin of effete red cells which are broken down in the RE system (Figs. 47.1, 47.2, and 47.3). It is known that bilirubin is not the only breakdown product of haem, but the alternative metabolic pathway is unknown. The fact that such an alternative pathway exists, however, helps explain why the blood bilirubin level becomes stable even when excretion by the liver is completely stopped. In animal studies in which ^{15}N-labelled glycine has been administered, it has been shown that of the labelled bilirubin, about 85 per cent is excreted at about 120 days. Glycine is

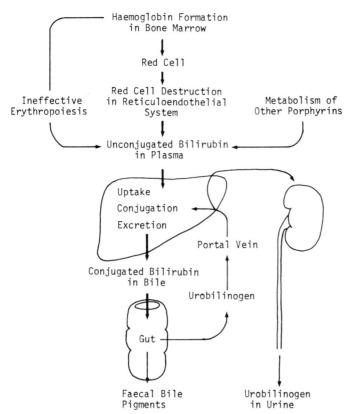

Figure 47.1
Metabolic pathways in the formation and excretion of bilirubin.

Figure 47.2
The structural formula of haem. Note the protoporphyrin ring structure which is composed of four pyrrole rings joined by methene (=CH—) bridges.

Figure 47.3
The structural formula of bilirubin. The iron has been split off, and the porphyrin ring has been opened. The pyrrole rings are now disposed in a straight line.

utilised in the synthesis of haemoglobin, and this excretion is as a result of the red-cell destruction. From 15 to 20 per cent of the labelled bilirubin is excreted within 10 days of the administered glycine. Some of this is derived from the bone marrow during the formation of haemoglobin (*ineffective erythropoiesis*). Although the amount of bilirubin formed in this way is small under normal circumstances, it may be increased in some diseases, e.g. thalassaemia and pernicious anaemia, and contribute to the jaundice. It has been described as a primary cause of jaundice in one family.[4] The early labelled bilirubin which is not derived from haemoglobin synthesis is produced during the metabolism of enzymes, such as the cytochromes, and possibly myoglobin.

Bilirubin is soluble in lipids but insoluble in water. It is kept in solution in the plasma by being tightly bound to albumin. It is removed from the circulation in the liver, where at the surface of the liver cells it is detached from the albumin. It is then bound by proteins in the liver. Two have been identified and designated Y and Z. Y protein is the principal binding protein, and it is quantitatively deficient in the newborn guinea-pig. The administration of phenobarbitone increases the amount of this protein. Z protein is less important, and is competitively inhibited by flavaspidic acid, the active agent in male fern used in the treatment of tape worm. Its administration can cause jaundice.[5] In the liver cell the bilirubin is conjugated into a water-soluble pigment, *bilirubin diglucuronide*, by a specific enzyme called bilirubin-UDP-glucuronyl transferase, which is located in the smooth endoplasmic reticulum. The amount of this enzyme can be increased by the administration of phenobarbitone or dicophane by a process of *enzyme induction*.[6] For this reason, and for the effect on protein Y, these drugs are useful in the treatment of enzyme-deficient jaundice (p. 564).

Some of the bilirubin diglucuronide in the liver cells is reconverted into bilirubin and excreted.[7] This has been demonstrated in the Gunn strain of rat. This animal lacks the necessary conjugating enzyme in the liver. If bilirubin is injected intravenously, none of the pigment appears in the bile. If bilirubin glucuronide is injected, both free and conjugated bilirubin appear in the bile.

The conjugated bilirubin is excreted *via* the bile-ducts into the intestine. It is excreted as a micellar complex with cholesterol, phospholipids, and bile salts. The large molecule of bilirubin diglucuronide is not absorbed in the gallbladder or small bowel, but in the colon it is hydrolysed to the unconjugated form by bacterial glucuronidases, and is then reduced to *stercobilinogen*, nearly all of which is passed in the faeces as stercobilin. Stercobilinogen pigment is well absorbed from the small bowel but minimally from the colon. That which is absorbed into the portal circulation is carried to the liver and re-excreted into the bile, apparently as bilirubin, since stercobilinogen has not been identified in the bile. There is therefore a considerable enterohepatic recirculation of bile pigments. The normal liver removes most of the stercobilinogen from the portal blood, and the little that escapes (1 to 2 mg a day) is excreted in the urine as *urobilinogen*. A damaged liver may fail to perform this function adequately, and an excess of urobilinogen appears in the urine. The normal daily excretion of stercobilinogen in the faeces is 40 to 280 mg.[8]

The differences between conjugated and unconjugated bilirubin. It is apparent that conjugated bilirubin gives a direct reaction with the diazo reagent because it is water soluble (polar). Unconjugated bilirubin is non-polar and cannot react until it is brought into aqueous solution by the presence of alcohol. The basis of its indirect reaction depends entirely on its insolubility in water.

Furthermore, conjugated bilirubin enters the glomerular filtrate with ease, and is excreted in the urine. Unconjugated bilirubin, being insoluble in water is bound to plasma albumin and cannot escape into the glomerular filtrate. This explains why haemolytic jaundice is 'acholuric', i.e. without bilirubin in the urine.

On the other hand, the lipid-solubility of unconjugated bilirubin has distinct dangers: when in high concentration it exhausts the binding capacity of the albumin, and it is then absorbed by lipid-rich areas in the brain. At a plasma concentration of about $340\ \mu$mol per litre (20 mg per dl) the basal ganglia may become deeply bile-stained, and there is irreparable damage to the neurons. The condition is called *kernicterus*. Bilirubin is indeed to be regarded as a toxic substance, and its conjugation is a part of the detoxifying function of the liver. Even the most severe obstructive jaundice is never complicated by kernicterus, because conjugated bilirubin is not soluble in lipids.

It is noteworthy that certain drugs, notably sulphonamides and salicylates, compete with bilirubin for albumin. The free, unbound, unconjugated bilirubin becomes redistributed in the tissues, and by traversing the blood-brain barrier can lead to kernicterus. The danger of giving such drugs in the early neonatal period is obvious. In this circumstance a plasma bilirubin level considerably below $340\ \mu$mol per litre can be dangerous.

It is also interesting that the blood-brain barrier against unconjugated bilirubin is poorly developed at birth, but that it increases considerably in childhood. In the Crigler–Najjar syndrome, which is mentioned later, if the infant is protected against kernicterus by early exchange transfusions, it may survive and develop normally. Despite high levels of plasma bilirubin, it does not develop subsequent kernicterus in later childhood. It therefore does not require repeated exchange transfusions.

Unconjugated bilirubin is very susceptible to photo-oxidation. The end-products are water soluble and not toxic, and this property has been utilised in the treatment of neonatal jaundice. Exposing the infant's body to bright blue or white light from a fluorescent lamp (phototherapy) lowers the plasma level of bilirubin, and it is usually harmless provided overheating is avoided.[9,10]

Types of Jaundice

Jaundice can conveniently be divided into three types: haemolytic, obstructive, and hepatocellular. The first two are relatively clear-cut, though there is invariably some hepatic dysfunction associated with them. Hepatocellular jaundice, on the other hand, can seldom be explained entirely in terms of a single mechanism.

Haemolytic jaundice. This is due to an increased bilirubin load consequent on an excessive breakdown of red cells, and perhaps augmented by ineffective erythropoiesis (see p. 562). The conditions that cause it are those associated with haemolytic anaemia, as described in Chapter 52. Though the cause of the jaundice is an excess of unconjugated bilirubin, there is an additional factor of hepatic dysfunction due to anaemia. The main biochemical features of a haemolytic jaundice are:

(i) An increased amount of indirectly-reacting bilirubin in the plasma.

(ii) An increased amount of stercobilinogen in the faeces.

(iii) An increased amount of urobilinogen in the urine. This is the result of the absorption of so much stercobilinogen from the bowel that some escapes hepatic metabolism.

(iv) An absence of bilirubin in the urine.

The jaundice is not often severe; the plasma bilirubin seldom rises above 85 to $170\ \mu$mol per litre (5 to 10 mg per dl), except in Rh-haemolytic disease of the newborn, in which intense jaundice and kernicterus are frequently encountered.

Obstructive jaundice. This occurs when there is an obstruction to the passage of conjugated bilirubin from the liver cells to the intestine. The condition is called *cholestasis*, and the obstruction may be intrahepatic or extrahepatic.

Extrahepatic cholestasis is very well recognised, because it comes into the category of 'surgical jaundice'. The best known examples of this are: (*a*) blockage of the common bile duct by gallstones; (*b*) occlusion of the duct by a carcinoma of the head of the pancreas; (*c*) pressure from without by enlarged lymph nodes in the porta hepatis; and (*d*) a carcinoma of the duct itself, either at the ampulla of Vater or else higher up. *Intrahepatic obstruction* occurs in *primary biliary cirrhosis*, which affects chiefly middle-aged women. There is a progressive obstructive jaundice which usually kills in about 5 years. The main bile ducts are normal, but there is destruction of the cholangioles, which are surrounded by a chronic inflammatory reaction: severe periportal fibrosis develops. The nature of the disease is obscure, but an autoimmune mechanism is important. The blood contains IgM antibodies active against bile-duct components as well as IgG antimitochondrial antibodies. The detection of the latter is a useful diagnostic test for primary biliary cirrhosis.

Intrahepatic cholestasis may occur from time to time in the absence of obstruction to the bile ducts; it is a rare complication of the last trimester of pregnancy, and is probably due to the effects of oestrogen. Some women who take the oral contraceptive have likewise exhibited cholestatic jaundice due to its oestrogen content.[11]

Intrahepatic cholestasis is produced by drugs, and is called *cholestatic drug jaundice*. There are two types: (*a*) that associated with chlorpromazine and other phenothiazine derivatives, and more rarely arsphenamine, para-aminosalicylic acid, erythromycin estolate (but not the free base or other salts), and thiouracil. About 1 per cent of patients on chloropromazine develop icterus after a month's therapy, irrespective of dosage. It is probable that drug allergy is responsible, for there is a heavy cellular infiltration containing many eosinophils in the portal tracts. *Halothane* occasionally causes hepatic damage,[12] and in fatal cases there is massive necrosis similar to that seen in viral hepatitis. Leucocytosis and eosinophilia occur, and hypersensitivity to the drug appears to be the explanation; (*b*) that associated with those steroids which have in common the substitution of an alkyl group in the C17 position; the most important is methyltestosterone (testosterone propionate has no effect). Steroid icterus affects all patients given a large enough dose, and does not produce portal-tract infiltrations.

In these conditions the liver cells are either normal or else show only minor degenerative changes. In all types of intrahepatic cholestasis abnormalities have been described, at electron-microscopic level, in the microvilli lining the bile canaliculi.

The main biochemical manifestations of an obstructive jaundice are:

(i) An increased amount of directly-reacting bilirubin in the plasma.

(ii) A decreased amount of stercobilinogen in the faeces, which are pale in colour, bulky, and offensive. Not only is bilirubin excluded from the bowel, but so also are the bile salts which are important in aiding the absorption of fat. In long-continued cases the patient may suffer from a malabsorption syndrome. In particular the absorption of the fat-soluble vitamins is impaired. Hypovitaminosis D eventually leads to osteomalacia, and the inadequate absorption of vitamin K to a bleeding tendency that can be remedied by the parenteral administration of the vitamin (see p. 568).

(iii) A complete absence of urobilinogen in the urine.

(iv) The presence of bilirubin and bile salts in the urine.

(v) A raised plasma alkaline phosphate (see p. 569).

Patients with cholestasis are subject to severe pruritus, which is closely related to plasma bile-salt concentration, and particularly to the presence of unconjugated bile salts in the skin (normally the bile salts are conjugated after synthesis in the liver with either glycine or taurine).

There is generally also hypercholesterolaemia, which is due to an overproduction by the liver itself rather than retention in the bile. If prolonged, the hypercholesterolaemia may lead to the formation of cutaneous xanthomata.

There is a rise in the level of low-density lipoproteins in the plasma, but the high-density fraction is decreased. An important low-density lipoprotein is an abnormal one called *lipoprotein X*, which contains a high proportion of unesterified cholesterol and phospholipid. The lipoproteins of cholestasis differ from those associated with atheroma, which is not a complication of obstructive jaundice.

In prolonged obstruction there is also hepatocellular damage due to the back-pressure of dammed-up bile.

Hepatocellular jaundice. In this type of jaundice the van den Bergh reaction usually shows both a directly and an indirectly-reacting type of bilirubin, and it is often called *biphasic*. This points both to a failure in the conjugating mechanism within the liver cells, and to an obstruction to the escape of conjugated bilirubin either from the cells into the canaliculi, or from the canaliculi themselves (which constitutes intrahepatic cholestasis). It is also well established that the time of red-cell survival is reduced in conditions of liver failure, so that there is the additional factor of an increased bilirubin load. Despite the complex nature of hepatocellular jaundice, it is helpful to note a few conditions in which the mechanism seems fairly definite.

Enzyme deficiency. During the first few days of life there is

a deficiency of glucuronyl transferase necessary for the conjugation of bilirubin. This is the primary cause of *icterus neonatorum*. In addition there is an increased bilirubin load because of haemolysis of some of the fetal red cells; the newborn infant produces bilirubin at a rate of about three times that of the adult. Furthermore, there may be a defective uptake of bilirubin by the Y protein, and hepatic excretion is probably impaired. This 'physiological' jaundice seldom exceeds a plasma bilirubin level of 204 μmol per litre (12 mg per dl), but all these effects are accentuated in premature infants. When Rh-haemolytic disease is added, kernicterus can easily follow. Severe bacterial infections in the newborn also cause jaundice that is predominantly haemolytic. It is occasionally severe enough to produce kernicterus.

Infants may develop jaundice when breast fed: the factor in milk appears to be an unusual steroid, 3α, 20β pregnanediol, which inhibits glucuronyl transferase. Another rare cause of neonatal jaundice is the familial *Lucey–Driscoll syndrome*; an unidentified factor present in the mother's serum is believed to be responsible.

A deficiency of the transferase enzyme is seen in the rare *Crigler–Najjar type of congenital jaundice*, which leads to severe jaundice and kernicterus. A similar condition is seen in the Gunn strain of rat. In some types of Crigler–Najjar jaundice there is a complete absence of the enzyme, but in others the defect is partial and they respond to the enzyme-inducing effect of phenobarbitone (p. 562).

A less severe variant is *Gilbert's disease*, which is the commonest form of unconjugated familial hyperbilirubinaemia.[13,14] It is probably inherited as a dominant characteristic, and is manifest as episodes of benign, intermittent jaundice starting from childhood. Needle biopsies have shown a considerable reduction of the conjugating enzyme; in addition there is probably also a defect in uptake of bilirubin into the cell and a mild degree of haemolysis associated with a slightly decreased red-cell survival time. Phenobarbitone induces the enzyme and relieves the jaundice; this also occurs in neonatal jaundice.

The Dubin–Johnson type of jaundice. This is a chronic, intermittent jaundice seen in young people. It is a benign condition and is often familial. The icterus is due to conjugated bilirubin (which escapes into the urine). An interesting, though obscure, feature is the presence of much brown pigment in the liver cells. Originally described as a lipofuscin, it is now thought to be a melanin. On electron microscopy it is seen to be associated with the lysosomes. Macroscopically the liver has a greenish-black colour. The defect appears to be one of failure of transport of conjugated bilirubin from the cells into the canaliculi. The canaliculi and bile ducts are normal.

A similar type of jaundice is seen in the *Rotor syndrome*, but here the liver cells do not show pigmentation. The Dubin–Johnson and Rotor syndromes are closely related and may occur in various members of a single family. Sometimes features of Gilbert's disease are mixed with those of the Dubin–Johnson and Rotor syndromes.

It is important to note that in jaundice due to enzyme deficiency only the bilirubin is retained in the blood; the bile salts are not affected.

Intrahepatic cholestasis complicating liver-cell damage. In some liver diseases, in addition to hepatocellular damage, there is also intrahepatic cholestasis. This may be due to defective transport of conjugated bilirubin into the canaliculi, as described in the Dubin–Johnson syndrome. Acute cholestasis may complicate viral hepatitis to such an extent that a laparotomy may be necessary to rule out the possibility of an organic obstruction to the bile ducts. The 'acute fatty liver' of the alcoholic may lead to obstructive jaundice, due perhaps to pressure on the canaliculi by the distended liver cells. An obstructive element may occur in the course of severe neonatal jaundice, and be due either to inspissated bile in the canaliculi or to frank hepatocellular damage leading to defective transport of conjugated bilirubin to the canaliculi.

It is obvious that in a common condition like viral hepatitis there may be several patterns of jaundice. In the early stage the obstructive element usually predominates. Later on it subsides, and the urine contains an excess of urobilinogen. In the absence of a haemolytic anaemia this is always a valuable sign of liver disease; it indicates that the liver is unable to cope with the absorbed stercobilinogen, which is passed straight on to the systemic circulation.

Cirrhosis is seldom associated with marked jaundice except during phases of acute exacerbation and terminally; indeed its presence is of evil omen. There is, however, a constant excess of urobilinogen in the urine.

Post-operative jaundice is not uncommon, but does not represent a separate entity since many factors can be involved. Amongst these are hepatic necrosis following a period of shock, hepatitis due to drugs or halothane, red-cell destruction in areas of bleeding, and haemolysis of transfused red cells.

THE PORTAL CIRCULATION IN LIVER DISEASE

The normal portal blood-flow is from 1000 to 1200 ml per minute. The pressure, normally 5 to 13 mm Hg, may be measured directly by the insertion of a catheter either through a patent umbilical vein[15] or directly into the vessel at operation. Two other methods are available:

The wedged hepatic venous pressure. Under fluoroscopic control a catheter is passed through an antecubital vein, past the heart, and into a radicle of the hepatic vein into which it is wedged. This gives a measure of the pressure at the venous end of the hepatic sinusoids (*postsinusoidal pressure*). It is normally 6 to 8 mm Hg.

The intrasplenic pressure. A thin needle is introduced through the skin into the splenic pulp. The pressure recorded is approximately the same as that in the portal vein, and is therefore a measure of the *presinusoidal pressure*. Splenic puncture may usefully be followed by the injection of diodone, which rapidly enters the portal vein and can be seen by radiography.

Portal Venous Occlusion

Mechanical obstruction of the portal blood-flow results in a rise in pressure (*portal hypertension*). The obstruction can occur in the portal vein itself, within the liver, or in the hepatic veins. However, from a functional point of view it is more useful to consider two types:

Postsinusoidal obstruction. This is seen in the Budd–Chiari syndrome, which may be either idiopathic or a result of hepatic-vein thrombosis related to trauma, polycythaemia,

tumour invasion, or contraceptive pills. Obstruction is also a feature of veno-occlusive disease.

Presinusoidal obstruction. This may be extrahepatic due to portal-vein thrombosis, or intrahepatic in conditions where there is fibrosis around the portal triads, as for instance in schistosomiasis.

In the common types of hepatic cirrhosis the obstruction is predominantly of the postsinusoidal type. In addition anastomoses develop between the small branches of the hepatic artery and the portal vein. This shunt contributes to the portal hypertension, as may be demonstrated by temporarily occluding the hepatic artery at operation and observing the fall in portal venous pressure.

Effects of Portal Hypertension

The abdominal viscera are engorged with blood, the portal vein and its tributaries are distended, and anastomoses develop between them and the systemic venous circulation.

Portal-systemic anastomoses. The most important site for these portal-systemic anastomoses is the lower end of the oesophagus, where the resulting varices may bleed and cause haematemesis. Not only is there an immediate danger of death from exsanguination, but it may also precipitate cholaemia either by causing shock and hepato-renal necrosis, or by adding to the alimentary protein load (p. 567). Anastomoses between the superior and inferior haemorrhoidal veins may result in the development of haemorrhoids. In practice this is not a common complaint in cirrhosis. A rare, but classical, sign is the *caput medusae* at the umbilicus, where veins of the abdominal wall drain blood from the umbilical vein, or if this is not patent, from the plexus that surrounds it. Other sites of anastomosis are lieno-phrenic, lieno-colic, lieno-renal, and in the retroperitoneal tissues around the duodenum. These may pose technical problems during surgery on patients with cirrhosis.

In advanced cirrhosis, most of the portal blood by-passes the liver and enters the systemic circulation, mostly *via* the azygos veins which in life are often demonstrably enlarged on a radiograph. The liver in these cases relies upon hepatic-artery blood, and is usually small.

Portal-pulmonary anastomoses. In addition to the portal-systemic anastomoses, branches of the left gastric vein may form portal-pulmonary communications. This shunt can result in some degree of arterial desaturation as well as contributing to the high cardiac output.

Congestive splenomegaly. An enlarged spleen is the single most important diagnostic sign of portal hypertension. The sinuses are dilated, and their walls show prominent lining cells and some increase in reticulin fibres. Splenic overactivity may result in depression of any or all of the circulating cells of the peripheral blood. It was indeed this aspect of cirrhosis that led to the original description of Banti's syndrome as a separate entity.

Atheromatous change in the portal vein with terminal thrombosis. This leads to rapid deterioration and intractably severe ascites.

Portal-systemic shunting of blood. The by-passing of the liver by the portal blood is an important feature of chronic liver disease:

1. Toxic substances from the intestine pass into the sys-

temic circulation and contribute to the *neuro-psychiatric manifestations* described on page 567.

2. *An oral glucose tolerance test is abnormal*, since the absorbed glucose passes directly into the systemic circulation.

3. *The ammonia tolerance is impaired*. If ammonium salts are administered by mouth, the liver normally converts the ammonia to urea, and the blood level of ammonia scarcely rises. Except as a terminal event liver disease is never severe enough to upset this mechanism. Hence any rise in blood ammonia in the test is due to portal-systemic shunting of blood rather than to hepatocellular damage.

4. Organisms from the gut can gain access to the general circulation and cause septicaemia. *Gram-negative endotoxic shock* is sometimes seen as a terminal manifestation.

5. *Peptic ulcer*. This is due apparently to the release of a gastric secretogogue, possibly histamine, from the bowel and its by-passing the liver, which would normally degrade it.

6. *Liver-cell failure* due to decreased hepatic blood flow. Hepatocellular necrosis is not uncommon as a terminal event in cirrhosis.

Hepatocellular Dysfunction

The main manifestations of dysfunction in hepatic disease are related to the processes of protein and carbohydrate metabolism and detoxification.

Disturbances of protein metabolism. The liver is responsible for the synthesis of most of the plasma proteins, the most notable exception being the immunoglobulins. It therefore follows that in progressive liver disease there is a fall in plasma albumin and sometimes in α and β-globulins also. The hypoalbuminaemia leads to a fall in the osmotic pressure of the plasma and is a considerable factor in producing the ascites of liver failure. Most liver disease is accompanied by hypergammaglobulinaemia, which is reflected by the empirical flocculation tests that were once in vogue but are now replaced by more accurate electrophoretic studies.

The cause of this hypergammaglobulinaemia is not entirely understood. Possible factors involved include antibodies against a causative organism or against necrotic liver cells (autoantibodies). It has also been found that patients with liver disease have high titres of antibodies against organisms that are normally resident in the bowel. It may be that antigens from these organisms pass directly into the systemic circulation *via* a portal-systemic shunt and stimulate antibody formation; normally such antigenic products would be removed by the Kupffer cells in the liver. Thus either a failure of Kupffer cells or a by-passing of them might lead to antibody formation and a consequent hypergammaglobulinaemia.[16] The most marked hypergammaglobulinaemia occurs in *chronic active hepatitis*.*

---

*The terminology of chronic hepatitis is confusing.[17–19] The essential histological feature is a chronic inflammatory reaction with fibrosis in the portal triads. The term *chronic persistent hepatitis* is used to describe the condition when there is good preservation of lobular structure and little or no hepatic-cell necrosis. Chronic persistent hepatitis may follow an attack of acute hepatitis and does not tend to progress to cirrhosis. In *chronic lobular hepatitis*, also called unresolved or protracted viral hepatitis, the lobules show patchy cellular inflammatory infiltrate, and occasional dead hepatocytes (acidophilic bodies) can be found. In chronic carriers of HBsAg some liver cells show a ground-glass appearance of the cytoplasm. These areas stain with orcein and have been

The liver is also responsible for the synthesis of most of the clotting factors, many of which are β-globulins. It is hardly surprising that liver disease is often accompanied by a haemorrhagic diathesis (see **Ch. 54**).

The liver is the principal seat of deamination of amino acids, and is probably the only organ that can convert the ammonia so produced into urea. In severe liver failure there may be an 'overflow' type of amino-aciduria as the result of increased blood levels of amino acids. This is to be contrasted with the renal type of amino-aciduria due to tubular defects (see **Ch. 46**).

Ammonia is also manufactured in the intestine by the bacterial decomposition of protein material. If the ammonia cannot be converted adequately into urea, the level of ammonia in the blood rises and it may interfere with cerebral metabolism. Ammonia intoxication is a possible cause of the neuro-psychiatric symptoms of cholaemia.

Disturbances of carbohydrate metabolism.[20] Following total hepatectomy in an experimental animal death is due to hypoglycaemia. Such is the hepatic reserve that hypoglycaemia is rarely a feature of human liver disease. It is occasionally seen in acute hepatic necrosis and following an acute episode of alcoholic debauchery. Impaired gluconeogenesis is the mechanism.

The impaired glucose tolerance in liver disease is due to portal-systemic shunting, and if hypoglycaemia occurs, the development of a hepatoma should be suspected, since this tumour is sometimes associated with hypoglycaemia. The mechanism is not clear, but it is usually assumed that the tumour metabolises glucose at a high rate. There is, however, some evidence that the tumour secretes an insulin-like substance.

Failure of detoxification. The usual method of detoxification is by conjugation, either with an organic or mineral acid, e.g. glucuronic acid or sulphuric acid, or with amino acids, e.g. glycine and glutamic acid. These conjugated products are then excreted in the bile or the urine. The conjugation of bilirubin is a classical example of this type.

---

shown to contain HBsAg (Figs 23.8 and 9). Such cells are common in chronic lobular hepatitis, but may also be found in other types of hepatitis and in cirrhosis. *Chronic active hepatitis*, also called chronic aggressive hepatitis, is characterised by a portal inflammatory infiltrate accompanied by necrosis of the adjacent liver cells (*piecemeal necrosis*). Necrosis can be much more extensive and extend between adjacent portal tracts and/or central veins (*bridging necrosis*). Chronic active hepatitis shows a great tendency to progress to cirrhosis. As first described, the condition occurred in young women, and recurrent attacks of hepatitis terminated in death from cirrhosis within 10 years. Hypergammaglobulinaemia is a characteristic feature, and both antinuclear and rheumatoid factors are usually present. Although the disease was originally called 'lupoid hepatitis', there is no evidence that the condition is related to lupus erythematosus itself. Nevertheless, over half the patients also have arthritis. Antibodies that react with smooth muscle are present in most cases, and the disease has a strong autoimmune component. The clinical syndrome and histological picture of chronic active hepatitis has now been extended to other groups of patients, and in these the autoimmune component is less striking. The various types of hepatitis described above should not be regarded as disease entities, but as reaction patterns to a variety of agents—viral infection, alcoholism, drug hypersensitivity, metabolic errors (Wilson's disease), and an abnormal or excessive immune response. The classification is based mainly on liver biopsy findings and has the advantage of being of prognostic value: chronic persistent hepatitis has a good prognosis, chronic active hepatitis a poor one.

Bromsulphalein is conjugated with glycine, glutamic acid, and as a mercaptide, and though it can be excreted in the bile without conjugation, its clearance from the plasma is an excellent test of liver function.

Morphine is conjugated as a glucuronide in the liver, and intolerance to this drug is an important feature of hepatocellular disease. A small dose may precipitate hepatic coma.

The steroid hormones are conjugated in the liver prior to being excreted in the urine. On the whole, their metabolism is not seriously impaired even in severe liver failure, but a few abnormalities are worth noting: (*a*) a reduced urinary output of 17-ketosteroids and 17-hydroxycorticoids; (*b*) an increased urinary output of aldosterone; apparently the liver cannot convert it into biologically inert substances; (*c*) a tendency towards oestrogen retention.

OTHER MANIFESTATIONS OF HEPATIC DYSFUNCTION

Although the liver plays an important role in *fat metabolism*, there is little significant disturbance in liver failure. There is evidence, however, that ketogenesis in response to starvation is reduced in patients with liver disease. The liver manufactures cholesterol, and low plasma levels are found in advanced liver failure.

Damaged liver cells release many of their chemical contents into the circulation. This accounts for the raised plasma levels of *enzymes*, e.g. transaminases, dehydrogenases, glucose 6-phosphatase, aldolase, and glutathione reductase, *iron*, and *vitamin B_{12}* encountered in hepatocellular disease.

Ascites

Ascites is a common manifestation of hepatic cirrhosis and its pathogenesis is complex. There is considerable controversy concerning the relative importance of the many factors involved. In the experimental animal ascites can be produced easily by obstructing the hepatic veins but not by ligating the portal vein. The blood in the hepatic sinusoids normally communicates with fluid in the space of Disse through pores between the endothelial cells. From here the fluid, virtually of the same composition as plasma, is drained by the hepatic lymphatics and reaches the thoracic duct. In cirrhosis the major vascular obstruction is postsinusoidal, and the *flow of lymph is considerably augmented*. The lymphatic vessels, including the thoracic duct, are dilated, but they nevertheless appear inadequate to deal with the increased volume of lymph. Fluid oozes from the liver surface, and while the patient suffers the liver weeps. It has been observed that if the thoracic duct is drained the ascites rapidly diminishes. Since external loss of protein-rich lymph is undesirable, the creation of a lymphatic-venous fistula is one approach to the treatment of ascites.

Other factors in the pathogenesis of ascites are *hypoalbuminaemia*, since if this is combined experimentally with portal-vein obstruction ascites develops, and *salt retention* due to hyperaldosteronism (this is more important in relation to the later generalised oedema). Finally there is the increased capillary pressure secondary to *portal obstruction*, but this appears to be of minor importance. It has been found that there is a rapid turnover of ascitic fluid, about 50 per cent being replaced every hour. Its protein content varies from 10 to 30 g per litre, and it must be concluded that ascites is a type of lymphoedema, with salt and water retention and hydrostatic forces acting as contributory factors.

The Systemic Circulation in Liver Disease

In hepatic failure the plasma volume is increased, but due to the pooling in the splanchnic area the effective volume is decreased. As described in Chapter 43 this causes water and salt retention. The latter may be aggravated by poor inactivation of aldosterone by the damaged liver. Salt retention is often marked in liver failure, and although it may be a factor in the production of ascites, it is probably of greater importance in causing the generalised oedema that occurs in the later stages of liver disease.

The cardiac output is increased in all forms of hepatocellular failure, and there is a hyperkinetic circulation. The hands are warm, the forearm veins dilated, and the pulses full. Interestingly, the renal blood flow is reduced.[1] Congestive cardiac failure of high output type occurs only rarely. The pathogenesis of these effects is complex and uncertain. The arteriovenous shunting in the liver and the portal-pulmonary anastomoses have already been described. The opening-up of many normally inactive arteriovenous anastomoses by a vasodilator material released from the damaged liver or inadequately detoxified by it has been suggested.

In progressive liver disease there sometimes develop numerous *vascular spiders* on the skin of the face, chest, and upper limbs. These consist of a central dilated arteriole from which emerges a leash of small vessels, and pressure on the central area causes blanching of the whole lesion. A few vascular spiders are not uncommon in healthy people. They are also found during pregnancy, disappearing within two months of delivery, and rarely in rheumatoid arthritis.

Another finding is *palmar erythema* (liver palms); the hands are warm and the palms bright red in colour. Many normal people have familial palmar flushing, unassociated with liver disease. Palmar erythema is also seen in rheumatoid arthritis and pregnancy, usually in association with vascular spiders. In liver disease they may also be present together, but are often independent of each other. Oestrogen excess has been suggested as a cause for these manifestations of liver disease, but the evidence is inconclusive. At present their aetiology remains unknown.

Neuro-psychiatric manifestations (portasystemic encephalopathy). These include abnormalities of behaviour, nocturnal ramblings, and attacks of screaming. Convulsions and coma may ensue. Ataxia and a characteristic 'flapping' tremor of the outstretched hands are also noteworthy accompaniments. The electroencephalograph shows changes typical of a metabolic disturbance of cerebral function. Sometimes the syndrome is acute, as in the course of massive necrosis or in advanced cirrhosis complicated by a precipitating factor like morphine intoxication, gastrointestinal haemorrhage, or even a heavy protein meal. On other occasions it is chronic, and may last intermittently for many years. It is this group of patients that is the most pathetic, for they exhibit personality changes, mental deterioration, and other neurological symptoms. It is one of the complications of portacaval shunt operations.

Animals with a portacaval (Eck) fistula become comatose

and die if given a meat meal ('meat intoxication'). It is believed that these manifestations are caused by nitrogenous substances which are formed in the bowel, perhaps as a result of bacterial action. They escape detoxification because of the portal-systemic shunt, and thereby reach the brain where they cause this *portasystemic encephalopathy*. A similar chain of events occurs clinically either spontaneously in liver disease or else following portacaval anastomosis.

The structural changes in the brain consist of characteristic abnormalities in the astrocytes.[21] One of these, probably caused by ammonia, appears to reside in the microtubules, and results in a mitotic defect similar to that produced by colchicine: cells entering mitosis do not divide, but instead form large tetraploid nuclei. As already mentioned, ammonia is the product chiefly incriminated for these effects. The liability to coma after gastrointestinal haemorrhage is explained by the large amount of extra protein in the bowel. The administration of broad-spectrum antibiotics, e.g. neomycin, reduces the severity of portasystemic encephalopathy by diminishing the bacterial activity in the intestine. It is in fact doubtful whether hepatic coma is attributable to any one single substance absorbed from the bowel.

It seems that the brain is peculiarly vulnerable to toxic and metabolic insults during the course of liver failure, and that such diverse factors as morphine, ammonia excess, electrolyte imbalance, infection, and hypoxia can all produce the non-specific picture of hepatic coma in susceptible subjects.

Foetor hepaticus. The offensive faecal odour of the breath of patients with liver disease is probably due to the passage of foul-smelling products from the gut into the systemic circulation, either through anastomotic channels or through a poorly-functioning liver. The nature of the offensive substances is unknown.

Endocrine changes. Signs of feminisation in men with cirrhosis—gynaecomastia, testicular atrophy, and loss of body hair—have been attributed to the over-production of oestrogen or a failure of the liver to detoxify it. In some of these patients the circulating level of oestrogen is high, but the pathogenesis is uncertain.[22, 23] Many of the patients are alcoholics, and may show feminisation before there is advanced liver damage. It may be that alcohol has a directly inhibiting action on the hypothalamus, pituitary, and the testis itself. The ingestion of alcohol reduces the blood levels of luteinising hormone releasing factor, luteinising hormone, and testosterone in healthy male volunteers.[24]

In women with liver disease endocrine changes are much less common, but there may be amenorrhoea and breast atrophy, the cause of which is obscure.

Fever. A low-grade pyrexia, uninfluenced by antibiotics or diet, is not uncommon during the course of progressive cirrhosis. Its cause is unknown; suggested factors are pyrogens liberated from necrotic cells and the failure of the liver to inactivate pyrogenic steroids, e.g. aetiocholanolone.

Anaemia. Patients with advanced liver disease are sometimes anaemic, and this is due to iron deficiency consequent on recurrent gastrointestinal haemorrhage, splenic overactivity, and a diminished rate of red-cell survival. Red-cell fragility is decreased and target cells may be present. A folic-acid deficiency megaloblastic anaemia is rarely present.

Bleeding tendencies. These are due to a failure of syn-thesis of such clotting factors as fibrinogen, prothrombin, Factor V, and Factor VII. Indeed, the only factor that is not made in the liver is Factor VIII (antihaemophilic globulin factor). Vitamin K given parenterally does not help, as it cannot be utilised. Other causes of a bleeding tendency are a *defibrination syndrome* sometimes encountered in liver failure, and *thrombocytopenia* secondary to splenic overactivity.

Hepatic osteodystrophy. This painful, terminal feature of liver disease, having features of osteoporosis and osteomalacia, is described on page 301.

Terminal manifestations of hepatic failure. As the patient's condition deteriorates, certain ill-understood biochemical disturbances may supervene. These consist of hyponatraemia and nitrogen retention. A fall in plasma sodium is common to many terminal states but in liver failure it is particularly severe. Unlike the low-sodium state that follows salt depletion, symptoms are not alleviated by the intravenous administration of saline solutions. On the contrary such treatment may hasten death. The hyponatraemia is not due to sodium loss, nor is there evidence that it is a dilutional effect secondary to water retention. It is probably due to the entry of sodium ions into damaged cells with a reciprocal escape of intracellular cations into the extracellular fluid. This has been called the 'sick-cell syndrome'.[25]

Terminal nitrogen retention, manifest by a rising plasma-urea level, is not uncommon, and the combination of renal failure with severe hepatic failure is known as the *hepato-renal syndrome*. Its existence as an entity is denied by some workers, but the frequency with which the combination occurs warrants its recognition. Nevertheless, the pathogenesis varies from case to case, and there is no constant finding to explain the renal failure. The following mechanisms may be postulated:

1. The agent causing the liver damage may also affect the kidneys, e.g. leptospirosis, carbon tetrachloride poisoning, and tetracycline overdosage.

2. Chronic liver disease may be accompanied by a chronic nephritis in which there is mesangial proliferation and eventual glomerular destruction. The pathogenesis is not known.

3. The renal blood flow is reduced in cirrhosis of the liver and this is usually associated with a redistribution of blood within the kidney, such that the flow through the outer cortex is reduced while that through the juxta-medullary cortex and medulla is maintained.[26] This may explain why patients with cirrhosis rapidly develop oliguric renal failure in response to a relatively minor reduction in blood volume.

4. Renal shut-down, terminating in renal tubular necrosis if the patient lives long enough, can complicate shock. This may be precipitated by haemorrhage, hypovolaemia secondary to rapid accumulation of ascitic fluid following paracentesis, septicaemia, or endotoxaemia. Renal shut-down is particularly common in jaundiced patients, and is a danger when operating on them. It is also common after cholecystectomy, and the infusion of mannitol to maintain renal perfusion is claimed to be of prophylactic value.

Another finding that usually heralds imminent death is the presence of large amounts of various amino acids in the urine. A rise in the level of plasma amino acids and their overflow into the urine is a sign of very severe hepatic dysfunction.

The patient gradually sinks into cholaemic coma in which deepening jaundice, haemorrhagic manifestations, ascites, remittent pyrexia, and circulatory collapse are the main features. A final haematemesis often precedes death.

TESTS OF LIVER FUNCTION

In the light of what has been discussed it is possible to adopt a rational approach to the testing of hepatic function. It is still as true as ever that most of the tests at our disposal assess only gross dysfunction. The following tests should be performed as a routine:

Estimation of the plasma bilirubin, together with an assessment of the bilirubin and urobilinogen contents of the urine, and an inspection of the faeces for stercobilinogen. By this procedure pure haemolytic jaundice can easily be distinguished from pure obstructive jaundice, as has already been described. It is seldom possible to distinguish between hepatocellular and obstructive jaundice on the basis of tests of pigment metabolism. As diagnostic aids in liver disease they are of limited value.

Estimation of plasma proteins with electrophoretic analysis. The changes in progressive liver disease are described on page 566. In cholestasis the lipoproteins (p. 583) migrate with the α_2- and β-globulins, which are therefore somewhat raised. In haemolytic jaundice the proteins are normal.

Bromsulphalein (BSP) clearance. In the absence of jaundice this is the best available test of liver function. A 5 per cent solution of BSP is injected slowly intravenously; the dose is 5 mg per kg body weight. Its concentration in the plasma is measured colorimetrically, and after 45 minutes there should be less than 3 per cent retention. In the presence of jaundice this test is rendered unreliable from a colorimetric point of view. In any case it is then unnecessary, since there is obvious retention in the plasma of another substance, bilirubin, normally conjugated in the liver and excreted into the bile. There is an increased BSP retention in nearly all cases of cirrhosis, except the most compensated. In heart failure, BSP excretion is generally within normal limits.

PLASMA ENZYMES IN LIVER DISEASE[27, 28]

Alkaline phosphatase. Various alkaline phosphatase isoenzymes may be found in the plasma, and they differ in their source, electrophoretic mobility, and stability to heating and urea. Five sources may be described:

1. *Bone.* This alkaline phosphatase is the least heat-stable, and is considered in Chapter 10.

2. *Liver.* This isoenzyme is usually the major component of plasma and is of intermediate stability.

3. *Intestine.* The amount of this stable enzyme depends on the diet. The highest quantity is found in people who are of blood groups B and O and who are also secretors and Le$^+$.

4. *Placental.* This is the most heat-stable, and is present during the third trimester.

5. *Tumour.* This type of alkaline phosphatase is indistinguishable from the placental type, and is most frequently found in patients with cancer of the lung.

The normal level of alkaline phosphatase in the plasma is 3 to 13 King-Armstrong units per dl.

In obstructive liver disease, the liver's content of alkaline phosphatase is increased due to overproduction. The enzyme regurgitates into the blood, and in obstructive jaundice values of over 30 units per 100 dl are the rule. In hepatocellular disease the level varies from 15 to 30 units, and normal values occur in haemolytic jaundice.

In bile-duct obstruction the alkaline phosphatase that is reabsorbed is in a macromolecular form and is not readily excreted. The conjugated bilirubin which is reabsorbed at the same time is easily excreted by the kidney. It follows therefore that if some of the bile ducts are obstructed, the plasma level of bilirubin can be normal whereas that of the alkaline phosphatase is raised. Any infiltrating lesion of the liver can produce this picture of a raised alkaline phosphatase level in the face of normal values for other tests of liver function. A common cause in practice is a tumour, either primary or secondary.

The plasma levels of two other enzymes, *5-nucleotidase* and *γ-glutamyl-transpeptidase*, correlate well with that of alkaline phosphatase.

Plasma transaminase activity. The liver is the second richest source of glutamate-oxaloacetate transaminase (GOT), and the richest of glutamate-pyruvate transaminase (GPT). It is not surprising that any marked necrosis of liver cells leads to an escape of these enzymes into the blood. In acute hepatitis both these enzymes are increased, sometimes ten or even a hundredfold. The increase affects the plasma GPT (normally 4 to 13 international units per litre) even more than the plasma GOT (normally 5 to 17 international units per litre), and these changes may precede the onset of clinical

TABLE 47.1 Liver function tests in the various types of jaundice

		Haemolytic jaundice	Hepatocellular jaundice	Obstructive jaundice
(a)	Pigment metabolism			
	Plasma bilirubin	Indirectly-reacting	Usually biphasic	Directly-reacting
	Faeces	Darkly coloured	Usually normal	Pale
	Urine	{ No bilirubin	{ Variable bilirubin	{ Bilirubin + +
		{ Urobilinogen + +	{ Urobilinogen + +	{ No urobilinogen
(b)	Plasma alkaline phosphatase			
	(in King–Armstrong units per dl)	3–13	15–30	>30
(c)	Plasma proteins	Normal	Increased γ-globulin. In progressive cases diminished albumin, α- and β-globulin	Slight rise in α_2- and β-globulins
(d)	Plasma transaminase	Normal	Great increase in acute necrosis Moderate increase in cirrhosis	Mild increase

jaundice. In cirrhosis and to a lesser extent obstructive jaundice there is also an increase in these transaminases. The rise is less pronounced than in acute necrosis, and the plasma GOT is somewhat higher than the plasma GPT. Glutamate-oxaloacetate is alternatively called aspartate aminotransferase (As-At) and glutamate-pyruvate alanine aminotransferase (Al-At).

Other enzymes. Other enzymes released from necrotic liver cells are *leucine aminopeptidase* and *isocitrate dehydrogenase*. More important is one of the isoenzymes of *lactate dehydrogenase*. LDH$_5$ is found in large amounts in the liver,

and the level in the plasma is raised in destructive liver disease (see also p. 513). Of all the enzymes liberated from disintegrating liver cells, these two—alanine aminotransferase and lactate dehydrogenase—are the most important diagnostically, as they occur predominantly in hepatic tissue.

In hepatocellular disease there is a fall in the *cholinesterase activity of the plasma*. This is in contrast to the other enzymes, the plasma levels of which rise after liver damage. Cholinesterase is a mucoprotein, an α-globulin, synthesised by the liver. Its level drops also in malnutrition.

GENERAL READING

SCHEUER, P. J. (1974) *Liver Biopsy Interpretation*, 2nd edn, 171 pp. London: Baillière, Tindall and Cassell.
SCHIFF, L. (Ed.) (1975) *Diseases of the Liver*, 4th edn, 1461 pp. Philadelphia and Toronto: Lippincott.
SHERLOCK, S. (1975) *Diseases of the Liver and Biliary System*, 5th edn, 821 pp. Oxford: Blackwell.

REFERENCES

1. WALKER, J. G. (1974) In *Clinical Physiology*, ed. Campbell, E. J. M., Dickinson, C. J. & Slater, J. D. H., 4th edn, p. 542. Oxford: Blackwell.
2. SCHMID, R. (1972) Bilirubin metabolism in man. *New England Journal of Medicine*, **287**, 703.
3. JAVITT, N. B. (1976) Hepatic bile formation. *New England Journal of Medicine*, **295**, 1464, and 1511.
4. ISRAELS, L. G. & ZIPURSKY, A. (1962) Primary shunt hyperbilirubinaemia. *Nature (London)*, **193**, 73.
5. LEVI, A. J., GATMAITAN, Z. & ARIAS, I. M. (1969) Two hepatic cytoplasmic protein fractions, Y and Z, and their possible role in the hepatic uptake of bilirubin, sulfobromophthalein, and other anions. *Journal of Clinical Investigation*, **48**, 2156; Deficiency of hepatic organic anion-binding protein as a possible cause of non-haemolytic unconjugated hyperbilirubinaemia in the newborn. (1969) *Lancet*, **2**, 139.
6. Leading Article (1969) Phenobarbitone and dicophane in jaundice. *Lancet*, **2**, 144.
7. OKOLICSANYI, L., MAGNENAT, P. & FREI, J. (1968) Deconjugation of bilirubin glucuronide by the liver. *Lancet*, **1**, 1173.
8. WINTROBE, M. M. *et al.* (1974) *Clinical Hematology*, 7th edn, p. 217. Philadelphia: Lea & Febiger.
9. Leading Article (1974) Management of neonatal jaundice. *British Medical Journal*, **1**, 469.
10. Leading Article (1974) Little light on phototherapy. *Lancet*, **2**, 1056.
11. Leading Article (1974) Oral contraceptives and the liver. *British Medical Journal*, **4**, 430.
12. Leading Article (1974) Halothane and liver damage. *British Medical Journal*, **3**, 589.
13. POWELL, L. W. *et al.* (1967) Idiopathic unconjugated hyperbilirubinemia (Gilbert's syndrome). *New England Journal of Medicine*, **277**, 1108.
14. BLACK, M. & BILLING, B. H. (1969) Hepatic bilirubin UDP-glucuronyl transferase activity in liver disease and Gilbert's syndrome. *New England Journal of Medicine*, **280**, 1266.
15. MALT, R. A., CORRY, R. J. & CHÁVEZ-PEÓN, F. (1968) Umbilical vein cannulation in portal-system disease. *New England Journal of Medicine*, **279**, 930.
16. Leading Article (1972) Bacterial antibodies in liver disease. *Lancet*, **1**, 80.
17. Leading Article (1971) Clarity and confusion in active chronic hepatitis. *British Medical Journal*, **4**, 126.
18. BAGENSTROSS, A. H. *et al.* (1972) Chronic active liver disease. *Human Pathology*, **3**, 183.
19. SCHEUER, P. J. (1977) Chronic hepatitis: a problem for the pathologist. *Histopathology*, **1**, 5.
20. Leading Article (1971) Hepatic hypoglycaemia. *British Medical Journal*, **2**, 416.
21. Leading Article (1971) The astrocyte in liver disease. *Lancet*, **2**, 1189.
22. Leading Article (1976) Endocrine disturbances in chronic hepatic disease. *British Medical Journal*, **2**, 1159.
23. Leading Article (1976) Feminisation in liver disease. *Lancet*, **2**, 408.
24. VAN THIEL, D. H. & LESTER, R. (1976) Sex and alcohol: a second peek. *New England Journal of Medicine*, **295**, 835.
25. Leading Article (1974) Sick cells and hyponatraemia. *Lancet*, **1**, 342.
26. KEW, M. C. *et al.* (1971) Renal and intrarenal blood-flow in cirrhosis of the liver. *Lancet*, **2**, 504.
27. KAPLAN, M. M. (1972) Alkaline phosphatase. *New England Journal of Medicine*, **286**, 200.
28. WIEME, R. J. & DEMEULENAERE, L. (1970) *Journal of Clinical Pathology*, **24**, Supplement (Association of Clinical Pathologists), **4**, 51.

Chapter 48. Amyloidosis

Amyloidosis was first described by Rokitansky in 1842. Virchow, who gave amyloid its name, found that, like the corpora amylacea of the brain, it stained violet with iodine and sulphuric acid, and he attributed this to its cellulose or starch-like nature. The salient feature of amyloidosis is the extracellular deposition of an eosinophilic hyaline material. Occasionally this occurs in an isolated area, but in most instances the deposits are widely distributed, though usually some organs, for example the liver, spleen, and kidneys, are more severely affected than others. The deposits tend to be adjacent to or within the walls of small blood vessels. Amyloid is a relatively inert substance, and its deposition excites little tissue response; rarely there is a foreign-body giant-cell reaction and even calcification in response to it. The parenchyma of the affected organ shows atrophy due perhaps to pressure, but more probably to direct interference with its blood supply.

CLASSIFICATION OF AMYLOIDOSIS[1,2]

The pathogenesis of amyloidosis is not well understood, and there is no acceptable classification which embodies all the known facts. As with tumours it is convenient to use several classifications, each based on a different facet of the disease.

Classification According to Staining Properties

Three empirical staining methods are in common use:

Iodine staining. This may be used either on the specimen itself or on a histological section. Amyloid is coloured mahogany brown, and if sulphuric acid is added may turn violet.

Methyl violet. This is a metachromatic histological stain because, whereas all other tissues become violet, amyloid appears rose pink.

Congo red. This dye is soluble in amyloid and can therefore be used to stain sections: the amyloid stains an orange colour, and when the stained slide is viewed in a polarising microscope a characteristic green birefringence is imparted. Apart from electron microscopy this is the most reliable method available for identifying amyloid.

Various other dyes have been used, but each lacks specificity. The fluorochrome *thioflavine-T* reacts strongly with amyloid, but it has been found to be more useful in demonstrating the juxtaglomerular apparatus of the kidney which also takes up the dye.

Amyloid which reacts characteristically with these stains is called *typical*, while if the stains are negative it is called *atypical*, or sometimes *paramyloid*. This classification is unsatisfactory, since the staining is dependent upon the way the sections are prepared and the precise technique used. Both methyl violet and Congo red stains work better on cryostat sections than on the usual paraffin ones.

Classification According to Organs or Tissues Involved

Typical generalised amyloid. The common type of severe generalised amyloid affects the *liver*, *spleen*, *kidneys*, and sometimes *intestine*, *adrenal*, *lung*, *lymph nodes*, and other sites to a lesser extent. This distribution is described as typical, the amyloid usually stains typically, and it is deposited external to the endothelial cells of the sinusoids and small blood vessels.

Atypical generalised amyloid. A less common severe generalised amyloidosis affects the collagenous connective tissue of heart, blood vessels, tongue, and gastrointestinal tract. The amyloid often shows atypical staining with methyl violet and iodine.

Localised amyloid deposits, or 'tumours'. Localised deposits of amyloid, either single or multiple, may occasionally be found in various sites—urethra, bladder, eye, lung, bronchi, larynx, and skin.

This classification is unsatisfactory because there is a considerable overlap between the various groups.

Classification According to Fibres Associated with Amyloid

It has been postulated that amyloid is deposited in tissue in relationship to pre-existing fibres. On this basis two types are described:

1. Perireticular, as when amyloid is deposited in spleen, liver, and kidney.

2. Pericollagenous, as in amyloid deposited in the adventitia of the blood vessels, heart, etc.

This classification has little to recommend it, since electron microscopy has shown amyloid deposition to be unrelated to collagenous fibrils. Furthermore, the two types described are in fact a reiteration of the classification proposed previously. Perireticular deposition corresponds to the type of amyloid described as of typical distribution, while the pericollagenous type corresponds to the localised tumours and amyloid of generalised atypical distribution.

Classification According to Associated Conditions

This is the most useful classification because the amyloidoses are grouped on a clinical basis.

Senile amyloid. In elderly people it is common to find amyloid in the brain as senile plaques, in the walls of arterioles of the heart, and in the islets of Langerhans. Amyloid may in fact be a substance which is laid down as part of the aging process. In the heart the deposits may lead to heart failure.

Primary amyloid. Amyloid may be deposited without any known preceding factors. Two types are described:

(i) Localised deposits forming tumour-like masses as described previously.

(ii) Generalised amyloidosis. Usually the distribution is atypical: involvement of the heart is sometimes a salient feature. Nevertheless, the typical distribution is not uncommon. In some cases of 'primary' amyloidosis Bence-Jones proteinuria may be found, and it is possible that these are atypical or occult cases of multiple myeloma. A diagnosis of primary amyloidosis should be made only after excluding myeloma, other gammopathies, and the causes of secondary amyloidosis.

Hereditary and familial amyloid.[3] Several syndromes are described:

Familial amyloid polyneuropathy. In the Portuguese type, inherited as an autosomal dominant trait, the amyloid is deposited in the blood-vessel walls of many tissues. The peripheral nerves, especially those of the legs, are affected most severely. Other types of familial polyneuropathy have been described in various parts of the world; each type has its own characteristic features. In some the heart, kidneys, and eyes are involved in addition to the nerves.

Amyloid nephropathy in familial Mediterranean fever. This is inherited as an autosomal recessive trait, and is found in people of Mediterranean stock, especially Sephardic Jews but also Arabs, Turks, and Armenians. Periodic attacks of fever and polyserositis (peritonitis is the most common manifestation) are associated with the development of generalised blood-vessel amyloid deposits. Renal involvement is marked and often leads to death. Curiously enough, the liver is spared.

Familial amyloid heart disease. One family in Denmark has been described.

Urticaria-deafness-nephropathy syndrome. This curious combination was first described in a family in Derbyshire. An urticarial rash and fever in adolescents is followed by deafness, glaucoma, and subsequent death in uraemia.

Familial cutaneous amyloid. Localised deposits of amyloid in the skin have been described in several families.

Lattice corneal dystrophy. This is inherited as a Mendelian dominant trait, and is characterised by the deposition of amyloid leading to progressive corneal opacity.

These various syndromes are rare; indeed, some have been described only in a few patients. Nevertheless, it is obvious that special attention should be paid to genetic factors whenever cases of primary amyloid are encountered.

Secondary amyloidosis. This is the common type of amyloid disease. At one time it was a not infrequent sequel to tertiary syphilis, chronic pulmonary tuberculosis, and chronic suppurative disease such as osteomyelitis and bronchiectasis. These conditions are now extremely uncommon, and amyloidosis is more often seen as a complication of *leprosy*[4] (the lepromatous type), *rheumatoid arthritis*[5] and *ankylosing spondylitis*, *chronic inflammatory bowel disease*, especially Crohn's disease, the *decubitus ulceration* and *suppurative pyelonephritis* that tend to develop in even the best treated victims of paraplegia,[6] and *malignant disease*, particularly carcinoma of the kidney and stomach and Hodgkin's disease. The amyloid disease that occurs in these conditions is usually generalised and of the typical distribution and staining. Nevertheless, involvement of any tissue may be the outstanding or presenting feature, e.g. heart failure or even involvement of the joints.[7]

Amyloidosis associated with multiple myeloma. This is often of atypical distribution and staining, thus closely resembling primary amyloidosis despite being secondary to a neoplastic condition.

Amyloid deposition in tumours. An extensive deposition of amyloid in the stroma of the medullary carcinoma of the thyroid is characteristic of this tumour, which may show a familial pattern and be associated with phaeochromocytoma and parathyroid adenoma as part of the type-2 multiple endocrine adenopathy syndrome (p. 452). Amyloid may also be found in pancreatic islet-cell tumours, and is common in the basal-cell carcinoma of the skin.

Specific Organ Involvement in Amyloid Disease

Spleen. The organ is enlarged and firm. The common type shows a focal distribution. Amyloid is laid down in the walls of the arterioles of the white pulp, and it subsequently replaces the malpighian bodies (Fig. 48.1). The cut surface of the spleen then presents the characteristic appearance of numerous translucent nodules scattered throughout the red pulp (*sago spleen*). A diffuse type of amyloid spleen is also recognised, in which the amyloid is laid down in the walls of the sinuses, and tends to spare the follicles.

Liver. The organ is enlarged, heavy, pale, and firm. Amyloid is deposited in the walls of the sinuses in the space of Disse between the endothelium and the liver cells, at first in the midzone, and later extending to the remainder of the lobule. The liver cells undergo atrophy (Fig. 48.2). The

Figure 48.1
Amyloidosis of spleen. This is part of a 'sago spleen', for the amyloid infiltration is confined to the malpighian bodies. × 160.

Figure 48.2
Amyloidosis of liver. There is an extensive deposition of amyloid in the space of Disse surrounding the sinusoids throughout the liver lobule. The adjacent liver cells are compressed and atrophied. × 120.

clinical effects of amyloidosis of the liver are often remarkably slight even in the presence of marked involvement. Signs of liver failure with an increased plasma bilirubin level may rarely occur; likewise portal hypertension with oesophageal varices has been described.

Kidney. Amyloid is deposited in the glomeruli, in the arterioles, and in the interstitial tissue between the tubules (Figs. 48.3 and 48.4). The organ is usually enlarged and pale, but in longstanding disease secondary ischaemic changes may result in a small scarred kidney. Renal involvement in amyloidosis is common and is the most serious manifestation, since its effects are often the presenting feature as well as the major cause of death. The common result of renal amyloidosis is a *nephrotic syndrome*. *Renal-vein thrombosis* is an occasional terminal manifestation. Persistent haematuria is sometimes seen, and occasionally the involvement of the medulla is sufficient to prevent water reabsorption; a clinical picture of nephrogenic diabetes insipidus then ensues.

Heart. Cardiac involvement is the major manifestation of primary amyloidosis and that which occurs in multiple myeloma. It usually occurs in elderly people. The heart is enlarged and its muscle is extremely rigid and firm. Histologically there is a widespread deposition of amyloid in the interstitial tissue surrounding and replacing muscle fibres as well as in the walls of small blood vessels. Clinically there is cardiomegaly with intractable heart failure. The rigidity of the muscle may lead to the condition mimicking constrictive pericarditis. Heart block and dysrhythmias are common, and

the patients are particularly susceptible to the effect of digitalis.

Gastrointestinal amyloidosis. An involvement of the gastrointestinal tract is common and may affect any part. Enlargement and rigidity of the tongue may cause dysphagia as may also involvement of the oesophagus. Plaque-like lesions of the bowel wall may occur at any level. The effects of gastrointestinal involvement include obstruction, ulceration, malabsorption, haemorrhage, protein loss, and diarrhoea.

Respiratory tract. Amyloidosis of the upper respiratory tract, although not common, may lead to the production of nodules which cause severe effects and even death when they occur in crucial anatomical locations. Amyloidosis of the lungs may produce multiple nodules; alternatively there may be diffuse involvement of the lung parenchyma and tracheobronchial tree. Haemoptysis and respiratory failure may result.

It is evident that the deposition of amyloid in any tissue can produce a variety of effects. The organ may become rigid, and this is particularly important if it has a mechanical function to perform, as for example the tongue or the heart. Amyloidosis produces atrophy of the parenchyma of the tissue, and while in an organ like the liver which has an abundant reserve this is unimportant, in the peripheral nerves the effects are severe. Affected vessels tend to bleed easily and therefore repeated haemorrhages are to be expected; thus purpura is a feature of amyloid deposits in the skin, while epistaxis, haemoptysis, haematemesis, melaena, and haematuria are not uncommonly seen when the respective systems are involved. Since almost any tissue can be affected in amyloidosis the clinical picture may be extremely varied, and the diagnosis should always be kept in mind when one is presented with an unusual case.

Diagnosis of Amyloid Disease in Life

Congo red test. A known quantity of Congo red is injected intravenously, and its concentration in the plasma measured at 4 minutes and again 60 minutes later. If over 80 per cent of the circulating Congo red has been removed from the plasma, amyloid disease may be diagnosed with confidence. Values between 60 and 80 per cent indicate that amyloid is probably present; below 40 per cent the test is negative. As with any test this investigation is not infallible. Furthermore, fatal anaphylactic reactions to Congo red have been reported, and the test is not popular.

Biopsy. Amyloid may be demonstrated in biopsy material obtained from bone marrow, spleen, liver, kidney, and intestine. Since the gastrointestinal tract is frequently involved in most types of amyloidosis, biopsy of the gingiva or rectal mucosa is a useful procedure, and has advantages over other sites in that, should haemorrhage occur, it can readily be controlled. As noted previously, tissue involved with amyloid disease has a tendency to bleed when subjected to trauma.

THE NATURE AND PATHOGENESIS OF AMYLOIDOSIS[1, 8, 9]

The current concept of the nature of amyloid is that it is a protein with a β-pleated configuration but of no fixed composition. Electron microscopy has revealed that amyloid material contains two filamentous components. The major component consists of *fibrils* (Fig. 48.5) that are composed of 1 to

Figure 48.3
Amyloidosis of kidney. Two adjacent glomeruli show almost complete infiltration with amyloid. × 80.

Figure 48.4
Amyloidosis of the kidney. The glomerulus shows extensive deposits of amyloid, but its capillaries are still patent. The cells of the proximal convoluted tubules show numerous hyaline droplets—a manifestation of the heavy proteinuria. × 500.

4 laterally aligned *filaments*, each 7·5 nm in diameter (Fig. 48.6). These filaments are themselves made up of 5 *protofibrils*, each 2·5 to 3·5 nm in diameter (Fig. 48.7). This filamentous structure is comparable to that of some other proteins of the body, for example keratin, and it is not in any way like that of antigen-antibody complexes. The fibrils have been extracted from amyloid and purified. They have the same staining reactions (e.g. with Congo red), and it is currently believed that they constitute the major, essential component of amyloid and are responsible for its unique staining and biological properties.

The second component of amyloid consists of rod-shaped structures, 10 nm in diameter, that are made up of pentagonal subunits piled one on top of another to give the fibre a 4 nm periodicity. These structures have the same chemical composition as an α_1-globulin (P-component) which is normally present in the blood and itself identical to a subunit of the first component of complement (C_1t). The relationship of these fibres to the major fibrillary component is not known, and indeed they may be an incidental constituent in much the same way that other complement components, fibrinogen, ground substance, and other tissue elements are also present to a limited extent in native amyloid.

Amyloid fibrils are very insoluble and resistant to digestion. This insolubility has greatly hindered investigations into their chemical nature. Nevertheless pure preparations of fibrils have been obtained, brought into solution, and subjected to peptide mapping and analysis of the sequence of amino acids in the molecule. Two major chemical types of amyloid have been identified, and both have been shown by X-ray diffraction analysis to have a β-pleated configuration.

Amyloid of immunoglobulin origin. The amyloid of

Figure 48.5
Amyloid-laden rabbit spleen. The amyloid fibrils (A) fill most of the space near the endothelial cell (END), whose plasma membrane bears an intricate relationship to the fibrils, especially in the areas marked by arrows. In several areas (Y) fibrils appear to be intracellular. Osmium-fixed, Epon-embedded tissue, stained with lead citrate. ×24 000. (*From Cohen, A. S.* (1965), in 'International Review of Experimental Pathology' vol. 4, p. 159, eds. Richter, G. W. and Epstein, M. A. New York and London: Academic Press)

Figure 48.6
Amyloid filaments stained negatively with phosphotungstate. In some portions fine linear structures, protofibrils, can be seen either beside the filaments (arrows) or on the filaments (circle) ×200 000. (*From Shirahama, T. and Cohen, A. S.* (1967), Journal of Cell Biology, **33**, 679).

primary amyloidosis, and that which accompanies multiple myeloma, consists of the light chains of immunoglobulin, or part of the light chain—always the amino-terminal fragment with the variable component of the polypeptide chain. Fibres with identical appearance and staining properties to that of native amyloid can be produced *in vitro* by limited proteolytic digestion (by pepsin) of Bence-Jones protein—particularly of the λ type. More recently it has been shown that similar fibrils can be produced by the breakdown of the protein found in patients with heavy-chain disease. The plasma of patients with primary amyloidosis or multiple myeloma contains an M-protein with identical amino-acid sequences to that of the amyloid deposits in that particular patient. As might be expected, amyloidosis is more common in cases of myeloma with λ type Bence-Jones protein than in those with the κ type. It should be noted that in amyloidosis of any type, all the deposits of amyloid present in a particular patient have the same chemical composition, but, of course, differ from the amyloid found in other patients.

Amyloid of unknown origin (AA). The amyloid of secondary amyloidosis, and that which accompanies familial Mediterranean fever, has no amino-acid sequences in common with immunoglobulin and is of unknown origin. It has a β-pleated configuration, and in any individual case there is a circulating plasma component, termed SAA, which is related in composition to the amyloid itself. This SAA may be a circulating precursor of the amyloid fibrils, and is found in all patients with amyloidosis. Indeed, it is found in all normal adults, but its concentration increases with age and also in some chronic diseases, for example tuberculosis, rheumatoid arthritis, and cancer. It has been found that the peptic digestion of many proteins, for example insulin, calcitonin, and glucagon, may yield products that *in vitro* will form typical amyloid fibrils.

It is therefore probable that amyloid fibrils can be formed *in vivo* from a variety of polypeptide fragments, derived either from immunoglobulin or from other protein. It may be that in a chronic destructive disease, such as osteomyelitis or tuberculosis, it is the tissue proteins themselves that provide the raw material for the formation of amyloid protein. It should be noted that some polypeptide fragments are more amyloidogenic than others: thus, as noted previously, the λ light chains form amyloid fibrils more readily than do the κ chains. Under some circumstances the formation of amyloid

Figure 48.7
(A) An amyloid filament about 7·5 mm wide (bottom half of the photomicrograph) has been dispersed into several (probably five) protofibrils (upper half of the picture) by treatment with urea. Negatively stained with phosphotungstate. × 320 000.
(B) A cross-section of an amyloid filament in a positively stained section. It measures 8 to 9 nm in diameter, and consists of five subunits of about 3 nm diameter, which are pentagonally arranged around an electron-lucent core of about 2 nm diameter. × 1 470 000.
(C) Same as (B), but five separate exposures have been given and superimposed on one another. Between each, the negative has been rotated through 72° around an axis in the centre of the filament. This confirms that the filaments contain five peripheral, evenly-spaced subunits. (*From Shirahama, T. and Cohen, A. S.* (1967), Journal of Cell Biology, **33**, 679).

appears to be a local affair and may be related to the partial breakdown of proteins by local reticuloendothelial cells. Thus the localised deposits of amyloid in medullary carcinoma of the thyroid may be derived from calcitonin, while the amyloidosis of the islets of Langerhans, and that found in some islet-cell tumours, could be explained by the formation of fibrils from polypeptide fragments of either insulin or glucagon.

In generalised amyloidosis it seems that an amyloidogenic protein, either immunoglobulin or SAA, is present in the blood-stream and is deposited in various sites. Even under these circumstances it is possible that the reticuloendothelial system plays some part, for the cells of this system could take up immunoglobulins, antigen-antibody complexes, or other proteins and produce the necessary polypeptides for the formation of amyloid fibrils. The raw material may thus be immunoglobulin, other plasma proteins, tissue proteins (perhaps altered in an inflammatory or neoplastic lesion), or exogenous protein (as in the casein-induced amyloidosis of mice).

proteins, and fibrin. It now appears that these are minor constituents, and that the essential component of amyloid is the fibril previously described. Amyloidosis occurs spontaneously in both the human being and animal, and exhibits many patterns of deposition, either localised or generalised. It can easily be induced in animals, for instance by the injection of sodium caseinate into mice. It is now clear that although amyloid has a characteristic appearance in routine paraffin sections and possesses specific staining properties, it cannot be considered to be a single substance. It is composed of proteins of varying chemical composition, but with a common structural configuration of β-pleating. At present two major types of protein have been identified—that of immunoglobulin origin and that of unknown origin—but it is likely that both components are present in many cases of amyloidosis, although in differing proportion. It is evident that instead of regarding amyloidosis as a disease and attempting to subdivide it, it would be more logical to regard amyloid deposition as occurring in a variety of different diseases—the *amyloidoses*.

Much research remains to be done before the reason why amyloid deposition occurs in some patients and not in others, or why it occurs in some sites and not in others, is known. It remains a possibility that amyloid is a normal constituent of the body, and that excessive accumulations occur as a result of defective removal. Experimentally it can be shown that amyloid deposits can be removed if the precipitating cause is withdrawn. However, the process is slow, the deposits in the kidneys being the most persistent. This has its clinical counterpart: amyloidosis of the kidney appears to be a non-reversible process, and it is often the cause of the patient's death.

SUMMARY

The reasons for the recurrent controversies that have raged over the composition and pathogenesis of amyloid disease are now becoming apparent. Amyloid can contain components of immunoglobulin, but it can also be free of them and contain other components. Two ultrastructural components have been identified in native amyloid, and these do not appear to be related to each other. Furthermore, native amyloid contains other components such as ground substance and substances derived from the blood-stream, such as complement, lipo-

REFERENCES

1. COHEN, A. S. (1967) Amyloidosis. *New England Journal of Medicine*, **277**, 522, 574, and 628.
2. STIRLING, G. A. (1975) In *Recent Advances in Pathology*, ed. Harrison, C. V. & Weinbren, K., number 9, p. 249. Edinburgh: Churchill Livingstone.

3. THOMAS, P. K. (1975) Genetic factors in amyloidosis. *Journal of Medical Genetics*, **12**, 317.
4. Leading Article (1975) Amyloidosis and leprosy. *Lancet*, **2**, 589.
5. COHEN, A. S. (1968) Amyloidosis associated with rheumatoid arthritis. *Medical Clinics of North America*, **52**, 643.
6. TRIBE, C. R. & SILVER, J. R. (1969) *Renal Failure in Paraplegia*, p. 54. London: Pitman Medical.
7. Leading Article (1974) Amyloid arthropathy. *British Medical Journal*, **1**, 297.
8. KATZ, A. & PRUZANSKI, W. (1976) Newer concepts in amyloidogenesis. *Canadian Medical Association Journal*, **114**, 872.
9. GLENNER, G. G. & PAGE, D. L. (1976) Amyloid, amyloidosis and amyloidogenesis. *International Review of Experimental Pathology*, **15**, 2.

Chapter 49. The Plasma Proteins

The only proteins of the body that are readily available for study in the human are those of the plasma. Although these, of course, represent but a small fraction of the total protein content of the body, they form an important group for both the pathologist and the clinician since their measurement provides a useful diagnostic aid.[1]

The plasma proteins have been classified in various ways. One approach has been to describe each protein in terms of its physico-chemical structure insofar as this is known. Alternatively, a plasma protein can be described in terms of its known function. Ideally a combination of both methods is used, but in practice this is not always possible.

Separation of Plasma Proteins on the Basis of Physico-Chemical Properties

The name attached to a plasma protein is often a reflection of the method used in its separation and identification. It is instructive therefore to outline how the present rather complex system has been evolved. *Fibrinogen* presents no great problem; it is a protein which during coagulation forms an insoluble fibrin clot. The remaining serum was thought, until the middle of the nineteenth century, to contain a single protein called 'albumin'. It was then shown that by half-saturation with ammonium sulphate, part of this could be precipitated (now called *globulin*) leaving the remainder in solution (the *albumin*). The normal levels are:

Albumin	40–57 g per litre
Globulin	13–30 g per litre
Fibrinogen	1– 5 g per litre
TOTAL	62–82 g per litre

A simple method of subdividing the globulin fraction depends upon *solubility in distilled water*. The *pseudoglobulins* are soluble, but the *euglobulins* are insoluble. This method of fractionation is not much used. A more complex separation was devised by Cohn. It involves the precipitation of many fractions by alteration of temperature and pH, and with differing ethanol concentrations. The method is used commercially for the preparation of plasma components.

For clinical practice a more useful separation is obtained by *electrophoresis*: many different components can be separated, but for most purposes recognition of albumin and the α_1, α_2, β, and γ-globulin fractions is sufficient (Fig. 1.7, p. 7). Many more components can be detected by the technique of immuno-electrophoresis (see Fig. 1.8, p. 8).

Molecular size has also been investigated. Fibrinogen has a molecular weight of 400 000 daltons, albumin 65 000 daltons, and the globulins range from 45 000 to several million daltons. A further separation can be made by means of the *ultracen-trifuge*. When human serum is centrifuged, three main components can be sedimented:

THE 4S FRACTION. This consists of albumin, the β-globulins, and some of the α-globulins.

THE 7S FRACTION. Composed by γ-globulins.

THE 19S FRACTION. Composed of α-globulins and γ-globulins.

The rapidly sedimenting material in the 19S fraction consists of large molecules, which are therefore called the *macroglobulins*.

Some proteins precipitate out of solution in the cold. These are called *cryoglobulins*.[2] Finally, some proteins may contain lipid or carbohydrate. The former are called *lipoproteins*, and the latter *glycoproteins*. These may also be divided electrophoretically into the conventional globulin fractions.

Separation of Plasma Proteins on the Basis of their Function[1]

Many proteins, or groups of proteins, can be recognised by virtue of their function:

Immunoglobulins. These proteins have antibody activity and have been described in Chapter 12. Most of them are γ-globulins, but some fall within the α and β range on electrophoresis. They may be further characterised by precipitin and other reactions as well as by the composition of their polypeptide chains.

The Proteins Concerned with Clotting.

The Proteins Concerned with Fibrinolysis.

The Components of Complement.

Hormones, e.g. of the anterior lobe of the pituitary.

Enzymes, e.g. alkaline phosphatase.

Carrier Proteins, e.g. caeruloplasmin (copper), transferrin (iron), haptoglobins (haemoglobin), haemopexin (haem), thyroxine-binding globulin, and corticosteroid-binding globulin. Albumin itself has an important carrier role, e.g. bilirubin, free fatty acid, and sulphonamides and many other drugs. The water-insoluble lipids, e.g. cholesterol and phospholipids, are combined with globulins to form the lipoproteins (see later).

It is evident from the above account that an individual protein may be described and named in various ways: a single substance can be labelled a macroglobulin, immunoglobulin, glycoprotein, β_2-globulin, or 19S-globulin.

Source of the Plasma Proteins[2]

The principal plasma proteins are all made in the liver, with the notable exception of the immunoglobulins, the protein hormones, and some enzymes. This has been elegantly demonstrated by experiments which showed that an isolated perfused rat's liver incorporated radioactive-labelled lysine into plasma albumin, α-globulin, β-globulin, and fibrinogen.

In the eviscerated rat, however, labelled lysine was incorporated into the γ-globulins, and to a lesser extent into the β-globulins, but not into the albumin.

The plasma immunoglobulins of the normal newborn child are of maternal origin, and their level diminishes after birth. Production of antibodies does not normally commence for some weeks (pp. 141 and 164).

Fate of the Plasma Proteins

There is a regular turnover of the plasma proteins but the sites of catabolism are poorly defined. The liver and probably other organs are concerned with the breakdown of γ-globulin, and there is good evidence that albumin is secreted into the gastrointestinal tract where it is broken down and its constituent amino acids reabsorbed.

Abnormalities of Plasma Proteins

There are three types of abnormality of any protein group. The level may either be raised or lowered, or else an abnormal form of the protein may be present. The term *dysproteinaemia* indicates that there is an imbalance between the proportions of the various plasma proteins. It is generally used to describe the conditions where the changes are marked, as when an M protein is present, or where a major component is absent (see dysgammaglobulinaemia, p. 171).

ALBUMIN

Albumin is the principal protein synthesised by the liver, and is passed directly into the blood stream.[3]

Hypoalbuminaemia

During *starvation* the protein reserves are metabolised, and the plasma protein level falls. This principally affects the albumin, the globulins remaining little altered. During *acute infections* and following *trauma* or *surgery* the albumin level drops due to its increased catabolism. This is accompanied by a rise in the α-globulins (especially the α_2-globulin), fibrinogen, and haptoglobin, and the appearance of C-reactive protein (see p. 581). This *acute reaction to stress* is nonspecific, and is probably mediated by the release of adrenal hormones. In *chronic liver disease* like cirrhosis, the plasma albumin falls due to a failure in its manufacture.

A low plasma albumin is also found whenever there is an excessive loss, e.g. the *nephrotic syndrome*, with rapidly accumulating exudates, and following haemorrhage and severe injury.

An uncommon cause of hypoproteinaemia is the syndrome of *protein-losing gastroenteropathy*.[4–6] Clinically this is characterised by oedema and a low plasma albumin level, but with no obvious source of protein loss. The syndrome is associated with a variety of local gastrointestinal lesions, e.g. gastric cancer, hypertrophic gastritis, Whipple's disease, Crohn's disease, steatorrhoea, ulcerative colitis, and intolerance to milk, and their cure may lead to its correction. Sometimes no such lesion is found, but instead the jejunum shows uniform thickening due to oedema. The lymphatics are dilated, and the gut wall is brown due to the presence of pigment within the muscle fibres and the phagocytes between the fibres (see

p. 591). Tracer techniques using [131]I- and ^{51}Cr-labelled albumin demonstrate the gastrointestinal loss, but the relationship between this and the organic lesions listed above is not clear.

The preponderance of albumin together with its low molecular weight makes this protein an important factor in the maintenance of the non-crystalloid osmotic pressure in plasma. A low plasma albumin level therefore contributes to oedema formation (see Ch. 43).

Analbuminaemia has been described as a rare genetic metabolic error. Curiously enough, symptoms (e.g. oedema) are remarkably slight.

Hyperalbuminaemia is seen in haemoconcentration.

Bisalbuminaemia.[7] In this rare condition, of which there are several variants, the plasma shows two closely adjacent peaks of albumin on electrophoresis instead of the usual one. In fact at least 11 variants of albumin have been found on electrophoresis, and are inherited as autosomal co-dominants. There is yet another form of inherited albumin variation, in which part of the albumin exists as a dimer.

THE GLOBULINS[8]

The globulins include a wide array of plasma proteins. The immunoglobulins form a major component, being present in the γ fraction and to a lesser extent the α and β. The normal level appears to be maintained by contact with micro-organisms. Thus in germ-free rats the γ-globulin level is reduced to about one-fifth. The α_2 and β fractions are also lowered. When the intestinal flora of such animals is restored, the plasma proteins return to normal. It is probable that even non-living antigens in the diet can stimulate antibody production.

Agammaglobulinaemia and **hypogammaglobulinaemia** are described in Chapter 13, since they are associated with various immunologically deficient states.

Hypergammaglobulinaemia

The immunoglobulins form the major component of the plasma globulin, and it follows that hyperglobulinaemia is invariably due to an increase in this fraction. Two main patterns are described.

Polyclonal gammopathy. This occurs whenever there is a prolonged and marked immune response, and is therefore common in chronic infections, e.g. tuberculosis, chronic osteomyelitis, leprosy, and kala-azar. It is also a feature of certain diseases which have an autoimmune component, such as systemic lupus erythematosus and rheumatoid arthritis. Whether this is part of the explanation of the hyperglobulinaemia of hepatic cirrhosis, chronic active hepatitis, and sarcoidosis is not known. Hypergammaglobulinaemia occasionally develops in the absence of detectable disease and is then labelled idiopathic.

The electrophoretic pattern in these conditions is that of a broad-based elevation of the γ globulins as well as some increase in the β and even the α fractions. There is an increase in many classes of immunoglobulin, and it is assumed that many clones of antibody-forming cells are involved, hence the term polyclonal gammopathy. A rise in the globulin level is sometimes seen when there is a marked hypoalbuminaemia, as in analbuminaemia and the nephrotic syndrome. In the latter there is sometimes a marked increase in the α_2 fraction, and this may simulate an M protein.[9]

Monoclonal gammopathy. In some cases of hyperglobulinaemia there is a marked increase in the level of one type of globulin, which appears as a heavy, narrow band on electrophoresis, or as a spike when the result is expressed graphically. The protein is homogeneous, and contains one type of heavy chain and one type of light chain. It is therefore postulated that only one clone of cells is involved in its production. The condition occurs commonly in *multiple myeloma*, Waldenström's *macroglobulinaemia*, as well as in a few cases of *malignant lymphoma*. The term *M protein** is aptly applied, but some writers use the term *paraprotein*, on the assumption that the protein is an abnormal one. In fact it is not known whether the appearance of an M protein is due to the production of an abnormal protein, or to the overproduction of one present normally but in low concentration.

Characteristics of the M proteins. An M protein belongs to one of the five classes of immunoglobulin, and is homogeneous in that it contains only one type of light chain. In the latter respect it differs from normal immunoglobulins, which occur as mixtures of K and L types. Rarely an M band consists of only light or heavy chains.

Effects of hypergammaglobulinaemia. Hypergammaglobulinaemia generally presents itself as a biochemical abnormality which requires further investigation. The patient's symptoms are those of the primary disease—commonly a tumour of lymphoid tissue or a myeloma when an M protein is present. Sometimes, however, the plasma-protein abnormality may directly lead to secondary effects:

Hyperviscosity syndrome.[10] The presence of a high concentration of protein, especially a macroglobulin, increases the viscosity of the blood and impedes the peripheral circulation. In the eye the retinal veins are dilated, and characteristically there are localised narrowings which give a 'link-sausage' appearance. Haemorrhage is common. Sudden paresis may occur, and can progress to coma and death when the cerebral vessels are involved. The heart, kidney, and digits may also suffer, and prompt and repeated plasmapheresis is indicated.

Cryoglobulinaemia. The presence of proteins which precipitate when the plasma is cooled may lead to Raynaud's syndrome through vascular blockage in the extremities. When the skin is involved, purpuric lesions appear. Cryoglobulinaemia has been described in macroglobulinaemia, multiple myeloma, kala-azar, malaria, systemic lupus erythematosus, and other connective-tissue diseases, all of which are associated with hypergammaglobulinaemia. Cryoglobulins may consist of immune complexes. Cryoglobulinaemia may also occur as an isolated idiopathic condition.

Haemolytic anaemia. Cold agglutinins directed against the I red-cell antigen are not uncommon in mycoplasmal and other infections, but they rarely lead to trouble. In macroglobulinaemia and lymphocytic lymphoma the antibody activity can be sufficiently marked to produce a severe haemolytic anaemia.

Bence-Jones proteinuria. The massive Bence-Jones proteinuria of multiple myeloma may so overload the resorptive capacity of the renal tubules that these structures are damaged. Protein casts form in the tubules, obstruct the lumen,

*It is not to be confused with the M protein of *Stept. pyogenes*.

and provoke a foreign-body reaction. The renal damage of multiple myeloma is due partly to this lesion, but other factors are also involved (p. 627).

Protein interactions. Abnormal proteins may interact and bind to other plasma components, such as calcium, platelets, and the proteins of the clotting system. A bleeding tendency may ensue.

Susceptibility to infection. Although M proteins belong to the immunoglobulins chemically, they have little if any antibody activity. Indeed, the production of antibody immunoglobulin is often inhibited, and this leads to an increased tendency to infection. Multiple myeloma often terminates in this manner.

Conditions under which M proteins are found. M proteins are found most commonly in *multiple myeloma* and *Waldenström's macroglobulinaemia*. In these two diseases there is an abnormal proliferation of cells of the plasma-cell series. Recently a third member has been added—*the heavy-chain diseases*. These are described below. In addition, M proteins may occur in other lymphoreticular proliferative disorders, most commonly lymphatic leukaemia. Occasional cases are encountered in which two or more M proteins are present in the same patient. These biclonal or triclonal gammopathies usually progress to a monoclonal state. Presumably one type of neoplastic cell replaces the others.

The routine screening of large numbers of sera has revealed subjects who have none of the diseases mentioned, but in whom an M protein is present. Some have other diseases, e.g. carcinoma, hepatic cirrhosis, or a collagen disease, while others appear healthy. In this latter group a number of cases subsequently develop multiple myeloma or macroglobulinaemia, but the residue remains healthy and has been called 'essential monoclonal benign hypergammaglobulinaemia'. Some cases appear to be familial. The level of M protein is generally low, and neither albumin nor normal γ-globulin is greatly reduced. Bence-Jones protein is not present in the urine, and the IgM is all present in a 19S form, there being no 7S IgM present. These features help to distinguish the benign condition from the malignant varieties, but a careful follow-up is essential.

Multiple Myeloma

Multiple myeloma is characterised by a neoplastic proliferation of the plasma-cell series. These cells produce an M protein which is usually of the IgG type (55 per cent of cases) or IgA (23 per cent). IgD type protein occurs in about 1 per cent of cases, while IgE myeloma is extremely rare, and in about 20 per cent of cases there are only light chains without a complete M protein in the plasma. By investigating myeloma proteins the classes of immunoglobulin have been delineated. IgD was discovered thus.

About 50 per cent of the patients excrete Bence-Jones protein in the urine. This substance has a molecular weight of about 22 000 daltons, and consists of light chains which are of the same type as those present in the M protein. It is recognised by its property of precipitating in urine heated to a temperature of 60 to 80°C, and then redissolving at higher temperatures. When cooled, it precipitates through the same temperature range, and then redissolves. Bence-Jones protein is produced by the myeloma cells, and since in any one patient it is homogeneous, the urine of patients with this disease is an invaluable source of light-chain polypeptide for chemical analysis.

Macroglobulinaemia of Waldenström

This condition is characterised by anaemia, hyperviscosity syndrome, and a tendency to haemorrhages from mucous membranes, especially the gingivae, either spontaneously or after dental extraction. Retinal haemorrhages also occur. Generalised lymphadenopathy, hepatomegaly, and splenomegaly are common. The disease is closely related to chronic lymphatic leukaemia, but it usually runs a more prolonged course than that condition and appears to be more benign. The serum has remarkable features: it is viscous, the globulin level is very high, and the albumin low. When a drop is allowed to sink in a cylinder of water, a heavy precipitate of euglobulin is formed (Fig. 49.1). This simple water dilution test is not specific, for it is also positive in some other hyperglobulinaemias, e.g. kala-azar. It is also called the *Sia test*. The ultracentrifuge shows a high level of macroglobulin due to the presence of an M protein of the IgM class. Monomer 7S IgM may also be found in the plasma both in this disease and in other examples of malignant monoclonal macroglobulinaemia.[11] Microscopically, the lymph nodes and bone marrow are crowded with lymphocytes or atypical plasma cells.

Heavy-Chain Disease[12,13]

The first of this group of diseases to be described was the γ variant, and was recorded by Franklin. It is characterised by painful enlargement of the lymph nodes with fever, splenomegaly, hepatomegaly, and recurrent bacterial infections. An odd feature is transient, though sometimes severe, oedema and erythema of the palate, accompanied by enlargement of the nodes of Waldeyer's ring, similar to that seen in infectious mononucleosis. In this condition, unlike multiple myeloma, skeletal lesions are not found, but the bone marrow and lymph nodes are crowded with atypical plasma cells. Both the serum and urine contain an abnormal peak on electrophoresis, which is in the fast γ or slow β region. It consists of a fragment of the γ chain resembling the Fc fragment (p. 142).

α heavy-chain disease is more common than γ heavy-chain disease, and was originally described in North Africa and in countries bordering on the Mediterranean in association with Mediterranean lymphoma—a malignant infiltrate of the intestinal tract consisting of lymphocytes and plasma cells and characterised by abdominal pain, malabsorption, steatorrhoea, and clubbing of the fingers. The disease has now been described in most countries and occurs in a younger age-group than the γ variant. Repeated remissions can occur with antibiotic and chemotherapeutic agents.

μ heavy-chain disease generally accompanies chronic lymphatic leukaemia. Bence-Jones protein is found in the urine, a point of difference from the other two types of heavy-chain disease.

C-reactive protein is so named because it reacts as a precipitin with the C-polysaccharide of the pneumococcus. Described originally as occurring in human serum in cases of

Figure 49.1
The water-dilution test. Left: normal serum; centre: macroglobulinaemic serum; right: kala-azar serum. Note the precipitation of euglobulin. (*From Waldenström, J.* (1958), Triangle, Sandoz Journal of Medical Science, **3**, 262).

pneumonia, it is found also in infections due to other organisms, in rheumatoid arthritis, and following trauma. The significance of this is not known. Its appearance is closely related to a rise in the ESR.

Genetic Variation in the Plasma Proteins[8]

The formation of the plasma proteins, like that of other proteins, is determined by genetic factors, and it is therefore not surprising that sometimes the structure of a protein of one person differs slightly from that of another. This variation, or polymorphism, may be detected by electrophoresis or immunoelectrophoresis, and although the various types of a particular protein do not seem to differ functionally, their detection is of considerable interest in anthropological studies. Some examples have already been described. Thus with the immunoglobulins, variations occur in both light and heavy chains, and are determined by alleles at each of the independent loci *Gm* and *Inv* (p. 143). Bisalbuminaemia is noted on page 579. Other examples are known in the group-specific component, haptoglobin, and transferrin (see below).

The group-specific component.[8,14] The α_2-globulin band contains several fractions whose function is unknown. Amongst these is a protein which shows polymorphism. This is the group-specific component, and its variants are directed by the genes Gc^1 and Gc^2 to give the three common phenotypes Gc 1-1 (fast), Gc 2-2 (slow), and Gc 2-1 (in which both fast and slow components are present).

Haptoglobin.[8] Three main types are known, Hp 1-1, Hp 2-1, and Hp 2-2, and are determined by the two alleles Hp^1

and Hp^2. Haptoglobin has the property of binding any free haemoglobin which is released in the circulation, and is further described on p. 606.

Transferrin.[8] The iron in plasma is bound to a β-globulin called transferrin, or siderophilin: each molecule binds two atoms of ferric iron. No less than seventeen variants are known and can be distinguished by their mobilities in starch-gel electrophoresis.

GLYCOPROTEINS[15,16]

The glycoproteins are proteins other than nucleoproteins, which contain more than 1 per cent of sugar. Certain well-known proteins, e.g. prothrombin, caeruloplasmin, haptoglobins, and the 19S macroglobulins, are included in this group, as are also some hormones—gonadotrophin, thyroid-stimulating hormone, and thyroglobulin. In general the carbohydrate is firmly bound to the protein, in contrast to the acid mucopolysaccharide-protein complex of connective tissue mucoproteins, which are only loosely bound. The plasma level of glycoproteins is raised in many conditions, including cancer, rheumatoid arthritis, acute rheumatic fever, and tuberculosis; the reason for this is unknown.

Glycoproteins are important components of the ground substance. They are not sulphated nor do they contain uronic acid, and have on this account been called neutral mucoproteins. However, this is a misnomer, because they contain the nine-carbon amino sugar sialic acid, which gives them acidic properties. Epithelial mucins and the blood-group substances belong to this general group.

LIPOPROTEINS[17,18]

The lipids of the blood form a heterogeneous group which includes phospholipids (such as lecithin), cholesterol and its esters, neutral fat (glyceryl triesters), free fatty acids, carotenoids, vitamin A, and vitamin E. They are carried in the blood as complexes with each other and with certain plasma proteins. Four proteins are involved:

Albumin, which is the carrier of free fatty acids.

The apoproteins. The apolipoproteins, usually shortened to apoproteins, form a group of proteins that occur in various concentrations and combinations to form the protein component of the lipoproteins. At least six have been characterised chemically, and their classification is under review.

The lipoproteins have been separated and characterised by three important techniques:

Chemical Analysis.

Density, as quantitated in the ultracentrifuge and measured in Svedberg units of flotation (Sf).

Electrophoresis.

Lipoproteins Found in the Blood

Free fatty acid is mostly combined with the albumin. This fraction is derived from the adipose tissues, and is the form in which lipid is transported from the fat depots to the tissues.

Chylomicrons. These are particles, over 0·1 μm in diameter, which on electrophoresis do not migrate from the point of application. They have a high neutral fat (triglyceride) content, and are formed in the intestine following the absorption of dietary fat.

Low density lipoproteins (density 1·006 to 1·063, Sf 0 to 20). These are β-lipoproteins and contain much cholesterol.

Very low density lipoproteins (density less than 1·006, Sf 20 to 400+). This fraction appears on paper electrophoresis between the α and the β bands. It is called the *pre-β-lipoprotein* fraction and contains much triglyceride of endogenous origin. It is made in the liver from carbohydrate or lipid sources, and is the form in which triglyceride is transported in the fasting individual.

High density lipoproteins (density 1·063 to 1·21). These are the α-lipoproteins and contain much phospholipid and fatty acid.

Abnormalities of the Plasma Lipoproteins

Hyperlipoproteinaemia is a common finding and indicates an increase in the level of one or more of the lipoprotein fractions described above. In *hypercholesterolaemia* there is an increase in the cholesterol content, due to a raised level of β-lipoproteins or the 'broad beta' lipoprotein (see below).

Two major groups of hyperlipoproteinaemia are recognised:

Primary, or familial, hyperlipoproteinaemia.

Secondary hyperlipoproteinaemia, in which the lipid abnormality is associated with some disease which is presumed to be its cause.

The first satisfactory subdivision of each group was that proposed by Fredrickson.[17] Five types, or patterns, were recognised, based on the lipoprotein fraction which was elevated. This classification has subsequently been modified by a committee of the WHO, which subdivided the original Type II into two subgroups depending on whether the elevated level of low-density lipoprotein occurred alone or was accompanied by an additional elevation of very low-density lipoprotein.[18,19] The memorandum also drew attention to a previously poorly-defined lipoprotein—the *sinking pre-β-lipoprotein*. This has pre-β mobility on electrophoresis, but unlike normal pre-β-lipoprotein, it has a density of 1·050 to 1·080 and is therefore relatively heavy. Its presence is unrelated to any hyperlipoproteinaemia and is found in about 11 per cent of subjects. It must be taken into account when interpreting the results of lipoprotein analyses. The current classification, which like its predecessor is to be regarded as provisional, is as follows:

Type I. Elevated chylomicron level.

Type II. (a) Elevated β-lipoproteins.

(b) Elevated β-lipoprotein and pre-β-lipoprotein.

Type III. Presence of an abnormal lipoprotein which appears as a broad band in the β region ('broad beta'). It is rich in both cholesterol and triglyceride, and is therefore of lower density than normal β-lipoprotein. It is also called 'floating beta' for this reason.

Type IV. Elevated pre-β-lipoproteins.

Type V. Elevated chylomicrons and pre-β-lipoproteins.

So far as the **primary group** is concerned, the five types have been recognised. Thus *type I*, or *familial fat-induced hyperlipaemia* is characterised by a raised triglyceride level, and there is a creamy, lipaemic plasma. It is a disease of infancy, and recurrent abdominal pain and pancreatitis are common. *Type II*, or *familial hyper-β-lipoproteinaemia* is the most common variety, and has a high plasma cholesterol. In this type, and also in types III and IV, there is a tendency for the patients to develop atherosclerosis at an early age.[20] They should therefore be remembered when a young person develops occlusive arterial disease or myocardial ischaemia. In all varieties of familial hyperlipoproteinaemia there is a tendency for focal collections of foam cells to occur in the skin or tendons. *Xanthomata* are therefore common particularly in type III. Eruptive xanthomata of the skin are invariably associated with a raised blood triglyceride level, and are therefore seen in types I and V.

It must be stressed that the lipoprotein pattern of an individual depends, to a considerable extent, on the diet immediately preceding the test. Abnormal patterns may be produced by an abnormal diet even in the absence of genetic error or associated disease. Before testing the lipoproteins therefore, a patient must be on a standard, reasonable diet and have the blood drawn after a sixteen-hour fast.[20] Types III, IV, and V have been called carbohydrate induced, because the abnormal lipid pattern is related to carbohydrate in the diet. An abnormal glucose tolerance is present, and there is often a family history of diabetes mellitus.

In **secondary hyperlipoproteinaemia**, apart from type III, the same spectrum of lipoprotein patterns is found. Thus, in obstructive jaundice there is an increase in plasma cholesterol and β-lipoproteins, whereas in diabetes mellitus it is the chylomicrons and pre-β-lipoproteins that are elevated. Other diseases characterised by hyperlipoproteinaemia are acute alcoholism, pancreatitis, hypothyroidism, and the nephrotic syndrome. As with the primary group the lipid pattern is influenced by diet, and there may be a change from one type to another.

Apart from correlating the various types of hyperlipoproteinaemia with the presence of arterial disease and various types of xanthomata, the classification is useful because it indicates a line of treatment.[18] Thus, if there is an increase in the level of chylomicrons containing triglyceride of exogenous origin, as in types I and V, limitation of dietary fat is indicated. If the pre-β-lipoprotein is elevated, as in type IV, carbohydrate restriction is likely to be effective. In hypercholesterolaemia (Types II) treatment with drugs is often necessary. In mixed types, IIb, III, and V, a combination of methods is required.

Lipoprotein Deficiency Syndromes

Three conditions are known in which one or more of the lipoproteins are either absent or in very low concentration. They are usually detected by the finding of a low plasma cholesterol level, a feature common to all three.

Tangier disease, or *familial alpha-lipoprotein deficiency*.[21] In this rare disease, named after Tangier Island (in Chesapeake Bay), which was the home of the first recognised case, there is an absence of the normal high-density, α-lipoprotein fraction. An abnormal, high-density lipoprotein is present in low con-

centration. Cholesterol esters are stored in the RE system, and this storage is responsible for the remarkable enlargement of the tonsils which have a characteristic orange colour—a unique and virtually diagnostic sign. Disabling peripheral neuropathy may develop later.

Abetalipoproteinaemia.[22] This syndrome is characterised by steatorrhoea, crenation of the red cells, retinitis pigmentosa, and cerebellar ataxia. The low-density lipoproteins, the very low-density lipoproteins, and the chylomicrons are absent.

Hypobetalipoproteinaemia. This condition has been described in several families, and is symptomless. The level of low-density lipoproteins is low.

THE ERYTHROCYTE SEDIMENTATION RATE (ESR)

When a column of blood mixed with anticoagulant is allowed to stand vertically, the red cells steadily gravitate downwards because their density is greater than that of plasma. The speed at which this sedimentation occurs is dependent upon many complex factors, chief of which are the degree of rouleaux formation and the extent of sludging. Both these phenomena are related to the composition of the plasma rather than to any change in the red cells themselves. Any increase in the plasma content of high-molecular-weight substances is found to increase the ESR. Thus an increase in fibrinogen or globulin (especially α and β fractions) has this effect; the 7S γ-globulins are the least effective, while excess albumin delays red-cell sedimentation. For this reason a raised ESR is particularly characteristic of macroglobulinaemia and myeloma, and also follows the infusion of high-molecular-weight dextrans. It is also raised in conditions of hypoalbuminaemia, e.g. the nephrotic syndrome.

The ESR is higher in normal women than in men, and it shows a significant rise with age. The upper limits of normal by the Westergren method may be taken as 15 mm per hour for men and 20 mm for women under the age of 50 years and 20 mm and 30 mm respectively for those over that age.[23,24] It is usually raised during infection and following tissue necrosis, e.g. myocardial infarction. Presumably an alteration in the balance between the plasma components is responsible, but the factors concerned are ill-defined. A raised ESR is usually accompanied by the appearance of C-reactive protein. The non-specific nature of the ESR limits its value in diagnosis, but nevertheless it is a useful investigation.

The presence of a raised ESR must always be taken to indicate disease, if anaemia and pregnancy are excluded—oral contraceptives are reported to raise it slightly.[25] However, a normal ESR does not rule out organic lesions. It is of value in following the course of a known disease, e.g. tuberculosis and rheumatoid arthritis.

It should be noted that the Westergren method is generally regarded as more meaningful than the Wintrobe method. For an account of various technical difficulties which attend the performance of the ESR a text book of haematology should be consulted.

GENERAL READING

PUTNAM, F. W. (1965) In *The Proteins*, 2nd edn, Vol. III, pp. 153–267. Ed. Neurath, H. New York & London: Academic Press.

REFERENCES

1. ALPER, C. A. (1974) Plasma protein measurements as a diagnostic aid. *New England Journal of Medicine*, **291**, 287.
2. HAUROWITZ, F. (1961) In *Functions of the Blood*, p. 527, ed. Macfarlane R. G. & Robb-Smith, A. H. T. Oxford: Blackwell.
3. ROTHSCHILD, M. A., ORATZ, M. & SCHREIBER, S. S. (1972) Albumin synthesis. *New England Journal of Medicine*, **286**, 748 and 816.
4. JARNUM, S. (1963) *Protein-Losing Gastroenteropathy*. Oxford: Blackwell.
5. DAWSON, A. M. (1965) In *Recent Advances in Gastroenterology*, p. 126 (Protein-losing enteropathy), ed. Badenoch, J. & Brooke, B. N. London: Churchill.
6. Leading Article (1967) Allergic gastroenteropathy. *British Medical Journal*, **3**, 510.
7. STANBURY, J. B., WYNGAARDEN, J. B. & FREDRICKSON, D. S. (1972) *The Metabolic Basis of Inherited Disease*, 3rd edn, p. 1629. New York: McGraw-Hill.
8. WALDMANN, T. A. (1969) Disorders of immunoglobulin metabolism. *New England Journal of Medicine*, **281**, 1170.
9. SUNDERMAN, F. W. (1964) In *Serum Proteins and the Dysproteinaemias*, p. 324, ed. Sunderman, F. W. & Sunderman, F. W. Jr. Philadelphia: Lippincott.
10. Leading Article (1971) Hyperviscosity syndrome. *British Medical Journal*, **2**, 184.
11. CARTER, P. M. & HOBBS, J. R. (1971) Clinical significance of 7S IgM in monoclonal IgM disease. *British Medical Journal*, **2**, 260.
12. FRANKLIN, E. C. (1970) Heavy-chain diseases. *New England Journal of Medicine*, **282**, 1098.
13. FRANKLIN, E. C. (1976) Some impacts of clinical investigation on immunology. *New England Journal of Medicine*, **294**, 531.
14. CLEVE, H. & BEARN, A. G. (1961) Inherited variations in human serum proteins: studies of the group-specific component. *Annals of the New York Academy of Sciences*, **94**, 218.
15. SHETLAR, M. R. (1961) Serum glycoproteins: their origin and significance. *Annals of the New York Academy of Sciences*, **94**, 44.
16. HEISKELL, C. L. *et al.* (1961) Serum glycoproteins in infectious and inflammatory diseases. *Annals of the New York Academy of Sciences*, **94**, 183.
17. FREDRICKSON, D. S., LEVY, R. I. & LEES, R. S. (1967) Fat transport in lipoproteins—an integrated approach to mechanisms and disorders. *New England Journal of Medicine*, **276**, 34, 94, 148, 215 and 273.
18. LEHMANN, H. & LINES, J. G. (1972) Hyperlipoproteinaemia classification: the optimum routine electrophoretic system and its relevance to treatment. *Lancet*, **1**, 557.
19. Leading Article (1971) Hyperlipoproteinaemias. *Lancet*, **2**, 806.
20. Leading Article (1971) Congenital hyperlipoproteinaemias and ischaemic heart-disease. *Lancet*, **1**, 117.
21. FREDRICKSON, D. S. (1972) Tonsils, apolipoproteins and enzymes. *New England Journal of Medicine*, **286**, 601.
22. OCKNER, R. K. (1971) Abetalipoproteinemia: rarity and relevance. *New England Journal of Medicine*, **284**, 848.
23. BÖTTIGER, L. E. & SVEDBERG, C. A. (1967) Normal erythrocyte sedimentation rate and age. *British Medical Journal*, **2**, 85.
24. BOYD, R. V. & HOFFBRAND, B. I. (1966) Erythrocyte sedimentation rate in elderly hospital in-patients. *British Medical Journal*, **1**, 901.
25. BURTON, J. L. (1967) Effect of oral contraceptives on erythrocyte sedimentation rate in healthy young women. *British Medical Journal*, **3**, 214.

Chapter 50. *Pigments of the Body and their Disorders*

The pigments of biological origin are frequently striking and of brilliant colour. Less marked in human beings than in many animals, they nevertheless exhibit obvious abnormalities in disease processes.[1,2]

The common pigments in the human body, e.g. melanin and haemoglobin, are manufactured by specialised cells: they are therefore termed *endogenous*, in contrast to other pigments, e.g. carbon and β-carotene, which are absorbed entire and are called *exogenous*.

Superficially satisfying, this classification is somewhat arbitrary, because exogenous pigments undergo some modification in the tissues. A good example of this is mercurial pigmentation, which is generally classified as exogenous. It is, in fact, produced after the absorbed mercury has been converted into mercuric sulphide.

In this chapter only the more important pigments will be considered in detail. Three main groups are found: the melanins, pigments derived from haemoglobin, and those associated with fat.

THE MELANINS[3]

Melanin gives colour to hair, skin, and the eye. It is also present in the leptomeninges, adrenal medulla, and certain nerve cells, e.g. those of the substantia nigra and the locus caeruleus. Limited areas of pigmentation are frequent in the juxtacutaneous mucous membranes, e.g. mouth and vagina, and are most obvious in dark-skinned individuals.

The pigment usually colours the tissue yellow-brown or, when in large quantities, black. It appears microscopically as brown intracellular granules. Under certain conditions its dispersion and situation may be such that it appears blue or even green.[1] This occurs in the iris of fair-haired individuals, in the sexual skin of certain baboons, and most strikingly of all in many fish.* Melanin reduces an ammoniacal silver-nitrate solution to metallic silver, and is stained black in a section. This forms the basis of the Masson–Fontana method. It is bleached by oxidising agents, such as hydrogen peroxide and potassium permanganate.

The function of melanin in nature appears to be largely protective. This is well exemplified by the 'ink' of the cuttle-fish and the changing colour of the chameleon. In the human subject the melanin of skin protects against sunlight. Thus the effects of sunlight are less severe in dark-skinned individuals than in the White races.

Site of melanin formation. In skin, melanin is formed in *melanocytes* or their precursors, the *melanoblasts*. These are

*Fish have additional reflecting cells, or iridocytes. These contain guanin instead of melanin, and are responsible for the beautiful iridescent metallic sheen of many fish.[1]

derived from the neural crest and migrate during development to their definitive position. In H. and E. sections of skin they appear as large clear cells in the basal layer of the epidermis, but special staining techniques reveal that they possess dendritic processes with which they make contact with a group of epithelial cells. It is through these processes that melanin is donated to the basal cells of the epidermis, which are thereby pigmented. A melanocyte and the group of keratinocytes with which it is associated is termed an *epidermal melanin unit*. The dermis of normal skin may also contain pigmented macrophages, or *melanophores*, which contain melanin but cannot produce it.

Melanocytes contain enzymes capable of bringing about the formation of melanin from tyrosine (see Fig. 50.1). The best defined of these is tyrosinase, a copper-containing enzyme which slowly oxidises tyrosine to dihydroxyphenylalanine (DOPA), and then more rapidly oxidises it to a quinone. After several further stages a closed-ring indol quinone is produced, which polymerises to melanin. This then combines with various proteins to form a melanoprotein (Fig. 50.1). The pigment therefore probably has a variable composition. Tyrosinase is synthesised in the rough endoplasmic reticulum, passes into the Golgi complex, and is finally released in membrane-bound structures called *melanosomes*. These develop a characteristic internal structure (Fig. 25.1), and undergo maturation as melanin is formed.

Although melanocytes contain tyrosinase, the enzyme is not always active and the cells do not always contain melanin. The presence of the enzyme can, however, be detected by incubating a section of tissue in a solution of either tyrosine or DOPA. The enzyme, if present, leads to a darkening of the cells due to the production of melanin. This *DOPA reaction* is occasionally of value in distinguishing an amelanotic melanoma from other anaplastic tumours. The reaction with tyrosine is more specific but slower than that with DOPA.

The distribution and extent of skin pigmentation are governed by many factors.

The type of melanin present. Although the precise composition of the melanins is unknown, it is convenient to divide them into two groups: the *eumelanins*, which are black or brown pigments, insoluble in most solvents, and resistant to chemical treatment, and the *phaeomelanins*, which vary in colour from red to yellow, and are soluble in dilute alkali solution. The tint in red hair is said to contain yet another type of pigment that contains iron.[4]

The *number of melanocytes* present varies from one site to another. Thus there are fewer in the palmar epidermis than in that of the dorsum of the hand.

The formation of tyrosinase in melanocytes appears to be controlled by *genetic factors*. In albinism the cells are present, but are DOPA-negative, and lack the ability to form melanin.

Figure 50.1
Stages in the formation of melanoprotein from tyrosine. The formulae of adrenaline and noradrenaline are shown for comparison with tyrosine. (*After Lerner, A. B.* (1955), American Journal of Medicine, **19,** 902)

The common freckles are also genetically determined. The degree of pigmentation is, of course, also racially determined; the increased pigmentation in dark-skinned races is due to the increased activity of the melanocytes rather than an increase in their number.

In view of the neural-crest origin of melanoblasts and the similarity in structure of adrenaline and melanin and its precursors, it is not surprising that pigmentary and *nervous abnormalities* may coexist. The best example of this is neurofibromatosis, in which there is an increased incidence of phaeochromocytoma as well as a tendency to focal pigmentation in the form of café-au-lait patches.

The depth of colouring of the skin depends not only upon the number of melanocytes and the type of melanin in them, but also upon the amount of melanin present and its distribution within these cells. This is related to certain *hormones* of the pituitary, and to a lesser extent of the gonads.

The pituitary (pars intermedia) of amphibians secretes a *melanocyte-stimulating hormone* (MSH), which is a polypeptide, and is capable of causing darkening of small, isolated pieces of frogs' skin. This it does by causing the melanin in melanocytes to become dispersed throughout the cytoplasm. This hormone probably regulates the rapid colour changes seen in reptiles: blanching is due to pigment concentrating around the nucleus. Adrenaline inhibits the action of MSH.

The role of this type of MSH, called α-MSH, in the human being is less certain.[5] There is no evidence that it exists in the circulation or has any pigmentary function in the normal individual. Although it can be obtained from the human pituitary, it is probably an artefact resulting from the degradation of corticotrophin during extraction. ACTH itself has melanocyte-stimulating activity, and shares an amino-acid sequence with α-MSH.

Another peptide with melanocyte-stimulating activity and containing a greater number of amino acids has also been identified in both the pituitary and the circulation of various animals and of human subjects. It is called β-MSH, but it too is not an independent hormone. It is formed from the enzymatic degradation of the much larger pituitary lipolytic hormones. Possibly β-MSH, which also has appreciable lipolytic activity, may be an important pigmentary hormone in the human being, being derived from the cleavage of the lipotrophins which act as prohormones.

The administration of ACTH causes hyperpigmentation; likewise diseases in which there is a raised level of plasma ACTH are associated with increased melanin pigmentation. These include those uncommon cases of *Cushing's syndrome* (properly called Cushing's disease) due to an ACTH-secreting tumour of the pituitary, the *ectopic ACTH syndrome* due to the inappropriate secretion of the hormone by a malignant tumour, *Nelson's syndrome*[6] (gross pigmentation due to an ACTH-secreting tumour of the pituitary developing after previous total bilateral adrenalectomy for Cushing's syndrome), and *Addison's disease*, where the normal feed-back mechanism is interrupted and the pituitary manifests overactivity. In Addison's disease glucocorticoids diminish the pigmentation; pallor is a feature of hypopituitarism. It is noteworthy that changes in plasma ACTH and β-MSH activity generally occur in parallel, but there are exceptions.

The sex hormones also play a part in the control of melanin pigmentation. *Progesterone* causes darkening of frogs' skin, but its role in the human subject is not known. *Oestrogen* also increases pigmentation if given systemically, as is seen in men treated with large doses for prostatic cancer. This might also explain the hyperpigmentation which sometimes occurs in chronic liver disease and pregnancy, and in women taking contraceptive pills. The action of oestrogen appears to be a direct one, for local application to a guinea-pig's nipples causes pigmentation.

In the male *androgens* are important for normal pigmentation. It is found that eunuchs are burnt by sunlight, but do not tan.

The most potent agent known to lighten the colour of frogs' skin is *melatonin*,[7] which like 5-HT, is found in the pineal gland, and has been identified as N-acetyl-5-methoxytryptamine. It acts by causing the melanin granules to aggregate around the nucleus. Whether it plays any part in the regulation of skin pigmentation in the human is not known.

Development of pigmentation. In the white races very little pigment is present in the skin at birth, and the hair is often fair. With increasing age progressive darkening occurs, usually reaching its maximum at puberty.

ABNORMALITIES IN PIGMENTATION[8]

Excessive Pigmentation

Generalised hyperpigmentation. A generalised increase in pigmentation is seen in a variety of conditions. In *Addison's disease* it is most marked in exposed parts and those areas normally pigmented. It is also conspicuous in areas of skin subject to repeated trauma, and is typically noted in the buccal mucosa. The hyperpigmentation seen in other conditions of ACTH oversecretion has already been mentioned.

Production of excessive pigmentation by oestrogens has already been mentioned. In pregnancy there is increased pigmentation of the nipples and genitalia, and sometimes a blotchy appearance of the face producing the 'pregnancy mask'. The term *chloasma* is applied to this condition, which is not uncommon in dark-complexioned women. In *chronic arsenical poisoning* a characteristic pigmentation with raindrop markings may occur, the mechanism of which is unknown. A generalised increase in skin pigmentation is quite often seen in *haemochromatosis*, and also in occasional cases of *chronic malnutrition, cachexia, rheumatoid arthritis* (especially in *Felty's syndrome*), *thyrotoxicosis*, and *pellagra*.

A curious melanosis may follow prolonged treatment with *chlorpromazine*.[9] It affects the eye (lens, cornea, conjunctiva, and retina) and also those areas of skin exposed to sunlight, which become violaceous or even slate-grey in colour. The substances deposited are melanin and a drug metabolite, and on occasions internal organs are also affected. The mechanism of chlorpromazine melanosis is unknown.

Focal hyperpigmentation. Scattered areas of pigmentation are common on the skin of normal people and are called freckles, or *ephelides*. There is an increased amount of pigment in the basal layer of the epidermis but the number of melanocytes is not increased.

Café-au-lait spots are large pigmented patches* which resemble freckles microscopically apart from a mild increase in the number of melanocytes. They are common in otherwise normal people, but multiple lesions form a component of two uncommon syndromes: (*a*) *neurofibromatosis* (see p. 354), and (*b*) *Albright's syndrome*, a non-hereditary condition which comprises a triad of polyostotic fibrous dysplasia, pigmentation, and precocity (sexual and skeletal).

---

*An area of altered skin that is not palpable is called a *macule* if it is less than 1·0 cm in diameter; if it is larger it is called a *patch*. Similar areas that are palpable are called *papules* if small, and *plaques* if over 1·0 cm in diameter.

Figure 50.2
Peutz-Jeghers syndrome. Linear streaks and brown spots of perioral pigmentation. (*Sheward, J. D.* (1962), British Medical Journal, **1**, 921)

Another rare condition associated with focal pigmentation is the *Peutz-Jeghers syndrome (familial gastrointestinal polyposis)*, inherited as an autosomal dominant characteristic and comprising multiple polyposis of the stomach and bowel, leading to transient, recurrent intussusception, and a brownish pigmentation peppered around the mouth and lips (Fig. 50.2), and sometimes in the skin elsewhere. The intestinal lesions do not become cancerous and are hamartomatous in nature. The condition is to be contrasted with polyposis coli, in which the polyps are confined to the colon, cancer invariably ensues, and there is no pigmentation.

Another focal pigmented lesion is the *lentigo*, which differs from the above in showing a great increase in the number of melanocytes in the basal layer of the epidermis. Syndromes of multiple symmetrical lentigenes have been described in association with electrocardiographic abnormalities or with obstructive cardiomyopathy.[10] *Lentigo senilis* is a common condition in the elderly, in which there are multiple, smooth 'liver spots' on the dorsa of the hands, the face, neck, and arms. *Lentigo maligna* also affects the elderly, but is usually solitary and on the face. There are many atypical melanocytes in the basal layer, and the condition is to be regarded as premalignant; about 25 per cent of cases develop invasive melanoma after some years (see p. 352). These tumours are less malignant than melanomata arising from junctional naevi or normal skin, but this is disputed.[11] The good prognosis may be merely an expression of the difficulty in distinguishing between lentigo maligna with marked cellular anaplasia and a malignant melanoma.

Finally, hyperpigmentation of a focal type follows exposure of the skin to ionising radiations, ultraviolet light (sun-tan), and heat. The last is called *erythema ab igne*, and is seen on the legs of people who habitually sit close to an open fire. Hyperpigmentation of the skin commonly accompanies dermatitis and other inflammatory dermatoses, particularly in patients with well-pigmented skin. It is a prominent feature of lichen planus and fixed drug eruptions. *Poikiloderma of Civatte* is a reticulated pigmentation with erythema and telangiectasia. It affects middle-aged women particularly, and is found on the sun-exposed parts of the face and neck; it is thought to be caused by photosensitisation induced by cosmetics.

Skin nodules commonly presenting as pigmented lesions are: naevocellular naevi, blue naevi, dermatofibromata, seborrhoeic keratoses, basal-cell carcinomata, and malignant melanomata.

Lack of Pigmentation

Generalised hypopigmentation. The most extreme example is *albinism*. In this defect characteristic dendritic melanocytes are present, but tyrosinase activity is defective, and little or no melanin is produced. Electron microscopy has confirmed the presence of melanocytes with non-pigmented melanosomes. In *universal albinism* the body contains no pigment-producing melanocytes, the skin is milk-white, the hair pale, the irides transparent, and the pupils pink. The condition occurs in animals, but no proven human case is known. In *generalised albinism* some melanin is produced in the iris and occasionally elsewhere; it is usually inherited as an autosomal recessive characteristic. The patient suffers from nystagmus and photophobia. In adult albinos the presence on the exposed parts of actinic keratoses, and squamous-cell and basal-cell carcinomata emphasises the importance of melanin as a protective agent.

Generalised pallor is a feature of panhypopituitarism, male eunuchoidism, and phenylketonuria. In the last condition the great excess of phenylalanine that accumulates probably competes for tyrosinase, and inhibits melanin formation. Thus pigment production in hair can be promoted either by increasing the intake of tyrosine or by lowering that of phenylalanine.

Focal hypopigmentation. A striking example is *cutaneous partial albinism*, variously called *congenital leucoderma* and *piebaldness*. It produces white patches on the skin which may be quite extensive (Fig. 50.3). It is usually inherited as an autosomal dominant character. Another type of localised albinism is *ocular albinism*, in which the eye alone is affected. It is inherited as a sex-linked recessive trait.

Acquired focal depigmentation is common in leprosy and following the healing of wounds—especially chemical burns. *Poikiloderma* is a term applied to the triad of *disturbed pigmentation* (areas of hyperpigmentation and hypopigmentation), *atrophy*, and *telangiectasia*. Chronic radiodermatitis and chronic discoid lupus erythematosus provide common examples.

However, by far the most common cause of focal depigmentation is *vitiligo*, a disease which is said to affect about 1 per cent of the population: there are sharply defined areas of depigmentation on the skin, commonly of the hands, face, and genital area. In the affected areas melanocytes are absent, and little or no melanin is present. The cause and pathogenesis are unknown, but in some cases a familial tendency is evident.

Pigments Related to Melanin

Ochronosis, first described by Virchow, is a condition in which a melanin-like pigment is present in the cartilages of

Figure 50.3
Cutaneous partial albinism. This reproduction of a painting in the Royal College of Surgeons of England shows a Black child. Note the segmental distribution of the areas of depigmentation, and the symmetry of the lesions on the forehead. The caption reads 'The true picture of Mary-Sabina, who was born on Oct. 12, 1736, at Matuna, a plantation belonging to ye Jesuits in ye city of Cartagena in America of two Negro slaves, named Martiniano and Patrona'. This rare type of cutaneous partial albinism should not be confused with the common vitiligo which usually first appears in early adult life.

the ear, larynx, trachea, and joints, in the tendons of the hand, and in ligaments and fibrous tissue generally. In the sclera it occurs midway between the cornea and the canthi.

Ochronosis generally occurs in alcaptonuria, and the pigment is presumably formed from homogentisic acid. A similar pigmentation also occurred in chronic phenol poisoning, in the days when this disinfectant was often applied to wounds.

Dubin-Johnson syndrome. The liver cells contain heavy deposits of a melanin pigment (see p. 564).

PIGMENTS DERIVED FROM HAEMOGLOBIN

Haemoglobin may form a variety of pigments:
1. Methaemoglobin and sulphaemoglobin are considered in Chapter 52. Carboxyhaemoglobin is a bright pink pigment produced from the combination of carbon monoxide and haemoglobin. These three pigments are all intracorpuscular.

2. The porphyrin moiety following haemoglobin breakdown is converted into bilirubin* (see jaundice, p. 561).

3. The porphyrins* in porphyria are described in Chapter 33.

4. The iron released following haemoglobin breakdown is stored in the body as either ferritin or haemosiderin (see below).

IRON-CONTAINING PIGMENTS[12,13]

Iron occurs in many forms in the body: it is present in such enzymes as the cytochromes and the peroxidases, but the largest quantities are present in the red cells as haemoglobin, in muscle as myoglobin, and in the RE system stores as ferritin and haemosiderin. The total body content of iron is about 4 g.

In order to remain in balance the normal adult male absorbs about 0.6 mg of iron daily, whereas the menstruating female requires about 1.2 mg. Since the diet contains about 15 mg, it is evident that the intestine plays a crucial part in preventing iron overloading. The mechanism is described on page 605.

Iron is normally stored in the ferric state and combined with a β-globulin (*apoferritin*) as *ferritin*,[14] a compound containing about 23 per cent ferric iron. On electron microscopy molecules of ferritin are visible as groups of four electron-dense particles. Ferritin cannot be seen under the light microscope in routine paraffin sections, and does not usually give a Prussian-blue reaction.

In this respect it is distinguished from *haemosiderin*, in which the proportion of iron is considerably higher (about 36 per cent, but varying from 24 to 45 per cent as opposed to 16 to 23 per cent in ferritin) and the Prussian-blue reaction is positive. In fact, a number of Prussian-blue positive, insoluble granules have been shown to contain ferritin (by electron microscopy), and it is now recognised that the distinction between ferritin and haemosiderin is not clear cut.[15] In most instances haemosiderin appears to be derived from ferritin, and ferritin polymers of various sizes may represent intermediates between ferritin and forms of haemosiderin. It seems that in the formation of haemosiderin, protein is lost by denaturation or proteolysis. Haemosiderin seems to represent a more stable and less available form of storage iron than ferritin. Haemosiderin appears as brown, insoluble granules that give the Prussian-blue reaction. It is found in any situation where excessive quantities of iron are being stored. This may occur as a local phenomenon or else be generalised.

Localised Haemosiderin Deposits

Whenever there is a haemorrhage, the iron from the broken-down red cells is found in the nearby macrophages in the form of haemosiderin (and also ferritin). This is seen around organising haematomata, haemorrhagic infarcts, fractures, etc. A brownish discoloration around a brain cyst is therefore good evidence of its origin from an infarct.

Another instance of localised haemosiderin deposition is important: the *sclerosing haemangioma* (p. 348), which is often

---

*Like haemoglobin, the porphyrins are composed of four substituted pyrrole nuclei joined to form a ring. In the bile pigments like bilirubin, the nuclei are joined to form a chain (see p. 562).

deeply pigmented and can be mistaken both clinically and pathologically for a malignant melanoma unless special stains are used. The epidermis overlying the lesion is frequently acanthotic and deeply pigmented with melanin; this is largely responsible for the pigmentation noted clinically. When the lesion is incised, the deeper haemosiderosis is apparent.

The cells of the renal tubules can also convert haemoglobin to haemosiderin. This pigment is therefore seen in the renal tubular cells after haemoglobinuria.

Pulmonary Haemosiderosis

The small haemorrhages which occur in the lungs in mitral stenosis and left ventricular failure are responsible for the formation of 'heart-failure cells'. These are alveolar macrophages containing haemosiderin. A mild diffuse fibrosis may occur in long standing cases to produce *brown induration*. In children and sometimes young adults pulmonary haemosiderosis may arise without obvious cause. This idiopathic haemosiderosis is manifested clinically by a progressive anaemia accompanied by miliary X-ray shadows in the lungs. One variety is accompanied by acute glomerulonephritis; it is called *Goodpasture's syndrome* and has an immunological basis (see p. 202).

Generalised Haemosiderosis

If the body is overloaded with iron, haemosiderin is formed in excessive amounts. Two patterns are seen.[13]

Parenchymatous deposition. When the overloading is due to excessive absorption from the intestine, the haemosiderin is deposited in the parenchymatous cells of the liver, pancreas, kidney, and heart, and considerable damage may be inflicted on these organs. This type of deposition is seen (*a*) when the normal regulating mechanism for iron absorption is impaired, as in haemochromatosis, (*b*) when there is increased erythropoietic activity, as in chronic haemolytic anaemia (especially thalassaemia), and (*c*) when there is a great increase in the iron content of the diet.[13]

Generalised haemosiderosis in refractory anaemias with a hyperplastic bone marrow is attributable to an increased rate of iron absorption from the bowel. The haemosiderosis is most severe in those conditions where few viable red cells are delivered to the circulation.

A similar type of haemosiderosis is met with in the Black South African, whose diet has a high iron content. Over 100 mg a day may be ingested, much being derived from the iron containers used in the preparation of alcoholic drinks.[13] In these conditions the haemosiderin distribution resembles that of haemochromatosis, but, for an unknown reason, causes less severe parenchymatous damage. Sometimes, however, hepatic cirrhosis and diabetes mellitus develop.[13]

RE Deposition. This is seen following parental iron administration or repeated blood transfusions. Haemosiderosis following transfusion affects the RE system primarily. However, the iron content of the body may exceed that attributable to the transfusion, in which case it is evident that there has been an excessive intestinal absorption.

Haemochromatosis.[13,16,17] Also known as 'bronzed diabetes', this disease is usually considered to be an inborn error of metabolism, and inherited as an autosomal dominant characteristic. It is postulated that there is some abnormality of the mechanism regulating the absorption of iron. This results in excessive absorption of iron (2 to 3 mg daily), and over a period of years the body builds up a large store of haemosiderin. The finding that many of the relatives of patients with haemochromatosis have an increased absorption of iron supports this genetic concept. It has been claimed that patients with haemochromatosis lack an iron-binding component present in the gastric juice, called gastroferrin, but the physiological importance of this substance, possibly a carbohydrate, remains to be demonstrated.[15]

Haemochromatosis most commonly affects men, women presumably being protected by their menstrual loss. The pigment is found in the liver cells, pancreas, heart, and other organs. The liver may contain over 50 g of iron. The pigment seems to cause damage, and in the fully-developed disease this results in hepatic cirrhosis, diabetes mellitus, and heart failure. A progressive polyarthritis occurs in about half the patients, usually starting in the small joints of the hand.[18,19] Other joints, e.g. the wrists, elbows, hips, knees, and ankles may become involved, the pattern somewhat resembling that of rheumatoid arthritis. In about half the cases there are X-ray changes of chondrocalcinosis (p. 464), and attacks of acute synovitis occur.

The plasma iron level is raised and the transferrin is almost completely saturated (see p. 605). The diagnosis is confirmed by liver biopsy or skin biopsy—the pigment is present in the cells of the sweat glands. It is interesting that these patients also show increased melanin pigmentation, and sometimes a lipofuscin pigmentation as well. The reason for this is unknown.

Not all workers accept the genetic basis of haemochromatosis.[20] The repeated failure to produce the disease in the experimental animal by iron overloading alone has led to the view that haemochromatosis is not a distinct entity, but merely represents cirrhosis of the liver in an iron-overloaded patient. Certainly alcoholism is common in haemochromatosis, and some beverages, for example wine, are rich in iron.

Haematin Pigmentation

When the ferrous iron of haem is oxidised to the ferric form, a bluish-black pigment, *haematin*, or *methaem*, is produced. As an intracorpuscular pigmentation, methaemoglobinaemia is described on page 617. Sometimes, however, particles of black pigment are found in macrophages and lying free in the connective tissue in chronic malaria and schistosomiasis, both infections in which the parasites live in the blood stream, and presumably utilise the red cells during their own metabolism (see Fig. 30.1, p. 392). This pigment is believed to be haematin—it does not give the Prussian-blue reaction, is bleached by formic acid, and is insoluble in strong acids, but is extracted by alkalies. It accounts for the blackish colour of malarial organs.

Formalin pigment, which is produced when tissue containing much blood is subjected to prolonged formalin fixation, is also believed to be haematin. The pigment is birefringent with polarised light; this provides a rapid method of distinguishing it from haemosiderin.

PIGMENTS ASSOCIATED WITH FAT

The term *lipopigment* is best applied to any pigment which is related to fat: it includes two main groups, the lipochromes and the lipofuscins.[*1]

The lipochromes, or carotenoids, are yellow pigments, soluble in fat and entirely exogenous, being derived from ingested vegetables. They are hydrocarbons, and constitute the colouring matter of beetroot,[21] carrots, tomatoes, etc. There are two groups: the *carotenes*, the best known of which are β-carotene and its isomer lycopene, and the *xanthophylls*, or *oxycarotenoids*. The pigments have attained considerable commercial importance since they are used as non-toxic, yellow or red, colouring additives in many foodstuffs.

These pigments are found dissolved in the fat of the body, and are responsible for the yellow colour of atheromatous plaques, the adrenal cortex, and corpora lutea, as well as that of the fat depots. The actual quantity and proportion of each carotenoid in the tissues depends upon the diet, and occasionally if excessive quantities of coloured vegetables are ingested, there is sufficient coloration of the plasma and skin to simulate jaundice.[22] This is said to occur also in diabetes mellitus, but in all probability it is due to a high dietary intake and not primarily to the disease itself.

Lipofuscins.[1] The brown pigments which are included under the name lipofuscins form an ill-defined group. Other names, like ceroid and haemofuscin, have been applied to some of them. They are all thought to be derived from lipids by oxidation, and are thus endogenous in origin. They are present in residual bodies (p. 24). They usually stain with the Sudan fat stains, and also retain basic fuchsin, i.e. they are acid fast.

The pigments tend to occur in old age and in atrophic conditions—whence the alternative name of 'wear and tear' pigment. One of the best examples is encountered in brown atrophy of the heart, which is seen in senility and severe wasting. The small muscle fibres contain caps of brown pigment in the cytoplasm at each pole of their centrally-placed nuclei. Although a small amount of pigment is normally found in this position, it is greatly increased in brown atrophy. Lipofuscins are found in the seminal vesicles and nerve cells in old age, and similar pigments are also found in the liver. 'Ceroid' is a pigment found in the liver cells of animals on deficient diets, and a similar pigment is often seen in hepatic cirrhosis. 'Haemofuscin' is found in haemochromatosis. Both are included in this rather vague group of pigments derived from fat.

The bowel sometimes shows lipofuscin pigmentation. The commonest example is *melanosis coli*,[23] a symptomless condition in which the mucous membrane of the colon has a brown or black colour. This is due to the presence of many macrophages laden with a brown pigment in the connective tissue of the mucosa. The pigment is a lipofuscin. The condition is related to the habitual ingestion of anthraquinone purgatives. It seems that these have a specific effect not only in increasing the number of macrophages in the bowel mucosa

---

*The suffix 'fuscin' is derived from the Latin *fuscus* meaning dark or sombre. It must not be confused with the fuchsin dyes, which are red in colour.

but also in intensifying the lysosomal activity within them; the lipofuscin is derived from the lysosomes.

Another, quite different, example of intestinal lipofuscin pigmentation is seen in some cases of protein-losing gastroenteropathy, in which the small intestine is pigmented due to the presence of lipofuscin in the muscle fibres and in the many macrophages found between the fibres.[24] The liver and skeletal muscles are also pigmented. Lipofuscin deposition can be produced in animals by a diet deficient in vitamin E.[2], but whether this is the cause of the lipofuscinosis of the bowel occasionally seen in cases of the malabsorption syndrome occurring in the human subject, e.g. in chronic pancreatitis, gluten-sensitive enteropathy, and Whipple's disease, is unknown.

MISCELLANEOUS PIGMENTS

Pigments Containing Copper[25]

The curious association between hepatic cirrhosis and degeneration of the basal ganglia found in Wilson's disease has stimulated research into copper metabolism. This metal, when given by mouth, is absorbed into the blood stream where it first becomes attached to albumin. Within 24 hours it is found more firmly bound to a specific copper-containing α_2-globulin fraction of the plasma proteins, which, because of its blue colour, is called *caeruloplasmin.*

In *Wilson's disease* copper absorption from the gut and its excretion in the urine are both increased. The plasma caeruloplasmin level is low, and the copper remains attached to albumin. Presumably this loosely-bound copper is more easily deposited in the basal ganglia and liver. There is no doubt that high levels of copper are found in these sites, and most likely account for the degeneration. Another metal, manganese, is also known to produce a similar type of brain and liver damage. Deposition of copper in the cornea produces the golden-brown *Kayser–Fleischer ring*, pathognomonic of the condition. The disease shows an autosomal recessive inheritance pattern and is to be regarded as an inborn error of metabolism. The basic defect appears to be an impaired production of the copper-binding globulin fraction of the plasma proteins.

Myoglobin[26]

Occasionally this pigment is released from the muscles, and is excreted in the urine. The mechanism is obscure. It may occur as the result of severe injury to muscle, following strenuous exercise in healthy people, after the ingestion of poisonous substances ('Haff disease'), in type V glycogenosis (p. 432), and finally as an acute idiopathic condition. The urine is a dark portwine colour, and gives the usual chemical tests for haemoglobin. The condition may be associated with acute renal failure secondary to vasoconstriction and tubular necrosis.

Pigmentation Due to Absorption of Heavy Metals

Silver and gold become deposited in the skin and produce permanent grey pigmentation. The silver pigmentation is called *argyria*, and was quite frequent in the days when silver nitrate was used as a disinfectant and in nasal drops.

Lead reacts with sulphides produced by bacteria around the gingival margin to form lead sulphide. This substance causes the characteristic 'blue line'. Mercury salts similarly produce a green gingival discoloration. It should be noted that the skin pigmentation of arsenical poisoning is due to melanin; it has a characteristic rain-drop appearance with most of the melanin disposed peripherally.

Pigmentation of the Lungs by Inhaled Particles

The lungs of most people, especially town-dwellers and tobacco-smokers, show black discoloration due to the accumulation of carbon. This is especially marked in coal-miners, and is called anthracosis. The brilliant brick-red discoloration of haematite-miner's lung also comes into this category. Haematite is an iron oxide ore (iron sesquioxide, Fe_2O_3).

Pigmentation of Skin by Topically Applied or Injected Dyes

Carbon and cinnabar are deliberately introduced into the dermis in the process of tattooing to produce blue and red colouring respectively. This is a true exogenous pigmentation, and it may occur accidentally when dirt is driven into wounds. The prolonged use of ointments containing mercury can lead to a slate-grey discoloration of the skin at the site of application.

REFERENCES

1. Fox, D. L. (1953) *Animal Biochromes and Structural Colours.* Cambridge University Press.
2. Wolman, M. (Ed.) (1969) *Pigments in Pathology.* New York and London: Academic Press.
3. Fitzpatrick, T. B. *et al.* (1971) In *Dermatology in General Practice*, (Biology of the melanin pigmentary system), ed. Fitzpatrick, T. B. *et al.*, p. 117. New York: McGraw-Hill.
4. Flesch, P. (1968) The epidermal iron pigments of red species. *Journal of Investigative Dermatology*, **51**, 337.
5. Leading Article (1977) Melanocyte-stimulating hormone? *British Medical Journal*, **1**, 533.
6. Cassar, J. *et al.* (1976) Treatment of Nelson's syndrome by pituitary implantation of yttrium-90 or gold-198. *British Medical Journal*, **2**, 269.
7. Annotation (1963) The pineal gland. *British Medical Journal*, **1**, 139.
8. Fitzpatrick, T. B. & Mihm, M. C. (1971) In *Dermatology in General Practice*, p. 591 (Abnormalities of the melanin pigmentary system), *loc. cit.*
9. Leading Article (1967) Chlorpromazine melanosis. *British Medical Journal*, **3**, 630.
10. Polani, P. E. & Moynahan, E. J. (1972) Progressive cardiomyopathic lentiginosis. *Quarterly Journal of Medicine*, **41**, 205.
11. Jackson, R., Williamson, G. S. & Beattie, W. G. (1966) Lentigo maligna and malignant melanoma. *Canadian Medical Association Journal*, **95**, 846.
12. Chanarin, I. (1970) In *Biochemical Disorders in Human Disease*, ed. Thompson, R. H. S. & Wootton, I. D. P., 3rd edn, p. 161. London: Churchill.
13. Charlton, R. W. & Bothwell, T. H. (1970) In *Biochemical Disorders in Human Disease*, p. 201, *loc. cit.*

14. CRICHTON, R. R. (1971) Ferritin: structure, synthesis and function. *New England Journal of Medicine*, **284**, 1413.
15. WINTROBE, M. M., LEE, G. R., BOGGS, D. R., BITHELL, T. C., ATHENS, J. W. & FOERSTER, J. (1974) In *Clinical Hematology*, 7th edn, p. 154 *et seq*. Philadelphia: Lea & Febiger.
16. POLLYCOVE, M. (1972) In *The Metabolic Basis of Inherited Disease*, ed. Stanbury, J. B., Wyngaarden, J. B. & Fredrickson, D. S., 3rd edn, p. 1051. New York: McGraw-Hill.
17. Leading Article (1967) Idiopathic haemochromatosis. *British Medical Journal*, **1**, 446.
18. Leading Article (1969) Bone and joint changes in haemochromatosis. *British Medical Journal*, **3**, 191.
19. Leading Article (1971) The arthropathy of haemochromatosis. *British Medical Journal*, **2**, 182.
20. MACDONALD, R. A. (1964) *Haemochromatosis and Haemosiderosis*. Springfield; Illinois: Thomas.
21. Annotation (1963) Beeturia. *British Medical Journal*, **2**, 948.
22. REICH, P., SHWACHMAN, H. & CRAIG, J. M. (1960) Lycopenemia. *New England Journal of Medicine*, **262**, 263.
23. STEER, H. W. & COLIN-JONES, D. G. (1975) Melanosis coli: studies of the toxic effects of irritant purgatives. *Journal of Pathology*, **115**, 199.
24. FOX, B. (1967) Lipofuscinosis of the gastrointestinal tract in man. *Journal of Clinical Pathology*, **20**, 806.
25. BEARN, A. G. (1972) In *The Metabolic Basis of Inherited Disease*, p. 1033, *loc. cit.*
26. Leading Article (1961) Myoglobinuria. *Lancet*, **1**, 704.

Chapter 51.   Calculi

A calculus is a mass of precipitated material derived from a secretion and deposited in an excretory duct. The mode of calculus formation is obscure. It is usually assumed that in any secretion the crystalloids are held in solution by adsorption on to colloidal particles,* and that when the concentration of crystalloids increases or the colloid content decreases, the crystalloids will precipitate out. The colloidal matrix in which the crystalloids of low molecular weight deposit varies according to the secretion; in urinary calculi it consists mostly of mucoprotein and mucopolysaccharide with smaller amounts of plasma proteins.

The important calculi are *urinary, biliary, salivary, pancreatic,* and *prostatic*. It is the calcium (and magnesium) content of a calculus that renders it radio-opaque; it follows that stones composed of the phosphate, carbonate, oxalate, or bilirubinate of calcium are revealed on a plain radiograph. Calculi composed of uric acid and xanthine can be detected only by the appearance of a filling defect during pyelography, and pure cholesterol stones are demonstrated similarly during cholecystography. Cystine and silica stones usually contain a sufficient amount of calcium to be faintly radio-opaque.

Causes of Calculus Formation

An increase in the crystalloid content of the secretion. The effect is a precipitation of some of the crystalloid, and the resulting calculus is called *primary*, or *metabolic*, i.e. it is formed without prior inflammation.

The presence of a solid mass acting as a nidus around which the crystalloids precipitate. Such a nidus may be formed by a foreign body, fibrin, necrotic epithelial cells, clumps of organisms, or a primary metabolic stone. This type of calculus is sometimes called *secondary*. It may also be called a *concretion*. Chemically it consists predominantly of calcium phosphate and calcium carbonate.

CALCULI OF THE URINARY TRACT

Bladder stones were once common in Europe and provided a livelihood for the lithotomist. Since the beginning of the twentieth century they have become extremely rare in Europe, and yet are still common in some developing countries. The reason for this remarkable change is not known.[1] The remainder of this section describes stone formation in the upper

*A colloid is a state of matter intermediate between a true solution and a suspension or emulsion. A colloidal solution (or sol) is one in which the dispersed particles have a diameter between 1 and 100 nm. The colloid is the discontinuous phase, and the medium the continuous phase (as distinct from solute and solvent). In a medium it is possible to separate crystalloid from colloid by means of a membrane, e.g. parchment or collodion, which is permeable to crystalloids only. This process is called *dialysis*.

urinary tract, a condition that appears to be on the increase. The stones are usually found in the renal pelves, occasionally in the ureter, and rarely in the bladder. The common primary calculi are:

Urate stones, composed of uric acid with sodium and ammonium urate. These are brown in colour, smooth and hard, and on section show concentric lamination.

Calcium oxalate stones, which vary in colour from a dirty yellow to a dark brown, and have rough surfaces which may be prolonged into sharp spikes that cause mucosal trauma and bleeding. They are very hard, and are laminated on section (Figs. 51.1, 51.2, and 51.3).

In addition three much rarer primary stones should be noted:

Cystine stones, which have a yellowish-brown colour resembling honey. They have a maple-sugar crystal surface, and are very firm.

Figure 51.1
Calcium oxalate calculus. The surface of this stone, which measured 7 cm in diameter, is light brown in colour and has an evenly granular contour. (*Reproduced by permission of the President and Council of the R.C.S. Eng.*)

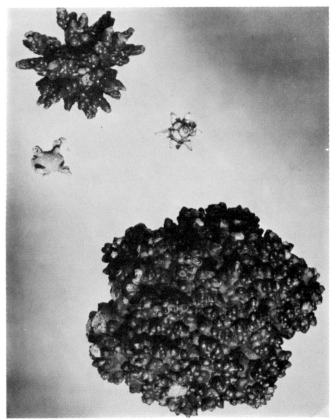

Figure 51.2
Calcium oxalate calculi. These stones of varying size all show the salient features of dark coloration and spiky irregularity of surface. (*Reproduced by permission of the President and Council of the R.C.S. Eng.*)

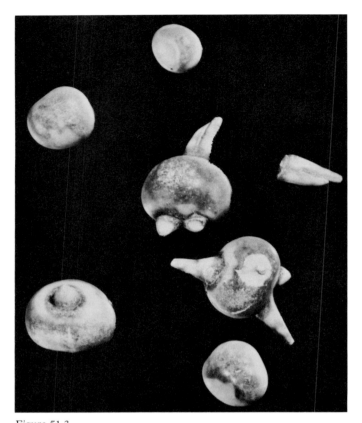

Figure 51.3
Small calcium oxalate calculi. The little spiky oxalate stones used to be called jackstones. Jackstones (also called checkstones, or dibstones) is a centuries-old children's game in which small round pebbles (or sheep's knuckle-bones) are tossed up in a small basket and caught again as they fall. These small calculi were presumably alleged to resemble the pebbles or knuckle-bones used in the game.

Some of the stones photographed are finely polished, and have a smooth contour. This is not unusual when the stones have been present for a long time. (*Reproduced by permission of the President and Council of the R.C.S. Eng.*)

Xanthine stones, which are reddish-brown or yellowish-brown in colour, smooth, round or oval, and friable. They are easily cut into, and are laminated on section.

Silica stones, which are white or yellow in colour, and are extremely hard.

Secondary calculi may arise *de novo* following infection of the urinary tract or the introduction of a foreign body into the bladder. In the course of time they also form around primary calculi, and the result is a *mixed stone*. They are composed of **calcium phosphate** and **magnesium ammonium phosphate** together with a variable amount of **calcium carbonate.** In appearance they are white and smooth, and have a soft, friable consistency (see Figs. 51.4 and 51.7).

Calculi composed of calcium salts, usually a mixture of oxalate and phosphate, are by far the most common in the urinary tract, and many are not due to infection. In conditions of hypercalciuria mentioned below it is this type of calculus that is formed. About 90 per cent of urinary calculi are composed of calcium salts, and 4 to 10 per cent of uric acid.

Aetiology of Primary Urinary Calculi[2]

The majority of primary urinary stones arise in an unknown way, but a few factors are worthy of consideration:

Increased content of crystalloids (or abnormal crystalloids) in urine. In the rare metabolic disorders of *xanthinuria* and *cystinuria* it is understandable that poorly soluble substances like cystine and xanthine should precipitate out of solution. Likewise, silica stones may follow the long-continued ingestion of magnesium trisilicate for indigestion.[3]

Hyperoxaluria.[4] An increased excretion of oxalate occurs if there is excessive oxalate ingestion (in green, leafy vegetables), in pyridoxine deficiency, and in patients with chronic ileal disease and steatorrhoea. *Primary oxaluria* is a rare condition, inherited as an autosomal recessive trait, in which there is increased oxalate synthesis in the body. The disease is usually evident before the age of 5 years, and terminates in uraemia. Deposits of oxalates are found in many tissues, including the kidney (*oxalosis*). Two separate types of the disease have been recognised biochemically. Although hyperoxaluria predisposes to the development of oxalate stones, the great majority of patients with such stones have no detectable abnormality of oxalate metabolism.

Hyperuricaemia. Uric-acid stones are not uncommon in

Figure 51.4
Staghorn calculus. This complex, branched, phosphate stone, which bears a somewhat fanciful resemblance to the horn of a stag, was found in a shrunken, fibrosed kidney that was removed surgically. It formed an accurate cast of the calyces, pelvis, and upper end of the ureter. (*Reproduced by permission of the President and Council of the R.C.S. Eng.*)

patients with *chronic gout*, and are related in part to the increased excretion of uric acid often found, but in addition gouty patients tend to secrete an unusually acid urine (see p. 434). Nevertheless, uric-acid stones are often found in patients with no obvious defect in uric-acid metabolism or any abnormality in acidification of the urine.

Hypercalciuria. An increased calcium excretion in the urine may also lead to calculus formation, e.g. in *hyperparathyroidism, sarcoidosis*, and in *patients immobilised in bed for a long time*, when the skeleton undergoes progressive demineralisation as the result of disuse atrophy. Such stones are composed of variable amounts of calcium phosphate and oxalate. About 20 per cent of cases of hyperparathyroidism, however, do not form calculi despite marked hypercalciuria. Conversely, many patients who form calculi repeatedly do not excrete calcium in excessive amounts.[2] There is also a syndrome of idiopathic hypercalciuria and renal lithiasis despite a normal plasma calcium level; sometimes the plasma phosphate level is reduced.[4, 5] It is possible that the cause of the hypercalciuria is an increased absorption of calcium from the bowel.[6] Another hypercalciuria syndrome associated with stones is *renal tubular acidosis* (see p. 559). An acquired type due

to chronic pyelonephritis may manifest itself with renal calculus.[7]

The mechanism of formation of calcium-containing calculi in those many instances in which there is no obvious abnormality in calcium metabolism is not known. It has been found that the concentration of calcium in the renal papilla is normally considerably greater than in the other parts of the kidney; in fact it is unknown how this high concentration of calcium is kept in solution. Hypercalciuria should be most dangerous in a hyperosmolal urine,[8] and indeed people who live in hot desert areas may develop renal stones. Likewise, stones are quite common in some tropical areas, but not in all of them. It has been found that the incidence of stone in Black South Africans is much less than that in those of White race. It has also been noted that the Bantu excretes much more sodium ions in his urine than does his fair-skinned neighbour, who excretes only a little more calcium than does the Bantu.[8] It would seem that hypercalciuria is dangerous in urine with a low sodium concentration, whereas an increase in the amount of both ions is relatively harmless. In fact, hypercalciuria is most dangerous in a hypo-osmolal urine. Thus the traditionally held deleterious effect of *dehydration* on stone formation needs reconsidering. While it probably is of importance, it is evident that the osmolality of the urine must also be considered when large amounts of water are prescribed as a prophylactic measure in those prone to calculus formation; this osmolality is mostly a function of sodium ions.[8] Whether other substances that hold calcium in solution are also present normally but deficient in those who form stones is not known—amongst such agents have been postulated citrate, amino acids, ascorbic acid, and pyrophosphate, but none has been substantiated.[2, 5]

Foci of calcification in the kidney (nephrocalcinosis) acting as a nidus for calculus formation. *Randall's plaques*. Randall described foci of dystrophic calcification in the renal papillae arising secondarily to injury; these ulcerated through the pelvic mucosa, and acted as a nidus for calculus formation. Such plaques are fairly common, but are usually not associated with stone formation. Conversely, stones may occur in kidneys without Randall's plaques. It is probable that these lesions are a result of the high calcium content of the papillary area of the kidney already noted.

Renal microliths. Small flecks of calcium salts are present in the interstitial tissue of all kidneys, and are probably situated in the renal lymphatics. It has been suggested that if the lymphatic system is blocked or overloaded, these microliths might coalesce to form calculi. They might then ulcerate into the pelvis, and form the nidus of an even larger calculus. Though interesting, this hypothesis lacks proof.

Stasis plays no part in the formation of primary stones with the probable exception of those calculi that develop in immobilised patients, in whom it is possible that the calcium salts may separate out in the calyces by a gravitational effect. In this example the stasis merely determines the site of stone formation. Obstruction leads to secondary calculus formation because it predisposes to infection.

Urinary pH. Uric-acid stones form in an acid urine, and patients who develop these calculi are often unable to secrete an adequate amount of ammonia in their distal renal tubules. Oxalate and cystine stones also precipitate in an acid urine.

On the other hand, the phosphates of calcium and magnesium ammonium deposit in an alkaline urine. The presence of urea-splitting organisms, notably *Proteus* species, in the urine leads to ammonia formation and alkalinity. It is not surprising that phosphate stones occur in severe urinary-tract infection. It is, however, interesting how seldom calculi are found in the very common condition of chronic pyelonephritis.

Vitamin-A deficiency may lead to renal stones in rats, but there is no evidence that it plays any part in human calculus formation.

Ureteric calculi are usually renal in origin, as are also many *vesical calculi*. Stones may also be produced in the bladder as the result of severe, persistent cystitis secondary to obstruction to the outflow of urine, or in narrow-necked diverticula. They also form around foreign bodies introduced from the outside, e.g. pieces of catheter and safety-pins. Such calculi are composed of calcium and magnesium ammonium phosphate.

BILIARY CALCULI

Gallstones are described classically as being either *primary* or *secondary*. There are three primary, or metabolic, types:

Cholesterol stones are characteristically solitary. They are pale yellow in colour, ovoid, and have a smooth surface. The cut surface shows a radiating, glistening, crystalline pattern. *Strawberry gallbladder*, or *cholesterolosis of the gallbladder*, in which the mucosa is thrown up into yellow plaques containing accumulations of fat-filled macrophages, is not usually accompanied by stones.

Calcium bilirubinate stones (pigment stones). These are multiple, jet-black in colour, irregular in shape, and rather friable in consistency.

Calcium carbonate stones are rare, and are chalky in appearance.

In fact, pure stones are not found, and the above classification is not regarded with favour by research workers, although it is of some clinical value. All stones contain variable amounts of bile pigments, cholesterol, calcium carbonate, and apatite, and their core usually consists of bile pigments or mucoprotein, which is secreted by the gallbladder epithelium.[9–11] The gallbladder is usually normal structurally.

Aetiology of Gallstones[12–14]

Cholesterol stones. The basis of the common cholesterol stone appears to be a precipitation of cholesterol which is not kept adequately in solution. Cholesterol, which is insoluble in water, is carried in solution in the bile in a mixed micelle consisting of bile salts, phospholipid, and the cholesterol itself. The micelle is a polymolecular aggregate comparable, in this instance, with a detergent molecule, and it is the bile salts, and to a lesser extent the phospholipid, that bring the cholesterol into solution.

Gallstones tend to form in bile in which the cholesterol cannnot be maintained in micellar form (*lithogenic bile*), either because of an increased secretion of cholesterol or a reduction in the total bile-salt pool. However, not all people with lithogenic bile develop gallstones, and some patients with gallstones do not appear to have lithogenic bile. The bile salts undergo an enterohepatic circulation, being reabsorbed chiefly in the terminal ileum. *Ileal disease or resection* eventually leads to a decreased biliary excretion of bile salts and phospholipids, and is associated with a high incidence of gallstones. The anion-exchange resin *cholestyramine* has a similar effect; it is used in patients with partial biliary obstruction who have severe pruritus, because it binds bile salts in the intestine so that they are eliminated in the faeces.

Drugs that increase the cholesterol content of the bile also predispose to gallstones, e.g. *clofibrate* used to reduce the hypercholesterolaemia in patients with ischaemic heart disease, and *oestrogen-progesterone combinations* used in the contraceptive pill. This hormonal effect probably explains why gallstones of the cholesterol type are twice as common in women as in men, especially below the age of 50.

Cirrhosis of the liver is frequently associated with gallstones, but these are usually pigment stones. In patients with cirrhosis there is a decreased excretion of bile salts, phospholipids, and cholesterol, so that the bile is usually not lithogenic. Indeed, it often has greater cholesterol-binding powers than in controls.

The population with the highest known incidence of gallstones is the American Indians, in whom the bile is supersaturated with cholesterol. Cholesterol stones are very common in the Western World, but decidedly uncommon in Esquimos, the Eastern peoples, and in Black Africans, except in those whose affluence is such as to encourage them to partake of Western diets.

The gallbladder plays a secondary part in allowing the cholesterol crystals to precipitate and form a stone. It may also provide a nidus for seeding in the form of mucous secretion, and stasis enhances the growth of the stone. This probably is another factor in the increased incidence of gallstones in women, since there is stasis during pregnancy, especially in the last trimester. Stones can form in the bile ducts of those who have undergone a cholecystectomy, thus proving that the gallbladder is not essential for stone production.

Attempts are being made to expand the bile-salt pool and thereby increase the bile-salt content of the bile. *Chenodeoxycholic acid* expands the pool and alters the bile composition towards favouring cholesterol solubility (cholic acid has no effect on the composition of the bile). It may be a means of dissolving cholesterol stones, thereby treating the condition medically. It will not dissolve calcareous material, and therefore an accurate assessment of the nature of the stone is important before the agent is given.[15,16]

Pigment stones are an important complication of some congenital haemolytic anaemias (see p. 615), but not of the acquired ones. They are much commoner in the Black African and the Asian than in the European. Apparently another factor, in addition to hyperbilirubinaemia, is operative in their production. Since most of the bile pigments are excreted as the soluble diglucuronide, increased activity of the enzyme β-glucuronidase may be a factor in promoting the release of bilirubin, which is subsequently precipitated as the calcium salt. An inhibitor of β-glucuronidase, identified as glucaro-1, 4-lactone, is present in the normal bile. Its activity may be overcome by the β-glucuronidase activity of *Esch. coli*, thereby providing another link between infection and calculus formation.[17]

Secondary biliary calculi are produced as the result of cholecystitis, which often occurs in a gallbladder that already harbours stones. Secondary infective stones are more obviously 'mixed' than the 'primary' cholesterol type; they consist of variable quantities of cholesterol, calcium bilirubinate, and calcium carbonate, which produce a predominantly brown colouring. Mixed stones are characteristically multiple, no doubt forming around organisms and necrotic inflammatory debris. It usually happens that a family of stones form at the same time, and as they grow at a regular rate, they tend to press on each other. This leads to the typically faceted surfaces of mixed stones (Fig. 51.5). On section the stones present a characteristic concentric laminated appearance, and it is of interest that the laminae are parallel to the surface even of the faceted stones. Their shape is therefore determined during growth, and is not produced by mechanical erosion of one stone against another.

A second type of mixed stone is the *mulberry stone*. Occasionally it is solitary, but more usually there are multiple stones of one or more generations.

Another type of secondary calculus is one that develops around a primary cholesterol stone. It enlarges progressively by the concentric precipitation of calcium salts, bile pigments, and cholesterol. It is called a *combination stone*, and may be accompanied by other stones of mixed type. Sometimes a combination stone remains solitary, and by its steady growth eventually fills and distends the gallbladder. This is called a *barrel stone* (Fig. 51.6).

A final type of mixed stone is earthy, soft, and laminated. It is formed in the bile ducts, and is smooth and egg-shaped or sausage-shaped. The formation of this type of stone is generally attributed to *stasis*.

SALIVARY CALCULI

Found most commonly in the submandibular duct, these consist of calcium phosphate and carbonate, i.e. they are of the secondary type. Their mode of formation is obscure, but it is probable that they form around a central nidus composed of desquamated epithelial cells and masses of organisms, e.g. actinomyces. Infection leads to calculus formation, and calculi predispose to infection. In this vicious circle it is impossible to decide which comes first.

PANCREATIC CALCULI

These are uncommon. They consist of calcium phosphate and carbonate. They are found in association with chronic pancreatitis, which is itself an obscure condition. The stones are found in the larger ducts, the epithelium of which shows squamous metaplasia. The mode of production of these stones is unknown.

Figure 51.5
A family of 'mixed' gallstones. They are all of approximately the same size, and their surfaces are smoothly faceted. Their predominantly dark colour testifies to the large amount of bile pigment present in them, while the pale areas are due to cholesterol. (*Reproduced by permission of the President and Council of the R.C.S. Eng.*)

Figure 51.6
Barrel stone. This large calculus forms a complete cast of an enlarged gallbladder. (*Reproduced by permission of the President and Council of the R.C.S. Eng.*)

Figure 51.7
Renal calculus. This is a hydronephrotic kidney, in the pelvis of which there is a large, round phosphatic calculus. It has been sectioned to show its laminated construction. It has been built up by the layering of successive deposits of phosphates on the original central phosphate piece. (U 25.3, *Reproduced by permission of the President and Council of the R.C.S. Eng.*)

PROSTATIC CALCULI

These are found not infrequently in the hyperplastic prostates of elderly men, and occur in the smaller ducts. They consist of calcium phosphate and carbonate. They are typically small and multiple. The secretions of the acini often become inspissated in the ducts to form *corpora amylacea*, and these are probably the nuclei around which the calcium salts precipitate. Sometimes necrotic inflammatory debris and blood clot also act as a central nidus.

EFFECTS OF CALCULI

Calculi are often silent, and are discovered accidentally during radiological or *post-mortem* examinations. They may, however, produce definite pathological effects:

Pain. The sudden distension or spasm of a hollow muscular viscus produced by a stone leads to pain. Spasm itself causes a typical colic. Urinary calculi, by abrading the mucosa, also cause **haemorrhage.**

Obstruction. A ureteric or renal calculus may obstruct the outflow or urine completely or partially. If obstruction is sudden and complete, the kidney stops secreting urine, and undergoes slow disuse atrophy. If obstruction is partial or intermittent, there is a dilatation of the ureter and pelvis proximal to the stone, so that a considerable hydronephrosis may eventually develop (Fig. 51.7).

Likewise an intermittent obstruction of the cystic duct leads to a mucocele of the gallbladder. A blockage of the common bile duct results in obstructive jaundice, which is characteristically intermittent and fluctuant in intensity. A barrel stone may rarely ulcerate through the wall of the gallbladder into the duodenum. In its subsequent passage down the bowel it may impact in the lumen, and lead to intestinal obstruction. The transient blockage of the ampulla of Vater by migrating gallstones is a possible cause of acute pancreatitis.[18]

A salivary calculus leads to a painful distension of the associated salivary gland, especially during mastication.

Infection. Where there is any element of stasis in an outflowing secretion, infection is bound to be superadded in due course. The organisms may come from the exterior, as in the salivary duct, or be derived from the excretion of the viscus itself, as in the kidney and liver. A pyonephrosis eventually complicates a hydronephrosis, and acute 'ascending' cholangitis stones in the common bile duct. An empyema of the gallbladder is a well-known sequel to a stone in the cystic duct. Suppurative sialadenitis is a frequent accompaniment of salivary calculi. The presence of infection leads to secondary calculus formation, and sets up a vicious circle.

Malignancy. Carcinoma of the gallbladder is very frequently superimposed on a chronically-inflamed organ that contains stones. On the other hand, it is an uncommon form of cancer, and there may well be little causal relationship between the stones and the subsequent malignancy (see Ch. 29).

Pancreatic and prostatic calculi seldom produce definite symptoms, and are usually discovered incidentally.

REFERENCES

1. Leading Article (1975) Bladder stone. *British Medical Journal*, **2,** 578.
2. McGeown, M. G. & Bull, G. M. (1957) Pathogenesis of urinary calculus formation. *British Medical Bulletin*, **13,** 53.
3. Joekes, A. M., Rose, G. A. & Sutor, J. (1973) Multiple renal silica calculi. *British Medical Journal*, **1,** 146.
4. Williams, H. E. & Smith, L. H. (1972) Primary hyperoxaluria, in *The Metabolic Basis of Inherited Disease*, ed. by Stanbury, J. B., Wyngaarden, J. B. & Fredrickson, D. S., 3rd edn, p. 196, New York: McGraw-Hill.
5. Leading Article (1963) Medical aspects of renal stones. *Lancet*, **1,** 34.
6. Peacock, M., Knowles, F. & Nordin, B. E. C. (1968) Effect of calcium administration and deprivation on serum and urine calcium in stone-forming and control subjects. *British Medical Journal*, **2,** 729.
7. Cochran, M. *et al.* (1968) Renal tubular acidosis of pyelonephritis with renal stone disease. *British Medical Journal*, **2,** 721.
8. Leading Article (1972) Calcium in the kidneys. *Lancet*, **1,** 825.
9. Annotation (1968) Classification of human gallstones. *Lancet*, **1,** 1416.

10. RUSSELL, I. S., WHEELER, M. B. & FREAKE, R. (1968) The composition of human gall-stones. *British Journal of Surgery*, 55, 161.
11. BOUCHIER, A. I. D. & FRESTON, J. W. (1968) The aetiology of gallstones. *Lancet*, 1, 340.
12. WALKER, J. G. (1974) In *Clinical Physiology*, ed. Campbell, E. J. M., Dickinson, C. J. & Slater, J. D. H., 4th edn, p. 568. Oxford: Blackwell.
13. SHERLOCK, S. (1975) *Diseases of the Liver and Biliary System*, 5th edn, p. 727. Oxford: Blackwell.
14. Leading Article (1976) Iatrogenic gallstones. *British Medical Journal*, 1, 859.
15. Leading Article (1972) Medical treatment of gallstone disease. *Lancet*, 1, 360.
16. Leading Article (1977) Choosing patients for chenodeoxycholic acid treatment. *British Medical Journal*, 2, 1119.
17. SMALL, D. M. (1968) Gallstones. *New England Journal of Medicine*, 279, 588.
18. ACOSTA, J. M. & LEDESMA, C. L. (1974) Gallstone migration as a cause of acute pancreatitis. *New England Journal of Medicine*, 290, 484.

Chapter 52.   Some Disorders of the Blood: The Red Cell

I—THE RED CELL

The science of haematology is now so complicated that many haematologists confine themselves to a single facet of the speciality, e.g. the haemolytic anaemias, the leukaemias, or the disorders of clotting, and relegate other aspects of blood disease to colleagues more expert than themselves. Despite this disheartening prospect it is still possible for the interested observer to learn a great deal about the common blood disorders through a grasp of elementary pathological principles. Once this has been achieved, the standard textbooks are at his disposal for further enlightenment.

THE NORMAL LIFE CYCLE OF THE RED CELL

Development

The original haematopoietic cell in the fetus is believed to be a migrating multipotential *stem cell* that arises in the yolk-sac and migrates to the liver, spleen, and bone marrow. In all these organs there is a period of haematopoiesis during fetal life, but at birth all blood formation is confined to the bone marrow, apart from small foci of haematopoiesis in the liver that disappear after a few days. The postnatal stem cell resides in the bone marrow and travels to distant sites from there. Whether this is the same stem cell that gives rise to all the cells mentioned in Chapter 30 seems unlikely.

If mice are lethally irradiated and then given an intravenous injection of marrow cells, macroscopic nodules of haemat-opoietic tissue are present on the surface of the animal's spleen ten days after the injection. These colonies are clonal, arising from a single cell. Such colonies may contain eryth-rocytes, neutrophils, megakaryocytes, and eosinophils, indicat-ing that the *colony-forming unit cell* is pluripotential for these cell lines. Cytogenetic data from patients with chronic myeloid leukaemia are compatible with the existence of such a cell in the human subject; when the Philadelphia chromosome abnor-mality is present it can be demonstrated in precursors of erythrocytes, leucocytes, eosinophils, and probably megaka-ryocytes, but not in lymphocytes or buccal mucosal cells. It may be present in the marrow fibroblast, suggesting a com-mon fibroblast-haematopoietic stem cell. This finding in-cidentally points to the clonal origin of chronic myeloid leukaemia (see Chapter 29).

Colonies grown on semi-solid media from human marrow or blood contain neutrophils, eosinophils, and monocytes. Since these colonies, at least in human beings, are also clonal in nature, this observation, in addition to the myeloblast-monoblast mixtures seen in some cases of acute myeloid leukaemia (see p. 624), suggests a common origin for neut-rophils, eosinophils, and monocytes.

Lymphocytes appear to form their own stem-cell compart-ment under steady-state conditions. Small lymphocytes under-go 'blastic' transformation and mitosis when necessary (see p. 151). The primitive stem cell can, however, give rise to lymphocytes in mice under conditions of extreme cellu-lar deprivation.

To summarise, there is a primitive stem cell (which may possibly be a special type of lymphocyte, as mentioned on p. 391) which is pluripotential for all blood cells. One of its progeny, the cell that forms spleen colonies in the mouse (the colony-forming unit cell) is in turn pluripotential for all cells except the lymphocyte. Differentiated stem-cell compartments replenish blood cells under normal circumstances; neutrophils, eosinophils, and monocytes share a common compartment.

If the differentiated stem-cell compartment is 'committed' to red-cell development, it passes through the following four stages:

Pronormoblast. A large cell with deeply basophilic cytoplasm and a large nucleus containing fine clumps of chromatin and several nucleoli.

Basophilic (early) normoblast. A slightly smaller cell with deeply basophilic cytoplasm. There are no nucleoli in its

Figure 52.1
Normoblasts in peripheral blood. The patient was a newborn infant with erythroblastosis fetalis due to Rh-haemolytic disease. One in-termediate normoblast and six late normoblasts are shown. × 960.

nucleus. Some authorities do not separate it from the pronormoblast.

Polychromatic (intermediate) normoblast. The cell is somewhat smaller, and the cytoplasm has a greenish tint due to the first appearance of haemoglobin. The nucleus is smaller and its chromatin is condensed into thick clumps (Fig. 52.1).

Pyknotic (late) normoblast. The cell is much smaller, and contains a dense pyknotic nucleus which is later extruded. The cytoplasm is usually reddish (orthochromatic) due to an abundance of haemoglobin.

It should be noted that the word 'erythroblast' refers to any nucleated red cell, both the normal normoblast series described above, and the megaloblast series typical of pernicious anaemia. A table illustrating the cellular components of the bone marrow and indicating their derivation is given in the next chapter (p. 619).

THE NORMAL RED CELL[1]

The mature red corpuscle appears greenish-yellow in unstained preparations, and is roughly circular in shape. Seen on edge it is a biconcave disc. It is brightly eosinophilic in blood films, using the usual Romanowsky techniques,* because of its content of haemoglobin. This is distributed uniformly throughout the cell, but the centre is somewhat paler than the periphery due to the biconcavity.

A young erythrocyte often contains remnants of the basophilic ribonucleic acid (RNA), which is very conspicuous in the cytoplasm of the early normoblast. Such a red cell may stain a bluish or greyish colour with Romanowsky dyes, and this is called *polychromasia* (or diffuse basophilia). Sometimes the RNA is aggregated in discrete granules, so producing *punctate basophilia* (or basophilic stippling). The most important appearance of this RNA, however, is as filamentous skeins that cannot be demonstrated by Romanowsky methods, which need preliminary fixation with methyl alcohol. If blood is stained supravitally with brilliant cresyl blue, these basophilic threads are outlined; they are the 'reticulum' of the *reticulocyte.* Polychromasia, punctate basophilia, and reticulocytosis are all manifestations of residual RNA in newly-formed red cells; the difference lies in the form that the RNA assumes and in the presence or absence of prior fixation. Electron microscopy shows it in the form of ribosomal aggregates.

In practice a *reticulocyte count* is the most accurate method of assessing an increase in the number of these young red cells; the range is 0·8 to 2·5 per cent in men and 0·8 to 4·1 per cent in women. A rise in the reticulocyte percentage indicates an accelerated rate of red-cell formation. This may be secondary to red-cell depletion, as after haemorrhage or haemolysis, or it may follow the successful treatment of a chronic anaemia like pernicious anaemia or iron-deficiency anaemia. In this

*The Romanowsky dyes (which include such well-known stains as Leishman, Jenner, May-Grünwald, and Giemsa) consist of a carefully blended mixture of methylene blue and eosin. Derivatives of the mixture stain the blood cells admirably. Acidic groupings in the nucleic acids of the nuclei and primitive cytoplasm take up variable amounts of basic methylene blue, while basic groupings on the haemoglobin molecule have an affinity for acidic eosin. An important derivative, *methylene blue azure,* stains the 'azurophil' granules of monocytes and promyelocytes, as well as the nuclei of malarial and other parasites, a reddish-purple colour.

case the reticulocytosis is temporary, and heralds a progressive increase in the red-cell count. Reticulocytes are larger than older red cells, therefore any condition accompanied by a reticulocytosis has a mildly macrocytic blood picture. In very severe haemolytic anaemias there may also be nucleated red cells in the peripheral blood, a feature especially typical of haemolytic disease of the newborn and thalassaemia major.

EXAMINATION OF THE RED CELL

The most useful method of examining red cells is to inspect them in a well-made, well-stained blood film. By this means an experienced haematologist can diagnose many common blood disorders. Quantitative indices are of value, but they merely state in figures what a trained eye can relate in form. A *haemoglobin estimation* is certainly essential in order to assess the presence and degree of anaemia. It is a simple and easily reproducible procedure. A *packed cell volume* is also useful and reliable, but it necessitates a venepuncture, whereas a blood film and haemoglobin estimation can be performed on capillary blood. A *red-cell count* has so great a margin of error that it cannot be recommended as a routine investigation, unless the laboratory is equipped with an electronic cell counter. There are three *absolute values*, which are of use provided accurate measurements are made.

Mean corpuscular volume (MCV), which is obtained thus:

$$\frac{\text{Volume packed red cells (l per l)} \times 1000}{\text{Red cell count } (\times 10^{12} \text{ per l})}$$

expressed in 10^{-15}l, or femtolitres (fl).

Mean corpuscular haemoglobin (MCH), obtained thus:

$$\frac{\text{Haemoglobin (g per l)}}{\text{Red cell count } (\times 10^{12} \text{ per l})}$$

expressed in 10^{-12}g, or picograms (pg).

Mean corpuscular haemoglobin concentration (MCHC), obtained thus:

$$\frac{\text{Haemoglobin (g per dl)}}{\text{Volume packed red cells (l per l)}}$$

expressed in grams of haemoglobin per decilitre of packed red cells (g per dl).

This index, unlike the MCH, assesses the degree of haemoglobinisation of the red cells irrespective of their size. Red cells cannot be over-haemoglobinised, but they can be deficient in haemoglobin, and the MCHC is particularly useful in assessing the extent of under-haemoglobinisation, thus confirming the appearance in a well-stained film.

Another investigation that is occasionally performed is a measurement of *mean corpuscular diameter* (MCD) using an eyepiece micrometer. It is a simple procedure but little more informative than a well-made blood film. The following table summarises the range of red-cell values in a normal man:

TOTAL RED-CELL COUNT	4·6 to 6·2 × 10^{12} per litre in SI units
	(4·6 to 6·2 million per μl, or mm³)
HAEMOGLOBIN	14 to 18 g per dl

PACKED CELL VOLUME	0·40 to 0·54 (no unit is necessary, but litre per litre is implied)
MEAN CORPUSCULAR VOLUME (MCV)	80 to 96 fl
MEAN CORPUSCULAR HAEMOGLOBIN (MCH)	27 to 31 pg
MEAN CORPUSCULAR HAEMOGLOBIN CONCENTRATION (MCHC)	32 to 36 g per dl
MEAN CORPUSCULAR DIAMETER (MCD)	6·7 to 7·7 μm*

There are some physiological variations in the levels of haemoglobin, total red cells, and packed cell volume. Thus, the newborn infant has a high level of circulating red cells, but there is such a precipitous drop within the first month of life that the subsequent level is distinctly below the adult standard. After the fifth year there is a steady rise to the adult level, which is finally attained at puberty. The red-cell count in women is about $0·5 \times 10^{12}$/litre (half a million cells per μl) less than in men, and the haemoglobin level is about 2 g per dl lower. Another important factor influencing the red-cell count is the barometric pressure. People who live at high altitudes have a moderate polycythaemia to compensate for the low oxygen tension of the surrounding air.

The normal red cell is described as *normocytic* and *normochromic*, i.e. it is normal in size and haemoglobin concentration as defined by the above table. If it is larger in volume than normal it is called a *macrocyte*, and if smaller, a *microcyte*. Marked variation in size of a population of red cells is called *anisocytosis*, and a marked variation in shape, *poikilocytosis*. Cells with a reduced concentration of haemoglobin are described as *hypochromic*, and in a stained film they are easily recognisable by their colourless centres, which may be so extensive that only a narrow rim of haemoglobin is left around the periphery ('pessary forms'). In addition, the cells may contain a small central aggregation of haemoglobin surrounded by the extensive colourless zone; these are called *target cells*. The term *leptocyte* is used to include all such abnormally thin, under-haemoglobinised red cells.

Although macrocytes often appear extremely well-coloured, they do not contain a greater concentration of haemoglobin than normal. The appearance is due to the increased cell thickness which obliterates the mild central pallor normally present. There is therefore no such condition as hyperchromia.

Another pathological type of red cell is the *spherocyte*, which appears on a blood film as a small, darkly-staining cell. It is almost perfectly spherical in shape, and although it seems small, its volume is normal because of an increased thickness. This accounts for its deep staining despite a normal concentration of haemoglobin.

'*Burr*' *cells*, or *acanthocytes*, are mature red cells which possess one or several spiky projections on their periphery. They are characteristic of those haemolytic anaemias in which

mechanical trauma is believed to damage the red cells, e.g. microangiopathic haemolytic anaemia. They are also found in uraemia and abetalipoproteinaemia (p. 583).

HAEMOGLOBIN

Haemoglobin is a conjugated protein. The molecule consists of four haem groups attached to the protein globin, which in turn is composed of two pairs of polypeptide chains, designated α and β respectively. A haem group is attached to each polypeptide chain (Fig. 52.2).

Haem is a metal complex. It consists of an iron (Fe^{2+}) atom in the centre of a porphyrin structure, which is in fact a protoporphyrin. Porphyrins are tetrapyrroles. The four pyrrole rings are united by four methene bridges to produce the porphin nucleus. The structural formula of haem is shown on page 562.

The biosynthesis of porphyrins starting with a simple acetate salt has been elucidated. It is a very complex process, and it is found that, in addition to the protoporphyrin bound in the haem group, there are two other by-products formed (see Fig. 33.8, p. 435). These are called *coproporphyrin* and *uroporphyrin*, because they were first discovered in the faeces and urine respectively. Coproporphyrin is excreted in small amounts both in the faeces and the urine. The amount is raised whenever there is increased erythropoiesis, and it is also high in chronic lead poisoning. Liver disease is associated with an increased urinary excretion and a diminished faecal excretion of coproporphyrin. Despite its name, uroporphyrin is present in the urine in an even smaller amount than coproporphyrin.* In the *porphyrias* there is a defect in pyrrole metabolism, which is either inherited or due to liver disease (see p. 434).

From a haematological point of view the *globin* moiety of haemoglobin is even more interesting than its haem group. An important group of blood dyscrasias is now known to be due to *abnormal haemoglobins* and the abnormality of these haemoglobins resides in their globin portion. The study of the *haemoglobinopathies*[2,3] is so specialised that it now forms a separate branch of haematology. Chemical analysis of the globin moiety has revealed that it consists of two pairs of polypeptide chains of which five types are known—α, β, γ, δ, and ε. Four normal types of haemoglobin have been recognised:

Haemoglobin A. This is the major component of normal adult human haemoglobin. Its globin consists of two α chains and two β chains, and the haemoglobin is therefore designated $\alpha_2^A \beta_2^A$.

Haemoglobin A_2. About 2 per cent of normal haemoglobin is designated Hb-A_2, and the β chains are replaced by δ. It is therefore $\alpha_2^A \delta_2^{A2}$.

Fetal haemoglobin. Hb-F is the normal haemoglobin found in the fetus and during early infancy. Its formation may continue abnormally in infancy as a result of any type of anaemia causing marrow overactivity. Hb-F is designated $\alpha_2^A \gamma_2^F$.

---

*This is the average red-cell diameter in a film. In an isotonic medium, the average red cell is 8·4 μm in diameter.[1]

*About 250 mg of porphyrin are made each day during haem synthesis. Nearly all of this is protoporphyrin. Less than 1 mg is excreted as coproporphyrin (about 300 μg in the faeces and 200 μg in the urine) and uroporphyrin (about 10 μg in the urine).

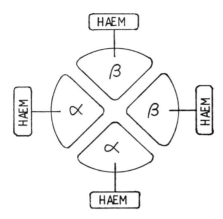

Figure 52.2
Diagrammatic representation of haemoglobin. The four polypeptide chains of globin are labelled α and β. (*After Wintrobe, M. M.* (1967), *Clinical Hematology, 6th ed., Fig.* 3–7, *p.* 139. *Philadelphia: Lea & Febiger*)

Embryonic haemoglobin. This is found only in the very early embryo and is depicted as $\alpha_2^A \varepsilon_2$; an ε_4 has also been described.

There are two types of inherited disorders of haemoglobin synthesis. There may be a structural abnormality in one of the polypeptide chains, usually the α or β chains of Hb-A. Thus Hb-S has a replacement of glutamic acid in the sixth position of the β chain by valine; a defect in mRNA is responsible. In the second type of abnormality, the thalassaemia syndromes, there is a gross reduction in the rate of synthesis of one of the globin subunits and overproduction of another. Thus in the common type of thalassaemia there is deficient β chain production, and an excess of Hb-F and Hb-A_2 is produced (p. 612). The actual structure of the haemoglobins is normal.

The various haemoglobins differ from the normal Hb-A in such physico-chemical attributes as electrophoretic mobility, resistance to alkali denaturation, solubility, and antigenicity. New variants were allotted a new letter, but this method of nomenclature soon proved inadequate (see later). The clinical effects of abnormal haemoglobins vary; some, such as Hb-G, Hb-J, and Hb-K are apparently symptomless. Others, by adding a new property, may have serious effects: the insolubility of Hb-S leads to the vascular occlusive effects of sickle-cell anaemia, which Hb-M leads to the formation of an abnormal methaemoglobin and so impairs the oxygen-carrying capacity of the red cells. The most important effect of abnormal haemoglobins is haemolytic anaemia (see p. 611).

The electrophoretic mobility of most abnormal haemoglobins is slower than that of normal adult haemoglobin, though a few rare ones are somewhat faster.

Normal adult haemoglobin (Hb-A) is rapidly denatured by an alkali, like potassium hydroxide, so that it cannot combine with oxygen any longer. Fetal haemoglobin (Hb-F) is much more resistant to alkali denaturation, and is easily distinguished from adult haemoglobin by this means. Hb-F is often present among the abnormal haemoglobins of different haemoglobinopathies, and is particularly conspicuous in β-thalassaemia major.

Haemoglobin-S, the abnormal haemoglobin of sickle-cell anaemia, is much more insoluble in its reduced state than as the oxy-compound. It is this property that enables sickling to be so easily demonstrable when the haemoglobin is reduced.

The abnormal haemoglobins are genetically determined; for instance large populations in Africa are heterozygous for Hb-S and often for Hb-C as well, whereas many South-East Asians are heterozygous for Hb-E. It has been well established that the Hb-S trait is associated with a relative immunity to *P. falciparum* malaria. The geneticist and the anthropologist are as interested in abnormal haemoglobins as is the haematologist.

The nomenclature of the haemoglobins is complicated. For a while capital letters were used according to the haemoglobin's electrophoretic mobility. If several haemoglobins occupied the same position on the strip, the geographical area where the abnormal haemoglobin was first found was appended, e.g. Hb-G(Baltimore), Hb-G(Honolulu), Hb-G(Norfolk), and Hb-G(Philadelphia).

It was finally decided to discontinue designating new variants by letter. New variants are named by the area or hospital where the haemoglobin was discovered, e.g. Hb-Dakar. The most logical nomenclature is to record the haemoglobin in terms of its structure; thus Hb-S is $\alpha_2^A \beta_2^S$ or better still, since the exact abnormality is known in this case, $\alpha_2^A \beta_2^{6glu \rightarrow val}$.

HAEMOGLOBIN AND OXYGEN CARRIAGE

Haemoglobin must be maintained in a reduced state to function as an oxygen carrier. However, in the presence of a high concentration of oxygen it is readily oxidised to methaemoglobin. This is useless for oxygen transport, but it can be reduced to haemoglobin by $NADH_2$, which itself is oxidised to NAD. The glycolytic, or Embden-Meyerhof, pathway (p. 48) provides the means whereby NAD is again reduced to $NADH_2$. The glycolytic pathway also results in the formation of ATP, a compound which provides the necessary source of energy for the red cell—particularly for the extrusion of sodium and the maintenance of a high level of intracellular potassium.

Another important pathway of glucose metabolism in the red cell is the oxidative hexosemonophosphate shunt (p. 24). In this NADP is reduced to NADPH, a co-enzyme necessary for the conversion of oxidised glutathione (GSSG) to the reduced state (GSH) through the glutathione reductase reaction. This GSH is a vital component of the red cell, for it helps to maintain the readily oxidisable SH groups of haemoglobin and red-cell enzymes. In the process GSH becomes oxidised to GSSG. The haemolytic anaemias related to genetic enzyme defects in both the glycolytic pathway and in the hexosemonophosphate shunt are described on page 612.

The important function of oxygen carriage by the haemoglobin of red cells has been found to be regulated by the concentration of 2,3-diphosphoglycerate (DPG) in the cells.[4] This substance complexes with reduced haemoglobin and inhibits its oxygen binding capacity; this facilitates the unloading of oxygen to the tissues. Variation in the DPG content of red cells is an important regulating mechanism, the details of which are not yet clear. Thus ascent to a high altitude causes a substantial increase in the DPG level, and oxygen is therefore made more readily available to the tissues. A similar increase occurs in other conditions of hypoxia such as in heart failure, chronic lung disease, and anaemia. The importance of DPG as a regulator is illustrated by comparing the well-tolerated anaemia of pyruvate-kinase deficiency, which has a high red-cell DPG level, with the poorly tolerated anaemia of hexo-kinase deficiency, in which DPG is deficient (see p. 612).

It has also been found that there are minor haemoglobin components consisting of complexes of haemoglobin A (and also haemoglobin A_2, which is less important because of the very small proportion in normal red cells) with glucose (HbA_{1c}), glucose phosphate (HbA_{1b}), pyridoxine, and glutathione. Although there is little difference in oxygen affinity between haemoglobins A and A_{1c} when they are stripped of 2,3-DPG, when DPG is added to haemoglobin A, the Po_2 at which the haemoglobin is half saturated (the P_{50}) is increased twofold, whereas the increase is only 23 per cent with HbA_{1c}. There is an increase in the proportion of these glycosylated haemoglobins, especially A_{1c}, in the red cells of patients with diabetes mellitus, and this has the effect of reducing the oxygen supply to the tissues. This is especially serious when there is diabetic angiopathy with ischaemia.[5,6]

REQUIREMENTS FOR RED-CELL PRODUCTION

Protein, including the essential amino acids.

Vitamin B. The essential factors are *folic acid (pteroylglutamic acid)* and *vitamin B_{12} (cobalamin)*. In the absence of either (or both) the red-cell precursors undergo a characteristic perversion of development called *megaloblastic erythropoiesis*. A *megaloblast* is a nucleated red cell which is tetraploid and therefore larger than a normoblast in the corresponding stage of development. It has a large nucleus containing chromatin arranged in a delicate, stippled pattern instead of the coarse clumps characteristic of a normoblast (Fig. 52.3). When the nucleus is finally extruded a macrocyte is produced. Pathological megaloblasts are very similar in appearance to the nucleated red cells seen in normal fetal marrow.

Folic acid is water-soluble and easily absorbed from the bowel. Vitamin B_{12} cannot be so absorbed, unless given in massive doses, except in the presence of *intrinsic factor*, a mucoprotein which is normally secreted by the epithelium of the stomach. Vitamin B_{12} is the *extrinsic factor*. The intrinsic factor-vitamin B_{12} complex is absorbed selectively by the terminal ileum; the vitamin enters the absorptive cell while the intrinsic factor apparently remains outside. Both vitamin B_{12} and folic acid are stored in the liver.

The metabolic functions of these two substances are still not well understood. Both are necessary for DNA biosynthesis. Nevertheless, an anaemia due to folic-acid deficiency does not respond well to vitamin B_{12}, and *vice versa*. Furthermore, the neurological complications of vitamin-B_{12} deficiency are aggravated by the administration of folic acid.

The most widely favoured hypothesis at present is that vitamin-B_{12} deficiency interferes with the metabolism or transport of folate.[7] It may well be that as in the case of megaloblast formation, the neurological manifestations of vitamin-B_{12} deficiency are due to a block in the metabolism of folic acid. Patients with neurological complications of vitamin-B_{12} deficiency have the highest level of plasma folate.[7]

The normal level of vitamin B_{12} in the plasma ranges from

Figure 52.3
A megaloblast. Note the large size of the cell and its stippled nuclear chromatin as compared with the much smaller normoblast and its pyknotic nucleus. The smear was from the marrow of a patient with pernicious anaemia. × 960.

200 to 900 ng per litre (pg per ml). In pernicious anaemia it is usually below 100 ng per litre. It is particularly low in subacute combined degeneration of the cord, which sometimes manifests itself before there is any anaemia.

The *Schilling test* is used to assess the absorption of vitamin B_{12} from the bowel. A test dose of the vitamin labelled with radioactive cobalt is given *orally*, and the patient is loaded with 1000 μg of *unlabelled vitamin intramuscularly* to prevent storage of any absorbed labelled vitamin. Hence all the absorbed labelled vitamin is excreted in the urine. The urine is collected for 24 hours, and the excretion of labelled vitamin measured. Normally more than 15 per cent is excreted. If the excretion is less than 5 per cent the test is repeated, this time mixing intrinsic factor with the labelled vitamin. If this restores excretion to normal, the defect is gastric (e.g. pernicious anaemia), but if it has no effect, there is an intestinal lesion. It is important first to exclude renal disease as a cause of poor excretion. It should be noted that the performance of the Schilling test involves the administration of large doses of vitamin B_{12}. Hence repeated blood counts should be performed lest a reticulocyte response be missed.

The normal plasma folate level is 5 to 21 μg per litre (ng per ml), and the red-cell folate is 160 to 640 μg per litre of packed cells. A plasma folate below 4 μg per litre and a red-cell folate below 140 μg per litre indicates folic-acid deficiency. Another useful test of folic-acid deficiency is the formiminoglutamic acid (Figlu) test. Histidine is degraded into Figlu when it is metabolised, and this in turn is acted on by folic acid. In cases of deficiency there is an accumulation of Figlu in the urine after an oral dose of histidine.

Pyridoxine (*vitamin* B_6) is also important in red-cell production. The cofactor pyridoxyl phosphate is essential for an early stage of porphyrin synthesis. Deficiency in animals leads to a hypochromic, microcytic anaemia despite great sideraemia and siderosis. In humans there is seldom any anaemia until the deficiency is very severe. Isoniazid therapy tends to interfere with the activity of pyridoxine, and may lead to symptoms of its deficiency.

Ascorbic acid. The part that vitamin C plays in erythropoiesis is still uncertain. Scurvy is usually attended by multiple deficiencies which complicate the blood picture. Ascorbic acid is necessary for the conversion of folic acid to folinic acid (citrovorum factor), which is also essential for nucleic-acid synthesis. Ascorbic acid deficiency may occasionally be associated with megaloblastic erythropoiesis especially in infancy, and cases are on record in which pernicious anaemia remained unresponsive to vitamin B_{12} until ascorbic acid was also administered. There may be a haemolytic element in the anaemia of scurvy.

Minerals

Iron.[8] This is obviously an essential mineral, as it forms an integral part of the haem group. Most iron is absorbed from the bowel in the ionic form, ferrous ions being more easily absorbed than ferric ions. The solubility of iron is decreased by phytates (present in cereals), phosphates, and an alkaline medium. It is for this reason that hydrochloric acid aids iron absorption, most of which occurs in the duodenum and upper portion of the small intestine, and little in the colon. Ascorbic acid also assists iron absorption, presumably because it reduces ferric iron to the ferrous state. In practice, however, neither hydrochloric acid nor ascorbic acid is necessary unless there is a considerable deficiency of iron in the diet.

Iron can also be absorbed directly from haem without prior digestion to an ionised form. This is derived from haemoglobin and myoglobin in the diet, and is important in Western diets. The haem appears to be absorbed into the mucosal cell as an intact porphyrin complex, and its absorption is not affected by gastric acidity, ascorbic acid, or phytate.

The mode of absorption of iron by the mucosal cells of the small intestine is still not certain, but it probably depends on the ferritin mechanism, which traps iron and prevents its further absorption into the body, and a second mechanism for the absorption of iron from the mucosal cells. It is believed that the amount of iron absorbed from the gut by the mucosal cells is determined by the iron content ('messenger iron') of the epithelial cells. This in turn is determined by the body's requirements at the time of the cell's formation in the crypts of Lieberkühn. This messenger iron may act by partially saturating a carrier essential to absorption.

It is suggested that the amount of messenger iron is increased in states of iron overload or depressed erythropoiesis, and decreased in iron-deficiency states or during accelerated phases of erythropoiesis. Depending on this 'message', iron taken up from the gut can either proceed into the plasma or be incorporated into ferritin to be sloughed at the end of the life span of the mucosal cell. The nature of the transport of the ferrous iron across the mucosal cell is not known.

Iron is carried in the blood in the ferric state bound to a globulin called *iron-binding protein, transferrin,* or *siderophilin.* The concentration of transferrin in the plasma is 1·2 to 2 g per litre, but more commonly transferrin is quantitated in terms of the total iron it will bind, the *total iron-binding capacity* (*TIBC*) *of the plasma*, which is 45 to 70 μmol per litre (250 to 400 μg per dl); the plasma is normally a third saturated with iron. The iron-binding capacity is increased in the latter part of pregnancy and in iron-deficiency anaemia, but it is reduced in chronic infection, rheumatoid arthritis, cancer, cirrhosis of the liver, and the nephrotic syndrome. The normal level of iron in the plasma is 13 to 32 μmol per litre (70 to 180 μg per dl), and it is much reduced in iron-deficiency anaemia (*sideropenia*), while in most other types of anaemia it is moderately or greatly raised (*sideraemia*). The plasma iron is also raised in liver necrosis (see p. 567), and especially in transfusional siderosis and haemochromatosis, in which two conditions the iron-binding capacity of the plasma is saturated.

Iron is stored as ferritin and haemosiderin in the RE cells of the liver, spleen, and bone marrow, and small amounts are also present in the parenchymal cells. It would appear that the function of transferrin is to transport iron from the RE cells to the red-cell precursors. In cases of absence of transferrin there is severe iron-deficiency anaemia and heavy siderosis. Apparently transferrin is not essential for the transport of iron from the bowel.

The iron is incorporated by the normoblasts into haemoglobin, but in from 20 to 60 per cent of normoblasts small granules of ferritin can be demonstrated by Prussian-blue staining. This number is decreased in sideropenic anaemias and increased in sideraemic ones. Siderotic normoblasts are called *sideroblasts*. Occasionally siderotic granules are found in mature red cells, which are then called *siderocytes*. These are seen especially after splenectomy (see p. 629).

Iron excretion is small in men, in whom minute losses occur from the faeces, urine, hair, and nails. In women greater losses occur during menstruation and pregnancy.

Copper. There is some experimental evidence that copper facilitates iron metabolism, but in clinical practice there is no convincing evidence that pure copper deficiency leads to anaemia.

Cobalt. Deficiency in animals leads to a severe anaemia, and excess cobalt may induce a polycythaemia. Its role in human nutrition is unknown. It is a constituent of vitamin B_{12}.

Hormonal Factors

Erythropoietin.[9] The glycoprotein erythropoietin is essential for the maintenance of the body's red-cell mass at an optimal physiological level, but how hypoxia, of whatever type, is translated by the body into augmented erythropoietin production is still not clear. The kidney is intimately involved, but attempts to extract an active erythropoietic substance from normal human kidney have often failed; it may be that the kidney secretes a precursor substance which acts on a plasma substrate to produce the hormone. Alternatively, the kidney may produce erythropoietin, which is then inhibited by a lipid present in renal tissue until activated by a factor in normal plasma. The cells involved are unknown. There are other sources of erythropoietin production, since a patient deprived of both kidneys can still mount a reticulocytosis in the face of blood loss or hypoxia. The liver is probably an important source of the hormone.

Volunteers who have undergone venesection have a high level of erythropoietin in their blood and urine, as do many patients with aplastic anaemia, but in other types of chronic anaemia the correlation between the haematocrit and the level of hormone is less convincing. This may be due to a defect in the erythropoietin system or to inadequate methods of hormone assay. The oxygen-delivering capacity of the blood is probably also important in determining the amount of circulating erythropoietin. Thus individuals with abnormal haemoglobins that possess an increased affinity for oxygen and in whom the Po_2 at which the haemoglobin is half saturated (this is called the P_{50}) is relatively low, show increased erythropoiesis, whereas those with abnormal haemoglobins that possess a decreased affinity for oxygen and in whom the P_{50} is high, seem to tolerate a low red-cell count without increased erythropoiesis or erythropoietin production. In a similar way some patients with chronic cor pulmonale are less polycythaemic than might be expected: respiratory acidosis decreases oxygen affinity and therefore tends to improve oxygen delivering capacity.

Erythropoietin appears to act on the stem cell, which once directed to erythroblastic differentiation, does not require any further erythropoietin stimulation. Erythropoietic depression occurs when there is a reduced demand for oxygen, e.g. after hypophysectomy and starvation.

Thyroxine. Lack of thyroxine decreases the rate of production of red cells, and there is a decreased use of iron for the synthesis of haemoglobin. Myxoedema sometimes causes a moderate normochromic, macrocytic anaemia with a hypocellular bone marrow. It is slowly reversed with thyroxine, which probably acts by altering the tissue demand for oxygen.

Androgen. This stimulates erythropoiesis, probably by potentiating the action of erythropoietin. It is useful in some types of aplastic anaemia, e.g. in myxoedema and hypopituitarism.

Glucocorticoids. These too stimulate erythropoiesis, but the mode of action is unknown. Polycythaemia may occur in Cushing's syndrome, and marrow aplasia in hypopituitarism. Addison's disease is associated with a normocytic, normochromic anaemia which is masked by the concomitant haemoconcentration.

The Disposal of the Red Cell

Two methods used to study the life-span of the red cell are *differential agglutination* using transfused compatible, though immunologically different, red cells, and *isotopic labelling* with radioactive elements, notably ^{51}Cr, which are incorporated metabolically into the patient's red cells. The cells are labelled with the chromate *in vitro*, and are then re-injected into the individual. Both these procedures indicate that the normal life-span of a red cell is about 120 days.

The manner in which the effete red cell is destroyed is still uncertain. The process of ageing precedes and is responsible for eventual destruction, and it is possible that the cell undergoes fragmentation in the circulation prior to its ultimate removal by the RE cells of the liver, bone marrow, and spleen.

Inside the RE cell the haemoglobin is broken down. The globin portion is released, degraded, and returned to the body's pool of amino acids. The porphyrin part of the haem molecule is converted into bilirubin (see Ch. 47), while the iron combines with apoferritin to form ferritin, and is then transported with transferrin to be used again.

Any free haemoglobin reaching the plasma is bound to an α_2-glycoprotein called *haptoglobin*. There are three main types of haptoglobins, and these are genetically distinct. Like the blood-group antigens and the abnormal haemoglobins, the haptoglobins are of anthropological and genetic interest. The plasma haptoglobin concentration (normally 0·4 to 2 g per litre) rises in inflammatory conditions similarly to the ESR.

If haemoglobin in excess of the haptoglobin binding capacity of the plasma is released, the free haemoglobin in the plasma is readily oxidised to methaemoglobin, which dissociates into haem and globin. Free haem is insoluble at the normal pH of the blood, but can be bound and maintained in a soluble form by two plasma proteins, haemopexin and albumin.

Haemopexin is a β_1-globulin (normal concentration 0·5 to 1 g per litre), and it has the greater affinity for haem, but when it is exhausted, its place is taken by *albumin*, which binds haem to form *methaemalbumin*. Both the haemopexin-haem and the methaemalbumin impart a coffee-brown colour to the plasma. With either, a spectral absorption band is observed at 620 to 630 nm, which will not (unlike a similar band in methaemoglobin) disappear if hydrogen peroxide is added. On the other hand, if ammonium sulphide is added, this band disappears and a band at 558 nm is formed. This is called *Schumm's test*, which is a reliable indication of an abnormal amount of intravascular haemolysis, since normally only traces of haemoglobin can be detected in the plasma. The haptoglobin, haemopexin, and albumin combinations are all metabolised in the body, principally in the liver, and none escapes into the urine.

Thus, after severe intravascular haemolysis haptoglobin is first lost from the circulation; then haemopexin disappears as the level of methaemalbumin increases. In acute haemorrhagic pancreatitis, extravasated haemoglobin is converted into haem which is absorbed into the circulation and forms complexes with haemopexin and albumin. The result is methaemalbuminaemia, a low haemopexin, and a *normal level of haptoglobin*; this finding has been described as a useful diagnostic test for the haemorrhagic variety of pancreatitis.[10]

Persistent haemoglobinaemia and haemoglobinuria occur only when all these binding proteins have been saturated. The tubular epithelium of the kidneys produces ferritin and haemosiderin from the free haemoglobin. *Haemosiderinuria* is therefore seen whenever there is persistent haemoglobinaemia. It is a common finding in patients with a heart-valve prosthesis.

THE ANAEMIAS

Anaemia may be defined as a condition in which there is a fall in the quantity of red cells or haemoglobin in a unit volume of blood in the presence of a low or normal total blood volume. In anaemia the total blood volume may be reduced due to a decrease in the number of red cells, but often, as in pernicious anaemia, this is offset by an absolute increase in the plasma volume. On the whole, the reduction in blood volume in anaemia is very small.

The question of blood volume and anaemia is important in relation to pregnancy. A moderate fall in the levels of red cells and haemoglobin is common during the latter part, and is followed by a slow recovery in the puerperium. There is a raised blood volume (due to a considerable increase in plasma volume) in pregnancy, and it is probable that much of the 'physiological anaemia' is due to simple haemodilution. However, there is often an additional element of iron deficiency.

There is no completely satisfactory classification of the anaemias. A *morphological classification* is extremely useful, but there is great overlapping, e.g. macrocytic anaemia is seen both in vitamin-B_{12} deficiency and in many haemolytic anaemias. Classifications based on *aetiology* or *pathogenesis* are also very helpful, but in some anaemias there are several mechanisms at work, e.g. pernicious anaemia has a haemolytic element as well as a maturation defect. Furthermore, some anaemias have no certain aetiology. The anaemia of chronic renal failure is described as 'toxic', but is probably secondary to deficient erythropoietin activity. The following classification is of practical value:

ACUTE POSTHAEMORRHAGIC ANAEMIA	Typically normochromic and normocytic. It is diagnosed clinically, and has been described on page 415.
IRON-DEFICIENCY ANAEMIA	Typically hypochromic and microcytic.
MEGALOBLASTIC ANAEMIA	Typically normochromic and macrocytic. The marrow contains megaloblasts.
HAEMOLYTIC ANAEMIA	Excessive red-cell destruction with subsequent regeneration (reticulocytosis) is the predominant feature.
ANAEMIA OF BONE-MARROW INADEQUACY	This is usually normocytic and normochromic, and there is little evidence of effective regeneration.

Anaemia results from the failure of the bone marrow to meet the demands of the body. This may be due to a massive haemorrhage depleting the blood mass too rapidly for it to be compensated, or to an absence of essential haematopoietic agents like iron, folic acid, or vitamin B_{12}, or else to excessive red-cell breakdown incompletely compensated by regeneration. In the anaemia of bone-marrow inadequacy there is reduced output, which can be assessed by studies of plasma and erythrocytic iron metabolism (ferrokinetics). The term *dyshaemopoietic anaemia* is not used, as it includes the iron-deficiency and megaloblastic group as well as some bone-marrow inadequacy states.

The main clinico-pathological features of anaemia are as follows:

Pallor, best detected in the conjunctiva, nail bed, or oral mucous membrane. Skin pallor, particularly of the face, is a deceptive sign. It may be absent in some patients with anaemia, and yet present in many pale-skinned, normal people.

Tiredness, easy fatigability, and *generalised muscular weakness* are common symptoms; their pathogenesis, however, is not clear. Such symptoms are also common in psychoneurotic patients who are not anaemic.

Shortness of breath, and *palpitations* are common. They are related to *tissue hypoxia* and an increased cardiac output. *Heart failure* can occur.

Angina pectoris, intermittent claudication, and *giddiness* are due to tissue hypoxia in organs in which the blood supply is already impaired by arterial disease.

The basal metabolic rate is raised, and in severe degrees of anaemia *pyrexia* is quite common. The cause of this is unknown.

The morbid anatomy of chronic anaemia is that of pallor and severe fatty change of the viscera. In days gone by, untreated pernicious anaemia was a frequent object of *post-mortem* study, and profound fatty change was described in the liver, kidneys, and even the heart. The 'thrush-breast', or 'tabby-cat', yellowish streaking of the papillary muscles, due to fatty change of the myocardium, was a classical finding. Nowadays death from chronic anaemia is very uncommon. Patients with incurable blood disorders, like aplastic anaemia and leukaemia, are kept at adequate haemoglobin levels by repeated red-cell transfusions until the final fatal episode.

IRON-DEFICIENCY ANAEMIA

Causes

Nutritional deficiency. In poor communities nutritional deficiency is the commonest cause of iron-deficiency anaemia. It is seen especially in infants, adolescent girls, middle-aged women, and the elderly.

Two historical conditions of iron deficiency are of interest.

(*a*) *Chlorosis*, which affected young girls between the ages of 14 and 17 years. The name derived from an alleged greenish pallor of the skin. The condition virtually disappeared after 1910 for reasons that are not readily apparent.

(*b*) *Idiopathic hypochromic anaemia*, which occurred predominantly in women in the fourth and fifth decades of life. There were usually severe epithelial changes due to the severity and chronicity of the iron deficiency. It was due to poor diets, multiple pregnancies, and menstrual irregularities. The condition is no longer recognised as a distinct entity; most cases, on investigation, prove to be due to chronic blood loss.

Inadequate absorption. Iron-deficiency anaemia is a common complication of *gastrectomy* and *vagotomy with gastroenterostomy* because of the rapid intestinal transit that follows the loss of the reservoir function of the stomach (intestinal hurry). This may lead to decreased absorption of iron, since the most active sites of iron absorption are in the duodenum (see p. 605). The lack of hydrochloric acid is a secondary factor. *Intestinal causes of malabsorption* often lead to severe iron deficiency.

Chronic blood loss. This is by far the most important cause of iron-deficiency anaemia in clinical practice. The source of blood loss may be *gastrointestinal*, e.g. from haemorrhoids, gastric and duodenal ulcers, oesophageal hiatal hernia, colonic diverticulosis and diverticulitis, and tumours of the stomach and intestines. Other important causes are *aspirin ingestion* leading to gastric erosions, and *hookworm infestation (ankylostomiasis)*. The worms attach to the upper small intestine and suck blood from the host. In most cases where there is severe anaemia, the inroads of poverty are major contributory factors, e.g. malnutrition and repeated pregnancies.

The other important source of blood loss is *reproductive*, e.g. menorrhagia, uterine fibroids, and metropathia haemorrhagica.

Haematological Findings

There is a moderate fall in red-cell count with a greater reduction in the haemoglobin level. The MCV, MCH, and MCHC are all reduced. Of these the MCHC is the most reliable, and is usually 25 to 30 g per dl. The red cells are microcytic and hypochromic, with a moderate degree of anisocytosis and poikilocytosis. Target cells are quite common (see Fig. 52.4). The reticulocyte count is normal or slightly increased. Rarely it is reduced.

The white cells and platelets are usually normal.

The bone marrow shows a mild to moderate degree of normoblastic hyperplasia. Less than 10 per cent of the normoblasts are sideroblasts, and the RE stores of iron are absent or severely reduced in the marrow (and liver).

Biochemical Findings

Reduced plasma iron, usually below $5 \cdot 6\,\mu$mol per litre ($30\,\mu$g per dl). The iron-binding capacity of the plasma is increased.

The plasma bilirubin is normal or low, for there is no increased haemolysis. There may be *achlorhydria* in some cases, especially in the idiopathic anaemia of the middle-aged.

Figure 52.4
Iron-deficiency anaemia. This film of peripheral blood contains red cells that are hypochromic. Quite a number show a target-like distribution of their haemoglobin. There are numerous platelets present. × 960.

Pathological Findings

Epithelial changes are important in longstanding cases of iron deficiency:

Mouth. Angular stomatitis.

Tongue. Atrophy of the filiform papillae. The tongue is red and sore, and burns when stimulated by food or drink.

Hypopharynx. Dysphagia due to web formation and strictures. Angular stomatitis, papillary atrophy of the tongue, and dysphagia together constitute the *Plummer-Vinson syndrome* (p. 375).

Stomach. Atrophic gastritis of varying degree, sometimes indistinguishable from that seen in pernicious anaemia. There may be severe hypochlorhydria as well as a reduction in the secretion of pepsin. The gastritis is both an accompaniment of chronic iron deficiency and a factor aggravating it.

Some patients with iron deficiency suffer from *pica* (derived from the Latin, and meaning a magpie), which is the habitual ingestion of unusual substances, e.g. earth or clay (geophagia)[11], laundry starch (amylophagia), or ice (pagophagia). The ingestion of clay or starch can both cause and aggravate iron deficiency by interfering with absorption (in the case of clay) or by constituting so much of the diet that iron and other nutriments are excluded (in the case of starch). Many forms of pica respond to iron therapy.

Nails. These become thinned, flattened, and eventually concave (spoon-shaped). This is called *kiolonychia*.

Hair. Diffuse loss of hair (alopecia) may be a feature of iron deficiency (as evidenced by low plasma iron levels) even in the absence of overt anaemia.

Other changes that may be seen in severe iron-deficiency anaemia are *an extension of red marrow into the shafts of the long bones* and *moderate enlargement of the spleen*. There are no specific pathological changes in the organ, and the pathogenesis of the enlargement is unknown.

MEGALOBLASTIC ANAEMIA[12]

Megaloblastic anaemias are characterised by disordered DNA synthesis. In the great majority of cases they are due to a deficiency of vitamin B_{12} or folic acid, either alone or in combination. Rarely they are due to drug-induced or inherited disorders of DNA synthesis.

Causes

Nutritional defects. It is noteworthy that a short period of dietary deprivation can lead to folate depletion, since the normal body folate stores remain adequate for only 2 to 4 months after the institution of an inadequate diet. By contrast, the stores of vitamin B_{12} can last for several years.

A nutritional megaloblastic anaemia is quite common in India, South-East Asia, and Africa. The diet contains much starches and grains with little animal protein or fresh, green vegetables. The condition has been called 'tropical macrocytic anaemia', although it can occur in temperate climates also, and it is due to folic-acid deficiency. If there is vitamin B_{12} deficiency also, the condition is considered to be caused by tropical sprue.

A true vitamin-B_{12}-deficiency anaemia has rarely been reported in vegans, strict vegetarians who do not eat any animal products. It is interesting that few vegans become anaemic despite the low level of plasma vitamin B_{12}.

Pregnancy. A nutritional megaloblastic anaemia is not uncommon in pregnant women living in temperate areas like Britain and the USA. It is due to folic-acid deficiency following poor intake and the demands of the fetus.

Megaloblastic anaemia has been noted in *infants*, and is once more due to a deficiency of folic acid.

Gastric defects. Since intrinsic factor is secreted by the gastric mucosa, it is to be expected that total gastrectomy would lead to megaloblastic anaemia. So great are the stores of vitamin B_{12} in the liver that it takes about 5 years for anaemia to develop. Partial gastrectomy may also lead to vitamin-B_{12} deficiency. The intestinal malabsorption due to intestinal hurry (see p. 441) acts together with the reduction in the amount of available intrinsic factor.

By far the most important gastric cause of megaloblastic anaemia is the mucosal atrophy that affects the upper two-thirds of the stomach in *pernicious anaemia*. This disease occurs most often in Northern Europeans, and shows a familial tendency. It is commonest in subjects of blood group A. It is probable that the tendency to mucosal atrophy is inborn, and that achylia gastrica (the absence of pepsin and hydrochloric acid in the gastric juice) is established before megaloblastic anaemia develops. In exceptional cases free hydrochloric acid is present in the gastric juice.

It is found that about 90 per cent of patients have antibodies (of IgA class) against parietal cells and 55 to 60 per cent have antibodies against intrinsic factor in their plasma. The presence of autoantibodies against intrinsic factor appears to be specific for pernicious anaemia, apart from rare cases of thyroid disease and atrophic gastritis. It has been suggested that pernicious anaemia is an autoimmune disease in which patients react abnormally to the frequent episodes of trauma to which the stomach is prone. The antibodies cause mucosal atrophy with an ensuing lack of secretion. On the other hand, it is possible that the autoantibodies are merely an indication of gastric disease. At any rate, an assessment of intrinsic factor antibodies is a useful diagnostic aid in some cases of pernicious anaemia. There is an increased incidence of disorders of a possibly 'autoimmune' type, e.g. thyroid disease, Addison's disease, vitiligo, and hypoparathyroidism, in near relatives, and some patients with pernicious anaemia have myxoedema or Graves's disease.

Cases of juvenile pernicious anaemia have been known in which there was no mucosal disease or autoantibodies. It is postulated that there is a genetic failure of the mucosal cells to produce intrinsic factor in these children.

Intestinal malabsorption. This, whether due to intrinsic mucosal disease or to conditions that lead to bacterial overgrowth in the small bowel, is often associated with megaloblastic anaemia.

Where there is bacterial overgrowth, as with strictures, fistulae, anastomoses, blind loops, and intestinal diverticulosis, vitamin B_{12} deficiency predominates. Apparently the organisms compete successfully for the vitamin, and they bind it so firmly that it becomes unavailable to the host. There is rarely any folate deficiency. The anaemia can be temporarily alleviated by the use of tetracyclines, which kill the organisms.

With intrinsic mucosal disease there may be a deficiency of both factors. In gluten-sensitive enteropathy folate deficiency is by far the commoner, since the ileum is often spared. In tropical sprue, which usually affects the whole of the small bowel, there tends to be an early folate deficiency with a later vitamin B_{12} deficiency, which may be quite severe.

Lesions affecting the ileum selectively, such as ileal resection, ileal bypass operations, and Crohn's disease, are often accompanied by a severe degree of vitamin B_{12} deficiency.

Fish-tapeworm infestation. This parasite, *Diphyllobothrium latum*, competes with its host for vitamin B_{12}. The megaloblastic anaemia is found only in Finland despite the wide distribution of the worm elsewhere in the world. The explanation for this is still not known.[13]

Drug-induced malabsorption. Megaloblastic anaemia due to the malabsorption of vitamin B_{12} is a rare complication of para-aminosalicylic acid (PAS) therapy.

Severe megaloblastic anaemia has been observed in patients taking anticonvulsants, notably primidone and phenytoin sodium, due to the malabsorption of folic acid. A similar defect in folate absorption has been reported in women taking oral contraceptives. The mechanism of these malabsorptions is not understood.

Hepatic cirrhosis. Megaloblastic anaemia due to folic-acid deficiency is sometimes seen in alcoholic cirrhosis of the liver. Plasma levels of vitamin B_{12} are normal or increased. The folate deficiency may be due to inadequate dietary intake, but there is also the possibility of disordered folate metabolism by the liver.

Rapid cellular proliferation. In many chronic haemolytic anaemias there is a relative folate deficiency sufficient to induce a megaloblastosis (see p. 615).

Drug-induced disorders of DNA synthesis. Megaloblastic anaemia is a predictable side-effect of cytotoxic drugs, e.g. cyclophosphamide, 6-mercaptopurine, 5-fluorouracil, cytosine arabinoside, and the folate antagonists (methotrexate). These drugs are used because they interfere with DNA synthesis and therefore inhibit the growth of rapidly dividing tissues. *Methotrexate* acts chiefly by competitive inhibition of dihydroxyfolate reductase. When this enzyme is inhibited, dietary folate cannot be converted into the active, tetrahydro form, and endogenous folate accumulates as the inactive dihydrofolate.

Trimethoprim also has an inhibitory effect on dihydroxyfolate reductase, but interferes with bacterial (or protozoal) enzyme more than with that of the host's cells. Combined with a sulphonamide, sulphamethoxazole (as 'co-trimoxazole' or 'septra'), there is a synergistic effect on bacterial folate metabolism that renders the mixture of use as a broad-spectrum antibacterial agent.[14] It is of particular use in *Pneumocystis carinii* lung infections. Anaemia is rarely a complication except in patients already prone to a megaloblastic anaemia for other reasons.

Inherited disorders affecting DNA synthesis. The most important example is orotic aciduria (p. 36). This is an inherited disorder of pyrimidine metabolism. There is a greatly reduced activity of two enzymes, orotidylic pyrophosphorylase and orotidylic decarbolase, both of which are required for the conversion of orotic acid to uridine-5'-phosphate. There is a megaloblastic anaemia and an excessive excretion of orotic acid in the urine. The condition does not respond to folate or vitamin B$_{12}$, but the administration of uridine leads to a haematological remission and a restoration of normal growth and development.

Haematological Findings

There is a considerable fall in red-cell count with a smaller reduction in the haemoglobin level. The MCV and MCH are greatly raised, but the MCHC is normal. The red cells are macrocytic and normochromic. Both anisocytosis and poikilocytosis are very marked (Fig. 52.5). Polychromasia and sometimes punctate basophilia may be noted, but the reticulocyte count is usually within normal limits. The peripheral blood often contains a few nucleated red cells. In the malabsorption syndrome there may be concomitant iron deficiency producing a 'dimorphic' blood picture.

There is a marked neutropenia, and some of the neutrophils are large and have multi-segmented nuclei (*macropolycytes*). A few myelocytes are often present in the peripheral blood.

The platelet count is reduced. Both the leucocyte and platelet abnormalities are more marked in pernicious anaemia than in the other megaloblastic anaemias.

The bone marrow shows megaloblastic hyperplasia, though normoblasts are also present in varying numbers. There is considerable myeloid hyperplasia also, and giant myelocytes are of diagnostic importance. Megakaryocytes may be reduced in number. It is evident that the dyshaematopoiesis of the megaloblastic anaemias is by no means confined to the red cells.

Biochemical Findings

There is a mild haemolytic process, which is most marked in

Figure 52.5
Megaloblastic anaemia. This film of peripheral blood contains well-haemoglobinized red cells which show considerable variation in size and shape. Large forms (macrocytes) predominate. × 800.

classical pernicious anaemia. This is manifested by a slightly raised plasma bilirubin (17 to 51 μmol per litre, or 1 to 3 mg per dl), an increased excretion of urobilinogen in the faeces, and moderate urobilinuria. The red-cell survival rate is considerably reduced, and in addition, the ineffective erythropoiesis adds to the bilirubin load. Patients given labelled glycine show an increased excretion of early labelled bilirubin (p. 562).

The plasma iron level is raised.

Achlorhydria is almost invariable in pernicious anaemia, but is inconstant in the other megaloblastic anaemias.

Pathological Findings

Severe fatty change of the liver, kidneys, and heart.

Marked haemosiderosis of the liver, bone marrow, kidneys, and spleen. This is due to a continued absorption of iron which is not adequately used for erythropoiesis.

The changes of subacute combined degeneration of the spinal cord: demyelination of the lateral and posterior columns without any gliosis. There may also be degenerative changes in the peripheral nerves and in the brain. It is taught that these neurological manifestations are peculiar to vitamin B$_{12}$ deficiency, but there is growing evidence that similar changes can occur in cases of folate deficiency.[15,16]

Atrophy of the mucosa of the tongue with disappearance of the filiform papillae. This is typical of pernicious anaemia, and produces the characteristic raw, beefy tongue. Glossitis is also seen in sprue, but is not constant in the other megaloblastic anaemias.

Atrophy of the gastric mucosa in pernicious anaemia has already been mentioned. It is the pathognomonic change of this disease.

Evidence of increased haematopoiesis: the marrow is deep red in colour, and extends into the shafts of the long bones where it replaces the fatty marrow. There may be extramedullary haematopoiesis in the spleen and liver. Moderate splenomegaly is typical of pernicious anaemia. In the malabsorption syndrome, on the other hand, splenic atrophy sometimes occurs.

There is evidence that a generalised cellular dystrophy attends folic-acid and vitamin-B$_{12}$ deficiency: many of the body's cells are larger than normal, and have a delicate chromatin network in their nuclei. This is seen not only in the cells of the bone marrow but also in the epithelial cells of the mouth and stomach (see p. 306).

THE HAEMOLYTIC ANAEMIAS[17]

Although there is a haemolytic component in many types of anaemia, in the haemolytic anaemias there is an increased rate of red-cell destruction with an unimpaired ability of the bone marrow to respond to the stimulus of anaemia. Under maximal stimulation the normal marrow is capable of undergoing hyperplasia until its production rate is increased from sixfold to eightfold. Thus with optimal marrow compensation it is theoretically possible for the survival of the red cells in the circulation to decrease from the normal 120 days to as little as 15 to 20 days without anaemia developing. This would be called *compensated haemolytic disease*, but when red-cell survival becomes so short that anaemia develops in spite of a vigorous erythropoietic response, the term *haemolytic anaemia* is appropriate.

The red-cell destruction is due either to some intrinsic defect in the red cells, or to some extracorpuscular factor acting on the red cells from without. If the defect is primarily corpuscular, the red cells of the patient will not survive long when transfused into a healthy recipient, whereas the patient's plasma will not destroy normal red cells. On the other hand, if the cause of the haemolysis is extracorpuscular, normal red cells will be eliminated in the same way as those of the patient, whereas the patient's red cells will survive well in a normal recipient. The diagnostic feature of a haemolytic anaemia is a persistent reticulocytosis in the absence of haemorrhage or bone-marrow replacement.

CORPUSCULAR DEFECTS

The most important of these are:

Hereditary spherocytosis (congenital acholuric jaundice). There is a spherocytic malformation of the red cell. The condition is inherited as an autosomal dominant characteristic, and is the most common hereditary haemolytic anaemia among people of Northern European stock. The abnormality lies in the cell membrane, but its underlying nature is obscure. Secondary effects on the membrane include a loss of phospholipid leading to spherocytosis, an abnormal permeability to sodium ions, and the change in shape predisposing to sequestration of the red cells in the spleen, where they are avidly phagocytosed and destroyed. Of all the haemolytic anaemias this one responds best to splenectomy. It is noteworthy that despite a dramatic amelioration of the anaemia and a greatly increased red-cell survival, the spherocytic malformation persists.

Hereditary elliptocytosis. This is another malformation inherited as an autosomal dominant characteristic. The red cells are oval in shape, and occasionally there is a moderate haemolytic anaemia. Splenectomy is of some value.

The Haemoglobinopathies[3]

The conditions associated with abnormal haemoglobins have been discussed on p. 602 and their ethnic significance stressed. If a patient inherits the gene from one parent only, i.e. if he is heterozygous, he shows minimal signs of the disease, but if he is homozygous, a haemolytic anaemia may result. Four haemoglobins, S, C, D Punjab, and E, are called the common haemoglobins, because each affects millions of people.

Sickle-cell anaemia. Haemoglobin S is the most common of all abnormal haemoglobins. It is found particularly in equatorial Africa in a broad zone extending from coast to coast, but the highest incidence occurs in the eastern part of the continent, where 40 to 50 per cent of the members of certain tribes are affected. In the USA the over-all prevalence of the trait among the Black population is about 8 per cent. There is a substitution of valine for glutamic acid in the sixth residue of the β polypeptide chain.

In a stained film sickled red cells are not conspicuous, but when a drop of blood is sealed under a cover-slip on a slide, and especially if a reducing agent such as sodium dithionite is added, bizarre sickling of the cells soon becomes apparent, a

phenomenon due to the insolubility of the reduced Hb-S. Clinically there is a *severe haemolytic anaemia, a tendency to vascular occlusion* (especially in the microcirculation and particularly in vascular beds that are characterised by slow flow and high oxygen extraction, such as the heart, spleen, bone marrow, and placenta), and *a susceptibility to infection*. This is most probably due to the ischaemia that follows vascular occlusion, but has been also attributed to impaired phagocytic function of the RE cells and complement dysfunction.

Even the sickle-cell trait is associated with a tendency to vascular occlusion when the subject is exposed to environmental hypoxia. Thus splenic infarction may occur after flying high in unpressurised aircraft. Asymptomatic bacteriuria, pyelonephritis, haematuria, and papillary necrosis are all more common in individuals with the trait than in the general population.[18]

Homozygous haemoglobin-C disease. Haemoglobin C is found in a comparatively small and sharply demarcated zone of Western Africa. About 28 per cent of the population in Northern Ghana harbour the gene. In Hb-C lysine replaces glutamic acid in position 6 of the β chain.

In a stained film target cells are conspicuous. There is a formation of haemoglobin aggregates and crystals, and the cells are very rigid. Clinically there is a rather mild haemolytic anaemia.

Homozygous haemoglobin-E disease. Haemoglobin E is most prevalent in South-East Asia. In Hb-E lysine replaces glutamic acid in position 26 of the β chain. There are many target cells, but the anaemia is minimal.

Haemoglobin-D Punjab. This is found in the greatest frequency (2 per cent) among the Sikhs of the Punjab of India. It has the same electrophoretic mobility at alkaline pH on conventional media as does Hb-S, but it does not cause sickling and its solubility is normal. People with the trait may occasionally have haematuria. Homozygous Hb-D disease is rare and often symptomless, but there may be a mild haemolytic anaemia.

Unstable haemoglobin disease (congenital Heinz-body haemolytic anaemia). There are a number of abnormal haemoglobins that exhibit reduced structural stability as evidenced by their tendency to precipitate intracellularly, forming inclusion bodies, and to precipitate with mild heating. Some, e.g. Hb-Southampton and Hb-Bristol, produce a severe haemolytic anaemia that does not respond to splenectomy, others, e.g. Hb-Boras and Hb-Istanbul, produce a moderate haemolytic anaemia that does improve after splenectomy, while others, e.g. Hb-Zürich and Hb-Köln, produce only a mild haemolytic anaemia except during crises, which may be precipitated by infection or the ingestion of drugs, notably sulphonamides. A few, e.g. Hb-Dakar and Hb-Toulouse, produce no clinical or haemolytic effects at all.

Apart from this last asymptomatic group, these abnormal haemoglobins are also associated with the formation of inclusion bodies, called Heinz bodies, in the red cells, and the excretion of a dark brown pigment in the urine. This pigment is thought to be a dipyrrole related to the mesobilifuscin group, which are brown pigments found in the colon and are probably anabolic by-products of haem synthesis. Heinz bodies are usually found only after splenectomy or during an acute haemolytic episode (see p. 614).

The thalassaemia syndromes. The one common denominator of all the thalassaemia syndromes is a decreased rate of synthesis of one or more polypeptide chains. This primary feature is a quantitative one, and contrasts with the qualitative changes in haemoglobin structure that characterise the other haemoglobinopathies. For this reason thalassaemia is often separated from the haemoglobinopathies into a special class of its own. Two types of thalassaemia are recognised according to whether the α or β chain synthesis is defective.

β-thalassaemia. This is the best known type, and is found in a broad belt extending from the Mediterranean basin through the Middle East to the Far East. It is very common in Italy and Greece. In *homozygous β-thalassaemia, Cooley's anaemia,* or *thalassaemia major,* there is a considerable increase in the amount of Hb-F, and the main effects are those of a very severe haemolytic anaemia. The poor synthesis of haemoglobin causes the red cells to be very hypochromic, and extreme leptocytosis is characteristic. The blood film resembles that of a severe iron-deficient anaemia. In *β-thalassaemia minor,* which is the heterozygous state, there is a mild anaemia and a tendency to develop gallstones. The level of Hb-A$_2$ is increased, as also may be that of Hb-F.

α-thalassaemia. This is especially common in South-East Asia. In the homozygous state there is a complete inability to produce α chains, and the major component is Hb-Bart's (γ$_4$). The condition of *α-thalassaemia major* is incompatible with life, but *α-thalassaemia minor,* found in individuals who are heterozygotes for the α-thalassaemia gene, is symptomless and difficult to detect. There is, however, another gene which alone is silent, but which when combined with one α-thalassaemia gene, leads to a mild anaemia. This is *Hb-H disease,* and the red cells contain Hb-H (β$_4$) together with some Hb-Bart's (γ$_4$).

Combinations of these haemoglobinopathies are quite common. The most important are sickle cell-Hb-C disease, sickle cell-thalassaemia, and Hb-C-thalassaemia. None of these conditions is as severe as sickle-cell anaemia or thalassaemia major.

The mechanism of haemolysis is largely mechanical in sickle-cell anaemia; the sickled cells are fragile and are destroyed in the circulation. In thalassaemia Heinz-body formation is the principal mechanism of haemolysis.

Paroxysmal nocturnal haemoglobinuria (PNH). This is an acquired, non-familial disease of adult life in which there is typically an episodic haemolytic anaemia manifested by attacks of haemoglobinuria occurring especially at night. In fact, the majority of cases present themselves with a chronic haemolytic anaemia; only a quarter have the classical haemoglobinuria, and many of these do not show nocturnal exacerbations. Nocturnal haemoglobinuria, when present, occurs as a result of an increase in haemolysis during sleep. Two important complications of PNH are a *tendency to thrombosis,* especially venous, which is often fatal, and a *susceptibility to infection,* which is probably due to leucopenia and leucocytic dysfunction.

The defect resides in clones of abnormal red cells, especially the young representatives (reticulocytes), which are abnormally susceptible to the lysis of complement *via* activation of the alternate pathway. PNH cells also show excessive lysis in acidified human serum (optimal pH for this reaction is 6·8 to 7·0).

Enzyme-deficient Red Cells

There are two basic types of enzyme deficiency in red cells that predispose to hereditary haemolytic anaemia (a) those associated with abnormalities in the *hexosemonophosphate oxidation pathway,* and (b) those associated with abnormalities in the *glycolytic pathway.*

Deficiencies involving the hexosemonophosphate pathway. The most important of this type is *glucose-6-phosphate dehydrogenase (G6PD) deficiency,*[19] which was first noted in Black Americans who were much more susceptible to the haemolytic effects of the antimalarial drugs pamaquine and primaquine than their White compatriots. Since then a vast number of G6PD variants have been discovered. They are transmitted as incomplete dominant sex-linked characteristics, and are found not only in Black people but also in many Mediterranean groups, especially Greeks and Italians.

The clinical manifestations may be episodic with complete recovery in the intervening period, as in the Black subjects exposed to primaquine, or they may be chronic, but often marked by periods of aggravation. Oxidant drugs like the two already mentioned, sulphones, sulphonamides, probenecid, acetanilide, aspirin, nitrofurans, isoniazid, and para-aminosalicylic acid are liable to induce haemolysis.

The acute haemolytic anaemia called *favism* that occasionally occurs after contact with or ingestion of fava beans (*Vicia faba*) is seen in Mediterranean groups; in addition to G6PD deficiency there appears to be some other factor required, since not all enzyme-deficient people, even sometimes in the same family, are susceptible.*

Another mode of presentation is as neonatal jaundice. Some patients have a chronic haemolytic anaemia from infancy or childhood, but in most cases haemolysis occurs only after the stress of infection or drug administration.

Other enzyme deficiencies involving the hexosemonophosphate pathway and glutathione metabolism are of *6-phosphogluconic dehydrogenase, glutathione reductase, glutathione peroxidase,* and *glutathione* itself. The last two are very probably related to a degree of haemolytic anaemia.

Deficiences involving the glycolytic pathway. The most important of this type is *pyruvate kinase (PK) deficiency.* This is inherited as an autosomal recessive trait, and occurs predominantly in people of Northern European descent. It is characterised by a non-spherocytic haemolytic anaemia usually commencing in early childhood. On the whole the anaemia is moderate, but death in childhood can occur in untreated cases. The condition responds fairly well to splenectomy, which may be necessary to preserve life; PK reticulocytes are particularly vulnerable to sequestration in the spleen. Even so, splenectomy is an imperfect form of therapy, as compared with its effect in hereditary spherocytosis, because a considerable degree of haemolysis persists; probably this takes place in the liver.

Other enzyme deficiencies involving the glycolytic pathway are of *hexokinase, glucose-phosphate isomerase, phosphofructokinase,* and *triosephosphate isomerase.* All may be associated with increased haemolysis of moderate degree.

---

*Pythagoras counselled his followers never to walk in bean fields, and is reputed to have suffered from favism.[19]

EXTRACORPUSCULAR FACTORS

The following conditions are important:

Autoantibodies[20] (see also Chapter 16). Autoantibodies against red cells usually arise idiopathically, but from time to time they occur during the course of another disease such as Hodgkin's disease or systemic lupus erythematosus, when they may lead to a secondary haemolytic anaemia. Some infective diseases, notably mycoplasmal pneumonia and syphilis, are occasionally attended by characteristic autoantibodies against the patient's red cells.

Most autoantibodies against red cells are agglutinins. Some of these agglutinate red cells in saline suspension, and are called *complete antibodies*; they are IgM. Others are *incomplete*, for although they coat the red cells and lead to their destruction in the body, they are incapable of agglutinating red cells *in vitro*. However, these coated red cells can be agglutinated *in vitro* by an antihuman-globulin serum. This is the basis of the *Coombs*, or *antiglobulin*, *test* which is described in detail on page 648. These antibodies are IgG.

The complete antibodies are amboceptors, and lead to *in-vitro* haemolysis in the presence of complement. There is indeed one antibody which acts primarily as a haemolysin, the *Donath-Landsteiner antibody*. By contrast, the incomplete antibodies are feebly haemolytic *in vitro*.

Some of these antibodies are most active at 37°C, and are called *warm antibodies*. Nearly all are incomplete IgG antibodies directed against Rh antigens. Clinically they are responsible for the most severe cases of autoimmune haemolytic anaemia. The autoantibodies that occasionally occur in systemic lupus erythematosus and lymphomata come into this category.

Cold antibodies are virtually inactive at 37°C, but become increasingly powerful *in vitro* as the temperature drops to 0°C. Such antibodies are complete IgM and usually anti-I. One type of chronic haemolytic anaemia caused by complete cold antibodies ('cold agglutinins') occurs predominantly in elderly subjects. The main features of this *cold-haemagglutinin syndrome* are a moderate anaemia, haemoglobinuria, and a Raynaud-like phenomenon. This follows blockage of the vessels of the extremities by red cells, which are agglutinated at the low surface temperature. A similar, though more acute, condition occasionally complicates mycoplasmal pneumonia, in which a raised titre of cold agglutinins is characteristic, and which has been known to lead to an acute haemolytic anaemia with renal failure.[21]

In paroxysmal cold haemoglobinuria, a rare disease which is usually a complication of tertiary syphilis, there are dramatic episodes of severe haemolysis occurring shortly after exposure to the cold. This is due to the Donath-Landsteiner cold haemolysin. It sensitises the red cells at a low temperature, but only when the temperature rises once more does gross haemolysis occur. The phenomenon is easily reproducible *in vitro*.

Clinically all these autoantibodies lead to rapid red-cell destruction. The level of complement in the plasma is lowered, since haemolysis involves its activation and consumption. These anaemias are sometimes accompanied by falsely positive serological reactions for syphilis, due presumably to autoantibodies formed against normal lipid constituents of the body.

The mode of red-cell destruction is largely due to complement activation in the intravascular types of haemolysis associated with cold-antibody haemoglobinuria. In the warm-antibody conditions red-cell destruction is extravascular, and it is the RE cells that remove the sensitised red cells rapidly from the circulation. Extravascular destruction may also be the major event in some cases of the cold-haemagglutinin syndrome; in these complement is fixed to the red cells, but for reasons which are not clear it fails to produce lysis. The spleen acts as the most sensitive filter, but the liver plays the dominant role in red-cell destruction when haemolysis is massive or when the spleen is overloaded or removed. The bone marrow is also active, accepting the overflow from liver and spleen. In the cold-antibody anaemias there is also prominent erythrophagocytosis in the RE cells, especially those of the liver.

Alloantibodies. These are discussed in Chapter 55. The common alloantibody anaemia is haemolytic disease of the newborn, in which the red cells of a Rhesus-positive infant are destroyed by antibodies from its Rhesus-negative mother, who has been sensitised beforehand either by a transfusion of Rh-positive blood or by a previously-conceived Rh-positive child. It is well established that fetal red cells commonly enter the maternal circulation during pregnancy. These can be demonstrated by the property of fetal haemoglobin to resist acid elution—fetal cells retain their haemoglobin in strong acid solution, whereas adult cells are decolorised. The most dangerous period is during parturition, especially if the labour is complicated. With a subsequent pregnancy, Rhesus antibodies (of a 'warm', incomplete type) cross the placenta. The infant's red cells, which give a positive Coombs test, are rapidly haemolysed. The clinical manifestations are anaemia, jaundice, and an enlarged liver and spleen. A great danger is bilirubin encephalopathy (kernicterus—see p. 563). In the worst cases the anaemia is so severe that it leads to heart failure with massive anasarca; this is called *hydrops fetalis*. The infant usually dies *in utero*, but if it survives, it seldom lives for more than a few hours.

An advance of great importance is the discovery that the administration of a γ-globulin containing incomplete anti-Rh of high activity can prevent the sensitisation of Rh-negative mothers by Rh-positive fetal cells provided it is given within 72 hours of delivery.

Rh-immune globulins are produced from the plasma of artificially immunised male volunteers or from highly sensitised Rh-negative women who may be hyperimmunised by the injection of Rh-positive cells if they can no longer bear children.

How the antibody suppresses the anti-Rh immune response is not known. There are several possibilities. (*a*) The Rh-positive cells are coated by antibody, and rapidly removed from the circulation by the RE system. No effective antigenic stimulus is therefore presented to the patient. This effect need not be specific, for the administration of an antibody directed against another antigen on the red cells would also block the formation of Rh antibody. There is evidence that this mechanism may indeed be involved. (*b*) The antigenic determinants are blocked or bound so that effective contact with antigen-sensitive cells is prevented. (*c*) The antibody directly suppresses the antigen-sensitive cells.

A group-A or group-B fetus may likewise be the victim of

anti-A or anti-B antibodies from its group-O mother. Although about 20 per cent of all pregnancies involve ABO incompatibilities of the type that could lead to haemolytic disease of the newborn, the incidence of significant haemolytic disease is only 1 in 150 births, and about 1 in 5 babies at risk develop jaundice. Only group-O mothers produce sufficient quantities of IgG anti-A or anti-B antibodies; the corresponding antibodies of mothers of groups A and B are confined to the IgM class, which does not cross the placenta. The matter is further discussed on p. 647.

Infective agents. These may produce haemolysis by the production of powerful toxins, e.g. *Cl. welchii* causing gas-gangrene or *Strept. pyogenes* producing septicaemia. Some organisms produce haemolysis secondarily to parasitisation of red cells, e.g. the parasites of malaria and Oroya fever. Blackwater fever is a fulminating intravascular haemolysis which occurs in chronically malarial subjects who have taken quinine fitfully; its mode of production is unknown.

Drugs. As has already been mentioned, the idiosyncratic haemolytic anaemias following many drugs are associated with a congenital enzyme deficiency in the red cells or an abnormal haemoglobin. There are, however, some agents which will produce haemolysis in any subject if given in a large enough dose, e.g. phenylhydrazine, methyl chloride, arsine, lead, and nitrobenzene. In drug-induced haemolytic anaemias, whether idiosyncratic or not, the red cells often contain inclusions of precipitated, denatured haemoglobin, which are called *Heinz bodies* and are useful evidence of exogenous intoxication. Heinz-body formation is also the principal mechanism of haemolysis in G6PD deficiency and related disorders, in unstable haemoglobin disease, and in the thalassaemias. These inclusions are not usually observed when ordinary staining procedures are employed. Supravital staining with crystal violet or brilliant cresyl blue (used also for reticulocytes) will reveal them.

Drugs may also cause haemolytic anaemia by immunological mechanisms. Three such mechanisms are recognised: (*a*) the drug, acting as a hapten, combines with red-cell proteins, and the antibodies formed lyse the cells by activating complement. High-dose penicillin therapy may act thus when the binding power of the plasma proteins is exhausted. (*b*) The red cell may be an 'innocent bystander' and be bound adventitiously by circulating antibodies to such drugs as stibophen, quinine, or phenacetin. These too act as haptens, but they combine with some body protein other than that of the red cell. When the red cell-antibody complex next meets antigen, complement is activated and lysis occurs. (*c*) Alpha-methyldopa is peculiar in stimulating antibodies that act specifically against red-cell antigens determined by the *Rh* locus. There is no drug binding as with penicillin. It would appear that the antibody produced by α-methyldopa is accidentally reactive to some of the host's antigens.

Extensive burns. The effect is a simple thermal damage to the red cells, which are then destroyed locally or else removed rapidly from the circulation by the spleen.

Red-cell fragmentation syndrome. Red cells that are subjected to excessive physical trauma in the circulation may undergo premature fragmentation and lysis. Sometimes the trauma may be so severe as to cause intravascular haemolysis with haemoglobinaemia, haemoglobinuria, haemosiderinuria,

and shortened red-cell survival. The hallmark of this type of haemolysis is the fragmented red cell, or *schistocyte*, which may take the form of crescents, helmets, triangles, and microspherocytes. The syndrome occurs under the following two conditions:

(*a*) *In association with abnormalities of the heart and great vessels.* This is important especially after the insertion of synthetic valvular prostheses and intracardiac patch repairs, but it has also been seen in unoperated valve disease and in coarctation of the aorta. The extreme turbulence common to all these conditions seems to be the operating factor.

(*b*) *In association with small vessel disease (microangiopathic haemolytic anaemia).* This type of anaemia is usually associated with one of two clinical findings: deposition of fibrin within the microvasculature or severe systemic hypertension or vasoconstriction. It is found in thrombotic thrombocytopenic purpura, disseminated intravascular coagulation, and the *haemolytic uraemic syndrome*, which is an acute condition occurring, in the great majority of cases, in infants and young children. There is acute haemolytic anaemia, thrombocytopenia, and acute renal failure, and the main pathological findings are in the kidneys which show focal infarction with hyaline thrombosis of the capillaries. The material deposited in the glomerular capillary wall consists, at least partially, of fibrin and its derivatives. The afferent arterioles show fibrinoid necrosis of their walls. The cause of this syndrome is obscure. It is often associated with bacterial or viral infections, with immunisations, and with immunological deficiency states, and there may well be an immunological mechanism responsible.

Microangiopathic haemolytic anaemia may also complicate malignant hypertension, eclampsia, giant haemangiomata, and disseminated carcinoma.

Other diseases. The list of diseases that may be complicated by haemolytic anaemia is quite impressive. Some, like Hodgkin's disease, chronic lymphatic leukaemia, and systemic lupus erythematosus, are usually associated with autoantibodies. Other conditions that may be complicated by haemolytic anaemia are carcinomatosis, ovarian tumours especially teratomata, thrombotic thrombocytopenic purpura, uraemia, liver failure, eclampsia, and sarcoidosis, and in these the cause of haemolysis varies.

Another important factor leading to haemolysis is splenic overactivity where there is splenomegaly, e.g. sarcoidosis, myelosclerosis, etc. (see p. 629).

Haematological Findings

There is a variable fall in red-cell count with a proportional drop in haemoglobin level. The red cells are typically normocytic and normochromic but the numerous reticulocytes produce a somewhat macrocytic picture. Anisocytosis and poikilocytosis are present in variable degree. In the congenital corpuscular defects there are characteristic malformations, e.g. spherocytes, leptocytes, and sickled forms. In the acquired anaemias due to autoimmune and alloimmune mechanisms there is also spherocytosis (Rh-haemolytic disease is an exception). Poikilocytosis is prominent in the schistocytosis of the red-cell fragmentation syndrome.

Polychromasia is conspicuous, and a reticulocytosis is invariable: it may exceed 30 per cent. Punctate basophilia is noteworthy in lead poisoning. Nucleated red cells may be present, especially in thalassaemia major and haemolytic disease of the newborn (erythroblastosis fetalis—Fig. 52.1, p. 601).

The red-cell osmotic-fragility test is an important investigation in cases of haemolytic anaemia. Normally the red cells start to haemolyse in a 0·45 to 0·50 g per dl saline solution, and nearly all are haemolysed in a 0·30 to 0·33 g per dl solution. The fragility is much increased when there is spherocytosis, and is decreased in the leptocytosis of thalassaemia major.

There is a neutrophil leucocytosis and often a thrombocytosis, especially in acute haemolytic anaemias. These changes are less pronounced in the chronic haemolytic processes. Leucopenia and thrombocytopenia are unusual except in paroxysmal nocturnal haemoglobinuria and the haemolytic anaemia that may accompany SLE.

The bone marrow shows intense normoblastic hyperplasia.

'*Crises*'. During the course of chronic, congenital, haemolytic diseases, e.g. hereditary spherocytosis, sickle-cell anaemia, and thalassaemia major, long periods of relatively asymptomatic disease may be punctuated by episodes of acute anaemia. An infection may precipitate a crisis.

The commonest of these is the *aplastic crisis*, in which there is a precipitate drop in the reticulocyte count and often a mild leucopenia and thrombocytopenia; the non-regenerative phase lasts from 5 to 12 days. Less common is the *haemolytic crisis*, in which there is increased jaundice and reticulocytosis, and the spleen may enlarge. The least common is the *megaloblastic crisis*, which is more gradual and not associated with infection. It is due to folate deficiency associated with cellular proliferation so rapid that the body's stores of folate cannot keep pace with it.

Biochemical Findings

There is a moderate or severe haemolytic jaundice with a raised plasma bilirubin, increased excretion of urobilinogen in the faeces, and a considerable urobilinuria (see Chapter 47). In most haemolytic anaemias there is methaemalbuminaemia even when there is no obvious evidence of intravascular haemolysis, and the level of haptoglobin is reduced, as the haemoglobin-haptoglobin complex is removed more rapidly than new haptoglobin can be synthesised. This is particularly well marked in sickle-cell anaemia and thalassaemia major.

Acute intravascular haemolysis is on occasions accompanied by dramatic symptoms, and fatal anuria may ensue. There is experimental evidence that large quantities of free haemoglobin in the circulation may lead to a decrease in the renal blood flow, but acting on its own it is probably insufficient to produce serious damage. Thus, patients with paroxysmal nocturnal haemoglobinuria may pass large amounts of haemoglobin in their urine, and yet usually have no specific renal symptoms; their complaints are those of severe anaemia. It will be recalled that in this condition there is destruction of abnormal red cells by the normal, complement-mediated, haemolytic mechanisms of the plasma.

When there is intravascular haemolysis as the result of antibodies acting on normal cells, the symptoms are more severe. There is pain in the back and calves, often accompanied by abdominal colic, headache, fever, and rigors. This is seen in paroxysmal cold haemoglobinuria. In conditions of very severe haemolysis, e.g. blackwater fever and incompatible blood transfusions, there is also marked renal vasoconstriction, and acute renal failure may ensue. It seems probable that an antigen-antibody reaction on the red cells is accompanied by the release of powerful vasoconstrictor substances that are responsible for the pain and renal effects. The matter is considered in greater detail with respect to blood-transfusion reactions in Chapter 55. Following massive intravascular haemolysis the binding power of plasma, due to haptoglobin, haemopexin, and albumin, is exhausted, and the plasma and urine are flooded with haemoglobin. This haemoglobinaemia and haemoglobinuria are accompanied by methaemalbuminaemia; jaundice and urobilinuria soon follow. In chronic cases there is haemosiderinuria as the result of the breakdown of haemoglobin by the proximal convoluted tubules.

Pathological Findings

The most pronounced pathological changes are seen in the chronic, congenital, haemolytic anaemias.

Skeletal changes. In adults the red marrow extends into the shafts of the long bones. In children these are already filled with red marrow, hence the tendency to widening of the marrow cavity and absorption of the cortex of the bone. Subperiosteal bone may also be laid down; in the skull this gives a 'hair-on-end' or 'brush' appearance on X-rays. These changes are seen most prominently in thalassaemia major and sickle-cell anaemia, in which there may be a tower-shaped skull and maxillary and dental abnormalities. In sickle-cell anaemia the vascular occlusion leads to bone-marrow infarction which may be complicated by pyogenic osteomyelitis due to *Salmonella* organisms or *Staph. aureus*.

Haemosiderosis, especially of the liver, spleen, kidneys, and bone marrow. The most marked haemosiderosis is seen in thalassaemia major, where iron deposits are also found in the lymph nodes, gastric mucosa, adrenal, thyroid, parathyroid, and pituitary glands, and in the heart muscle. In children requiring regular transfusion and surviving to puberty, a characteristic hepatic cirrhosis and myocardial degeneration are seen. Sickle-cell anaemia is also associated with severe haemosiderosis and fibrosis.

In PNH the haemosiderosis is largely confined to the kidneys, which may be brown in colour.

Splenomegaly. This is a common finding in haemolytic anaemias, but the histological findings are seldom remarkable. The red pulp is often crowded with erythrocytes. In thalassaemia major there is considerable extramedullary haematopoiesis and also hyperplasia of the RE cells. In sickle-cell anaemia the sinusoids are dilated, and there is RE-cell hyperplasia; erythrophagocytosis is a prominent feature, as is also the case in the autoimmune types of anaemia.

Splenic infarction and *atrophy* is usual in sickle-cell anaemia, so that splenomegaly is not a feature of this haemoglobinopathy except in the early stages.

There may also be moderate *hepatomegaly* due to RE-cell hyperplasia and extramedullary haematopoiesis.

Gallstones. These are seen only in the chronic, congenital, haemolytic anaemias. They are pigment stones (calcium bilirubinate), and are presumably the result of the persistently excessive bilirubin load presented to the gallbladder. They are rare before puberty, but about 85 per cent of adults with hereditary spherocytosis are affected.

Chronic leg ulcers. These too are peculiar to the chronic, congenital, haemolytic anaemias. They are often bilateral, and affect the malleolar areas of the lower legs. If the haemolytic process is arrested, e.g. by splenectomy in hereditary spherocytosis, the ulcers tend to heal. The cause is unknown.

ANAEMIAS OF BONE MARROW INSUFFICIENCY

This group includes those anaemias which are usually normocytic and normochromic and show no evidence of increased red-cell regeneration.

The anaemia of chronic disease (e.g. chronic infection, rheumatoid arthritis, leukaemia, and some cases of cancer) though usually normocytic and normochromic, may show mild microcytosis and hypochromia. The plasma iron is low, the iron-binding capacity is reduced, and the level of saturation of transferrin is low. The percentage of sideroblasts in the marrow is reduced, yet the RE cells are crowded with haemosiderin. Thus there is sideropenia in the presence of a surfeit of iron. The basic dysfunction is not clear; the two most likely defects are impaired erythropoietin production and a reduced red-cell survival time.

The anaemia of renal failure.[22] This rather similar anaemia occurs in chronic renal failure. An important factor, if not the major one, in its aetiology is the decrease in renal production of erythropoietic factor directly consequent upon the reduction in functioning renal mass. There is also a degree of reduced red-cell survival in uraemia, and the haemorrhagic diathesis may lead to iron deficiency. The haemoglobin level tends to remain at about 8 g per dl despite all treatment.

Endocrine anaemias, especially those of hypopituitarism, myxoedema, and Addison's disease, have been noted on page 606.

The anaemia of bone-marrow replacement—leucoerythroblastic anaemia—is described on p. 630.

The anaemia of bone-marrow aplasia—aplastic anaemia—is described on p. 627.

Sideroblastic anaemia. In this condition there is a hypochromic anaemia with abnormal sideroblasts in the marrow. Not only are the sideroblasts increased in number, but they also contain increased amounts of iron in the cytoplasm, characteristically in a conspicuous ring around the nucleus in association with the mitochondria. There is also increased iron in the RE cells, and the plasma iron is usually high. The level of transferrin is reduced, but it is almost fully saturated.

A hereditary sex-linked type of sideroblastic anaemia is described, but most cases are acquired. An important cause is pyridoxine deficiency after using the antituberculous drugs isoniazid, cycloserine, and pyrazinamide. Lead poisoning and chronic alcoholism occasionally lead to a sideroblastic anaemia, which has also been described in the malabsorption syndrome (no doubt through pyridoxine lack). Some cases complicate lymphomata, leukaemia, and myelosclerosis. One type is idiopathic. The nature of the dysfunction is not known.

POLYCYTHAEMIA

Polycythaemia is a condition in which the quantity of red cells is raised in a unit volume of blood in the presence of an increased total blood volume. It must be distinguished from the haemoconcentration that follows sodium and water deficiency (see Chapter 38). In polycythaemia the total blood volume is notably raised owing to a considerable increase in the red-cell mass. The plasma volume is normal or low, therefore the viscosity of the blood is greatly increased. In polycythaemia the ESR is decreased, whereas in anaemia it is increased.

Polycythaemia secondary to other conditions is called *erythrocytosis*, when the red-cell count, haemoglobin content of the blood, and packed cell volume are all increased, but the white-cell and platelet counts are not raised. It occurs in the following conditions:

Hypoxia due to chronic pulmonary disease, cyanotic congenital heart disease, methaemoglobinaemia, and sulphaemoglobinaemia. A marked polycythaemia is found in those who live at high altitudes. There are a number of abnormal haemoglobins with an increased affinity for oxygen, e.g. Hb-Chesapeake, Hb-Capetown, and Hb-Yakima. The resulting tissue hypoxia evokes a polycythaemia, which is hereditary. No significant untoward effects have been observed with this haemoglobinopathy.

Miscellaneous conditions. The occasional occurrence of polycythaemia with renal lesions, mostly clear-cell carcinoma and sometimes polycystic disease and hydronephrosis, has led to the suggestion that these lesions may promote the secretion of an erythropoietin-like factor. Indeed, such a factor has been isolated from some tumours and cysts. More rarely polycythaemia may complicate cerebellar angioma, uterine myoma, hepatoma, and Wilms's tumour. Once again an erythropoiesis stimulating factor has sometimes been found in these tumours, the removal of which leads to a haematological remission.

Cushing's syndrome.

In the primary type of polycythaemia, called **polycythaemia vera** or **erythraemia**,[23] there is a monoclonal neoplastic process involving the normoblastic element of the marrow. This is typically a disease of later life, and is much less common among the Black population than the Caucasian group; Jews are amongst the most frequent victims of this condition.

There is a great rise in the red-cell count, sometimes up to 10×10^{12} per litre, (10 million per μl), with a comparable or less marked rise in the level of haemoglobin. The cells are normocytic and usually normochromic (though after a therapeutic venesection there may be temporary hypochromia); a few polychromatic and nucleated red cells are also present in the blood. In most cases there is a considerable neutrophil leucocytosis with a shift to the left, and also a thrombocytosis. These changes indicate a general proliferative change in the bone marrow, but in some cases the increase is confined to the erythroblastic element, when the condition can scarcely be distinguished from an erythrocytosis.

The pathological features of polycythaemia vera are those of intense venous engorgement which is manifested in the ruddy, plethoric, cyanotic appearance of victims of the disease. There is considerable splenomegaly, and both the spleen and liver may contain foci of extramedullary haematopoiesis. There is a marked tendency to thrombotic complications, e.g. cerebral and coronary thrombosis, and mesenteric venous thrombosis, which are probably related to the high platelet count and the increased viscosity of the blood. Surprisingly, haemorrhagic manifestations also occur, and there is no satisfactory explanation. Hypertension is not unduly common in polycythaemic subjects despite the increased viscosity of the blood. Peptic ulceration occurs more frequently than usual, and has been ascribed to thrombosis of the vessels in the gastric and duodenal mucosa.

Occasionally chronic myeloid leukaemia or myelosclerosis develops. In such an instance the polycythaemia is replaced by a normocytic, normochromic anaemia.

DISORDERS OF HAEMOGLOBIN ACCOMPANIED BY CYANOSIS

There are two such conditions, methaemoglobinaemia and sulphaemoglobinaemia. In *methaemoglobinaemia* the ferrous iron of normal haemoglobin is converted into the ferric form, and as such it cannot combine with oxygen. There is therefore tissue hypoxia, and a secondary polycythaemia may result. The condition is usually produced by oxidant drugs e.g. nitrates, sulphonamides, phenacetin, acetanilide, aniline, and nitrobenzene. These may also cause haemolytic anaemia. NADPH cannot act as a hydrogen donor and reduce methaemoglobin to haemoglobin except in the presence of methylene blue. This dye, or the reducing agent ascorbic acid,

is therefore a useful therapeutic agent in the treatment of methaemoglobinaemia (p. 603). Methaemoglobinaemia may also be due to congenital defects in the red cells. An example of this is a haemoglobinopathy due to Hb-M, which is oxidised abnormally easily. In this type of methaemoglobinaemia reducing agents are powerless. Another cause of hereditary methaemoglobinaemia is a deficiency of the enzyme NADH-methaemoglobin reductase in the red cells. This type of methaemoglobinaemia does respond to methylene blue.

In *sulphaemoglobinaemia* an abnormal compound is formed by the further oxidation of haemoglobin. Sulphaemoglobin itself has not yet been completely characterised, but it is a form of irreversibly denatured haemoglobin. Additional oxidation leads to a rupture of the haem-globin linkage and the intracellular precipitation of Heinz bodies, which are removed by the spleen. Any of the oxidant drugs causing methaemoglobinaemia can also lead to sulphaemoglobinaemia, but in practice acetanilide and phenacetin are usually responsible. Since this pigment cannot be reversed by reducing agents, time has to elapse before it is eliminated from the body.

The clinical manifestation of these disorders is a slate-blue cyanosis in the absence of dyspnoea. Spectroscopic examination is essential to identify these two abnormal intracorpuscular pigments and to distinguish them from reduced haemoglobin.

GENERAL READING FOR CHAPTERS 52–54

HARDISTY, R. M. & WEATHERALL, D. J. (Eds.) (1974) *Blood and its Disorders*, 1540 pp. Oxford: Blackwell.
WINTROBE, M. M., LEE, G. R., BOGGS, D. R., BITHELL, T. C., ATHENS, J. W. & FOERSTER, J. (1974) *Clinical Hematology*, 7th edn, 1896 pp. Philadelphia: Lea & Febiger.

REFERENCES

1. BIRD, G. W. G. (1972) The red cell. *British Medical Journal*, 1, 293.
2. LEHMANN, H. & HUNTSMAN, R. G. (1972) The hemoglobinopathies. In *The Metabolic Basis of Inherited Disease*, ed. Stanbury, J. B., Wyngaarden, J. B. & Fredrickson, D. S., 3rd edn, p. 1398 *et seq.* New York: McGraw-Hill.
3. WEATHERALL, D. J. (1974) Molecular basis for some disorders of haemoglobin synthesis. *British Medical Journal*, 4, 451 and 516.
4. FINCH, C. A. & LENFANT, C. (1972) Oxygen transport in man. *New England Journal of Medicine*, 286, 407.
5. Leading Article (1977) Glycosylated haemoglobins and disease. *Lancet*, 2, 22.
6. CERAMI, A., KOENIG, R. & PETERSON, C. M. (1978) Haemoglobin A_{1c} and diabetes mellitus. *British Journal of Haematology*, 38, 1.
7. REYNOLDS, E. H. (1976) The neurology of vitamin B_{12} deficiency. *Lancet*, 2, 832.
8. Leading Article (1971) Iron. *Lancet*, 2, 475.
9. Leading Article (1977) Erythropoietin. *Lancet*, 1, 1137.
10. NORTHAM, B. E., WINSTONE, N. E. & BANWELL, J. G. (1965) In *Recent Advances in Gastroenterology*, ed. Badenoch, J. A. & Brooke, B. N., p. 349. London: Churchill.
11. Leading Article (1978) Clay eating. *Lancet*, 2, 614.
12. CHANARIN, I. (1969) *The Megaloblastic Anaemias*. Oxford: Blackwell.
13. Leading Article (1976) Pathogenesis of the tapeworm anaemia. *British Medical Journal*, 2, 1028.
14. Leading Article (1973) Co-trimoxazole and blood. *Lancet*, 2, 950.
15. Leading Article (1976) Folate deficiency and the nervous system. *British Medical Journal*, 2, 71.
16. Leading Article (1976) Folic acid and the nervous system. *Lancet*, 2, 836.
17. DACIE, J. V. (1960), (1962) and (1967) *The Haemolytic Anaemias*, 2nd edn, parts 1, 2, 3 and 4. London: Churchill. An exhaustive account of the subject.
18. Leading Article (1976) Sickle cell trait. *British Medical Journal*, 1, 1359.
19. Leading Article (1969) Glucose-6-phosphate-dehydrogenase deficiency and favism. *Lancet*, 2, 1177.
20. DACIE, J. V. (1970) Autoimmune haemolytic anaemias. *British Medical Journal*, 2, 381.
21. LAWSON, D. H. *et al.* (1968) Acute renal failure in the cold-agglutination syndrome. *Lancet*, 2, 704.
22. Leading Article (1975) Anaemia in chronic renal failure. *Lancet*, 1, 959.
23. BECK, W. S. (1976) New outpost on the trail of polycythemia vera. *New England Journal of Medicine*, 295, 951.

Chapter 53.   *Some Disorders of the Blood: The White Cells*

II. THE WHITE CELLS, BONE MARROW, AND SPLEEN

THE CONSTITUENT CELLS

A differentiated stem-cell which is developing into a granulocytic leucocyte passes through the following stages:

Myeloblast. This is the most primitive of the granulocytic series. It is a large cell, very similar in appearance to a pronormoblast. It has a scanty basophilic cytoplasm and a large round nucleus containing fine strands of chromatin and several prominent nucleoli.

Promyelocyte. This cell is transitional between a myeloblast and a myelocyte. It is smaller than the myeloblast, and has few, if any, nucleoli. On the other hand, it does not contain specific cytoplasmic granules, though a few non-specific azurophil granules may be present.

Myelocyte. This is smaller, and the specific neutrophil, eosinophil, or basophil granules are present in the cytoplasm. The nucleus is smaller and may be indented.

Metamyelocyte. A somewhat smaller cell in which the specific cytoplasmic granulation is fully developed. The nucleus is kidney-shaped and its chromatin is condensed into clumps. A later 'band' form stage is described, in which the nucleus has assumed a sausage shape, but there are no constrictions.

The mature granulocyte, i.e. neutrophil, eosinophil, and basophil polymorphonuclears. In these mature cells, which are 10 to 15 μm in diameter, the fine lilac-coloured granules of the neutrophil, the large red granules of the eosinophil, and the very coarse purple granules which overlie the nucleus of the basophil, are the typical features, and are well shown in Romanowsky-stained films. The mature neutrophil polymorphonuclear in fact contains two types of granules. The *azurophil*, or *primary*, *granules* are large and electron dense; they contain lysosomal enzymes—acid phosphatase, cationic proteases, myeloperoxidase, and some lysozyme. The smaller *specific granules* are less dense; they contain alkaline phosphatase, lysozyme, and lactoferrin. They contain neither lysosomal hydrolases nor peroxidase. In H. and E. sections only the granules of the eosinophil are clearly stained.

The nuclei are separated into two or three lobes joined by fine chromatin strands. It is the peculiarly shaped nucleus that gives rise to the name 'polymorph'. The neutrophil leucocytes play an essential part in many acute inflammatory processes, but the function of the eosinophils and basophils is less certain (see pp. 97 and 186).

The other leucocytes seen in the marrow and the peripheral blood are the lymphocyte and the monocyte. Neither contains specific granules in its cytoplasm.

The lymphocyte is a small round cell about 10 μm in diameter with a large round or indented nucleus containing dark clumps of chromatin. Its cytoplasm is scanty and basophilic. A larger form (up to 20 μm in diameter) is also seen, in which there is much more cytoplasm but a similar darkly-staining nucleus. Its precursor is the *lymphoblast*, a cell almost indistinguishable from the myeloblast, but said to have fewer nucleoli and a coarser chromatin pattern. Lymphoblasts are found in lymphoid tissue. They are not normally recognisable in a marrow film, but they predominate in acute lymphatic leukaemia.

The monocyte is an irregularly-shaped cell 12 to 20 μm in diameter with abundant muddy-blue cytoplasm, which is often filled with dust-like azurophilic granules. Its nucleus is large, central, and irregular in shape. Its chromatin is disposed in lace-like strands. Precursor cells called *promonocytes* and *monoblasts* are described. These are larger and have nucleoli, but they retain the typical monocytic morphology. They are not normally recognisable in the marrow, but are predominant in acute monoblastic leukaemia.

A cell that is regularly present in the marrow, but not normally seen in the peripheral blood is the *plasma cell*. It is large and pear-shaped, and has deeply basophilic cytoplasm and an eccentric nucleus containing clumps of chromatin arranged like a cart wheel. The current view is that it arises from the lymphocyte. Neoplastic plasma cells are seen in the marrow in multiple myeloma.

The monocytes form the second phagocytic system of the blood. The part played by these cells, the lymphocytes, and the plasma cells in the immune response is described in Chapter 12. The relationship of the lymphocyte to the 'stem cell' is discussed in Chapter 30.

It will be noted that the leucoblastic elements of the marrow predominate over the erythroblastic ones in the ratio of about 2:1 (see Table 53.1). This is called the *myeloid-erythroid ratio*; it is decreased and even reversed in normoblastic and megaloblastic hyperplasia of the marrow, whereas it is increased when there is leucoblastic (myeloid) proliferation, e.g. in acute pyogenic infections and leukaemia.

From the description of the development of the red and white cells it is apparent that as a blood cell matures, so it undergoes the following changes:

(*a*) It becomes smaller.

(*b*) Its nucleus becomes smaller, the chromatin becomes condensed, and the nucleoli disappear.

(*c*) The cytoplasm becomes less basophilic, except with the plasma cell.

(*d*) The specific cytoplasmic constituents, e.g. haemoglobin and granules, appear.

THE NORMAL WHITE-CELL COUNT

The total white-cell count of the peripheral blood varies

TABLE 53.1 The cellular constituents of the normal bone marrow

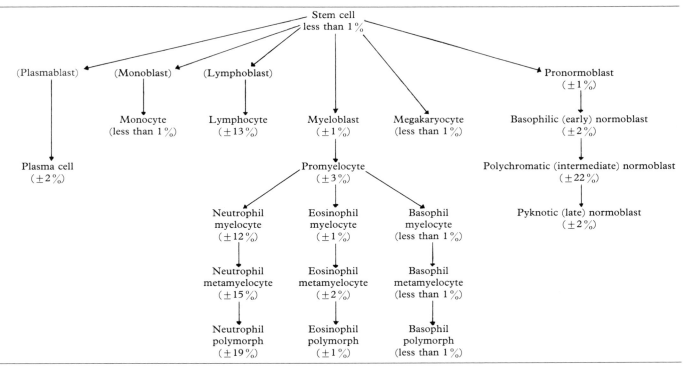

The percentages are a rough average of the normal range of the cells. Plasmablasts, monoblasts, and lymphoblasts are not normally present.

from 4 to 11×10^9 per litre (4000 to 11 000 per μl). The range of the differential leucocyte count in a healthy adult is as follows:

NEUTROPHIL POLYMORPHONUCLEARS	40 to 75% ($2\cdot0$ to $7\cdot5 \times 10^9$ per litre or 2000 to 7500 per μl)
EOSINOPHIL POLYMORPHONUCLEARS	1 to 5% ($0\cdot05$ to $0\cdot4 \times 10^9$ per litre, or 50 to 400 per μl)
BASOPHIL POLYMORPHONUCLEARS	0 to 1% (up to $0\cdot1 \times 10^9$ per litre, or 100 per μl)
LYMPHOCYTES	20 to 45% ($1\cdot5$ to 4×10^9 per litre, or 1500 to 4000 per μl)
MONOCYTES	3 to 7% ($0\cdot2$ to $0\cdot8 \times 10^9$ per litre, or 200 to 800 per μl)

The figures in brackets are the range of absolute counts, and are much more significant than a mere percentage figure. With neutropenia there is often an apparent, or 'relative', increase in the lymphocyte count, when the absolute figure is normal or even lowered. Normally a small percentage of the neutrophils have unsegmented nuclei. These are called juvenile, or 'band', forms. In conditions of neutrophil leucocytosis their proportion increases, and there may be numbers of metamyelocytes and even myelocytes in the circulation. At one time a classification of the maturity of leucocytes based on their nuclear segmentation was very much in vogue. Arneth devised an exhaustive system in which the most primitive cells were tabulated on the left-hand side of a page and the most mature cells on the right-hand side. Though the Arneth count is now obsolete, the term 'a shift to the left' is still useful in denoting an increase in the blood of young forms of polymorphs. The most extreme example of such a shift is the leukaemoid reaction which is occasionally encountered in severe infections and intoxications. A 'shift to the right' is characteristic of pernicious anaemia with its multi-segmented

macropolycyte, though there is also a tendency for a few myelocytes to enter the blood in this condition.

In the newborn infant there is a moderate neutrophil leucocytosis which usually drops to nearly normal within the first week. From then on there is a relative lymphocytosis until the fourth year, when neutrophil and lymphocyte counts are almost equal. The normal adult count is attained at puberty. Strenuous exercise, convulsions, paroxysmal tachycardia, emotional stress, and ether anaesthesia are all associated with a transient neutrophil leucocytosis. During parturition this is very marked.

VARIATIONS IN THE WHITE-CELL COUNT

A total and differential white-cell count is a basic diagnostic procedure in clinical medicine. It is often an eloquent commentary on the body's reaction to infectious agents of various types, and is therefore a valuable guide in pointing to the cause of an undiagnosed pyrexial illness.

Neutrophil Leucocytosis (Neutrophilia)

The commonest alteration in the white-cell count is a

leucocytosis due to an increase in the number of neutrophils. It is encountered in the following pathological conditions:

Infection (*a*) Pyogenic, both acute, e.g. staphylococcal, and chronic, e.g. actinomycotic, (*b*) other bacterial diseases, e.g. anthrax, plague, diphtheria, scarlet fever, and leptospiral jaundice (Weil's disease), and (*c*) viral disease after the prodromal period, e.g. smallpox, poliomyelitis, and zoster.

Metabolic disorders. Uraemia, acute gout, diabetic ketosis, and eclampsia.

Intoxications. Lead (especially chronic lead poisoning), mercury, digitalis, potassium chlorate, and insect venoms.

With some hypersensitivity reactions, e.g. serum sickness, acute rheumatic fever, and acute glomerulonephritis.

After acute haemorrhage especially into a serous cavity, e.g. ruptured ectopic pregnancy.

In acute haemolytic anaemia.

In the catabolic phase of convalescence after injury.

In conditions of massive necrosis, e.g. myocardial infarction.

In rapidly-growing malignant tumours, e.g. cancer of the liver, lung, or colon, and Hodgkin's disease.

In chronic myeloid leukaemia and *polycythaemia vera.*

In most of these conditions, especially the acute pyogenic group, there is a variable 'shift to the left'. This becomes very marked in severe infections, when metamyelocytes and even myelocytes may enter the blood. *Leukaemoid blood pictures* are an extreme manifestation of this tendency. They are occasionally encountered in (*a*) severe infections, e.g. pneumonia, meningitis, plague, septicaemia, and especially miliary tuberculosis, (*b*) sudden acute haemolysis, (*c*) eclampsia, (*d*) widespread malignant disease without skeletal metastases, and (*e*) conditions associated with bone-marrow replacement (see p. 630). The peripheral blood picture may closely resemble that of myeloid leukaemia, both chronic and acute. An assessment of the *leucocyte alkaline phosphatase* level in the neutrophils may be of value in the differential diagnosis. The activity of the enzyme is moderately increased in the leucocytosis of infection and in the leukaemoid reaction, whereas it is characteristically low in chronic myeloid leukaemia.

A test of limited value in assessing the origin of a neutrophil leucocytosis is the *nitroblue-tetrazolium test*, which depends on the ability of neutrophils to reduce the colourless soluble dye nitroblue tetrazolium and produce a blue-black formazan precipitate. Normally less than 10 per cent of circulating neutrophils have this ability, but the percentage is much greater in systemic bacterial and fungal infections associated with a neutrophilia. It was originally believed that no such increase occurred in viral infections, allergic diseases, or traumatic inflammation, but many false positive results have since become apparent.[1,2] The main use of this test is in the diagnosis of chronic granulomatous disease in children, in whom the neutrophils show no reaction at all. There is a reduction in the reaction in carriers of this condition. A further possible use for the test may lie in the early disclosure of infection in patients who are particularly at risk, e.g. those who are immunosuppressed.[1]

In severe infections the fine lilac granulation of the neutrophils may be replaced by irregular bluish granules, a condition called *toxic granulation*.

Regulation of the neutrophil count.[3,4] The neutrophil count can be altered by two regulatory mechanisms:

(1) *Release of neutrophils from the reserves.* Of the neutrophils in the blood stream, over half are in a 'marginated pool' adherent to the walls of blood vessels, particularly in the lungs. These can be released rapidly; this release accounts for the leucocytosis occurring with exercise and following the administration of adrenaline. The second reserve is in the bone marrow, where the number of neutrophils sequestered is about 10 times the total number of cells present in the blood. The mechanism of their release is poorly understood. Various neutrophil-releasing factors have been described; one of them is a cleavage fragment of C3.

(2) *Increased production of neutrophils in the bone marrow.* Granulocyte precursors can be cultured *in vitro* in semi-solid agar or methyl cellulose to form colonies, but this occurs only in the presence of stimulating substances. Such *colony-stimulating substances* have been isolated from many sources, e.g. macrophages, fibroblasts, and lymphocytes. An inhibitory granulocyte chalone has also been described. The role, if any, of these agents in the regulation of the neutrophil count in health or disease is unknown.

Leucopenia

This is invariably due to a fall in the neutrophil count, i.e. neutropenia. It is less common than a neutrophilia, and is seen in the following conditions:

Infections (*a*) Certain specific bacterial diseases, e.g. typhoid fever and brucellosis, (*b*) viral disease especially in the prodromal period, e.g. influenza, smallpox, chickenpox, dengue, yellow fever, sandfly fever, viral hepatitis, and also rickettsial disease, e.g. typhus and Rocky Mountain spotted fever, (*c*) chronic protozoal disease, e.g. malaria, leishmaniasis, and trypanosomiasis, and (*d*) overwhelming bacterial infection, e.g. miliary tuberculosis, septicaemia, and pneumonia, when it is of very serious prognostic import.

Some conditions associated with splenomegaly (*hypersplenism*), e.g. Felty's syndrome, hepatic cirrhosis (Banti's syndrome), primary splenic neutropenia, and Gaucher's disease.

In pernicious anaemia, and occasionally in chronic iron-deficiency anaemia.

Systemic lupus erythematosus.

Bone-marrow aplasia (see p. 627). If the neutrophils alone are involved, the condition is called *agranulocytosis*.

Acute leukaemia. In the subleukaemic and aleukaemic forms (p. 624).

In anaphylactic shock and after the parenteral injection of foreign protein or endotoxin. This occurs during the first few hours, and is probably due to an accumulation of marginated neutrophils in the internal organs, especially the lungs. A neutrophilia soon follows.

Neutropenia is almost always accompanied by a relative lymphocytosis. Occasionally the lymphocytosis may be so great that the total white-cell count is within normal limits despite the severe neutropenia.

Lymphocytosis

An absolute lymphocytosis, i.e. lymphocytic leucocytosis, is met with in a few specific conditions:

Whooping-cough. White cell counts of over 50×10^9 per litre (50 000 per μl) have been reported.

Infectious mononucleosis (*glandular fever*). This common disease, seen most often in children and young adults, is infective in origin. The classical condition with heterophile antibodies to sheep red cells, which are discussed below, is caused by the EB virus, a herpes virus which has been noted on pages 290 and 380. It seems that primary infection in childhood is usually subclinical, and is followed by antibody production and life-long carriage of the virus in the naso-pharyngeal lymphoid tissue; the virus is present in the buccal secretions.[5] Primary infection in adolescents and young adults results in infectious mononucleosis in from one-half to two-thirds of those exposed; perhaps the large dose of virus acquired during kissing is related to this response. Since childhood infection is commonest in low socio-economic conditions, infectious mononucleosis is rare in the developing countries, e.g. in Africa, but is prevalent in the privileged groups in Western society. In later life the few remaining individuals without antibodies to the EB virus may acquire a primary infection, but, as with young children, this is rarely accompanied by clinical symptoms.[5]

The symptoms of infectious mononucleosis are protean, and important features are a prolonged pyrexia, enlarged painful lymph nodes, sore throat, and an enlarged spleen. Its course is typically benign, but complications like splenic rupture, hepatic necrosis, encephalitis, and oedema of the glottis may rarely cause death.

The leucocytosis is due to the presence of variable numbers of abnormal lymphocytes in the blood. These vary in size, and have a vacuolated or foamy basophilic cytoplasm. The nucleus varies in shape, and its chromatin is disposed in coarse clumps and strands. Though the nuclear shape may resemble that of a monocyte, the chromatin lacks the lacy disposition so typical of this cell. Sometimes the white-cell count may exceed 40 × 10^9 per litre (40 000 per μl).

Another characteristic finding is the presence of *heterophile antibodies* in the patient's plasma, which are capable of agglutinating sheep's red cells in high titre (*Paul-Bunnell test*). A rather similar antibody is found to low titre in normal people, especially after the injection of horse serum (Forssman antibody, see p. 139). It is distinctive in being absorbed by a suspension of guinea-pig kidney, which is rich in Forssman antigen, and not by ox red cells. The glandular-fever antibody, on the other hand, is absorbed by ox red cells but not by guinea-pig kidney. Differential absorption followed by a sheep red-cell agglutination test serves to distinguish between the two antibodies.

A disease clinically and haematologically indistinguishable from the EB virus infectious mononucleosis, but without heterophile antibodies, may occur in young adults with cyto-megalic inclusion disease and toxoplasmosis.

Acute infectious lymphocytosis. This is an uncommon, benign, febrile disease of childhood in which there is a lymphocytosis of up to 100 × 10^9 per litre (100 000 per μl). The cells are mature, and the titre of heterophile antibodies is not increased.

Chronic infections, e.g. secondary and congenital syphilis and healing tuberculosis.

Endocrine conditions. Thyrotoxicosis may be accompanied by an inconstant lymphocytosis.

Chronic lymphatic leukaemia and less constantly in lymphocytic lymphoma and heavy-chain disease.

Waldenström's macroglobulinaemia. As a terminal event the atypical lymphocytes may appear in the blood-stream. These cells, which produce the abnormal immunoglobulin, have a copious basophilic cytoplasm rich in carbohydrate which stains with the PAS method.

Occasionally a reactive lymphocytosis may be marked enough to mimic lymphatic leukaemia. This *lymphocytic leukaemoid reaction* has been described in whooping-cough, infectious mononucleosis, infectious lymphocytosis, miliary tuberculosis, and carcinoma of the stomach.

Lymphopenia

This is not common, and the fall in lymphocytes is seldom great enough to lead to a leucopenia. It is seen in the following conditions:

After whole-body irradiation (see Ch. 31).

In response to ACTH or glucocorticoids.

In Hodgkin's disease. The usual white-cell picture in this condition is a moderate neutrophilia. Sometimes there may also be an absolute fall in the lymphocyte count.

Monocytosis

A rise in the monocyte count may be found in:

Infections. (*a*) Chronic bacterial diseases, e.g. tuberculosis, subacute infective endocarditis, and brucellosis. It is said to indicate activity in tuberculosis, and was regarded as an unfavourable sign in the pre-antibiotic era. (*b*) Protozoal and rickettsial disease, e.g. malaria, leishmaniasis and trypanosomiasis, where it is a characteristic finding, and also typhus and Rocky Mountain spotted fever. (*c*) In the later stages of acute pyogenic infection. It declines once resolution has occurred, but persists if chronic inflammation develops.

Tetrachlorethane poisoning.

Monocytic variant of acute leukaemia.

Lymphomata. It is found in about one-third of cases of Hodgkin's disease and less often in the other lymphomata.

Eosinophilia

T lymphocytes are necessary for the development of eosinophilia in mice and rats infected with *Trichinella spiralis*; the mechanism is not understood (see p. 97). In human pathology eosinophilia is found in:

Hypersensitivity of atopic type, e.g. bronchial asthma, hayfever, and urticaria. Eosinophils are present in large numbers in the sputa or nasal discharges of such patients. Wherever eosinophils are being broken down Charcot-Leyden crystals are found; they are protein in nature, and are probably derived from lysosomes.

Interestingly, eosinophilia is not a feature of generalised anaphylaxis, though there may be some eosinophils in the exudates in the tissues. Likewise, serum sickness does not usually lead to eosinophilia except, to an extent, around the lesions in the tissues. Delayed-type hypersensitivity is not associated even with eosinophils in the local lesions, except for the rather strange retest phenomenon (see p. 186).

Certain chronic skin diseases, e.g. pemphigus vulgaris and bullous pemphigoid.

Infections. Eosinophilia is characteristic of all helminthic infestations which invade the tissues, e.g. schistosomiasis, trichinosis, hydatid disease, and filariasis.

Loeffler's syndrome is a transient pulmonary infiltration accompanied by a marked eosinophilia. It is probably a hypersensitivity reaction, and is seen most often in connexion with helminthic infestations, e.g. ankylostomiasis, ascariasis, and trichinosis. It has also been described in tuberculosis, brucellosis, and coccidioidomycosis. A related hypersensitivity of a longer duration and relapsing course has also been described. Another hypersensitivity syndrome with pulmonary infiltration, asthmatic symptoms, weight loss, and moderate splenomegaly is called *tropical eosinophilia*, because it was first described in South-East Asia. It is a reaction to various parasites, usually microfilariae (see also p. 182).

Intestinal worm infestation is less commonly accompanied by eosinophilia. It is in the early stages of ascariasis and ankylostomiasis that the blood change occurs.

During most acute infections the eosinophil count drops as a result of the increased output of adrenal cortical hormones. Recovery is often heralded by an eosinophilia. *Scarlet fever* and *chorea* are sometimes associated with a marked eosinophilia.

Polyarteritis nodosa is attended by an eosinophilia in about 20 per cent of cases.

Diseases of the bone marrow. In chronic myeloid leukaemia there is an absolute eosinophilia which is overshadowed by the neutrophilia. A special 'eosinophilic leukaemia' has been described. Polycythaemia vera and Hodgkin's disease are sometimes associated with a considerable eosinophilia, and so occasionally are widely metastasising tumours.

Plasma Cells and Atypical Lymphoid Cells in the Blood

Plasma cells are not commonly present in the peripheral blood. They occur typically in *rubella*, and rather less constantly in *measles* and *chickenpox*. They may occasionally be present in multiple myeloma, and are very numerous in the rare *plasma-cell leukaemia*.

Atypical lymphoid cells with very basophilic cytoplasm and resembling the immunoblasts seen in active lymph nodes are found in small numbers in the blood from time to time in *bacterial infections*, and during *immunological reactions*. The Türk cell is probably of this nature. A rare condition in which there are many abnormal lymphocytic cells in the blood is the *Sézary syndrome* (see p. 400).

Table 53.2 relates white-cell patterns with diseases which often present themselves clinically as a prolonged *pyrexia of unknown origin*. Such pyrexia may be due to the following factors:

Infections. *Bacterial*, e.g. deep-seated suppuration, typhoid fever, subacute infective endocarditis, miliary tuberculosis, and brucellosis.

Protozoal, e.g. malaria, leishmaniasis, and trypanosomiasis.

Helminthic, e.g. trichinosis and schistosomiasis.

Due to other agents, e.g. Q-fever, mycoplasmal pneumonia, and infectious mononucleosis.

Widespread or deep-seated malignancy, e.g. clear-cell carcinoma of the kidney, carcinoma of the lung and liver, and tumours of the lymphoreticular system, especially Hodgkin's disease.

Diseases in which hypersensitivity is a factor, e.g. systemic lupus erythematosus and polyarteritis nodosa.

HAEMATOLOGICAL ASPECTS OF THE LEUKAEMIAS

Leukaemia is a condition in which there is a widespread proliferation of the leucocytes and their precursors throughout the tissues of the body, with a variable circulating component. Its aetiology is unknown, and its course is nearly always fatal. As a neoplastic condition of the haematopoietic tissues it has been mentioned in Chapter 30, and it is now necessary to consider its haematological manifestations in some detail. It is

TABLE 53.2 The leucocytic response to some of the agents causing a prolonged pyrexia

Blood picture	Possible cause of pyrexia
Neutrophilia	a. Hidden pus, e.g. subphrenic or perinephric abscess
	b. Widespread malignancy including Hodgkin's disease
	c. Polyarteritis nodosa (frequent)
Neutropenia with relative lymphocytosis	a. Typhoid fever
	b. Brucellosis
	c. Systemic lupus erythematosus
	d. Chronic protozoal disease
Absolute lymphocytosis	a. Infectious mononucleosis—abnormal lymphocytes
Eosinophilia	a. Early helminthic infestations
	b. Polyarteritis nodosa (occasional)
	c. Hodgkin's disease (uncommon)
Monocytosis	a. Protozoal disease
	b. Subacute infective endocarditis (occasional)
	c. Active tuberculosis (occasional)
Normal	a. Subacute infective endocarditis. This is the usual white-cell count; sometimes there is a moderate leucopenia or leucocytosis
	b. Tuberculosis. Usually the white-cell count is normal, though all pictures from agranulocytosis to a leukaemoid reaction are possible
	c. Q-fever and mycoplasmal pneumonia
	d. Widespread malignancy including Hodgkin's disease (less common than neutrophilia)
	e. Polyarteritis nodosa (less common than neutrophilia)
	f. Systemic lupus erythematosus (less common than neutropenia)

worth recalling that, although the aetiology is unknown, there are a few suggestive factors:[6]

Viruses in fowl and mouse leukaemia (see Ch. 29).

Ionising radiation in human leukaemia (see Ch. 31).

Chemical agents. Myeloid leukaemia, usually acute, has been described as a complication of benzene ingestion, and acute leukaemia has occasionally been known to follow the use of phenylbutazone. Patients with multiple myeloma occasionally develop acute myeloid leukaemia after several years' treatment with alkylating agents, especially melphalan.[7] Nevertheless, there is little evidence that any drug predisposes to leukaemia.

Congenital chromosomal abnormalities. Acute leukaemia, usually myeloid, is 20 times commoner in children with Down's syndrome than in normal children. There is also an increased incidence of acute leukaemia in Fanconi's hypoplastic anaemia, mentioned on page 627, in which cultured blood cells show a high frequency of chromosomal breakage and rearrangement (see also p. 31).

Immunological deficiency syndromes are not infrequently complicated by lymphoma and leukaemia, see page 170.

Classification

The important factors are the rapidity of the process and the type of cell involved. The more acute the process, the more primitive is the predominant cell. Nowadays acute leukaemias are often successfully checked, though in due course a relapse is to be expected. Thus a case of acute leukaemia may sometimes survive as long as some chronic leukaemias. The difference in the cell type and the clinical picture make a distinction quite easy in practice. The following classification is recommended:

CHRONIC LEUKAEMIA (*a*) Myeloid (myelocytic)
                (*b*) Lymphatic (lymphocytic)
ACUTE LEUKAEMIA (*a*) Myeloid (myeloblastic)
                (*b*) Lymphatic (lymphoblastic).

The names in brackets allude to the predominant cell in the blood.

Acute myeloid leukaemia has several variants: acute myelomonoblastic leukaemia of Naegeli, acute monoblastic leukaemia of Schilling, acute promyelocytic leukaemia, and several syndromes associated with the name of the Italian haematologist di Guglielmo, in which there is an erythroblastic proliferation with or without myeloblasts in addition.

Whether monoblastic leukaemia is a distinct entity or represents merely one end of the morphological spectrum of acute myeloid leukaemia is uncertain, but it is known that the myeloblast and the monocyte have a common stem cell (see p. 600).

Chronic Myeloid Leukaemia

This disease has its maximum incidence in early and middle adult life. The organs principally involved are the bone marrow and the spleen. Lymph-node involvement occurs late in the disease, and is seldom conspicuous. The liver is frequently enlarged, and skin lesions are occasionally present.

Blood picture. *The most prominent finding is an enormous increase in the white-cell count*, a figure of 1000 × 10⁹ per litre (1 million per μl) being occasionally attained. The greatest white-cell counts are found in this disease, but sometimes the leucocytosis is smaller. The predominant cells are neutrophil polymorphs with a variable admixture of metamyelocytes and myelocytes. Myeloblasts are present only in very small numbers. There is also an increase in the number of eosinophils, basophils, and their myelocyte precursors. The blood film, on cursory inspection, resembles a normal marrow film. As the disease progresses to a fatal termination, the proportion of promyelocytes and myeloblasts increases markedly.

Occasionally rare morphological variants are seen in which there is a striking eosinophilia, basophilia, or monocytosis, but the course of the disease is unaltered.

If the leucocytes are grown in tissue culture, in from 70 to 90 per cent of cases the abnormal Philadelphia (Ph') chromosome is found (see p. 44).

The red cells may be little reduced in number in the early stages (occasionally a mild polycythaemia is encountered), but later on a severe normocytic, normochromic anaemia develops. There is some polychromasia, and a mild reticulocytosis is quite common. Nucleated red cells are present in small numbers. The cause of the anaemia is complex. There is usually a haemolytic element, and the bone marrow itself is inadequate.

The platelet count may be normal or raised in the early stages, but later on there is a moderate thrombocytopenia. These changes in the red cells and platelets are valuable in distinguishing chronic myeloid leukaemia from a leukaemoid blood picture.

The bone marrow is very hypercellular due to leucoblastic proliferation. The cells present are similar to those seen in the blood, but slightly less mature forms predominate. The normoblastic element is relatively reduced, but the megakaryocytes are often increased in number until the final stages of the disease.

Chronic Lymphatic Leukaemia

The maximum incidence of this disease is in the middle-aged and elderly. The organ principally involved is the lymph node, and generalised painless lymphadenopathy is the main clinical feature. The bone marrow and spleen are affected later in the course of the disease, and the degree of involvement is seldom as great as in the myeloid variety. The liver is often enlarged, and cutaneous lesions are commoner than in myeloid leukaemia. The tonsils, salivary glands, eyes, stomach, and gut are also sometimes affected.

Since chronic lymphatic leukaemia is a neoplastic condition of the B lymphocytes, there is often impaired immunoglobulin formation, which results in hypogammaglobulinaemia and a susceptibility to infection by pyogenic organisms; pneumonia is a common complication. More rarely there is a monoclonal gammopathy, and the picture of multiple myeloma has been known to supervene as a terminal complication.

Blood picture. *There is a considerable leucocytosis* varying from 20 to 250 × 10⁹ per litre (20 000 to 250 000 per μl), a figure lower than that of the myeloid variety. The most important feature is an absolute lymphocytosis, about 90 per cent of the cells being mature, small lymphocytes. Large lymphocytes are not infrequent, but lymphoblasts are very uncommon. There is a relative reduction in the granulocytic polymorph elements.

The red cells and platelets are reduced in number as in the myeloid variety. In chronic lymphatic leukaemia there is seldom the early increase in the red-cell and platelet counts sometimes noted in the myeloid type. On the other hand, the ensuing anaemia develops rather more slowly. Acute haemolytic anaemia is common, and there may be autoantibodies in the blood.

The bone marrow may show no changes at all at first, but later on there is an absolute increase in the number of lymphocytes, which may crowd out the other cells in the terminal stages.

Course of chronic leukaemia. The average duration of life in the myeloid type from the onset of symptoms is from 3 to 4 years. About 20 per cent survive for 5 years, but very few reach the ten-year mark. The presence of the Ph′ chromosome is associated with an improved prognosis, and if the cultured cells lack a Y chromosome in addition, so that they may be designated 45, XO, Ph′, the outlook is even better. A few such cases have survived over 10 years.

Chronic lymphatic leukaemia runs a considerably more benign course. The average case survives from 4 to 6 years, but many live for over 10 years. Indeed, the full survival time is often unknown, since many of the patients are elderly and liable to die of intercurrent disease.

In myeloid leukaemia the end is nearly always heralded by an acute exacerbation in which the blood is flooded with myeloblasts. This does not occur in the lymphatic type, where death is usually the result of uncontrolled infection.

Acute Leukaemia

This condition can occur at any age, and it is encountered quite frequently in the first five years of life. In childhood most acute leukaemia is of the lymphatic type, during adolescence the lymphatic and myeloid types occur with equal frequency, but in adult life there is a progressive predominance of the myeloid type; the lymphatic type is rare in people over the age of 45 years.

The onset of acute leukaemia is usually sudden and fulminating, but there is sometimes a prodromal period of malaise lasting a few months, during which there may be an obscure thrombocytopenia or anaemia. The condition is called 'preleukaemia'.

The disease is heralded by a rapidly-developing anaemia, necrotic lesions in the mouth and throat, and generalised bleeding manifestations. A high remittent fever is so common that an infective disease is often mimicked. There is usually some enlargement of the lymph nodes, spleen, and liver, though never so marked as in chronic leukaemia. Skeletal lesions are often sufficiently severe to produce bone tenderness and joint pains.

It is not possible to distinguish clinically between acute lymphatic and myeloid leukaemia. However, gingival infiltration with swollen, spongy gums is particularly common in *myelomonoblastic and monoblastic leukaemias* (this may be due to the ability of some immature, leukaemic monocytes, not shared by myeloblasts, to migrate into inflammatory exudates). *Promyelocytic leukaemia* is commonly associated with hypofibrinogenaemia and bleeding, especially when the cells contain large, abnormal azurophil granules.[8]

The white cell count varies from a severe leucopenia of less than 1×10^9 per litre (1000 per μl) to a leucocytosis of more than 100×10^9 per litre (100 000 per μl). The leucocyte count is elevated in rather more than half of the patients, but even when it is low, blast cells can nearly always be seen in the peripheral blood, although these can easily be classed as lymphocytes by the inexperienced worker. This type of leukaemia may be called 'subleukaemic'. A frankly 'aleukaemic leukaemia' in which there are absolutely no blast cells present in the blood does occur, but it is very uncommon. These patients are extremely leucopenic, but the diagnosis is made clear by bone-marrow examination.

It is often extremely difficult to distinguish between myeloblasts and lymphoblasts. The best criterion is a study of the other white cells, because a 'blast' cell is known by the company it keeps, e.g. the presence of myelocytes and neutrophils would suggest that the cell is a myeloblast, whereas a number of mature lymphocytes would indicate the lymphoblastic nature of an unidentified primitive cell.

There are often very few mature cells, in which case histochemistry may be useful in identifying the 'blast' cells.

(*a*) *The peroxidase test*, which demonstrates the presence of peroxidase in the azurophil granules of neutrophils and monocytes (and their precursors). Lymphocytes are peroxidase-negative. In practice this method is seldom helpful, because the 'blast' cells are usually too primitive to contain any granules.

(*b*) *The PAS stain*, which may show coarse masses of glycogen in cells of the lymphoid series. Myeloblasts do not contain any, but glycogen is plentiful in mature polymorphs.

(*c*) *Sudan black staining*, which shows up lipid material in myeloblasts and monoblasts. Lymphoblasts do not show sudanophilia.

In the acute myeloid leukaemic variants there may be a predominance of myeloblasts with some monocytic characteristics (acute myelomonoblastic leukaemia of Naegeli), or the cells may all have the characteristics of immature monocytes (acute monoblastic leukaemia of Schilling). In promyelocytic leukaemia most of the cells have cytoplasmic granules which are peroxidase positive.

A leukaemia composed of cells so immature that it cannot be classified is called a 'stem-cell leukaemia'.

There is a severe normochromic, normocytic anaemia. Anisocytosis and poikilocytosis are not conspicuous (this applies also to the chronic types), and the reticulocyte count is reduced. There are nucleated red cells in the peripheral blood.

There is a profound thrombocytopenia.

The bone marrow is always crowded out with these primitive cells, except, of course, during a remission.

Di Guglielmo first described a condition characterised by neoplasia of both erythroblastic and leucoblastic tissues, and this he called *erythroleukaemia*. Later he described *acute erythraemic myelosis*, in which there is a generalised proliferation of erythroblasts analogous to the leucocytic proliferation of leukaemia. The blood contains erythroblasts in all stages of maturation with a predominance of the most immature forms. There is a slight leucopenia, but only occasional myelocytes and metamyelocytes, as well as RE cells, are present in the peripheral blood. The bone marrow is crowded with erythropoietic elements, and basophilic forms predominate. Primitive erythroblasts and RE cells are present in the blood-forming organs, the kidneys, adrenals, and other organs.

Both erythroleukaemia and acute erythraemic myelosis follow a course indistinguishable from that of acute myeloid leukaemia.

A *chronic erythraemic myelosis* is also described; here the erythroblasts are more mature and there is only moderate thrombocytopenia and no leucopenia. But it tends to develop into an acute myeloid leukaemic type of disease, and it is best regarded as a preleukaemic manifestation.

Course of acute leukaemia. Untreated cases usually die within a few weeks to 6 months of the onset of symptoms. Spontaneous remissions are not uncommon, and exceptionally these have lasted a number of years, but most soon relapse. Death is due in most cases to infection (resulting from neutropenia) and massive haemorrhage, especially into the brain or the gastrointestinal tract (resulting from thrombocytopenia). Occasionally the lethal factor is a leukaemic infiltration into a vital organ like the heart, liver, lung, or kidney, or into the meninges.

Therapy has increased the average survival period considerably.[9] Acute lymphatic leukaemia in children has by far the best prognosis, and even before modern combination therapy was used, nearly 3 per cent had survived for 5 years. Patients who do survive this length of time show less tendency to die later, so that after 10 to 11 years there is no greater likelihood of death in this group than in the general population.

With intensive combination chemotherapy in association with prophylactic measures (radiotherapy and intrathecal methotrexate) against infiltration of the central nervous system actively pursued for three years, five-year survivals are now being achieved in as many as 50 per cent of patients in some centres. It would seem that disease-free survival for 4 to 5 years carries a very good chance of cure. Perhaps one-third of children with acute lymphatic leukaemia can now be cured.

At present it is not known which children are liable to respond best to chemotherapy, but lymphoblasts with T-cell features form a sub-group with a very poor prognosis.[10] The cells of most cases of acute lymphatic leukaemia have neither B nor T characteristics.[11] Adults with acute lymphatic leukaemia have a worse prognosis than the more usual childhood subject.

Chemotherapy has a much less impressive effect in acute myeloid leukaemia, but some cases have survived for over two years.

PATHOLOGICAL FEATURES OF LEUKAEMIA

The invariable feature of leukaemia is a monotonous infiltration of various organs with the primitive cells. The spleen, liver, bone marrow, and lymph nodes are particularly severely affected, but no organ is exempt. On the whole, the infiltrations of acute leukaemia are more circumscribed than those of chronic leukaemia, and there is a greater tendency for a single organ, e.g. intestine, lung, kidney, or gonad, to be massively involved.

In chronic myeloid leukaemia the *spleen* is enormously enlarged, and its architecture is submerged by an accumulation of myelocytes and more mature leucocytes, whereas in chronic lymphatic leukaemia there is a diffuse infiltration of lymphocytes. In acute leukaemia there is a similar infiltration of 'blast' cells.

The *lymph nodes* are affected more severely in acute leukaemia and chronic lymphatic leukaemia than in the chronic myeloid variety.

In chronic myeloid leukaemia the *liver* is diffusely infiltrated throughout its sinusoids by myelocytes (Fig. 53.1), whereas in chronic lymphatic leukaemia the lymphocytic infiltration is usually more marked around the portal tracts (Fig. 53.2).

The *marrow* of the long bones is increased in amount, and is pinkish-grey in colour. Bone destruction is uncommon, but subperiosteal leukaemic infiltrations are not infrequent in acute leukaemia. A rare manifestation is *chloroma*, in which there are extensive leukaemic deposits under the periosteum of the bones. The skull (especially the orbital regions) is typically the site of these tumour deposits, and exophthalmos may be a presenting symptom. The condition is peculiar to acute myeloid leukaemia. Excised chloroma tumours have a greenish tinge which fades rapidly on exposure to air. The nature of the pigmentation is unknown.

The other pathological features of the leukaemias are due to the effects of *thrombocytopenia* and *agranulocytosis*, and the *blockage of blood vessels* by leukaemic cells. Vascular occlusion produces the priapism which may be so troublesome during life, and is also the cause of the areas of infarction so typical of leukaemic spleens. Foci of necrosis and haemorrhage are common in the brain, and are often the immediate cause of death. Other frequent *post-mortem* findings are purpura and haemorrhagic extravasations into the tissues. There is almost

Figure 53.1
Chronic myeloid leukaemia. There is a diffuse infiltration of leukaemic cells throughout the sinusoids of the liver. × 120.

Figure 53.2
Chronic lymphatic leukaemia. The infiltration of leukaemic cells is much more dense around the portal tracts than in the sinusoids of the liver. × 100.

Figure 53.3
Multiple myeloma. This section of vertebral bone marrow shows almost complete replacement of haematopoietic tissue by neoplastic plasma cells. × 200.

invariably severe bacterial infection, e.g. pneumonia, tonsillitis, and enterocolitis, which is aggravated by the cytotoxic drugs used therapeutically.

MULTIPLE MYELOMA

Multiple myeloma is a monoclonal gammopathy, and as such is described on page 580. There is a neoplastic proliferation of plasma cells, called *myeloma cells*, scattered throughout the skeleton (Fig. 53.3). Myeloma cells are large (15 to 30 μm in diameter), and have a prominent eccentric nucleus with a coarse chromatin pattern which is reminiscent of that of the plasma cell. The tumours so produced are intramedullary, unlike chloroma, and they cause destruction of the surrounding cortex, seen radiologically as areas of translucency (Fig. 53.4). Pathological fracture is the usual sequel.

The disease is predominantly one of the later years of life. The tumours are found usually in those bones containing red marrow, such as the vertebrae, pelvis, ribs, sternum, clavicles, skull, and the proximal portions of the humerus and femur. Multiple myeloma, unlike the leukaemias, is usually not associated with extraskeletal lesions, but sometimes the lymph nodes, liver, spleen, and other organs are involved.

Solitary plasma-cell tumours have also been found in patients who appear otherwise healthy; a bone lesion is the most usual manifestation of solitary myeloma, but solitary, soft-tissue plasma-cell tumours may occur in the submucosa of the

Figure 53.4
Multiple myeloma. This radiograph of the skull shows numerous osteolytic tumour deposits that produce a typical moth-eaten appearance resulting from the punched-out areas where bone has been destroyed. An appearance similar to this can be produced by secondary carcinoma. (*Photograph by courtesy of Dr. D. E. Sanders.*)

upper air passages and the oral cavity. More rarely such tumours have been reported in the kidney, ovary, stomach and intestine, spleen, and breast.[12] These single lesions tend to terminate in multiple myeloma, and cannot be regarded as innocent.

Apart from the pain, deformity, and neurological effects of its skeletal lesions, multiple myeloma also causes profound metabolic changes. The demineralisation of the skeleton may cause *hypercalcaemia* and renal failure (this occurs especially with IgA myeloma). The disturbances in protein metabolism, considered in detail on page 580, also produce clinical effects. Thus the *Bence-Jones protein*, present in about half the cases, may precipitate in the tubules, blocking them, and inducing a foreign-body reaction. The tubular obliteration and fibrosis lead to progressive renal failure—the condition is called *myeloma kidney*. In fact, the renal failure so common in multiple myeloma may be due to a combination of several factors: protein deposition, amyloid infiltration, pyelonephritis due to a generalised susceptibility to infection, and hypercalcaemia. The *cryoglobulinaemia* sometimes present leads to vascular occlusion in cold surroundings, and the *hyperglobulinaemia* increases the viscosity of the blood and is important in causing bleeding tendencies similar to those found in macroglobulinaemia. *Amyloidosis* occurs in about 10 per cent of cases, especially those with heavy Bence-Jones proteinuria. The abnormal globulin formation also leads to an impaired production of other immunoglobulins, and *susceptibility to infection by pyogenic organisms* is another complication. It is seen most often in IgG myelomata.

Blood picture. *The red cells* are moderately or severely reduced in number, and are normochromic and normocytic (or often macrocytic). There is usually little evidence of increased formation. The hyperglobulinaemia leads to marked rouleaux formation (and sludging), and is responsible for the raised ESR so characteristic of the condition.

The white-cell count shows no constant change, but there may occasionally be evidence of marrow replacement. Plasma cells may be present in small numbers in the blood, but any great invasion is rare. A few cases are associated with a high plasma-cell count, and these have been called 'plasma-cell leukaemia'.

The platelets are reduced in the later stages of the disease.

With the use of alkylating agents the median survival time is between 2 and 4 years from the onset of treatment. Occasional cases live for more than 10 years.

The commonest cause of death is infection, and this is followed by chronic renal failure. Other important factors are progressive anaemia and pathological fracture of the spinal column with compression of the cord and paraplegia.

BONE-MARROW APLASIA[13]

In the conditions about to be considered there is a depression in the formation of blood cells in the marrow. This most commonly affects all three elements. *Aplasia* is a word with two different connotations in pathology (see p. 299); it is preferably applied specifically to the bone marrow, when it means a sudden cessation of division of the blood-cell precursors. These are usually destroyed by some noxious agent, but sometimes they persist and yet fail to develop into more mature forms. The mature elements in the blood are destroyed in the normal way, and are not replaced.

Pure red-cell aplasia is unusual; in the commoner *agranulocytosis* the aplasia is confined to the granulocytic precursors. Whether a *pure platelet aplasia* occurs is doubtful; in idiopathic thrombocytopenic purpura the platelets are destroyed after they are released from the bone marrow (p. 639). A marked reduction in numbers of all three elements of the blood is called **pancytopenia**, and is met with under the following circumstances:

Acute aleukaemic leukaemia. Bone-marrow examination makes the diagnosis clear.

Splenic overactivity. This is described separately.

Congenital pancytopenia. Fanconi has described a familial disease (not in any way related to the renal tubular defect he also described, see p. 559) in which the bone marrow is congenitally hypoplastic and there is a moderate pancytopenia. There are also multiple congenital abnormalities of the skeleton, central nervous system, and other organs. It is better to reserve the word *hypoplasia* for conditions in which an organ or tissue does not attain full, mature size. In such a connotation Fanconi's anaemia is indeed hypoplastic, as it is a developmental defect. Its liability to be complicated by leukaemia has already been noted (see p. 623).

Bone-marrow aplasia. This is also called *aplastic anaemia*.

Causes of Bone-Marrow Aplasia

Ionising radiation. Both whole-body irradiation, as in the Hiroshima victims, and continuous skeletal irradiation, as in the girls who swallowed luminous watch-paint (see Ch. 31), may be associated with bone-marrow aplasia.

Drugs. Some substances lead to aplasia in all individuals, provided a large enough dose is given. Examples of these are benzene, antimetabolites, and alkylating agents. On the other hand, a large number of drugs act unpredictably on only a few unfortunate individuals. In these cases the mysterious factor of idiosyncrasy* has to be invoked. Examples of this type of drug are chloramphenicol, organic arsenicals like arsphenamine, sulphonamides (a rather uncommon side-effect), phenylbutazone, quinacrine, gold salts, and the anticonvulsants methoin and troxidone.

Infections. Traditionally miliary tuberculosis may lead to aplastic anaemia, but this is very rare nowadays. Some viral infections are more important causes of a marrow aplasia that may last some time and is often fatal. Viral hepatitis has been complicated by aplasia on numerous occasions; it usually occurs a few months after the hepatitis.[14]

Hypopituitarism, and occasionally myxoedema.

'Idiopathic' aplastic anaemia. Despite exhaustive investigations, no immediate cause can be found for about 50 per cent of cases of aplastic anaemia. The possibility of preleukaemia or paroxysmal nocturnal haemoglobinuria must always be borne in mind.

Mechanism in marrow aplasia.[15] It is not known whether the damaging agents act on the stem cell or on the microenvironment, e.g. the sinusoids of the marrow, so as to

---

*A qualitatively abnormal drug reaction is termed *idiosyncrasy*, e.g. haemolytic anaemia with primaquine. It is to be distinguished from (a) *intolerance*, which is an excessive, though normal, reaction to a small dose, e.g. morphine in liver failure, and (b) *hypersensitivity*, in which an immunological reaction is involved.

destroy the medullary microcirculation. Probably, at least in the human subject, a direct action on the stem cell is the more important of the two mechanisms. Intravenous infusions of syngeneic marrow cells to patients with acquired aplastic anaemia of whatever cause usually lead to a complete restoration of haematopoietic function. There may also be an immunological mechanism mediated by the lymphocytes in the marrow.

Blood picture. All three elements are greatly reduced in number.

The red cells are normocytic and normochromic. There is little anisocytosis or poikilocytosis, and there is no evidence of regeneration—the reticulocyte count is very low.

The severe leucopenia is accompanied by a relative lymphocytosis, but in the worst cases there may also be a lymphopenia.

The thrombocytopenia is severe.

The bone marrow is very hypocellular, and many of the nucleated cells present may be lymphocytes. Sometimes the cellularity is normal or even increased, and it would appear that the failure of division occurs in the later stages of haematopoiesis. On the other hand, the aplasia itself may be patchy, and the marrow may have been taken fortuitously from a normal or hypercellular area; several areas of marrow should be examined. Sometimes there is a failure in maturation, or *maturation arrest.*

Biochemical changes. The plasma iron is raised, and the iron-binding protein may be saturated. There is an increased percentage of sideroblasts, and the RE cells also contain granules of haemosiderin. This siderosis becomes extreme in patients kept alive for long periods with transfusions.

Prognosis. This is grave. The worst cases (over the age of 40 years and with severe leucopenia and thrombocytopenia) usually die within 12 months, but others survive for longer periods, even many years, in a continuing state of severe anaemia or else in partial remission before they finally recover or else succumb.

The advent of marrow transplantation has improved the prognosis greatly.[16—18] Indeed, those patients fortunate to have an identical twin can look forward to complete recovery after syngeneic grafting. Allografts, even from a sibling donor compatible for the major histocompatibility complex, present formidable technical problems in terms of graft rejection, graft-versus-host disease, and overwhelming infection in an immunosuppressed patient, but they have proved successful and will no doubt be used more often in the future when more special centres are built.

Pathological features. *Haemorrhages* due to the thrombocytopenia.

Infective lesions due to the agranulocytosis.

Replacement of the red marrow by yellow fatty material, except when there is maturation arrest.

Lymphoid atrophy. The spleen may be small, and it often shows atrophy of the malpighian bodies. The liver, spleen, and lymph nodes are not usually enlarged in aplastic anaemia; an increase in size suggests that the diagnosis is wrong.

Individual Aplasias

Pure red-cell aplasia. In this condition the white cells and platelets are normal. It is rare, but is well recognised as an occasional accompaniment of *thymic tumours.* These are usually benign thymomata, and there may be an associated myasthenia gravis; an immunological mechanism is probably responsible. A *congenital hypoplastic anaemia* involving the red cells alone has been described by Diamond and Blackfan. It develops insidiously during the later neonatal period, and there is no evidence of red-cell regeneration. The bone marrow is deficient in normoblasts.

Acute red-cell aplasia may occur during the *crises* of hereditary spherocytosis and sickle-cell anaemia (see p. 615).

Agranulocytosis. This is a very important condition which occurs both as a component of marrow aplasia and as a separate disease in which the defect is confined to the white cells.

The white-cell count is below 2×10^9 per litre (2000 per μl) and it may drop to less than 0.1×10^9 per litre (100 per μl). Of the cells present only 1 to 2 per cent are granulocytes. There is thus a relative lymphocytosis and monocytosis. In pure agranulocytosis the red-cell and platelet counts are normal. The marrow shows a great reduction of myelocytes and granulocytes, with variable numbers of myeloblasts and promyelocytes and usually an increase in lymphocytes and plasma cells.

The agents that may lead to agranulocytosis are grouped into those that will produce it regularly if a sufficient dose is given, i.e. the agents already mentioned in relation to marrow aplasia such as ionising radiations and benzene, and those in which the condition is an occasional unpredictable occurrence (idiosyncrasy). The list of such drugs is very large: the most important are amidopyrine (the most notorious of all), thiouracil and its derivatives, phenylbutazone, chlorpromazine and other phenothiazine derivatives, sulphonamides, troxidone, pyribenzamine, and dinitrophenol. The drugs that may occasionally lead to marrow aplasia can obviously be included in the list.

The mechanism of production of agranulocytosis is uncertain, and probably there is more than one process. A leucocyte-agglutinating globulin has been found in the sera of patients sensitive to amidopyrine. This drug is particularly apt to lead to a rapid disappearance of granulocytes from the blood, and it may well be that they are destroyed in the capillaries after agglutination. Such leucocyte agglutinins are true autoantibodies, but the matter is not as simple as this, because similar antibodies are also found in the sera of people who have received blood transfusions. In chlorpromazine agranulocytosis no agglutinins are present; instead there is a temporary leucocytic aplasia of the marrow. The same may be seen after sulphonamides and amidopyrine. It is probable that toxic action on the proliferating cells in the marrow and a destructive action on the mature circulating granulocytes both play their part in producing agranulocytosis.

The pathological effects of agranulocytosis are those of severe infection. Necrotic lesions of the skin, mouth, throat, vagina, and gastrointestinal tract are common, and there is usually confluent bronchopneumonia. In all these lesions there is a conspicuous absence of polymorphs, only lymphocytes and plasma cells being present together with masses of bacteria. In the liver, spleen, and lymph nodes foci of necrosis are common. Perhaps they are due to the effect of infection.

Idiopathic thrombocytopenic purpura. (See Ch. 54.)

The Prevention of Drug-Induced Marrow Aplasia

The best way to obviate the danger of aplasia is to use drugs that are relatively safe. The performance of routine blood counts may lull one into a false sense of security. When aplasia strikes, it tends to do so out of the blue. In those exposed in the course of their work to ionising radiations it is more helpful to control the doses received than to perform routine blood counts.

SPLENIC OVERACTIVITY

The functions of the spleen. These are incompletely understood. It is well known that splenectomy is followed by no obvious ill-effects, though there are minor haematological changes.

New cell formation. Except in fetal life the human spleen plays no part in haematopoiesis, but if the bone marrow is destroyed, it is capable of taking over its role. In other animals, e.g. mice, the spleen is normally a haematopoietic organ even in the adult, and the animal can survive whole-body ionising irradiation if the spleen is shielded from the radiation (see Ch. 31).

Effect on haematopoiesis. It is possible that the spleen exerts some inhibitory effect on leucocyte production in the marrow, but the evidence for inhibition of erythropoiesis and platelet production is unconvincing.

Phagocytosis and removal of defective red cells. As noted in Chapter 52, the effete red cell is removed from the circulation by phagocytic RE cells in the liver, bone marrow, and spleen. Of these three organs the spleen plays the greatest part. The spleen also has a special capacity for trapping even mildly damaged red cells, such as those treated with small amounts of antibody, low doses of oxidant drugs, or incomplete antibodies, which are then destroyed, a process called 'culling'. Spherocytes are particularly susceptible to this process.

By contrast to this phagocytic process that results in the destruction of the whole cell, the spleen also has the capacity to remove particles from the intact red cell without destroying it. This is called 'pitting', and is the means by which Heinz bodies are removed from red cells. Probably the siderotic granules of siderocytes are removed in the same way, as are also Howell–Jolly bodies and larger nuclear remnants, and intracellular organisms, e.g. those of malaria and Oroya fever. The sticky surface of reticulocytes, which makes them agglutinate easily, is modified by the spleen, possibly by its pitting function.

The splenic reservoir. The blood reservoir of the spleen is useful in lower animals but not in humans; the average adult spleen holds 20 to 40 ml of red cells only. It is probable, however, that the spleen acts as a reservoir for platelets, lymphocytes, plasma cells, and monocytes.

The production of antibodies. Since the lymphoid tissue of the spleen plays a part in the immune response in regard to the formation of both immunoglobulins and lymphocytes, it is to be expected that it is of some importance in antibody production. Although it is not indispensable to antibody formation, there is a delay in appearance and a lower peak of antibody titres after splenectomy.

Defence against infection.[19] The spleen plays an important role against blood-borne infection, and splenectomised patients are liable to develop septicaemia. The organisms most often responsible are the meningococcus, pneumococcus, and *Haemophilus influenzae*, and the septicaemia or meningitis they produce is likely to be fulminating and fatal within 24 hours. Less commonly the infecting organism is a streptococcus, staphylococcus, or Gram-negative intestinal organism (including salmonellae). Apart from bacterial infections, splenectomised individuals are at risk from *Plasmodium falciparum* malaria and the protozoa of the genus *Babesia*. Human babesiosis is transmitted to human subjects from cattle and rodents by ticks, and presents as a fulminating haemolytic anaemia with intravascular haemolysis.[20] It resembles blackwater fever, and indeed the intra-erythrocytic 'rings' resemble malarial parasites.

It is generally agreed that children are at greater risk than are adults, and the first three years after splenectomy are the most hazardous. Healthy individuals who have undergone splenectomy for trauma are also at risk, but less so than those who have had the operation for haematological disease.

The basis of the spleen's effect against blood-borne infection is probably a function of its phagocytic role and the ability of the RE cells to remove intra-erythrocytic organisms.

Blood changes following splenectomy. As the spleen removes imperfectly-formed *red cells* from the circulation, it is not surprising that after splenectomy (or with splenic atrophy or agenesis) the blood contains numbers of nucleated red cells, most of which have Howell–Jolly bodies rather than complete nuclei. Siderocytes are also numerous. It seems that the spleen in some way ensures that red cells have a normal shape, for after splenectomy thin target cells (leptocytes) are conspicuous. Howell–Jolly bodies, siderocytes, and target cells persist indefinitely, and afford valuable evidence of splenectomy. There is an early reticulocytosis, because the normal spleen traps reticulocytes, which are sticky and easily agglutinated. There is no constant change in the red-cell count, both a mild, transient anaemia and polycythaemia having been reported.

There is an immediate *neutrophil leucocytosis* greater than can be attributed merely to a surgical procedure, and this is followed by a mild increase in lymphocytes, monocytes, eosinophils, and basophils. These later changes may last for a long time.

There is also a *thrombocytosis* maximal about 3 weeks after splenectomy, and this too may persist for some time. It is probably due to the removal of the normal storehouse for about one-third of the blood platelets.

The relationship between the spleen and anaemia. In *hypersplenism* there is an alleged splenic overactivity which is associated with increased destructive changes in the peripheral blood. As has been noted, the haematological functions of the spleen are obscure, and it is not certain that any of these changes is due entirely to splenic activity. Nevertheless, it is clinically well recognised that some blood dyscrasias respond favourably to splenectomy.

Splenic overactivity is suggested by the following findings taken together:

(*a*) A fall in the count of any or all of the three elements of the blood, or else a haemolytic type of anaemia.

(*b*) A normal or hypercellular marrow.

(c) Splenomegaly.

(d) Cure following splenectomy.

The enlarged spleen probably acts by sequestering large numbers of red cells, granulocytes, and platelets, which may then be damaged or destroyed there. The hyperactive marrow is probably merely a response to the deficiency of cells in the peripheral blood.

Splenic overactivity may be primary or secondary. *Primary hypersplenism* is a somewhat controversial condition. It has two possible manifestations, 'primary splenic pancytopenia' and 'primary splenic neutropenia'. These are chronic diseases in which there is a persistent or cyclical aplastic type of anaemia or agranulocytosis of moderate severity. There is an associated splenomegaly and a hyperplastic bone marrow. Splenectomy sometimes produces a slow improvement. The conditions are rare, and it is by no means certain that the spleen is the culprit.

Secondary hypersplenism is more definite, for it is well known that in the course of many diseases associated with splenomegaly there is a tendency towards pancytopenia or haemolytic anaemia. The marrow is usually hyperplastic, and splenectomy often relieves the blood manifestations even when having no effect on the primary condition.

The best-known example of this type of disease is *chronic congestive splenomegaly (Banti's syndrome)*, in which there is a greatly enlarged spleen secondary to portal hypertension. This usually follows hepatic cirrhosis, but may also be due to a malformation of the splenic vein. A severe 'splenic anaemia' follows, in which there is a normocytic, normochromic anaemia, a leucopenia, and a moderate thrombocytopenia. Recurrent haematemeses lead to an additional iron-deficiency anaemia. A splenectomy, while relieving the pancytopenia, does not diminish the portal hypertension in cases secondary to cirrhosis.

A similar type of blood picture occurs in *Felty's syndrome*, in which chronic rheumatoid arthritis is associated with splenomegaly. Here it is the red cells and leucocytes that bear the brunt of the splenic overactivity. Gaucher's disease, schistosomiasis (Egyptian splenomegaly), and leishmaniasis may also produce anaemia and leucopenia.

Sometimes there is an acute haemolytic anaemia instead of an aplastic one, and this may occasionally be accompanied by autoantibodies. Acute haemolytic anaemia occurring during the course of chronic lymphatic leukaemia, Hodgkin's disease, sarcoidosis, and myelosclerosis may be due to splenic overactivity, and a splenectomy may relieve this complication while having no effect on the primary condition.

It can be seen that the term hypersplenism is imprecise and has the effect of laying too great an emphasis on the spleen's part in disease processes that have their primary cause elsewhere. Probably even the 'primary' types have a basic origin in some other organ of the body. Therefore it is better to state exactly how the spleen is affecting the cells of the blood, e.g. by sequestration or destruction, rather than to use the vague concept of hypersplenism.

INDICATIONS FOR SPLENECTOMY IN BLOOD DISEASE

Hereditary spherocytosis, the indication *par excellence*.

Acquired haemolytic anaemia due to autoantibodies. It is effective in about 50 per cent of cases.

Idiopathic thrombocytopenic purpura.

Hodgkin's disease, and perhaps some of the other lymphomata, for the purpose of staging prior to starting treatment in selected cases. The value of this procedure is debatable; it is not favoured by all workers.

'Hypersplenism', especially chronic congestive splenomegaly. Many surgeons believe that splenectomy should not be attempted in this condition unless the surgeon is prepared to undertake a venous-shunting operation at the same time, since this may be the only opportunity to construct a satisfactory shunt.

Other conditions. These are controversial, and only acceptable under special conditions. Splenectomy does have an ameliorative effect in hereditary elliptocytosis and in the anaemia associated with pyruvate kinase deficiency, but it should not be performed unless there is severe anaemia.

THE SYNDROME OF BONE-MARROW REPLACEMENT

The normal bone marrow may be replaced by fibrous tissue, bone, or some foreign element like tumour tissue. In each case a characteristic blood picture is produced, and it is called *leuco-erythroblastic anaemia* because of the presence of many primitive white and red cells in the blood.

Causes of Leuco-erythroblastic Anaemia

Tumour destruction of the bone marrow. Metastatic carcinoma is the commonest cause of this condition. Of the various cancers that frequently metastatise to bone (p. 361), it is the prostatic lesion that is especially liable to produce a leuco-erythroblastic anaemia, because its metastases are typically osteosclerotic: much of the marrow is replaced with new bone in which clumps of cancer cells are present. Five per cent of cases of multiple myeloma produce it, and so occasionally does Hodgkin's disease.

Replacement of marrow by lipid-filled macrophages in Gaucher's disease and Niemann-Pick disease (see Ch. 30).

Myelofibrosis (myelosclerosis). This is an interesting disease of later life in which the bone marrow is replaced by fibrous or even bony tissue. The cortex is normal, but in the medulla there is either cellular fibrous tissue or else a thickening of bone with a laying down of new trabeculae. Such changes may be recognisable radiologically, and the condition is then called osteosclerosis. Of all the bone-marrow replacement diseases this one is the most chronic, and there is widespread myeloid metaplasia of many organs, especially the spleen and liver. This has led to confusion, and a plethora of synonyms has arisen, e.g. 'agnogenic myeloid metaplasia', 'myeloid megakaryocytic hepato-splenomegaly', and 'aleukaemic megakaryocytic myelosis'.

The nature of the condition is uncertain. In many cases there is hyperplasia of the marrow early in the disease even though there is also marked extramedullary haematopoiesis. Later on the cellular elements of the marrow become sparser and fibrosis develops. Finally there is complete fibrous or bony replacement. The condition has much in common with polycythaemia vera and haemorrhagic thrombocythaemia; in all three there is a proliferation of red-cell, white-cell, and platelet precursors, and there are borderline cases in which all three overlap. Thus these three diseases can be grouped together as the *myeloproliferative disorders.*[21] It is better not to include chronic myeloid leukaemia among them because of the frankly malignant nature of the cellular proliferation and its much worse prognosis. Why some cases of myeloproliferative disorder should proceed to fibrosis is not clear. But it is evident that the extramedullary haematopoiesis cannot be attributed simply to the bone-marrow replacement; while this no doubt accentuates the extramedullary blood formation, it also often follows it.

Marble-bone disease of Albers-Schönberg (osteopetrosis). This is a congenital disease in which there is a failure of removal of bony trabeculae and their replacement by marrow spaces. The bones are enormously thick and sclerotic, and are uniformly radio-opaque. The manifestations of this condition include spontaneous fractures, various cranial nerve palsies, hydrocephalus, and in about 25 per cent of cases, a leuco-erythroblastic anaemia.

Blood picture. *There is a variable degree of anaemia,* though in the early stages the red-cell count may be normal or even raised. The cells are normochromic and are mostly normocytic. Anisocytosis is usual and often marked, and poikilocytosis is characteristic, many of the red cells having a teardrop shape in myelofibrosis. There are considerable numbers of nucleated red cells in the blood and often a moderate reticulocytosis.

The white-cell count varies from a moderate leucopenia to a leucocytosis of up to 50×10^9 per litre (50 000 per μl). There are numerous myelocytes in the blood and even a few myeloblasts. The picture may resemble chronic myeloid leukaemia, but the white-cell count is seldom as high as in that condition.

The platelet count is normal or reduced. Abnormally large, bizarre platelets are common, especially in myelofibrosis.

A bone-marrow examination is essential; it is the only method by which tumour cells or lipid-filled macrophages can be demonstrated. In myelofibrosis the marrow feels gritty, and hardly any can be aspirated. Sometimes, however, it may be

normal or even hyperplastic. To confirm a diagnosis of myelofibrosis a surgical biopsy should be performed. Stained sections are necessary in order to study the architecture of the marrow and assess the degree of fibrosis.

In some of these conditions there may be splenic overactivity producing thrombocytopenic purpura or haemolytic anaemia.

Pathology. The most profound pathological changes are encountered in myelofibrosis. There is enormous splenomegaly, and the spleen shows marked *myeloid metaplasia* i.e. the red pulp contains all the marrow elements including many megakaryocytes (Fig. 53.5). Its architecture, including the malpighian bodies, is not destroyed. In the enlarged liver the haematopoietic cells are present in the sinusoids, as is seen in chronic myeloid leukaemia and fetal haematopoiesis. The lymph nodes and connective tissue may also be sites of extramedullary haematopoiesis.

The bone marrow is replaced by fibrous tissue or bony trabeculae. Some haematopoietic tissue persists, and in it megakaryocytes are often plentiful.

In secondary carcinoma the marrow contains foci of tumour tissue surrounded by zones of active blood formation. Extramedullary haematopoiesis is seldom conspicuous, because the patient rarely survives long enough for this to occur.

In myelosclerosis the leuco-erythroblastosis is apparently due to the spleen and other organs augmenting the marrow's function. Such organs lack the regulatory mechanism of the marrow, and are unable to prevent primitive cells from entering the blood. It is logical to regard the enlarged spleen as vital to the patient's well-being, as it is a major blood-forming organ. In practice, however, splenectomy is usually followed by no ill-effects, and the patient may actually improve if there has been an aspect of splenic overactivity in his blood condition. Obviously the other foci or haematopoiesis take over the spleen's function quite satisfactorily.

The mechanism of the leuco-erythroblastosis accompanying bone-marrow metastases is unknown. There is a decreased red-cell survival time in conditions of bone-marrow replace-

Figure 53.5
Myeloid metaplasia of spleen. The red pulp is crowded with haematopoietic tissue including a number of large megakaryocytes. The patient suffered from myelosclerosis, and the spleen was removed because of evidence of over-activity. × 200.

ment, and it is evident that haematopoiesis does not adequately compensate for the cellular destruction.

BONE-MARROW EXAMINATION

A bone-marrow examination is useful for the following purposes:

1. To assess the over-all cellularity of the marrow as well as the development of its individual elements.

2. To determine whether erythropoiesis is normoblastic or megaloblastic.

3. To detect foreign elements in the marrow, e.g. tumour cells, myeloma cells, or lipid-filled macrophages.

4. To assess whether there is fibrous or bony replacement of functioning tissue. A surgical biopsy is necessary for this.

5. To detect (and if necessary culture) blood-borne organisms, e.g. leishmania, histoplasma, malarial plasmodia, and typhoid bacilli.

REFERENCES

1. Leading Article (1974) Another look at the N.B.T. test. *Lancet*, **1**, 664.
2. NATHAN, D. G. (1974) NBT reduction by human phagocytes. *New England Journal of Medicine*, **290**, 280.
3. RYAN, G. B. & MAJNO, G. (1977) Acute inflammation. *American Journal of Pathology*, **86**, 183.
4. GOLDE, D. W. & CLINE, M. J. (1974) Regulation of granulopoiesis. *New England Journal of Medicine*, **291**, 1388.
5. EPSTEIN, M. A. & ACHONG, B. G. (1973) Various forms of Epstein-Barr virus infection in man: established facts and a general concept. *Lancet*, **2**, 836.
6. Leading Article (1972) Epidemiology of leukaemia. *Lancet*, **1**, 82.
7. TURSZ, T. *et al.* (1974) Simultaneous occurrence of acute myeloblastic leukaemia and multiple myeloma without previous chemotherapy. *British Medical Journal*, **2**, 642.
8. GOLDMAN, J. M. (1974) Acute promyelocytic leukaemia. *British Medical Journal*, **1**, 380.
9. Leading Article (1975) Long survival from acute leukaemia in childhood. *British Medical Journal*, **1**, 111.
10. CATOVSKY, D. *et al.* (1974) T-lymphoblastic leukaemia: a distinct variant of acute leukaemia. *British Medical Journal*, **2**, 643.
11. GELFAND, E. W. & CHECHIK, B. E. (1976) Unmasking the heterogeneity of acute lymphoblastic leukemia. *New England Journal of Medicine*, **294**, 275.
12. WILTSHAW, E. (1976) The natural history of extramedullary plasmacytoma and its relation to solitary myeloma of bone and myelomatosis. *Medicine (Baltimore)*, **55**, 217.
13. LEWIS, S. M. (1971) Aplastic anaemia. *British Journal of Hospital Medicine*, **6**, 593.
14. Leading Article (1971) Infectious hepatitis and aplastic anaemia. *Lancet*, **1**, 844.
15. Leading Article (1976) Mechanisms in aplastic anaemia. *Lancet*, **2**, 1179.
16. Leading Article (1975) Bone-marrow grafting for aplastic anaemia. *Lancet*, **1**, 22.
17. Leading Article (1975) Prognosis in aplastic anaemia. *British Medical Journal*, **4**, 126.
18. Leading Article (1977) Changed outlook in aplastic anaemia. *British Medical Journal*, **1**, 63.
19. Leading Article (1976) Infective hazards of splenectomy. *Lancet*, **1**, 1167.
20. Leading Article (1976) Human babesiosis. *Lancet*, **1**, 1001.
21. WARD, H. P. & BLOCK, M. H. (1971) The natural history of agnogenic myeloid metaplasia (AMM) and a critical evaluation of its relationship with the myeloproliferative syndrome. *Medicine (Baltimore)*, **50**, 357.

Chapter 54. *Some Disorders of the Blood: The Platelets*

III. THE PLATELETS AND CLOTTING FACTORS

The precursor of the platelet is the megakaryocyte, an extremely large cell ranging from 40 to 160 μm in diameter, with an irregularly lobed, ring-shaped or doughnut-shaped nucleus and a light blue cytoplasm packed with fine azurophilic granules. It arises from the pluripotential stem-cell, which when committed to differentiation along the megakaryocyte line, undergoes a process of endomitosis in which the nuclear material reduplicates but the nucleus does not divide. Such a cell cannot be called a giant cell, since it has only one nucleus, which, however, is extremely complex. It is indeed polyploid inasmuch as each division produces a doubling of the total nuclear material. Thus the megakaryocyte has a polyploid nucleus, and is different from a true giant cell, like the osteoclast, which is a multinucleate cell.

As the megakaryocyte develops, so it also becomes larger and its basophilic cytoplasm develops granules. While nuclear endomitosis is taking place, the cytoplasm develops strings of vesicles which fuse to form a pronounced network of double membranes. Clefts form between these membranes, and the cytoplasm fragments into individual, single, membrane-covered platelets.

In the fetus megakaryocytes are found successively in the liver, spleen, and bone marrow, whereas in adult mammals they are present in the bone marrow, lung, and spleen (to a negligible degree in the healthy human spleen). Whether those present in the lungs represent effete cells in the process of destruction, or whether they constitute an important supply of platelets is still an unsettled problem. It is certain that the main source of platelets is the marrow.

Platelets[1,2] are formed by the fragmentation and detachment of delicate processes from the cytoplasm of megakaryocytes. Their morphology and function are described in Chapter 39.

The normal platelet count varies from 140 to 440 $\times$ 10^9 per litre (140 000 to 440 000 per μl) with an average of 250 $\times$ 10^9 per litre (250 000 per μl). A count below 100 $\times$ 10^9 per litre (100 000 per μl) can be taken as a thrombocytopenia. There are comparatively few physiological variations in platelet count; neither the newborn infant nor the menstruating woman has any alteration in count. It tends to be reduced in later pregnancy, but during the puerperium there is a moderate rise in count. The administration of adrenaline produces an immediate increase in count up to 50 per cent, and is presumably due to splenic release, since it does not occur in individuals without a spleen. On the other hand, the increased count that follows exercise is unaffected by splenectomy, and may be the result of the release of platelets from the lungs. The pathological causes of an increased count (thrombo-cytosis) have been considered on page 489. The opposite condition (thrombocytopenia) is associated with a bleeding tendency, and is discussed later.

The normal life span of a platelet varies from 9 to 12 days in the human being. Damaged and effete platelets are sequestered principally in the spleen, where they are destroyed.

The Functions of Platelets in Haemostasis

(*a*) They seal the injured vessel by adhering to the damaged area and aggregating to form a mass known as a *haemostatic plug*. The platelet lipoprotein surface catalyses the intrinsic clotting system, and the fibrin which is formed consolidates the plug. Finally the fibrin clot retracts. The mechanism is uncertain, but it is established that the adhesion of platelets to fibrin is an essential preliminary step. The mechanical work of clot retraction is carried out by *thrombosthenin*, a contractile protein complex present in platelets and which is apparently identical with the actomyosin system of muscle.

Thrombin released during coagulation causes further platelet deposition as well as fibrin formation. Defects in the intrinsic system of blood clotting, such as in haemophilia, do not prevent the formation of a haemostatic plug, and therefore the bleeding time is normal (p. 637). However, the plug is not stable, and re-bleeding may occur later.

(*b*) When exposed to stimuli, such as collagen, antigen-antibody complexes, and bacterial endotoxin, they release a number of chemical agents (*platelet release reaction*).[3] These include *ADP*, which causes the platelets to swell, throw out pseudopods, and adhere together, *5-HT*, which is a vasoconstrictor and plays a minor part in haemostasis, and *lipoprotein*, which plays a part in clotting. Aspirin inhibits the platelet release reaction, but does not prevent ADP-induced platelet aggregation.

(*c*) They are necessary for proper clot retraction.

THE CLOTTING MECHANISM

The object of the very complex clotting mechanism is the conversion of the plasma protein fibrinogen into the insoluble network of fibres which is called fibrin. In order to systematise the bewildering number of clotting factors that have been discovered, the International Committee for the Nomenclature of Blood Clotting Factors has decreed that each factor should be designated by a Roman numeral, starting with fibrinogen as Factor I. It therefore comes about that the clotting process is best described by starting at the final stage, and then working backwards. As the most recently discovered factors, other than Factor XIII, are all concerned with the initial stages of the process, this is less unreasonable than would appear at first sight. The platelet lipoprotein factors are designated by Arabic numerals; in practice the only important one is factor 3.

When plasma clots, the fluid that is subsequently expressed is called serum, and it is completely lacking in *fibrinogen* (**Factor I**). This conversion of fibrinogen to fibrin is brought about by thrombin, which is normally present as an inert precursor called **prothrombin** (**Factor II**). *Thrombin*, also called *Factor IIa* to denote that it is activated Factor II, is a proteolytic enzyme that splits off two peptide fragments, fibrinopeptides A and B, from a molecule of fibrinogen; these peptides cause smooth muscle to contract. The remainder of the fibrinogen molecule is capable of spontaneous polymerisation with its fellows; in this way the fibrin monomer forms orderly molecular aggregates which reach a sufficient size to make up the network of fibres called a clot. This is easily disrupted until **Factor XIII, fibrin-stabilising factor,** creates covalent bonds between the aggregates, so converting soluble fibrin into insoluble, or stabilised, fibrin; the clot becomes a firm gel which is resistant to urea.

Prothrombin, like fibrinogen, is a glycoprotein. It migrates with the α_2 or β-globulins. Prothrombin is converted into thrombin by *prothrombinase*.

Prothrombinase (also called prothrombin activator) is formed by the interaction of activated Factor X (designated Xa) with Factor V, platelet factor 3, and calcium ions.

This sequence is called the *common pathway*, and can be initiated by two completely separate mechanisms, the *intrinsic (blood) system* and the *extrinsic (tissue) system* (Figs 54.1 and 54.2)

In the *intrinsic system* contact with an abnormal surface leads to the activation of Factor XII and the sequential interaction of Factors XI, IX, VIII, and (with calcium ions and platelet factor 3) Factor X.

In the *extrinsic system* tissue damage results in the release of a **tissue factor** rich in lipoproteins, phosphatides, and cholesterol. It is called **Factor III**, or thromboplastin, and is found in large amounts in the brain, extracts of which are used as a source of it in some laboratory tests, such as the prothrombin time. It too, in interacting with Factor VII, activates Factor X, which, as already described, is involved in the formation of prothrombinase *via* the common pathway.

The two pathways of blood clotting are both important, for a derangement of either leads to a serious defect in haemostasis. The intrinsic system develops much more slowly than the extrinsic one, but both are initiated by tissue damage, either by releasing tissue factor or providing an abnormal

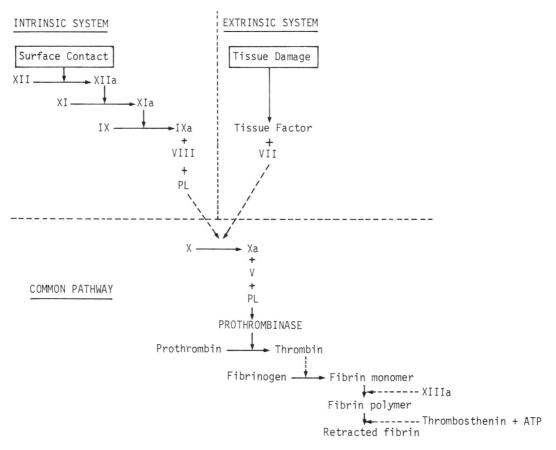

Figure 54.1

A simplified diagrammatic representation of the blood clotting mechanism. The three pathways are separated by interrupted lines. Solid arrows indicate transformation, interrupted arrows denote actions. PL denotes platelet factor 3. There is evidence that platelets in conjunction with Factor XII can form a platelet 'tissue-factor' and thereby initiate the extrinsic system. The importance of this *in vivo* is debatable. Not shown in the diagram is the ionic calcium which is required for most of the steps shown. (After Marcus, A. J. (1969), *New Engl. J. Med.*, 280, 1213).

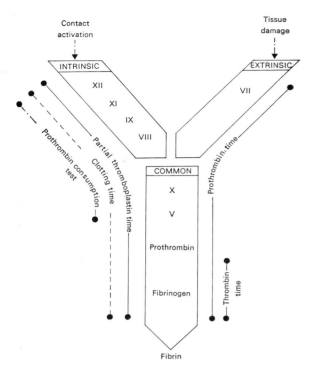

Figure 54.2
The interpretation of screening tests of blood clotting. (*From Bithell, T. C. and Wintrobe, M. M.* (1970), *in* Harrison's Principles of Internal Medicine, *6th ed., Fig. 62.3, p. 323, New York. McGraw-Hill.*)

surface. In both systems there is activation of Factor X, and from then on there is a final *common pathway* involving Factor V, platelet factor 3, calcium ions, prothrombin, and fibrinogen.

In all the phases leading up to the formation of thrombin from prothrombin, **calcium ions (Factor IV)** are necessary, with the exception of the contact phases involving Factors XII and XI and the enzymatic effect of thrombin on fibrinogen and on Factor XIII. Its mode of action is uncertain; it is possible that it acts in an adsorbed rather than in an ionic form. Clinical conditions of hypocalcaemia are never severe enough to interfere with clotting.

Factors Involved in the Clotting Mechanism

Factor V, also called **proaccelerin** and **labile factor.** This is present in normal plasma even when treated with aluminium hydroxide, but is not found in serum. The term Factor VI, which originally referred to the activated form of Factor V, has been abandoned. Factor V migrates electrophoretically as an albumin.

Factor VII, also called **proconvertin** and **stable factor.** This is present in normal serum, from which it is adsorbed by aluminium hydroxide. Unlike Factor V, it is resistant to heat and survives storage. It migrates electrophoretically as an α or β-globulin.

Factor VIII, also called **antihaemophilic factor** or **antihaemophilic globulin (AHG),** is an α_2 or β-globulin present in alumina-treated plasma but not in serum (like Factor V).

Factor IX, also called **Christmas factor** after a patient in whom a deficiency was first noted, is an imperfectly characterised protein present in serum but not in alumina-treated plasma (like Factors VII and X). It is also called **plasma thromboplastin component (PTC).**

Factor X, also called **Stuart–Prower factor** after the two patients in whom a deficiency was first described, is another imperfectly characterised protein which is present in serum but not in alumina-treated plasma.

Factor XI, also called **plasma thromboplastin antecedent (PTA),** migrates electrophoretically as a β or γ-globulin. It is present both in serum and alumina-treated plasma.

Factor XII, also called **Hageman factor** after a patient, also migrates electrophoretically as a β or γ-globulin. It too is present both in serum and alumina-treated plasma. Deficiency of this factor is peculiar in having little clinical effect despite producing a greatly prolonged clotting time.

Platelet factor 3. It is probable that this does not exist as a distinct entity, but is the altered lipoprotein surface of the platelets which catalyses at least two steps in clotting. Nevertheless, the term may usefully be employed to denote this activity.

It should be noted that Factors II, VII, IX, X, XI, XII, and XIII are all enzymes; they are of a class called serine proteases. Digestive enzymes and complement enzymes are also members of this class. Characteristically they are all stored as an inactive precursor, activated by a given stimulus, and then undergo a cascade-like activation. Thus the activation of the various factors involved in clotting is believed to follow a *cascade sequence*, many of the factors being substrates that are activated by a preceding enzyme. The original theory was described independently by Macfarlane in England and Davie and Ratnoff in the USA, but since then a number of modifications have been discovered (Fig. 54.1).

Factor XII is first activated by the contact of blood with a foreign surface, the product being Factor XIIa. This activates Factor XI, and Factor XIa activates Factor IX. Factor IXa forms a complex with Factor VIII, calcium ions, and platelet Factor 3, and the complex activates Factor X. Factor Xa now forms a complex with Factor V, calcium ions, and platelet Factor 3, and this complex activates Factor II (prothrombin) to Factor IIa (thrombin). The thrombin then converts fibrinogen to fibrin which is stabilised by Factor XIII, itself first activated by thrombin.

The earliest phase of the intrinsic system is slow. However, once thrombin is formed the process is greatly accelerated—indeed, there is a real cascade, for thrombin potentiates the activity of Factors V and VIII. It also causes platelets to aggregate and so increases the amount of Factor 3. This is called the *autocatalytic action of thrombin*. Interestingly, thrombin also destroys Factors V and VIII after potentiating their reactivity; in this way fibrin formation is stopped when a high concentration of thrombin has been achieved.

THE PHYSIOLOGICAL INHIBITION OF INTRAVASCULAR CLOTTING

The first natural mode of inhibition of intravascular clotting is the slowness of thrombin formation due to the exclusion of tissue factor and the almost complete absence of prothrombinase, which is attributable to the stability of the various clotting factors. Once the vascular endothelium is damaged and tissue fluids enter the blood, there is a great tendency for clotting to occur intravascularly. Furthermore, the autocatalytic action of thrombin has an amplifying effect on clotting, which could soon become extensive. To obviate this danger, there are a number of inhibitors, or anticoagulants, present in the blood. Several antithrombins have been described and designated with Roman numerals; of these only two are of considerable importance.

Fibrin. Fibrin, at one time called antithrombin I, is a natural antithrombin, in that the thrombin is removed as a result of its affinity for the fibrin surface. The fibrin threads with the adsorbed thrombin are filtered off in the capillaries and destroyed.

Antithrombin III. Antithrombin III is by far the most important natural constraint to coagulation. It combines with, and inactivates, most serine proteases. This combination is enhanced by heparin. In fact, antithrombin III is the factor through which heparin exerts its effects. For this reason it is called the *heparin cofactor.*

Heparin. This is a sulphated mucopolysaccharide found in most tissues of the body, and prominent in the granules of mast cells. These cells are distributed typically around small vessels and capillaries. The anticoagulant effects of heparin involve a preliminary interaction with plasma proteins called *heparin cofactors.* The most important of these is antithrombin III. Heparin inhibits many of the interactions involved in the clotting mechanism. In particular it aids the adsorption of thrombin on fibrin threads, and inhibits the autocatalytic action of thrombin as well as the action of this enzyme on fibrinogen. The effects of heparin are counteracted by protamine. Platelet factor 4 is an antiheparin agent, and like factor 3 is liberated by platelet aggregating agents.

Fibrinopeptides may also act as antithrombins.

CLOT DISSOLUTION (FIBRINOLYSIS)

Fibrin formed *in vitro* from normal blood usually remains intact for days or weeks provided bacterial contamination is avoided. In extravascular situations in the body large deposits may be found in the form of haematomata and inflammatory exudates, and these too are fairly stable. They are ultimately removed in the demolition phase which precedes resolution or organisation. In both instances digestion is brought about by proteolytic enzymes derived most probably from the polymorphs. There is, however, a proteolytic enzyme which is formed from the constituents of the blood, and this acts intravascularly. Although called a fibrinolysin, it can also slowly digest fibrinogen and other plasma proteins.

Plasminogen, a normal plasma protein, can be activated in a variety of ways to produce the active fibrinolytic enzyme **plasmin**. These plasminogen activators, previously called kinases,* have now been identified with *kallikrein*, an enzyme that is present in an inert precursor form, *prekallikrein* (see

---

*A *kinase* is a substance which activates an enzyme. It usually forms the suffix of the word indicating what is being activated, e.g. thrombokinase (now called prothrombinase) activates thrombin from prothrombin. However, in regard to fibrinolysis the word kinase is used in the context described above.

p. 82). This is concentrated in the lysosomes of most tissue cells, especially those of the small veins and the renal vasculature; it has also been isolated from leucocytes and platelets. Prekallikrein can be activated by Factor XIIf and also by plasmin. Possibly streptokinase and staphylokinase also activate prekallikrein, but this is uncertain.

Trace amounts of kallikrein are present in the plasma, from which it is rapidly removed by the liver. It has been isolated from the urine as 'urokinase', probably following local synthesis rather than excretion from the blood.

Plasmin, unlike thrombin, has a wide spectrum of proteolytic activity, and is comparable in this respect to trypsin. In addition to fibrin and fibrinogen, it degrades other clotting factors as well as many other plasma proteins, e.g. complement and various hormones. When blood clots, plasminogen is adsorbed on to the fibrin, and it is at this site that activation occurs rather than in the blood itself.

Most of the stimuli that lead to the release of kallikrein *in vivo* are vasoactive and presumably precipitate the release of prekallikrein from the endothelial cells of the small blood vessels. The stimuli include exercise, physical stress, adrenaline, histamine, bacterial pyrogen, ischaemia, and hypoxia. Lysosomal prekallikrein from other cells may also be released under physiological circumstances and in states of shock and tissue damage. Plasmin activity probably accounts for the persistent fluidity of the blood which is so frequent a *post-mortem* finding after sudden death, haemorrhage, shock, and asphyxia. It was indeed noted by John Hunter that the blood of two deer chased to exhaustion failed to clot.

There are at least two plasma proteins that specifically neutralise free plasmin (*antiplasmins*). They are an α_2-macroglobulin, which neutralises plasmin rapidly, and a slowly acting α_1-globulin (α_1-antitrypsin). Antiplasmins have also been isolated from platelets and from mesothelium and endothelium. A number of chemical agents also inhibit fibrinolysis, and some have therapeutic value in the human subject, e.g. epsilon-aminocaproic acid.

It seems apparent that the plasmin content of the blood is increased in a wide range of conditions, and is presumably a defence mechanism contrived to balance the clotting mechanism. One might postulate that an imbalance between the two systems leads to intravascular clotting on the one hand and afibrinogenaemia on the other (see disseminated intravascular coagulation syndrome, p. 643).

A reduction in the quantity of kallikrein, or the presence of an inhibitor, have been suggested as factors concerned in the fibrin accumulation found in the lungs of patients with uraemia or subjected to thoracic radiation. They may possibly play a subsidiary role in hyaline-membrane disease of the newborn.

TESTS OF IMPORTANCE IN THE BLEEDING DISEASES

There is no single test which will evaluate the integrity of the complex haemostatic mechanisms of blood. Many tests are available, and an outline of the commonly used ones will be given. When evaluating the tests for clotting defects, it is convenient to consider whether the test is measuring the intrinsic system, the extrinsic system, the common pathway, or a combination of these (see Fig. 54.2). The *sensitivity* of each test must also be remembered. Thus the commonly used clotting time can be normal when one of the clotting factors involved is as low as 1 or 2 per cent of normal.

Bleeding time. This is the time taken for a small skin puncture to stop bleeding. It varies from 1 to 9 minutes. An increased bleeding time is due to inadequate platelet activity in sealing the puncture, or to a failure of vascular contraction; in practice both are often combined. It is invariable in thrombocytopenia and usual with defective platelet function (*thrombocytopathia*) and in von Willebrand's disease.

Capillary fragility test (Hess's test). This test assesses the degree of fragility of the capillaries to a sustained rise of blood pressure (between systolic and diastolic for 5 minutes), and a positive result is manifested by a purpuric eruption on the skin of the arm below the applied tourniquet. Presumably the capillaries are mildly damaged by the sudden rise in pressure, and become more permeable. The platelets cover the endothelium, and so protect it.

The test is positive in severe thrombocytopenia, but the results correlate poorly with the platelet count. Indeed, some normal people develop a considerable number of petechiae when tested. This test is also positive when there is vascular damage, e.g. scurvy, scarlet fever, and hypertension.

Platelet count has already been mentioned.

Clotting time. This is the time taken before a specimen of whole blood clots. It is important to exclude tissue factors, therefore the venepuncture must be 'clean'. The blood is placed in an unsiliconised tube at a temperature of 37°C, and clotting should occur within 5 to 15 minutes. If a siliconised tube is used the clotting time is 20 to 60 minutes. The clotting time is prolonged if there is a deficiency of any of the factors concerned in the *intrinsic clotting system* or in the *common pathway*. The test is insensitive, and the clotting time is significantly prolonged only in severe deficiencies of the various factors involved in the intrinsic and common pathways; indeed, it is usually normal when these factors are present in amounts exceeding 1 per cent of the normal plasma levels. Relatively little prothrombinase is needed to produce a normal clotting time. The test is not affected by the level of Factor VII (extrinsic system), but is prolonged when a circulating anticoagulant such as heparin is present in excess. The test is widely used to control heparin therapy, but the partial thromboplastin time is a better method. With thrombocytopenia there is usually a normal clotting time despite a prolonged bleeding time. This is because clotting requires only a very small amount of platelet factor 3 for its initiation.

Prothrombin consumption test. The clotting time can be normal even though a small amount of prothrombinase is produced (see above). However, much unused prothrombin will remain and this can be measured in the prothrombin consumption test. The test measures only those factors required for prothrombin production in the intrinsic system (XII, XI, IX, VIII, X, and V), and is more sensitive than the clotting time. It is also affected by platelet abnormality and thrombocytopenia.

Clot retraction. In the absence of platelets the clot is soft and jelly-like; it lacks the firmness and adhesiveness of a normal clot, and is less effective in producing permanent haemostasis. Measurements of clot retraction are not done as a routine procedure. Normal blood starts retracting 30 to 60 minutes after being drawn. Associated with thrombocytopenia there is a defective retraction of the clot, and this contributes to the bleeding tendency.

Prothrombin time. In this test equal amounts of brain extract (containing tissue factor), calcium-chloride solution, and test plasma are incubated at 37°C, and the time taken for clotting to occur is recorded. A control must be put up at the same time, and this should clot in 10 to 16 seconds. The test is a measure of the factors concerned in the *extrinsic system* (Factor VII) and in the *common pathway* (Factors X, V, prothrombin, and fibrinogen). The intrinsic pathway is by-passed.

This test was introduced as an indicator of prothrombin deficiency, but it is now known that deficiencies of the other factors mentioned above also serve to prolong the prothrombin time. It is nevertheless of great value in controlling anti-coagulant therapy in thrombotic disorders, because the commonly-used anticoagulants of the coumarin and phenylin-danedione types depress Factors VII and X as well as prothrombin. These anticoagulants also depress the level of Factor IX, and unfortunately the test is of no value in assessing a deficiency of this factor.

Where the prothrombin time is greatly prolonged, there is also a prolonged clotting time. The clotting time may, however, be normal despite a significantly increased prothrombin time, e.g. during the administration of anticoagulants, and the patient's life is in jeopardy.

Plasma thrombin time. This is the time taken for plasma to clot when thrombin is added. It is a measure of the fibrinogen level, and is also affected by excess heparin and other anticoagulants.

The Fi test. This is a rapid test for hypofibrinogenaemia. Latex particles coated with antibody to human fibrinogen are mixed with plasma. Normally there is aggregation, and a failure of this to occur indicates afibrinogenaemia.

Partial thromboplastin time (PTT). This is the time taken for plasma to clot under the following three conditions:

(*a*) The test is carried out in a glass tube—the surface causes activation of Factor XII.

(*b*) A fraction of brain extract called 'cephalin' is added.* This provides excess phospholipid, and makes the test independent of the platelet count.

(*c*) Calcium chloride is added.

The PTT is a sensitive measure of the factors concerned in the *intrinsic system and common pathway* (see Fig. 54.2). It is increased if any of the factors are below 15 to 20 per cent of normal, and is also prolonged by heparin and other inhibitors. Sometimes kaolin is added to the mixture to aid the activation of Factor XII: this is then called the *activated partial thromboplastin time.*

Thromboplastin generation test. This invaluable test assesses the factors that are of importance in *the intrinsic system*, and it depends on the fact that some of these are contained in normal plasma adsorbed with aluminium hydroxide, and others are present in normal serum. These

---

*This extract is soluble in ether but not in acetone. It is not the same as the water-soluble extract used in the prothrombin time. It is indeed a 'partial thromboplastin' when compared to the complete thromboplastin used in the prothrombin time.

factors produce prothrombinase (which was originally called thromboplastin, a name now reserved for tissue factor in the new nomenclature) in the presence of platelet factor 3 and ionic calcium. The prothrombinase reacts with prothrombin and leads to clotting.

Normally the test is carried out in two stages. In the first a mixture of serum, adsorbed plasma, and platelets has ionic calcium added to it. In the second stage the prothrombinase formed is assayed by adding a portion of the complete mixture to normal plasma which contains normal amounts of prothrombin and fibrinogen. The prothrombinase content of the mixture, if serially determined, increases with time, and within 3 to 5 minutes reaches a maximal level, so that the clotting time of the substrate plasma is from 8 to 15 seconds. If the result is abnormal, the deficient factor can be determined by replacing in turn the patient's plasma, serum, and platelets with normal adsorbed plasma, serum, and platelets (or a platelet substitute), and repeating the test.

Table 54.1 indicates the presence or absence of the various clotting factors in serum and alumina-treated plasma. Although Factor VII is included in the table, it plays no part in the thromboplastin generation test.

Table 54.1

Factor	Serum	Alumina-treated plasma
V	Absent	Present
VII	Present	Absent
VIII	Absent	Present
IX	Present	Absent
X	Present	Absent
XI	Present	Present
XII	Present	Present

If normal adsorbed plasma induces the rapid formation of **prothrombinase but normal serum has no effect, the deficiency is one of Factors V or VIII. These two can be distinguished by means of the prothrombin time which is normal in Factor-VIII deficiency and prolonged in Factor-V deficiency.**

If the defect is relieved by normal serum but not by normal adsorbed plasma, there is a deficiency of Factor IX or Factor X. Factor-X deficiency leads to a prolonged prothrombin time, which is normal in Factor-IX deficiency.

If the defect is relieved both by normal adsorbed plasma and normal serum, the deficiency is one of Factors XI or XII, and as already mentioned, Factor-XII deficiency does not usually cause any clinical symptoms.

If the defect is present even when normal adsorbed plasma and normal serum are used, the fault lies in the patient's platelets, which are deficient in function.

In practice, there are specialised laboratories which keep plasma of patients known to be deficient in these individual factors. Depending on whether or not such a plasma can be corrected by that of a fresh case, a diagnosis of specific factor deficiency can be confirmed.

The four tests which can most easily be carried out as an initial investigation of a patient with a bleeding disease are the *platelet count*, the *bleeding time*, the *partial thromboplastin time* (*PTT*), and the *prothrombin time* (*PT*). If both PTT and PT are normal, the defect is probably in the vessels or the platelets. If either PTT or PT is prolonged, there is probably a defect in the clotting system. If both PTT and PT are abnormal, the defect is most likely in the common pathway. If the PTT is prolonged and the PT is normal, it is the intrinsic system which is most probably at fault. A prolonged PT and a normal PTT is rare, and indicates a deficiency of Factor VII (see Fig. 54.2).

THE HAEMORRHAGIC DISEASES

A haemorrhagic tendency may be due to one or more of three factors:

(*a*) A defect in or damage to the blood vessels.

(*b*) A decreased number of platelets (or inadequately functioning platelets).

(*c*) A defect in the clotting mechanism.

The clinical manifestation of these diseases is an increased tendency to bleed. This may occur after obvious trauma, like bruising or a surgical incision, or it may take place apparently spontaneously as haemorrhages into the skin, mucous membranes, and viscera. Haemorrhages less than 2 mm in diameter are called *petechiae*. Diffuse flat haemorrhages larger than this are *ecchymoses*, and if there is a definite swelling the lesion is called a *haematoma*. *Purpura* is defined as any condition in which there is bleeding into the skin.

Purpura is peculiar to states of vascular damage and platelet inadequacy. It is rare in the disorders of clotting. Not all purpuric lesions are evidence of a generalised bleeding tendency. Quite a large number of purpuras are due to local vascular damage, and these should be separated from the generalised purpuras which are clearly important manifestations of a haemorrhagic diathesis. Localised purpuric lesions include (*a*) *senile purpura*; (*b*) *cachectic purpura*, in both of which the blood vessels are poorly protected against trauma in the atrophic skin and subcutaneous tissue; (*c*) *orthostatic purpura* on the legs of people who stand for long periods of time; (*d*) *mechanical purpura*, which may occur in whooping-cough, convulsions, and traumatic asphyxia, due to the rupture of many capillaries; (*e*) *purpura in women who bruise easily*, probably due to excessively fragile capillaries; (*f*) *purpura in certain rare skin diseases*, e.g. the Ehlers-Danlos syndrome,* where there is inadequate support for the capillaries;[4] (*g*) *corticosteroid purpura*, due to the mechanical rupture of poorly supported blood vessels in the atrophic skin which results from the prolonged local or systemic use of glucocorticoids.

The generalised purpuric diseases may be divided into those due to *platelet abnormalities*, and those due primarily to *vascular damage*.

HAEMORRHAGIC DISEASES DUE TO PLATELET ABNORMALITIES

Thrombocytopenia[5]

The main features of the bleeding tendency that is as-

---

*This consists of hyperelasticity of the skin and hyperextensibility of the joints, and is apparently due to a congenital defect of the collagen, which is sparse and thin. The skin is very fragile, and haematoma formation is a conspicuous feature.

sociated with thrombocytopenia is superficial haemorrhage and haemorrhage into mucous membranes. Purpura is characteristic, and there are often multiple, small, superficial ecchymoses, but deeper haematomata are unusual. Mucosal bleeding from the gingivae and nose (epistaxis) is common, as is also haematuria, menorrhagia, and bleeding from the gastrointestinal tract. A serious hazard is intracranial haemorrhage, which is rare in idiopathic thrombocytopenic purpura but not in the severe thrombocytopenia associated with acute leukaemia or bone-marrow aplasia. There may also be retinal haemorrhages.

Persistent, often profuse, bleeding occurs from superficial cuts and scratches, and haemorrhage after trauma and operations is an important feature. Delayed bleeding and spontaneous haemarthrosis are both extremely unusual.

Bleeding is seldom troublesome or purpura profuse until the platelet count drops to 30×10^9 per litre (30 000 per μl). Severe thrombocytopenia is associated with (*a*) a prolonged bleeding time, (*b*) a positive capillary fragility test, and (*c*) poor clot retraction.

Thrombocytopenia may be due to three factors, (*a*) increased platelet destruction, (*b*) increased platelet consumption, and (*c*) a failure of platelet production.

Increased platelet destruction. The most important condition in this group is *idiopathic thrombocytopenic purpura*. It occurs as an acute, self-limiting disease in children from the age of 2 to 6 years, and as a more chronic condition with episodic or even cyclical exacerbations lasting days or weeks, usually in older children and young adults. In the chronic type there is a female preponderance. One interesting variant of acute thrombocytopenia is *onyalai*, which affects young adult Black males in Africa and is associated with haemorrhagic bullae in the mouth and on other mucous surfaces. The acute type of disease in young children often occurs about three weeks after an acute infectious fever, e.g. chickenpox, measles, rubella, and occasionally infectious mononucleosis and cytomegalovirus infection. It tends to resolve within a few weeks in most cases. The chronic condition can persist with partial remissions for many years. It usually runs a benign course, and intracranial haemorrhage is rare.

Apart from the thrombocytopenia, the blood picture is normal unless there has been severe enough bleeding to produce a post-haemorrhagic anaemia. The bone marrow contains an excess of megakaryocytes, which are larger than normal and of abnormal morphology. Young forms predominate.

It is accepted that idiopathic thrombocytopenic purpura is due to an autoantibody of IgG class against platelets. The spleen sequesters the sensitised platelets and then destroys them, as it does in autoimmune haemolytic anaemia. Splenectomy is of value in this condition because of the destructive effect of the spleen on the sensitised platelets, and glucocorticoids may be of use against the autoantibodies.

Thrombocytopenia due to immunological platelet destruction can also occur in the *newborn*, either through the passive transfer of autoantibodies present in the maternal circulation as the result of chronic idiopathic thrombocytopenic purpura, or from the active immunisation of the mother by fetal platelet alloantigens in a way similar to haemolytic disease of the newborn. On the whole, the bleeding manifestations are mild. Other causes of immunological platelet destruction are *systemic lupus erythematosus* with its many autoantibodies, and *drug-induced antibodies*. Selective thrombocytopenia can be produced by almost any drug in therapeutic amounts in immunologically susceptible people; some drugs are especially involved, e.g. quinidine, stibophen, the thiazides, some sulphonamides, digitoxin, and a notorious hypnotic called Sedormid (allylisopropylacetyl carbamide) which was once widely used.

A different mechanism of platelet destruction is seen in conditions of *splenic overactivity (hypersplenism)* described on page 629.

Increased platelet consumption. This occurs in *cardiopulmonary by-pass surgery* and also in *disseminated intravascular coagulation* described on page 643. A noteworthy example of this type of thrombocytopenia is *thrombotic thrombocytopenic purpura*, also called *thrombotic microangiopathy* and *Moschcowitz's syndrome*. It is characterised by haemolytic anaemia, thrombocytopenia, neurological signs, renal failure, and fever. It occurs mostly in young adults, affects many organ systems, and has an acute course and a very high mortality rate. At necropsy the terminal arterioles and capillaries of many organs, especially the heart, brain, kidneys, pancreas, and adrenals are occluded by material in which there is fibrin and entrapped platelets. The aetiology of the condition is not understood, but it may be that there is an obscure damage to the vessel walls and secondary fibrin deposition and thrombosis.

The anaemia is of the microangiopathic haemolytic type, and the platelets are used in the formation of thrombus, as they are in the other two examples mentioned. Their gratuitous consumption on the walls of blood vessels or in the circulation around fragments of blood clot leads to a severe depletion in the peripheral blood.

Failure of platelet production. Good examples of this type of thrombocytopenia are seen in *bone-marrow aplasia*, *acute leukaemia*, *conditions of extensive bone-marrow replacement* (especially in myelofibrosis, multiple myeloma, and secondary carcinoma), and to a considerably milder extent in the *megaloblastic anaemias*.

Other Causes of Thrombocytopenia

Some *viruses* may impair platelet production by invading the megakaryocytes, e.g. live measles vaccine. Others may destroy circulating platelets; this has been reported in rubella and influenza. Most viruses act against platelets by the stimulation of antigen-antibody complexes, as described in acute idiopathic thrombocytopenic purpura. The thrombocytopenia that develops in association with most severe *bacterial infections* is the result of disseminated intravascular coagulation; perhaps damaged vascular surfaces add their quota to the increased platelet consumption.

Drugs act mostly by an immunological mechanism or by suppressing platelet production as part of the marrow aplasia they produce. Chlorothiazide, in addition to stimulating the formation of platelet antibodies, also has a directly suppressive effect on the development of the megakaryocyte. Ristocetin, an antibiotic now no longer used therapeutically, has a directly toxic effect on the platelet.

Other causes of thrombocytopenia are the *administration of massive blood transfusions*, in which the haemorrhage has resulted in the external loss of viable platelets and the blood administered merely replaces them with non-viable platelets (see p. 653) and certain *hereditary conditions*, notably the Wiskott-Aldrich syndrome mentioned on page 171.

Giant haemangiomata in infants are occasionally complicated by thrombocytopenia, which is relieved when the lesion is removed. Probably the lesion sequesters large numbers of platelets; in addition there may be increased consumption of platelets due to local clotting in the abnormal blood vessels, and a microangiopathic haemolytic anaemia may occur.

Thrombocytopathia[2]

In thrombocytopathia there is defective platelet function but a normal platelet count. The following conditions are worthy of note; in some there is also a concomitant thrombocytopenia:

Glanzmann's thrombasthenia. The platelets do not aggregate in the presence of ADP and the clot retraction is deficient; the bleeding time is prolonged. The disease is inherited as an autosomal recessive trait, and it is believed that the defect is in the platelet membrane. There is epistaxis, gingival bleeding, menorrhagia, and sometimes striking generalised ecchymoses. In contrast to most other disorders of platelet function, spontaneous bleeding may be disabling, and post-traumatic and postoperative haemorrhage may be severe.

'*Storage pool disease*'. The response to ADP is normal, but the platelet release reaction is deficient. Its pattern of inheritance is probably as an autosomal dominant trait, and there is mild mucocutaneous bleeding. Petechiae are uncommon, and sometimes the only complaint is one of easy bruising.

Bernard–Soulier syndrome. There is a mild thrombocytopenia as well as severely defective function, the nature of which is not well characterised. There are giant platelets, a prolonged bleeding time, and variable abnormalities in platelet-factor 3 activity. Clinically there is moderate to severe bleeding with purpura, bruising, menorrhagia, and epistaxis. It is inherited as an autosomal recessive trait.

Wiskott–Aldrich syndrome. In addition to marked thrombocytopenia, there is also deficient platelet function: aggregation induced by ADP, adrenaline, and collagen is deficient, and the platelet storage pool of adenine nucleotides is deficient.

Other hereditary disorders that may be associated with deficient platelet function are albinism, glycogen-storage disease, hereditary afibrinogenaemia, the mucopolysaccharidoses, Marfan's syndrome, and the Ehlers-Danlos syndrome.

Acquired disorders of platelet function. Among the more important *drugs* interfering with platelet function are aspirin and indomethacin, which impair the release reaction; they inhibit the production of prostaglandin E_2 by platelets, an effect which may underlie the interference with the release reaction. The aggregation induced by secondary agents (i.e. those apart from ADP), for example adrenaline and collagen, may be abnormal. The bleeding time may sometimes be slightly prolonged, but there is no clinical evidence of bleeding, apart from a mild purpura that is sometimes seen with chronic aspirin ingestion.

In *uraemia* there may be mild thrombocytopenia, but the main defect is one of dysfunction, involving especially the release reaction. The bleeding time is variably prolonged, and platelet-factor 3 activity is usually deficient. A dialysable factor in the plasma appears to be responsible, but its nature is still not known.

The monoclonal gammopathies, especially Waldenström's macroglobulinaemia, are associated with various platelet dysfunctions, such as deficient factor-3 activity, reduced adhesiveness, and poor aggregation, and these may be due to the abnormal protein coating the platelet membrane.

Scurvy may be associated with significant bleeding, and the platelets may show an abnormality in the release reaction.

Thrombocythaemia

In the rare disease *haemorrhagic thrombocythaemia* the platelet count may reach over $10\,000 \times 10^9$ per litre ($10\,000\,000$ per μl), yet there is a severe bleeding tendency marked by gastrointestinal bleeding, and occasionally haematuria, haemoptysis, menorrhagia, and postoperative haemorrhage. The platelets vary in size and show evidence of dysfunction, for example impaired release reaction and impaired liberation of factor 3. There is also a moderate leucocytosis and sometimes a slight polycythaemia, but the bleeding may lead to anaemia. The disease bears some relationship to polycythaemia vera; there is splenomegaly, and furthermore it may be complicated by venous thrombosis despite the tendency to haemorrhagic manifestations.

HAEMORRHAGIC DISEASE DUE TO VASCULAR DAMAGE

This group comprises the non-thrombocytopenic purpuras. The haematological findings are negative. The capillary fragility test is sometimes positive.

'Anaphylactoid' ('allergic') purpura of Henoch-Schönlein[6] This is a disease especially of children, which is characterised clinically by multiform skin lesions such as urticarial weals, bullae, and purpuric spots, and also arthritic pains, severe abdominal colic, and haematuria. The abdominal symptoms are due to extravasations of blood into the bowel wall. This may simulate intussusception clinically, and also precipitate it. The joint pains are due to peri-articular lesions; haemarthrosis is not encountered.

The renal symptoms are due not merely to haemorrhages into the kidney, but are also often a manifestation of acute glomerulonephritis. This is in fact the great danger of the condition, and is the cause of death in the occasional fatal cases. The haemorrhagic manifestations do not jeopardise life on account of blood loss, and there is no tendency towards excessive bleeding after injury or operation.

The characteristic finding in the lesions of this disease is an acute vasculitis involving the arterioles and venules. Immunofluorescent studies have shown variable deposits of IgA, IgG, complement components (especially C3), and fibrin in glomeruli and capillary walls in cutaneous and renal-biopsy specimens. Although the aetiology of Henoch-Schönlein purpura remains unknown, it would seem to be a hypersensitivity reaction (of immune-complex type) to bacteria and viruses.

Scurvy. See page 439.

Infections. Many severe infections are accompanied by purpura, e.g. haemorrhagic smallpox, viral haemorrhagic fevers, scarlet fever, chickenpox, measles, diphtheria, and typhus. Direct endothelial damage by the organism or its toxins is the probable explanation, as there is seldom a marked thrombocytopenia in these conditions. Another possibility is the defibrination syndrome, which may occur in fulminating infections, causing both infarction and diffuse haemorrhage.[7] This is the most likely explanation of the *Waterhouse–Friderichsen syndrome* that characteristically complicates meningococcal septicaemia ('spotted fever') and more rarely staphylococcal, *Esch. coli*, and *H. influenzae* septicaemias. The massive adrenal haemorrhage is probably a haemorrhagic infarct.

In some infections bacterial embolism may play a part in the purpuric eruption, e.g. subacute infective endocarditis with its splinter haemorrhages into the nail-beds and typhoid fever with its rose spots on the abdomen.

Drugs and chemical agents. These include iodides, belladonna, quinine, aspirin, phenacetin, sulphonamides, and procaine penicillin. Viperine snake venom produces petechial haemorrhages into many organs as the result of the diffuse vascular damage it produces.

Macroglobulinaemia. The bleeding in this condition has not been adequately explained. Vascular damage secondary to an infiltration of the wall by the abnormal protein is one possible factor. Interference by the protein with platelet function (see p. 640) and with the clotting mechanism may occur. Hyperviscosity of the plasma (p. 580) and precipitates of cryoglobulin are other mechanisms.

Hereditary Haemorrhagic Telangiectasia

Although this is not a purpuric condition, it merits consideration because it leads to severe haemorrhages from many areas of the body. The disease is essentially a malformation of the capillaries and venules, which has the characteristics of a generalised hamartomatous dysplasia. The telangiectases, which consist of dilated capillaries and defective venules, usually appear in adult life, though the defect is no doubt already present in childhood. There is recurrent bleeding from the nose, mouth, and stomach, and also from damaged telangiectases in the skin. There are no conspicuous haematological findings. Capillary fragility is usually normal, though a few cases are on record in which the tourniquet test was positive. The disease is inherited as an autosomal dominant characteristic; in some individuals the manifestations are so mild that they are missed until carefully sought. Pulmonary arteriovenous fistulae and aneurysms of the splenic artery have been described in association with this condition, thereby stressing once again the generalised nature of the angiomatous malformation (see Ch. 27).

HAEMORRHAGIC DISEASE DUE TO DEFECTS IN THE CLOTTING MECHANISM

The pattern of haemorrhage from disorders of clotting, especially the hereditary ones, differs from that encountered in thrombocytopenia. Petechial haemorrhages are rare, and although there may be superficial ecchymoses, these tend to be large and solitary. Deep haematomata which dissect the tissues are characteristic. Haemarthrosis is common in the hereditary clotting disorders that produce severe bleeding. Although superficial bleeding from cuts and scratches is minimal, delayed bleeding following trauma is very common, and the haemorrhage may persist for days, weeks, or even months.

Hereditary Clotting Disorders

With the exception of fibrinogen and prothrombin, the clotting factors are trace proteins, and as such have been difficult to study by chemical methods. It used to be assumed that the hereditary clotting disorders were the result of a quantitative deficiency of trace plasma proteins. However, the use of immunological techniques has established that the absence of clotting activity in many patients with these disorders may result from either *deficient biosynthesis* of a requisite protein, or else *defective biosynthesis*, leading to the production of normal amounts of functionally inactive or functionally abnormal analogues. Thus most cases of haemophilia are due to defective biosynthesis of Factor VIII leading to a functionally inactive form; this applies also to Christmas disease, except that here there may also be a functionally abnormal form of Factor IX produced as well as an inactive one.

Haemophilia (haemophilia A). This is by far the most common of the hereditary clotting disorders, and is the classical example of a disease inherited as a sex-linked recessive characteristic; the affected males exhibit the disease while the females merely transmit it to the next generation. It can rarely affect a female if she is the offspring of an affected father and a mother who carries the trait, and the disease is no more severe than in the male subject. There is a quantitative deficiency or qualitative defect in the production of Factor VIII which can be of all grades of severity, from mild (when the active level of the factor is from 5 to 25 per cent of normal) to very severe (when the level is less than 2 per cent).

The features of haemophilic bleeding have already been described. Noteworthy findings are bleeding from the mucous membranes (leading to epistaxis, gastrointestinal haemorrhage, and haematuria) and into the tissues (producing large retroperitoneal, intrapsoas, and sometimes intracranial haematomata), severe, somewhat delayed, bleeding after trauma and operation (from the deeper vessels), and *recurrent haemarthrosis*, which often appears to be spontaneous or else to follow a negligible injury. The joint is progressively destroyed by the chronic inflammation induced by the residual blood clot, the cavity is obliterated by fibrous adhesions or bony ankylosis, and the adjacent bone shows severe destructive changes.

The blood picture is normal apart from the clotting defect (there may be post-haemorrhagic anaemia). The tests that are specifically abnormal are the clotting time, partial thromboplastin time, and the thromboplastin generation test. Of these, the clotting time is the least valuable, as it tends to be normal except in severe cases. The partial thromboplastin time is variable in mild cases, but prolonged in moderate and severe ones. A positive thromboplastin generation test with a normal prothrombin time is virtually diagnostic of haemophilia in a patient with a hereditary disorder.

Christmas disease (haemophilia B). This hereditary clotting defect is clinically indistinguishable from haemophilia, except that severe cases (with factor levels of less than 2 per cent of normal) are less common. Its mode of inheritance is also as a sex-linked recessive characteristic. As in haemophilia there is more often a qualitative defect than a quantitative deficiency in the production of the clotting factor, which is Factor IX. The thromboplastin generation test distinguishes Christmas disease from haemophilia.

von Willibrand's disease.[8,9] This is probably the second most common of the hereditary clotting disorders, and bears a close relationship to haemophilia. There is a mild to moderate deficiency in Factor VIII but in addition a prolonged bleeding time, which is exceptional in a pure clotting disorder. It is now recognised that Factor VIII may exist *in vivo* as a complex of at least two related proteins. Three functionally distinct components have been recognised as part of the Factor VIII system: (*a*) a clot-promoting activity that corrects the clotting abnormality of plasma from a haemophiliac patient, (*b*) an antigen that can be detected by immunological techniques, which is decreased in the plasma of patients with von Willebrand's disease but is normal in haemophilia, and (*c*) von Willebrand factor that corrects a platelet-function defect in von Willebrand's disease. There are two *in-vitro* defects in platelet function in this condition: they are not retained normally in glass-bead columns, and they do not aggregate in the presence of the antibiotic ristocetin (as do normal platelets). It has been shown that this defective function is not due to thrombocytopathia but to the deficiency of a humoral factor, which is in fact the von Willebrand factor.

In the classical, severe von Willebrand's disease all three functional components of the Factor-VIII system, which is synthesised by the vascular endothelial cells, are proportionally decreased, but there are variants in which the von Willebrand factor is discordantly reduced as compared with the other two. A qualitatively abnormal Factor VIII antigen may also be produced.

The disease was first described by von Willebrand in a family living in the Åland Islands (in the Baltic Sea). It is inherited as an incompletely dominant autosomal characteristic. It is evident therefore that the Factor VIII complex consists of a combination of autosomally determined antigen and the clotting factor situated on the X chromosome. Presumably the von Willebrand factor is also autosomally determined.

Clinically the disease has the features of a combined platelet and clotting-factor defect. Thus mucosal bleeding from the nose, gastrointestinal tract, and genito-urinary system (especially menorrhagia) is considerably more common than in haemophilia, and cutaneous bleeding is frequent, although petechiae are rare. But in severe cases there may also be dissecting intramuscular haematomata and haemarthroses. Post-traumatic and postoperative bleeding is an important feature.

In von Willebrand's disease the infusion of normal plasma usually produces a gradual and sustained rise in the level of Factor VIII in the recipient. Plasma devoid of Factor VIII, and even serum, produce comparable results, therefore the effect cannot be attributed to the Factor VIII present in the plasma. By contrast, in haemophilia such an infusion of normal plasma produces a maximal immediate effect with a rapid diminution of activity consistent with the short *in-vivo* survival time of Factor VIII. Apparently the antigen is a precursor of Factor-VIII synthesis. Whereas haemophilic serum produces an alleviation in von Willebrand's disease, the phenomenon is not reciprocal; the infusion of plasma from a case of von Willebrand's disease into a haemophiliac produces no new synthesis of Factor VIII.

Other hereditary clotting disorders. These are all rare. *Factor XI and Factor XII deficiencies* are both inherited as autosomal recessive characteristics, but whereas that of Factor XI produces definite, but comparatively mild, bleeding symptoms, Factor XII deficiency is nearly always symptomless. Both *Factor V and Factor VII* deficiency are inherited as autosomal recessive characteristics, and can be associated in some cases with severe haemorrhage; since Factor VII is concerned only in the extrinsic system of clotting, it is apparent that this system is extremely important in haemostasis. The manifestations of *Factor X deficiency* resemble those of Factor VII deficiency, and it is inherited in the same way.

Hereditary prothrombin deficiency is extremely rare, and is inherited as an autosomal dominant characteristic; the bleeding diathesis is usually mild.

Hereditary afibrinogenaemia is inherited as an autosomal recessive characteristic. The blood is incoagulable, and there are severe bleeding manifestations present from birth. Nevertheless the patients survive well, haemarthrosis is uncommon, and the menses are often normal. The condition causes less disability than does haemophilia. In the less severe *hereditary, or constitutional, hypofibrinogenaemia,* inherited either as an autosomal dominant or recessive characteristic, bleeding is infrequent and rarely severe. In *hereditary dysfibrinogenaemia,* inherited as an autosomal dominant characteristic, various qualitatively abnormal fibrinogens are produced. The condition may be symptomless or associated with mild bleeding.

Factor XIII deficiency is often associated with a serious bleeding tendency which may first show itself in the newborn when the umbilical cord separates. Ecchymoses, haematomata, post-traumatic and postoperative bleeding, and haemorrhage into the central nervous system may all occur; indeed intracranial bleeding, which is often fatal, is commoner in this condition than in any of the other hereditary clotting disorders. It is inherited as an autosomal recessive characteristic. All the usual clotting tests are normal in Factor XIII deficiency, but the condition can be diagnosed by clot solubility tests; normal clots are insoluble in 5 M urea or 1 per cent monochloracetic acid.

An interesting feature seen in both hereditary fibrinogen deficiency and Factor XIII deficiency is delayed wound healing and a tendency to wound dehiscence after operations. This does not appear to complicate the other clotting disorders, and it has been suggested that a deficiency of fibrinogen or Factor XIII may result in abnormal or deficient fibroblastic proliferation.

Treatment of hereditary clotting disorders. This is essentially replacement therapy. For most of the disorders stored plasma is adequate, but for Factor V deficiency the plasma must be fresh or fresh frozen. For haemophilia plasma cryoprecipitates, freeze-dried concentrates of Factor VIII, or in an emergency fresh or fresh-frozen plasma are used. For von Willebrand's disease cryoprecipitate seems to be the best replacement, or else fresh or fresh-frozen plasma. Purified fibrinogen or cryoprecipitate are best in fibrinogen deficiencies. See also page 650.

Acquired Clotting Disorders

Hypoprothrombinaemia. The basis of acquired hypoprothrombinaemia is a deficiency of vitamin K, which is necessary for the hepatic synthesis not only of prothrombin but also of Factors VII, IX, and X. It therefore follows that the term hypoprothrombinaemia embraces an acquired deficiency of all four clotting factors. The prothrombin time is always prolonged and so also is the partial thromboplastin time. The clotting time is usually normal except in haemorrhagic disease of the newborn.

Vitamin-K deficiency is only occasionally due to nutritional deficiency[10] because the vitamin is derived both from the diet and the synthetic activity of the intestinal bacterial flora.

Malabsorption is an important cause, because the vitamin is fat soluble, and therefore depends on the pancreatic lipase as well as the bile salts for its absorption from the gut. *Obstructive jaundice* is an extremely important surgical cause of hypoprothrombinaemia.

Liver disease leads to hypoprothrombinaemia since the associated clotting factors are synthesised in that organ. However, hypoprothrombinaemia is only one aspect of a much more severe bleeding diathesis associated with hepatic failure. Every clotting factor, apart from Factor VIII, is synthesised there. Fibrinolysis is also an important cause of bleeding in liver disease (see below).

Haemorrhagic disease of the newborn[11] is a hypoprothrombinaemia that usually shows itself on the second or third day of life. It is more frequent in premature infants. Even in normal newborn infants there is a moderate deficiency of vitamin K-dependent clotting factors, which persists for about a week before a rise occurs; normal adult levels are attained by about three months. This deficiency is attributed to hepatic immaturity, and it is not influenced by vitamin K therapy. The secondary deficiency that is associated with haemorrhagic disease of the newborn is corrected by vitamin K, and has been attributed to inadequate dietary intake, maternal deficiency of vitamin K, and delayed colonisation of the gut by bacteria. The bleeding is severe and often fatal unless treated at once; there is melaena, bleeding from the umbilical stump, cephalhaematomata, ecchymoses, intramuscular haemorrhages, and intracranial bleeding.

Anticoagulants of the coumarin and indanedione groups antagonise the action of vitamin K and produce an identical clotting abnormality.

Hypofibrinogenaemia

Acquired hypofibrinogenaemia may be seen in severe liver failure as a result of impaired synthesis of fibrinogen, but the most important and dramatic type of acquired fibrinogen deficiency occurs in the **defibrination syndrome**. This occurs under two circumstances:

The fibrinolytic syndrome, also called *fibrinogenolysis*.

Disseminated intravascular coagulation, also called *consumptive coagulopathy*.

The fibrinolytic syndrome. Activation of the plasmin system can occur when large amounts of tissue activator are released into the blood stream, for example during major operations especially those involving the lungs and heart, in obstetrical accidents such as abruptio placentae, and in certain tumours, particularly carcinoma of the prostate and acute leukaemia. It also occurs in *liver disease* and congenital heart disease. The plasmin which is formed can be detected in the blood; it digests fibrinogen as well as other clotting factors, and the blood eventually becomes incoagulable. Fibrin de-

gradation products can be detected in the blood, and are of importance because they are inhibitors of thrombin (the thrombin time is increased), they interfere with the polymerisation of fibrin, and they impair platelet aggregation. *The platelet count remains normal.* Bleeding, e.g. from an operation site, is the salient clinical feature. Treatment consists of eliminating the cause, replacing clotting factors, and administering a fibrinolytic inhibitor such as epsilon-aminocaproic acid.

Disseminated intravascular coagulation. This condition occurs under two circumstances which may be found separately or in combination:

(*a*) The release of clotting factors into the blood stream.

(*b*) Extensive endothelial damage.

The result is the formation of fibrin in the circulation and this produces vascular obstruction and micro-infarction. In addition, the extensive intravascular coagulation consumes the coagulation factors so that *afibrinoginaemia and thrombocytopenia* are characteristic features. Moreover, the formation of fibrin leads to the activation of the fibrinolytic system; while this is beneficial in that it removes some of the obstructing fibrin, it also has the detrimental effect of causing further degradation of the clotting factors and the formation of anticoagulant fibrinogen breakdown products, as noted in the fibrinolytic syndrome. Thus the two effects of consumptive coagulopathy are a severe bleeding tendency and a tendency to infarction, primarily microscopic in extent but becoming larger when fibrinolysis is inadequate. The syndrome of disseminated intravascular coagulation is seen under many circumstances:

(*a*) In abruptio placentae with amniotic-fluid embolism, when placental material enters the circulation.

(*b*) Intrauterine retention of a dead fetus.

(*c*) In incompatible blood transfusion reactions.

(*d*) After severe trauma, fat embolism, open-heart surgery with an extracorporeal circulation, and extensive lung operations.

(*e*) In the newborn after abruptio placentae, birth asphyxia, hypothermia, and Rhesus immunisation. It must be differentiated from Vitamin K deficiency by the tests mentioned below.

(*f*) Severe infections. This has been discussed on page 419; the Waterhouse-Friderichsen syndrome is probably caused in this way. So also is the generalised Shwartzman reaction described on page 417. In the Shwartzman reaction it would seem that the first dose of endotoxin initiates clotting, but the RE cells are able to clear the endotoxin complexes and clotting intermediates. The second dose likewise initiates clotting, but the complexes cannot be removed by a blocked RE system.

(*g*) Purpura fulminans,[12] a rare bleeding disease with extensive infarction particularly of the skin occurring usually about a week after an acute streptococcal infection. It may represent an antigen-antibody reaction in the blood. It resembles the localised Shwartzman reaction in histology.

(*h*) Metastatic cancer, usually of the prostate, and occasionally of the lung, pancreas, and stomach. This is a rare complication of disseminated cancer.

(*i*) Acute leukaemia, especially the promyelocytic variety.

(*j*) Certain vascular disorders, e.g. giant haemangiomata, aneurysms of the aorta and other large vessels, and cyanotic congenital heart disease. It may be that hypoperfusion of local vascular beds is important in producing this syndrome in the first two conditions. The hypoxia of congenital heart disease may have the same effect, but its association is obscure.

Clinically there is bleeding, ecchymosis, and haemorrhage from the body's orifices. In addition to the severe hypofibrinogenaemia with increased fibrin breakdown products there is a fall in the level of Factors V and VIII due to the large amount of thrombin formed (see p. 635). A thrombocytopenia is also characteristic. There may also be a mild haemolytic anaemia (see p. 614). The condition is an emergency and is treated with transfusions of fresh blood or fibrinogen. Heparin should be administered to prevent further intravascular clotting. The fibrinolysin inhibitor ε-aminocaproic acid can be given at the same time as the heparin.

Therapeutic defibrination. From the venom of the Malayan pit viper a purified coagulant fraction called *ancrod* has been prepared. By converting fibrinogen into a fibrin-like substance it leads to defibrination and incoagulability of the blood. Its use as a therapeutic anticoagulant has been encouraging, but it does not seem to have any notable advantages over heparin.

Circulating Anticoagulants

Pathological circulating anticoagulants prevent the formation of prothrombinase, but seldom interfere with its action on prothrombin. The most important inhibitors of clotting are antibodies to various clotting factors; those against Factor VIII are the most common and produce the most severe bleeding. They may arise in haemophiliacs who are under treatment, but sometimes they are found in association with various unrelated conditions, such as rheumatoid arthritis, systemic lupus erythematosus, ulcerative colitis, and sometimes in the absence of apparent underlying disease, as in the elderly or after a pregnancy. The bleeding diathesis resembles that of haemophilia. A unique type of inhibitor is found in systemic lupus erythematosus; it is an immunoglobulin, but does not appear to be an antibody. It seems to act specifically against prothrombinase.

CONCLUSIONS

It is clear that an abnormal bleeding tendency may be due to a bewilderingly large variety of conditions. Nevertheless, certain clinical observations can assist in the elucidation of the nature of the disorder.

1. The commonest cause of regional haemorrhage is local vascular disease. Severe postoperative bleeding is much more likely to be due to badly-ligated blood vessels or secondary infection than to any of the generalised bleeding disorders. Similarly, recurrent epistaxis is usually due to a vascular abnormality in the nose, and haematuria is usually a symptom of a lesion in the urinary tract.

2. Severe postoperative bleeding may be due to a deficiency in the platelets (either quantitative or qualitative) or to an impairment of the clotting mechanism, but is not caused by generalised vascular damage acting on its own.

3. Purpura is typical of conditions of generalised vascular damage and platelet inadequacy, but is uncommon in the clotting disorders.

4. Recurrent haemarthrosis is very suggestive of Factor VIII or IX deficiency. It is not a feature of the platelet and vascular disorders.

5. A family history should always be carefully elicited. Many of the clotting diseases and also hereditary haemorrhagic telangiectasia have a strongly familial tendency.

REFERENCES

1. MARCUS, A. J. (1969) Platelet function. *New England Journal of Medicine*, **280**, 1213, 1278, and 1330.
2. WEISS, H. J. (1975) Platelets: physiology and abnormalities of function. *New England Journal of Medicine*, **293**, 531 and 580.
3. MUSTARD, J. F. & PACKHAM, M. A. (1970) Platelet aggregation and the platelet release reaction in thromboembolism. *Canadian Medical Association Journal*, **103**, 859.
4. MCKUSICK, V. A. (1972) *Heritable Disorders of Connective Tissue*, 4th edn., p. 292. St. Louis: Mosby.
5. BARKHAN, P. (1974) Thrombocytopenia. *British Medical Journal*, **2**, 324 and 376.
6. Leading Article (1977) Henoch–Schönlein purpura. *British Medical Journal*, **1**, 190.
7. CRONBERG, S. & NILSSON, I. M. (1970) Pneumococcal sepsis with generalised Shwartzman reaction. *Acta medica scandinavica*, **188**, 293.
8. Leading Article (1976) Von Willebrand's disease. *British Medical Journal*, **2**, 715.
9. NACHMAN, R. L. (1977) Von Willebrand's disease and the molecular pathology of hemostasis. *New England Journal of Medicine*, **296**, 1059.
10. COLVIN, B. T. & LLOYD, M. J. (1977) Severe coagulation defect due to a dietary deficiency of vitamin K. *Journal of Clinical Pathology*, **30**, 1147.
11. Leading Article (1978) Vitamin K and the newborn. *Lancet*, **1**, 755.
12. ANTLEY, R. M. & MCMILLAN, C. W. (1967) Sequential coagulation studies in purpura fulminans. *New England Journal of Medicine*, **276**, 1287.

Chapter 55. *Blood Grouping and Blood Transfusion*

Attempts to transfuse blood from one individual to another, both in animals and humans, were made from the fifteenth century onwards. One of the early experimenters was Dr C. Wren, who is better known for creating the famous landmark in the City of London than for his work on blood transfusion. It was fortunate that the clotting of blood frustrated many of these early attempts.

The human red cell is a veritable mosaic of blood-group antigens. With the major exception of the ABO and Rhesus antigens these are weak, and when once methods were devised for matching individuals with respect to the ABO and Rhesus groups, blood transfusion became a practical and useful procedure. Antibodies are produced against leucocytes and platelets, but these are rarely a cause of serious trouble. The term 'blood groups' is applied to the genetically determined antigens which can be detected on the red-cell surface by specific antibodies.

With the exception of one X-linked system (Xg), the locus for each blood group system is situated on an autosome. For example, the *Rhesus* locus is on chromosome number 1; the *ABO* locus is on chromosome number 9. It is unfortunate that the notation used to describe the blood-group genes and antigens has evolved haphazardly.

Blood-group notation. Three types of notation are used:
1. Alleles may be designated by capital letters, e.g. *A* and *B*, *M* and *N*.
2. Alleles may be designated by capital and lower-case letters, e.g. *S* and *s*, *C* and *c*. The use of the lower case does not imply that the trait is recessive.
3. Alleles may be designated by a symbol (sometimes derived from the name of the person in whom the antibody was first detected) with superscript, e.g. Lu^a and Lu^b, Fy^a and Fy^b,

Blood-Group Systems

The ABO system is by far the most important in clinical medicine because the associated antibodies occur naturally. The Rhesus system is the next most important because of the danger of anti-Rh being formed following the introduction of Rh-positive cells into Rh-negative persons. Other well-defined systems are MNSs, P, Lutheran (Lu), Kell, Lewis (Le), Duffy (Fy), Kidd (Jk), Diego (Di), Dombrock (Do), Colton (Co), and Xg. Many other red-cell antigens are known, and more no doubt remain to be discovered. Some, such as Chido and Rodgers,* are present in almost all individuals, while others are restricted to a few individuals (*private antigens*).

*It has been shown that Chido and Rodgers blood groups are antigenic components of human complement C4. It therefore follows that C4-deficient patients lack the Chido and Rodgers antigens.

Blood-Group Antibodies

Antibodies to blood-group antigens not possessed by the individual are termed *alloantibodies*. They are capable of reacting with the red cells of people of a different blood group, but do not react with the individual's own red cells.

In the ABO system, *naturally-occurring antibodies* are almost always present, and may also be accompanied by other naturally-occurring antibodies, e.g. anti-P_1. They are predominantly IgM, and react more strongly at lower temperatures than at 37°C.

Naturally-occurring antibodies are generally capable of agglutinating red cells in saline suspension, and for this reason have been called *complete antibodies*, or direct agglutinins. Antibodies which are formed as a result of a known antigenic stimulus, e.g. pregnancy, blood transfusion, or the injection of red-cell antigens, are called *immune antibodies*. They are generally IgG, most active at 37°C, and often fail to agglutinate red cells in saline suspension. In contrast to the naturally-occurring antibodies they are therefore called *incomplete antibodies*.

Relationship between Blood Groups and Susceptibility to Disease

There is statistical evidence that cancer of the stomach is more common in group-A subjects than in the general population, and that duodenal ulceration is likewise commoner in people of group O. Pernicious anaemia is also found most frequently in group-A people. Secretor status has also been related to disease: non-secretors are more liable to duodenal ulceration and acute rheumatic fever than are secretors. The significance of these findings is not understood.

The Duffy blood-group system has recently attracted interest because of its relationship to malaria. The majority (about 70 per cent) of Black Americans are naturally resistant to *Plasmodium vivax* infection, and are Duffy negative [Fy(a−b−)]. In contrast, White Americans are susceptible to infection; the phenotype Fy(a−b−) is extremely rare in White populations. Experimental work has shown that *Plasmodium knowlesi*, which has much in common with *Plasmodium vivax*, can enter red cells that carry either Fy^a or Fy^b antigens, but it cannot enter cells lacking both antigens. Whether these Duffy antigens act as receptors for the parasite or whether some closely related gene product is involved is not known.

THE ABO AND RELATED BLOOD GROUPS

The ABO blood groups are determined by genes which govern the presence of antigens on the cells, in particular the red cells. There are four major ABO blood groups, as Table 55.1 shows.

Table 55.1

Genotype	Phenotype (blood group)	Antibody normally present in serum
AA or *AO*	A	anti-B
BB or *BO*	B	anti-A
AB	AB	none
OO	O	anti-A and anti-B

The serum of each person generally contains antibodies to those antigens which he does not possess. The prefix *iso-* has been used previously in connexion with these antibodies. Unfortunately *iso-* and *syn-* are now used in transplantation immunology to indicate genetic identity. Individuals of a species who differ genetically are called allogeneic, therefore antibodies formed by one individual against antigens possessed by another should be called alloantibodies, alloagglutinins, etc. This terminology has now been adopted by Mollison. Alloantibodies must be distinguished from *autoantibodies*, which are capable of reacting with the individual's own red cells (see Ch. 52).

The anti-A and anti-B antibodies are naturally occurring. Those present in an infant at birth are passively acquired from the mother. The child begins to develop his own antibodies at the age of 3 to 6 months. It is unknown how such antibodies can develop in the absence of the appropriate antigenic stimulus. It may be that these agglutinins develop as a response to substances which are antigenically similar to the human blood-group substances, and which are inhaled or ingested. Such antigens are widely distributed in nature, being present in animal tissues, e.g. horse serum, and in bacteria.* It has been noted that chicks reared in a germ-free environment do not develop heteroagglutinins against human B cells, such as are found in chicks reared normally. This might be related to the finding that many Gram-negative bacteria have high concentrations of blood-group specific substances. If this is the correct explanation, the term 'naturally-occurring antibody' is a misnomer, since the antibody is specifically stimulated. Nevertheless, the matter is by no means settled, and it is convenient to retain the term.

Subgroups of group A. About 80 per cent of the White population of group A or AB belong to the subgroup A_1 or A_1B, and there is a specific antibody (anti-A_1) which reacts with these cells. The remaining 20 per cent of group A and AB individuals belong to the subgroups A_2 or A_2B. The difference between A_1 and A_2 red cells is related to the number of A antigenic sites on the cell membrane. Thus, an A_1 red cell has approximately 10^6 sites, whereas an A_2 cell has about 250 000. Hence only a potent anti-A serum will agglutinate both A_1 and A_2 cells, whereas a weaker serum (anti-A_1)

will agglutinate A_1 but not A_2 cells. There is no specific anti-A_2 serum.

The importance of this subgrouping is that A_2 cells, and particularly A_2B cells, sometimes react weakly with an anti-A serum and are therefore mislabelled as group O or group B respectively. The serum of an A_2 or an A_2B subject often contains anti-A_1. An A_1B or an A_1 individual's serum may contain anti-H, which agglutinates O and A_2 cells.

Nature of the ABO blood-group substances. Ovarian-cyst fluid has provided a rich source of human ABH and Lewis blood-group substances for chemical analysis. The soluble ABH and Lewis antigens are glycoproteins which consist of a protein backbone with many short polysaccharide side-chains; the composition of the side-chains determines specificity.

A glycoprotein precursor substance is converted into H substance under the influence of the *H* gene. Nearly all individuals are of genotype *HH* or *Hh*,* and their red cells contain H substance. The *ABO* genes are at a different locus, and by their presence some H substance is converted into A or B substance. *O* is an amorph and leaves H unchanged. Each step in the sequence: precursor glycoprotein→H substance→A or B substance, involves the addition of a single sugar, e.g. N-acetylgalactosamine for A specificity and D-galactose for B specificity. Likewise, the production of the Lewis antigens involves the addition of a sugar unit. Since each of these steps is determined genetically, it is evident that the red-cell antigens are not the direct gene products. Each gene gives rise to a specific glycosyltransferase; these enzymes are present in the plasma and secretions.

The ABO group of the red cells is thus determined by the presence of an immunodominant sugar (e.g. D-galactose for B) carried by glycoproteins and glycolipids on the cell membrane. These blood-group antigens are also present on the membranes of all vascular endothelial cells and some epithelial cells. Hence the importance of ABO matching with renal and other allografts (p. 196).

Secretor status. About 80 per cent of the population possess the secretor gene *Se* (genotype *SeSe* or *Sese*), and are able to form water-soluble glycoproteins which have the antigenic specificity of H substance (as well as that of A and B, if the *A* and *B* genes are also present). Such people are called 'secretors', and have H (and A and B) antigens in their secretions such as saliva and gastric juice. 'Non-secretors', who lack the *Se* gene (genotype *sese*), do in fact secrete a glycoprotein, but it has no H, A, or B activity. Le^a is secreted if the Lewis gene *Le* is present (see below). The classification of secretor status ignores the presence of Lewis substances and of non-specific glycoprotein; only ABH antigens are considered. See Table 55.2.

The Lewis antigens. The two Lewis antigens are known, Le^a and Le^b, together with the corresponding antibodies anti-Le^a and anti-Le^b. The antigens are found primarily in the body fluids such as plasma and saliva, and are taken up from the plasma on to red

---

*It is interesting to note that agglutinins are found in extracts of the seeds of certain plants, e.g. Lima beans. These agglutinins are called *lectins*. One of them is useful in being highly specific for A_1 cells. Antibodies to blood-group antigens are found in high concentration in certain animal tissues. For example, a few snail eggs can provide enough anti-A to type blood donors in a city the size of Bristol! Since most bacteria contain A substance, it has been suggested that these antibodies have a protective role—hence they are called *protectins*. Salmon eggs contain anti-B.

---

h (like *O* and *le*) is an amorph, i.e. a gene which has no detectable product. The cells of an individual of genotype *hh* therefore do not contain H, A, or B antigen. The serum contains anti-H, anti-A, and anti-B. This very rare condition was first described in two people in Bombay, and is therefore called the 'Bombay', or Oh, phenotype.

TABLE 55.2 ABH antigens in secretors and non-secretors

ABO group	Antigens of secretors Red cells	Secretions	Antigens of non-secretors Red cells	Secretions
O	H	H	H	—
A	A	A and H	A	—
B	B	B and H	B	—
AB	A and B	A, B, and H	A and B	—

cells and white cells. The formation of the Lewis antigens is dependent upon the presence of a single gene *Le* (genotype *LeLe* or *Lele*) sometimes acting in conjunction with the *Se* gene(see above).

The *Le* gene acting alone leads to the formation of Le^a antigen, found in the plasma, saliva, and on the red cells, which are therefore of phenotype Le(a+b−). *Such people never secrete A, B, or H substances in their saliva.* The *Le* gene in conjunction with the secretor gene (genotype *SeSe* or *Sese*) leads to the formation of Le^b in plasma and thus to the red-cell phenotype Le(a−b+). Such a person secretes Le^b, and also some Le^a and H substance. If the *A* and *B* genes are present there is also A and B substance in the saliva of Le(a−b+) persons. The gene *le* is an amorph, and individuals of the genotype *lele* form no Lewis antigen, and their red cells are of group Le(a−b−). They secrete H (and A and B) if the *Se* gene (with the *A* and *B* genes) is present.

Immune anti-A and anti-B. If a patient is transfused with blood of an incompatible A or B group, a high titre of *immune anti-A or anti-B* will develop. This antibody is normally present only in traces, but its titre rises after an incompatible transfusion or after the injection of A or B substance obtained from the tissues of certain animals, e.g. pigs. Preparations of diphtheria and tetanus toxoid are particularly liable to stimulate these antibodies, apparently because the medium on which the organisms are grown contains peptone derived from hog's stomach, which is very rich in these substances. Immune anti-A and anti-B are stronger agglutinins at 37°C than are their naturally-occurring counterparts, and furthermore haemolyse red cells in the presence of complement. It therefore follows that grouping sera are always heated to inactivate complement before being issued by blood transfusion centres, because haemolysis is less easy to interpret than agglutination.

Some of these immune antibodies are IgM, but others are IgG and IgA. The IgG antibodies traverse the placenta (see p. 614) and can cause a neonatal haemolytic anaemia, but usually only when the mother is group O and the fetus group A. Unlike Rh-haemolytic disease, ABO-disease commonly affects the firstborn, some of whose group A cells have entered the mother's circulation during pregnancy and acted as a booster to the already present maternal anti-A antibody. Although 1 in 5 A (or B) infants born to group O mothers show some signs of a mild haemolytic process, only rarely is the anaemia severe enough to require treatment.

THE RHESUS (Rh) SYSTEM

If the red-cells of *Rhesus* monkeys are injected into other animals, an anti-Rhesus serum is produced which will agglutinate the red cells of about 85 per cent of white-skinned people.* These cells are designated Rh-positive. Subsequent investigations have shown that the gene involved in the Rhesus groups is complex and is responsible for the formation of several different antigens, one of which (D or Rh$_o$) is the antigen present in Rhesus-positive cells. There are two main theories concerning the nature of the Rhesus groups, and these have led to two separate systems of nomenclature.

The *linked gene theory* of Fisher and Race supposes that there are three very closely linked loci occupied by the genes *C*, *D*, and *E* or their alleles *c*, *d*, and *e*. These genes give rise to the red-cell antigens C, D, E, c, and e. There is no d antigen, but it is convenient to use the symbol *d* in writing Rh genotypes. Each person inherits one trio of genes from each parent. Thus an individual of the genotype *CDe/cdE* inherited *CDe* from one parent and *cdE* from the other. The antigens C, c, D, E, and e are present on the red cells. Since the genes are very close together (i.e. they are linked), crossing over almost never occurs. The Fisher–Race nomenclature has the asset of simplicity. Cells containing D are termed Rhesus (Rh) positive, and those which lack it Rh negative. In practice D-negative donors are also tested with anti-C and anti-E, and donations from *Cde/cde* or *cdE/cde* subjects are identified accordingly.

The Rhesus antigens are more complex than the above account would suggest. There are other alleles as well, e.g. four of C (C^w, C^v, C^u, and C^x), one of D (D^u), and two of E (E^u and E^w), and these are associated with corresponding antigens. Furthermore, genes in combination on one chromosome (e.g. *Cde*) sometimes produce a compound antigen (e.g. Ce). The antibody to this antigen (anti-Ce) reacts with a sample of *Cde/cDE* cells but not *CDE/cde* cells.

The second theory is that of Wiener, and it supposes that there is a single locus which can be occupied by any of a large number of alleles. This *multiple allele theory* supposes that a single gene can give rise to several antigens of different specificities. In the Wiener classification the common antigens are called rh′ (C), hr′ (c), rh″ (E), hr″ (e), and Rh$_o$ (D). In brackets are the corresponding antigens of the Fisher–Race nomenclature. Table 55.3 shows a comparison of Rh gene nomenclature according to the two theories. Thus the allele R^1 gives rise to the antigens Rh$_o$, rh′, and hr″; these correspond to D, C, and e. The Wiener theory is more difficult to learn and work with, but its main assertion, that the Rh antigens are determined by

*This discovery was made in 1940 by Landsteiner and Wiener, but the antibodies they discovered are now known to be distinct from, though closely related to, those now called Rhesus antibodies. The *LW* gene (named after the discoverers) leads to the production of the LW antigen. This reacts with true anti-Rhesus antibody—i.e. serum from a guinea-pig immunised against *Rhesus*-monkey red cells. Both LW and Rhesus antigens are probably derived from a common substrate under the influence of the *LW* and *Rh* genes.

TABLE 55.3 The common Rh genes

Wiener notation	Fisher–Race notation
R^1	CDe
r	cde
R^2	cDE
R^0	cDe
r''	cdE
r'	Cde
R^z	CDE
r^y	CdE

Table showing the Rhesus genes arranged in descending order of frequency. The first column shows the symbols for the genes based on the notation of Wiener. The corresponding genes of the *CDE* notation are shown in the second column. It should be noted that the capital *R* always indicates the presence of the gene responsible for the antigen D; *r* implies its absence. The most common genotypes in a Caucasian population are *CDe/cde*, *CDe/CDe*, and *cde/cde*. There is some evidence that the actual order of the genes is *DCE* rather than *CDE*.

a series of alleles at a single locus, is probably correct. Nevertheless, the simple Fisher–Race nomenclature is commonly used and is adequate for most purposes. It has the great advantage of being the only notation readily useful for communicating information between workers in blood-transfusion laboratories. For research work a numerical nomenclature has been described. Each phenotype is defined in terms of the reaction of the red cells with specific antisera, to which numbers have been assigned.

In practice it is the D antigen that is of crucial importance in causing haemolytic disease of the newborn and transfusion reactions. Occasionally reactions occur as a result of anti-c and anti-E; anti-C and anti-e are rarely involved.

The Rh antigens appear to be confined to the red cells; evidence of their presence in white cells, platelets, and body secretions is not convincing. The chemical nature of the Rh antigens is not known.

Rhesus Antibodies

Naturally-occurring Rhesus antibodies are rare, though a number of cases of anti-E and anti-C^w have been reported. Such antibodies are usually more active at lower temperatures than at 37°C.

On the other hand, *immune Rhesus antibodies* are commonly formed following the introduction of Rh-positive cells into an Rh-negative subject by: (*a*) transfusion, or (*b*) the transplacental passage of fetal cells.

Early in the course of Rh sensitisation IgM antibodies are formed. These are not passed across the placenta. Later on they are succeeded by IgG antibodies, which are actively transferred across the placenta. These IgG antibodies act best at 37°C, and are *incomplete*, that is, incapable of agglutinating red cells in saline suspension, but detectable in other ways (see antiglobulin test later). Haemolytic disease of the newborn due to the formation of Rh antibodies by the mother is described on page 613.

RED CELL-ANTIBODY INTERACTIONS

Red-cell agglutination. It has been found that red cells possess a surface negative charge and that they normally repel one another. This electrical property is due to the carboxyl group of sialic acid: treatment with proteolytic enzymes such as trypsin or papain liberates a sialomucopeptide. The result is a great reduction in negative charge, and incomplete antibodies are helped in their agglutinating action. A colloid medium like albumin also reduces the electric repulsion between red cells and so facilitates their agglutination.

Most IgG are incomplete antibodies—those against A and B antigens are exceptions—whereas most IgM are complete. It will be recalled that IgG antibodies have 2 binding sites and IgM probably 10. Because the antigens are spaced on the red-cell surface, both IgG and IgM antibodies probably attach to a red cell only by a single binding site. Presumably IgM, being larger than IgG, can bridge a larger gap between cells, and thus facilitate agglutination. Thus an IgG molecule can bind sites which are up to 14 nm apart, whereas an IgM molecule has a maximum span of 35 nm. IgG incomplete antibodies can prevent the agglutinating action of complete antibodies of the same specificity, and are an example of a blocking antibody (see p. 147); in fact, incomplete anti-Rh was first discovered by this blocking effect.

In summary then, incomplete antibodies react specifically with red cells containing the appropriate antigen, but do not agglutinate them. They may be detected, directly or indirectly, in the following ways:

(*a*) The red cells are suspended in a colloid medium before the serum is added. A suitable medium is provided by a concentrated protein solution such as 30 per cent bovine albumin.

(*b*) The red cells are treated with such enzymes as trypsin, ficin (from figs), or papain before the addition of the serum.

(*c*) The red cells are first incubated at 37°C with the serum, then washed three times to remove all traces of serum proteins, and finally mixed with an antiglobulin serum prepared by injecting human globulin into a rabbit. This is called the *indirect Coombs test*, or *indirect antiglobulin test*.

The most sensitive procedure of all is an indirect antiglobulin test on enzyme-treated red cells.

Antiglobulin (Coombs) Test

In the antiglobulin test, as outlined above, the antibody combines with the cells *in vitro*. This is the *indirect test*; it detects incomplete antibody in the patient's serum, and is invaluable in cross-matching blood.

In haemolytic anaemia due to warm antibodies, the patient's red cells have already been exposed to the incomplete antibody *in vivo*, and they will undergo agglutination *in vitro* once they have been washed and then mixed with an antiglobulin serum. This is the *direct test*; it detects globulin already on the cells. In the direct antiglobulin test all that needs to be done is to mix the washed cells with the antiglobulin reagent, whereas in the indirect test the cells have first to be incubated with the patient's serum.*

*The antiglobulin test is in fact more complex than is described above. The reagent commonly used contains antibodies of two separate specificities: anti-human IgG and anti-human complement. The anticomplement antibodies are directed against C3 and its activated and breakdown products (e.g. C3b and C3d) as well as C4.

The anti-IgG agglutinates red cells coated with IgG antibody; the reaction may be inhibited by free IgG in the solution. Certain incomplete antibodies, commonly IgM, fix complement, which is thereby attached to red cells. Such cells are agglutinated by the anticomplement in the antiglobulin reagent. This reaction is inhibited by the C3 and C4 components of complement, but not by IgG. Some antibodies of the Kidd and Duffy systems sensitise cells to anti-IgG and to anticomplement.

BLOOD GROUPING

ABO grouping. The ABO grouping of a blood sample is performed on a tile or in tubes, preferably at room temperature. 2 drops of a 2 per cent red-cell suspension in normal saline are mixed with 1 drop of potent anti-A and anti-B serum respectively, and the development of agglutination is noted. If this occurs with anti-A, the cells are group A, and with anti-B, group B. If both sera agglutinate the red cells, they are group AB, and if there is no agglutination with either, they are group O. An additional safeguard is to test the cells with a group O serum (containing anti-A and anti-B). This agglutinates all cells which are not group O, and is a safeguard against mistaking an A_2 subject for group O. Agglutination is easily recognisable with the naked eye, but should be confirmed microscopically. As a routine procedure the patient's serum is tested with group A, B, and O cells to confirm the presence of the expected alloagglutinins, anti-A and anti-B, according to the table on page 646. This is termed 'reverse grouping'.

The anti-A and anti-B sera are prepared by blood transfusion centres. They are collected from blood donors, and are selected for their potency. It is most important to be sure that the anti-A serum will reliably detect the weak forms of the A antigen.

Apart from alloagglutination, the red cells may be clumped under the following conditions:

Pseudoagglutination. This is the clumping of red cells by non-immunological means, and is due to rouleaux formation such as occurs in multiple myeloma and macroglobulinaemia.

Autoagglutination due to cold agglutinins. The effect could be overcome by carrying out the reverse grouping at 37°C. However, this is technically difficult since 'cold' agglutinins can act up to 30°C. This difficulty can be overcome by carrying out the grouping on red cells that have been washed several times in warm saline.

Panagglutination. This is a non-specific agglutination of *contaminated red cells*, particularly liable to occur in old blood samples. The agglutination is due to the unmasking of an antigen (T antigen) which is present in all human red cells. Such 'changed' red cells are agglutinated by normal human serum which contains anti-T. The change can be brought about by bacteria *in vitro*, and it may rarely occur *in vivo*. Cells which have become panagglutinable (also called polyagglutinable) can readily be detected by the use of an anti-T lectin extracted from peanuts.

Rhesus grouping. Powerful anti-D sera are obtained from women who have already been sensitised during previous pregnancies. A complete anti-D serum is particularly desirable, as it can be used with saline-suspended cells, but often an incomplete serum has to suffice.

1 drop of a 5 per cent red-cell suspension in saline is added to a drop of complete anti-D serum in a serological tube, and the mixture is incubated at 37°C for 1 hour, after which the tube is centrifuged and examined for agglutination. If an incomplete anti-D serum is used, a drop of 30 per cent bovine albumin is added to the tube, and the rest is carried out as above. If the controls give the expected results, agglutination indicates that the cells are Rh-positive. The antiglobulin technique is un-

necessary for Rh grouping, unless the antigen D^u is being investigated.*

Rhesus grouping is also performed on a slide by mixing 1 drop of a 50 per cent suspension of red cells in serum with 1 drop of incomplete anti-D serum. The test is read for agglutination in 2 minutes, and the result should agree with that obtained by the tube method outlined above. In the negative control the anti-D is replaced by a drop of albumin.

In Rhesus grouping it is essential to use the proper controls. Thus known Rh-positive and Rh-negative cells should give the expected results. Furthermore, the cells to be tested should be mixed with albumin without anti-D, because the cells from a patient with autoimmune incomplete antibodies may agglutinate in albumin alone as well as in albumin mixed with anti-D. Hence an Rh-negative person may be grouped erroneously as Rh-positive, and subsequently given Rh-positive blood, thereby becoming sensitised.

INDICATIONS FOR BLOOD TRANSFUSION

A sudden reduction of blood volume after haemorrhage. Not only is *whole-blood transfusion* mandatory after severe haemorrhage, but it is also used during major operative procedures. The most spectacular example is the use of large quantities of blood in the elaborate extracorporeal circulations set up during open-heart surgery. It is now common, particularly in the large medical centres, to use red-cell concentrates instead of whole blood. This practice not only avoids circulatory overload but also permits the other components of blood to be harvested.

An inadequate concentration of circulating haemoglobin which cannot be relieved by specific therapy, e.g. vitamin B_{12} or iron. All severe anaemias are potentially eligible for packed red-cell transfusion, but only rarely do the megaloblastic or iron-deficiency types require it. A special circumstance may, of course, necessitate transfusion of these patients, e.g. parturition or a surgical operation. The demand of some surgeons, that the haemoglobin concentration be 'normal' prior to surgery, is misconceived. Often the patient has become adjusted to the new haemoglobin level, and a transfusion merely disturbs the equilibrium for the time being. It should be remembered that transfusions are not free from risk, and the more anaemic the patient, the more carefully should blood be administered.

Transfusions need rarely be used in autoimmune haemolytic anaemia, and should be reserved for acutely anaemic patients awaiting splenectomy or a response to glucocorticoids. In haemolytic disease of the newborn *exchange transfusion* is often imperative to prevent a rise in the plasma level of unconjugated bilirubin by removing cells that have been damaged by antibody. In addition the anaemia can also be corrected (see also p. 653).

In aplastic anaemia the patient may be tided over by transfusions for a long time in the hope of ultimate recovery. There is also an important role for transfusions in leukaemia,

---

*Phenotype cD^ue masquerades as cde, and the antigen D^u may be missed in the albumin test, especially if the anti-D is not very strong. The phenotype is not uncommon in Black people, and is of importance when Rh-negative donors are being selected. Obviously a D^u donor is Rh-positive.

particularly the acute variety. The anaemia of chronic renal failure may be relieved, but the effect is only temporary, for the haemoglobin soon falls to its previous low level.

Blood Component Therapy

When whole blood has been lost, it is logical to replace it by whole blood. If, however, the circulating blood is lacking certain components, it is logical to supply those components only. Many are now available from transfusion centres.

Packed red cells. These, prepared by removing about 85 per cent of the plasma, are ideal for use in correcting anaemia, especially when there is a danger of circulatory overload. In addition, the plasma is available for the preparation of other components.

Platelet transfusions. These are useful in patients with severe thrombocytopenia due to the failure of platelet production. The commonest indication is acute leukaemia and generalised bone-marrow aplasia. A temporary increase in the platelet count sufficient to prevent or arrest bleeding may be achieved by this treatment. Although intact platelets are readily detectable in stored blood, their survival after transfusion is much impaired. Platelet transfusions are ineffective in four groups of patients:

(*a*) Those who have had multiple transfusions; the platelets are rapidly eliminated by alloantibodies.

(*b*) In thrombocytopenia due to autoantibodies.

(*c*) In disseminated intravascular coagulation or any type of consumptive process, including that due to infection.

(*d*) In patients with splenomegaly.

Granulocyte transfusions. With special equipment large numbers of granulocytes can be harvested from normal donors using methods involving differential centrifugation, gravity sedimentation, or reversible leucoadhesion. The transfusion of granulocytes is helpful in neutropenic patients with bacterial infections, and may prevent infections in patients receiving chemotherapy that induces neutropenia, such as cytotoxic drugs for malignant disease.

Fresh frozen plasma. This is prepared by removing plasma from fresh blood and freezing it at $-20°C$ to preserve labile clotting factors. It is used in the treatment of Christmas disease (haemophilia B). Factor IX concentrates are also available and effective; unfortunately the risk of viral hepatitis is high. Fresh frozen plasma must be transfused as quickly as possible after thawing, and cannot then be refrozen.

Cryoprecipitated anti-haemophilic factor. When fresh frozen plasma is thawed at 4°C, the Factor VIII precipitates as a cryoglobulin. Such *cryoprecipitates* are used in the treatment of haemophilia A: 1 unit of cryoprecipitate raises the Factor VIII level of the average adult by 2 per cent. Progressively more use is now made of dried Factor VIII concentrates although they are more expensive than cryoprecipitate.

Other plasma fractions. *Albumin.* This is available for the treatment of haemoconcentration and shock as may follow extensive burns, intestinal obstruction, and acute pancreatitis. Supplies are limited, and albumin is of no value in treating the hypoalbuminaemia of chronic renal disease.

Fibrinogen. 1 gram vials are available, and the usual adult dose is 4 to 8 grams. It is of value in congenital hypofibrinogenaemia, but there is a great risk of viral hepatitis.

Gamma-globulin. This is useful in the prophylaxis or attenuation of some viral diseases and in the treatment of hypogammaglobulinaemia.

Rh (D) immune globulin (human). This is used in the prevention of Rh sensitisation of Rh-negative women after the delivery of an Rh-positive baby or fetus (see p. 613), or after a miscarriage of a fetus of unknown Rhesus type. The usual intramuscular injection contains 200 to 300 μg of anti-D.

THE STORAGE OF BLOOD

Blood is collected aseptically from donors, and is stored in plastic bags. The anticoagulant usually employed is 'ACD', a mixture of citric *a*cid, trisodium *c*itrate, and *d*extrose. Dextrose appears to decrease the rate of hydrolysis of ester phosphate during storage. The acidification increases the preserving power of the solution.

Stored red cells have an increased affinity for oxygen, and are less ready to release oxygen than are fresh cells. This affinity for oxygen increases with the age of the banked blood. A number of organic phosphate esters, ATP, ADP, and especially *2:3 diphosphoglycerate (DPG)*, lower the oxygen affinity regardless of oxygen tension (see p. 603). It has been found that the concentration of 2:3 diphosphoglycerate in the red cells declines on storage, and this is probably the reason for their increased affinity for oxygen. It is useless adding these phosphates to the extracellular medium as they cannot enter the cells, but the effect can be arrested and reversed by adding nucleosides, such as inosine and adenosine. It may be that these are broken down to purine bases and ribose-1-phosphate, which is then converted to 2:3 diphosphoglycerate. Some blood banks add inosine weekly to banked blood to prevent this oxygen-binding effect.

Another anticoagulant solution containing citrate, phosphate, and dextrose (CPD) is less acid than ACD, and the preservation of red-cell DPG is better. It is steadily replacing ACD, particularly when the blood is to be stored.

Blood should be kept stored at a temperature of about 4°C. It has been found that at temperatures above 10°C there is a rapid deterioration of the red cells. On the other hand, slow freezing is to be avoided at all costs. Much of the damage inflicted is due to the residual hypertonic fluid. Once thawing occurs, there is haemolysis when the cells are exposed once more to the isotonic solution. Much research has been done on blood which is frozen very rapidly in liquid nitrogen, and thawed equally rapidly. It has been found that the red cells survive slow freezing only when glycerol is added to the anticoagulant mixture. At a temperature of $-50°C$ there may be no impairment in survival rate even after a year's storage.

The post-transfusion survival of red cells in blood stored at 4°C for various periods, using ACD as the anticoagulant, has been investigated. After 14 days' storage from 6 to 10 per cent of the red cells are destroyed within 24 hours of transfusion, but the remainder survive almost as well as do fresh cells. After 28 days' storage there is a 30 per cent destruction within 24 hours, and the remainder show a considerably more rapid rate of disappearance than normal. It is advisable not to use blood stored longer than 21 days.

Components of a unit of blood. 1 unit (pint) of blood contains approximately 450 ml of blood and 67·5 ml of

ACD. The number of red cells is such that the transfusion of 1 unit should raise the haemoglobin concentration of the average adult by approximately 1 g per dl. At 21 days' storage, the maximum storage time, 70 to 80 per cent of red cells survive following transfusion. As noted previously, the granulocytes are not viable in stored blood, and in fresh blood there are too few to be effective. White-cell transfusions are available in specialised centres only. Platelets are viable only if the blood is less than 24 hours old.

Each unit contains approximately 10 g albumin, 2 g gammaglobulin, and 0·7 g fibrinogen. These are relatively stable when stored at 4°C. Prothrombin and Factors VII, IX, and X are also stable. Factors V and VIII are not stable at 4°C, but are stable in fresh plasma and cryoprecipitates stored frozen at −22°C.

PREPARATIONS FOR BLOOD TRANSFUSION

Routinely the entire blood grouping and cross-matching procedure takes at least 2 hours, even if no difficulties are encountered.

Blood grouping. The patient's red cells are tested with anti-A, anti-B, and anti-A plus-B (group O) sera as described. The serum is tested for the presence of the expected alloagglutinins.

The red cells are tested with anti-Rh (D) by two methods (p. 649).

Antibody screening. *Donor.* Blood issued by transfusion services has been screened for the presence of irregular antibodies (e.g. anti-K, anti-c) in the donor's plasma.

Recipient. Trouble due to antibodies can usually be met in advance of cross-matching tests by 'screening' the sera of patients likely to require transfusion. Many laboratories use a 'pool' of antigens (prepared by mixing the red cells of two or three selected donors) to test the patient's serum for irregular antibodies. A preliminary screening test is particularly helpful in patients anticipating surgery. Irregular antibodies are then identified by further tests, which may require several hours or days to complete.

Cross-matching of blood. Once the ABO and Rhesus blood groups of donor and recipient are known, it is necessary to proceed with cross-matching before a transfusion can be performed. Having chosen blood of the same ABO and Rhesus groups as the recipient, the donor's red cells must be tested against the recipient's serum. The donor's serum is much less important, because any antibodies it may contain should be so diluted by the recipient's plasma as to become insignificant. Cross-matching is always necessary even if the ABO and Rhesus blood groups of donor and recipient are identical, because (*a*) there may be an error in sample identification, and (*b*) the recipient's serum may contain antibodies other than anti-A, anti-B, anti-D. Approximately 1 per cent of hospital patients possess antibodies outside the ABO and Rhesus systems.

Group O donors were often referred to as 'universal donors', and there was a temptation to administer uncross-matched, group O, Rh-negative blood indiscriminately in times of emergency. While this procedure may be justified in a particular circumstance when the patient might have died of exsanguination had he been kept waiting until a standard cross-matching had been performed, it must be understood that the casual use of group O blood is not free from risk. Occasionally severe haemolytic reactions follow, and these are due to high-titre immune antibodies (usually anti-A) in the donor's plasma reacting with the recipient's red cells despite the very considerable diluting effect of the recipient's plasma. Even the administration of uncross-matched, Rh-negative blood to Rh-positive recipients is not entirely innocuous, because the patient may have formed antibodies such as anti-c, anti-Jk^a, or anti-Fy^a, which react with the red cells of most donors, whether Rh-negative or Rh-positive. Preliminary cross-matching would expose this danger. In practice the use of uncross-matched group O blood is justifiable *only* for emergency transfusions, e.g. following trauma. In all other cases there should be sufficient time to select donor blood of the same ABO and Rhesus groups as those of the recipient, and to perform a 15-minute cross-marching test.

The Technique of Cross-Matching

The aim is to detect antibodies in the *recipient's serum* against the *donor's red cells*. These antibodies may be detected directly by a simple agglutination test or indirectly by the antiglobulin test.

(a) Agglutination test. Equal volumes of a 2 per-cent saline suspension of donor cells and recipient serum are mixed and left at room temperature for 1 hour. The sedimented cells are then examined for agglutinates. This test detects saline agglutinins such as anti-P$_1$; it also provides a further check that group A or group B blood is not being matched for a group O recipient.

As with ABO grouping, difficulty may be encountered because of pseudoagglutination and autoagglutination. The former is seen in patients with multiple myeloma and macroglobulinaemia, and can hardly be distinguished from true agglutination by microscopy. Dilution with saline breaks up the clumps to some extent. Agglutination due to cold auto-agglutinins is prevented by performing the test at 37°C after pre-warming the donor's cell suspension and the patient's serum.

(b) Indirect antiglobulin test. 6 drops of the patient's serum are mixed with 2 drops of a 2 per cent suspension of the donor's cells. After incubation at 37°C for 30 to 60 minutes, the cells are washed three times in large volumes of saline and drained. A drop of antiglobulin serum is added to the final cell button, and the mixture is lightly centrifuged. Agglutination occurs if the cells are 'coated' with globulin (antibody).

Although in cross-matching the most important component of an antiglobulin reagent is anti-gammaglobulin, the reagent usually also contains antibodies against C3 and C4 components of complement, and will react with the complement bound by some antibodies (e.g. Anti-Le^a and anti-Jk^a). In relatively few blood-group systems can the antibodies be detected as agglutinins in saline or albumin. However, the indirect antiglobulin test, when properly performed, will detect antibodies of almost all blood-group systems.

In general, cells which react with the patient's serum *in vitro* at 37°C do not survive well after transfusion. However, when there is doubt about the interpretation of serological tests, a direct measurement of red-cell compatibility can be made by following the survival of 1 ml of the prospective donor's chromium-labelled (^{51}Cr) cells in the patient over a period of several hours.

Patients with acquired haemolytic anaemia are a special problem, since the serum may contain a mixture of alloantibodies and autoantibodies. In these and other difficult cases, a sample of the patient's blood should be sent to a Transfusion Centre or Reference Laboratory for further investigation.

THE ADVERSE EFFECTS OF BLOOD TRANSFUSION

These effects can be classified into those which occur immediately and those which are delayed.

Immediate Reactions

Immediate simple febrile reactions. These reactions may occur either during or shortly after a transfusion. Most often they can be attributed to the presence of white-cell antibodies formed by the recipient as a result of previous transfusions or pregnancies. Febrile reactions may be quite severe but usually last only a few hours. Nevertheless, although not dangerous they must be investigated, since fever is also a component of the haemolytic reaction (see below). Aspirin will usually alleviate the symptoms, but antihistamine drugs are not effective. If febrile reactions are troublesome in patients who require further transfusions, they may usually be avoided by giving blood from which the white cells have been removed ('buffy-coat poor' blood).

Febrile reactions may also be due to the presence of Gram-negative endotoxin in either the transfusion fluid or the apparatus. Modern disposable apparatus and properly prepared fluids have largely eliminated this complication.

Allergic reactions. Urticarial reactions are usually due to sensitising antibodies in the recipient interacting with an exogenous antigen, e.g. milk or egg protein, in the plasma of the donor. Reactions are therefore most common in patients who suffer from atopic diseases such as asthma or hay-fever. The development of an urticarial reaction is comparatively common; it is usually harmless, and is easily controlled by oral or parenteral antihistamine drugs. Very rarely the reaction has features of generalised anaphylaxis, and can be fatal.

Immediate-type hypersensitivity reactions occur when the transfused plasma (or blood product) contains plasma proteins with antigenic determinants which are lacking in the patient's own plasma proteins and to which he has previously been exposed. Severe anaphylactic reactions can occur due to *anti-IgA* formed as a result of previous transfusion in subjects who either lack IgA or who belong to a different IgA subclass. Similarly, reactions are occasionally seen following the injection of the immunoglobulin in patients with agammaglobulinaemia.

Allergic reactions may also occur as a result of the passive transfer of a hypersensitive state from the donor to the recipient. A reaction develops if the recipient happens to come into contact with the relevant antigen. Donors with a history of striking hypersensitivity should not be accepted.

Haemolytic transfusion reactions. These are usually due to the rapid destruction of donor red cells by antibodies in the recipient's plasma, and are generally the result of transfusion of ABO incompatible blood, for example group A red cells in a group O recipient. These mishaps are almost always due to an error in the identification of the patient, a specimen, or the unit of blood, rather than a technical failure to detect incompatibility.

The patient, usually soon after the transfusion has begun, complains of a sensation of heat and pain along the transfused vein, and this is followed by facial flushing, rigors, fever, severe pain in the loins, and a feeling of constriction in the chest. Hypotension and shock may follow and terminate in death. In severe cases there is intravascular haemolysis of red cells with haemoglobinaemia, haemoglobinuria, lowering of the haptoglobin level, and the appearance of methaemalbumin in the plasma. Jaundice takes several hours to develop. Oliguria may develop and be followed by acute renal failure. There is little doubt that these dramatic symptoms are due to the substances released as a result of an antigen–antibody reaction, because a similar amount of haemolysed compatible blood does not have such severe effects. Activation of complement probably plays an important part.

The most serious effect is progressive oliguria, which is due to intense renal vasoconstriction. As mentioned on page 615, the presence of much free haemoglobin in the circulation does cause a degree of interference with the renal blood flow, but acting on its own it is inadequate to produce much damage. In this type of intravascular haemolysis there are the two additional important factors: liberated vasoconstrictor substances and the primary condition that necessitated transfusion in the first place.

After incompatible transfusion there is often leucopenia and thrombocytopenia. The lysis of red cells leads to the liberation of clotting substances which cause disseminated intravascular coagulation (p. 643). The incoagulability of the blood causes a generalised bleeding tendency. In anaesthetised patients, whose subjective responses have been abolished, this bleeding tendency is a very important indication of incompatibility. The other suspicious finding is persistent hypotension despite the transfusion.

With other antibodies, especially those of the Rhesus system, red-cell destruction is usually slower and less dramatic. It is nearly always extravascular, occurring in the RE system, especially the spleen (p. 613). Symptoms are usually milder in degree, although haemoglobinaemia may occur with a severe degree of red-cell destruction. Renal failure and a fatal outcome rarely occurs after extravascular haemolysis.

In the mildest incompatibility reactions there are no obvious symptoms or signs. The anaemia is merely not improved as much as would be hoped, so that another transfusion has to be administered sooner than expected.

Haemolysis also results from transfusion of blood rendered non-viable by faulty storage (freezing or heating), over-long storage, or bacterial contamination.

Circulatory overload. Congestive heart failure and pulmonary oedema may be precipitated by the excessive or too rapid administration of blood, plasma, or other intravenous fluids, particularly in patients with severe anaemia or pre-existing heart disease.

In susceptible patients it is wise to limit transfusion to two units of packed cells over 24 hours, each unit taking 4 hours (never more) to transfuse. The patient must be examined frequently throughout the transfusion for evidence of elevated jugular venous pressure and pulmonary oedema. Exchange transfusion or intraperitoneal injection are alternative approaches.

Intraperitoneal injection of blood. Intraperitoneal blood is absorbed by the lymphatics in the diaphragm and travels thence *via* the lymph ducts to the blood. This route is useful in children and in patients with very severe anaemia in whom intravenous transfusion is dangerous. In haemolytic disease of the newborn intraperitoneal blood transfusions have been given to the fetus *in utero* in order to correct the anaemia which is the cause of early fetal death (hydrops fetalis). To avoid the risk of a graft-versus-host reaction in the newborn infant, the blood should be irradiated (1000 r) before transfusion.

Bacterial contamination of blood is due to accidental introduction of organisms during collection or storage. The dangerous ones are cold-growing Gram-negative bacilli of the *Pseudomonas* genus and also certain coliform organisms. After a brief latent period there is profound shock associated with fever and abdominal pain. Death may ensue within a few hours (see p. 418). As a general rule, *a unit of blood should be given within 4 hours*, for prolonged storage at room temperature encourages the growth of contaminating bacteria.

Biochemical upsets following massive transfusions. With storage there is an increased amount of potassium in the plasma and a decreased amount in the red cells. It sometimes happens that massive transfusions, e.g. exchange transfusions in infants, may be accompanied by transient hyperkalaemia of sufficient severity to produce ECG changes and sudden death. Hyperkalaemia in adults may be avoided by the use of packed red cells.

Another danger of this type of transfusion is citrate intoxication, which produces the effects of hypocalcaemia. It is probable that citrate intoxication is not due entirely to hypocalcaemia, because transfused hypocalcaemic blood does not have the same effect as citrate. Nevertheless, the effects are reversed by calcium salts. The effects of hyperkalaemia and citrate intoxication tend to potentiate one another.

The plasma of stored blood has an increased content of ammonia, which may be dangerous in patients with liver failure. The context of organic acids also rises, and the pH falls.

Generalised bleeding tendency. *Thrombocytopenia* is an occasional complication of rapidly repeated large transfusions, and can result in a serious haemorrhagic state. The mechanism is dilutional, since the platelets in the transfused blood are non-viable.

In some cases platelet antibodies are formed against incompatible transfused platelets, and it seems that the antibodies can also damage the recipient's own platelets. Occasionally potent anti-platelet antibodies in the donor's plasma may be incriminated.

The generalised bleeding tendency which results from hypofibrinogenaemia has already been described.

Air embolism. The introduction of air through ill-fitting tubing, especially when blood is introduced under pressure, may result in air embolism; the use of plastic bags has virtually eliminated this danger. In terms of experimental work on animals, it would seem that a considerable amount of air (about 200 ml) should be tolerated by humans, but there is clinical evidence that as little as 40 ml can have serious results, particularly in severely ill patients.

Delayed Reactions

Sensitisation. The transfusion of red cells, white cells, or platelets carrying antigens not present on the recipient's cells may stimulate the production of alloantibodies directed against the foreign antigen. These alloantibodies may complicate future transfusions or pregnancies. Sensitisation to plasma protein antigens, particularly IgA, has already been noted on pp. 143 and 652.

Delayed haemolytic transfusion reactions. In patients who have become sensitised through transfusion or pregnancy, the titre of the alloantibody may with time fall to such a low level as to be undetectable. During later transfusions blood may be given which appears to be compatible, but which restimulates antibody production. The antibody then causes sudden destruction of the transfused cells, usually within 3 to 7 days following transfusion.

A delayed haemolytic reaction should be suspected when jaundice appears some days after transfusion, or when the haemoglobin concentration fails to rise by the expected amount (p. 651) or drops unexpectedly. Often the irregular antibody is suspected only when further blood is cross-matched, or when the patient's direct antiglobulin (Coombs) test is found to be positive.

Infection introduced from the donor. Syphilis, malaria, brucellosis, and, in tropical Africa and South America, trypanosomiasis may be transmitted by transfusion. The most important hazard, however, is hepatitis due either to virus A or virus B (see p. 284).

Virus B hepatitis is by far the more important, and the presence of the infective agent is related to the presence of the surface antigen HBsAg.

HBsAg. This antigen can be detected by a variety of methods involving the use of serum known to contain high-titre antibody. Immunodiffusion, counter-immuno-electrophoresis* (immunoelectro-osmophoresis), inhibition of haemagglutination, complement fixation, radio-immunoassay, and electron microscopy have all been used. These vary in sensitivity and ease of performance. At the present time counter-immunoelectrophoresis is commonly used to screen all blood donors. Radio-immunoassay is, however, approximately a hundred times more sensitive, and has been introduced for routine testing of blood donors by the American Red Cross Transfusion Service. The incidence of HBsAg-positivity varies from one community to another and also with the sensitivity of the method used to detect the antigen. Thus in Canada the incidence is 0·063 per cent in North Alberta and 0·484 per cent in West Quebec. It is high in the inmates of institutions, particularly prisons (0·903 per cent), and in patients with lepromatous leprosy, Down's syndrome, and immunological deficiency states, patients on renal haemodialysis, those who have had multiple transfusions, and people who have had virus B hepatitis. The incidence of antigen is approximately 0·1 per cent in unpaid blood donors in Britain and the USA, but with professional

---

*When placed in an electric field, antigen having a negative charge migrates towards the anode. Antibody under the influence of endosmotic flow migrates towards the cathode. By placing the antigen and antibody in separate wells, a current is passed in such a direction that the antigen and antibody flow towards each other and interact to produce a precipitate. The method is faster and more sensitive than simple double diffusion.

donors the incidence is 10 times higher. It has been estimated that about 50 per cent of people who receive HBsAg-positive blood develop hepatitis. If the sensitivity of the test employed is known, the expected incidence of hepatitis can be calculated. At present about 1 in 4 carriers are detected, and the incidence of hepatitis is about 0·15 per cent following a transfusion from a single donor, assuming that HBsAg-positive donors are excluded. The figures quoted are from Mollison (1972) and Moore *et al.* (1972).

Some cases of long-incubation-period, post-transfusion hepatitis appear to be due neither to virus A nor virus B. For the time being these cases are classified as non-A, non-B.

Another complication that appears to be infective in nature is the *post-perfusion*, or *post-transfusion, syndrome*. It develops 3 to 5 weeks after the transfusion of fresh blood, often in large amounts as for open-heart surgery, and its main features are fever, splenomegaly, and atypical lymphocytes in the blood. The condition is a variety of infectious mononucleosis, but the Paul-Bunnell reaction is negative. Some cases are associated with cytomegalovirus infection.

Multiple microembolism. Blood and transfusion fluids have been found to contain particulate matter—particles of rubber bungs, glass particles, and cellulose fibres as well as debris consisting of aggregated platelets and white cells. These may cause significant pulmonary microembolism in a seriously ill patient.

Toxic substances in plastic. Another transfusion hazard is the presence of plasticisers (usually phthalate derivatives) which are leached by blood from the plastic of the bag and tubing. Although toxic to minnows, the effects of these substances in human recipients is less well defined.

Transfusional haemosiderosis. This is a hazard of repeated transfusions given over many years for a chronic condition like aplastic anaemia. The iron deposited in the tissues is derived not only from the blood, but also from the diet (see p. 589).

Thrombophlebitis. This is due to the needle or cannula of the infusion set damaging the vein wall. Factors which influence the development of this complication are the period of transfusion (it is progressively more frequent after 12 hours' infusion), the tubing used (rubber is more damaging than plastic tubing), and the administration of autoclaved glucose solutions, which are strongly acid. The practice of giving glucose through a set previously used for blood is also said to predispose to thrombophlebitis, perhaps because the red cells lyse in contact with the glucose solution.

Indwelling plastic catheters left *in situ* for over 48 hours are frequently contaminated, and can lead to *septic thrombophlebitis* and fatal septicaemia. Indwelling catheters must therefore be changed, ideally every 8 hours.

Graft-versus-host reaction. This rare complication occurs when viable white cells are transfused into an immunologically deficient host (see pp. 171 and 195).

THE HAEMATOLOGICAL HAZARDS OF EXTRACORPOREAL CIRCULATIONS

Extracorporeal circulations maintain a flow of blood through the tissues while the cardiac action is suspended during open-heart surgery. The underlying principle is that blood, rendered incoagulable with heparin and passed through an oxygenator, is pumped into a large artery (usually the femoral), perfused through the tissues, and then returned to the circuit *via* the venae cavae.

Apart from such immediate mechanical hazards as leakage of blood and inadequate perfusion leading to tissue hypoxia and subsequent metabolic acidosis, a serious, though fortunately rather infrequent, complication is severe post-operative bleeding. The main factors involved are (*a*) the presence of residual heparin in the circulation, (*b*) an early activation of clotting leading to disseminated intravascular coagulation, and (*c*) thrombocytopenia, which is probably due to a sequestration of platelets in the tissues and their use in badly-damaged areas; in addition some platelet clumps may be removed by the filters or else become adherent to the oxygenator screen. The first two factors appear to be more relevant to the bleeding tendency than does the platelet deficiency. Another possibility is that some patients have a minor degree of a specific clotting defect, e.g. haemophilia, Christmas disease, or von Willebrand's disease, and under the stress of extracorporeal circulation this is made overt. Specific assay systems would reveal the defect pre-operatively, whereas routine screening would miss it (see also p. 40). Bleeding may occasionally be due to extensive vascular damage caused by hypoxia or sludging.

Another potential hazard is extensive mechanical haemolysis during perfusion; in practice this does not seem to cause much harm.

PRECAUTIONS TO BE TAKEN BEFORE AND DURING BLOOD TRANSFUSION

(1) The donor must be carefully selected. A history of malaria, syphilis, or jaundice should exclude a potential donor.

(2) Thorough grouping and cross-matching of donor and recipient bloods must be carried out. Whenever possible the recipient should be given blood of his own ABO and Rh group. Group O blood cannot be considered universally suitable.

(3) The container must be correctly and distinctly labelled, to minimise the chance of the recipient being given the wrong blood.

(4) The blood should be kept at 4°C, and not used for transfusion after 3 weeks' storage.

(5) Obviously haemolysed blood should not be used.

(6) If there is any question of contamination, a Gram stain of the blood should be performed before it is administered. Packed red cells should not be used later than 24 hours after removing the plasma from the whole blood, unless the manoeuvre has been performed at a transfusion centre under aseptic conditions.

(7) The recipient should be observed so that manifestations of incompatibility, overloading, and allergy can be detected and treated as soon as possible. If there is any question of incompatibility, the transfusion must be stopped at once. The next specimen of urine passed should be examined for free haemoglobin, and the patient's plasma for haemoglobin, methaemalbumin, and bilirubin. If the evidence points to an incompatibility reaction, the cross-matching should be re-

peated; a sample of the recipient's blood should be sent with the unit of donor blood to the hospital's transfusion laboratory. If there is no obvious error, it may be worth seeking the advice of a Transfusion Centre or Reference Laboratory. Meanwhile some of the blood should be cultured to rule out the possibility of contamination.

GENERAL READING

BOORMAN, K. E., DODD, B. E. & LINCOLN, P. J. (1977) *Blood Grouping Serology*, 5th ed., 495 pp. Edinburgh: Churchill Livingstone.

DACIE, J. V. & LEWIS, S. M. (1975) *Practical Haematology*, 5th edn, 629 pp. Edinburgh: Churchill Livingstone.

GIBLETT, E. R. (1969) *Genetic Markers in Human Blood*, 629 pp. Oxford: Blackwell.

MOLLISON, P. L. (1978) *Blood Transfusion in Clinical Medicine*, 6th edn, Oxford: Blackwell.

MOORE, B. P. L., HUMPHREYS, P. & LOVETT-MOSELEY, C. A. (1972) *Serological and Immunological Methods, Technical Manual of the Canadian Red Cross Blood Transfusion Service*, 7th edn, 450 pp. Toronto: Canadian Red Cross Society.

O'NEILL, G. J. *et al.* (1978) Chido and Rodgers blood groups are distinct antigenic components of human complement C4. *Nature (London)*, **273**, 668.

RACE, R. R. & SANGER, R. (1975) *Blood Groups in Man*, 6th edn, 659 pp. Oxford: Blackwell.

THOMPSON, J. S. & THOMPSON, M. W. (1973) *Genetics in Medicine*, pp. 202–240. Philadelphia: Saunders.

WALLACE, J. (1977) *Blood Transfusion for Clinicians*, 392 pp. Edinburgh: Churchill Livingstone.

Appendix 1. The Principles of Disinfection

Sterilisation is a process whereby all living organisms, including spores, are destroyed. It is to be contrasted with **disinfection**, a process which destroys only the vegetative forms of organisms, but which leaves intact any spores that may be present. In practice it often suffices, because spore-bearing organisms are often not an important hazard. For example, the skin could never be sterilised without its own destruction, but it can be satisfactorily disinfected with an iodine solution. The terms 'germicide', 'antiseptic', and 'disinfectant' refer to chemical agents which kill organisms or prevent their growth. Though there are subtle theoretical differences in the meanings of these three words, in practice the term *disinfectant* can be used quite conveniently to describe any chemical substance with either a bactericidal or a bacteriostatic action.

Asepsis is the technique employed to prevent the contamination of wounds and other susceptible sites by ensuring that only sterile material makes contact with them and that the air-borne transmission of organisms is minimised. The prevention of hospital infection, described in Chapter 19, is a vital part of asepsis.

There are two methods of disinfection, physical and chemical. Of these, the physical ones are by far the more important, as they alone can be relied on to ensure the sterilisation of articles used in the treatment of patients.

PHYSICAL METHODS OF DISINFECTION

The most important physical agent is heat which may be either dry or moist.

Dry Heat

The surest form of heat sterilisation is incineration, as is practised by the bacteriologist when flaming a wire-loop.

Hot-air oven. For the sterilisation of instruments a hot-air oven is used. Hot-air is an inefficient sterilising agent because it is a poor conductor of heat and it penetrates feebly. It is therefore necessary that the oven be fitted with fans to circulate the air through the chamber around the assembled load. A temperature of 160°C will sterilise the contents after 1 hour. Such a high temperature damages fabrics and melts rubber; therefore hot-air sterilisation is used only for:

Glassware, especially syringes, in which moisture is a nuisance.

Oily fluids, which are impenetrable to steam.

Powders, which would cake in the presence of moisture.

Metallic objects may be sterilised in the hot-air oven, but the autoclave is preferred. Some sharp instruments used in ophthalmic surgery may be damaged by moist heat, and so are preferably sterilised in the hot-air oven.

Infra-red radiation. Infra-red radiation has been used as a method of sterilisation by dry heat. Heating to 200°C *in vacuo* has been employed as a means of sterilising surgical instruments.

Moist Heat

Moist heat is a much more valuable sterilising agent than is dry heat because it is effective at a lower temperature for a shorter period of time. For less ambitious disinfection moist heat is also useful.

Pasteurisation. Milk is pasteurised by being held in water at 63°C for 30 minutes. Instruments that cannot withstand great heat can likewise be disinfected by hot water, for instance endoscopes. If a cystoscope is held in water at 75°C for 10 minutes all vegetative organisms will be destroyed. Admittedly spores will survive, but they are not of importance in urinary-tract infection.

Boiling. An advantage of boiling over pasteurisation is that it is efficacious in destroying the viruses of hepatitis. These are very resistant to heat, but are said to be killed after 30 minutes' boiling at 100°C. Boiling will not destroy spores.

In consulting-room practice syringes and other instruments are disinfected quite satisfactorily by boiling. Admittedly there is a hazard of anaerobic wound infection, but it is not a very real danger in these circumstances. In operating theatres, however, such a risk should never be tolerated. In this respect the ward 'sterilisers' are really only 'boilers'. They do not sterilise. Indeed, pathogenic clostridia have on occasion been isolated from them.

Tyndallisation. This is the steaming of a solution for 20 minutes on 3 successive days. After the first steaming only spores are left behind. These germinate in the medium, and are destroyed by the next steaming. Any that survive should be killed after the third steaming. Tyndallisation is, in fact, a true sterilising process, but is applicable only to media in which the spores can germinate and grow as vegetative organisms. It fails when applied to drugs, suture material, and instruments.

Steaming Under Pressure (Autoclaving)

This is the most important method of sterilisation at our disposal, and it is necessary to understand the principles involved. Because water boils when its vapour pressure is equal to that of the surrounding atmosphere, it follows that the boiling point of water can be increased by raising the atmospheric pressure. At normal (sea-level) atmospheric pressure (760 mm Hg or 14·7 lb per square inch) water boils at 100°C, and this pressure is referred to as 'zero' on the pressure gauge. If the pressure is increased by 10 lb per square inch, the water boils at 115°C, and if the pressure is 15 lb per square inch, the boiling point rises to 121°C. If material is held under pure steam at a temperature of 121°C for 15 minutes, sterilisation can be guaranteed. At 126°C, 10 minutes suffices, and at 134°C sterilisation is complete within 3 minutes.

The great superiority of steam over hot air as a steriliser is due to the following factors:

(*a*) Moist heat kills by its effect in denaturing and coagulating enzymes and proteins, whereas dry heat acts by virtue of a destructive oxidation of cell constituents. Moist heat kills more rapidly and at a far lower temperature than dry heat.

(*b*) As steam condenses, it liberates a wealth of latent heat to the surface. The latent heat of vaporisation of water is 540 calories per gram, and 1 ml of water vaporises to produce 1700 ml of steam at 100°C. It is obvious that when steam condenses, not only is a large amount of heat emitted, but there is also a great contraction in its volume. This produces a negative pressure, and brings more steam to the same site. Very soon the temperature of the surface is raised to that of the surrounding steam. Therefore steam acts much more quickly in heating exposed articles than does hot air. A simple proof of this is afforded by placing a finger in a jet of steam from a kettle, and comparing the effect with that produced by the atmosphere of a hot oven!

(*c*) Finally steam penetrates much better than does hot air. This is due in part to its density being only half that of air, and in part to the negative pressure, as already described. Penetration is, of course, of importance only with respect to porous articles.

The all-important factor is the quality of the steam. It must be (*a*) *dry*, i.e. it must not carry suspended droplets of water, because water soaks porous surfaces, thereby interfering with the removal of air and the final drying of the load, (*b*) *close to its point of condensation*, because if it is superheated it does not condense well, its latent heat is not emitted, and its penetrating power vitiated. In fact, superheated steam behaves exactly like hot air and damages fabrics, and (*c*) *free from air*, because the temperature at any pressure is lower when air is mixed with the steam. Air also hinders the penetration of steam, and by virtue of its greater density forms a separate cooler layer at the bottom of the autoclave, thus preventing the steam reaching the articles there.

The autoclave. A steriliser that contains steam under pressure is called an *autoclave*. The simplest type, which still has some use in small laboratories, contains its own water which is boiled under pressure like a domestic pressure-cooker. The steam produced expels the residual air. This type of instrument is quite unsuitable for hospital purposes because of its small size and the inadequacy of air expulsion.

All modern sterilising units are equipped with capacious autoclaves which consist of large, steam-jacketed, metal cylinders fastened by bolted swing-doors. The steam enters the roof of the cabinet from a central supply, from which it emerges under considerable pressure (about 60 lb per square inch). Before entering the autoclave the pressure is reduced to about 20 lb per square inch. This in itself removes excess water from the steam. Some of the steam enters the jacket directly, so that the side walls of the autoclave are heated independently of the steam in the chamber itself. This prevents the loss of heat from the chamber with consequent condensation of water on its walls.

As steam is lighter than air, the air is displaced downwards and is expelled together with the condensed steam through an outlet in the floor of the cabinet. A thermostatic valve, called the *balanced pressure steam trap*, or *near-to-steam trap*, is present in the outlet channel, and controls the discharge through it. At a definite temperature, usually 121°C, it expands sufficiently to occlude the outlet. A thermometer is situated just above this steam trap, which is the coolest part of the autoclave.

This steriliser is called the *downward displacement autoclave*, because air is displaced downwards by the emerging steam. In up-to-date autoclaves there is also fitted a vacuum pump which removes as much air as possible before the steam is admitted. High-vacuum, downward displacement autoclaves are very efficient because the air is removed so expeditiously that the required temperature is reached very rapidly.

In this respect the new *high-vacuum high-temperature autoclaves* are worthy of mention. In them a very high preliminary vacuum (below 20 mm Hg absolute) is first produced, and then steam at a pressure of 32 lb per square inch introduced. A temperature of 134°C is attained, and sterilisation is complete within 3 minutes. It is used widely for porous loads containing dressings, rubber, and wrapped instruments.

Another modification is the *high-vacuum low-temperature autoclave*, in which steam at a temperature of 70 to 80°C is used. Heat-sensitive material, fabrics, plastics, rubber endoscopes, and electrical equipment can be disinfected in this way, but if formalin is added to the steam, sterility can be assured in 2 hours.

In order to operate an autoclave, the following procedures are carried out:

1. The articles are placed in the cabinet and the doors are bolted.

2. A considerable vacuum is first applied in order to evacuate as much air as possible.

3. Steam is then admitted at a pressure of about 15 lb per square inch, and when the thermometer registers the required temperature, say 121°C, sterilisation will have commenced.

4. Sterilisation is continued for the required time, say 15 minutes, and then the steam is turned off.

5. If the articles comprise bottles of fluid, they can simply be left to cool. The steam gradually dissipates, and cooling follows. If the material is porous, it must be quite dry before it is removed from the cabinet, because organisms penetrate moist wrappings with great ease. This drying is carried out by re-applying a vacuum to evacuate the steam, and then by introducing dry, filtered air into the cabinet. This air comes from the outside and it is sterilised by being drawn (by the negative pressure) through an inlet-pipe which is provided with two filters. The drying should continue for about 15 minutes. This air is warmed by its contact with the sides of the autoclave, which are directly heated by the residual steam in the surrounding jacket.

The autoclave is used in the sterilisation of most surgical equipment, e.g. dressings, theatre apparel, rubber material, and metal instruments. It is also used in the sterilisation of water, glucose solutions, and saline solutions used parenterally. Some solutions used in microbiology are similarly treated.

Failures in sterilisation may be due to any of the following factors:

Improper packing of the load. If dressings or theatre garments are to be autoclaved, they must be arranged so loosely that the steam can circulate intimately around them. The use of metal drums is now outdated, and paper packs which may contain the instruments for quite complicated procedures are dispensed from the *central sterile supply department* of most modern hospitals. These packs may contain operating theatre items, such as the usual instruments used in routine operations. Others are prepared for use in the ward, e.g. renal or liver biopsy sets, local anaesthetic sets, and many others.

Defects in the autoclave. With the development of modern autoclaves, the inefficient ones of past years have been removed from service. Nevertheless, the perfect autoclave has still not appeared. The snag is the presence of air mixed with the steam; none of the modifications has yet eliminated this nuisance. It may leak in through the door seal or the valves, or it may enter with the steam supply. The door seals and valves must be carefully overhauled, and efficient air pumps must be employed. Various preliminary manoeuvres have been suggested to eliminate as much air as possible, e.g. a double pre-vacuum with steam introduced between each phase, or a continuous influx of steam during the pre-vacuum phase, but none is completely effective.

Defects in the steam. Over-saturated and superheated steam have already been discussed. If the jacket is too warm, the steam inside the cabinet will become superheated.

Faulty operation of the autoclave. It is regrettable that in some hospitals the operation of the autoclave is still left to completely untrained staff like porters, who have other duties to perform. Until a fully-trained staff is employed, no expenditure on modern equipment will ensure safety. The responsibility for efficient sterilisation must remain now as always with those who use the finished product, namely the surgeons themselves.

Tests of Efficiency for Heat Sterilisation

The thermocouple. This is by far the most reliable gauge of efficiency, and proper thermometric testing is essential before a new steriliser is put into commission. One recording is taken from a thermocouple placed inside a test pack of towels and another from one in the chamber drain. Comparison between the two recordings gives a good guide to the speed at which steam penetrates the load.

Browne's tubes. These are ampoules that contain a patent chemical indicator which changes from red through amber to green at a specific temperature. Various types are available for use in autoclaves and hot air ovens, each changing colour at a specific temperature.

Autoclave tape. This is a tape printed with a sensitive ink that undergoes a colour change at a specific temperature. It forms the basis of the *Bowie–Dick test* for high-vacuum autoclaves. In the middle of a test pack of towels there is placed a square of paper on to which has been stuck two strips of a specified autoclave tape (3M brand No. 1222) in the shape of a St. Andrew's Cross (diagonally). A temperature of 134°C is applied for $3\frac{1}{2}$ minutes. There should be a uniform development of bars throughout the length of the strips. This indicates that the steam has passed freely and rapidly to the centre of the load.

Spores of a non-pathogenic organism. The aerobic spore-bearer *Bacillus stearothermophilus* is used; its spores are killed at 121°C after 15 minutes. Test samples are put through the autoclave and an attempt is subsequently made to culture them. Unfortunately growth is often slow, so that when a positive culture is obtained the load has probably already been used. The method is therefore of little value for routine use, but it still has a place in the testing of new equipment. A similar type of test can be used for ethylene-oxide sterilisation.

Other Physical Methods

Light. If a spectrum is thrown out on to an inoculated plate, it can be shown that most of the bactericidal activity resides in the ultraviolet band. Unfortunately ultraviolet light cannot penetrate to any extent. It can be used to disinfect surfaces. As an air disinfectant it is useful in virological laboratories, but it is unreliable in the presence of large particles of dust. These must first be filtered off, e.g. by electrostatic precipitation.

Ionising radiation. Both γ-rays and β-particles are used. This is a good method of sterilisation, for penetration is satisfactory and closed packs can be used. It is still outside the realm of hospital sterilisation, but is employed with increasing frequency commercially for plastics, rubber, and fabrics. Equipment containing metal, polythene, polyvinyl chloride, nylon, terylene, polystyrene, paper, wool, and cotton is usually unaffected. Rubber varies in its response to ionising radiation; butyl and chlorinated rubbers are not suitable for this type of sterilisation. The types of hospital equipment most eligible for sterilisation by ionising radiation are disposable rubber gloves, plastic syringes, blood transfusion sets, and needles. Since the material is discarded after it has been used, there is no danger of it transmitting the viruses of hepatitis.

Filtration is used by microbiologists to sterilise fluids containing sera and amino acids, which would be denatured by heating. The most commonly-used filters are made either of asbestos discs, e.g. Seitz filters, or of finely-ground glass, fused sufficiently to make the small particles adhere (sintered-glass filters). Filtration is also used in the sterilisation of air in operating theatres. For this purpose disposable fabric and oiled mesh are the most satisfactory.

CHEMICAL DISINFECTANTS

A vast number of these have been tried, but mention will be made only of those in current use. A satisfactory agent should have the following qualities:

(*a*) It should be active against a wide range of organisms and spores. Only a few chemical agents are true sterilisers.

(*b*) It should have a rapid action.

(*c*) It should not be vitiated by organic matter like blood, pus, and faeces. In practice most chemicals combine indifferently with organisms and organic matter, and this impairs their disinfectant powers.

(*d*) It should not be toxic or irritating, or induce hypersensitivity.

Inorganic Disinfectants

Of these the only useful ones are the *halogens*. They have a rapid action against both vegetative organisms and spores, i.e.

they are true sterilisers. A grave disadvantage is the ease whereby their action is annulled by foreign organic matter. The halogens of greatest use are iodine and chlorine.

The most important **iodine** disinfectant is the tincture (Weak Iodine Solution, BP), which contains 2·5 per cent iodine and 2·5 per cent potassium iodide in approximately 90 per cent ethanol. It is the best skin disinfectant, but is irritating to raw areas and may induce an allergic contact dermatitis. More recent additions are the *iodophors*, which are solutions of iodine in non-ionic detergents. The iodine is complexed with surface-active agents, e.g. polyvinyl-pyrrolidone-iodine (povidone-iodine or betadine). They are less irritating and stain less than does the tincture, but their activity is equivalent to the available, as compared with the bound, iodine content. As skin disinfectants they are inferior to the tincture, but can be used in 'scrubbing up' before operations. They have also been used on floors with a mop, and are quite effective in disinfecting fomites.

Chlorine is a powerful disinfectant, and is used to sterilise water. Hypochlorite solutions are very useful in the disinfection of the hospital environment and fomites. They are particularly active against viruses, including those of hepatitis. Strong hypochlorite solutions, e.g. 'Chloros', are too corrosive for general use, but if a dilute solution is mixed with a compatible detergent, it will reliably disinfect clean surfaces. Weaker solutions, e.g. 'Milton', can be used diluted for disinfecting infant feeding bottles. Abrasive powders containing hypochlorite, e.g. 'Vim' and 'Ajax', are useful for scouring baths and sinks.

Organic Disinfectants

Alcohols. It is interesting that, whereas pure ethanol is useless as a disinfectant, *70 per cent ethanol* is quite effective against vegetative organisms, but not spores. A 50 to 70 per cent solution of *isopropyl alcohol* is particularly useful as a skin disinfectant.

Aldehydes. *Commercial formalin*, a 37 to 41 per cent solution of formaldehyde gas in water, is a powerful disinfectant and a true steriliser. Its action is rather slow, and it penetrates organic matter slowly. Obvious disadvantages are its irritating odour and a tendency to produce sensitisation due to a residue of paraformaldehyde. Amongst other aldehydes, *glutaraldehyde* deserves special mention. As a 25 per cent aqueous solution diluted to 2 per cent with sodium bicarbonate solution it is of use as a steriliser for instruments that cannot be autoclaved. It is not volatile, and is less irritant and more rapidly sterilising than formalin.

Phenols. Phenol itself is a fairly efficient disinfectant, though neither it nor any of its many derivatives are true sterilisers. A great advantage of these substances is their continued activity in the presence of organic matter, which makes them admirable for the disinfection of faeces. Phenol itself is far too toxic and expensive to be used as a disinfectant, but closely-related substances, the cresols, are extensively used in routine hospital practice. *Lysol* is a solution of cresols in soap, and 'Sudol' is another powerful phenolic compound. They are relatively cheap, and are somewhat less poisonous than pure phenol. They too are active in the presence of organic matter. Their disadvantages are the objectionable odour and irritant effect on the skin. Both are too corrosive

for general use, but there are related clear-soluble phenolic compounds, such as 'Hycolin', 'Stericol', and 'Clearsol', which are less corrosive, and are recommended for the disinfection of fomites.

Another class of phenolic disinfectants is *chloroxylenol* and its compounds, of which 'Dettol' is the best known. These are much less irritating and toxic than the others, but their efficiency is also considerably less. They are inactivated by foreign organic matter. Probably the attached halogen group is responsible for this drawback.

More recently two phenolic derivatives of great importance have been introduced, chlorhexidine and hexachlorophane. *Chlorhexidine*, better known in Britain as 'Hibitane', is an extremely powerful disinfectant against most vegetative organisms, especially Gram-positive ones, but not spores. It is of low toxicity. The parent substance is an odourless, white, crystalline powder. It can be incorporated into watery or alcoholic solutions, and it provides an admirable disinfectant for the skin. It has been used as a bladder irrigant during cystoscopy. Incorporated in a cream it is often used in obstetrics, and it has also been employed to reduce the staphylococcal population of the hands of nurses.

Hexachlorophane (in the United States Pharmacopoeia it is called hexachlorophene) is a whitish crystalline powder which often has a faint phenolic odour. Unlike chlorhexidine it is very insoluble in water and even in alcohol, but it can be incorporated into soap. A 1 per cent hexachlorophane soap is powerfully destructive to Gram-positive organisms but much less so to Gram-negative ones, so that *Pseudomonas* species have been cultured from a stock bottle of 3 per cent hexachlorophane. Its use on several consecutive occasions cuts down the staphylococcal population of the skin quite remarkably, an effect due in some measure to its capacity to remain on the skin. It is a very useful tool both in the preoperative toilet of a patient and in cutting down the residual staphylococcal flora on the hands of nursing attendants. A preparation of hexachlorophane mixed with a detergent is available as 'pHiso-MED'.

Rats given hexachlorophane orally may develop cerebral lesions resembling the rare 'spongy degeneration' found in infants. Although there is no evidence that this condition is due to hexachlorophane, it has been found that infants treated with the disinfectant (to reduce staphylococcal infection) sometimes have high blood levels of it. Certainly such infants should be thoroughly rinsed to diminish parenteral absorption of the disinfectant. Another hazard is the development of Gram-negative infections, unresponsive to hexachlorophane, in these infants. Because of the misgivings over the value of hexachlorophane and the possibility of its having toxic effects, this compound has been removed from many non-prescription medications.

Cationic surface-active agents. These dissociate in aqueous solution into a large, complex cation which is responsible for the surface activity, and a smaller inactive anion. The cation usually contains a pentavalent nitrogen atom which is often present as a quaternary ammonium group, and so these types of disinfectants are usually referred to as *quaternary ammonium compounds*. They have the usual emulsifying and detergent properties associated with surface-active agents, but in addition they are moderately bactericidal. The one that is best known and most widely used is *cetrimide*; this is a mixture of dodecyl-, tetradecyl-, and hexadecyl-trimethylammonium bromides, and is also known as 'CTAB' or 'Cetavlon'. These compounds are colourless, odourless, non-irritating, and non-toxic in bactericidal doses. They do not act well in acid solutions, and are incompatible with soap, which is an anionic surface-active agent. They are moderately effective against Gram-positive organisms, but often less so than would appear at first sight. Their surface activity produces a delusive absence of organisms in a fluid medium; in fact many bacteria will be found adhering to free surfaces, e.g. the sides of the container. Against Gram-negative organisms this group of disinfectants is particularly ineffectual. Indeed, *Pseudomonas* organisms survive in bottles containing these compounds, after being introduced into them from bark corks used as stoppers. A particular danger with these agents is that they are adsorbed by fabrics. Hence if swabs are repeatedly dipped or soaked in a solution of cetrimide, the active agent is removed and virtually all that remains is a bottle of contaminated water.

While these agents can be used as preliminary detergents in the pre-operative toilet of skin, they should not be relied on for disinfection.

GASEOUS DISINFECTANTS

Formaldehyde gas. The sterilising power of formaldehyde has already been noted. Cold formaldehyde does not penetrate well and is adsorbed by fabrics, but hot formaldehyde is much more useful, as it penetrates fabrics with greater ease. Since 3 to 4 per cent of people are sensitive to paraformaldehyde, formolisation cannot be regarded as a satisfactory commercial undertaking.

Ethylene oxide. This is a colourless fluid which boils at 12°C. It is a powerful steriliser, and has many advantages. Unlike formalin it *penetrates extremely well*, even going through plastics. It can be *used at a low temperature, leaves no residue, is a deodoriser,* and *is comparatively non-toxic.* It must be used at a relative humidity of about 33 per cent, and unfortunately it is explosive and inflammable. This hazard is averted if it is used as a 10 per cent mixture with CO_2 or a halogenated hydrocarbon. At 20 to 25°C sterilisation takes 18 hours, but if the temperature is raised to 50 to 60°C the period is reduced to 4 hours. Ethylene oxide has been used with effect in hospitals to sterilise fabrics, plastics, endoscopes, and electrical equipment, but the process is difficult to control and requires bacteriological monitoring. It is not to be used when alternative methods, such as sub-atmospheric steam (steam at a lower atmospheric pressure than normal) and formaldehyde, are available (see p. 657).

PRACTICAL STERILISATION

The present tendency in hospitals is to use pre-sterilised, disposable equipment whenever possible, e.g. rubber gloves, scalpel blades, needles, syringes, biopsy punches, haemodialysis equipment, etc. Nevertheless, there are occasions when sterilisation must be performed on the spot, and it is useful to consider the disinfection of a few articles in common hospital use.

Dressings, theatre apparel, and gloves, should all be autoclaved. Provided the autoclave is working properly, there is no reason why gloves should perish in it. Destruction is due to oxidation, and if the air is completely expelled this cannot happen.

Surgical instruments. These too should be autoclaved. Some surgeons object to the heating of sharp-edged instruments because of the alleged blunting that follows. This is due to oxidation, and should not occur in a properly functioning autoclave.

Chemical sterilisation of cutting instruments cannot be relied on, and should be abolished. There is, however, a place for disinfectants in regard to endoscopes.

Catheters. Rubber and plastic catheters can be boiled (spore-bearing organisms do not cause urinary-tract infections). Silk-web (gum-elastic) catheters are most difficult to sterilise. The usual method is suspension in formaldehyde gas, but this is quite inefficient, and in addition does not penetrate properly. If they are immersed in glutaraldehyde or mercuric chloride solutions, they will certainly be disinfected, but the agents have then to be removed prior to the use of the catheter. This is very difficult without an elaborate rinsing of the lumen. More recently 0·2 per cent chlorhexidine solution has been tried. Ethylene oxide vapour is another possibility. In fact no method is really satisfactory, and we must hope that disposable catheters, which are sterilised commercially by γ-radiation, will soon be available in bulk.

Cystoscopes and other endoscopes. These instruments do not tolerate heat well, but many can be adequately disinfected by pasteurisation in water at 75°C; alternatively low-temperature steam can be used, with or without the addition of formaldehyde.

The chemical disinfectants that can be used are glutaraldehyde (2 per cent) or alcoholic chlorhexidine (0·5 per cent).

Polythene tubing. Heat causes softening; ionising radiation or ethylene oxide are the best sterilisers.

Anaesthetic face-masks. The mask with its rubber tubing is best disinfected by pasteurisation in water at 75°C. Chemical disinfectants may damage the skin of the face of the next patient.

Suture material. Catgut is now prepared under licence by a special patent process in order to prevent the possibility of surgical tetanus. If it is rendered unsterile, it can be re-sterilised by immersion in Lugol's iodine solution for 1 week. All other suture materials can be autoclaved. The heat causes shrinkage, so the spools should be loosely wound.

Syringes. Plastic disposable syringes are commonly used, but if not available, the all-glass type should be acquired. If the nozzle and shoulder is of metal, it should be attached to the glass body by a cement that can withstand a high temperature. If the cement is of poor quality, the syringe will have to be boiled. In practice it is best to discard all such syringes. Autoclaving is not as satisfactory as dry heat in a hot-air oven, because the steam has to penetrate right through the syringe for sterilisation to be complete. This is impossible if a lubricated plunger is placed in position beforehand. In any case some moisture is bound to remain. This will cause haemolysis if the syringe is used to collect blood for diagnostic purposes.

Fomites. *Urinals and bed-pans*, if not of the disposable variety, should be disinfected by heat. The carrier for a disposable bed-pan should be washed and dried after use, or disinfected with a strong phenolic compound, e.g. 'Hycolin', 'Stericol', or 'Clearsol', if it has been used by an infected patient. A similar type of phenolic disinfectant can be used for urinals as an alternative to heat.

Bowls should be autoclaved if used surgically. Those used for washing should be cleaned with a detergent. If they are used by infected patients they should be disinfected with heat or a phenolic compound, as already mentioned.

Oral thermometers should be disinfected in an iodine solution, e.g. 1 per cent iodine in 70 per cent ethanol, or in a phenolic compound. They are rinsed and stored dry.

Bedding. Sheets, cotton blankets, and bed-covers are boiled in the laundering process. Mattresses and pillows should be completely enclosed in plastic covers. Then a mere washing outside the cover with soap and water is adequate; a phenolic disinfectant can be added if the patient has an infection.

If the mattress or pillow is itself contaminated it will have to be disinfected with low-temperature steam or formaldehyde.

Rooms. A contaminated room should be disinfected with hot formalin vapour. A less drastic procedure is a washing of all surfaces, including furniture, with a detergent solution and hypochlorite.

Disinfection of skin. As already mentioned, there is no effective method of skin sterilisation. An excellent agent for the pre-operative treatment of skin is tincture of iodine; a patch test should be performed before the operation to detect the hypersensitive patient. Dilute (70 per cent) ethanol on its own is satisfactory, but cetrimide cannot be relied on. Another good skin disinfectant is 0.5 per cent chlorhexidine in 70 per cent ethanol, but povidone-iodine containing 1 per cent available iodine is better. For surgical personnel an alcoholised chlorhexidine solution is valuable. The continual use of hexachlorophane liquid soap, preferably containing a phenolic preservative chlorocresol (0.3 per cent), is slightly less effective.

The ritual of applying an antiseptic to the skin for a few seconds before taking a blood sample or giving an injection, although commonly practised, is of limited value, and its omission does not seem to result in local infection. When complete asepsis is required, as with intra-articular or intrathecal manipulations, a thorough skin preparation is necessary.

After attending an infected patient, the hands should be thoroughly scrubbed, and then immersed in an alcohol or hypochlorite solution.

GENERAL READING

For further information the following sources are recommended:

CRUICKSHANK, R., DUGUID, J. P., MARMION, B. P. & SWAIN, R. H. A. (1973) *Medical Microbiology*, 12th edn, Vol. 1 (*Microbial Infections*). See chapter 5: Sterilization and Disinfection. Edinburgh: Churchill Livingstone.
LOWBURY, E. J. L., AYLIFFE, G. A. J., GEDDES, A. M. & WILLIAMS, J. D. (1975) *Control of Hospital Infection*. London: Chapman and Hall.
WILSON, G. S. & MILES, A. A. (1975) Topley and Wilson's *Principles of Bacteriology, Virology and Immunity*, 6th edn, pp. 144–186. London: Arnold. This gives a good account of the principles of disinfection with special regard to chemical agents.

Appendix 2.   The Principles of Bacteriological Diagnosis

THE GENERAL PROPERTIES OF BACTERIA

CONSTITUTION

Although bacteria are generally unicellular, they are often found attached one to another in the form of clusters, chains, or, in the higher *Actinomyces* organisms, an elaborate mass of filaments.

Bacteria vary in size: staphylococci and streptococci are 0·75 to 1·25 μm in diameter, while one of the largest bacilli, *Bacillus anthracis*, is 1 to 1·25 μm thick and 3 to 8 μm long. *Haemophilus influenzae* is a very small bacterium, measuring 0·2 to 0·4 μm × 0·7 to 1·5 μm.

The bacterial body is contained in a rigid cell wall 10 to 25 nm thick, which encloses a thin cytoplasmic membrane 5 to 10 nm thick, composed of lipoprotein. On electron microscopy the bacterial cytoplasm is homogeneous and granular. This granularity is due to innumerable ribosomes which contain RNA and manufacture the bacterial proteins and enzymes. There is no endoplasmic reticulum and no mitochondria. The enzymes are present in the cytoplasmic membrane.

The bacterial DNA is contained in the nuclear body. This has no nuclear membrane, nucleolus, or separate chromosomes. It appears that all the bacterial genes are contained by a single linkage group, or chromosome. It is probably a long fibre folded on itself in the form of a skein. There is usually only one nuclear body in each bacterium, but as its division precedes that of the bacterial cell, there is often the suggestion of two, four, or even more.

Bacteria divide by simple binary fission which involves the nuclear body also. There is no evidence of mitosis. The cell divides into two by constriction with or without primary septation. A few groups exhibit sexual conjugation.

ASSOCIATED STRUCTURES

Intracellular granules. Many organisms contain granular aggregations of metabolic substances in their cytoplasm, e.g. volutin, lipid, and starch. *Volutin granules* are particularly important. They stain metachromatically with toluidine blue, turning a violet colour. The nature of volutin granules is obscure; they are said to contain polymerised inorganic polyphosphate which may act as a reserve of energy for cell metabolism. They are of importance in the identification of *Corynebacterium diphtheriae*.

Capsules. A capsule is a gelatinous layer 0·2 μm or more in width which covers the wall of a bacterium. It is usually composed of polysaccharide, but sometimes it is of polypeptide or protein nature. Capsules are of the greatest importance in contributing to the virulence of an organism, and are also of use in typing procedures; both these features are, of course, due to the specific antigens or haptens contained in them. Important capsulated bacteria are the pneumococcus,

Clostridium welchii, *B. anthracis*, and *Klebsiella pneumoniae*.

Flagella. These are filamentous appendages which act as organs of locomotion, and are possessed by all motile bacteria except spirochaetes, whose motility is apparently a function of the bacterial body itself. Flagella originate in the cytoplasm, and protrude through the cell wall. They contain a protein called *flagellin*, which is related to *myosin*, the contractile protein of muscle.

Fimbriae. These too are filamentous appendages. They are shorter and thinner than flagella, and have nothing to do with locomotion, since they are found in non-motile organisms. It is possible that they act as organs of adhesion to free surfaces.

Spores. A spore is a highly resistant resting phase of a bacterium. It is formed within the body of the organism, i.e. it is an endospore, and eventually the whole organism is converted into a single, thick-walled mass which is round or oval in shape, and highly refractile.

Sporulation in bacteria is not a process of multiplication; it is merely a method of survival during unfavourable circumstances, e.g. starvation, desiccation, extremes of temperature, and unsuitable atmospheric conditions. It incorporates some of the chromatin material as well as the bacterial cytoplasm. Spores are characteristic of only a few genera, e.g. *Bacillus* and *Clostridium*. They appear either subterminally, terminally, or equatorially in relation to the bacterial body, and eventually the remainder of the organism disintegrates. The free spore survives, and germinates when conditions are propitious.

L-forms. These are degenerate bacterial variants, first described in the Lister Institute, London (hence the letter L), which are seen in connexion with cocci, bacilli, and vibrios. They lack a rigid cell wall and therefore vary greatly in size and shape—the largest are 10 to 20 μm long and the smallest only 0·1 μm in diameter. They are resistant to the action of penicillin regardless of the sensitivity of the parent organism. L-forms can be isolated from patients with bacterial infections especially if on penicillin or cephalosporin treatment, and can also be induced in culture by drugs, lysozyme, nutritional deficiency, or the action of amboceptor and complement. A variant of L-form obtained from Gram-positive organisms by the action of penicillin or lysozyme is called the *protoplast*. It contains no cell wall, and differs from the usual L-forms in that it can survive only in a hypertonic environment and usually fails to grow in artificial media. Similar spherical variants of Gram-negative organisms have a cell wall which is defective due to the absence of a strengthening mucoprotein. These are called *spheroplasts*. Protoplasts and spheroplasts are laboratory artefacts. L-forms, unlike protoplasts and spheroplasts, can multiply on an artificial medium, on which characteristic tiny 'fried-egg' colonies are produced.

Some L-forms revert to the normal bacterial form especially if the inducing agent, e.g. penicillin, is removed. Others however, are stable and do not revert. These resemble myco-plasma in appearance, but tend to be somewhat larger. They are said to be non-pathogenic to animals, and their re-lationship to disease is not known (see p. 93).

DEMONSTRATION OF BACTERIA

Unstained preparations are of limited value. The general shape and motility can be ascertained in fluid preparations viewed between a glass slide and a cover-slip. Some or-ganisms, e.g. the spirochaetes, are so slender and feebly refractile that only dark-ground illumination can reveal their presence (Fig. 1.1, p. 2).

Staining. *Organisms can be made visible with simple stains* like methylene blue and basic fuchsin.

The Gram technique is of greater value, because it helps to distinguish between different groups of organisms. It is de-scribed later on. A Gram-positive organism resists decol-orisation by alcohol or acetone after it has been stained with a pararosaniline dye, e.g. crystal violet or methyl violet, and then treated with an iodine solution. A Gram-negative or-ganism is decolorised, and takes up the red counter-stain.

This difference in Gram-staining is fundamental, and is reflected in basic differences in the reaction of the organism to antibiotics and disinfectants. Its mechanism is uncertain. It is established that Gram-positivity depends on the integrity of the cellular structure and the presence in the cell of a specific magnesium ribonucleate-protein complex. If the magnesium ribonucleate is removed, a Gram-positive organism becomes Gram-negative. What part the cell wall plays in aiding (or preventing) decolorisation is unknown; it is possible that the wall of a Gram-positive organism is less permeable to the decoloriser than that of a Gram-negative organism.

Flagella and capsules can be demonstrated only by special techniques,* and fimbriae are revealed by means of the electron microscope. Spores appear as clear spaces within Gram-stained organisms; they do not take up the stain, no doubt because of their thick walls.

Ziehl-Neelsen staining. This is also described later on. It depends on the fact that a few organisms, notably the genus *Mycobacterium*, are particularly rich in lipids. These not only prevent the entry of the usual stains, but also retain any concentrated stain that may have been forced into them by the process of heating. Even strong acid will then not decolorise these organisms. If the lipids are extracted with fat solvents, this *acid-fastness* is lost.

SHAPE

The following shapes are recognised:

Cocci—spherical (or nearly spherical) cells, e.g. *Staphylococcus aureus.*

Bacilli—straight and rod-shaped cells, e.g. *Escherichia coli.*

Vibrios—curved and rod-shaped cells—'comma-shaped', e.g. *Vibrio cholerae.*

Capsules are best demonstrated by 'negative' or 'relief' staining, in which a smear of the organisms is stained with India ink. The unstained capsular areas contrast with the refractile organism and the diffusely stained background.
Flagella are so thin that they can be made visible with the light microscope only after a thick layer of stain has been deposited on them. A mixture of basic fuchsin and tannic acid is efficacious.

Spirilla—spirally-twisted rods which are not capable of bending, e.g. *Spirillum minus.*

Spirochaetes—these resemble spirilla, but have an intrin-sic bending motion, e.g. *Treponema pallidum.*

Actinomycetes—simple branching filaments aggregated into compact colonies, e.g. *Actinomyces bovis.*

NUTRITIONAL DEMANDS

Nearly all bacteria can grow on artificial cell-free media (*Myco. leprae* and *Tr. pallidum* are exceptions). The nut-ritional requirements are:

(*a*) A source of energy for such metabolic processes as growth and motility.

(*b*) A source of carbon, nitrogen, various inorganic salts, e.g. sulphates and phosphates of sodium, potassium, calcium, and iron, and finally certain *accessory growth factors*. These are 'bacterial vitamins', and are necessary for the synthesis of essential metabolites in certain organisms.

Some non-parasitic bacteria are able to utilise CO_2 as a source of carbon, while energy is obtained from the oxidation of inorganic chemicals or directly from sunlight. Most bac-teria, however, including all the parasitic ones, require organic nutrients such as carbohydrate, amino acids, and lipids. Some, e.g. *Esch. coli*, are able to synthesise their own amino acids from a source of inorganic nitrogen such as nitrates or ammonium salts.

Most of the pathogens are very exacting in their demands, and require a wide range of amino acids, e.g. tryptophan, methionine, and histidine, and growth factors, e.g. purines and pyrimidines, for nucleic-acid synthesis, and most of the vitamin-B group as precursors for the formation of co-enzymes.

In addition, bacteria vary widely in their oxygen require-ments. Obligatory anaerobes cannot tolerate the presence of oxygen, perhaps because they are damaged by the peroxides they produce. Normally these are destroyed by the enzyme catalase, but anaerobes are lacking in it.

GROWTH PHASES

When bacteria are inoculated into a sterile fluid culture medium and serial counts are performed on viable organisms, the following four phases of multiplication are noted:

Lag phase, which lasts about 2 hours. There is no change in number, though the size of the bacteria increases.

Logarithmic phase, which lasts up to eight hours in optimal conditions. There is a regular, maximal proliferation of bacteria increasing in geometrical progression per unit time.

Stationary phase, which lasts for several hours to a few days. There is no increase in numbers, as the death rate is as great as that of reproduction.

Phase of decline, which is completed from a few days to some months. The viable count gradually diminishes until the culture becomes sterile once more. The cause of the decline is presumably a combination of exhaustion of nutriment and an accumulation of toxic waste matter.

THE DIAGNOSIS OF INFECTIVE DISEASE

This is based on three postulates originally laid down by Koch (*Koch's postulates*).

1. *The organism should be found in the lesion in a quantity adequate to account for its effects.* In toxic bacterial infections, e.g. due to *C. diphtheriae* and *Cl. tetani*, the remote effects are due to exotoxins, and the organism is present only in the local lesion. Organisms that act by hypersensitivity, e.g. *Myco. tuberculosis* and *Tr. pallidum*, are sometimes very scanty in the lesions they produce, e.g. gummata. On the other hand, carriers may transmit pathogenic organisms in the absence of overt pathological lesions.

2. *The organism from the lesion should be cultivated in a pure state on an artificial medium.* Most bacteria fulfil this requirement; *Myco. leprae* and *Tr. pallidum* are exceptions. The cultivation of viruses requires living cells (see Ch. 22).

3. *The organism grown in artificial culture should be capable of producing a similar lesion in another member of the species.* Theoretically this would entail human transference, which is impracticable except in volunteers. Animal inoculation is used instead of this. As regards viruses the second and third postulates merge when the animal provides the living cells necessary for viral growth. On the whole, animal inoculation does not play an important part in routine bacteriological diagnosis; tuberculosis is an exception. Other bacterial infections in which animal inoculation is necessary for diagnosis are diphtheria, anthrax, plague, glanders, and leptospiral jaundice.

A fourth postulate was added after Koch's time: *the presence in the circulation of antibodies against the organism in the later stages of the illness and during convalescence.*

It therefore follows that in routine bacteriological diagnosis the organism should be isolated from the pathological material:

(*a*) by demonstrating it directly using Gram's or Ziehl-Neelsen's stains.

(*b*) by culturing it on suitable media. Animal inoculation is seldom necessary.

If the organism is scanty, e.g. in the blood, it may be demonstrable only by culture methods. Direct examination is seldom successful.

PRACTICAL BACTERIOLOGY

COLLECTION OF SPECIMENS

Pus. This may be taken on a swab, which should then be tightly inserted into a test-tube, so that it does not undergo desiccation. Large amounts of pus are conveniently collected in screw-capped universal containers.

Exudates, e.g. pleural fluid, are collected in universal containers. If a cytological examination is required, an anti-coagulant, e.g. potassium oxalate, should be added.

Urine. In both sexes a midstream specimen should be taken. Catheterisation should be avoided (see p. 234). The urine is collected in a universal container.

Sputum and faeces are collected in waxed or plastic cartons which are burnt and destroyed after use.

In the collection of specimens care must be taken to avoid (*a*) desiccation; (*b*) contamination of the specimen; (*c*) infection of personnel handling the material.

If the patient is some distance away from the laboratory, the organism may die before it can be cultured. Various transport media are available to prevent the organisms from drying and being overgrown by contaminants. Some contain charcoal to neutralise the possible effects of toxic lipoproteins on cotton swabs. A special medium is available for the gonococcus; it is called *Stuart's holding medium*, and consists of a soft agar base in which there is an anaerobic salt solution containing thioglycollic acid and also a methylene-blue solution. To protect the gonococcus during the period between collection and culture, the pus is collected on specially prepared swabs, which are then inserted into the medium. This is cultured on to the basic medium when it reaches the laboratory.

THE STAINING OF BACTERIA

The pus or exudate is transferred on to a clean slide, and a film is made. After drying, it is fixed on to the slide by passing it rapidly through a flame. Staining is then carried out:

Gram's stain. (i) 0·5 per cent methyl violet for about 1 minute.

(ii) Wash off with Lugol's or Gram's iodine, and apply more iodine solution for about 2 minutes.

(iii) Decolorise with ethanol until the stain ceases to come out of the preparation.

(iv) Wash with water, and counter-stain with 0·1 per cent neutral red for about 2 minutes.

Gram-positive organisms, e.g. staphylococci, streptococci, pneumococci, clostridia, anthrax bacilli, diphtheria bacilli, actinomyces, and fungi, stain blue, whereas *Gram-negative organisms*, e.g. *Neisseria* organisms and intestinal bacilli of the coli-typhoid type, stain red. The nuclei of pus cells are also Gram-negative.

Ziehl-Neelsen stain. This is reserved for *Mycobacteria*, the waxy content of which is impermeable to Gram's stain.

(i) Flood strong carbol fuchsin on to the slide, and keep it steaming for 5 minutes.

(ii) Wash with water, and then apply 20 per cent sulphuric acid. This is washed off after about a minute, and reapplied several times until no more stain comes out of the preparation.

(iii) Wash with water, and apply absolute ethanol for 2 minutes.*

(iv) Wash with water, and counter-stain with 1 per cent methylene blue or malachite green for about 20 seconds.

Acid-fast material stains red; everything else is blue or green. *Myco. leprae* is less acid fast than *Myco. tuberculosis*, and the preparation should either be decolorised with 5 per cent sulphuric acid or some other modification used, e.g. the Fite stain. Some *Nocardia* species are also acid fast, and so are the granules of lipofuscin. These granules are sometimes a source of confusion, particularly when present in a lesion of sarcoidosis. The Ziehl-Neelsen method also stains keratin and chitin, and can be used to demonstrate the hooklets found in echinococcal cysts and the chitinous shells of *Schistosoma* ova.

THE CULTIVATION OF BACTERIA

Culture media are divided into 2 classes, fluid and solid:

Fluid media. The basic medium is called *nutrient broth*, which is a mixture of meat extract (Lab-Lemco), commercial

---

*3 per cent HCl in 95 per cent ethanol may be substituted for (ii) and (iii).

bacteriological peptone (a mixture of peptones, amino acids, vitamins, and salts, obtained from the enzymatic breakdown of lean meat and other protein material), sodium chloride, and water.

Some laboratories make up their own broth by extracting lean beef or ox heart muscle in watery solution and then adding peptone and salt (*infusion broth*), or by digesting the meat with trypsin (*digest broth*), in which case peptone does not need to be added. A special fluid medium is *Robertson's meat medium* (cooked meat broth), which is useful for culturing anaerobes (see Ch. 18).

Fluid media are useful for promoting the growth of bacteria when these are scanty, but they have two disadvantages:

(i) They are of little value in identifying individual organisms.

(ii) They are of no use in separating mixtures of organisms.

Solid media. The usual solidifying element in solid media is agar, a polysaccharide substance derived from certain seaweeds, and the basic solid medium is *nutrient agar*. This consists of nutrient broth solidified by the addition of agar (1·2 to 2 per cent depending on the type). It forms a gel, stable at temperatures well above 37°C.

Nutrient agar can support the growth of some organisms, e.g. staphylococci, but others, like streptococci and *Neisseria* organisms, require the presence of blood or serum products. This is described as *enrichment* of a medium. Although nutrient agar melts at about 95°C, it remains fluid on subsequent cooling down to a temperature as low as 40°C. Therefore blood or serum can be incorporated into molten nutrient agar at about 45°C, at which temperature there is no denaturation of its proteins.

Solid media are usually distributed in flat plastic plates called Petri dishes. They may also be placed in small bottles, universal containers, or test-tubes. The molten medium is allowed to solidify while the container is tilted at an angle. This is a 'slope' culture medium.

Blood agar. This consists of 5 to 10 per cent horse blood in nutrient agar. It is the standard solid medium used in bacteriological laboratories.

Serum agar. This consists of 10 per cent animal serum in nutrient agar. It is useful for the cultivation of gonococci and meningococci, and for demonstrating the volutin granules of *C. diphtheriae*.

Chocolate agar. This is blood agar which is heated to boiling point for about a minute. The breakdown products of haemoglobin, especially haematin ('X Factor'), are useful for the growth of *H. influenzae*.

Solid media enable individual bacteria to grow into discrete, recognisable colonies, and are essential for the identification of organisms. If there are few bacteria in a specimen, it is wise to start with a fluid medium and then to subculture some of this on to a solid medium.

Selective media. If certain substances are added to a fluid or solid medium, they may promote the growth of a particular type of bacterium while inhibiting that of all other organisms. The following selective media are commonly used:

MacConkey's medium. This consists of a peptone solution solidified with agar, to which is added a bile salt (sodium taurocholate), lactose, and a neutral-red indicator. The bile salt inhibits most organisms, but promotes the growth of the Gram-negative intestinal group. *Esch. coli* ferments lactose, and turns the indicator pink (see Ch. 17).

Deoxycholate-citrate-agar. This works on the same principle as the MacConkey's medium, but sodium deoxycholate is used instead of sodium taurocholate, and sodium citrate, sodium thiosulphate, and ferric ammonium citrate are included. These salts inhibit the growth of *Esch. coli* while promoting that of *Salmonella* and *Shigella* organisms. This medium is used for the bacteriological examination of faeces, because even in the presence of a typhoid or dysentery infection there is such a predominance of *Esch. coli* that a MacConkey plate would be overgrown with this organism at the expense of all others.

Tetrathionate broth and selenite-F enrichment medium. These two fluid media contain sodium tetrathionate and sodium selenite respectively. These salts are particularly inhibitory to coliform organisms, while allowing *Salmonella* organisms to grow freely. If faeces contain scanty numbers of these organisms, it is best to culture them initially in these selective fluid media, and then to subculture them a day later on to deoxycholate-citrate-agar.

Potassium tellurite media. A considerable number of media containing this salt are in use for the selective growth and identification of *C. diphtheriae*. They inhibit the growth of most of the other organisms found in the throat.

Sodium chloride is useful for the selective cultivation of staphylococci. It is conveniently incorporated into Robertson's meat medium in a 10 per cent concentration.

Sabouraud's medium. This simple medium contains only glucose and peptone as its nutrients, and the low pH and high sugar content make it selective for fungi as against bacterial contaminants. Antibacterial agents, usually chloramphenicol and cycloheximide, are often added.

Temperature. Nearly all pathogenic organisms grow best at body temperature (37°C). *Myco. ulcerans* and *Myco. marinum* are exceptions, growing best at 31 to 33°C. Rhinoviruses also need a temperature of 33°C, while some pathogenic fungi grow at room temperature.

Atmospheric conditions. Most organisms flourish well in air, but a few are strict anaerobes (e.g. clostridia). If their presence is suspected, the medium must be incubated in a *McIntosh and Fildes anaerobic jar*. Alternatively, Robertson's meat medium can be used. Gonococci demand an atmosphere containing 5 per cent CO_2, and *Brucella abortus* one of 10 per cent CO_2.

EXAMINATION OF INDIVIDUAL SPECIMENS

PUS

The usual organisms to be expected in pus are:

Pyogenic cocci, i.e. staphylococci and streptococci.

Gram-negative intestinal bacilli.

Clostridial organisms in infected wounds. These organisms seldom occur alone, but are found together with the others.

Myco. tuberculosis and *Actino. israeli* in chronic lesions.

Smear and Gram-stain. In true pus there are numerous pus cells and usually groups of causative organisms among them. If there is only amorphous debris, it is suggestive of tuberculosis.

Culture on blood agar aerobically and anaerobically. Anaerobic culture is essential in all pus from infected wounds, and some of the material must also be inoculated into Robertson's meat medium in case the anaerobic technique is faulty. The meat medium can be subcultured on to blood-agar the next day. In pus from abdominal wounds MacConkey's medium may be used in addition to blood agar because of the probability of infection with Gram-negative intestinal bacilli.

After 24 hours the plates are examined. Staphylococci are coagulase tested, and β-haemolytic streptococci may be Lancefield grouped (see Ch. 17). The Gram-negative intestinal group may need further investigation. If clostridia are isolated, a Nagler test (see Ch. 18) is worth performing. Antibiotic sensitivities are carried out on all pathogenic organisms.

If *tuberculosis* is suspected, a Ziehl-Neelsen stain should be done on the pus (it is usually negative), and some of the material should be inoculated on to Löwenstein-Jensen medium, and some injected into a guinea-pig (see Ch. 20). Six weeks may elapse before a positive result is forthcoming.

If *actinomycosis* is suspected, the pathognomonic sulphur granules must be isolated by shaking up the pus in sterile water. The granules sink rapidly to the bottom, and are easily removed by suction with a Pasteur pipette. They are then crushed between two slides and stained. Some are inoculated on to blood agar and incubated anaerobically (see Ch. 20).

URINE

The usual infecting organisms are:

(*a*) Gram-negative intestinal bacilli.

(*b*) *Strept. faecalis.*

(*c*) *Myco. tuberculosis*, an important cause of 'sterile' pyuria.

Centrifuge some of the urine at about 2000 revolutions per minute for 5 to 10 minutes, and examine a drop of the unstained deposit under the low power of a microscope at once. The presence of white cells ('pus cells'), red cells, and casts is to be noted. Sometimes motile organisms can be seen among the cells. Gram-staining is not necessary as a routine measure.

More than one white cell per high power field is abnormal, and then the urine should be cultured on blood agar. Anaerobic culture is not necessary. MacConkey's medium can also be used.

The urine normally contains a small number of bacteria that are merely an expression of contamination by organisms resident in the urethra. A Gram stain on a smear of *fresh uncentrifuged* urine should be examined, and if organisms are seen a urinary-tract infection is generally present. A more precise investigation is the *bacterial count*. Urinary-tract infections are associated with a count of above 100 000 per ml.

Another test of some value is the *white-cell excretion rate*; if above 200 000 cells per hour it is probably abnormal. Unfortunately it is difficult to distinguish between leucocytes and epithelial cells, but it is less crude than the centrifugation method.

In the investigation of *tuberculosis* it is best to collect three consecutive early-morning specimens of urine, centrifuge them, and stain and culture the sediments.

PLEURAL AND PERITONEAL EXUDATES

The infecting organisms may be pyogenic cocci, e.g. pneumococci, or else *Myco. tuberculosis.*

Smear and Gram-stain of centrifuged deposit.

Culture on to blood agar. It is advisable to culture some of the specimen in nutrient broth, because organisms tend to be scanty in exudates. The broth is subcultured on to blood agar the next day.

If *tuberculosis* is suspected, it is useful to examine the cells in some detail. A tuberculous effusion contains a large number of lymphocytes. The sediment is then stained and cultured.

CEREBROSPINAL FLUID

The important infecting organisms are (*a*) meningococci, (*b*) pneumococci, (*c*) *H. influenzae*, (*d*) *Esch. coli* (in the neonatal period), and (*e*) *Myco. tuberculosis.* The first four produce a purulent fluid, whereas that of tuberculous meningitis is clear and colourless. A 'spider-web clot' tends to form as the tuberculous fluid sediments in the universal container.

Cell count. This is normally not more than 3 lymphocytes per μl.

Biochemistry. The normal range is:

Protein   0·15 to 0·4 g per litre
Glucose   2·8 to 3·9 mmol per litre (50 to 70 mg per dl)
Chloride   120 to 127 mmol per litre

The protein content is raised in all types of meningitis (including viral ones). Both sugar and chloride levels are reduced in all types of bacterial meningitis especially the tuberculous variety.

Smear and Gram-stain of centrifuged deposit. In tuberculous cases some of the spider-web clot is spread on to a slide and stained by the Ziehl-Neelsen method.

Culture on to blood agar; serum agar is useful for meningococci, and chocolate agar for *H. influenzae.* If tuberculosis is suspected, the sediment is carefully collected and cultured.

A fungal meningitis closely resembling the tuberculous variety both in cellular reaction and biochemistry is caused by *Cryptococcus neoformans.* The capsules of the organisms are sometimes small, and the cryptococci can easily be mistaken for lymphocytes if the diagnosis is not considered. Wet films mixed with India ink show up the capsules by contrast. The fluid should be cultured on Sabouraud's medium as well as blood agar, and the cultures should be retained for at least 2 weeks before being reported as negative.

The term *aseptic meningitis* is applied to clinical conditions of meningitis in which the cerebrospinal fluid contains an excess of cells (mostly lymphocytes) and protein, but is bacteriologically sterile. It is usually caused by viruses, e.g. (*a*) enteroviruses including polioviruses, (*b*) lymphocytic choriomeningitis virus, (*c*) togaviruses, (*d*) bunyaviruses, (*e*) herpes-simplex virus, (*f*) occasionally as a complication of zoster, vaccinia, mumps (which causes a specific encephalitis), measles, influenza, and chickenpox.

BLOOD CULTURE

The important organisms are *Strept. viridans* in subacute

infective endocarditis; *Salmonella typhi* and *S. paratyphi A, B, and C*; *Staph. aureus* and *Strept. pyogenes*; Gram-negative pyogenic intestinal bacilli; *Brucella* organisms.

About 5 to 10 ml of blood is collected aseptically from a forearm vein, and is cultured in 50 to 100 ml of nutrient or digest broth. A large amount of blood is needed, because organisms are usually very scanty even in pronounced septicaemias. A large amount of medium is used in order to dilute natural bactericidal and bacteriostatic substances present in the blood. Trypsin or 'Liquoid' (sodium polyanethol sulphonate) is often incorporated into the broth to annul any such bactericidal activity. In cases of suspected typhoid fever some of the blood should be inoculated into broth containing 0·5 per cent sodium taurocholate. Penicillinase may be added if the patient has been treated with penicillin.

Occasionally subacute infective endocarditis is caused by an anaerobic streptococcus or *Bacteroides*; it is therefore advisable to inoculate some of the blood anaerobically in a suitable medium, e.g. cooked-meat broth.

Coxiella burneti is another cause of endocarditis. If this is suspected, some of the blood must be inoculated into the yolk-sac of a fertile egg.

The broth is incubated for 24 hours, and then films of it are made and stained with Gram's stain. Some of it is subcultured on to blood agar (and MacConkey's medium, if typhoid fever is likely). This procedure is repeated for 4 consecutive days and after the first and second weeks. After 14 days the culture may be discarded except if brucellosis is suspected, when at least 3 weeks should elapse before a negative result is reported. For *Br. abortus* the blood culture must be incubated in an atmosphere of 10 per cent CO_2.

Under unusual circumstances, as following open-heart surgery or in patients on immunosuppressive therapy, endocarditis may be caused by almost any organism, including some like *Staph. albus* that are generally considered to be non-pathogenic, and also fungi. The repeated culture of an organism from the blood-stream should not be lightly dismissed as due to contamination.

SPUTUM

This contains a large number of organisms, e.g. staphylococci, streptococci, pneumococci, Gram-negative intestinal bacilli, and *H. influenzae*. These are isolated quite easily by aerobic culture on blood agar. Colonies of *H. influenzae* tend to aggregate around staphylococcal colonies, a feature called *satellitism*. This is because staphylococci synthesise a factor (the 'V factor') which is essential for the growth of *H. influenzae*.

The most important bacterium to be sought in sputum is *Myco. tuberculosis*. When present it should be easily detectable on direct examination. A purulent portion is selected and stained by the Ziehl-Neelsen technique, or else fluorescence microscopy can be used after staining with auramine. In this case the auramine is simply substituted for strong carbol fuchsin. Under the fluorescence microscope the organisms are yellow and luminous against a black background.

In culturing for *Myco. tuberculosis* the sputum must first be homogenised in alkaline or acid solutions, which destroy other organisms while leaving the tubercle bacilli intact. Guinea-pig inoculation should not often be required; direct examination confirmed by Löwenstein-Jensen culture is generally adequate and indeed essential if atypical mycobacteria are to be identified. Culture is important to assess the sensitivity of the organism to antituberculous agents.

FAECES

The important pathogenic bacteria in faeces are the *Salmonella* and *Shigella* species. Enteropathogenic *Esch. coli* may cause epidemics of infantile diarrhoea.

Emulsify a suspicious portion of the faeces with saline, and examine it microscopically (unstained). The presence of pus cells suggests a bacillary type of dysentery, but ulcerative colitis and carcinoma of the colon may produce a similar appearance. The presence of amoebae, cysts, and parasitic ova is also noted.

Some of the faeces are inoculated directly on to deoxycholate-citrate-agar, and some into tetrathionate and selenite-F enrichment media.

The next day colourless colonies are sought on the solid medium, and at the same time the fluid enrichment media are subcultured on to deoxycholate-citrate-agar. They are examined the next day.

Colourless colonies are picked off and subcultured in peptone water.

About 6 hours later the peptone water is subcultured into other peptone waters containing various sugars (e.g. lactose, glucose, mannitol, and saccharose) and a pH indicator. Into the fluid medium there is placed a small inverted tube called a *Durham fermentation tube*. Within 24 hours the organism will have formed acid (with or without gas, which accumulates in the Durham tube) with some, all, or none of the sugars. The table below gives an indication of how the fermentation reactions help in the identification of these organisms.

Other tests of value are indole formation in peptone water (in some *Shigella* species) and urea decomposition to ammonia (which excludes *Proteus* organisms).

Finally, identification is performed by means of agglutination reactions, using specific antisera prepared from rabbits immunised against these organisms.

For enteropathogenic *Esch. coli*, MacConkey's medium is used. It is impossible to distinguish between enteropathogenic and non-enteropathogenic strains by their colonial appearance. All that can be done is to pick off a number of colonies from the plate and perform agglutination tests using specific antisera obtained by immunising rabbits against known enteropathogenic strains.

Organism	Lactose	Glucose	Mannitol	Saccharose
Salmonella typhi	Nil	Acid only	Acid only	Nil
Salmonella typhimurium	Nil	Acid and gas	Acid and gas	Nil
Shigella sonnei	Delayed acid only	Acid only	Acid only	Delayed acid only
Shigella dysenteriae	Nil	Acid only	Nil	Nil

Table showing fermentation reactions of some common intestinal Gram-negative organisms.

THROAT SWAB. Important organisms to be sought are *Strept. pyogenes* and *C. diphtheriae*.

Smear and Gram-stain is useful for demonstrating *Borrelia vincenti*, *Fusobacterium fusiforme*, and *Candida albicans*.

Culture. (i) Blood agar for streptococci and *Candida albicans*.

(ii) Serum agar is excellent for stimulating the development of volutin granules in *C. diphtheriae*.

(iii) Tellurite selective media of the solid type not only favour the growth of *C. diphtheriae*, but also show colonial differences between the three types of the organism—gravis, intermedius, and mitis.

If suspicious colonies appear on the tellurite plate, sugar reactions (using serum-water) are carried out to differentiate between harmless diphtheroid organisms and diphtheria bacilli, which ferment glucose but not sucrose.

Finally, pathogenicity tests are performed on guinea-pigs.

GENERAL READING

For further information the following sources are recommended:

WILSON, G. S. & MILES, A. A. (1975) Topley and Wilson's *Principles of Bacteriology, Virology, and Immunity*, 6th edn, pp. 24–143. London: Arnold. This constitutes a comprehensive account of bacterial morphology, metabolism, and growth.

CRUICKSHANK, R., DUGUID, J. P., MARMION, B. P., & SWAIN, R. H. A. (1973) *Medical Microbiology*, 12th edn, Vol. 1, 667 pp. *Microbial Infections*, and (1975) Vol. 2, 587 pp. *The Practice of Medical Microbiology*. Edinburgh: Churchill Livingstone.

DAVIS, B. D., DULBECCO, R., EISEN, H. N., GINSBERG, H. S., & WOOD, W. B. (1973) *Microbiology*, 2nd edn, 1562 pp. New York: Harper and Row.

YOUMANS, G. P., PATERSON, P. Y. & SOMMERS, H. M. (1975) *The Biologic and Clinical Basis of Infectious Diseases*. See Chapter 10. The laboratory diagnosis of bacterial and fungal infections. Philadelphia: Saunders.

Appendix 3. The Physics of Ionising Radiation

One pictures an atom as composed of a central nucleus surrounded by a cloud of orbiting *electrons*. Practically all the mass of the atom resides in its nucleus, which (with the exception of hydrogen) consists of a densely-packed assembly of *protons* and *neutrons*. These two particles are of equal mass (1.66×10^{-24} g), the proton having a unit positive electrical charge and the neutron having none. An electron has a unit negative charge, but its mass is only about 1/2000 of that of a proton or neutron.

The so-called *atomic number* Z of an element is defined as the number of protons in the nucleus. With the atom in its normal state there is an equal number of orbiting electrons, so that as a whole the atom is electrically neutral. The chemical nature of an element is decided by the number Z. Thus an atom of atomic number Z has Z protons and Z electrons. The *mass number* is the total number of protons and neutrons present in the nucleus.

Hydrogen atom
Atomic Number 1
Mass Number 1

Deuterium atom
Atomic Number 1
Mass Number 2

Tritium atom
Atomic Number 1
Mass Number 3

Figure A3.1

Hydrogen (Z = 1, the lightest atom) is exceptional, in that in its most common form there are no neutrons in its nucleus but only a single proton, and there is but one orbiting electron. It therefore has the simplest possible atomic structure. It can also exist in two further forms, or *isotopes*.* Chemically these are identical, but they differ in those physical properties which are related to mass.

Atoms of higher atomic number have their electrons arranged in definite orbits, or shells, each of which can contain only a precise maximum number of electrons. Thus, the inner shell (K) can contain only two, as in helium.

Helium
Atomic Number 2
Mass Number 4

Hydrogen Molecule

Figure A3.2
Both the helium atom and the hydrogen molecule are stable.

*Many elements exist in nature as a mixture of isotopes each with the same atomic number Z, but with different mass numbers. The average of the mass numbers is the atomic weight. Thus, chlorine exists as a mixture of $^{35}_{17}Cl$ and $^{37}_{17}Cl$ in the proportion of almost exactly three to one, so that its atomic weight is 35.5.

The chemical stability of an atom depends upon the number of electrons in its outer shell. With the first shell two electrons give stability. The helium atom is stable, while hydrogen is not: the latter in fact usually exists as a molecule of two atoms, the one sharing its electron with the other. Oxygen (atomic number 8) has two electrons in its inner but six in its outer shell (maximum number in this shell is eight). With the exception of hydrogen and helium, atoms are most stable when their outer shells contain eight electrons, and they can attain this configuration in two ways. Firstly, one atom may donate an electron to another. As an example, $^{23}_{11}Na$ and $^{35}_{17}Cl$ (sodium and chlorine) combine as follows:

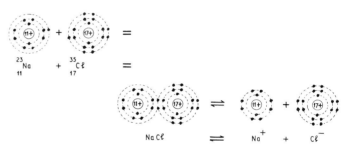

Figure A3.3
The atom of sodium is unstable because it has one electron in its outer shell. Likewise the chlorine atom is unstable due to its seven outer electrons. By donating an electron stable sodium chloride is formed. In solution this molecule may split to produce two charged and stable ions.

The sodium, by donating an electron, and chlorine, by acquiring an electron, both attain a stable configuration to form a molecule of sodium chloride. In solution they may exist as stable charged ions. The chemical properties of these ions, depending upon the number of electrons, are, of course, very different from those of the parent atoms. A second method of attaining stability is by way of a covalent linkage: in this, electrons are shared, not donated. For instance, water is:

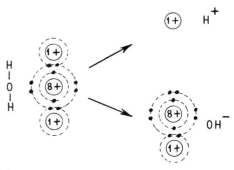

Figure A3.4

This molecule can be dissociated to form the two stable but charged ions: H^+, the positive hydrogen ion, and OH^-, the negative hydroxyl ion. It should be noted that the ions so far described in aqueous solution are stable, and facilitate the conduction of an electric current. The ions produced by the radiations to be described are of a different type, but nevertheless also increase electrical conductivity, e.g. in a gas.

Nature of Ionising Radiations

Certain naturally-occurring elements, like radium, continually emit radiations which may be of one or more of three types:

1. α-'rays'. These are, in fact, helium nuclei with mass of 4 and two positive charges.

2. β-'rays', which are electrons of negligible mass, but with one negative charge.

3. γ-'rays'. Electromagnetic waves of short wavelength, generally similar to X-rays.

X-rays. Electrons are emitted when a wire is heated, but normally do not escape because of their charge. As they have a negative charge, they can be drawn away by applying a strong electric field provided by a positive charge. This must be done in a vacuum, because they are readily stopped by any matter in their path (Fig. A3.5).

These streams of electrons are in fact similar to the naturally-occurring β-rays. Their energy is dependent upon the voltage applied. It is measured in electron volts, and with electrons is numerically equal to the voltage used to accelerate them. If the electrons hit a 'target', much of their energy is transformed into heat, the remainder appearing as electromagnetic radiations (X-rays) of varying wavelengths. The shortest wavelength of the spectrum produced in this way is dependent upon the energy of the electrons. When 20 kV is used in an X-ray tube, the rays have a long wavelength and relatively

poor penetrating power ('soft'). For many years machines with a 'harder' ray generated at about 250 kV were used. Nowadays X-rays generated at several million volts can be produced, and are commonly used in the treatment of cancer. The naturally-emitted γ-rays do not differ from these high energy X-rays. Thus the rays from ^{60}Co are the same as the hardest X-rays generated at about 1·2 MeV.*

Streams of electrons, protons, neutrons, and the charged nuclei of heavier atoms can be generated in various ways, and are being used in radiotherapy.

Changes Induced in Matter by the Passage of Ionising Radiation

The changes that occur have been studied mostly in gases, and it is assumed that liquids and solids behave in a similar manner.

β-Particles. Because of their charge and negligible mass they are rapidly slowed down, giving up their energy to atoms through which they pass. Electrons at 2 MeV have a maximum range of about 1 cm in water.

α-Particles. These have a double positive charge and a mass of 4. Because of their high charge and relatively low velocity, they have little penetrating power.

Protons. With mass of 1 and charge of +1 they are intermediate between γ-rays and β-particles in their power of penetration.

Neutrons. These particles with no charge and a mass of 1 can readily penetrate tissue, and are impeded only when they collide with atomic nuclei. With fast neutrons a proton is knocked out of the nucleus, and the effects are due to this released particle. With slow neutrons no proton is ejected, but the nucleus traps the neutron. In this way the atom increases its mass number by one, and frequently the isotope so formed is radioactive. It may then emit either β- or γ-rays or both, and (rarely) α-particles. Neutron-induced radioactivity is used in atomic reactors for manufacturing isotopes, and is one of the sources of the radioactivity following nuclear explosions. Electromagnetic radiation and β-particles of very high energy, e.g. over 8 MeV, may also induce radioactivity.

Gamma and X-rays. These electromagnetic radiations have great penetrating power; the shorter the wavelength, the greater their penetration. It should be noted that the particulate radiations have a definite range in matter: electromagnetic radiations, on the other hand, are merely reduced in quantity. Thus, a particular thickness of a material (the *half-value thickness*) will reduce the intensity by half, a further thickness by another half, etc. When they traverse matter, they give up quanta of energy which cause atoms to emit high-energy electrons. In this way a positive ion is formed. The electrons then behave like β-particles, causing other atoms to eject further electrons. These slower electrons are more readily deflected, and finally are caught in the orbit of some atom to produce a negative ion. For each electron ejected an ion pair is formed, and the *density of this ionisation* varies with the different radiations. The density of ionisation for charged particles is directly proportional to the square of their charge and inversely proportional to their velocity.

Figure A3.5
Diagrammatic representation of an X-ray tube. The filament is heated by a small electric current which can be varied. The emitted electrons are drawn to the target (anode) where they are stopped, and their energy converted into heat and X-radiation. A cooling mechanism is therefore required to dissipate the heat, while a suitable lead shield allows the X-rays to pass through only one controlled gap. The tube current (i.e. the electron stream between cathode and target) determines the quantity of X-rays generated. It is measured in milliamperes, mA, and is itself related to the temperature of the filament. The energy (i.e. wavelength) of the X-rays is related to the kilovoltage applied, and in the above diagram 250 kV is shown.

*The maximum energy of such X-rays is 1·2 MeV (million electron-volts). ^{60}Co emits 2 γ-rays of energy 1·17 and 1·33 MeV.

Electrons and protons of equal velocity produce the same ion density, but as they slow down, the density increases. Alpha-particles, on the other hand, with their double charge and slow velocity, produce dense ionisation. Gamma and X-rays of high energy (short wavelengths) produce fewer ionisations than do low-energy rays.

Ion Formation

The ions formed by radiation are not the same as those of salts in solution, e.g. Na^+, Cl^-, OH^-, etc. If a molecule of water ejects an electron, the ion H_2O^+ is formed:

$$H_2O \rightarrow H_2O^+ + e$$

The electron may be captured by another molecule of water

$$H_2O + e \rightarrow H_2O^-$$

These charged ions are unstable and decompose immediately:

$$H_2O^+ \rightarrow H^+ + OH\dot{}$$
$$H_2O^- \rightarrow H\dot{} + OH^-$$

The radicals $OH\dot{}$ and $H\dot{}$, although electrically neutral, are highly unstable and reactive, because they have an odd number of outer orbiting electrons.

Although there can be little doubt that when aqueous solutions are irradiated, the hydroxyl radical $OH\dot{}$ is formed, because oxidative reactions predominate, there is some doubt about the $H\dot{}$ radical (or hydrogen atom). It has been suggested that H_2O^- breaks down as follows:

$$H_2O^- + H_2O \rightarrow H_2 + OH\dot{} + OH^-$$

HO˙   H˙

Figure A3.6
Ionising radiations lead to the formation of the free radicals $OH\dot{}$ and $H\dot{}$ (the hydrogen atom). Although electrically neutral these radicals are highly unstable because of the seven outer electrons in the case of the $OH\dot{}$ radical and the odd electron in the hydrogen atom. By convention a dot is placed after these radicals to distinguish them from the charged ions OH^- and H^+.

In the presence of oxygen further powerfully oxidising radicals are formed:

$$H_2O + O_2 \xrightarrow[\text{radiation}]{\text{ionising}} OH\dot{} + HO_2\dot{}$$

$$H\dot{} + O_2 \rightarrow HO_2\dot{}$$
$$HO_2\dot{} + HO_2\dot{} = H_2O_2 + O_2$$

Oxidising compounds are certainly formed; many of them are in a very active state as free radicals, and have an existence of only a small fraction of a second.

Although most work has been directed to the effects of radiation on water, other substances are also changed. In addition to the formation of free radicals, some molecules are 'excited' by a change in the energies of their electrons. Much has yet to be learned even about the changes occurring in simple solutions on irradiation.

Radioactive Elements

Some elements, like radium, are not stable, but show a continuous loss of energy and mass due to the emission of radiations of some kind. Alpha, beta, or gamma radiations are given off either singly or in combination, each radioactive element having its own characteristic properties. The energy of each radiation also varies from one element to another. For instance, tritium, ^3_1H, emits β-particles of 0.018 MeV, while $^{131}_{53}I$ emits β-particles (0.605 MeV) and γ-rays of two separate energies.

The activity of any portion of a radioactive material is measured by the number of atoms which disintegrate each second. In 1 gram of radium there are 3.7×10^{10} disintegrations every second, and this is arbitrarily taken to be one unit—the Curie. *One Curie* is thus that amount of any element which produces 3.7×10^{10} disintegrations per second. The actual weight of material will vary from micrograms to tons, depending upon the speed at which the element decays.

Measurement of Radiations

The Roentgen. Since the radiations produce ion pairs in air, a convenient unit of measurement is dependent upon this ionisation, which can be measured by a change in the electrical conductivity of air. *One Roentgen* (r) may be described as that amount of radiation, which under specified conditions produces in 1 ml of air at NTP, 1 ESU* of electricity of either charge.

The effect of radiation is dependent upon the energy actually absorbed by the substance radiated. A more logical unit of measurement is, therefore, dependent upon energy absorbed. *One Rad* is a dose which equals an absorption of 100 ergs per gram of substance irradiated. A unit that has recently been introduced is the *Gray*, named after Dr Gray for his work on the oxygen effect. One Gray is equal to 100 Rad.

When 1 gram of water or soft tissue is exposed to a dose of 1 r of X-radiation, the absorbed dose is almost equal to 1 rad. When, however, other radiations are used, e.g. neutrons, or when bone is irradiated, much more energy is absorbed.

Another unit which has been suggested is the *rep* (*Roentgen equivalent physical*), which is that quantity of radiation which releases the same amount of energy in water as 1 r of X-rays. The unit is now obsolete.

In radiobiology it is the effect on cells which is important. Even with an equal amount of energy absorption, the different radiations produce different biological effects. The *relative biological efficiency* (*RBE*) is a measure of this. Thus the RBE for neutrons compared with X-rays is about 10, when considering the lethal effect on the mouse. This means that if 500 rad of X-rays causes death, then 50 rad of neutrons produces the same effect.

*Electrostatic Unit.

An alternative method of expressing this is to use the *rem* (*Roentgen equivalent man*). The dose in rems = Rads × RBE. Thus in the above example 500 rem of X-rays (500 rad × RBE, i.e. 500 × 1) produces the same effect as 500 rem of neutrons (50 rad × RBE, i.e. 50 × 10).

When considering other biological effects, e.g. chromosomal damage, the RBE is different. In general the RBE is greatest for those radiations which produce the densest ionisation. It should be noted that the RBE is merely a method of comparing the ability of one type of radiation with another to produce a particular biological effect. It is not an absolute figure.

General Reading. See Chapter 31.

Appendix 4.   *The HLA Histocompatibility Antigens*

The HLA (human leucocyte antigen) system comprises a complex group of antigens which are present on the cell membranes, not only of human leucocytes, but of all other tissue cells other than erythrocytes. It was the result of studies on the sera of patients who had suffered from febrile, non-haemolytic reactions after the transfusion of whole blood that drew attention to the existence of antibodies to several white-cell antigens. From 1960 onwards it was recognised that antigens present on human leucocytes might provide part of the explanation of allograft rejection. Thus it comes about that this ubiquitous system of tissue antigens is called the human leucocyte antigen system.

In the mouse a somewhat related system of tissue antigens is called the H-2 system. Both HLA and H-2 antigens are glycoproteins; in the intact cell they are integrated into the cell membrane. The molecular weight of antigens HLA-A, HLA-B, and HLA-C is about 55 000 daltons. They comprise a glycosylated polypeptide chain of about 43 000 daltons molecular weight that is non-covalently associated with a β_2-microglobulin*, a non-glycosylated polypeptide of about 12 000 daltons molecular weight. The alloantigenic activity appears to be determined by the 43 000 daltons molecular-weight polypeptide. The newly defined HLA-DRw antigens comprise one each of 2 glycosylated polypeptides of molecular weights 33 000 and 28 000 daltons that are not covalently linked.

Inheritance of HLA

The HLA system is a highly polymorphic one, and five major gene loci are at present recognised (on the short arm of chromosome 6). These are called *HLA-A, HLA-B, HLA-C, HLA-D,* and the recently described *HLA-DR,* which is closely related to the *HLA-D* locus. Each of these loci contains a considerable number of alleles; Table A4.1 gives the situation in 1978, but new alleles are continually being discovered. The development of our knowledge of the HLA system has been greatly helped by a series of international collaborative workshops called the International Histocompatibility Workshops, the first of which was convened in 1964 and the seventh in 1977. The names given to newly-discovered HLA antigens by these workshops are communicated to the WHO nomenclature committee for approval. The letter w (for workshop) has always been included in HLA nomenclature as the first step in official recognition by the WHO committee.

Every individual inherits one antigen from each series from each parent. At present most laboratories have antisera for the A (first) and B (second) series only, and so an individual is typed according to two A series and two B series antigens.

*β_2-microglobulin is a small protein, the amino-acid sequence of which closely resembles that of regions of the IgG molecule.

TABLE A4.1 The nomenclature of the HLA system (*Reproduced from Bodmer, W. F. (1978) British Medical Bulletin,* **34,** *215*).

Locus A	Locus B	Locus C	Locus D	Locus DR
HLA-A1	HLA-B5	HLA-Cw1	HLA-Dw1	HLA-DRw1
HLA-A2	HLA-B7	HLA-Cw2	HLA-Dw2	HLA-DRw2
HLA-A3	HLA-B8	HLA-Cw3	HLA-Dw3	HLA-DRw3
HLA-A9	HLA-B12	HLA-Cw4	HLA-Dw4	HLA-DRw4
HLA-A10	HLA-B13	HLA-Cw5	HLA-Dw5	HLA-DRw5
HLA-A11	HLA-B14	HLA-Cw6	HLA-Dw6	HLA-DRw6
HLA-Aw19	HLA-B15		HLA-Dw7	HLA-DRw7
HLA-Aw23	HLA-Bw16		HLA-Dw8	
HLA-Aw24	HLA-B17		HLA-Dw9	
HLA-A25	HLA-B18		HLA-Dw10	
HLA-A26	HLA-Bw21		HLA-Dw11	
HLA-A28	HLA-Bw22			
HLA-A29	HLA-B27			
HLA-Aw30	HLA-Bw35			
HLA-Aw31	HLA-B37			
HLA-Aw32	HLA-Bw38			
HLA-Aw33	HLA-Bw39			
HLA-Aw34	HLA-B40			
HLA-Aw36*	HLA-Bw41			
HLA-Aw43*	HLA-Bw42*			
	HLA-Bw44			
	HLA-Bw45			
	HLA-Bw46†			
	HLA-Bw47			
	HLA-Bw48			
	HLA-Bw49			
	HLA-Bw50			
	HLA-Bw51			
	HLA-Bw52			
	HLA-Bw53			
	HLA-Bw54†			
	HLA-Bw4			
	HLA-Bw6			

*Found so far only in Black populations.
†Found so far only in Mongoloid populations.

The C and D loci are closely linked to the A and B loci, and the probable order of these four loci on the chromosome is D, B, C, and A from the centromere peripherally.

It may be, for instance, that a person inherits HLA-A1 and HLA-B8 from his mother and HLA-A2 and HLA-B12 from his father. In this case he has four different antigens, and is heterozygous at both A and B loci. If both parents contribute, say, HLA-B8, he has only three different antigens, since he is homozygous at the B locus. If both parents were to contribute HLA-A1 and HLA-B8, he would have only two different antigens, being homozygous at both the A and B loci.

The C locus antigens are studied by the cytotoxic tests used for the A and B loci, but the D locus antigens are studied by the mixed lymphocyte culture reaction, in which lymphocytes from different individuals grown together in tissue culture show a proliferative response (pp. 151 and 197).

Another completely different system involved with the immune response to other agents is closely associated with the HLA-D antigens. This system, the *Ia (immune associated) antigen system*, also called the *B-cell antigen system* because the antigens are found predominantly on B lymphocytes, has its Ia antigen counterpart in the mouse, where it is controlled by the *Ir (immune response)* genes that are closely linked to the *H-2* locus. The genetic region controlling this human Ia antigen system is very closely related to the *D* locus on chromosome 6, and is called the *HLA-DR* locus. The antigens associated with this locus are now called HLA-DRw antigens, and are listed in Table A4.1. These antigens can be detected by cytotoxic tests, and it is hoped that these may eventually be used for the HLA-Dw antigens also, since the mixed lymphocyte culture reaction is very cumbersome to perform.

The *HLA* gene locus also controls the expression of some serum complement components; the region includes the structural genes for the C2 and C4 components of complement as well as for factor B of the alternative pathway.

An important genetic factor in understanding how HLA correlations work is *linkage disequilibrium*. This is the tendency in a population for some alleles at closely linked loci to occur together in the same haplotype* more often than expected by chance. One striking example of this in the HLA system is the association of HLA-A1 (A-locus allele number 1) and HLA-B8 (B-locus allele number 8), which occur together at a higher frequency than would be expected from their individual frequencies in a Caucasian population. In fact, some antigens can be differently associated in different populations. For example, HLA-B8 is more frequently associated with HLA-Aw30 than with HLA-A1 in Black Zambians. The principle of linkage disequilibrium may explain the correlation between HLA antigens and particular characteristics, such as a disease state. Over 90 per cent of individuals with ankylosing spondylitis have HLA-B27. This disease-predisposing genetic factor is separate from the HLA specificity, but is in linkage disequilibrium with it.

HLA Typing

There are a number of methods of 'tissue typing'. The earliest technique was *leucoagglutination*, in which antiserum was mixed with a crude leucocyte preparation, incubated for $1\frac{1}{2}$ hours at 37°C, and then the degree of leucoagglutination recorded. Another method is *complement fixation*, using platelets as a source of HLA antigen. A third is the *mixed lymphocyte culture reaction* already alluded to.

The most important method is *complement-mediated lymphocytotoxicity*, which is nowadays performed by a microlymphocytotoxicity test. This consists of preparing an almost pure lymphocyte suspension from a blood sample taken as recently as possible and either defibrinated or else anticoagulated with heparin or ACD. To the blood there are added dextran, which sediments the erythrocytes, and carbonyl iron, which is taken up by the phagocytes; these are attracted to the bottom of the container when it is placed on a magnet. The supernatant fluid, which consists largely of plasma, lymphocytes, and

*The *haplotype* is the haploid genetic composition of a chromosomal region: a series of alleles in a defined segment of a chromosome that are usually transmitted from parent to offspring as a unit; two haplotypes, one from each parent, constitute the genotype.

platelets, is layered on Ficol/Triosil and centrifuged; this concentrates the lymphocytes, which are then washed at low centrifuge speeds to remove the platelets. A suspension of lymphocytes in the proper concentration (about 1 000 000 cells per ml) is prepared and equal parts of this and the antiserum (2 μl of each) are placed in the well of a plastic microtyping tray (which has about 60 similar wells). A pool of complement-high serum is prepared immediately before use, and 4 μl is added to each well containing the lymphocyte-antiserum mixture. The tray is incubated at room temperature for an hour, after which the supernatant fluids are carefully removed, and 1 μl of a trypan-blue solution, followed by 1 μl of bovine albumin and 1 μl of 5 per cent acetic acid, are added to each well. The tests are read by an inverted microscope; killed cells stain blue, and are larger than those not killed. A large number of killed cells with a well-defined antiserum indicates that the cell possesses the antigen for that antibody.

Production of Antisera

Anti-HLA sera produced in lower mammals have an anti-human component that is difficult to remove without also removing the specific activity. Chimpanzees can be successfully used to produce antisera of some specificities, but in practice human antisera are employed. These are obtained from the following sources:

(*a*) Recipients of multiple blood transfusions.

(*b*) Multiparous women. These are the main source (see p. 194).

(*c*) Recipients of rejected kidney grafts.

(*d*) Volunteers who have been immunised deliberately by the injection of leucocytes and/or skin grafting.

Good anti-HLA sera are scarce; few are truly monospecific (reacting only with one antigen), but many useful reagents are duospecific, for example reacting with HLA-B27 and HLA-B7 or HLA-A1 and HLA-B8. A large number of antisera are multispecific, reacting with 50 per cent or more of a cell panel (a group of unrelated cells) in a way which shows no clear specificity. It is for this reason that a continuous search is made for useful HLA antisera to meet the growing demand for tissue typing.

HLA and Disease

As mentioned above, certain genes controlling the genetic predisposition to disease have been linked with the HLA system and have been marked mainly by HLA-A, HLA-B, HLA-Dw and HLA-DRw antigens. These individual antigens or combinations of antigens may contribute to a hyporeactive or hyper-reactive state of that individual, or may confer a survival advantage. Some studies, for example, have suggested that long-surviving patients with Hodgkin's disease have a predominance of HLA-B8, and long-term survivors of acute lymphatic leukaemia of HLA-A2, but other workers have not confirmed this.

It is most likely that the *HLA-DR* genes provide the basis for disease associations. It is therefore not surprising that efforts have shifted to identifying the linkage disequilibrium between disease states and the DRw antigens. However, up to the present most of the disease associations in human subjects are with alleles of the HLA-A and HLA-B loci. Thus, as noted previously, there is a strikingly high frequency of the **antigen HLA-B27** in patients with ankylosing spondylitis (p. 208). More than 90 per cent of patients carry this antigen as compared with 5 to 6 per cent of a control population. Nevertheless it is reckoned that fewer than 5 per cent of individuals with HLA-B27 will develop ankylosing spondylitis, and even within affected families the disease does not show 100 per cent linkage with the antigen. Other conditions associated with HLA-B27 are Reiter's disease, anterior uveitis, and the frozen-shoulder syndrome. While there is no relationship between uncomplicated ulcerative colitis, Crohn's disease, or *Yersinia enterocolitica* dysentery and HLA-B27, if these conditions are complicated by sacro-iliitis or frank ankylosing spondylitis, there is a very significant association.

Antigen HLA-Cw6 is associated with psoriasis. There is also a secondary association between psoriasis and antigens HLA-B13, -B17, and -B37. This is due to the probability of their 3 alleles being in linkage disequilibrium with allele *HLA-Cw6*. It is noteworthy that cases of psoriatic arthropathy also show a strong association with antigen HLA-B27, but not so uncomplicated psoriasis.

Antigens HLA-B8, HLA-Dw3, and HLA-DRw3 are significantly associated with some diseases that have an immunological component: gluten-sensitive enteropathy (coeliac disease) and the clinically related dermatitis herpetiformis, Graves's disease, Addison's disease, HBsAg-negative chronic active hepatitis, and myasthenia gravis (those cases without a thymoma). The primary association is with alleles -*Dw3* and -*DRw3* which are in linkage disequilibrium with allele -*B8*.

Juvenile-onset diabetes mellitus is associated with these same antigens, but **HLA-Dw4** and **-DRw4** may also be involved. Rheumatoid arthritis is associated with antigens -Dw4 and -DRw4. It is noteworthy that the Japanese lack antigens -B8, Dw3, and DRw3, and that Japanese patients with juvenile-onset diabetes mellitus and myasthenia gravis show a close association with antigens -Dw4 and -DRw4.

Antigens -Dw2 and -DRw2 are associated with multiple sclerosis. There is a secondary association with antigens -A3 and -B7 due again to the fact of linkage disequilibrium between the respective alleles.

Antigen HLA-A3 is closely related to haemochromatosis. There is a strong secondary association with antigen HLA-B7

and also one with antigen -B14 in what may be another expression of the disease.

A very interesting feature of the HLA antigens is their racial incidence. Thus in Northern European Caucasoid groups multiple sclerosis tends to be associated with antigens HLA-Dw2 and HLA-DRw2. There is, however, a steady decrease in the strength of the association from Northern to Southern Europe, and specifically different associations are found in Mediterranean and Japanese populations of patients with this disease.

The association between antigen HLA-B27 and ankylosing spondylitis is close in Caucasoid and Japanese groups but not in Black populations or American Indians. Indeed, in Pima Indians the risk of acquiring sacro-iliitis is essentially the same with or without -B27 antigen. In Black groups the association is present but comparatively weak as compared with Caucasoids.

In the Japanese, apart from the absence of certain antigens noted above, Graves's disease is accompanied by an increased frequency of antigen HLA-Bw35. Nasopharyngeal carcinoma, which occurs with unusual frequency among the Chinese and related groups, is associated with antigen HLA-Bw46, an antigen which seems to be peculiar to the Chinese race, being found rarely, if at all, in other groups. There is likewise an increased frequency of antigen HLA-B40 in Turkish–Mongol groups with oesophageal carcinoma, a disease with a remarkably limited, circumscribed geographical incidence (p. 385).

It would seem that an individual's 'tissue type' is a marker to an aspect of his genetic make-up, which provides a setting that determines how he will react to disease-producing factors in his environment. As Rosenberg and Kidd suggest, the disease-associated HLA antigen may be thought of as an innocent but visible witness to a health 'crime' rather than the actual culprit.

HLA and Transplantation

This is considered in greater detail in Chapter 15. It should be noted that the lymphocyte-definable (LD) determinants recognised in the mixed lymphocyte culture test are probably as important as the serologically definable (SD) antigens for determining graft survival.

GENERAL READING

ROSENBERG, L. E. & KIDD, K. K. (1977) HLA and disease susceptibility: a primer. *New England Journal of Medicine*, **297**, 1060.
    Various Authors (1978) The HLA system. *British Medical Bulletin*, **34**, 213–316.

Index